SIXTH EDITION

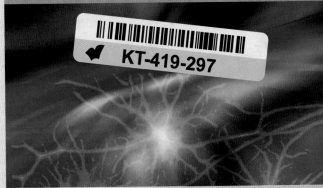

RANG AND DALE'S
Pharmacology

Commissioning Editor: Kate Dimock
Development Editors: Stephen McGrath/Louise Cook
Project Manager: Gemma Lawson
Design Manager: Erik Bigland
Illustration Manager: Bruce Hogarth
Illustrator: Peter Lamb and Antbits
Marketing Manager(s) (UK/USA): Amy Hey/John Gore

SIXTH EDITION

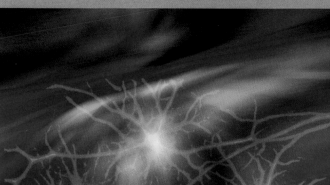

RANG AND DALE'S
Pharmacology

H P Rang MB BS MA DPhil FMedSci FRS

Emeritus Professor of Pharmacology
University College London, London, UK

M M Dale MB BCh PhD

Senior Teaching Fellow, Department of Pharmacology, University of Oxford
Honorary Lecturer, Department of Pharmacology, University College London, UK

J M Ritter DPhil FRCP FMedSci FBPharmacolS

Professor, Department of Clinical Pharmacology, School of Medicine,
King's College London, UK

R J Flower PhD DSc FBPharmacolS FMedSci FRS

Professor, Biochemical Pharmacology, The William Harvey Research Institute,
Barts and the London, Queen Mary's School of Medicine and Dentistry, London, UK

CHURCHILL
LIVINGSTONE

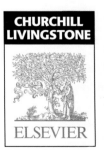

ELSEVIER

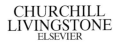

© 2007, Elsevier Limited. All rights reserved.

First edition 1987
Second edition 1991
Third edition 1995
Fourth edition 1999
Fifth edition 2003
Sixth edition 2007

The right of H P Rang, M M Dale, J M Ritter and R J Flower to be identified as authors of this work has been asserted by them in accordance with the Copyright, Designs and Patents Act 1988.

Main edition ISBN: 9780443069116
  Reprinted 2008 (three times)
International edition ISBN: 9780808923541
  Reprinted 2008 (twice)

British Library Cataloguing in Publication Data
A catalogue record for this book is available from the British Library

Library of Congress Cataloging in Publication Data
A catalog record for this book is available from the Library of Congress

Notice

ELSEVIER your source for books, journals and multimedia in the health sciences
www.elsevierhealth.com

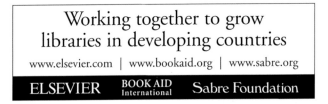

Working together to grow libraries in developing countries

www.elsevier.com | www.bookaid.org | www.sabre.org

ELSEVIER   BOOK AID International   Sabre Foundation

The publisher's policy is to use **paper manufactured from sustainable forests**

Printed in China

Contents

General principles

Chemical mediators

Drugs affecting major organ systems

CONTENTS

Preface

In this edition, as in its predecessors, we set out not just to describe what drugs do but to emphasise the *mechanisms* by which they act. This entails analysis not only at the cellular and molecular level, where knowledge and techniques are advancing rapidly, but also at the level of physiological mechanisms and pathological disturbances. Pharmacology has its roots in therapeutics, where the aim is to ameliorate the effects of disease, so we have attempted to make the link between effects at the molecular and cellular level and the range of beneficial and adverse effects that humans experience when drugs are used for therapeutic or other reasons. Therapeutic agents have a high rate of obsolescence, and new ones appear each year. An appreciation of the mechanisms of action of the class of drugs to which a new agent belongs provides a good starting point for understanding and using a new compound intelligently.

Pharmacology is a lively scientific discipline in its own right, with an importance beyond that of providing a basis for the use of drugs in therapy, and we are aware that some of our readers may be studying to be not doctors but scientists or practitioners of other disciplines. We have therefore, where appropriate, included brief coverage of the use of drugs as probes for elucidating cellular and physiological functions, even when the compounds have no clinical use.

Names of mediators are established through usage and sometimes there is more than one name in common use. When mediators are formulated as medicines, these are prescribed by their recommended international non-proprietary, name (rINN), as are other medicinal substances. We use the rINN in the context of therapeutic use, but (where relevant) the common name in the setting of endogenous mediator, e.g. ; 'prostaglandin I$_2$' becomes 'epoprostenol' (rINN) and 'corticotrophin' becomes 'corticotropin' (rINN). Sometimes English and American usage varies (as with adrenaline/epinephrine and noradrenaline/norepinephrine). Adrenaline and noradrenaline are the official names in EU member states and related clearly to terms such as 'noradrenergic', 'adrenoceptor' and 'adrenal gland' and we prefer them for these reasons.

Drug action can be understood only in the context of what else is happening in the body. So at the beginning of most chapters, we briefly discuss the physiological and biochemical processes relevant to the action of the drugs described in that chapter. As regards the *chemical structures of drugs*, we have included these only where this information helps in understanding how those drugs act.

Small print sections have been included in many chapters. These contain more detailed, sometimes speculative material, which can be skipped by the reader in a hurry without losing the main thread, but will be of interest to readers wishing to go into a particular topic in greater depth.

There are three new chapters.

- One on cannabinoids (Ch. 15). This topic, previously concerned mainly with the social use of marijuana, has moved into the pharmacological mainstream, reflecting the growing importance of cannabinoids as endogenous mediators and potential therapeutic agents. (Enthusiasm should be curbed; it's early days yet.)
- One on lifestyle drugs and drugs in sport (Ch. 54). This chapter discusses the growing use of drugs for non-medical purposes, particularly to enhance sporting performance.
- One on biopharmaceuticals and developments in gene therapy (Ch. 55). These subjects reflect the impact of biotechnology on the development of therapeutic agents, an impact that is likely to assume major importance in tomorrow's pharmacology.

All other chapters have been extensively revised and updated since the fifth edition, and new information has been inserted. In particular, the following aspects are new:

- nuclear receptors and related signal transduction mechanisms (Ch. 3)
- a discussion of tissue regeneration and the possibility of facilitating this pharmacologically (Ch. 5)
- animal models of disease, and principles of clinical trials (Ch. 6)
- a section on pulmonary hypertension (Ch. 19) and its treatment—which, you may be surprised to learn, includes sildenafil (Viagra) (Ch. 30)
- cholesterol absorption inhibitors in atherosclerosis therapy (Ch. 20)
- protein misfolding and aggregation as a common feature in neurodegenerative diseases, with implications for future therapeutic strategies (Ch. 35)
- an updated discussion of drug addiction and dependence (Ch. 43)
- the significance of the negative regulation of T cells by apoptosis-inducing surface receptors for the future treatment of chronic viral infections (e.g. HIV) and some cancers (Ch. 5, also Ch. 47)
- information about the regulatory hurdles involved in the introduction of new drugs (Ch. 56).

In selecting new material for inclusion, we have taken into account not only new agents but also recent extensions of basic knowledge that presage further drug development. And where possible, we have given a brief outline of new treatments in the pipeline.

For new readers, we draw attention to two particular aspects of the book.

- There are two chapters on *cellular mechanisms* (Chs 4 and 5), which bring together, update and extend information usually scattered throughout most pharmacology textbooks. They are intended to establish the common ground on which many, at first sight very different, drug effects are based, not only drugs in use but drugs in development or being planned.
  — Chapter 4 deals with mechanisms involved in *short-term reactions* such as excitation, contraction and secretion, which underlie the rapid actions of many drugs that affect the cardiovascular, nervous, respiratory and endocrine systems.
  — Chapter 5 deals with *reactions that occur rather more slowly*: cell proliferation and apoptosis. These are involved in more gradually developing phenomena such as inflammation, immune responses, tissue repair and malignancies—conditions that are affected by drugs used over longer periods.
- There is a general chapter on *Drugs used in the treatment of infections and cancer*. This chapter gives an overview of the basic mechanisms of drug action common both to agents acting on various bacterial, viral and parasitic infections, and to anticancer drugs. It is aimed primarily at non-medical students studying pharmacology who need a bird's-eye view of these topics but do not have sufficient background in microbiology, parasitology and cancer pathology to be able to cope with the following more detailed chapters.

Finally, a *References and further reading* section is given at the end of each chapter. These sections are fairly extensive, because most medical and science curricula stress project work and the preparation of special study modules. To make these easier for students to use, short descriptions have been added to most references, summarising the main aspects covered.

We are grateful to the readers who have taken the trouble to write to us with constructive comments and suggestions on the fifth edition. We have done our best to incorporate these. Comments on the new edition will be welcome.

ACKNOWLEDGEMENTS

We would like to thank the following for their help and advice in the preparation of this edition: Professor J. Mandelstam, Professor Chris Corrigan, Professor George Haycock, Professor Jeremy Pearson, Dr Tony Wierzbicki, Professor Martin Wilkins and Professor Ignac Fogelman.

We would like to put on record our appreciation of the team at Elsevier who worked on this edition: Alex Stibbe and her replacement, Kate Dimock (commissioning editor), Louise Cook and Stephen McGrath (development editors), Gemma Lawson (project manager), Bruce Hogarth (illustration manager), Peter Lamb and Antbits (freelance illustrators), Kim Howell (freelance copyeditor), Pat Pole (freelance proofreader) and Susan Boobis (freelance indexer).

London 2007

H. P. Rang
M. M. Dale
J. M. Ritter
R. J. Flower

Abbreviations and acronyms

α-Me-5-HT	α-methyl 5-hydroxytrypamine	Arg	arginine
α-MSH	α-melanocyte-stimulating hormone	ARND	alcohol-related neurodevelopmental disorder
12-S-HETE	12-S-hydroxyeicosatetraenoic acid	ASCI	ATP-sensitive Ca^{2+}-insensitive
2-AG	2-arachidonoyl glycerol	ASCOT	Anglo-Scandinavian Cardiac Outcomes Trial
2-Me-5-HT	2-methyl-5-hydroxytrypamine	ASIC	acid-sensing ion channel
4S	Scandinavian Simvastatin Survival Study	AT	angiotensin
5-CT	5-carboxamidotryptamine	AT_1	angiotensin II receptor subtype 1
5-HIAA	5-hydroxyindoleacetic acid	AT_2	angiotensin II receptor subtype 2
5-HT	5-hydroxytryptamine [serotonin]	ATIII	antithrombin III
8-OH-DPAT	8-hydroxy-2-(di-*n*-propylamino) tetraline	ATP	adenosine triphosphate
AA	arachidonic acid	AUC	area under the curve
AC	adenylate cyclase	AV	atrioventricular
ACAT	acyl coenzyme A: cholesterol acyltransferase	AZT	zidovudine
AcCoA	acetyl coenzyme A	BARK	β-adrenoceptor kinase
ACE	angiotensin-converting enzyme	BDNF	brain-derived neurotrophic factor
ACh	acetylcholine	B_{max}	binding capacity
AChE	acetylcholinesterase	BMI	body mass index
ACTH	adrenocorticotrophic hormone	BMPR-2	bone morphogenetic protein receptor type 2
AD	Alzheimer's disease	BNP	B-type natriuretic peptide
ADH	antidiuretic hormone	BSE	bovine spongiform encephalopathy
ADHD	attention deficit–hyperactivity disorder	BuChE	butyrylcholinesterase
ADMA	asymmetric dimethylarginine	CaC	calcium channel
ADME	absorption, distribution, metabolism and elimination [studies]	CAD	coronary artery disease
		cADPR	cyclic ADP-ribose
ado-B_{12}	5′-deoxyadenosylcobalamin	CaM	calmodulin
ADP	adenosine diphosphate	cAMP	cyclic 3′,5′-adenosine monophosphate
AF1	activation function 1	CAR	constitutive androstane receptor
AF2	activation function 2	CARE	Cholesterol and Recurrent Events [trial]
AGEPC	acetyl-glyceryl-ether-phosphorylcholine	CAT	choline acetyltransferase
AGRP	agouti-related protein	CBG	corticosteroid-binding globulin
Ah	aromatic hydrocarbon	CCK	cholecystokinin
AIDS	acquired immunodeficiency syndrome	cdk	cyclin-dependent kinase
AIF	apoptotic initiating factor	cDNA	circular deoxyribonucleic acid
ALA	δ-amino laevulinic acid	CETP	cholesteryl ester transfer protein
ALDH	aldehyde dehydrogenase	CFTR	cystic fibrosis transport [transmembrane conductance] regulator
AMP	adenosine monophosphate		
AMPA	α-amino-5-hydroxy-3-methyl-4-isoxazole propionic acid	cGMP	cyclic guanosine monophosphate
		CGRP	calcitonin gene-related peptide
ANF	atrial natriuretic factor	ChE	cholinesterase
ANP	atrial natriuretic peptide	CHO	Chinese hamster ovary [cell]
AP	adapter protein	CICR	calcium-induced calcium release
Apaf-1	apoptotic protease-activating factor-1	CIP	cdk inhibitory proteins
APC	antigen-presenting cell	CJD	Creutzfeldt–Jakob disease
APP	amyloid precursor protein	*CL*	total clearance of a drug
APTT	activated partial thromboplastin time	CNP	C-natriuretic peptide
AR	aldehyde reductase; androgen receptor	CNS	central nervous system

CO	carbon monoxide
CoA	coenzyme A
COMT	catechol-O-methyl transferase
COPD	chronic obstructive pulmonary disease
COX	cyclo-oxygenase
CREB	cAMP response element–binding protein
CRF	corticotrophin-releasing factor
CRH	corticotrophin-releasing hormone
CRLR	calcitonin receptor–like receptor
CSF	cerebrospinal fluid; colony-stimulating factor
C_{ss}	steady-state plasma concentration
CTL	cytotoxic T lymphocyte
CTZ	chemoreceptor trigger zone
CYP	cytochrome P450 [system]
DAAO	d-amino acid oxidase
DAG	diacylglycerol
DAGL	diacylglycerol lipase
DAT	dopamine transporter
DBH	dopamine-β-hydroxylase
DDAH	dimethylarginine dimethylamino hydrolase
DHFR	dihydrofolate reductase
DHMA	3,4-dihydroxymandelic acid
DHPEG	3,4-dihydroxyphenylglycol
DIT	diiodotyrosine
DMARD	disease-modifying antirheumatic drug
DMPP	dimethylphenylpiperazinium
DNA	deoxyribonucleic acid
DOH	oxidised [hydroxylated] drug
DOPA	dihydroxyphenylalanine
DOPAC	dihydroxyphenylacetic acid
DSI	depolarisation-induced suppression of inhibition
DTMP	2-deoxythymidylate
DUMP	2-deoxyuridylate
EAA	excitatory amino acid
EC_{50}/ED_{50}	concentration/dose effective in 50% of the population
ECG	electrocardiogram
ECM	extracellular matrix
ECP	eosinophil cationic protein
ECT	electroconvulsive therapy
EDHF	endothelium-derived hyperpolarising factor
EDRF	endothelium-derived relaxing factor
EEG	electroencephalography
EET	epoxyeicosatetraenoic acid
EGF	epidermal growth factor
EG-VEGF	endocrine gland–derived vascular endothelial growth factor
E_{max}	maximal response that a drug can produce
EMBP	eosinophil major basic protein
EMT	endocannabinoid membrane transporter
ENaC	epithelial sodium channel
eNOS	endothelial nitric oxide synthase [NOS-III]
epp	endplate potential
EPS	extrapyramidal side effects
epsp	excitatory postsynaptic potential
ER	endoplasmic reticulum; (o)estrogen receptor
FA kinase	focal adhesion kinase

FAAH	fatty acid amide hydrolase
FAD	flavin adenine dinucleotide
FAS	fetal alcohol syndrome
FDUMP	fluorodeoxyuridine monophosphate
Fe^{2+}	ferrous iron
Fe^{3+}	ferric iron
FeO^{3+}	ferric oxene
FEV_1	forced expiratory volume in 1 second
FGF	fibroblast growth factor
FH_2	dihydrofolate
FH_4	tetrahydrofolate
FKBP	FK-binding protein
FLAP	five-lipoxygenase activating protein
FMN	flavin mononucleotide
formyl-FH_4	formyl tetrahydrofolate
FSH	follicle-stimulating hormone
FXR	farnesoid [bile acid] receptor
G6PD	glucose 6-phosphate dehydrogenase
GABA	gamma-aminobutyric acid
GAD	glutamic acid decarboxylase
GC	guanylate cyclase
G-CSF	granulocyte colony-stimulating factor
GDP	guanosine diphosphate
GFR	glomerular filtration rate
GH	growth hormone
GHB	γ-hydroxybutyrate
GHRF	growth hormone–releasing factor
GHRH	growth hormone–releasing hormone
GI	gastrointestinal
GIP	gastric inhibitory polypeptide
GIRK	G-protein–sensitive inward-rectifying potassium [channel]
GIT	gastrointestinal tract
Gla	γ-carboxylated glutamic acid
GLP	glucagon-like peptide
Glu	glutamic acid
GM-CSF	granulocyte–macrophage colony-stimulating factor
GnRH	gonadotrophin-releasing hormone
GP	glycoprotein
GPCR	G-protein–coupled receptor
GPL	glycerophospholipid
GR	glucocorticoid receptor
GRE	glucocorticoid response element
GRK	GPCR kinase
GSH	glutathione
GSSG	glutathione, oxidised
GTP	guanosine triphosphate
GUSTO	Global Use of Strategies to Open Occluded Coronary Arteries [trial]
H_2O_2	hydrogen peroxide
HAART	highly active antiretroviral therapy
HCG	human chorionic gonadotrophin
HCl	hydrochloric acid
HDAC	histone deacetylase
HDL	high-density lipoprotein
HDL-C	high-density lipoprotein cholesterol

HER2	human epidermal growth factor receptor 2		**LSD**	lysergic acid diethylamide
HERG	human ether-a-go-go related gene		**LT**	leukotriene
HETE	hydroxyeicosatetraenoic acid		**LTP**	long-term potentiation
hGH	human growth hormone		**LXR**	liver oxysterol receptor
HIT	heparin-induced thrombocytopenia		**lyso-PAF**	lysoglyceryl-phosphorylcholine
HIV	human immunodeficiency virus		**mAb**	monoclonal antibody
HLA	histocompatibility antigen		**MAC**	minimal alveolar concentration
HMG-CoA	3-hydroxy-3-methylglutaryl-coenzyme A		**mAChR**	muscarinic acetylcholine receptor
HnRNA	heterologous nuclear RNA		**MAGL**	monoacyl glycerol lipase
HPA	hypothalamic–pituitary–adrenal [axis]		**MAO**	monoamine oxidase
HPETE	hydroperoxyeicosatetraenoic acid		**MAOI**	monoamine oxidase inhibitor
HRT	hormone replacement therapy		**MAP**	mitogen-activated protein
HSP	heat shock protein		**MAPK**	mitogen-activated protein kinase
HVA	homovanillic acid		**MCP**	monocyte chemoattractant protein
IAP	inhibitor of apoptosis protein		**M-CSF**	macrophage colony-stimulating factor
IC$_{50}$	concentration causing 50% inhibition in the population		**MDMA**	methylenedioxymethamphetamine ['ecstasy']
ICAM	intercellular adhesion molecule		**MeNA**	methylnoradrenaline
ICE	interleukin-1–converting enzyme		**methyl-FH$_4$**	methyltetrahydrofolate
ICSH	interstitial cell–stimulating hormone		**MGluR**	metabotropic glutamate receptor
IDDM	insulin-dependent diabetes mellitus [*now known as type 1 diabetes*]		**MHC**	major histocompatibility complex
IFN	interferon		**MHPEG**	3-methoxy, 4-hydroxyphenylglycol
Ig	immunoglobulin		**MHPG**	3-hydroxy-4-methoxyphenylglycol
IGF	insulin-like growth factor		**MIT**	monoiodotyrosine
IL	interleukin		**MLCK**	myosin light-chain kinase
Ink	inhibitors of kinases		**MPTP**	1-methyl-4-phenyl-1,2,3,5-tetrahydropyridine
iNOS	inducible nitric oxide synthase		**MR**	mineralocorticoid receptor
INR	international normalised ratio		**mRNA**	messenger ribonucleic acid
IP	inositol phosphate		**MRSA**	methicillin-resistant *Staphylococcus aureus*
IP$_3$	inositol trisphosphate		**MSH**	melanocyte-stimulating hormone
IP$_3$R	inositol trisphosphate receptor		**N$_2$O**	nitrous oxide
IP$_4$	inositol tetraphosphate		**NA**	noradrenaline [norepinephrine]
ipsp	inhibitory postsynaptic potential		**NAADP**	nicotinic acid dinucleotide phosphate
IRS	insulin receptor substrate		**NaC**	voltage-gated sodium channel
ISI	international sensitivity index		**nAChR**	nicotinic acetylcholine receptor
ISIS	International Study of Infarct Survival		**NAD**	nicotinamide adenine dinucleotide
ISO	isoprenaline		**NADH**	nicotinamide adenine dinucleotide, reduced
IUPHAR	International Union of Pharmacological Sciences		**NADPH**	nicotinamide adenine dinucleotide phosphate, reduced
JRA	juvenile rheumatoid arthritis		**NANC**	non-noradrenergic non-cholinergic
K$_{ACh}$	potassium channel		**NAPBQI**	*N*-acetyl-*p*-benzoquinone imine
K$_{ATP}$	ATP-sensitive potassium [activator, channel]		**NAPE**	*N*-acyl-phosphatidylethanolamine
KIP	kinase inhibitory protein		**NASA**	National Aeronautics and Space Administration
LA	local anaesthetic		**NAT**	*N*-acyl-transferase
LC	locus coeruleus		**NCX**	Na$^+$-Ca^{2+} exchange transporter
LCAT	lecithin cholesterol acyltransferase		**NET**	norepinephrine transporter
LD$_{50}$	dose that is lethal in 50% of the population		**NF**	nuclear factor
LDL	low-density lipoprotein		**NFκB**	nuclear factor kappa B
LDL-C	low-density lipoprotein cholesterol		**NGF**	nerve growth factor
LGC	ligand-gated cation channel		**nGRE**	negative glucocorticoid response element
LH	luteinising hormone		**NIDDM**	non-insulin-dependent diabetes mellitus [*now known as type 2 diabetes*]
LMWH	low-molecular-weight heparin		**NIS**	Na$^+$/I$^-$ symporter
L-NAME	N^G-nitro-L-arginine methyl ester		**NK**	natural killer
L-NMMA	N^G-monomethyl-L-arginine		**NM**	normetanephrine
LQT	long QT [channel, syndrome]		**NMDA**	*N*-methyl-D-aspartic acid
			nNOS	neuronal nitric oxide synthase [NOS-I]

NNT	number needed to treat		**PPADS**	pyridoxal-phosphate-6-azophenyl-2′, 4′-disulfonate
NO	nitric oxide		**PPAR**	peroxisome proliferator-activated receptor
NOS	nitric oxide synthase			
NPR	natriuretic peptide receptor		**PR**	progesterone receptor; prolactin receptor
NPY	neuropeptide Y		**PRF**	prolactin-releasing factor
NRM	nucleus raphe magnus		**PRIF**	prolactin release–inhibiting factor
NRPG	nucleus reticularis paragigantocellularis		**Pro-CCK**	procholecystokinin
NSAID	non-steroidal anti-inflammatory drug		**pS**	picosiemens
ODQ	1H-[1,2,4]-oxadiazole-[4,3-α]-quinoxalin-1-one		**PT**	prothrombin time
			PTH	parathyroid hormone
OPG	osteoprotegerin		**PTZ**	pentylenetetrazol
oxLDL	oxidised low-density lipoprotein		**PUFA**	polyunsaturated fatty acid
PA	partial agonist; phosphatidic acid		**PUVA**	psoralen plus ultraviolet A
PABA	*p*-aminobenzoic acid		**QALY**	quality-adjusted life year
P_ACO_2	partial pressure of carbon dioxide in arterial blood		**R & D**	research and development
			RA	rheumatoid arthritis
PAF	platelet-activating factor		**RAMP**	receptor activity–modifying protein
PAG	periaqueductal grey		**RANK**	receptor activator of nuclear factor kappa B
PAH	*p*-aminohippuric acid		**RANKL**	RANK ligand
PAI	plasminogen activator inhibitor		**RANTES**	regulated on activation normal T-cell expressed and secreted
PAMP	pathogen-associated molecular pattern			
P_AO_2	partial pressure of oxygen in arterial blood		**RAR**	retinoic acid receptor
PAR	protease-activated receptor		**Rb**	retinoblastoma
PARP	poly-[ADP-ribose]-polymerase		**REM**	rapid eye movement [sleep]
PC	phosphorylcholine		**RGS**	regulator of G-protein signalling
PCPA	*p*-chlorophenylalanine		**RIMA**	reversible inhibitor of the A-isoform of monoamine oxidase
PD	Parkinson's disease			
PDE	phosphodiesterase		**RNA**	ribonucleic acid
PDGF	platelet-dependent growth factor		**RNAi**	ribonucleic acid interference
PDS	pendrin; paroxysmal depolarising shift		**ROS**	reactive oxygen species
PE	phosphatidylethanolamine		**rRNA**	ribosomal ribonucleic acid
PECAM	platelet endothelium cell adhesion molecule		**RTI**	reverse transcriptase inhibitor
			RTK	receptor tyrosine kinase
PEFR	peak expiratory flow rate		**RXR**	retinoid X receptor
PEG	polyethylene glycol		**RyR**	ryanodine receptor
PG	prostaglandin		**SA**	sinoatrial
PGE	prostaglandin E		**SAH**	subarachnoid haemorrhage
PGI₂	prostacyclin [prostaglandin I_2]		**SCF**	stem cell factor
PI	phosphatidylinositol		**SCID**	severe combined immunodeficiency
PIN	protein inhibitor of nNOS		**SERCA**	sarcoplasmic/endoplasmic reticulum APTase
PIP₂	phosphatidylinositol bisphosphate		**SERM**	selective (o) estrogen receptor modulator
PKA	protein kinase A			
PKC	protein kinase C		**SERT**	serotonin transporter
PKK	cGMP-dependent protein kinase		**SG**	substantia gelatinosa
PL	phospholipid		**SH**	sulfhydryl [e.g. –SH group]
PLA₂	phospholipase A_2		**siRNA**	small [short] interfering ribonucleic acid (*see also* **sRNAi** *below*)
PLC	phospholipase C			
PLCβ	phospholipase Cβ		**SLE**	systemic lupus erythematosus
PLD	phospholipase D		**SNAP**	*S*-nitrosoacetylpenicillamine
Plk	Polo-like kinase		**SNOG**	*S*-nitrosoglutathione
PLTP	phospholipid transfer protein		**SNRI**	serotonin/noradrenaline reuptake inhibitor
PMCA	plasma membrane Ca^{2+}-ATPase		**SOC**	store-operated calcium channel
PMN	polymodal nociceptor		**SOD**	superoxide dismutase
PNMT	phenylethanolamine *N*-methyl transferase		**SP**	substance P
PNS	peripheral nervous system		**SR**	sarcoplasmic reticulum
Po_2	partial pressure of oxygen		**sRNAi**	small ribonucleic acid interference (*see also* **siRNA** *above*)
POMC	prepro-opiomelanocortin			
			SRS-A	slow-reacting substance of anaphylaxis

SSRI	selective serotonin reuptake inhibitor	**TRP**	transient receptor potential [channel]
STX	saxitoxin	**TRPV1**	transient receptor potential vanilloid receptor 1
SUR	sulfonylurea receptor		
SVT	supraventricular tachycardia	**TSH**	thyroid-stimulating hormone
SXR	xenobiotic receptor	**TTX**	tetrodotoxin
T₃	triiodothyronine	**TX**	thromboxane
T₄	thyroxine	**TXA₂**	thromboxane A₂
TBG	thyroxine-binding globulin	**TXSI**	TXA₂ synthesis inhibitor
TC	tubocurarine	**UCP**	uncoupling protein
TCA	tricyclic antidepressant	**UDP**	uridine diphosphate
TEA	tetraethylammonium	**UDPGA**	uridine diphosphate glucuronic acid
TF	transcription factor	**UMP**	uridine monophosphate
TGF	transforming growth factor	**vCJD**	variant Creutzfeldt–Jakob disease
Th	T-helper [cell]	**Vd**	volume of distribution
THC	Δ^9-tetrahydrocannabinol	**VDCC**	voltage-dependent calcium channel
Thp	T-helper precursor [cell]	**VDR**	vitamin D receptor
TIMI	Thrombolysis in Myocardial Infarction [trial]	**VEGF**	vascular endothelial growth factor
		VGCC	voltage-gated calcium channel
TIMPs	tissue inhibitors of metalloproteinases	**VHeFT**	Vasodilator Heart Failure Trial
TLR	Toll receptor	**VIP**	vasoactive intestinal peptide
TNF	tumour necrosis factor	**VLA**	very late antigen
TNFR	tumour necrosis factor receptor	**VLDL**	very low-density lipoprotein
tPA	tissue plasminogen activator	**VMA**	vanillylmandelic acid
TR	thyroid receptor	**VMAT**	vesicular monoamine transporter
TRAIL	tumour necrosis factor-α–related apoptosis-inducing ligand	**VOCC**	voltage-operated calcium channel
		WHO	World Health Organization
TRH	thyrotrophin-releasing hormone	**WOSCOPS**	West of Scotland Coronary Prevention Study
tRNA	transfer ribonucleic acid		

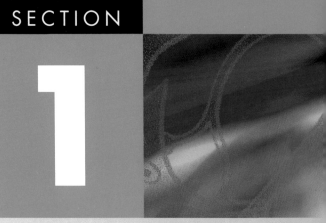

GENERAL PRINCIPLES

What is pharmacology?

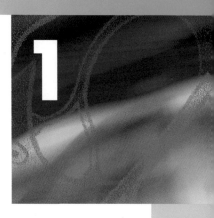

OVERVIEW

In this introductory chapter, we explain how pharmacology came into being and evolved as a scientific discipline, and describe the present day structure of the subject and its links to other biomedical sciences. The structure that has emerged forms the basis of the organisation of the rest of the book. Readers in a hurry to get to the here-and-now of pharmacology can safely skip this chapter.

WHAT IS A DRUG?

For the purposes of this book, a drug can be defined as *a chemical substance of known structure, other than a nutrient or an essential dietary ingredient, which, when administered to a living organism, produces a biological effect.*

A few points are worth noting. Drugs may be synthetic chemicals, chemicals obtained from plants or animals, or products of genetic engineering. A *medicine* is a chemical preparation, which usually but not necessarily contains one or more drugs, administered with the intention of producing a therapeutic effect. Medicines usually contain other substances (excipients, stabilisers, solvents, etc.) besides the active drug, to make them more convenient to use. To count as a drug, the substance must be administered as such, rather than released by physiological mechanisms. Many substances, such as insulin or thyroxine, are endogenous hormones but are also drugs when they are administered intentionally. Many drugs are not used in medicines but are nevertheless useful research tools. In everyday parlance, the word *drug* is often associated with addictive, narcotic or mind-altering substances—an unfortunate negative connotation that tends to bias opinion against any form of chemical therapy. In this book, we focus mainly on drugs used for therapeutic purposes but also describe important examples of drugs used as experimental tools. Although poisons fall strictly within the definition of drugs, they are not covered in this book.

ORIGINS AND ANTECEDENTS

Pharmacology can be defined as the study of the effects of drugs on the function of living systems. As a science, it was born in the mid-19th century, one of a host of new biomedical sciences based on principles of experimentation rather than dogma that came into being in that remarkable period. Long before that—indeed from the dawn of civilisation—herbal remedies were widely used, pharmacopoeias were written, and the apothecaries' trade flourished, but nothing resembling scientific principles was applied to therapeutics. Even Robert Boyle, who laid the scientific foundations of chemistry in the middle of the 17th century, was content, when dealing with therapeutics (*A Collection of Choice Remedies*, 1692), to recommend concoctions of worms, dung, urine, and the moss from a dead man's skull. The impetus for pharmacology came from the need to improve the outcome of therapeutic intervention by doctors, who were at that time skilled at clinical observation and diagnosis but broadly ineffectual when it came to treatment.[1] Until the late 19th century, knowledge of the normal and abnormal functioning of the body was too rudimentary to provide even a rough basis for understanding drug effects; at the same time, disease and death were regarded as semisacred subjects, appropriately dealt with by authoritarian, rather than scientific, doctrines. Clinical practice often displayed an obedience to authority and ignored what appear to be easily ascertainable facts. For example, cinchona bark was recognised as a specific and effective treatment for malaria, and a sound protocol for its use was laid down by Lind in 1765. In 1804, however, Johnson declared it to be unsafe until the fever had

---

[1]Oliver Wendell Holmes, an eminent physician, wrote in 1860: '...firmly believe that if the whole materia medica, as now used, could be sunk to the bottom of the sea, it would be all the better for mankind and the worse for the fishes.' (see Porter, 1997).

3

subsided, and he recommended instead the use of large doses of calomel (mercurous chloride) in the early stages—a murderous piece of advice, which was slavishly followed for the next 40 years.

The motivation for understanding what drugs can and cannot do came from clinical practice, but the science could be built only on the basis of secure foundations in physiology, pathology and chemistry. It was not until 1858 that Virchow proposed the cell theory. The first use of a structural formula to describe a chemical compound was in 1868. Bacteria as a cause of disease were discovered by Pasteur in 1878. Previously, pharmacology hardly had the legs to stand on, and we may wonder at the bold vision of Rudolf Buchheim, who created the first pharmacology institute (in his own house) in Estonia in 1847.

In its beginnings, before the advent of synthetic organic chemistry, pharmacology concerned itself exclusively with understanding the effects of natural substances, mainly plant extracts—and a few (mainly toxic) chemicals such as mercury and arsenic. An early development in chemistry was the purification of active compounds from plants. Friedrich Sertürner, a young German apothecary, purified morphine from opium in 1805. Other substances quickly followed, and, even though their structures were unknown, these compounds showed that chemicals, not magic or vital forces, were responsible for the effects that plant extracts produced on living organisms. Early pharmacologists focused most of their attention on such plant-derived drugs as quinine, digitalis, atropine, ephedrine, strychnine and others (many of which are still used today and will have become old friends by the time you have finished reading this book).[2]

PHARMACOLOGY IN THE 20TH AND 21ST CENTURIES

Beginning in the 20th century, the fresh wind of synthetic chemistry began to revolutionise the pharmaceutical industry, and with it the science of pharmacology. New synthetic drugs, such as barbiturates and local anaesthetics, began to appear, and the era of antimicrobial chemotherapy began with the discovery by Paul Ehrlich in 1909 of arsenical compounds for treating syphilis. Further breakthroughs came when the sulfonamides, the first antibacterial drugs, were discovered by Gerhard Domagk in 1935, and with the development of penicillin by Chain and Florey during the Second World War, based on the earlier work of Fleming.

These few well-known examples show how the growth of synthetic chemistry, and the resurgence of natural product chemistry, caused a dramatic revitalisation of therapeutics in the first half of the 20th century. Each new drug class that emerged gave pharmacologists a new challenge, and it was then that pharmacology really established its identity and its status among the biomedical sciences.

In parallel with the exuberant proliferation of therapeutic molecules—driven mainly by chemistry—which gave pharmacologists so much to think about, physiology was also making rapid progress, particularly in relation to chemical mediators, which are discussed in depth elsewhere in this book. Many hormones, neurotransmitters and inflammatory mediators were discovered in this period, and the realisation that chemical communication plays a central role in almost every regulatory mechanism that our bodies possess immediately established a large area of common ground between physiology and pharmacology, for interactions between chemical substances and living systems were exactly what pharmacologists had been preoccupied with from the outset. The concept of 'receptors' for chemical mediators, first proposed by Langley in 1905, was quickly taken up by pharmacologists such as Clark, Gaddum, Schild and others and is a constant theme in present day pharmacology (as you will soon discover as you plough through the next two chapters). The receptor concept, and the technologies developed from it, have had a massive impact on drug discovery and therapeutics. Biochemistry also emerged as a distinct science early in the 20th century, and the discovery of enzymes and the delineation of biochemical pathways provided yet another framework for understanding drug effects. The picture of pharmacology that emerges from this brief glance at history (Fig. 1.1) is of a subject evolved from ancient prescientific therapeutics, involved in commerce from the 17th century onwards, and which gained respectability by donning the trappings of science as soon as this became possible in the mid-19th century. Signs of its carpetbagger past still cling to pharmacology, for the pharmaceutical industry has become very big business and much pharmacological research nowadays takes place in a commercial environment, a rougher and more pragmatic place than the glades of academia.[3] No other biomedical 'ology' is so close to Mammon.

ALTERNATIVE THERAPEUTIC PRINCIPLES

Modern medicine relies heavily on drugs as the main tool of therapeutics. Other therapeutic procedures such as surgery, diet, exercise, etc. are also important, of course, as is deliberate

---

[2]A handful of synthetic substances achieved pharmacological prominence long before the era of synthetic chemistry began. Diethyl ether, first prepared as 'sweet oil of vitriol' in the 16th century, and nitrous oxide, prepared by Humphrey Davy in 1799, were used to liven up parties before being introduced as anaesthetic agents in the mid-19th century (see Ch. 36). Amyl nitrite (see Ch. 18) was made in 1859 and can claim to be the first 'rational' therapeutic drug; its therapeutic effect in angina was predicted on the basis of its physiological effects—a true 'pharmacologist's drug' and the smelly forerunner of the nitrovasodilators that are widely used today. Aspirin (Ch. 14), the most widely used therapeutic drug in history, was first synthesised in 1853, with no therapeutic application in mind. It was rediscovered in 1897 in the laboratories of the German company Bayer, who were seeking a less toxic derivative prof salicylic acid. Bayer commercialised aspirin in 1899 and made a fortune.

[3]Some of our most distinguished pharmacological pioneers made their careers in industry: for example, Henry Dale, who laid the foundations of our knowledge of chemical transmission and the autonomic nervous system; George Hitchings and Gertrude Elion, who described the antimetabolite principle and produced the first effective anticancer drugs; and James Black, who introduced the first β-adrenoceptor and histamine H_2-receptor antagonists. It is no accident that in this book, where we focus on the scientific principles of pharmacology, most of our examples are products of industry, not of nature.

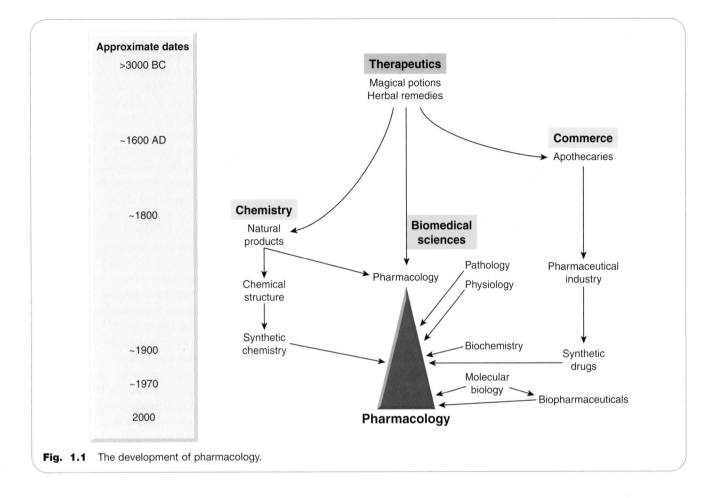

Fig. 1.1 The development of pharmacology.

non-intervention, but none is so widely applied as drug-based therapeutics.

Before the advent of science-based approaches, repeated attempts were made to construct systems of therapeutics, many of which produced even worse results than pure empiricism. One of these was allopathy, espoused by James Gregory (1735–1821). The favoured remedies included blood letting, emetics and purgatives, which were used until the dominant symptoms of the disease were suppressed. Many patients died from such treatment, and it was in reaction against it that Hahnemann introduced the practice of homœopathy in the early 19th century. The guiding principles of homœopathy are:

- like cures like
- activity can be enhanced by dilution.

The system rapidly drifted into absurdity: for example, Hahnemann recommended the use of drugs at dilutions of $1:10^{60}$, equivalent to one molecule in a sphere the size of the orbit of Neptune.

Many other systems of therapeutics have come and gone, and the variety of dogmatic principles that they embodied have tended to hinder rather than advance scientific progress. Currently, therapeutic systems that have a basis which lies outside the domain of science are actually gaining ground under the general banner of 'alternative' or 'complementary' medicine. Mostly, they reject the 'medical model', which attributes disease to an underlying derangement of normal function that can be defined in bio-

chemical or structural terms, detected by objective means, and influenced beneficially by appropriate chemical or physical interventions. They focus instead mainly on subjective malaise, which may be disease-associated or not. Abandoning objectivity in defining and measuring disease goes along with a similar departure from scientific principles in assessing therapeutic efficacy and risk, with the result that principles and practices can gain acceptance without satisfying any of the criteria of validity that would convince a critical scientist, and that are required by law to be satisfied before a new drug can be introduced into therapy. Public acceptance, alas, has little to do with demonstrable efficacy.

THE EMERGENCE OF BIOTECHNOLOGY

Since the 1980s, biotechnology has emerged as a major source of new therapeutic agents in the form of antibodies, enzymes and various regulatory proteins, including hormones, growth factors and cytokines (see Buckel, 1996; Walsh, 2003). Although such products (known as *biopharmaceuticals*) are generally produced by genetic engineering rather than by synthetic chemistry, the pharmacological principles are essentially the same as for conventional drugs. Looking further ahead, gene- and cell-based therapies (Ch. 55), although still in their infancy, will take therapeutics into a new domain. The principles governing the design, delivery and control of functioning artificial genes introduced into cells, or of engineered cells introduced into the body, are very different from those of drug-based therapeutics and will require a different conceptual framework, which texts such as this will increasingly need to embrace if they are to stay abreast of modern medical treatment.

PHARMACOLOGY TODAY

As with other biomedical disciplines, the boundaries of pharmacology are not sharply defined, nor are they constant. Its exponents are, as befits pragmatists, ever ready to poach on the territory and techniques of other disciplines. If it ever had a conceptual and technical core that it could really call its own, this has now dwindled almost to the point of extinction, and the subject is defined by its purpose—to understand what drugs do to living organisms, and more particularly how their effects can be applied to therapeutics—rather than by its scientific coherence.

Figure 1.2 shows the structure of pharmacology as it appears today. Within the main subject fall a number of compartments (neuropharmacology, immunopharmacology, pharmacokinetics, etc.), which are convenient, if not watertight, subdivisions. These topics form the main subject matter of this book. Around the edges are several interface disciplines, not covered in this book, which form important two-way bridges between pharmacology and other fields of biomedicine. Pharmacology tends to have more of these than other disciplines. Recent arrivals on the fringe are subjects such as pharmacogenomics, pharmacoepidemiology and pharmacoeconomics.

Biotechnology. Originally, this was the production of drugs or other useful products by biological means (e.g. antibiotic production from microorganisms or production of monoclonal antibodies). Currently in the biomedical sphere, biotechnology refers mainly to the use of recombinant DNA technology for a wide variety of purposes, including the manufacture of therapeutic proteins, diagnostics, genotyping, production of transgenic animals, etc. The many non-medical applications include agriculture, forensics, environmental sciences, etc.

Pharmacogenetics. This is the study of genetic influences on responses to drugs. Originally, pharmacogenetics focused on familial idiosyncratic drug reactions, where affected individuals show an abnormal—usually adverse—response to a class of drug (see Nebert & Weber, 1990). It now covers broader variations in drug response, where the genetic basis is more complex.

Pharmacogenomics. This recent term overlaps with pharmacogenetics, describing the use of genetic information to guide the choice of drug therapy on an individual basis. The underlying principle is that differences between individuals in their response to therapeutic drugs can be predicted from their genetic make-up. Examples that confirm this are steadily accumulating (see Ch. 51). So far, they mainly involve genetic polymorphism of drug-metabolising enzymes or receptors (see Weinshilboum & Wang,

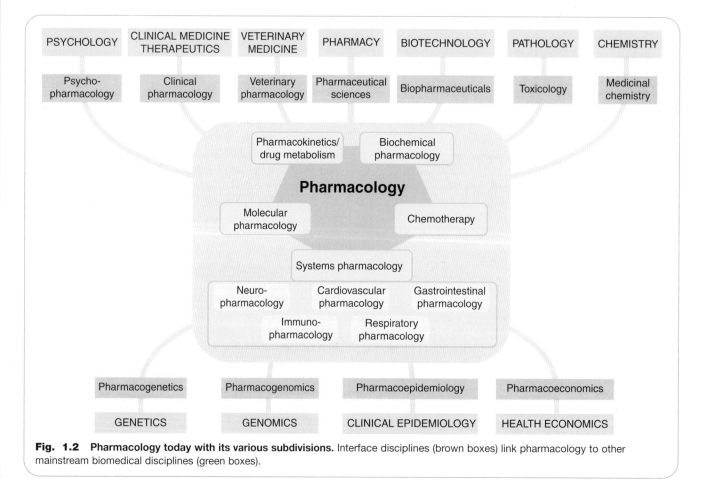

Fig. 1.2 Pharmacology today with its various subdivisions. Interface disciplines (brown boxes) link pharmacology to other mainstream biomedical disciplines (green boxes).

2004). Ultimately, linking specific gene variations with variations in therapeutic or unwanted effects of a particular drug should enable the tailoring of therapeutic choices on the basis of an individual's genotype. The consequences for therapeutics will be far-reaching.[4]

Pharmacoepidemiology. This is the study of drug effects at the population level (see Strom, 1994). It is concerned with the variability of drug effects between individuals in a population, and between populations. It is an increasingly important topic in the eyes of the regulatory authorities who decide whether or not new drugs can be licensed for therapeutic use. Variability between individuals or populations has an adverse effect on the utility of a drug, even though its mean effect level may be satisfactory. Pharmacoepidemiological studies also take into account patient compliance and other factors that apply when the drug is used under real-life conditions.

Pharmacoeconomics. This branch of health economics aims to quantify in economic terms the cost and benefit of drugs used therapeutically. It arose from the concern of many governments to provide for healthcare from tax revenues, raising questions of what therapeutic procedures represent the best value for money. This, of course, raises fierce controversy, because it ultimately comes down to putting monetary value on health and longevity. As with pharmacoepidemiology, regulatory authorities are increasingly requiring economic analysis, as well as evidence of individual benefit, when making decisions on licensing. For more information on this complex subject, see Drummond et al. (1997).

---

[4]An interesting recent example concerns a newly introduced anticancer drug, gefitinib, which is highly effective in treating lung cancer but works in only about 10% of cases. Responders have mutations in the receptor tyrosine kinase (see Ch. 3) that is the target of this drug, and can be identified in advance by genotyping (see Lynch et al., 2004).

REFERENCES AND FURTHER READING

Buckel P 1996 Recombinant proteins for therapy. Trends Pharmacol Sci 17: 450–456 (*Thoughtful review of the status of, and prospects for, protein-based therapeutics*)

Drews J 1998 In quest of tomorrow's medicines. Springer-Verlag, New York (*An excellent account of the past, present and future of the drug discovery process, emphasising the growing role of biotechnology*)

Drummond M F, O'Brien B, Stoddart G I, Torrance G W 1997 Methods for the economic evaluation of healthcare programmes. Oxford University Press, Oxford (*Coverage of the general principles of evaluating the economic costs and benefits of healthcare, including drug-based therapeutics*)

Evans W E, Relling M V 1999 Pharmacogenomics: translating functional genomics into rational therapeutics. Science 286: 487–501 (*A general overview of pharmacogenomics*)

Lynch T J, Bell D W, Sordella R et al. 2004 Activating mutations in the epidermal growth factor receptor underlying responsiveness of non–small-cell lung cancer to gefitinib. N Engl J Med 350: 2129–2139 (*An important early example of a genetic determinant of therapeutic efficacy depending on mutations affecting the drug target—a likely pointer to what is to come*)

Nebert D W, Weber W W 1990 Pharmacogenetics. In: Pratt W B, Taylor P (eds) Principles of drug action, 3rd edn. Churchill-Livingstone, New York (*A detailed account of genetic factors that affect responses to drugs, with many examples from the pregenomic literature*)

Porter R 1997 The greatest benefit to mankind. Harper-Collins, London (*An excellent and readable account of the history of medicine, with good coverage of the early development of pharmacology and the pharmaceutical industry*)

Strom B L (ed) 2000 Pharmacoepidemiology, 3rd edn. Wiley, Chichester (*A multiauthor book covering all aspects of a newly emerged discipline, including aspects of pharmacoeconomics*)

Walsh G 2003 Biopharmaceuticals: biochemistry and biotechnology. Chichester, Wiley (*Good introductory textbook covering many aspects of biotechnology-based therapeutics*)

Weinshilboum R, Wang L 2004 Pharmacogenomics: bench to bedside. Nat Rev Drug Discov 3: 739–748 (*Discusses, with examples, the growing importance of the correlation between genetic make-up and response to therapeutic drugs*)

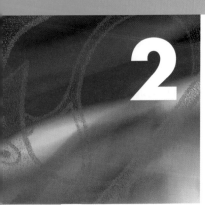

2

How drugs act: general principles

OVERVIEW

The emergence of pharmacology as a science came when the emphasis shifted from describing what drugs do to explaining how they work. In this chapter, we set out some general principles underlying the interaction of drugs with living systems (Ch. 3 goes into the molecular aspects in more detail). The interaction between drugs and cells is described, followed by a more detailed examination of different types of drug–receptor interaction. We are still far from the holy grail of being able to predict the pharmacological effects of a novel chemical substance, or to design *ab initio* a chemical to produce a specified therapeutic effect; nevertheless, we can identify some important general principles, which is our purpose in this chapter.

THE BINDING OF DRUG MOLECULES TO CELLS

To begin with, we should gratefully acknowledge Paul Ehrlich for insisting that drug action must be explicable in terms of conventional chemical interactions between drugs and tissues, and

for dispelling the idea that the remarkable potency and specificity of action of some drugs put them somehow out of reach of chemistry and physics and required the intervention of magical 'vital forces'. Although many drugs produce effects in extraordinarily low doses and concentrations, low concentrations still involve very large numbers of molecules. One drop of a solution of a drug at only 10^{-10} mol/l still contains about 10^{10} drug molecules, so there is no mystery in the fact that it may produce an obvious pharmacological response. Some bacterial toxins (e.g. diphtheria toxin) act with such precision that a single molecule taken up by a target cell is sufficient to kill it.

One of the basic tenets of pharmacology is that drug molecules must exert some chemical influence on one or more constituents of cells in order to produce a pharmacological response. In other words, drug molecules must get so close to these constituent cellular molecules that the two interact chemically in such a way that the function of the latter is altered. Of course, the molecules in the organism vastly outnumber the drug molecules, and if the drug molecules were merely distributed at random, the chance of interaction with any particular class of cellular molecule would be negligible. Pharmacological effects, therefore, require, in general, the non-uniform distribution of the drug molecule within the body or tissue, which is the same as saying that drug molecules must be 'bound' to particular constituents of cells and tissues in order to produce an effect. Ehrlich summed it up thus: '*Corpora non agunt nisi fixata*' (in this context, 'A drug will not work unless it is bound').[1]

These critical binding sites are often referred to as 'drug targets' (an obvious allusion to Ehrlich's famous phrase 'magic bullets' describing the potential of antimicrobial drugs). The mechanisms by which the association of a drug molecule with its target leads to a physiological response constitute the major thrust of pharmacological research. Most drug targets are protein molecules. Even general anaesthetics (see Ch. 36), which were long thought to produce their effects by an interaction with membrane lipid, now appear to interact mainly with membrane proteins (see Franks & Lieb, 1994). All rules need exceptions, and many antimicrobial and antitumour drugs (Chs 45 and 51), as well as mutagenic and carcinogenic agents (Ch. 51), interact directly with DNA rather

---

[1]There are, if one looks hard enough, exceptions to Ehrlich's dictum—drugs that act without being bound to any tissue constituent (e.g. osmotic diuretics, osmotic purgatives, antacids, and heavy metal chelating agents). Nonetheless, the principle remains true for the great majority.

than protein; bisphosphonates, used to treat osteoporosis (Ch. 31), bind to calcium salts in the bone matrix, rendering it toxic to osteoclasts, much like rat poison.

PROTEIN TARGETS FOR DRUG BINDING

Four main kinds of regulatory protein are commonly involved as primary drug targets, namely:

- receptors
- enzymes
- carrier molecules (transporters)
- ion channels.

A few other types of protein are known to function as drug targets, and there exist many drugs with sites of action that are not yet known. Furthermore, many drugs are known to bind (in addition to their primary targets) to plasma proteins (see Ch. 5), and to a variety of cellular proteins, without producing any obvious physiological effect. Nevertheless, the generalisation that most drugs act on one or other of the four types of protein listed above serves as a good starting point.

Further discussion of the mechanisms by which such binding leads to cellular responses is given in Chapters 3–5.

DRUG RECEPTORS

WHAT DO WE MEAN BY RECEPTORS?

▼ As emphasised in Chapter 1, the concept of receptors is central to pharmacology, and the term is most often used to describe the target molecules through which soluble physiological mediators—hormones, neurotransmitters, inflammatory mediators, etc.—produce their effects. Examples such as acetylcholine receptors, cytokine receptors, steroid receptors, and growth hormone receptors abound in this book, and generally the term *receptor* indicates a recognition molecule for a chemical mediator.

'Receptor' is sometimes used to denote *any* target molecule with which a drug molecule (i.e. a foreign compound rather than an endogenous mediator) has to combine in order to elicit its specific effect. For example, the voltage-sensitive sodium channel is sometimes referred to as the 'receptor' for **local anaesthetics** (see Ch. 44), or the enzyme dihydrofolate reductase as the 'receptor' for **methotrexate** (Ch.14). The term *drug target* is preferable in this context.

In the more general context of cell biology, the term receptor is used to describe various cell surface molecules (such as T-cell receptors, integrins, Toll receptors, etc.) involved in the immunological response to foreign proteins and the interaction of cells with each other and with the extracellular matrix. These have many important roles in cell growth and migration (see Ch.5), and are also emerging as drug targets. These receptors differ from conventional pharmacological receptors in that they respond to proteins attached to cell surfaces or extracellular structures, rather than to soluble mediators.

Various carrier proteins are often referred to as receptors, such as the *low-density lipoprotein receptor* that plays a key role in lipid metabolism (Ch.19) and the *transferrin receptor* involved in iron absorption (Ch.21). These entities have little in common with pharmacological receptors.

RECEPTORS IN PHYSIOLOGICAL SYSTEMS

Receptors form a key part of the system of chemical communication that all multicellular organisms use to coordinate the activities of their cells and organs. Without them, we would be no better than a bucketful of amoebae.

Some fundamental properties of receptors are illustrated by the action of **adrenaline** (epinephrine) on the heart. Adrenaline first binds to a receptor protein (the β adrenoceptor, see Ch. 11) that serves as a recognition site for adrenaline and other catecholamines. When it binds to the receptor, a train of reactions is initiated (see Ch. 3) leading to an increase in force and rate of the heartbeat. In the absence of adrenaline, the receptor is functionally silent. This is true of most receptors for endogenous mediators (hormones, neurotransmitters, cytokines, etc.), although there are now several examples (see Ch. 3) of receptors that are 'constitutively active'—that is, they exert a controlling influence even when no chemical mediator is present.

There is an important distinction between *agonists*, which 'activate' the receptors, and *antagonists*, which may combine at the same site without causing activation, and block the effect of agonists on that receptor. The distinction between agonists and antagonists only exists for receptors with this type of physiological regulatory role; we cannot usefully speak of 'agonists' for the more general class of drug targets, such as the noradrenaline (norepinephrine) transporter, the voltage-sensitive sodium channel or dihydrofolate reductase, or for entities such as the transferrin receptor.

The characteristics of pharmacological receptors, and the descriptors that are conventionally used for them, are described in a review by Neubig et al. (2003). The origins of the receptor concept and its pharmacological significance are discussed by Rang (2006).

Targets for drug action

- A drug is a chemical applied to a physiological system that affects its function in a specific way.
- With few exceptions, drugs act on target proteins, namely:
  —receptors
  —enzymes
  —carriers
  —ion channels.
- The term *receptor* is used in different ways. In pharmacology, it describes protein molecules whose function is to recognise and respond to endogenous chemical signals. Other macromolecules with which drugs interact to produce their effects are known as drug targets.
- Specificity is reciprocal: individual classes of drug bind only to certain targets, and individual targets recognise only certain classes of drug.
- No drugs are completely specific in their actions. In many cases, increasing the dose of a drug will cause it to affect targets other than the principal one, and this can lead to side effects.

DRUG SPECIFICITY

For a drug to be useful as either a therapeutic or a scientific tool, it must act selectively on particular cells and tissues. In other words, it must show a high degree of binding site specificity. Conversely, proteins that function as drug targets generally show a high degree of ligand specificity; they will recognise only ligands of a certain precise type and ignore closely related molecules.

These principles of binding site and ligand specificity can be clearly recognised in the actions of a mediator such as **angiotensin** (Ch. 19). This peptide acts strongly on vascular smooth muscle, and on the kidney tubule, but has very little effect on other kinds of smooth muscle or on the intestinal epithelium. Other mediators affect a quite different spectrum of cells and tissues, the pattern in each case being determined by the specific pattern of expression of the protein receptors for the various mediators. A small chemical change, such as conversion of one of the amino acids in angiotensin from L to D form, or removal of one amino acid from the chain, can inactivate the molecule altogether, because the receptor fails to bind the altered form. The complementary specificity of ligands and binding sites, which gives rise to the very exact molecular recognition properties of proteins, is central to explaining many of the phenomena of pharmacology. It is no exaggeration to say that the ability of proteins to interact in a highly selective way with other molecules—including other proteins—is the basis of living machines. Its relevance to the understanding of drug action will be a recurring theme in this book.

Finally, it must be emphasised that no drug acts with complete specificity. Thus tricyclic antidepressant drugs (Ch. 39) act by blocking monoamine transporters but are notorious for producing side effects (e.g. dry mouth) related to their ability to block various receptors. In general, the lower the potency of a drug, and the higher the dose needed, the more likely it is that sites of action other than the primary one will assume significance. In clinical terms, this is often associated with the appearance of unwanted side effects, of which no drug is free.

Since the 1970s, pharmacological research has succeeded in identifying the protein targets of many different types of drug. Drugs such as opiate analgesics (Ch. 41), cannabinoids (Ch. 15), and benzodiazepine tranquillisers (Ch. 37), with actions that were described in exhaustive detail for many years, are now known to target well-defined receptors, which have been fully characterised by gene-cloning techniques (see Ch. 3).

RECEPTOR CLASSIFICATION

▼ Where the action of a drug can be associated with a particular receptor, this provides a valuable means for classification and refinement in drug design. For example, pharmacological analysis of the actions of histamine (see Ch. 13) showed that some of its effects (the H_1 effects, such as smooth muscle contraction) were strongly antagonised by the competitive histamine antagonists then known. Black and his colleagues suggested in 1970 that the remaining actions of histamine, which included its stimulant effect on gastric secretion, might represent a second class of histamine receptor (H_2). Testing a number of histamine analogues, they found that some were selective in producing H_2 effects, with little H_1 activity. By analysing which parts of the histamine molecule conferred this type of specificity, they were able to develop selective antagonists, which proved to be potent in blocking gastric acid secretion, a development

of major therapeutic significance (Ch. 25). Two further types of histamine receptor (H_3 and H_4) were recognised later.

Receptor classification based on pharmacological responses continues to be a valuable and widely used approach. Newer experimental approaches have produced other criteria on which to base receptor classification. The direct measurement of ligand binding to receptors (see p.11) has allowed many new receptor subtypes to be defined that could not easily be distinguished by studies of drug effects. Molecular cloning (see Ch.3) provided a completely new basis for classification at a much finer level of detail than can be reached through pharmacological analysis. Finally, analysis of the biochemical pathways that are linked to receptor activation (see Ch.3) provides yet another basis for classification.

The result of this data explosion has been that receptor classification has suddenly become very much more detailed, with a proliferation of receptor subtypes for all the main types of ligand; more worryingly, alternative molecular and biochemical classifications began to spring up that were incompatible with the accepted pharmacologically defined receptor classes. Responding to this growing confusion, the International Union of Pharmacological Sciences (IUPHAR) convened expert working groups to produce agreed receptor classifications for the major types, taking into account the pharmacological, molecular and biochemical information available (see http://www.iuphar.org). These wise people have a hard task; their conclusions will be neither perfect nor final but are essential to ensure a consistent terminology. To the student, this may seem an arcane exercise in taxonomy, generating much detail but little illumination. There is a danger that the tedious lists of drug names, actions and side effects that used to burden the subject will be replaced by exhaustive tables of receptors, ligands and transduction pathways. In this book, we have tried to avoid detail for its own sake and include only such information on receptor classification as seems interesting in its own right or is helpful in explaining the actions of important drugs. A useful summary of known receptor classes is now published annually (Alexander et al., 2006).

DRUG–RECEPTOR INTERACTIONS

Occupation of a receptor by a drug molecule may or may not result in *activation* of the receptor. By activation, we mean that the receptor is affected by the bound molecule in such a way as to elicit a tissue response. The molecular mechanisms associated with receptor activation are discussed in Chapter 3. Binding and activation represent two distinct steps in the generation of the

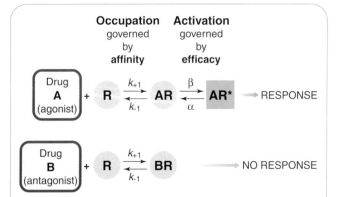

Fig. 2.1 The distinction between drug binding and receptor activation. The rate constants k_{+1}, k_{-1}, β and α, which apply to the binding and activation reactions, respectively, are referred to in the text (pp. 15-20). Ligand A is an agonist, because it leads to activation of the receptor (R), whereas ligand B is an antagonist.

receptor-mediated response by an agonist (Fig. 2.1). If a drug binds to the receptor without causing activation and thereby prevents the agonist from binding, it is termed a *receptor antagonist*. The tendency of a drug to bind to the receptors is governed by its *affinity*, whereas the tendency for it, once bound, to activate the receptor is denoted by its *efficacy*. These terms are defined more precisely below (p. 12). Drugs of high potency will generally have a high affinity for the receptors and thus occupy a significant proportion of the receptors even at low concentrations. Agonists will also possess high efficacy, whereas antagonists will, in the simplest case, have zero efficacy. Drugs with intermediate levels of efficacy, such that even when 100% of the receptors are occupied the tissue response is submaximal, are known as *partial agonists*, to distinguish them from *full agonists*, the efficacy of which is sufficient that they can elicit a maximal tissue response. These concepts, even though we now see them as an oversimplified description of events at the molecular level (see Ch. 3), provide a useful basis for characterising drug effects.

We now discuss certain aspects in more detail, namely drug binding, agonist concentration–effect curves, competitive antagonism, partial agonists and the nature of efficacy, and spare receptors. Understanding these concepts at a qualitative level is sufficient for many purposes, but for more detailed analysis a quantitative formulation is needed (see p. 20).

THE BINDING OF DRUGS TO RECEPTORS

▼ The binding of drugs to receptors can often be measured directly by the use of drug molecules labelled with one or more radioactive atoms (usually ^3H, ^{14}C or ^{125}I). The main requirements are that the radioactive ligand (which may be an agonist or antagonist) must bind with high affinity and specificity, and that it can be labelled to a sufficient specific radioactivity to enable minute amounts of binding to be measured. The usual procedure is to incubate samples of the tissue (or membrane fragments) with various concentrations of radioactive drug until equilibrium is reached. The tissue is then removed, or the membrane fragments separated by filtration or centrifugation, and dissolved in scintillation fluid for measurement of its radioactive content.

In such experiments, there is invariably a certain amount of 'non-specific binding' (i.e. drug taken up by structures other than receptors), which obscures the specific component and needs to be kept to a minimum. The amount of non-specific binding is estimated by measuring the radioactivity taken up in the presence of a saturating concentration of a (non-radioactive) ligand that inhibits completely the binding of the radioactive drug to the receptors, leaving behind the non-specific component. This is then subtracted from the total binding to give an estimate of specific binding (Fig. 2.2). The *binding curve* (Fig. 2.2B)

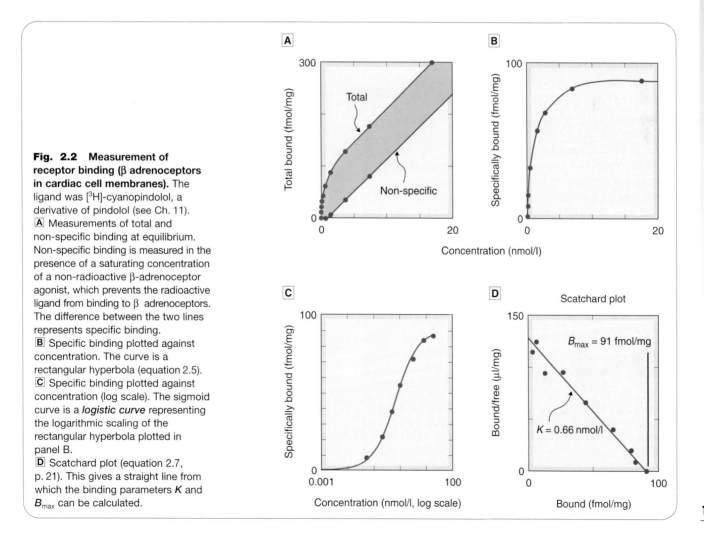

Fig. 2.2 Measurement of receptor binding (β adrenoceptors in cardiac cell membranes). The ligand was [^3H]-cyanopindolol, a derivative of pindolol (see Ch. 11). **A** Measurements of total and non-specific binding at equilibrium. Non-specific binding is measured in the presence of a saturating concentration of a non-radioactive β-adrenoceptor agonist, which prevents the radioactive ligand from binding to β adrenoceptors. The difference between the two lines represents specific binding. **B** Specific binding plotted against concentration. The curve is a rectangular hyperbola (equation 2.5). **C** Specific binding plotted against concentration (log scale). The sigmoid curve is a *logistic curve* representing the logarithmic scaling of the rectangular hyperbola plotted in panel B. **D** Scatchard plot (equation 2.7, p. 21). This gives a straight line from which the binding parameters K and B_{max} can be calculated.

defines the relationship between concentration and the amount of drug bound (B), and in most cases it fits well to the relationship predicted theoretically (see Fig. 2.12, below), allowing the affinity of the drug for the receptors to be estimated, as well as the *binding capacity* (B_{max}), representing the density of receptors in the tissue.

Autoradiography can also be used to investigate the distribution of receptors in structures such as the brain, and direct labelling with ligands containing positron-emitting isotopes is now used to obtain images by positron emission tomography of receptor distribution in humans. This technique has been used, for example, to measure the degree of dopamine receptor blockade produced by antipsychotic drugs in the brains of schizophrenic patients (see Ch. 38). When combined with pharmacological studies, binding measurements have proved very valuable. It has, for example, been confirmed that the spare receptor hypothesis (p. 15) for muscarinic receptors in smooth muscle is correct; agonists are found to bind, in general, with rather low affinity, and a maximal biological effect occurs at low receptor occupancy. It has also been shown, in skeletal muscle and other tissues, that denervation leads to an increase in the number of receptors in the target cell, a finding that accounts, at least in part, for the phenomenon of denervation supersensitivity. More generally, it appears that receptors tend to increase in number, usually over the course of a few days, if the relevant hormone or transmitter is absent or scarce, and to decrease in number if it is in excess, a process of adaptation to drugs or hormones resulting from continued administration (see p. 17).

Binding curves with agonists are more difficult to interpret than those with antagonists, because they often reveal an apparent heterogeneity among receptors. For example, agonist binding to muscarinic receptors (Ch. 10) and also to β-adrenoceptors (Ch. 11) suggests at least two populations of binding sites with different affinities. This may be because the receptors can exist either unattached or coupled within the membrane to another macromolecule, the G-protein (see Ch. 3), which constitutes part of the transduction system through which the receptor exerts its regulatory effect. Antagonist binding does not show this complexity, probably because antagonists, by their nature, do not lead to the secondary event of G-protein coupling. Agonist affinity has proved to be an elusive concept, a fact that has generated an algebraic paper-chase in the pharmacological literature, with many enthusiastic followers.

Although binding can be measured directly, it is usually a biological response, such as a rise in blood pressure, contraction or relaxation of a strip of smooth muscle in an organ bath, or the activation of an enzyme, that we are interested in, and this is often plotted as a *concentration–effect* or *dose–response curve*, as in Figure 2.3. Such curves allow us to estimate the maximal response that the drug can produce (E_{max}), and the concentration or dose needed to produce a 50% maximal response (EC_{50} or ED_{50}), parameters that are useful for comparing the potencies of different drugs that produce qualitatively similar effects (see Ch. 4). Although they look similar to the binding curves in Figure 2.2, concentration–effect curves cannot be used to measure the affinity of agonist drugs for their receptors, because the physiological response produced is not, as a rule, directly proportional to occupancy. For an integrated physiological response, such as a rise in arterial blood pressure produced by adrenaline (epinephrine), many factors interact. Adrenaline (see Ch. 11) increases cardiac output and constricts some blood vessels while dilating others, and the change in arterial pressure itself evokes a reflex response that modifies the primary response to the drug. The final effect will clearly not be a direct measure of receptor occupancy in this instance, and the same is true of most drug-induced effects.

In interpreting concentration–effect curves, it must be remembered that the concentration of the drug at the receptors may differ from the known concentration in the organ bath. Agonists may be subject to rapid enzymic degradation or uptake by cells as they diffuse from the surface towards their site of action, and a steady state can be reached in which the agonist concentration at the receptors is very much less than the concentration in the bath. In the case of acetylcholine, for example, which is hydrolysed by cholinesterase present in most tissues (see Ch. 10), the concentration reaching the receptors can be less than 1% of that in the bath, and an even bigger difference has been found with noradrenaline (norepinephrine), which is avidly taken up by sympathetic nerve terminals in many tissues (Ch. 11). Thus, even if the concentration–effect curve, as in Figure 2.3, looks just like a facsimile of the binding curve (Fig. 2.2C), it cannot be used directly to determine the affinity of the agonist for the receptors.

PARTIAL AGONISTS AND THE CONCEPT OF EFFICACY

So far, we have considered drugs either as agonists, which in some way activate the receptor when they occupy it, or as antagonists, which cause no activation. However, the ability of a drug molecule to activate the receptor is actually a graded, rather than an all-or-nothing, property. If a series of chemically related agonist drugs acting on the same receptors is tested on a given biological system, it is often found that the maximal response (the largest response that can be produced by that drug in high concentration) differs from one drug to another. Some compounds (known as *full agonists*) can produce a maximal response (the largest response that the tissue is capable of giving), whereas others (*partial agonists*) can produce only a submaximal response (Fig. 2.4). The difference between full and partial agonists lies in the relationship between receptor occupancy and response.

Figure 2.5 shows schematically the relationship between occupancy and concentration for two drugs that have the same affinity for receptors, producing 50% occupancy at a concentration of

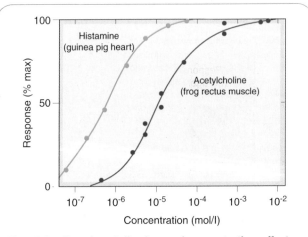

Fig. 2.3 Experimentally observed concentration–effect curves. Although the lines, drawn according to the binding equation 2.5, fit the points well, such curves do not give correct estimates of the affinity of drugs for receptors. This is because the relationship between receptor occupancy and response is usually non-linear.

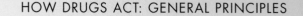

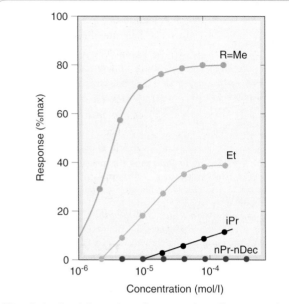

Fig. 2.4 Partial agonists. Concentration–effect curves for substituted methonium compounds on frog rectus abdominis muscle. The compounds were members of the decamethonium series (Ch. 7), $RMe_2N^+(CH_2)_{10}N^+Me_2R$. The maximum response obtainable decreases (i.e. efficacy decreases) as the size of R is increased. With R = nPr or larger, the compounds cause no response and are pure antagonists. (Results from Van Rossum J M 1958 Pharmacodynamics of cholinometic and cholinolytic drugs. St Catherine's Press, Bruges.)

occupancy is much smaller for the partial agonist, which cannot produce a maximal response even at 100% occupancy. This can be expressed quantitatively in terms of *efficacy* (*e*), a parameter originally defined by Stephenson (1956) that describes the 'strength' of the agonist–receptor complex in evoking a response of the tissue. In the simple scheme shown in Figure 2.1, efficacy describes the tendency of the drug–receptor complex to adopt the active (AR*), rather than the resting (AR) state. A drug with zero efficacy (e = 0) has no tendency to cause receptor activation, and causes no tissue response. A drug with maximal efficacy (e = 1) is a full agonist, while partial agonists lie in between.

▼ Subsequently, it was appreciated that characteristics of the tissue (e.g. the number of receptors that it possesses and the nature of the coupling between the receptor and the response; see Ch.3), as well as of the drug itself, were important, and the concept of *intrinsic efficacy* was developed (see Jenkinson, 1996; Kenakin, 1997). The relationship between occupancy and response can thus be represented:

$$\text{Response} = f\left(\frac{\varepsilon N_{tot} x_A}{x_A + K_A}\right)$$

In this equation, f (the transducer function) and N_{tot} (the total number of receptors) are characteristics of the tissue; ε (the intrinsic efficacy) and K_A (the equilibrium constant, see p. 20) are characteristics of the agonist. The importance of this formal representation is that it explains how differences in the transducer function and the density of receptors in different tissues can result in the same agonist, acting on the same receptor, appearing as a full agonist in one tissue and as a partial agonist in another. By the same token, the relative potencies of two agonists may be different in different tissues, even though the receptor is the same.

For a more detailed discussion of drug–receptor interactions, see Jenkinson (1996) and Kenakin (1997).

1.0 µmol/l. Drug **a** is a full agonist, producing a maximal response at about 0.2 µmol/l, the relationship between response and occupancy being shown by the steep curve in B. Comparable plots for a partial agonist (**b**) are shown as the shallow curves in A and B, the essential difference being that the response at any given

It would be nice to be able to explain what efficacy means in physical terms, and to understand why one drug may be an agonist while another, chemically very similar, is an antagonist. We are beginning to understand the molecular events underlying receptor

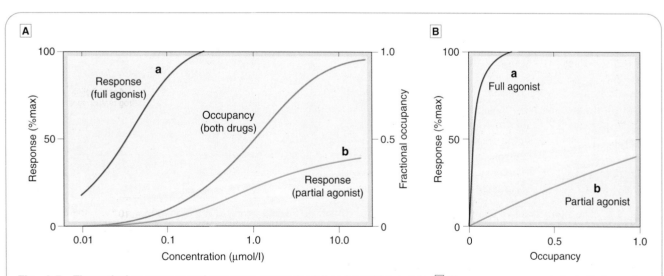

Fig. 2.5 Theoretical occupancy and response curves for full and partial agonists. **A** The occupancy curve is for both drugs, the response curves a and b are for full and partial agonist, respectively. **B** The relationship between response and occupancy for full and partial agonist, corresponding to the response curves in A. Note that curve a produces maximal response at about 20% occupancy, while curve b produces only a submaximal response even at 100% occupancy.

activation (described in Ch. 3) but can still give no clear answer to the question of why some ligands are agonists and some are antagonists, although the simple theoretical two-state model described below provides a useful starting point.

Despite its uncertain theoretical status, efficacy is a concept of great practical importance. Adrenaline (epinephrine) and propranolol have comparable affinities for the β-adrenoceptor but differ in efficacy. Woebetide the doctor—and the student, for that matter—who confuses them. Efficacy matters!

CONSTITUTIVE RECEPTOR ACTIVATION AND INVERSE AGONISTS

▼ Although we are accustomed to thinking that receptors are activated only when an agonist molecule is bound, there are examples (see De Ligt et al., 2000; Teitler et al., 2002) where an appreciable level of activation may exist even when no ligand is present. These include receptors for **benzodiazepines** (see Ch. 37), **cannabinoids** (Ch. 15), **serotonin** (Ch. 12) and several other mediators. Furthermore, receptor mutations occur—either spontaneously, in some disease states or experimentally created (see Ch. 4)—that result in appreciable activation in the absence of any ligand (*constitutive activation*). Resting activity may be too low to have any effect under normal conditions but become evident if receptors are overexpressed, a phenomenon clearly demonstrated for β-adrenoceptors (see Bond et al., 1995), a result that may prove to have major pathophysiological implications. Thus if, say, 1% of receptors are active in the absence of any agonist, in a normal cell expressing perhaps 10 000 receptors, only 100 will be active. Increasing the expression level 10-fold will result in 1000 active receptors, producing a significant effect. Under these conditions, it may be possible for a ligand to *reduce* the level of

constitutive activation; such drugs are known as *inverse agonists* (Fig.2.6; see De Ligt et al., 2000) to distinguish them from simple competitive antagonists, which do not by themselves affect the level of activation. Inverse agonists can be regarded as drugs with negative efficacy, to distinguish them from agonists (positive efficacy) and competitive antagonists (zero efficacy). New examples of constitutively active receptors and inverse agonists are emerging with increasing frequency (mainly among G-protein–coupled receptors; see Daeffler & Landry, 2000; Seifert & Wenzel-Seifert, 2002). Kenakin (2002) reported that over 80% of G-protein receptor antagonists reported in the literature are actually inverse agonists when tested in systems showing constitutive receptor activation. However, most receptors—like cats—seem to have a strong preference for the inactive state, and for these there is no practical difference between a competitive antagonist and an inverse agonist. It has been suggested, however, that inverse agonism at serotonin receptors may be relevant for antipsychotic drugs (see Ch. 38), but it remains to be seen whether the inverse agonist principle will prove to be generally important in therapeutics. So far, nearly all the examples come from the family of G-protein–coupled receptors (see Ch. 3, review by Costa & Cotecchia, 2005), and it is not clear whether similar phenomena occur with other receptor families.

The two-state model described below explains normal and inverse agonism in terms of the relative affinity of different ligands for the resting and activated states of the receptor. Constitutive activation is a relatively recent discovery, however, and may prove to be of greater pharmacological significance than is realised at present (see Milligan et al., 1995).

The two-state receptor model

▼ As illustrated in Figure 2.1, agonists and antagonists both bind to receptors, but only agonists activate them. How can we express this difference in theoretical terms? The simplest formulation (see Fig. 2.1) envisages that the occupied receptor can switch from its 'resting' (R) state

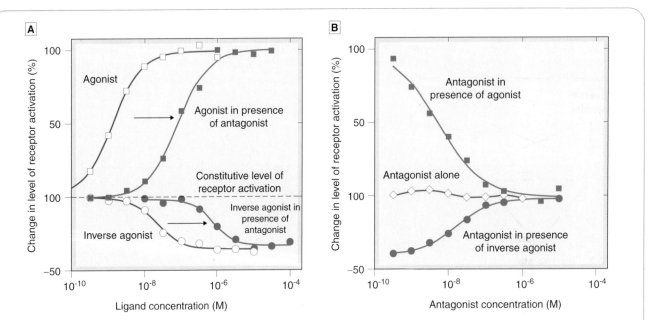

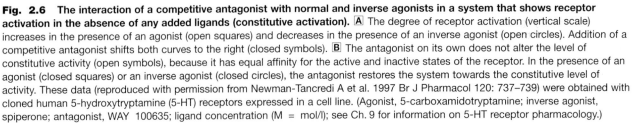

Fig. 2.6 **The interaction of a competitive antagonist with normal and inverse agonists in a system that shows receptor activation in the absence of any added ligands (constitutive activation).** **A** The degree of receptor activation (vertical scale) increases in the presence of an agonist (open squares) and decreases in the presence of an inverse agonist (open circles). Addition of a competitive antagonist shifts both curves to the right (closed symbols). **B** The antagonist on its own does not alter the level of constitutive activity (open symbols), because it has equal affinity for the active and inactive states of the receptor. In the presence of an agonist (closed squares) or an inverse agonist (closed circles), the antagonist restores the system towards the constitutive level of activity. These data (reproduced with permission from Newman-Tancredi A et al. 1997 Br J Pharmacol 120: 737–739) were obtained with cloned human 5-hydroxytryptamine (5-HT) receptors expressed in a cell line. (Agonist, 5-carboxamidotryptamine; inverse agonist, spiperone; antagonist, WAY 100635; ligand concentration (M = mol/l); see Ch. 9 for information on 5-HT receptor pharmacology.)

to an activated (R*) state, R* being favoured by binding of an agonist but not an antagonist molecule.

The tendency for the occupied receptor, AR, to convert to the activated form, AR*, will depend on the equilibrium constant for this reaction, β/α.

For a pure antagonist, $\beta/\alpha = 0$, implying that there is no conversion to the activated state, whereas for an agonist, $\beta/\alpha > 0$ and will be different for different drugs. Suppose that for drug X, β/α is small, so that only a small proportion of the occupied receptors will be activated even when the receptor occupancy approaches 100%, whereas for drug Y, β/α is large and most of the occupied receptors will be activated. The constant β/α is, therefore, a measure of efficacy (see p. 12). As we now know, receptors may show constitutive activation (i.e. the R* conformation can exist without any ligand being bound, so the added drug encounters an equilibrium mixture of R and R* (Fig. 2.7). If it has a higher affinity for R* than for R, the drug will cause a shift of the equilibrium towards R* (i.e. it will promote activation and be classed as an agonist). If its preference for R* is very large, nearly all the occupied receptors will adopt the R* conformation and the drug will be a full agonist (positive efficacy); if it shows no preference, the prevailing R:R* equilibrium will not be disturbed and the drug will be a competitive antagonist (zero efficacy), whereas if it prefers R it will shift the equilibrium towards R and be an inverse agonist (negative efficacy). We can therefore think of efficacy as a property determined by the relative affinity of a ligand for R and R*, a formulation known as the *two-state hypothesis*, which is useful in that it puts a physical interpretation on the otherwise mysterious meaning of efficacy.

A major problem with the two-state model is that, as we now know, receptors are not actually restricted to two distinct states but have much greater conformational flexibility, so that there is more than one inactive and active conformation. The different conformations that they can adopt may be preferentially stabilised by different ligands, and may produce different functional effects by activating different signal transduction pathways (see Ch. 3). Redefining efficacy for such a multistate model is difficult, however, and will require a more complicated state transition theory than that described here.

SPARE RECEPTORS

▼ Stephenson (1956), studying the actions of acetylcholine analogues in isolated tissues, found that many full agonists were capable of eliciting maximal responses at very low occupancies, often less than 1%. This means that the mechanism linking the response to receptor occupancy has a substantial reserve capacity. Such systems may be said to possess *spare receptors*, or a *receptor reserve*. This is common with drugs that elicit smooth muscle contraction but less so for other types of receptor-mediated response, such as secretion, smooth muscle relaxation or cardiac stimulation, where the effect is more nearly proportional to receptor occupancy. The existence of spare receptors does not imply any functional subdivision of the receptor pool, but merely that the pool is larger than the number needed to evoke a full response. This surplus of receptors over the number actually needed might seem a wasteful biological arrangement. It means, however, that a given number of agonist–receptor complexes, corresponding to a given level of biological response, can be reached with a lower concentration of hormone or neurotransmitter than would be the case if fewer receptors were provided. Economy of hormone or transmitter secretion is thus achieved at the expense of providing more receptors.

DRUG ANTAGONISM

Frequently, the effect of one drug is diminished or completely abolished in the presence of another. One mechanism, competitive antagonism, was discussed earlier; a more complete classification includes the following mechanisms:

- chemical antagonism
- pharmacokinetic antagonism
- antagonism by receptor block
- non-competitive antagonism, i.e. block of receptor–effector linkage
- physiological antagonism.

CHEMICAL ANTAGONISM

Chemical antagonism refers to the uncommon situation where the two substances combine in solution; as a result, the effect of the active drug is lost. Examples include the use of chelating agents (e.g. **dimercaprol**) that bind to heavy metals and thus reduce their toxicity, and the use of neutralising antibodies against protein mediators, such as cytokines and growth factors, a strategy recently applied for therapeutic use (see Ch. 14).

PHARMACOKINETIC ANTAGONISM

Pharmacokinetic antagonism describes the situation in which the 'antagonist' effectively reduces the concentration of the active drug at its site of action. This can happen in various ways. The rate of metabolic degradation of the active drug may be increased (e.g. the reduction of the anticoagulant effect of **warfarin** when an agent that accelerates its hepatic metabolism, such as **phenobarbital**, is given; see Chs 8 and 52). Alternatively, the rate of absorption of the active drug from the gastrointestinal tract may be reduced, or the rate of renal excretion may be increased. Interactions of this sort can be important in the clinical setting and are discussed in more detail in Chapter 52.

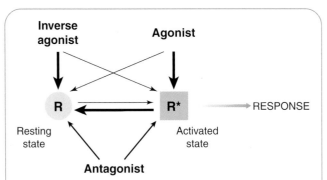

Fig. 2.7 The two-state model. The receptor is shown in two conformational states, 'resting' (R) and 'activated' R*, which exist in equilibrium. Normally, when no ligand is present, the equilibrium lies far to the left, and few receptors are found in the R* state. For constitutively active receptors, an appreciable proportion of receptors adopt the R* conformation in the absence of any ligand. Agonists have higher affinity for R* than for R, so shift the equilibrium towards R*. The greater the relative affinity for R* with respect to R, the greater the efficacy of the agonist. An inverse agonist has higher affinity for R than for R* and so shifts the equilibrium to the left. A 'neutral' antagonist has equal affinity for R and R* so does not by itself affect the conformational equilibrium but reduces by competition the binding of other ligands.

ANTAGONISM BY RECEPTOR BLOCK

Receptor block antagonism involves two important mechanisms:

- reversible competitive antagonism
- irreversible, or non-equilibrium, competitive antagonism.

Competitive antagonism

Competitive antagonism describes the common situation whereby a drug binds selectively to a particular type of receptor without activating it, but in such a way as to prevent the binding of the agonist. There is often some similarity between the chemical structures of the agonist and antagonist molecules. The two drugs compete with each other, because the receptor can bind only one drug molecule at a time. At a given agonist concentration, the agonist occupancy will be reduced in the presence of the antagonist. However, because the two are in competition, raising the agonist

concentration can restore the agonist occupancy (and hence the tissue response). The antagonism is therefore said to be *surmountable*, in contrast to other types of antagonism (see below) where increasing the agonist concentration fails to overcome the blocking effect. A simple theoretical analysis (see p. 21) predicts that in the presence of a fixed concentration of the antagonist, the log concentration–effect curve for the agonist will be shifted to the right, without any change in slope or maximum—the hallmark of competitive antagonism. The shift is expressed as a *dose ratio* (the ratio by which the agonist concentration has to be increased in the presence of the antagonist in order to restore a given level of response). Theory predicts that the dose ratio increases linearly with the concentration of the antagonist (see p. 21). These predictions are often borne out in practice (see Fig. 2.8), and examples of competitive antagonism are very common in pharmacology. The surmountability of the block by the antagonist may be important

---

Agonists, antagonists and efficacy

- Drugs acting on receptors may be *agonists* or *antagonists*.
- Agonists initiate changes in cell function, producing effects of various types; antagonists bind to receptors without initiating such changes.
- Agonist potency depends on two parameters: *affinity* (i.e. tendency to bind to receptors) and *efficacy* (i.e. ability, once bound, to initiate changes that lead to effects).
- For antagonists, efficacy is zero.
- Full agonists (which can produce maximal effects) have high efficacy; partial agonists (which can

produce only submaximal effects) have intermediate efficacy.
- According to the two-state model, efficacy reflects the relative affinity of the compound for the resting and activated states of the receptor. Agonists show selectivity for the activated state; antagonists show no selectivity. This model, although helpful, fails to account for the complexity of agonist action.
- Inverse agonists show selectivity for the resting state of the receptor, this being of significance only in unusual situations where the receptors show constitutive activity.

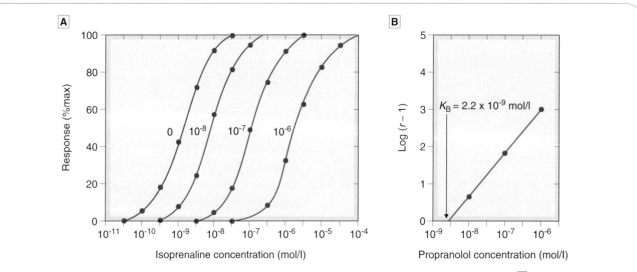

Fig. 2.8 Competitive antagonism of isoprenaline by propranolol measured on isolated guinea pig atria. Ⓐ Concentration–effect curves at various propranolol concentrations (indicated on the curves). Note the progressive shift to the right without a change of slope or maximum. Ⓑ Schild plot (equation 2.10). The equilibrium constant (*K*) for propranolol is given by the abscissal intercept 2.2×10^{-9} mol/l. (Results from Potter L T 1967 J Pharmacol 155: 91.)

Competitive antagonism

- Reversible competitive antagonism is the commonest and most important type of antagonism; it has two main characteristics:
  - in the presence of the antagonist, the agonist log concentration–effect curve is shifted to the right without change in slope or maximum, the extent of the shift being a measure of the dose ratio
  - the dose ratio increases linearly with antagonist concentration; the slope of this line is a measure of the affinity of the antagonist for the receptor.
- Antagonist affinity, measured in this way, is widely used as a basis for receptor classification.

in practice, because it allows the functional effect of the agonist to be restored by an increase in concentration. With other types of antagonism (see below), the block is usually insurmountable.

The salient features of competitive antagonism are:

- shift of the agonist log concentration–effect curve to the right, without change of slope or maximum
- linear relationship between agonist dose ratio and antagonist concentration
- evidence of competition from binding studies.

Competitive antagonism is the most direct mechanism by which one drug can reduce the effect of another (or of an endogenous mediator), and several examples are listed in Table 3.1; other mechanisms that are commonly encountered are discussed below.

The characteristics of reversible competitive antagonism described above reflect the fact that the rate of dissociation of the antagonist molecules is sufficiently high that a new equilibrium is rapidly established on addition of the agonist. In effect, the agonist

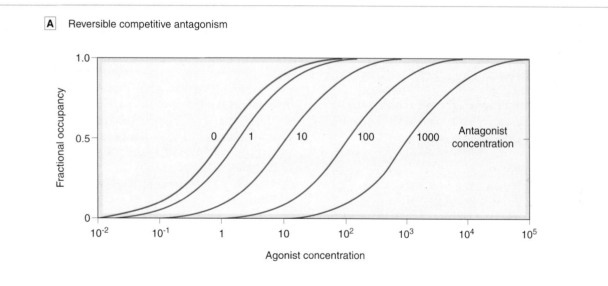

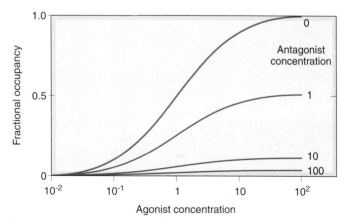

Fig. 2.9 Hypothetical agonist concentration–occupancy curves in the presence of reversible and irreversible competitive antagonists. The concentrations are normalised with respect to the equilibrium constants, K, (i.e. 1.0 corresponds to a concentration equal to K and results in 50% occupancy). **A** Reversible competitive antagonism. **B** Irreversible competitive antagonism.

is able to displace the antagonist molecules from the receptors, although it cannot, of course, evict a bound antagonist molecule. Displacement occurs because, by occupying a proportion of the vacant receptors, the agonist reduces the rate of association of the antagonist molecules; consequently, the rate of dissociation temporarily exceeds that of association, and the overall antagonist occupancy falls.

Irreversible, or non-equilibrium, competitive antagonism occurs when the antagonist dissociates very slowly, or not at all, from the receptors, with the result that no change in the antagonist occupancy takes place when the agonist is applied.[2]

The predicted effects of reversible and irreversible antagonists are compared in Figure 2.9.

▼ In some cases (Fig. 2.10A), the theoretical effect is accurately reproduced, but the distinction between reversible and irreversible competitive antagonism (or even non-competitive antagonism; see below) is not always so clear. This is because of the phenomenon of spare receptors (see p. 15); if the agonist occupancy required to produce a maximal biological response is very small (say 1% of the total receptor pool), then it is possible to block irreversibly nearly 99% of the receptors without reducing the maximal response. The effect of a lesser degree of antagonist occupancy will be to produce a parallel shift of the log concentration–effect curve that is indistinguishable from reversible competitive antagonism (Fig. 2.10B). In fact, it was the finding that an irreversible competitive antagonist of histamine was able to reduce the sensitivity of a smooth muscle preparation to histamine nearly 100-fold without reducing the maximal response that first gave rise to the spare receptor hypothesis.

Irreversible competitive antagonism occurs with drugs that possess reactive groups that form covalent bonds with the receptor. These

are mainly used as experimental tools for investigating receptor function, and few are used clinically. Irreversible enzyme inhibitors that act similarly are clinically used, however, and include drugs such as **aspirin** (Ch. 14), **omeprazole** (Ch. 25) and **monoamine oxidase inhibitors** (Ch. 39).

Non-competitive antagonism

Non-competitive antagonism describes the situation where the antagonist blocks at some point the chain of events that leads to the production of a response by the agonist. For example, drugs such as **verapamil** and **nifedipine** prevent the influx of Ca^{2+} through the cell membrane (see Ch. 19) and thus block non-specifically the contraction of smooth muscle produced by other drugs. As a rule, the effect will be to reduce the slope and maximum of the agonist log concentration–response curve as in Figure 2.10B, although it is quite possible for some degree of rightward shift to occur as well.

PHYSIOLOGICAL ANTAGONISM

Physiological antagonism is a term used loosely to describe the interaction of two drugs whose opposing actions in the body tend to cancel each other. For example, histamine acts on receptors of the parietal cells of the gastric mucosa to stimulate acid secretion, while omeprazole blocks this effect by inhibiting the proton pump; the two drugs can be said to act as physiological antagonists.

DESENSITISATION AND TACHYPHYLAXIS

Often, the effect of a drug gradually diminishes when it is given continuously or repeatedly. *Desensitisation* and *tachyphylaxis*

---

[2]This type of antagonism is sometimes called *non-competitive*, but that term is best reserved for antagonism that does not involve occupation of the receptor site.

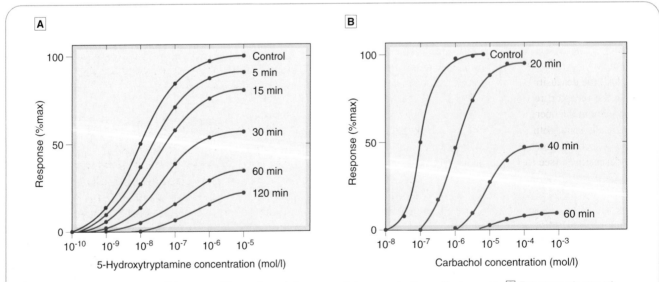

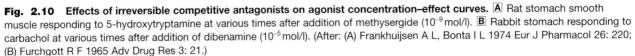

Fig. 2.10 **Effects of irreversible competitive antagonists on agonist concentration–effect curves.** **A** Rat stomach smooth muscle responding to 5-hydroxytryptamine at various times after addition of methysergide (10^{-9} mol/l). **B** Rabbit stomach responding to carbachol at various times after addition of dibenamine (10^{-5} mol/l). (After: (A) Frankhuijsen A L, Bonta I L 1974 Eur J Pharmacol 26: 220; (B) Furchgott R F 1965 Adv Drug Res 3: 21.)

are synonymous terms used to describe this phenomenon, which often develops in the course of a few minutes. The term *tolerance* is conventionally used to describe a more gradual decrease in responsiveness to a drug, taking days or weeks to develop, but the distinction is not a sharp one. The term *refractoriness* is also sometimes used, mainly in relation to a loss of therapeutic efficacy. *Drug resistance* is a term used to describe the loss of effectiveness of antimicrobial or antitumour drugs (see Chs 45 and 51). Many different mechanisms can give rise to this type of phenomenon. They include:

- change in receptors
- loss of receptors
- exhaustion of mediators
- increased metabolic degradation of the drug
- physiological adaptation
- active extrusion of drug from cells (mainly relevant in cancer chemotherapy; see Ch. 51).

CHANGE IN RECEPTORS

Among receptors directly coupled to ion channels, desensitisation is often rapid and pronounced. At the neuromuscular junction (Fig. 2.11A), the desensitised state is caused by a conformational change in the receptor, resulting in tight binding of the agonist molecule without the opening of the ionic channel (see Changeux et al., 1987). Phosphorylation of intracellular regions of the receptor protein is a second, slower mechanism by which ion channels become desensitised (see Swope et al., 1999).

Most G-protein–coupled receptors (see Ch. 3) also show desensitisation (see Fig. 2.11B). Phosphorylation of the receptor interferes with its ability to activate second messenger cascades, although it can still bind the agonist molecule. The molecular mechanisms of this 'uncoupling' are described by Lefkowitz et al. (1998) and considered further in Chapter 3. This type of desensitisation usually takes a few minutes to develop, and recovers at a similar rate when the agonist is removed.

It will be realised that the two-state model in its simple form, discussed earlier, needs to be further elaborated to incorporate additional 'desensitised' states of the receptor.

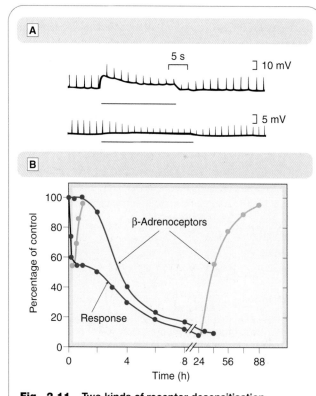

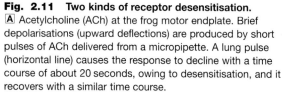

Fig. 2.11 **Two kinds of receptor desensitisation.**
[A] Acetylcholine (ACh) at the frog motor endplate. Brief depolarisations (upward deflections) are produced by short pulses of ACh delivered from a micropipette. A lung pulse (horizontal line) causes the response to decline with a time course of about 20 seconds, owing to desensitisation, and it recovers with a similar time course.
[B] β-Adrenoceptors of rat glioma cells in tissue culture. Isoprenaline (1 μmol/l) was added at time zero, and the adenylate cyclase response and β-adrenoceptor density measured at intervals. During the early uncoupling phase, the response (blue line) declines with no change in receptor density (red line). Later, the response declines further concomitantly with disappearance of receptors from the membrane by internalisation. The green and orange lines show the recovery of the response and receptor density after the isoprenaline is washed out during the early or late phase. (From: (A) Katz B, Thesleff S 1957 J Physiol 138: 63; (B) Perkins J P 1981 Trends Pharmacol Sci 2: 326.)

LOSS OF RECEPTORS

Prolonged exposure to agonists often results in a gradual decrease in the number of receptors expressed on the cell surface, as a result of *internalisation* of the receptors. This is shown for β-adrenoceptors in Figure 2.11B and is a slower process than the uncoupling described above. In studies on cell cultures, the number of β-adrenoceptors can fall to about 10% of normal in 8 hours in the presence of a low concentration of isoprenaline, and recovery takes several days. Similar changes have been described for other types of receptor, including those for various peptides. The internalised receptors are taken into the cell by *endocytosis* of patches of the membrane, a process that also depends on receptor phosphorylation. This type of adaptation is common for hormone receptors and has obvious relevance to the effects produced when drugs are given for extended periods. It is generally an unwanted complication when drugs are used clinically, but it can be exploited. For example, **gonadotrophin-releasing hormone** (see Ch. 30) is used to treat endometriosis or prostatic cancer; given continuously, this hormone paradoxically inhibits gonadotrophin release (in contrast to the normal stimulatory effect of the physiological secretion, which is pulsatile).

EXHAUSTION OF MEDIATORS

In some cases, desensitisation is associated with depletion of an essential intermediate substance. Drugs such as **amphetamine,** which acts by releasing amines from nerve terminals (see Chs 11 and 32), show marked tachyphylaxis because the amine stores become depleted.

ALTERED DRUG METABOLISM

Tolerance to some drugs, for example **barbiturates** (Ch. 37) and **ethanol** (Ch. 43), occurs partly because repeated administration of the same dose produces a progressively lower plasma concentration, because of increased metabolic degradation. The degree of tolerance that results is generally modest, and in both of these examples other mechanisms contribute to the substantial tolerance that actually occurs. On the other hand, the pronounced tolerance to **nitrovasodilators** (see Chs 17 and 19) results mainly from *decreased* metabolism, which reduces the release of the active mediator, nitric oxide.

PHYSIOLOGICAL ADAPTATION

Diminution of a drug's effect may occur because it is nullified by a homeostatic response. For example, the blood pressure–lowering effect of **thiazide diuretics** is limited because of a gradual activation of the renin–angiotensin system (see Ch. 19). Such homeostatic mechanisms are very common, and if they occur slowly the result will be a gradually developing tolerance. It is a common experience that many side effects of drugs, such as nausea or sleepiness, tend to subside even though drug administration is continued. We may assume that some kind of physiological adaptation is occurring, presumably associated with altered gene expression resulting in changes in the levels of various regulatory molecules, but little is known about the mechanisms involved.

QUANTITATIVE ASPECTS OF DRUG–RECEPTOR INTERACTIONS

▼ Here we present some aspects of so-called receptor theory, which is based on applying the Law of Mass Action to the drug–receptor interaction and which has served well as a framework for interpreting a large body of quantitative experimental data.

The binding reaction

▼ The first step in drug action on specific receptors is the formation of a reversible drug–receptor complex, the reactions being governed by the Law of Mass Action. Suppose that a piece of tissue, such as heart muscle or smooth muscle, contains a total number of receptors, N_{tot}, for an agonist such as adrenaline (epinephrine). When the tissue is exposed to adrenaline at concentration x_A and allowed to come to equilibrium, a certain number, N_A, of the receptors will become occupied, and the number of vacant receptors will be reduced to $N_{tot} - N_A$. Normally, the number of adrenaline molecules applied to the tissue in solution greatly exceeds N_{tot}, so that the binding reaction does not appreciably reduce x_A. The magnitude of the response produced by the adrenaline will be related (even if we do not know exactly how) to the number of receptors occupied, so it is useful to consider what quantitative relationship is predicted between N_A and x_A. The reaction can be represented by:

$$\begin{array}{ccccc} A & + & R & \underset{k_{-1}}{\overset{k_{+1}}{\rightleftharpoons}} & AR \\ \text{drug} & + & \text{free receptor} & & \text{complex} \\ (x_A) & & (N_{tot}-N_A) & & (N_A) \end{array}$$

The Law of Mass Action (which states that the rate of a chemical reaction is proportional to the product of the concentrations of reactants) can be applied to this reaction.

$$\text{Rate of forward reaction} = k_{+1}x_A(N_{tot} - N_A) \qquad (2.1)$$

$$\text{Rate of backward reaction} = k_{-1}N_A \qquad (2.2)$$

At equilibrium, the two rates are equal:

$$k_{+1}x_A(N_{tot} - N_A) = k_{-1}N_A \qquad (2.3)$$

The proportion of receptors occupied, or occupancy (p_A), is N_A/N_{tot}, which is independent of N_{tot}.

$$P_A = \frac{x_A}{x_A + k_{-1}/k_{+1}} \qquad (2.4)$$

Defining the equilibrium constant for the binding reaction, $K_A = k_{-1}/k_{+1}$, equation 2.4 can be written:

$$P_A = \frac{x_A/K_A}{x_A/K_A+1} \qquad (2.5)$$

▼ This important result is known as the Hill–Langmuir equation.[3]

The equilibrium constant,[4] K_A, is a characteristic of the drug and of the receptor; it has the dimensions of concentration and is numerically equal to the concentration of drug required to occupy 50% of the sites at equilibrium. (Verify from equation 2.5 that when $x_A = K_A$, $p_A = 0.5$.) The higher the affinity of the drug for the receptors, the lower will be the value of K_A. Equation 2.5 describes the relationship between occupancy and drug concentration, and it generates a characteristic curve known as a rectangular hyperbola, as shown in Figure 2.12A. It is common in pharmacological work to use a logarithmic scale of concentration; this converts the hyperbola to a symmetrical sigmoid curve (Fig. 2.12B).

The same approach is used to analyse data from experiments in which drug binding is measured directly (see p. 11, Fig. 2.2). In this case, the relationship between the amount bound (B) and ligand concentration (x_A) should be:

$$B = B_{max}x_A/(x_A + K_A) \qquad (2.6)$$

---

[3] A. V. Hill first published it in 1909, when he was still a medical student. Langmuir, a physical chemist working on gas adsorption, derived it independently in 1916. Both subsequently won Nobel prizes. Until recently, it was known to pharmacologists as the Langmuir equation, even though Hill deserves the credit.

[4] The equilibrium constant is sometimes called the dissociation constant. Some authors prefer to use the reciprocal of K_A, referred to as an affinity constant, in these expressions, which can cause confusion to the unwary.

Binding of drugs to receptors

- Binding of drugs to receptors necessarily obeys the Law of Mass Action.
- At equilibrium, receptor occupancy is related to drug concentration by the Hill–Langmuir equation (2.7).
- The higher the affinity of the drug for the receptor, the lower the concentration at which it produces a given level of occupancy.
- The same principles apply when two or more drugs compete for the same receptors; each has the effect of reducing the apparent affinity for the other.

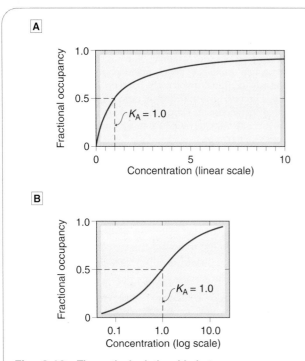

Fig. 2.12 Theoretical relationship between occupancy and ligand concentration. The relationship is plotted according to equation 2.5. **A** Plotted with a linear concentration scale, this curve is a rectangular hyperbola. **B** Plotted with a log concentration scale, it is a symmetrical sigmoid curve.

where B_{max} is the total number of binding sites in the preparation (often expressed as pmol/mg of protein). To display the results in linear form, equation 2.6 may be rearranged to:

$$B/x_A = B_{max}/K_A - B/K_A \qquad (2.7)$$

A plot of B/x_A against B (known as a Scatchard plot; Fig. 2.2C) gives a straight line from which both B_{max} and K_A can be estimated. Statistically, this procedure is not without problems, and it is now usual to estimate these parameters from the untransformed binding values by an iterative non-linear curve-fitting procedure.

To this point, our analysis has considered the binding of one ligand to a homogeneous population of receptors. To get closer to real-life pharmacology, we must consider (a) what happens when more than one ligand is present, and (b) how the tissue response is related to receptor occupancy.

Binding when more than one drug is present

▼ Suppose that two drugs, A and B, which bind to the same receptor with equilibrium constants K_A and K_B, respectively, are present at concentrations x_A and x_B. If the two drugs *compete* (i.e. the receptor can accommodate only one at a time), then, by application of the same reasoning as for the one-drug situation described above, the occupancy by drug A is given by:

$$P_A = \frac{x_A/K_A}{x_A/K + x_B/K_B + 1} \qquad (2.8)$$

Comparing this result with equation 2.5 shows that adding drug B, as expected, reduces the occupancy by drug A. Figure 2.9A shows the predicted binding curves for A in the presence of increasing concentrations of B, demonstrating the shift without any change of slope or maximum that characterises the pharmacological effect of a competitive antagonist (see Fig. 2.8). The extent of the rightward shift, on a logarithmic scale, represents the ratio (r_A, given by x_A'/x_A where x_A' is the increased concentration of A) by which the concentration of A must be increased to overcome the competition by B. Rearranging 2.8 shows that

$$r_A = (x_B/K_B) + 1 \qquad (2.9)$$

Thus r_A depends only on the concentration and equilibrium constant of the competing drug B, not on the concentration or equilibrium constant of A.

If A is an agonist, and B is a competitive antagonist, and we assume that the response of the tissue will be a function of p_A (not necessarily a linear function), then the value of r_A determined from the shift of the agonist concentration–effect curve at different antagonist concentrations can be used to estimate the equilibrium constant K_B for the antagonist. Such pharmacological estimates of r_A are commonly termed *agonist dose ratios* (more properly *concentration ratios*, although most pharmacologists use the older, improper term). This simple and very useful equation (2.9) is known as the *Schild equation*, after the pharmacologist who first used it to analyse drug antagonism.

Equation 2.9 can be expressed logarithmically in the form:

$$\log (r_A - 1) = \log x_B - \log K_B \qquad (2.10)$$

Thus a plot of $\log (r_A - 1)$ against $\log x_B$, usually called a Schild plot (as in Fig. 2.8), should give a straight line with unit slope and an abscissal intercept equal to $\log K_B$. Following the pH and pK notation, antagonist potency can be expressed as a pA_2 value; under conditions of competitive antagonism, $pA_2 = -\log K_B$. Numerically, pA_2 is defined as the negative logarithm of the molar concentration of antagonist required to produce an agonist dose ratio equal to 2. As with pH notation, its principal advantage is that it produces simple numbers, a pA_2 of 6.5 being equivalent to a K_B of 3.2×10^{-7} mol/l.

This analysis of competitive antagonism shows the following characteristics of the dose ratio r:

- it depends only on the concentration and equilibrium constant of the antagonist, and not on the size of response that is chosen as a reference point for the measurements
- it does not depend on the equilibrium constant for the agonist
- it increases linearly with x_B, and the slope of a plot of ($r_A - 1$) against x_B is equal to $1/K_B$; this relationship, being independent of the characteristics of the agonist, should be the same for all agonists that act on the same population of receptors.

These predictions have been verified for many examples of competitive antagonism (Fig. 2.8).

In this section, we have avoided going into great detail and have oversimplified the theory considerably. As we learn more about the actual

Drug effects

- Drugs act mainly on cellular targets, producing effects at different functional levels (e.g. biochemical cellular, physiological and structural).
- The direct effect of the drug on its target produces acute responses at the biochemical cellular or physiological levels.
- Acute responses generally lead to delayed long-term effects, such as desensitisation or down-regulation of receptors, hypertrophy, atrophy or remodelling of tissues, tolerance, dependence and addiction.
- Long-term delayed responses result from changes in gene expression, although the mechanisms by which the acute effects bring this about are often uncertain.
- Therapeutic effects may be based on acute responses (e.g. the use of bronchodilator drugs to treat asthma; Ch. 23) or delayed responses (e.g. antidepressants; Ch. 39).

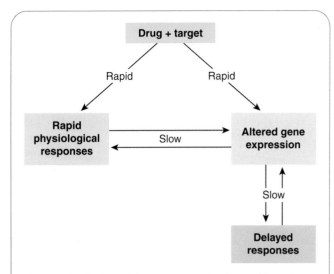

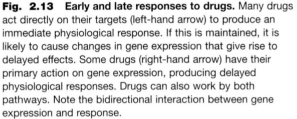

Fig. 2.13 Early and late responses to drugs. Many drugs act directly on their targets (left-hand arrow) to produce an immediate physiological response. If this is maintained, it is likely to cause changes in gene expression that give rise to delayed effects. Some drugs (right-hand arrow) have their primary action on gene expression, producing delayed physiological responses. Drugs can also work by both pathways. Note the bidirectional interaction between gene expression and response.

molecular details of how receptors work to produce their biological effects (see Ch. 3), the shortcomings of this theoretical treatment become more obvious. Particular complications arise when we include the involvement of G-proteins (see Ch. 3) in the reaction scheme, and when we allow for the fact that receptor 'activation' is not a simple on–off switch, as the two-state model assumes, but may take different forms. It is as though the same receptor can turn on a tap or a light bulb, depending on which agonist does the talking. Attempts by theoreticians to allow for such possibilities lead to some unwieldy algebra and fancy three-dimensional graphics, but somehow the molecules always seem to remain one step ahead. Despite its shortcomings, the two-state model remains a useful basis for developing quantitative models of drug action. The book by Kenakin (1997) is recommended as an introduction, and his later review (Kenakin, 2002) presents a more elaborate theoretical approach.

THE NATURE OF DRUG EFFECTS

In discussing how drugs act in this chapter, we have focused mainly on the consequences of receptor activation. Details of the receptors and their linkage to effects at the cellular level are described in Chapter 3. We now have a fairly good understanding at this level. It is important, however, particularly when considering drugs in a therapeutic context, that their direct effects on cellular function generally lead to secondary, delayed effects, which are often highly relevant in a clinical situation in relation

to both therapeutic efficacy and harmful effects (see Fig. 2.13). For example, activation of a β-adrenoceptor in the heart (see Chs 3 and 18) causes rapid changes in the functioning of the heart muscle, but also slower (minutes to hours) changes in the functional state of the receptors (e.g. desensitisation), and even slower (hours to days) changes in gene expression that produce long-term changes (e.g. hypertrophy) in cardiac structure and function. Similarly, antidepressant drugs, which have immediate effects on transmitter metabolism in the brain (see Ch. 39) take weeks to produce therapeutic benefit. Opiates (see Ch. 41) produce an immediate analgesic effect but, after a time, tolerance and dependence ensue, and in some cases long-term addiction. In these, and many other examples, the nature of the intervening mechanism is unclear, although as a general rule any long-term phenotypic change necessarily involves alterations of gene expression. Drugs are often used to treat chronic conditions, and understanding long-term as well as acute drug effects is becoming increasingly important. Pharmacologists have traditionally tended to focus on short-term physiological responses, which are much easier to study, rather than on delayed effects. The focus is now clearly shifting.

REFERENCES AND FURTHER READING

General

Alexander SP, Mathie A, Peters JA 2006 Guide to receptors and channels, 2nd edition. Br J Pharmacol 147 (suppl 3):S1

Changeux J-P, Giraudat J, Dennis M 1987 The nicotinic acetylcholine receptor: molecular architecture of a ligand-regulated ion channel.

Trends Pharmacol Sci 8: 459–465 (*One of the first descriptions of receptor action at the molecular level*)

Franks N P, Lieb W R 1994 Molecular and cellular mechanisms of general anaesthesia. Nature 367: 607–614 (*A review of changing ideas about the site of action of anaesthetic drugs*)

Jenkinson D H 1996 Classical approaches to the study of drug–receptor interactions. In: Foreman J C, Johansen T (eds) Textbook of receptor pharmacology. CRC Press, Boca Raton (*Good account of pharmacological analysis of receptor-mediated effects*)

Kenakin T 1997 Pharmacologic analysis of drug–receptor interactions, 3rd edn. Lippincott-Raven,

New York (*Useful and detailed textbook covering most of the material in this chapter in greater depth*)

Neubig R, Spedding M, Kenakin T, Christopoulos A 2003 International Union of Pharmacology Committee on receptor nomenclature and drug classification: XXXVIII. Update on terms and symbols in quantitative pharmacology. Pharmacol Rev 55: 597–606. (*Summary of IUPHAR-approved terms and symbols relating to pharmacological receptors—useful for reference purposes*)

Rang H P 2006 The receptor concept: Pharmacology's Big idea. Br J Pharmacol 147 (Supp 1): 9–16 (*Short review of the origin and status of the receptor concept*)

Stephenson R P 1956 A modification of receptor theory. Br J Pharmacol 11: 379–393 (*Classic analysis of receptor action introducing the concept of efficacy*)

Teitler M, Herrick-Davis K, Purohit A 2002 Constitutive activity of G-protein coupled receptors: emphasis on serotonin receptors. Curr Top Med Chem 2: 529–538.

Receptor mechanisms: agonists and efficacy

Bond R A, Leff P, Johnson T D et al. 1995 Physiological effects of inverse agonists in transgenic mice with myocardial overexpression of the β_2-adrenoceptor. Nature 374: 270–276 (*A study with important clinical implications, showing that overexpression of β adrenoceptors results in constitutive receptor activation*)

Costa T, Cotecchia S 2005 Historical review: negative efficacy and the constitutive activity of G-protein–coupled receptors. Trends Pharmacol Sci 26: 618–624. (*A clear and thoughtful review of ideas relating to constitutive receptor activation and inverse agonists*)

Daeffler L, Landry Y 2000 Inverse agonism at heptahelical receptors: concept, experimental approach and therapeutic potential. Fundam Clin Pharmacol 14: 73–87

De Ligt R A F, Kourounakis A P, Ijzerman A P 2000 Inverse agonism at G protein-coupled receptors: (patho)physiological relevance and implications for drug discovery. Br J Pharmacol 130: 1–12 (*Useful review article giving many examples of constitutively active receptors and inverse agonists, and discussing the relevance of these concepts for disease mechanisms and drug discovery*)

Kenakin T 2002 Drug efficacy at G protein-coupled receptors. Annu Rev Pharmacol Toxicol 42: 349–379. (*A theoretical treatment that attempts to take into account recent knowledge of receptor function at the molecular level*)

Milligan G, Bond R A, Lee M 1995 Inverse agonism: pharmacological curiosity or potential therapeutic strategy? Trends Pharmacol Sci 16: 10–13 (*Excellent review of the significance of constitutive receptor activation and the effects of inverse agonists*)

Seifert R, Wenzel-Seifert K 2002 Constitutive activity of G-protein–coupled receptors: cause of disease and common properties of wild-type receptors. Naunyn-Schmiedeberg's Arch Pharmacol 366: 381–416 (*Detailed review article emphasising that constitutively active receptors occur commonly and are associated with several important disease states*)

Desensitisation

Lefkowitz R J, Pitcher J, Krueger K, Daaka Y 1998 Mechanisms of β-adrenergic receptor desensitization and resensitization. Adv Pharmacol 42: 416–420

Swope S L, Moss S I, Raymond I A, Huganir R L 1999 Regulation of ligand-gated ion channels by protein phosphorylation. Adv Second Messenger Phosphoprotein Res 33: 49–78 (*Comprehensive review article describing the role of phosphorylation in desensitisation*)

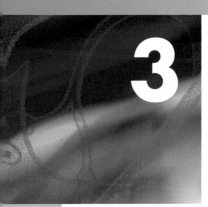

3 How drugs act: molecular aspects

OVERVIEW

In this chapter, we move from the general principles of drug action outlined in Chapter 2 to the molecules that are involved in recognising chemical signals and translating them into cellular responses. Molecular pharmacology has advanced rapidly in recent years. This new knowledge is not only changing our understanding of drug action, it is also opening up many new therapeutic possibilities, further discussed in other chapters.

First, we consider the types of target proteins on which drugs act. Next, we describe the main families of receptors and ion channels that have been revealed by cloning and structural studies. Finally, we discuss the various forms of receptor–effector linkage (signal transduction mechanisms) through which receptors are coupled to the regulation of cell function. The relationship between the molecular structure of a receptor and its functional linkage to a particular type of effector system is a principal theme. In the next two chapters, we see how these molecular events alter important aspects of cell function—a useful basis for understanding the effects of drugs on intact living organisms. We go into more detail than is necessary for understanding today's pharmacology at a basic level, intending that students can, if they wish, skip or skim these chapters without losing the thread; however, we are confident that tomorrow's pharmacology will rest solidly on the advances in cellular and molecular biology that are discussed here.

TARGETS FOR DRUG ACTION

The protein targets for drug action on mammalian cells (Fig. 3.1) that are described in this chapter can be broadly divided into:

- receptors
- ion channels
- enzymes
- carrier molecules (transporters).

The great majority of important drugs act on one or other of these types of protein, but there are exceptions. For example **colchicine** (Ch. 14) interacts with the structural protein *tubulin*, while several immunosuppressive drugs (e.g. **ciclosporin**, Ch. 14) bind to cytosolic proteins known as *immunophilins*. Therapeutic antibodies that act by sequestering cytokines (protein mediators involved in inflammation, see Ch. 14) are also used. Targets for chemotherapeutic drugs (Chs 45–51), where the aim is to suppress invading microorganisms or cancer cells, include DNA and cell wall constituents as well as other proteins.

Receptors

Receptors (Fig. 3.1A) are the sensing elements in the system of chemical communications that coordinates the function of all the different cells in the body, the chemical messengers being the various hormones, transmitters and other mediators discussed in Section 2. Many therapeutically useful drugs act, either as agonists or antagonists, on receptors for known endogenous mediators. Some examples are given in Table 3.1. In most cases, the endogenous mediator was discovered before—often many years before—the receptor was characterised pharmacologically and biochemically, but there are examples of receptors for synthetic drug molecules (e.g. **benzodiazepines**, Ch. 33; and **sulfonylureas**, Ch. 26) for which no endogenous mediator has been identified. Receptors are discussed in more detail below (p. 27).

Ion channels[1]

Some ion channels (known as *ligand-gated ion channels* or *ionotropic receptors*) incorporate a receptor and open only when the receptor is occupied by an agonist; others (see p. 48) are gated by different mechanisms, *voltage-gated ion channels* (see p. 49) being particularly important. In general, drugs can affect ion channel function by interacting either with the receptor site of ligand-gated channels, or with other parts of the channel molecule. The interaction can be indirect, involving a G-protein and other intermediaries (see below), or direct, where the drug itself binds to the channel protein and alters its function. In the simplest case, exemplified by the action of local anaesthetics on the voltage-gated sodium channel (see Ch. 44), the drug molecule plugs the channel physically (Fig. 3.1B), blocking ion permeation.

Examples of drugs that bind to accessory sites on the channel protein and thereby affect channel gating include:

- vasodilator drugs of the **dihydropyridine** type (see Ch. 19), which inhibit the opening of L-type calcium channels (see Ch. 4).
- **benzodiazepine tranquillisers** (see Ch. 37). These drugs bind to a region of the GABA receptor–chloride channel complex (a ligand-gated channel; see above), this region being distinct from the GABA binding site. Most benzodiazepines facilitate the opening of the channel by the inhibitory neurotransmitter GABA (see Ch. 33), but some *inverse agonists* are known that have the opposite effect, causing anxiety rather than tranquillity.
- **Sulfonylureas** (see Ch. 26) used in treating diabetes, which act on ATP-sensitive potassium channels of pancreatic β-cells and thereby enhance insulin secretion.

A summary of the different ion channel families and their functions is given below (p. 50).

Enzymes

Many drugs are targeted on enzymes (Fig. 3.1C), examples being given in Table 3.1. Often, the drug molecule is a substrate analogue that acts as a competitive inhibitor of the enzyme (e.g. **captopril,** acting on angiotensin-converting enzyme; Ch. 19); in other cases, the binding is irreversible and non-competitive (e.g. **aspirin,** acting on cyclo-oxygenase; Ch. 14). The immunophilin to which ciclosporin binds (see above) has enzymic activity as an isomerase that catalyses the *cis–trans* isomerisation of proline residues in proteins, a reaction that is important in allowing expressed proteins to fold correctly. Inhibition of this enzymic activity is one of the mechanisms by which ciclosporin causes immunosuppression. Drugs may also act as *false substrates*, where the drug molecule undergoes chemical transformation to form an abnormal product that subverts the normal metabolic pathway. An example is the anticancer drug **fluorouracil**, which replaces

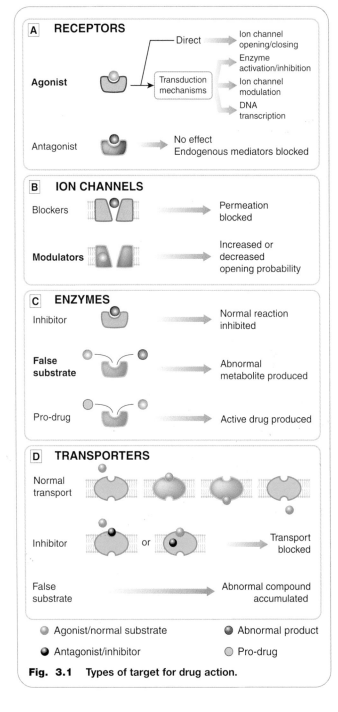

Fig. 3.1   Types of target for drug action.

uracil as an intermediate in purine biosynthesis but cannot be converted into thymidylate, thus blocking DNA synthesis and preventing cell division (Ch. 51).

It should also be mentioned that drugs may require enzymic degradation to convert them from an inactive form, the *prodrug* (see Ch. 8), to an active form. Examples are given in Table 8.3. Furthermore, as discussed in Chapter 53, drug toxicity often results from the enzymic conversion of the drug molecule to a reactive metabolite. As far as the primary action of the drug is concerned, this is an unwanted side reaction, but it is of major practical importance.

---

[1]Ion channels and the electrical properties they confer on cells are involved in every human characteristic that distinguishes us from the stones in a field.' (Armstrong C M 2003 Voltage-gated K channels http://www.stke.org).

Table 3.1   Some examples of targets for drug action[a]

Type of target	Effectors		Chapter(s) to refer to
Receptors	**Agonists**	**Antagonists**	
Nicotinic ACh receptor	Acetylcholine	Tubocurarine	10
	Nicotine	α-Bungarotoxin	
β-Adrenoceptor	Noradrenaline (norepinephrine)	Propranolol	11
	Isoprenaline		
Histamine (H₁ receptor)	Histamine	Mepyramine	18
Opiate (μ receptor)	Morphine	Naloxone	41
Dopamine (D₂ receptor)	Dopamine	Chlorpromazine	35 and 38
	Bromocriptine		
Oestrogen receptor	Ethinylestradiol	Tamoxifen	30
Epidermal growth factor receptor		Trastuzumab	55
Ion channels	**Blockers**	**Modulators**	
Voltage-gated sodium channels	Local anaesthetics	Veratridine	44
	Tetrodotoxin		
Renal tubule sodium channels	Amiloride	Aldosterone	24
Voltage-gated calcium channels	Divalent cations (e.g. Cd^{2+})	Dihydropyridines	18 and 19
		Opioids	41
ATP-sensitive potassium channels	ATP	Sulfonylureas	26
GABA-gated chloride channels	Picrotoxin	Benzodiazepines	33
Enzymes	**Inhibitors**	**False substrates**	
Acetylcholinesterase	Neostigmine	–	10
Cyclo-oxygenase	Aspirin	–	14
Angiotensin-converting enzyme	Captopril	–	19
HMG-CoA reductase	Simvastatin	–	20
Monoamine oxidase-A	Iproniazid	–	39
Phosphodiesterase type V	Sildenafil	–	30
Dihydrofolate reductase	Trimethoprim	–	46
	Methotrexate	–	14 and 51
Thymidine kinase	Aciclovir	–	47
HIV protease	Saquinavir	–	47
Carriers	**Inhibitors**	**False substrates**	
Noradrenaline transporter	Tricyclic antidepressants	–	39
	Cocaine	–	11 and 53
	–	Amphetamine	11 and 42
	–	Methyldopa	19
Weak acid carrier (renal tubule)	Probenecid	–	24
$Na^+/K^+/2Cl^-$ cotransporter (loop of Henle)	Loop diuretics	–	24
Proton pump (gastric mucosa)	Omeprazole	–	25

Table 3.1 (cont'd)   Some examples of targets for drug action[a]

Type of target	Effectors		Chapter(s) to refer to
Others			
Immunophilins	Ciclosporin	–	17
	Tacrolimus	–	17
Tubulin	Colchicine	–	17
	Taxol	–	50

HMG-CoA, 3-hydroxy-3-methylglutaryl-coenzyme A.
[a]These are representative examples and by no means a complete list. Other biochemical targets for drugs used in chemotherapy are discussed in Chapters 44–51.

Carrier molecules

The transport of ions and small organic molecules across cell membranes generally requires a carrier protein, because the permeating molecules are often too polar (i.e. insufficiently lipid-soluble) to penetrate lipid membranes on their own. There are many examples of such carriers (Fig. 3.1D), including those responsible for the transport of glucose and amino acids into cells, the transport of ions and many organic molecules by the renal tubule, the transport of Na^+ and Ca^{2+} out of cells, and the uptake of neurotransmitter precursors (such as choline) or of neurotransmitters themselves (such as noradrenaline, 5-hydroxytryptamine [5-HT], glutamate, and peptides) by nerve terminals. The amine transporters belong to a well-defined structural family, distinct from the corresponding receptors. In most cases, the transport of organic molecules is coupled to the transport of ions (usually Na^+), either in the same direction (*symport*) or in the opposite direction (*antiport*), as discussed in Chapter 24. The carrier proteins embody a recognition site that makes them specific for a particular permeating species, and these recognition sites can also be targets for drugs whose effect is to block the transport system. Some examples are given in Table 3.1.

RECEPTOR PROTEINS

ISOLATION AND CLONING OF RECEPTORS

In the 1970s, pharmacology entered a new phase when receptors, which had until then been theoretical entities, began to emerge as biochemical realities following the development of receptor-labelling techniques (see Ch. 2), which made it possible to extract and purify the receptor material. This approach was first used successfully on the nicotinic acetylcholine receptor (see Ch. 7), where advantage was taken of two natural curiosities. The first was that the electric organs of many fish, such as rays (*Torpedo* sp.) and electric eels (*Electrophorus* sp.) consist of modified muscle tissue in which the acetylcholine-sensitive membrane is extremely abundant, and these organs contain much larger amounts of acetylcholine receptor than any other tissue. The second was that the venom of snakes of the cobra family contains polypeptides that bind with very high specificity to nicotinic acetylcholine receptors. These substances, known as α-toxins, can be labelled and used to assay the receptor content of tissues and tissue extracts. The best known is **α-bungarotoxin**, the main component of the venom of the Malayan banded krait (*Bungarus multicinctus*).[2] Treatment of muscle or electric tissue with non-ionic detergents renders the membrane-bound receptor protein soluble, and it can then be purified by the technique of affinity chromatography. Similar approaches have now been used to purify a great many hormone and neurotransmitter receptors, as well as ion channels, carrier proteins, and other kinds of target molecules.

▼ Once receptor proteins were isolated and purified, it was possible to analyse the amino acid sequence of a short stretch, allowing the corresponding base sequence of the mRNA to be deduced and full-length DNA to be isolated, by conventional cloning methods, starting from a cDNA library obtained from a tissue source rich in the receptor of interest. The first receptor clones were obtained in this way, but subsequently *expression cloning* and cloning strategies based on sequence homologies, which do not require prior isolation and purification of the receptor protein, were widely used, and now several hundred receptors of all four structural families (see below) have been cloned. Endogenous ligands for many of these 'receptor-like' molecules identified by gene cloning are so far unknown, and they are described as 'orphan receptors'.[3] Identifying ligands for these presumed receptors is often difficult. However, there are examples (e.g. the cannabinoid receptor; see Ch. 15) where important ligands have been linked to hitherto orphan receptors, and it is likely that this pool of unclaimed receptors will yield many more receptors of physiological and therapeutic significance.

Much information has been gained by introducing the cloned DNA encoding individual receptors into cell lines, producing

---

[2]Nature has had the good sense to keep these heavily armed fishes and snakes well apart. Ironically enough, *B. multicinctus* is now officially an endangered species, threatened by scientists' demand for its venom. Evolution for survival can go one step too far.

[3]An oddly Dickensian term that seems inappropriately condescending, because we can assume that these receptors play defined roles in physiological signalling—their 'orphanhood' reflects our ignorance, not their status.

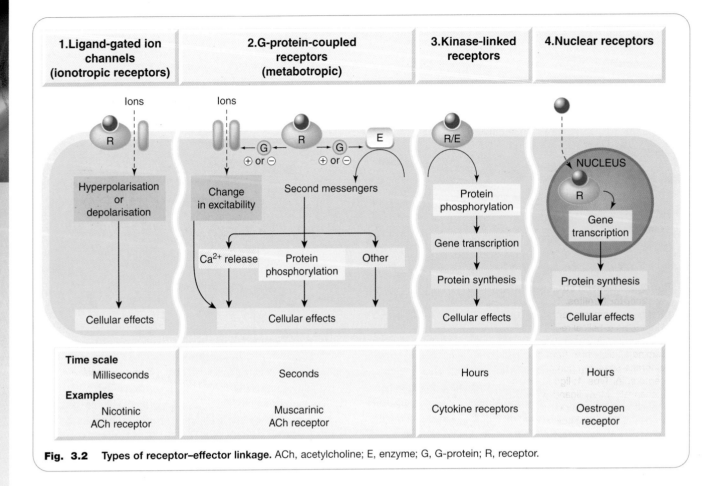

Fig. 3.2   Types of receptor–effector linkage. ACh, acetylcholine; E, enzyme; G, G-protein; R, receptor.

cells that express the foreign receptors in a functional form. Such engineered cells allow much more precise control of the expressed receptors than is possible with natural cells or intact tissues, and the technique is widely used to study the binding and pharmacological characteristics of cloned receptors.

The cloning of receptors revealed many molecular variants (subtypes) of known receptors, which had not been evident from pharmacological studies. This produced some taxonomic confusion, but in the long term molecular characterisation of receptors is essential. Barnard, one of the high priests of receptor cloning, was undaunted by the proliferation of molecular subtypes among receptors that pharmacologists had thought that they understood. He quoted Thomas Aquinas: 'Types and shadows have their ending, for the newer rite is here'. The newer rite, Barnard confidently asserted, was molecular biology. Analysis of the human and other mammalian genomes suggests that many hundreds of receptor-like genes are present, of which only a minority so far have a pharmacological identity. Now that most of the genes have been clearly identified, and the full molecular inventory established, the emphasis has shifted to characterising the receptors pharmacologically and determining their physiological functions.

TYPES OF RECEPTOR

Receptors elicit many different types of cellular effect. Some of them are very rapid, such as those involved in synaptic transmission,

operating within milliseconds, whereas other receptor-mediated effects, such as those produced by thyroid hormone or various steroid hormones, occur over hours or days. There are also many examples of intermediate timescales—catecholamines, for example, usually act in a matter of seconds, whereas many peptides take rather longer to produce their effects. Not surprisingly, very different types of linkage between the receptor occupation and the ensuing response are involved. Based on molecular structure and the nature of this linkage (the transduction mechanism), we can distinguish four receptor types, or superfamilies (see Figs 3.2 and 3.3 and Table 3.2).

- Type 1: **ligand-gated ion channels** (also known as **ionotropic receptors**).[4] These are membrane proteins with a similar structure to other ion channels, and incorporate a ligand-binding (receptor) site, usually in the extracellular domain. Typically, these are the receptors on which fast neurotransmitters act. Examples include the nicotinic acetylcholine receptor (nAChR; see Ch. 10); $GABA_A$ receptor (see Ch. 33); and glutamate receptors of the NMDA, AMPA and kainate types (see Ch. 33).

---

[4]Here, focusing on receptors, we consider ligand-gated ion channels as an example of a receptor family. Other types of ion channels are described later (p. 48); many of them are also drug targets, although not receptors in the strict sense.

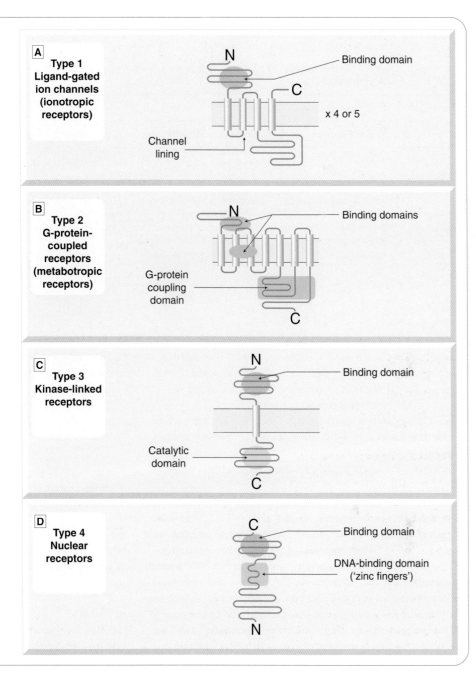

Fig. 3.3 General structure of four receptor families. The rectangular segments represent hydrophobic α-helical regions of the protein comprising approximately 20 amino acids, which form the membrane-spanning domains of the receptors. **A** Type 1: ligand-gated ion channels. Many ligand-gated ion channels comprise four or five subunits of the type shown, the whole complex containing 16–20 membrane-spanning segments surrounding a central ion channel. Other structural types are shown in Fig. 3.16. **B** Type 2: G-protein–coupled receptors. **C**. Type 3: kinase-linked receptors. Most growth factor receptors incorporate the ligand-binding and enzymatic (kinase) domains in the same molecule, as shown, whereas cytokine receptors lack an intracellular kinase domain but link to cytosolic kinase molecules. Other structural variants also exist. **D** Type 4: nuclear receptors that control gene transcription.

- Type 2: **G-protein–coupled receptors** (GPCRs). These are also known as **metabotropic receptors** or **7-transmembrane-spanning (heptahelical) receptors**. They are membrane receptors that are coupled to intracellular effector systems via a G-protein (see below). They constitute the largest family,[5] and include receptors for many hormones and slow transmitters, for example the muscarinic acetylcholine receptor (mAChR;

see Ch. 10), adrenergic receptors (see Ch. 11) and chemokine receptors (see Ch. 16).
- Type 3: **kinase-linked and related receptors**. This is a large and heterogeneous group of membrane receptors responding mainly to protein mediators. They comprise an extracellular ligand-binding domain linked to an intracellular domain by a single transmembrane helix. In many cases, the intracellular domain is enzymic in nature (with protein kinase or guanylyl cyclase activity). Type 3 receptors include those for insulin and for various cytokines and growth factors (see Chs 16 and 26); the receptor for atrial natriuretic factor (ANF, Chs 18 and 19) is the main example of the guanylyl cyclase type. The two kinds are very similar structurally, even though their transduction mechanisms differ.

---

[5]There are probably more than 1000 human GPCRs, comprising roughly 3% of the genome. About half of these are believed to be odorant receptors involved in smell and taste sensations, the remainder being receptors for known or unknown endogenous mediators—enough to keep pharmacologists busy for some time yet.

Table 3.2 The four main types of receptor

	Type 1: ligand-gated ion channels	Type 2: G-protein–coupled receptors	Type 3: receptor kinases	Type 4: nuclear receptors
Location	Membrane	Membrane	Membrane	Intracellular
Effector	Ion channel	Channel or enzyme	Protein kinases	Gene transcription
Coupling	Direct	G-protein	Direct	Via DNA
Examples	Nicotinic acetylcholine receptor, GABA$_A$ receptor	Muscarinic acetylcholine receptor, adrenoceptors	Insulin, growth factors, cytokine receptors	Steroid receptors
Structure	Oligomeric assembly of subunits surrounding central pore	Monomeric dimericor structure comprising seven transmembrane helices	Single transmembrane helix linking extracellular receptor domain to intracellular kinase domain	Monomeric structure with separate receptor- and DNA-binding domains

- Type 4: **nuclear receptors**. These are receptors that regulate gene transcription. The term *nuclear receptors* is something of a misnomer, because some are actually located in the cytosol and migrate to the nuclear compartment when a ligand is present. They include receptors for steroid hormones (see Ch. 28), thyroid hormone (Ch. 29), and other agents such as retinoic acid and vitamin D.

MOLECULAR STRUCTURE OF RECEPTORS

The molecular organisation of typical members of each of these four receptor superfamilies is shown in Figure 3.3. Although individual receptors show considerable sequence variation in particular regions, and the lengths of the main intracellular and extracellular domains also vary from one to another within the same family, the overall structural patterns and associated signal transduction pathways are very consistent. The realisation that just four receptor superfamilies provide a solid framework for interpreting the complex welter of information about the effects of a large proportion of the drugs that have been studied has been one of the most refreshing developments in modern pharmacology.

Receptor heterogeneity and subtypes

Receptors within a given family generally occur in several molecular varieties, or subtypes, with similar architecture but significant differences in their sequences, and often in their pharmacological properties.[6] Nicotinic acetylcholine receptors are typical in this respect; distinct subtypes occur in different brain regions, and these differ from the muscle receptor. Some of the known pharmacological differences (e.g. sensitivity to blocking agents) between muscle and brain acetylcholine receptors correlate with specific sequence differences; however, as far as we know, all nicotinic acetylcholine receptors respond to the same physiological mediator and produce the same kind of synaptic response, so why many variants should have evolved is still a puzzle.

▼ Much of the sequence variation that accounts for receptor diversity arises at the genomic level, i.e. different genes give rise to distinct receptor subtypes. Additional variation arises from *alternative mRNA splicing*, which means that a single gene can give rise to more than one receptor *isoform*. After translation from genomic DNA, the mRNA normally contains non-coding regions (*introns*) that are excised by mRNA splicing before the message is translated into protein. Depending on the location of the splice sites, splicing can result in inclusion or deletion of one or more of the mRNA coding regions, giving rise to long or short forms of the protein. This is an important source of variation, particularly for GPCRs (see Kilpatrick et al., 1999), which produces receptors with different binding characteristics and different signal transduction mechanisms, although its pharmacological relevance remains to be clarified. Another process that can produce different receptors from the same gene is *mRNA editing*, which involves the mischievous substitution of one base in the mRNA for another, and hence a small variation in the amino acid sequence of the receptor.

Molecular heterogeneity of this kind is a feature of all kinds of receptors—indeed of functional proteins in general. New receptor subtypes and isoforms are continually being discovered, and regular updates of the catalogue are available (Alexander et al., 2004; *IUPHAR Receptor Database and Channel Compendium*). The problems of classification, nomenclature and taxonomy resulting from this flood of data have been mentioned earlier (p. 28). From the pharmacological viewpoint, where our concern is to understand individual drugs and what they do to living organisms, and to devise better ones, it is important that we keep molecular pharmacology in perspective. The 'newer rite' has proved revelatory in many ways, but the sheer complexity of the ways in which molecules behave means that we have a long way to go before reaching the reductionist Utopia that molecular biology promises. When we do, this book will get much shorter. In the meantime, we try to pick out the general principles without getting too bogged down in detail.

We will now describe the characteristics of each of the four receptor superfamilies.

---

[6]Receptors for 5-HT (see Ch. 12) are currently the champions with respect to diversity, with 14 cloned subtypes.

TYPE 1: LIGAND-GATED ION CHANNELS

MOLECULAR STRUCTURE

These molecules have structural features in common with other ion channels, described on p. 50 (see Ashcroft, 2000). The nicotinic acetylcholine receptor (Fig. 3.3A), the first to be cloned, has been studied in great detail (see Karlin, 1993). It is assembled from four different types of subunit, termed α, β, γ and δ, each of M_r 40–58 kDa. The four subunits show marked sequence homology, and analysis of the hydrophobicity profile, which determines which sections of the chain are likely to form membrane-spanning α helices, suggests that they are inserted into the membrane as shown in Figure 3.4. The pentameric structure (α_2, β, γ, δ) possesses two acetylcholine binding sites, each lying at the interface between one of the two α subunits and its neighbour. Both must bind acetylcholine molecules in order for the receptor to be activated. This receptor is sufficiently large to be seen in electron micrographs, and Figure 3.4 shows its structure, based mainly on a high-resolution electron diffraction study (Unwin 1993, 1995; Miyazawa et al., 2003). Each subunit spans the membrane four times, so the channel comprises no less than 20 membrane-spanning helices surrounding a central pore.

▼ The two acetylcholine-binding sites lie on the extracellular parts of the two α subunits. One of the transmembrane helices (M_2) from each of the five subunits forms the lining of the ion channel (Fig. 3.4). The five M_2 helices that form the pore are sharply kinked inwards halfway through the membrane, forming a constriction. When acetylcholine molecules bind, the α subunits twist, causing the kinked M_2 segments to swivel out of the way, thus opening the channel (Miyazawa et al., 2003).

The use of site-directed mutagenesis, which enables short regions, or single residues, of the amino acid sequence to be altered, has shown (see Galzi & Changeux, 1994) that a mutation of a critical residue in the M_2 helix changes the channel from being cation-selective (hence excitatory in the context of synaptic function) to being anion-selective (typical of receptors for inhibitory transmitters such as GABA). Other mutations affect properties such as gating and desensitisation of ligand-gated channels.

Receptors for some other fast transmitters, such as the $GABA_A$ receptor (Ch. 33), the $5\text{-}HT_3$ receptor (Ch. 12) and the glycine receptor (Ch.33) are built on the same pattern, and some show considerable sequence homology with the nicotinic acetylcholine receptor; the number of subunits that go to make up a functional receptor varies somewhat but is usually four or five. However, other ligand-gated ion channels have a somewhat different architecture, in which the pore is built from loops rather than transmembrane helices (see p. 50), in common with many other (non ligand-gated) ion channels. ATP receptors of the P_{2X} type (see Ch. 12) and glutamate receptors (see Ch. 33), whose structures are shown in Figure 3.18, are of this type.

THE GATING MECHANISM

Receptors of this type control the fastest synaptic events in the nervous system, in which a neurotransmitter acts on the postsynaptic membrane of a nerve or muscle cell and transiently increases its permeability to particular ions. Most excitatory neurotransmitters, such as acetylcholine at the neuromuscular junction (Ch. 10) or glutamate in the central nervous system (Ch. 33), cause an increase

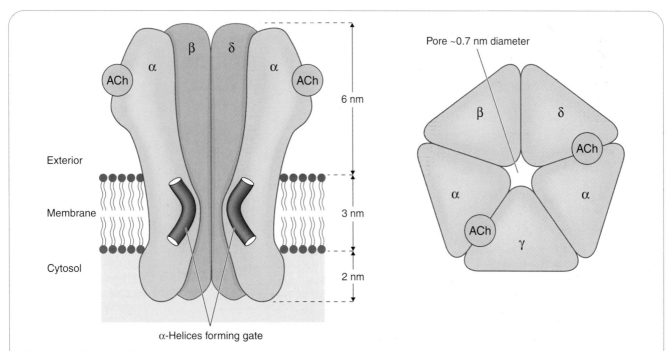

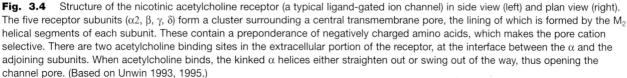

Fig. 3.4 Structure of the nicotinic acetylcholine receptor (a typical ligand-gated ion channel) in side view (left) and plan view (right). The five receptor subunits (α2, β, γ, δ) form a cluster surrounding a central transmembrane pore, the lining of which is formed by the M_2 helical segments of each subunit. These contain a preponderance of negatively charged amino acids, which makes the pore cation selective. There are two acetylcholine binding sites in the extracellular portion of the receptor, at the interface between the α and the adjoining subunits. When acetylcholine binds, the kinked α helices either straighten out or swing out of the way, thus opening the channel pore. (Based on Unwin 1993, 1995.)

in Na⁺ and K⁺ permeability. This results in a net inward current carried mainly by Na⁺, which depolarises the cell and increases the probability that it will generate an action potential. The action of the transmitter reaches a peak in a fraction of a millisecond, and usually decays within a few milliseconds. The sheer speed of this response implies that the coupling between the receptor and the ionic channel is a direct one, and the molecular structure of the receptor–channel complex (see above) agrees with this. In contrast to other receptor families (see below), no intermediate biochemical steps are involved in the transduction process.

▼ A breakthrough by Katz and Miledi in 1972 made it possible for the first time to study the properties of individual ligand-gated channels by the use of *noise analysis*. Studying the action of acetylcholine at the motor endplate, they observed that small random fluctuations of membrane potential were superimposed on the steady depolarisation produced by acetylcholine (Fig.3.5). These fluctuations arise because, in the presence

of an agonist, there is a dynamic equilibrium between open and closed ion channels. In the steady state, the rate of opening balances the rate of closing, but from moment to moment the number of open channels will show random fluctuations about the mean. By measuring the amplitude of these fluctuations, the conductance of a single ion channel can be calculated, and by measuring their frequency (usually in the form of a spectrum in which the noise power of the signal is plotted as a function of frequency) the average duration for which a single channel stays open (mean open time) can be calculated. In the case of acetylcholine acting at the endplate, the channel conductance is about 20 picosiemens (pS), which is equivalent to an influx of about 10^7 ions per second through a single channel under normal physiological conditions, and the mean open time is 1–2 milliseconds. The magnitude of the single channel conductance confirms that permeation occurs through a physical pore through the membrane, because the ion flow is too large to be compatible with a carrier mechanism. The channel conductance produced by different acetylcholine-like agonists is the same, whereas the mean channel lifetime varies.

The simple scheme shown in Fig. 2.1 is a useful model for ion channel gating. The conformation R*, representing the open state of the ion channel, is thought to be the same for all agonists, accounting for the finding that the channel conductance does not vary. Kinetically, the mean open time is determined mainly by the closing rate constant, α, and this varies from one drug to another. As explained in Chapter 2, an agonist of high efficacy that activates a large proportion of the receptors that it occupies will be characterised by $\beta/\alpha \gg 1$, whereas for a drug of low efficacy β/α has a lower value.

The patch clamp recording technique, devised by Neher and Sakmann, allows the very small current flowing through a single ionic channel to be measured directly (Fig. 3.6), and the results have fully confirmed the interpretation of channel properties based on noise analysis. This technique provides a view, unique in biology, of the physiological behaviour of individual protein molecules in real time, and has given many new insights into the gating reactions and permeability characteristics of both ligand-gated channels and voltage-gated channels (see p. 49). Single-channel recording has shown that many agonists cause individual channels to open to one or more of several distinct conductance levels. In the case of glutamate-activated channels, it appears that different agonists produce different receptor conformations

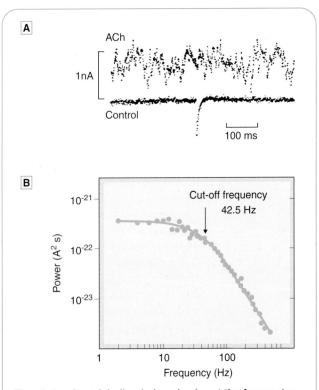

Fig. 3.5 Acetylcholine-induced noise at the frog motor endplate. **A** Records of membrane current recorded at high gain under voltage clamp. The upper noise record was recorded during the application of acetylcholine (ACh) from a micropipette. The lower record was obtained in the absence of ACh, the blip in the middle being caused by the spontaneous release of a packet of ACh from the motor nerve. The steady (DC) component of the ACh signal has been removed by electronic filtering, leaving the high-frequency noise signal. **B** Power spectrum of ACh-induced noise recorded in a similar experiment to that shown above. The spectrum is calculated by Fourier analysis and fitted with a theoretical (Lorentzian) curve that corresponds to the expected behaviour of a single population of channels whose lifetime varies randomly. The cut-off frequency (at which the power is half of its limiting low-frequency value) enables the mean channel lifetime to be calculated. (From: (A) Anderson C R, Stevens C F 1973 J Physiol 235: 655; (B) Ogden D C et al. 1981 Nature 289: 596.)

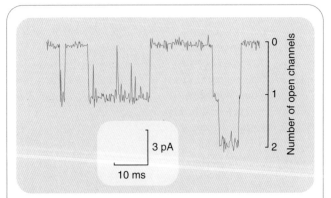

Fig. 3.6 Single acetylcholine-operated ion channels at the frog motor endplate recorded by the patch clamp technique. The pipette, which was applied tightly to the surface of the membrane, contained 10μmol/l ACh. The downward deflections show the currents flowing through single ion channels in the small patch of membrane under the pipette tip. Towards the end of the record, two channels can be seen to open simultaneously. The conductance and mean lifetime of these channels agrees well with indirect estimates from noise analysis (see Fig. 3.5). (Figure courtesy of D Colquhoun and D C Ogden.)

associated with different channel conductances (Jin et al., 2003). Desensitisation of ligand-gated ion channels also involves one or more additional agonist-induced conformational states. These findings necessitate some elaboration of the simple scheme of Fig. 2.1, in which only a single open state, R*, is represented, and are an example of the way in which the actual behaviour of receptors makes our theoretical models look a little threadbare.

TYPE 2: G-PROTEIN–COUPLED RECEPTORS

The abundant GPCR family comprises many of the receptors that are familiar to pharmacologists, such as mAChRs, adrenoceptors, dopamine receptors, 5-HT receptors, opiate receptors, receptors for many peptides, purine receptors and many others, including the chemoreceptors involved in olfaction and pheromone detection, and also many 'orphans' (see Pierce et al., 2002). For most of these, quantitative pharmacological studies with different agonists and antagonists have revealed a variety of subtypes. Many GPCRs have been cloned, revealing a strikingly coherent pattern of their molecular structure.

Many neurotransmitters, apart from peptides, can interact with both GPCRs and with ligand-gated channels, allowing the same molecule to produce a wide variety of effects. Individual peptide hormones, on the other hand, generally act either on GPCRs or on kinase-linked receptors (see below), but rarely on both, and a similar choosiness applies to the many ligands that act on nuclear receptors.[7]

The human genome includes genes encoding about 400 GPCRs (excluding odorant receptors; see Ben-Shlomo et al., 2003). GPCRs constitute the commonest single class of targets for therapeutic drugs, and it is thought that many promising therapeutic drug targets of this type remain to be identified. For a short review, see Hill (2006).

MOLECULAR STRUCTURE

The first GPCR to be fully characterised was the β-adrenoceptor (Ch. 11), which was cloned in 1986. Subsequently, molecular biology caught up very rapidly with pharmacology, and most of the receptors that had been identified by their pharmacological properties have now been cloned. What seemed revolutionary in 1986 is now commonplace, and nowadays any aspiring receptor has to be cloned before it is taken seriously.

G-protein–coupled receptors consist of a single polypeptide chain of up to 1100 residues whose general anatomy is shown in Figure 3.3B. Their characteristic structure comprises seven transmembrane α helices, similar to those of the ion channels discussed above, with an extracellular N-terminal domain of varying length, and an intracellular C-terminal domain. GPCRs are divided into three distinct families (see Schwartz, 1996).

> **Ligand-gated ion channels**
>
> - These are sometimes called ionotropic receptors.
> - They are involved mainly in fast synaptic transmission.
> - There are several structural families, the commonest being heteromeric assemblies of four or five subunits, with transmembrane helices arranged around a central aqueous channel.
> - Ligand binding and channel opening occur on a millisecond timescale.
> - Examples include the nicotinic acetylcholine, GABA type A (GABA$_A$), and 5-hydroxytryptamine type 3 (5-HT$_3$) receptors.

There is considerable sequence homology between the members of one family, but none between different families. They share the same seven-helix (heptahelical) structure, but differ in other respects, principally in the length of the extracellular N terminus and the location of the agonist binding domain (Table 3.3). Family A is by far the largest, comprising most monoamine, neuropeptide and chemokine receptors. Family B includes receptors for some other peptides, such as calcitonin and glucagon (see Ch. 14). Family C is the smallest, its main members being the metabotropic glutamate and GABA receptors (Ch. 33) and the Ca^{2+}-sensing receptors[8] (see Ch. 31).

The understanding of the function of receptors of this type owes much to studies of a closely related protein, *rhodopsin*, which is responsible for transduction in retinal rods. This protein is abundant in the retina, and much easier to study than receptor proteins (which are anything but abundant); it is built on an identical plan to that shown in Figure 3.3 and also produces a response in the rod (hyperpolarisation, associated with inhibition of a Na$^+$ conductance) through a mechanism involving a G-protein (see below). The most obvious difference is that a photon, rather than an agonist molecule, produces the response. In effect, rhodopsin can be regarded as incorporating its own inbuilt agonist molecule, namely *retinal*, which isomerises from the *trans* (inactive) to the *cis* (active) form when it absorbs a photon.

Site-directed mutagenesis experiments show that the long third cytoplasmic loop is the region of the molecule that couples to the G-protein, because deletion or modification of this section results in receptors that still bind ligands but cannot associate with G-proteins or produce responses. Usually, a particular receptor subtype couples selectively with a particular G-protein, and

---

[7]Examples of promiscuity are increasing, however. Steroid hormones, normally faithful to nuclear receptors, make the occasional pass at ion channels and other targets (see Falkenstein et al., 2000), and some eicosanoids act on nuclear receptors as well as GPCRs. Nature is quite open-minded, although such examples are liable to make pharmacologists frown and students despair.

[8]The Ca^{2+}-sensing receptor (see Conigrave et al., 2000) is an unusual GPCR that is activated, not by conventional mediators, but by extracellular Ca^{2+} in the range of 1–10 mM—an extremely low affinity in comparison with other GPCR agonists. It is expressed by cells of the parathyroid gland, and serves to regulate the extracellular Ca^{2+} concentration by controlling parathyroid hormone secretion (Ch. 31). This homeostatic mechanism is quite distinct from the mechanisms for regulating intracellular Ca^{2+} discussed in Chapter 4.

Table 3.3 G-protein–coupled receptor families[a]

Family	Receptors[b]	Structural features
A: rhodopsin family	The largest group. Receptors for most amine neurotransmitters, many neuropeptides, purines, prostanoids, cannabinoids, etc.	Short extracellular (N terminal) tail. Ligand binds to transmembrane helices (amines) or to extracellular loops (peptides).
B: secretin/glucagon receptor family	Receptors for peptide hormones, including secretin, glucagon, calcitonin.	Intermediate extracellular tail incorporating ligand-binding domain.
C: metabotropic glutamate receptor/calcium sensor family	Small group. Metabotropic glutamate receptors, $GABA_B$ receptors, Ca^{2+}-sensing receptors.	Long extracellular tail incorporating ligand binding domain.

[a]A fourth distinct family includes many receptors for pheromones but no pharmacological receptors.
[b]For full lists, see http://www.iuphar-db.org.

swapping parts of the cytoplasmic loop between different receptors alters their G-protein selectivity.

For small molecules, such as noradrenaline (norepinephrine), the ligand-binding domain is buried in the cleft between the α-helical segments within the membrane (Fig. 3.3B), similar to the slot occupied by retinal in the rhodopsin molecule. Peptide ligands, such as substance P (Ch. 16) bind more superficially to the extracellular loops, as shown in Figure 3.3B. By single-site mutagenesis experiments, it is possible to map the ligand-binding domain of these receptors, and the hope is that it may soon be possible to design synthetic ligands based on knowledge of the receptor site structure—an important milestone for the pharmaceutical industry, which has relied up to now mainly on the structure of endogenous mediators (such as histamine) or plant alkaloids (such as morphine) for its chemical inspiration.[9] So far, GPCRs cannot be obtained in crystalline form, so the powerful technique of X-ray crystallography cannot yet be used to define the molecular structure of these receptors in detail. Until then, designing new GPCR ligands will remain a somewhat hit-or-miss business.

ALTERNATIVE MECHANISMS OF RECEPTOR ACTIVATION

▼ Although activation of GPCRs is normally the consequence of agonist binding, it can occur by other mechanisms. Rhodopsin, mentioned earlier, is activated by light-induced *cis–trans* isomerisation of prebound retinal. Another example is that of the *protease-activated receptors* (*PARs*), of which four have so far been identified (see Vergnolle et al., 2001). Many proteases, such as thrombin (a protease involved in the blood-clotting cascade, see Ch. 21), activate PARs by snipping off the end of the extracellular N-terminal tail of the receptor (Fig. 3.7). The exposed N-terminal residues then bind to receptor domains in the extracellular loops, functioning as a 'tethered agonist'. Receptors of this type occur in many tissues (see Ossofskaya & Bunnett, 2004, Vergnolle, 2004), and they appear to play a role in inflammation and other responses to tissue damage where tissue proteases are released. One of the family of PARs, PAR-2, is activated by

a protease released from mast cells, and is expressed on sensory neurons. It is thought to play a role in inflammatory pain (see Ch. 41). One consequence of this type of activation is that the receptor can be activated only once, because the cleavage cannot be reversed, so continuous resynthesis of receptor protein is necessary. Inactivation occurs by desensitisation, involving phosphorylation (see below), after which the receptor is internalised and degraded, to be replaced by newly synthesised protein.

Several human disease states have been described (see below) that are associated either with spontaneous receptor mutations that result in constitutive activation of receptors, or with the production of autoantibodies directed against the extracellular domain of receptors, which mimic the effect of agonists.

G-proteins and their role

G-proteins comprise a family of membrane-resident proteins whose function is to recognise activated GPCRs and pass on the message to the effector systems that generate a cellular response. They represent the level of middle management in the organisational hierarchy, intervening between the receptors—choosy mandarins alert to the faintest whiff of their preferred chemical—and the effector enzymes or ion channels—the blue collar brigade that gets the job done without needing to know which hormone authorised the process. They are the go-between proteins, but were actually called G-proteins because of their interaction with the guanine nucleotides, GTP and GDP. For more detailed information on the structure and functions of G-proteins, see reviews by Offermanns (2003) and Milligan and Kostenis (2006). G-proteins consist of three subunits: α, β and γ (Fig. 3.8). Guanine nucleotides bind to the α subunit, which has enzymic activity, catalysing the conversion of GTP to GDP. The β and γ subunits remain together as a βγ complex. All three subunits are anchored to the membrane through a fatty acid chain, coupled to the G-protein through a reaction known as *prenylation*. G-proteins appear to be freely diffusible in the plane of the membrane, so a single pool of G-protein in a cell can interact with several different receptors and effectors in an essentially promiscuous fashion. In the 'resting' state (Fig. 3.8), the G-protein exists as an unattached αβγ trimer, with GDP occupying the site on the α subunit. When a GPCR is activated by an agonist molecule, a conformational change occurs, involving the cytoplasmic domain

---

[9]Many lead compounds in recent years have come from screening huge chemical libraries (see Ch. 56). No inspiration is required, just robust assays, large computers and efficient robotics.

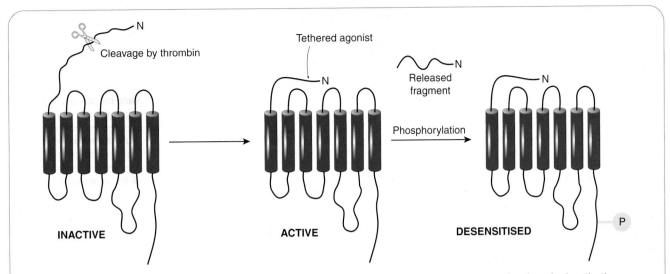

Fig. 3.7 **Activation of the thrombin receptor by proteolytic cleavage of the N-terminal extracellular domain.** Inactivation occurs by phosphorylation. Recovery requires resynthesis of the receptor.

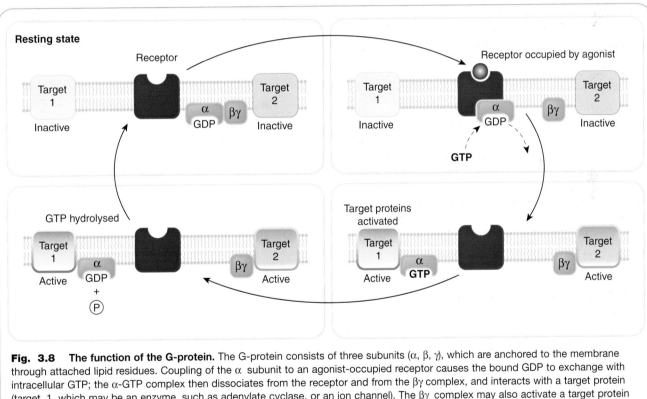

Fig. 3.8 **The function of the G-protein.** The G-protein consists of three subunits (α, β, γ), which are anchored to the membrane through attached lipid residues. Coupling of the α subunit to an agonist-occupied receptor causes the bound GDP to exchange with intracellular GTP; the α-GTP complex then dissociates from the receptor and from the $\beta\gamma$ complex, and interacts with a target protein (target 1, which may be an enzyme, such as adenylate cyclase, or an ion channel). The $\beta\gamma$ complex may also activate a target protein (target 2). The GTPase activity of the α subunit is increased when the target protein is bound, leading to hydrolysis of the bound GTP to GDP, whereupon the α subunit reunites with $\beta\gamma$.

of the receptor (Fig. 3.3B), causing it to acquire high affinity for $\alpha\beta\gamma$. Association of $\alpha\beta\gamma$ with the receptor causes the bound GDP to dissociate and to be replaced with GTP (GDP–GTP exchange), which in turn causes dissociation of the G-protein trimer, releasing α-GTP and $\beta\gamma$ subunits; these are the 'active' forms of the G-protein, which diffuse in the membrane and can associate with various enzymes and ion channels, causing

activation of the target (Fig. 3.8). It was originally thought that only the α subunit has a signalling function, the $\beta\gamma$ complex serving merely as a chaperone to keep the flighty α subunits out of range of the various effector proteins that they might otherwise excite. However, the $\beta\gamma$ complexes actually make assignations of their own, and control effectors in much the same way as the α subunits (see Clapham & Neer, 1997). In general, it appears that

35

Table 3.4 The main G-protein subtypes and their functions[a]

Subtypes	Associated receptors	Main effectors	Notes
Gα subunits			
Gα_s	Many amine and other receptors (e.g. catecholamines, histamine, serotonin)	Stimulates adenylyl cyclase, causing increased cAMP formation.	Activated by cholera toxin, which blocks GTPase activity, thus preventing inactivation.
Gα_i	As for Gα_s, also opioid, cannabinoid receptors	Inhibits adenylyl cyclase, decreasing cAMP formation.	Blocked by pertussis toxin, which prevents dissociation of $\alpha\beta\gamma$ complex.
Gα_o	As for Gα_s, also opioid, cannabinoid receptors	?Limited effects of α subunit (effects mainly due to $\beta\gamma$ subunits).	Blocked by pertussis toxin. Occurs mainly in nervous system.
Gα_q	Amine, peptide and prostanoid receptors	Activates phospholipase C, increasing production of second messengers inositol trisphosphate and diacylglycerol (see p. 38).	–
G$\beta\gamma$ subunits	All GPCRs	As for Gα subunits (see above). Also: • activate potassium channels • inhibit voltage-gated calcium channels • activate GPCR kinases (p. 40) • activate mitogen-activated protein kinase cascade.	Many G$\beta\gamma$ isoforms identified, but specific functions are not yet known. G$\beta\gamma$-mediated effects probably require higher levels of GPCR activation than Gα-mediated effects.

GPCR, G-protein-coupled receptor.
[a]This table lists only those isoforms of major pharmacological significance. Many more have been identified, some of which play roles in olfaction, taste, visual transduction and other physiological functions (see Offermanns, 2003).

higher concentrations of $\beta\gamma$ complex than of α subunits are needed, so $\beta\gamma$-mediated effects occur at higher levels of receptor occupancy than α-mediated effects. Association of α subunits with target enzymes can cause either activation or inhibition, depending on which G protein in involved (see Table 3.4).

Signalling is terminated when the hydrolysis of GTP to GDP occurs through the GTPase activity of the α subunit. The resulting α-GDP then dissociates from the effector, and reunites with $\beta\gamma$, completing the cycle. Attachment of the α subunit to an effector molecule actually increases its GTPase activity, the magnitude of this increase being different for different types of effector. Because GTP hydrolysis is the step that terminates the ability of the α subunit to produce its effect, regulation of its GTPase activity by the effector protein means that the activation of the effector tends to be self-limiting. The mechanism results in *amplification* because a single agonist–receptor complex can activate several G-protein molecules in turn, and each of these can remain associated with the effector enzyme for long enough to produce many molecules of product. The product (see below) is often a 'second messenger', and further amplification occurs before the final cellular response is produced.

How is specificity achieved so that each kind of receptor produces a distinct pattern of cellular responses? With a common pool of promiscuous G-proteins linking the various receptors and effector systems in a cell, it might seem that all specificity would be lost, but this is clearly not the case. For example, mAChRs and β-adrenoceptors, both of which occur in cardiac muscle cells, produce opposite functional effects (Chs 10 and 11). The main reason

is molecular variation within the α subunits, of which more than 20 subtypes have been identified[10] (see Wess, 1998; Table 3.4). Four main classes of G-protein (G$_s$, G$_i$, G$_o$ and G$_q$) are of pharmacological importance. As summarised in Table 3.4, they show selectivity with respect to both the receptors and the effectors with which they couple, having specific recognition domains in their structure complementary to specific G-protein–binding domains in the receptor and effector molecules. G$_s$ and G$_i$ produce, respectively, stimulation and inhibition of the enzyme adenylyl cyclase (Fig. 3.9). The G-proteins can be thought of as the intramembrane managers, bustling between receptors and effectors, controlling this microcosm but communicating very little with the world outside.

The α subunits of these G-proteins differ in structure. One functional difference that has been useful as an experimental tool to distinguish which type of G-protein is involved in different situations, concerns the action of two bacterial toxins, cholera toxin and pertussis toxin (see Table 3.4). These toxins, which are enzymes, catalyse a conjugation reaction (ADP ribosylation) on the α subunit of G-proteins. Cholera toxin acts only on G$_s$, and it causes persistent activation. Many of the symptoms of cholera, such as the excessive secretion of fluid from the gastrointestinal

---

[10]As well as more than 20 known subtypes of Gα, there are 6 of Gβ and 12 of Gγ, providing, in theory, about 1500 variants of the trimer. We know little about the role of different α, β, γ subtypes, but it would be rash to assume that the variations are functionally irrelevant. By now, you will be unsurprised (even if somewhat bemused) by such a display of molecular heterogeneity, for it is the way of evolution.

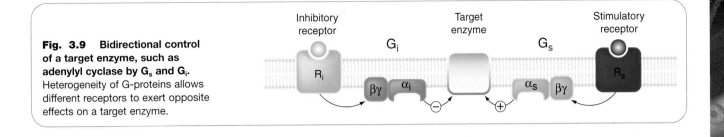

Fig. 3.9 Bidirectional control of a target enzyme, such as adenylyl cyclase by G$_s$ and G$_i$. Heterogeneity of G-proteins allows different receptors to exert opposite effects on a target enzyme.

epithelium, are due to the uncontrolled activation of adenylyl cyclase that occurs. Pertussis toxin specifically blocks G$_i$ and G$_o$ by preventing dissociation of the G-protein trimer.

TARGETS FOR G-PROTEINS

The main targets for G-proteins, through which GPCRs control different aspects of cell function (see Milligan, 1995; Gudermann et al., 1996; Nahorski, 2006; Table 3.4), are:

- *adenylyl cyclase*, the enzyme responsible for cAMP formation
- *phospholipase C*, the enzyme responsible for inositol phosphate and diacylglycerol (DAG) formation
- *ion channels*, particularly calcium and potassium channels
- *Rho A/Rho kinase,* a system that controls the activity of many signalling pathways controlling cell growth and proliferation, smooth muscle contraction, etc.

The adenylyl cyclase/cAMP system

The discovery by Sutherland and his colleagues of the role of cAMP (cyclic 3′,5′-adenosine monophosphate) as an intracellular mediator demolished at a stroke the barriers that existed between

> ### G-protein–coupled receptors
>
> - These are sometimes called metabotropic receptors.
> - Structures comprise seven membrane-spanning α-helices, often linked as dimeric structures.
> - One of the intracellular loops is larger than the others and interacts with the G-protein.
> - The G-protein is a membrane protein comprising three subunits (α, β, γ), the α subunit possessing GTPase activity.
> - When the trimer binds to anagonist-occupied receptor, the α subunit dissociates and is then free to activate an effector (a membrane enzyme or ion channel). In some cases, the βγ subunit is the activator species.
> - Activation of the effector is terminated when the bound GTP molecule is hydrolysed, which allows the α subunit to recombine with βγ.
> - There are several types of G-protein, which interact with different receptors and control different effectors.
> - Examples include muscarinic acetylcholine receptors, adrenoceptors, neuropeptide and chemokine receptors, and protease-activated receptors.

biochemistry and pharmacology, and introduced the concept of second messengers in signal transduction. cAMP is a nucleotide synthesised within the cell from ATP by the action of a membrane-bound enzyme, adenylyl cyclase. It is produced continuously and inactivated by hydrolysis to 5′-AMP, by the action of a family of enzymes known as *phosphodiesterases* (*PDEs*). Many different drugs, hormones and neurotransmitters act on GPCRs and produce their effects by increasing or decreasing the catalytic activity of adenylyl cyclase, thus raising or lowering the concentration of cAMP within the cell. There are several different molecular isoforms of the enzyme, some of which respond selectively to Gα$_s$ or Gα$_i$ (see Simonds, 1999).

Cyclic AMP regulates many aspects of cellular function including, for example, enzymes involved in energy metabolism, cell division and cell differentiation, ion transport, ion channels, and the contractile proteins in smooth muscle. These varied effects are, however, all brought about by a common mechanism, namely the activation of *protein kinases* by cAMP. Protein kinases regulate the function of many different cellular proteins by controlling protein phosphorylation (see p. 43). Figure 3.10 shows how increased cAMP production in response to β-adrenoceptor activation affects enzymes involved in glycogen and fat metabolism in liver, fat and muscle cells. The result is a coordinated response in which stored energy in the form of glycogen and fat is made available as glucose to fuel muscle contraction.

Other examples of regulation by cAMP-dependent protein kinases include the increased activity of voltage-activated calcium channels in heart muscle cells (see Ch. 18). Phosphorylation of these channels increases the amount of Ca^{2+} entering the cell during the action potential, and thus increases the force of contraction of the heart.

In smooth muscle, cAMP-dependent protein kinase phosphorylates (thereby inactivating) another enzyme, myosin–light-chain kinase, which is required for contraction. This accounts for the smooth muscle relaxation produced by many drugs that increase cAMP production in smooth muscle (see Ch. 19).

As mentioned above, receptors linked to G$_i$ rather than G$_s$ inhibit adenylyl cyclase, and thus reduce cAMP formation. Examples include certain types of mAChR (e.g. the M$_2$ receptor of cardiac muscle; see Ch. 10), α$_2$-adrenoceptors in smooth muscle (Ch. 11), and opioid receptors (see Ch. 41). Adenylyl cyclase can be activated directly by certain agents, including forskolin and fluoride ions, agents that are used experimentally to study the role of the cAMP system.

Cyclic AMP is hydrolysed within cells by *phosphodiesterases* (PDEs), an important and ubiquitous family of enzymes (see Beavo, 1995, for review). Many PDE subtypes exist, of which some (e.g.

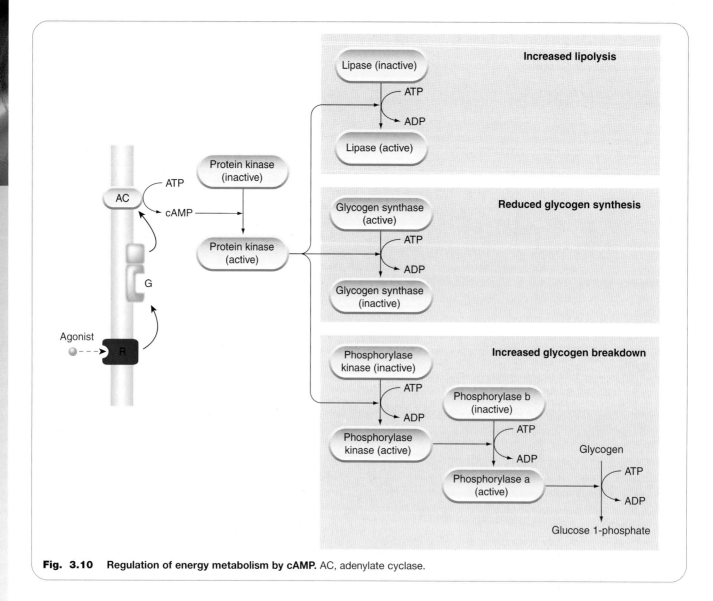

Fig. 3.10 **Regulation of energy metabolism by cAMP.** AC, adenylate cyclase.

PDE$_3$ and PDE$_4$) are cAMP-selective, while others (e.g PDE$_5$) are cGMP-selective. Most are weakly inhibited by drugs such as methylxanthines (e.g. **theophylline** and **caffeine**; see Chs 23 and 42). **Rolipram** (used to treat asthma, Ch. 23) is selective for PDE$_4$ expressed in inflammatory cells; **milrinone** (used to treat heart failure, Ch. 18) is selective for PDE$_4$, which is expressed in heart muscle; **sildenafil** (better known as Viagra, Ch. 30) is selective for PDE$_5$, and consequently enhances the vasodilator effects of NO and drugs that release NO, whose effects are mediated by cGMP (see Ch. 17). The similarity of some of the actions of these drugs to those of catecholamines probably reflects their common property of increasing the intracellular concentration of cAMP. Selective inhibitors of the various PDEs are being developed, mainly to treat cardiovascular and respiratory diseases (Chs 19 and 23).

The phospholipase C/inositol phosphate system

The phosphoinositide system, an important intracellular second messenger system, was first discovered in the 1950s by Hokin and Hokin, whose recondite interests centred on the mechanism

of salt secretion by the nasal glands of seabirds. They found that secretion was accompanied by increased turnover of a minor class of membrane phospholipids known as *phosphoinositides* (collectively known as PIs; Fig. 3.11). Subsequently, Michell and Berridge found that many hormones that produce an increase in free intracellular Ca^{2+} concentration (which include, for example, muscarinic agonists and α-adrenoceptor agonists acting on smooth muscle and salivary glands, and vasopressin acting on liver cells) also increase PI turnover. Subsequently, it was found that one particular member of the PI family, namely phosphatidylinositol (4,5) bisphosphate (PIP$_2$), which has additional phosphate groups attached to the inositol ring, plays a key role. PIP$_2$ is the substrate for a membrane-bound enzyme, phospholipase Cβ (PLCβ), which splits it into DAG and inositol (1,4,5) trisphosphate (IP$_3$; Fig. 3.12), both of which function as second messengers as discussed below. The activation of PLCβ by various agonists is mediated through a G-protein (G$_q$, see Table 3.4). After cleavage of PIP$_2$, the status quo is restored as shown in Figure 3.12, DAG being phosphorylated to form phosphatidic acid (PA), while the IP$_3$ is dephosphorylated and then recoupled with PA to form PIP$_2$

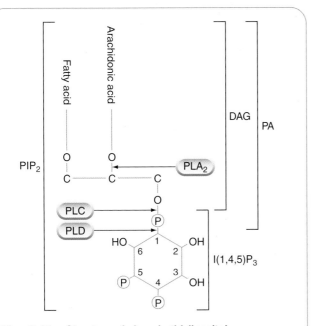

Fig. 3.11 **Structure of phosphatidylinositol bisphosphate (PIP$_2$), showing sites of cleavage by different phospholipases to produce active mediators.** Cleavage by phospholipase A$_2$ (PLA$_2$) yields arachidonic acid. Cleavage by phospholipase C (PLC) yields inositol trisphosphate (I(1,4,5)P$_3$) and diacylglycerol (DAG). PA, phosphatidic acid; PLD, phospholipase D.

once again.[11] **Lithium**, an agent used in psychiatry (see Ch. 39) blocks this recycling pathway (see Fig. 3.12).

Inositol phosphates and intracellular calcium

Inositol (1,4,5) trisphosphate is a water-soluble mediator that is released into the cytosol and acts on a specific receptor—the IP$_3$ receptor—which is a ligand-gated calcium channel present on the membrane of the endoplasmic reticulum. The main role of IP$_3$, described in more detail in Chapter 4, is to control the release of Ca^{2+} from intracellular stores. Because many drug and hormone effects involve intracellular Ca^{2+}, this pathway is particularly important. IP$_3$ is converted inside the cell to the (1,3,4,5) tetraphosphate, IP$_4$, by a specific kinase. The exact role of IP$_4$ remains unclear (see Irvine, 2001), but there is evidence that it too is involved in Ca^{2+} signalling. One possibility is that it facilitates Ca^{2+} entry through the plasma membrane, thus avoiding depletion of the intracellular stores as a result of the action of IP$_3$.

Diacylglycerol and protein kinase C

Diacylglycerol is produced as well as IP$_3$ whenever receptor-induced PI hydrolysis occurs. The main effect of DAG is to activate a membrane-bound protein kinase, *protein kinase C* (PKC), which catalyses the phosphorylation of a variety of intracellular proteins (see Nishizuka, 1988; Walaas & Greengard, 1991). DAG, unlike the inositol phosphates, is highly lipophilic and remains within the membrane. It binds to a specific site on the PKC molecule, which migrates from the cytosol to the cell membrane in the presence of DAG, thereby becoming activated. There are 10 different mammalian PKC subtypes, which have distinct cellular distributions and phosphorylate different proteins. Most are activated by DAG and raised intracellular Ca^{2+}, both of which are produced by activation of GPCRs. PKCs are also activated by **phorbol esters** (highly irritant, tumour-promoting compounds produced by certain plants), which have been extremely useful in studying the functions of PKC. One of the subtypes is activated by the lipid mediator arachidonic acid (see Ch. 13) generated by the action of phospholipase A$_2$ on membrane phospholipids, so PKC activation can also occur with agonists that activate this enzyme. The various PKC isoforms, like the tyrosine kinases discussed below (p. 43) act on many different functional proteins, such as ion channels, receptors, enzymes (including other kinases) and cytoskeletal proteins. Kinases in general play a central role in signal transduction, and control many different aspects of cell function. The DAG–PKC link provides a channel whereby GPCRs can mobilise this army of control freaks.

Ion channels as targets for G-proteins

G-protein–coupled receptors can control ion channel function directly by mechanisms that do not involve second messengers such as cAMP or inositol phosphates. This was first shown for cardiac muscle, but it now appears that direct G-protein–channel interaction may be quite general (see Wickham & Clapham, 1995). Early examples came from studies on potassium channels. In cardiac muscle, for example, mAChRs are known to enhance K$^+$ permeability (thus hyperpolarising the cells and inhibiting electrical activity; see Ch. 18). Similar mechanisms operate in neurons, where many inhibitory drugs such as opiate analgesics reduce excitability by opening potassium channels (see Ch. 41). These actions are produced by direct interaction between the βγ subunit of G$_0$ and the channel, without the involvement of second messengers.

The Rho/Rho kinase system

▼ This recently discovered signal transduction pathway (see Bishop & Hall, 2000) is activated by certain GPCRs (and also by non-GPCR mechanisms), which couple to G-proteins of the G$_{12/13}$ type. The free G-protein α subunit interacts with a *guanosine nucleotide exchange factor*, which facilitates GDP–GTP exchange at another GTPase, Rho. Rho–GDP, the resting form, is inactive, but when GDP–GTP exchange occurs, Rho is activated, and in turn activates Rho kinase. Rho kinase phosphorylates many substrate proteins and controls a wide variety of cellular functions, including smooth muscle contraction and proliferation, angiogenesis and synaptic remodelling. By enhancing hypoxia-induced pulmonary artery vasoconstriction, activation of Rho kinase is thought to be important in the pathogenesis of pulmonary hypertension (see Ch. 19). Specific Rho kinase inhibitors are in development for a wide range of clinical indications—an area to watch.

The main postulated roles of GPCRs in controlling enzymes and ion channels are summarised in Figure 3.13.

Desensitisation

▼ As described in Chapter 2, desensitisation is a feature of all GPCRs, and the mechanisms underlying it have been extensively studied. Two main processes are involved (see Koenig & Edwardson, 1997; Krupnick & Benovic, 1998; Ferguson, 2001):

---

[11]Alternative abbreviations for these mediators are PtdIns (PI), PtdIns (4,5)-P$_2$ (PIP$_2$), Ins (1,4,5)-P$_3$ (IP3), and Ins (1, 2, 4, 5)-P4 (IP$_4$).

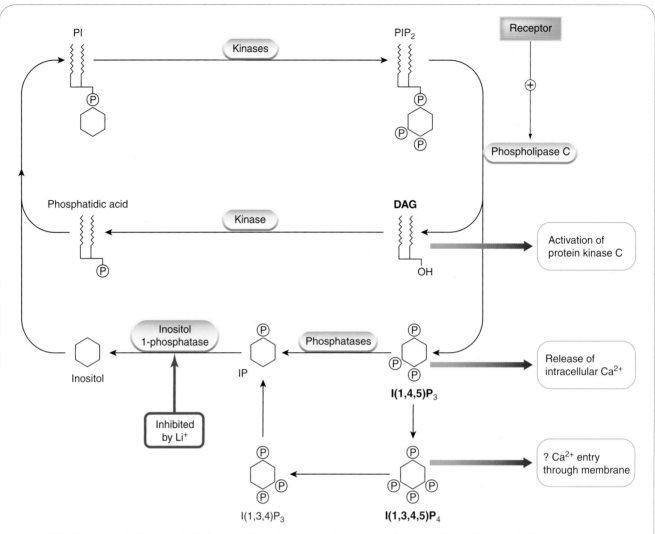

Fig. 3.12   The phosphatidylinositol (PI) cycle. Receptor-mediated activation of phospholipase C results in the cleavage of phosphatidylinositol bisphosphate (PIP$_2$), forming diacylglycerol (DAG) (which activates protein kinase C) and inositol trisphosphate (IP$_3$) (which releases intracellular Ca^{2+}). The role of inositol tetraphosphate (IP$_4$), which is formed from IP$_3$ and other inositol phosphates, is unclear, but it may facilitate Ca^{2+} entry through the plasma membrane. IP$_3$ is inactivated by dephosphorylation to inositol. DAG is converted to phosphatidic acid, and these two products are used to regenerate PI and PIP$_2$.

- receptor phosphorylation
- receptor internalisation (endocytosis).

The sequence of GPCRs includes certain residues (serine and threonine), mainly in the C-terminal cytoplasmic tail, which can be phosphorylated by kinases such as protein kinase A (PKA), PKC, and specific membrane-bound GPCR kinases (GRKs).

Phosphorylation by PKA and PKC, which are activated by many GPCRs, generally leads to impaired coupling between the activated receptor and the G-protein, so the agonist effect is reduced. These kinases are not very selective, so receptors other than that for the desensitising agonist will also be affected. This effect, whereby one agonist can desensitise other receptors, is known as *heterologous desensitisation*, and is generally weak and short-lasting (see Fig. 3.14).

Phosphorylation by GRKs (see Krupnick & Benovic, 1998; Fig. 3.14) is receptor-specific to a greater or lesser degree, and affects mainly receptors in their activated (i.e. agonist-bound) state, resulting in *homologous desensitisation*. The residues that IGRKs phosphorylate are different from those targeted by other kinases, and the phosphorylated receptor serves as a binding site for *arrestins*, intracellular proteins that block the interaction with G-proteins and also target the receptor for endocytosis, producing a more profound and long-lasting desensitisation. The first GRK to be identified was the β-adrenoceptor kinase, BARK, but several others have since been discovered, and this type of desensitisation seems to occur with most GPCRs.

SOME RECENT DEVELOPMENTS

▼ Our knowledge of GPCR biology is expanding rapidly. Here we describe some recent developments that may have important implications for pharmacology in the future (see review by Pierce et al., 2002). Those wishing to stick to the basic story of GPCR function can safely skip this section.

GPCR dimerisation

▼ The conventional view that GPCRs exist and function as monomeric proteins (in contrast to ion channels, which generally form multimeric complexes; see p. 50) was first overturned by work on the GABA$_B$ receptor. Two subtypes of this GPCR exist, encoded by different genes, and the functional receptor consists of a heterodimer of the two. It now seems

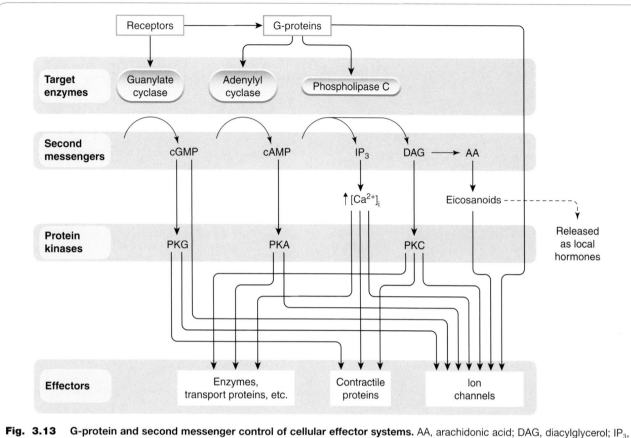

Fig. 3.13 **G-protein and second messenger control of cellular effector systems.** AA, arachidonic acid; DAG, diacylglycerol; IP$_3$, inositol trisphosphate.

likely that most, if not all, GPCRs exist as oligomers (Angers et al., 2002). Within the opioid receptor family (see Ch. 41), stable and functional dimers of κ and δ receptors have been found whose pharmacological properties differ from those of either parent. More diverse GPCR combinations have also been found, such as that between dopamine (D$_2$) and somatostatin receptors, on which both ligands act with increased potency. Roaming even further afield in search of functional assignations, the dopamine receptor D$_5$ can couple directly with a ligand-gated ion channel, the GABA$_A$ receptor, inhibiting the function of the latter without the intervention of any G-protein (Liu et al., 2000). These interactions have so far been studied mainly in engineered cell lines, and their importance in native cells is uncertain. There is evidence, however (AbdAlla et al., 2001), that functional dimeric complexes between angiotensin (AT$_1$) and bradykinin (B$_2$) receptors occur in human platelets and show greater sensitivity to angiotensin than 'pure' AT$_1$ receptors. In pregnant women suffering from hypertension (pre-eclamptic toxaemia), the number of these dimers increases due to increased expression of B$_2$ receptors, resulting—paradoxically— in increased sensitivity to the vasoconstrictor action of angiotensin. This is the first instance of the role of dimerisation in human disease.

It is too early to say what impact this newly discovered versatility of GPCRs in linking up with other receptors to form functional combinations will have on conventional pharmacology and therapeutics, but it could be considerable.

Constitutively active receptors

▼ G-protein–coupled receptors may also be constitutively (i.e. spontaneously) active in the absence of any agonist (see Ch. 2, review by Costa & Cotecchia, 2005). This was first shown for the β-adrenoceptor (see Ch. 11), where mutations in the third intracellular loop, or simply overexpression of the receptor, result in constitutive receptor activation. There are now many examples of native GPCRs that show constitutive activity when expressed in vitro (see Teitler et al., 2002). The histamine H$_3$ receptor also shows constitutive activity in vivo, and this may prove to be a quite general phenomenon. It means that inverse agonists, which suppress this basal activity, may exert effects distinct from those of neutral antagonists, which block agonist effects without affecting basal activity.

Agonist specificity

▼ It was thought that the linkage of a particular GPCR to a particular signal transduction pathway depends mainly on the structure of the receptor, particularly in the region of the third intracellular loop, which confers specificity for a particular G-protein, from which the rest of the signal transduction pathway follows. This would imply, in line with the two-state model discussed in Chapter 2, that all agonists acting on a particular receptor stabilise the same activated (R*) state and should activate the same signal transduction pathway, and produce the same type of cellular response. It is now clear that this is an oversimplification. In many cases, for example with agonists acting on opiate receptors, or with inverse agonists on β-adrenoceptors, the cellular effects are qualitatively different with different ligands, implying the existence of more than one—probably many—R* states (sometimes referred to as *agonist trafficking* or *protean agonism*, see Kenakin, 2002). How general this will prove to be is not yet clear, but it may have profound implications— indeed heretical to many pharmacologists, who are accustomed to think of agonists in terms of their affinity and efficacy, and nothing else. If substantiated, it will add a new dimension to the way in which we think about drug efficacy and specificity.

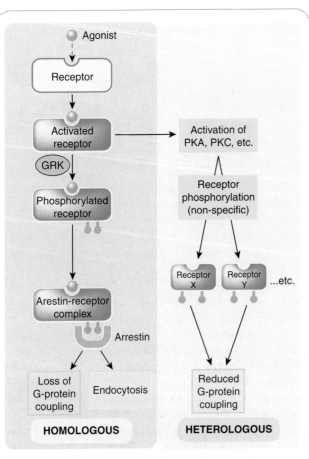

Fig. 3.14 Desensitisation of G-protein–coupled receptors (GPCRs). Homologous (agonist-specific) desensitisation involves phosphorylation of the activated receptor by a specific kinase (GPCR kinase, GRK). The phosphorylated receptor (P-R) then binds to *arrestin*, causing it to lose its ability to associate with a G-protein, and to undergo endocytosis, which removes the receptor from the membrane. Heterologous (cross-)desensitisation occurs as a result of phosphorylation of one type of receptor as a result of activation of kinases by another. PKA and PKC, protein kinase A and C, respectively.

RAMPs and RGS proteins

▼ Receptor activity–modifying proteins (RAMPs) are a family of membrane proteins that associate with GPCRs and alter their functional characteristics. They were discovered in 1998 when it was found that the functionally active receptor for the neuropeptide *calcitonin gene–related peptide* (CGRP) (see Ch. 13) consisted of a complex of a GPCR—called calcitonin receptor–like receptor (CRLR)—that by itself lacked activity, with another membrane protein (RAMP1). More surprisingly, CRLR when coupled with another RAMP (RAMP2) showed a quite different pharmacology, being activated by an unrelated peptide, adrenomedullin. In other words, the agonist specificity is conferred by the associated RAMP as well as by the GPCR itself. Whether this type of modulation occurs with other GPCR families is not yet known.

Regulators of G-protein signalling (RGS) proteins (see review by Hollinger & Hepler, 2002) are a large and diverse family of cellular proteins that possess a conserved sequence that binds specifically to Gα subunits. They increase greatly the GTPase activity of the active GTP–Gα complex, thus hastening the hydrolysis of GTP and inactivating the complex. They thus exert an inhibitory effect on G-protein signalling, a

mechanism that is thought to have a regulatory function in many situations. RAMPs and RGS proteins are two examples (see Pierce et al., 2002) where protein–protein interactions influence the pharmacological behaviour of the receptors in different ways.

G-protein–independent signalling

▼ In using the term G-protein–coupled receptor to describe the class of receptors characterised by their heptahelical structure, we are following conventional textbook dogma but neglecting the fact that G-proteins are not the only link between GPCRs and the various effector systems that they regulate. The example of direct linkage between GPCRs and ion channels was mentioned above. There are also many examples where the various 'adapter proteins' that link receptors of the tyrosine kinase type to their effectors (see below) can also interact with GPCRs (see Brzostowski & Kimmel, 2001), allowing the same effector systems to be regulated by receptors of either type. In this context, the specific receptor kinases that are involved in desensitisation (see above) may also contribute to signal transduction, because phosphorylation of the C-terminal region of the GPCR produces a recognition site for molecules of the signal transduction pathway, analogous to the functioning of the kinase-linked receptors (see below; review by Bockaert & Pin, 1999).

In summary, the simple dogma that underpins much of our current understanding of GPCRs, namely,

one GPCR gene—one GPCR protein—
one functional GPCR—one G-protein—one response

is beginning to show signs of wear. In particular:

- one gene, through alternative splicing, RNA editing, etc., can give rise to more than one receptor protein
- one GPCR protein can associate with others, or with other proteins such as RAMPs, to produce more than one type of functional receptor
- different agonists may affect the receptor in different ways and elicit qualitatively different responses
- the signal transduction pathway does not invariably require G-proteins, and shows cross-talk with tyrosine kinase–linked receptors (see below).

G-protein–coupled receptors are evidently versatile and adventurous molecules around which much modern pharmacology revolves, and nobody imagines that we have reached the end of the story.

TYPE 3: KINASE-LINKED AND RELATED RECEPTORS

These membrane receptors are quite different in structure and function from either the ligand-gated channels or the GPCRs. They mediate the actions of a wide variety of protein mediators, including growth factors and cytokines (see Ch. 16), and hormones such as insulin (see Ch. 26) and leptin (Ch. 27), whose effects are exerted mainly at the level of gene transcription. Most of these receptors are large proteins consisting of a single chain of up to 1000 residues, with a single membrane-spanning helical region, associated with a large extracellular ligand-binding domain, and an intracellular domain of variable size and function. The basic structure is shown in Fig. 3.3C, but many variants exist (see below). Over 100 such receptors have been cloned, and many structural variations exist. For more detail, see reviews by Barbacid (1996),

Two key pathways are controlled by receptors via G-proteins. Both can be activated or inhibited by pharmacological ligands, depending on the nature of the receptor and G-protein.

- Adenylyl cyclase/cAMP:
  - adenylyl cyclase catalyses formation of the intracellular messenger cAMP
  - cAMP activates various protein kinases that control cell function in many different ways by causing phosphorylation of various enzymes, carriers and other proteins.
- Phospholipase C/inositol trisphosphate (IP$_3$)/diacylgcerol (DAG):
  - catalyses the formation of two intracellular messengers, IP$_3$ and DAG, from membrane phospholipid
  - IP$_3$ acts to increase free cytosolic Ca^{2+} by releasing Ca^{2+} from intracellular compartments
  - increased free Ca^{2+} initiates many events, including contraction, secretion, enzyme activation and membrane hyperpolarisation
  - DAG activates protein kinase C, which controls many cellular functions by phosphorylating a variety of proteins.

Receptor-linked G-proteins also control:

- phospholipase A$_2$ (and thus the formation of arachidonic acid and eicosanoids)
- ion channels (e.g. potassium and calcium channels, thus affecting membrane excitability, transmitter release, contractility, etc.).

activate, a cytosolic tyrosine kinase, such as Jak (the Janus kinase) or other kinases. Ligands for these receptors include cytokines such as interferons and colony-stimulating factors involved in immunological responses.

- *Guanylyl cyclase–linked receptors.* These are similar in structure to RTKs, but the enzymic moiety is guanylyl cyclase and they exert their effects by stimulating cGMP formation. The main example is the receptor for ANF (see Ch. 18).

PROTEIN PHOSPHORYLATION AND KINASE CASCADE MECHANISMS

One of the major principles to emerge from recent studies (see Cohen, 2002) is that *protein phosphorylation* is a key mechanism for controlling the function of proteins (e.g. enzymes, ion channels, receptors, transport proteins) involved in regulating cellular processes. Phosphorylation and dephosphorylation are accomplished by *kinases* and *phosphatases*, respectively—enzymes of which several hundred subtypes are represented in the human genome—which are themselves subject to regulation dependent on their phosphorylation status. Much effort is currently being invested in mapping the complex interactions between signalling molecules that are involved in drug effects and pathophysiological processes such as oncogenesis, neurodegeneration, inflammation and much else. Here we can present only a few pharmacologically relevant aspects of what has become an enormous subject.

In many cases, ligand binding to the receptor leads to *dimerisation*. The association of the two intracellular kinase domains allows a mutual autophosphorylation of intracellular tyrosine residues to occur. The phosphorylated tyrosine residues then serve as high-affinity docking sites for other intracellular proteins that form the next stage in the signal transduction cascade. One important group of such 'adapter' proteins is known as the *SH2 domain proteins* (standing for Src homology, because it was first identified in the Src oncogene product). These possess a highly conserved sequence of about 100 amino acids, forming a recognition site for the phosphotyrosine residues of the receptor. Individual SH2 domain proteins, of which many are now known, bind selectively to particular receptors, so the pattern of events triggered by particular growth factors is highly specific. The mechanism is summarised in Figure 3.15.

What happens when the SH2 domain protein binds to the phosphorylated receptor varies greatly according to the receptor that is involved; many SH2 domain proteins are enzymes, such as protein kinases or phospholipases. Some growth factors activate a specific subtype of phospholipase C (PLCγ), thereby causing phospholipid breakdown, IP$_3$ formation and Ca^{2+} release (see above). Other SH2-containing proteins couple phosphotyrosine-containing proteins with a variety of other functional proteins, including many that are involved in the control of cell division and differentiation. The end result is to activate or inhibit, by phosphorylation, a variety of transcription factors that migrate to the nucleus and suppress or induce the expression of particular genes. For more detail, see Pawson (2002). *Nuclear factor kappa B (NFκB)* is a transcription factor that plays a key role in inflammatory responses (see Ch. 13; Karin et al., 2004). It is normally present in the cytosol complexed with an inhibitor (IκB).

Ihle (1995), and Schenk & Snaar-Jakelska (1999). They play a major role in controlling cell division, growth, differentiation, inflammation, tissue repair, apoptosis and immune responses, discussed further in Chapters 5 and 13.

The main types are as follow.

- *Receptor tyrosine kinases (RTKs).* These receptors have the basic structure shown in Fig. 3.15A, incorporating a tyrosine kinase moiety in the intracellular region. They include receptors for many growth factors, such as epidermal growth factor and nerve growth factor, and also the group of Toll-like receptors that recognise bacterial lipopolysaccharides and play an important role in the body's reaction to infection (see Ch. 13 and review by Cook et al., 2004). The insulin receptor (see Ch. 26) also belongs to the RTK class, although it has a more complex dimeric structure.
- *Serine/threonine kinases.* This smaller class is similar in structure to RTKs but phosphorylate serine and/or threonine residues rather than tyrosine. The main example is the receptor for transforming growth factor (TGF).
- *Cytokine receptors.* These receptors (Fig. 3.15B) lack intrinsic enzyme activity. When occupied, they associate with, and

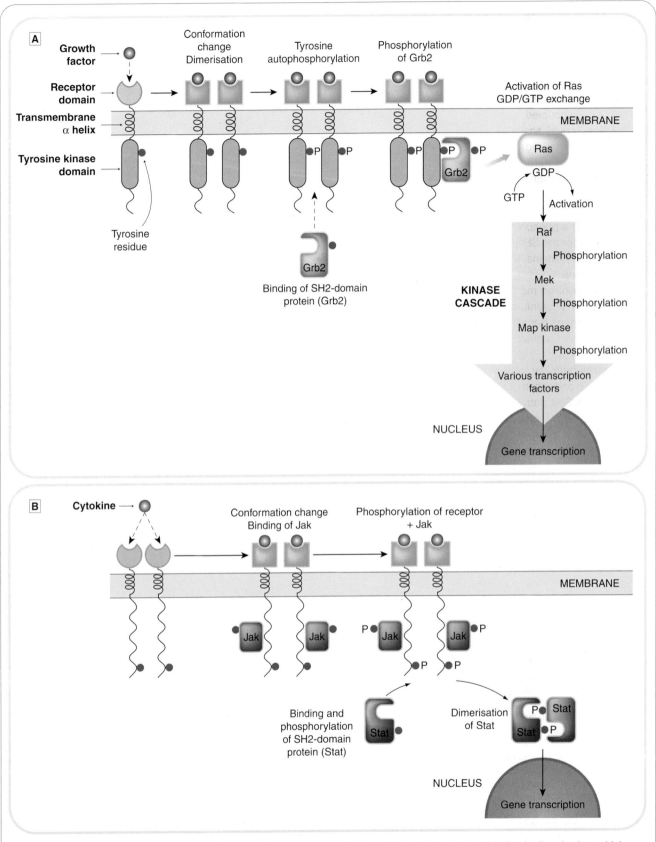

Fig. 3.15 Transduction mechanisms of kinase-linked receptors. The first step following agonist binding is dimerisation, which leads to autophosphorylation of the intracellular domain of each receptor. SH2 domain proteins then bind to the phosphorylated receptor and are themselves phosphorylated. Two well-characterised pathways are shown: **A** The growth factor (Ras/Raf/mitogen-activated protein [MAP] kinase) pathway (see also Ch. 5); **B** the cytokine (Jak/Stat) pathway (see also Ch. 13). Several other pathways exist, and these phosphorylation cascades interact with components of G-protein systems.

Kinase-linked receptors

- Receptors for various growth factors incorporate tyrosine kinase in their intracellular domain.
- Cytokine receptors have an intracellular domain that binds and activates cytosolic kinases when the receptor is occupied.
- The receptors all share a common architecture, with a large extracellular ligand-binding domain connected via a single membrane-spanning helix to the intracellular domain.
- Signal transduction generally involves dimerisation of receptors, followed by autophosphorylation of tyrosine residues. The phosphotyrosine residues act as acceptors for the SH2 domains of a variety of intracellular proteins, thereby allowing control of many cell functions.
- They are involved mainly in events controlling cell growth and differentiation, and act indirectly by regulating gene transcription.
- Two important pathways are:
  - the Ras/Raf/mitogen-activated protein (MAP) kinase pathway, which is important in cell division, growth and differentiation
  - the Jak/Stat pathway activated by many cytokines, which controls the synthesis and release of many inflammatory mediators.
- A few hormone receptors (e.g. atrial natriuretic factor) have a similar architecture and are linked to guanylate cyclase.

Phosphorylation of IκB occurs when a specific kinase (IKK) is activated in response to various inflammatory cytokines and GPCR agonists. This results in dissociation of IκB from NFκB and migration of NFκB to the nucleus, where it switches on a wide variety of proinflammatory genes.

▼ Two well-defined signal transduction pathways are summarised in Figure 3.15. The Ras/Raf pathway (Fig. 3.15A) mediates the effect of many growth factors and mitogens. Ras, which is a proto-oncogene product, functions like a G-protein, and conveys the signal (by GDP/GTP exchange) from the SH2 domain protein, Grb, which is phosphorylated by the RTK. Activation of Ras in turn activates Raf, which is the first of a sequence of three serine/threonine kinases, each of which phosphorylates, and activates, the next in line. The last of these, mitogen-activated protein (MAP) kinase, phosphorylates one or more transcription factors that initiate gene expression, resulting in a variety of cellular responses, including cell division. This three-tiered *MAP kinase cascade* forms part of many intracellular signalling pathways (see Garrington & Johnson, 1999) involved in a wide variety of disease processes, including malignancy, inflammation, neurodegeneration, atherosclerosis and much else. The kinases form a large family, with different subtypes serving specific roles. They are thought to represent an important target for future therapeutic drugs. Many cancers are associated with mutations in the genes coding for proteins involved in this cascade, leading to activation of the cascade in the absence of the growth factor signal (see Chs. 5 and 51). For more details, see reviews by Marshall (1996), Schenk & Snaar-Jakelska (1999), and Chang & Karin (2001).

A second pathway, the Jak/Stat pathway (Fig. 3.15B) is involved in responses to many cytokines. Dimerisation of these receptors occurs when the cytokine binds, and this attracts a cytosolic tyrosine kinase unit (Jak) to associate with, and phosphorylate, the receptor dimer. Jaks belong to a family of proteins, different members having specificity for different cytokine receptors. Among the targets for phosphorylation by Jak are a family of transcription factors (Stats). These are SH2 domain proteins that bind to the phosphotyrosine groups on the receptor–Jak complex, and are themselves phosphorylated. Thus activated, Stat migrates to the nucleus and activates gene expression (see Ihle, 1995).

Recent work on signal transduction pathways has produced a bewildering profusion of molecular detail, often couched in a jargon that is apt to deter the faint-hearted. Perseverance will be rewarded, however, for there is no doubt that important new drugs, particularly in the areas of inflammation, immunology and cancer, will come from the targeting of these proteins (see Cohen, 2002). A recent breakthrough in the treatment of chronic myeloid leukaemia was achieved with the introduction of the first specific kinase inhibitor, **imatinib**, a drug that inhibits a specific tyrosine kinase involved in the pathogenesis of the disease (see Ch. 51).

The membrane-bound form of guanylyl cyclase, the enzyme responsible for generating the second messenger cGMP in response to the binding of peptides such as atrial natriuretic peptide (see Chs 16 and 18), resembles the tyrosine kinase family and is activated in a similar way by dimerisation when the agonist is bound (see Lucas et al., 2000).

Figure 3.16 illustrates the central role of protein kinases in signal transduction pathways in a highly simplified and schematic way. Many, if not all, of the proteins involved, including the receptors and the kinases themselves, are substrates for kinases, so there are many mechanisms for feedback and cross-talk between the various signalling pathways. Given that there are over 500 protein kinases, and similarly large numbers of receptors and other signalling molecules, the network of interactions can look bewilderingly complex. Dissecting out the details has become a major theme in cell biology. For pharmacologists, the idea of a simple connection between receptor and response, which guided thinking throughout the 20th century, is undoubtedly crumbling, although it will take some time before the complexities of signalling pathways are assimilated into a new way of thinking about drug action.

TYPE 4: NUCLEAR RECEPTORS

The fourth type of receptors we will consider belong to the *nuclear receptor family*. By the 1980s, it was clear that receptors for steroid hormones such as oestrogen and the glucocorticoids were present in the cytoplasm of cells and translocated into the nucleus after binding with their steroid partner. Other hormones, such as the thyroid hormone T_3 (Ch. 29) and the fat-soluble vitamins D and A (retinoic acid) and their derivatives that regulate growth and development, were found to act in a similar fashion. Genome and protein sequence data revealed a close relationship between these receptors and led to the recognition that they were members of a much larger family of related proteins. As well as the glucocorticoid and retinoic acid receptor whose ligands were well characterised, the nuclear receptor family (as it became known) included a great many *orphan receptors*—receptors with no known well-defined ligands. The first of these to be described, in the 1990s, was *RXR*, a receptor cloned on the basis of its similarity

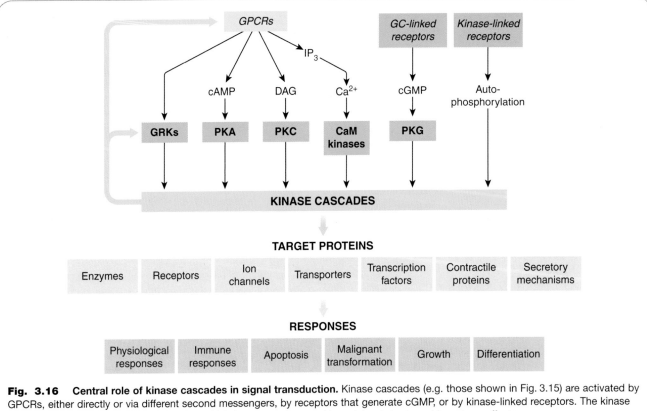

Fig. 3.16 **Central role of kinase cascades in signal transduction.** Kinase cascades (e.g. those shown in Fig. 3.15) are activated by GPCRs, either directly or via different second messengers, by receptors that generate cGMP, or by kinase-linked receptors. The kinase cascades regulate various target proteins, which in turn produce a wide variety of short- and long-term effects.
CaM kinase, Ca^{2+}/calmodulin-dependent kinase; DAG, diacylglycerol; GC, guanylate cyclase; GRK, GPCR kinase; IP_3, inositol trisphosphate; PKA, cAMP-dependent protein kinase; PKC, protein kinase C; PKG, cGMP-dependent protein kinase.

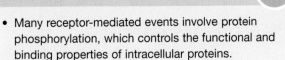

Protein phosphorylation in signal transduction

- Many receptor-mediated events involve protein phosphorylation, which controls the functional and binding properties of intracellular proteins.
- Receptor-linked tyrosine kinases, cyclic nucleotide–activated tyrosine kinases, and intracellular serine/threonine kinases comprise a 'kinase cascade' mechanism that leads to amplification of receptor-mediated events.
- There are many kinases, with differing substrate specificities, allowing specificity in the pathways activated by different hormones.
- Desensitisation of G-protein–coupled receptors occurs as a result of phosphorylation by specific receptor kinases, causing the receptor to become non-functional and to be internalised.
- There is a large family of phosphatases that act to reverse the effects of kinases.

with the vitamin A receptor and that was subsequently found to bind the vitamin A derivative 9-*cis*-retinoic acid. Over the intervening years, binding partners have been identified for many, although by no means all, of these receptors, but some authors continue to use the terminology 'orphan receptor' even when a ligand has been identified or 'adopted' (as in the case of RXR). It is now clear that there are at least 48 members of the nuclear receptor family in the human genome, and while this represents a rather small proportion of all receptors (less than 10% of the total number of GPCRs), the nuclear receptors are important drug targets and play a vital role in endocrine signalling as well as metabolic regulation.

Today, it is convenient to regard the entire nuclear receptor family as *ligand-activated transcription factors* that transduce signals by modifying gene transcription. Unlike the receptors described in the preceding sections of this chapter, the nuclear receptors are not embedded in membranes but are present in the soluble phase of the cell. Some, such as the steroid receptors, become mobile in the presence of their ligand and can translocate from the cytoplasm to the nucleus, while others such as the RXR probably dwell mainly within the nuclear compartment. Many nuclear receptors act as lipid sensors and are intimately involved in the regulation of lipid metabolism within the cell. In this way, they are crucial links between our dietary and metabolic status and the expression of genes that regulate the metabolism and disposition of lipids. Pharmacologically, this entire family of nuclear receptors is very important; they can recognise an extraordinarily diverse group of substances. They regulate many drug metabolic enzymes and transporters and are responsible for the biological effects of approximately 10% of all prescription drugs. There are also many illnesses associated with malfunctioning of the nuclear receptor system, including inflammation, cancer, diabetes, cardiovascular disease, obesity and reproductive disorders (see Murphy & Holder, 2000, and Kersten et al., 2000).

STRUCTURAL CONSIDERATIONS

▼ The nuclear receptors share a broadly similar structural design comprised of four modules (see Fig. 3.17 and Bourguet et al., 2000, for further details). The *N-terminal domain* displays the most heterogeneity. It harbours the *AF1* (activation function 1) site that binds to other cell-specific transcription factors in a ligand-independent way and modifies the binding or activity of the receptor itself. Alternative splicing of genes may yield several receptor isoforms each with slightly different N-terminal regions. The *core domain* of the receptor is highly conserved and consists of the structure responsible for DNA recognition and binding. At the molecular level, this comprises two *zinc fingers*—cysteine- (or cystine/histidine) rich loops in the amino acid chain that are held in a particular conformation by zinc ions. The main function of this portion of the molecule is to recognise and bind to the *hormone response elements* located in genes that are sensitive to regulation by this family of receptors, but it plays a part in regulating receptor dimerisation as well.

A highly flexible *hinge region* in the molecule allows it to dimerise with other nuclear receptors and also to exhibit DNA binding in a variety of configurations. Finally, the *C-terminal domain* contains the ligand-binding module and is specific to each class of receptor. A highly conserved *AF2* region is important in ligand-dependent activation. Also located near the C-terminal are motifs that contain nuclear localisation signals and others

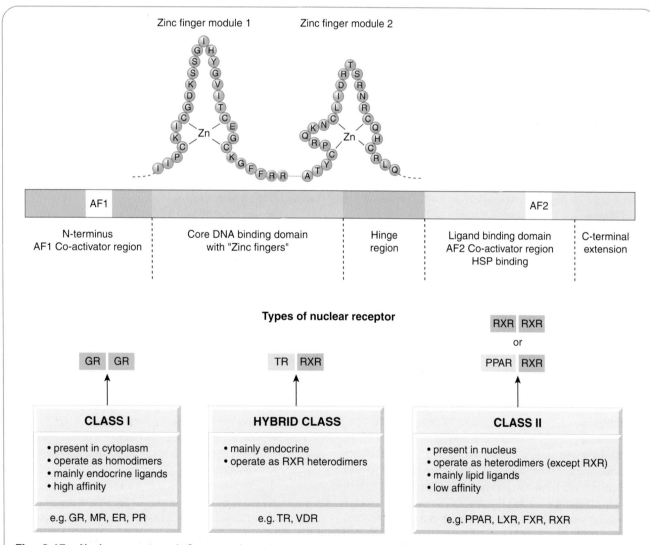

Fig. 3.17 Nuclear receptors. A. Structure of a nuclear receptor, showing the different domains. The partial structure of the 'zinc fingers' is shown above using the single-letter amino acid code. Residues in yellow actually contact DNA. B. The two main classes of nuclear receptors.
ER, oestrogen receptor; FXR, farnesoid receptor; GR, glucocorticoid receptor; LXR, liver oxysterol receptor; MR, mineralocorticoid receptor; PPAR, peroxisome proliferator receptor; PR, prolactin receptor; RXR, retinoid receptor; TR, thyroid receptor; VDR, vitamin D receptor.

that may, in the case of some receptors, bind *accessory heat shock* and other proteins.

CLASSIFICATION OF NUCLEAR RECEPTORS

The nuclear receptor superfamily consist of two *main* classes—together with a third that shares some of the characteristics of both (see Fig. 3.17 and Novac & Henzel, 2004, for further details). Class I consists largely of receptors for the steroid hormones, including the glucocorticoid and mineralocorticoid receptors (GR and MR, respectively), as well as the oestrogen, progesterone and androgen receptors (ER, PR, and AR, respectively). In the absence of their ligand, these receptors are predominantly located in the cytoplasm, complexed with heat shock and other proteins and possibly reversibly attached to the cytoskeleton or other structures. Following diffusion (or possibly transportation) of their ligand partner into the cell and high-affinity binding, these receptors generally form homodimers and translocate to the nucleus, where they can *transactivate* or *transrepress* genes by binding to 'positive' or 'negative' *hormone response elements* (see Ch. 28). Large numbers of genes can be regulated in this way by a single ligand. For example, it is estimated that the activated GR itself can regulate up to 1% of the genome either directly or indirectly. Class I receptors generally recognise hormones that act in a negative feedback fashion to control biological events (see Ch. 28 for more discussion on this topic).

Class II nuclear receptors function in a slightly different way. Their ligands are generally lipids already present to some extent within the cell. This group includes the *peroxisome proliferator-activated receptor (PPAR)* that recognises fatty acids; the *liver oxysterol (LXR) receptor* that recognises and acts as a cholesterol sensor, the *farnesoid (bile acid) receptor (FXR)*, a *xenobiotic receptor (SXR*; in rodents the PXR) that recognises a great many foreign substances, including therapeutic drugs, and the constitutive *androstane receptor (CAR)*, which not only recognises the steroid androstane but also some drugs such as **phenobarbital** (see Ch. 40). These latter receptors are akin to airport security guards who alert the bomb disposal squad when suspicious luggage is found. They induce drug-metabolising enzymes such as CYP3A (which is responsible for metabolising about 60% of all prescription drugs; see Ch. 8 and Synold et al., 2001), and also bind some prostaglandins and non-steroidal drugs, as well as the antidiabetic **thiazolidinediones** (see Ch. 26) and **fibrates** (see Ch. 20). Unlike the receptors in class I, these receptors almost always operate as heterodimers together with the retinoid receptor (RXR). They tend to mediate positive feedback effects (e.g. occupation of the receptor amplifies rather than inhibits a particular biological event). When class II monomeric receptors bind to RXR, two types of heterodimer may be formed: a *non-permissive heterodimer*, which can be activated only by the RXR ligand itself, and the *permissive heterodimer*, which can be activated either by retinoic acid itself or by its partner's ligand.

A third group of nuclear receptors is really a subgroup of class II in the sense that they form obligate heterodimers with RXR, but rather than sensing lipids, they too play a part in endocrine signalling. The group includes the *thyroid hormone receptor (TR)*, the *vitamin D receptor (VDR)* and the *retinoic acid receptor (RAR)*.

CONTROL OF GENE TRANSCRIPTION

▼ Hormone response elements are the short (four or five base pairs) sequences of DNA to which the nuclear receptors bind to modify gene transcription. They are usually present symmetrically in pairs or *half sites*, although these may be arranged together in different ways (e.g. simple repeats or inverted repeats). Each nuclear receptor exhibits a preference for a particular *consensus sequence* but because of the family homology, there is a close similarity between these sequences.

In the nucleus, the ligand-bound receptor recruits further proteins including *coactivators* or *corepressors* to modify gene expression through its AF1 and AF2 domains. Some of these coactivators are enzymes involved in chromatin remodelling such as *histone acetylase* which, together with other enzymes, regulates the unravelling of the DNA to facilitate access by polymerase enzymes and hence gene transcription. Corepressor complexes are recruited by some receptors and comprise *histone deacetylase* and other factors that cause the chromatin to become tightly packed, preventing further transcriptional activation. Some unliganded class II receptors such as TR and VDR are constitutively bound to these repressor complexes in the nucleus, thus 'silencing' the gene. The complex dissociates on ligand binding, permitting an activator complex to bind. The case of CAR is particularly interesting; like some types of G-proteins described earlier in this chapter, CAR also forms a constitutively active complex that is terminated when it binds its ligand.

The discussion here must be taken only as a broad guide to the action of this family of nuclear receptors, as many other types of interaction have also been discovered. For example, some members may bring about non-genomic actions by directly interacting with factors in the cytosol, or they may be covalently modified by phosphorylation or by protein–protein interactions with other transcription factors and their function altered as a result (see Falkenstein et al., 2000). In addition, there is good evidence for separate membrane and other types of receptor that can bind some steroid hormones such as oestrogen (see Walters & Nemere, 2004). This intricate network of receptors and their nuclear and cytosolic interactions serves as a subtle regulator of blood lipids as well as transducing the effects of hormones that have arrived from distant tissues. Much remains to be discovered about this interesting and complex family of receptor proteins.

ION CHANNELS AS DRUG TARGETS

We have discussed ligand-gated ion channels as one of the four main types of drug receptor. There are many other types of ion channel that represent important drug targets, even though they are not generally classified as 'receptors' because they are not the immediate targets of fast neurotransmitters.[12]

Here we discuss the structure and function of ion channels at the molecular level; their role as regulators of cell function is described in Chapter 4.

---

[12]In truth, the distinction between ligand-gated channels and other ion channels is an arbitrary one. In grouping ligand-gated channels with other types of receptor in this book, we are respecting the historical tradition established by Langley and others, who first defined receptors in the context of the action of acetylcholine at the neurosmuscular junction. The advance of molecular biology may force us to reconsider this semantic issue in the future, but for now we make no apology for upholding the pharmacological tradition.

Nuclear receptors

- A family of 48 soluble receptors that sense lipid and hormonal signals and modulate gene transcription.
- Two main categories:
  - those that are present in the cytoplasm, form homodimers in the presence of their partner, and migrate to the nucleus. Their ligands are mainly endocrine in nature (e.g. steroid hormones).
  - those that are generally constitutively present in the nucleus and form heterodimers with the retinoid X receptor. Their ligands are usually lipids (e.g. the fatty acids).
  - A third subgroup transduce mainly endocrine signals but function as heterodimers with retinoid X receptor (e.g. the thyroid hormone).
- The liganded receptor complexes initiate changes in gene transcription by binding to hormone response elements in gene promoters and recruiting coactivator or corepressor factors.
- The receptor family is responsible for the pharmacology of approximately 10%, and the pharmacokinetics of some 60%, of all prescription drugs.

Ions are unable to penetrate the lipid bilayer of the cell membrane, and can get across only with the help of membrane-spanning proteins in the form of channels or transporters. The concept of ion channels was developed more than 50 years ago on the basis of electrophysiological studies on the mechanism of membrane excitation (see below). Electrophysiology, particularly the *voltage clamp* technique (see Ch. 4) remains an essential tool for studying the physiological and pharmacological properties of ion channels. Since the mid-1980s, when the first ion channels were cloned by Numa in Japan, a highly productive collaboration between electrophysiologists and molecular biologists has revealed many details about the structure and function of these complex molecules. The use of tight-seal ('patch clamp') recording, which allows the behaviour of individual channels to be studied in real time, has been particularly valuable in distinguishing channels on the basis of their conductance and gating characteristics. Accounts by Hille (2001), Ashcroft (2000), and Catterall (2000) give more information.

Ion channels consist of protein molecules designed to form water-filled pores that span the membrane, and can switch between open and closed states. The rate and direction of ion movement through the pore is governed by the electrochemical gradient for the ion in question, which is a function of its concentration on either side of the membrane, and of the membrane potential. Ion channels are characterised by:

- their *selectivity* for particular ion species, determined by the size of the pore and the nature of its lining
- their *gating* properties (i.e. the nature of the stimulus that controls the transition between open and closed states of the channel)
- their molecular architecture.

SELECTIVITY

Channels are generally either cation-selective or anion-selective. Cation-selective channels may be selective for Na^+, Ca^{2+} or K^+, or non-selective and permeable to all three. Anion channels are mainly permeable to Cl^-, although other types also occur. The effect of modulation of ion channels on cell function is discussed in Chapter 4.

GATING

Voltage-gated channels

These channels open when the cell membrane is depolarised. They form a very important group because they underlie the mechanism of membrane excitability (see Ch. 4). The most important channels in this group are selective sodium, potassium or calcium channels.

Commonly, the channel opening (*activation*) induced by membrane depolarisation is short-lasting, even if the depolarisation is maintained. This is because, with some channels, the initial activation of the channels is followed by a slower process of *inactivation*.

The role of voltage-gated channels in the generation of action potentials and in controlling other cell functions is described in Chapter 4.

Ligand-gated channels

These (see above) are activated by binding of a chemical ligand to a site on the channel molecule. Fast neurotransmitters, such as glutamate, acetylcholine, GABA and ATP (see Chs 10, 12, and 33) act in this way, binding to sites on the outside of the membrane. The vanilloid receptor TRPV1 mediates the pain-producing effect of **capsaicin** on sensory nerves (see Ch. 41).

Some ligand-gated channels in the plasma membrane respond to intracellular rather than extracellular signals, the most important being the following.

- Calcium-activated potassium channels, which occur in most cells, and open, thus hyperpolarising the cell, when $[Ca^{2+}]_i$ increases.
- ATP-sensitive potassium channels, which open when the intracellular ATP concentration falls because the cell is short of nutrients. These channels, which are quite distinct from those mediating the excitatory effects of extracellular ATP, occur in many nerve and muscle cells, and also in insulin-secreting cells (see Ch. 26), where they are part of the mechanism linking insulin secretion to blood glucose concentration.

Other examples of channels that respond to intracellular ligands include arachidonic acid–sensitive potassium channels and DAG-sensitive calcium channels, whose functions are not well understood.

Calcium release channels

These are present on the endoplasmic or sarcoplasmic reticulum rather than the plasma membrane. The main ones, IP_3 and ryanodine receptors (see Ch. 4) are a special class of ligand-gated calcium channels that control the release of Ca^{2+} from intracellular stores.

Store-operated calcium channels

When the intracellular Ca^{2+} stores are depleted, channels in the plasma membrane open to allow Ca^{2+} entry. The mechanism by which this linkage occurs is poorly understood (see Barritt, 1999), but store-operated calcium channels (SOCs) are important in the mechanism of action of many GPCRs that elicit Ca^{2+} release. The opening of SOCs allows $[Ca^{2+}]_i$ to remain elevated even when the stores are running low, and also provides a route through which the stores can be replenished (see Ch. 4).

MOLECULAR ARCHITECTURE

▼ Ion channels are large and elaborate molecules. Their characteristic structural motifs have been revealed as knowledge of their sequence and structure has accumulated since the mid-1980s, when the first ligand-gated channel (the nicotinic acetylcholine receptor) and the first voltage-gated sodium channel were cloned. The main structural subtypes are shown in Figure 3.18. All consist of several (often four) domains, which are similar or identical to each other, organised either as an oligomeric array of separate subunits, or as one large protein. Each subunit or domain contains a bundle of two to six membrane-spanning helices. Most ligand-gated channels have the basic structure shown in Figure 3.18A, comprising a pentameric array of non-identical subunits, each consisting of four transmembrane helices, of which one—the M₂ segment—from each subunit lines the pore. The large extracellular N-terminal region contains the ligand-binding region. Several exceptions to this simple design for ligand-gated channels have emerged recently. They include (see Fig. 3.18) the **glutamate NMDA receptor** (Ch. 33), the **purine P₂ₓ receptor** (Ch. 12) and the **vanilloid receptor** (a channel that responds not only to chemicals of the vanilloid class, but also to heat and protons; see Ch. 41). In these, as in many other

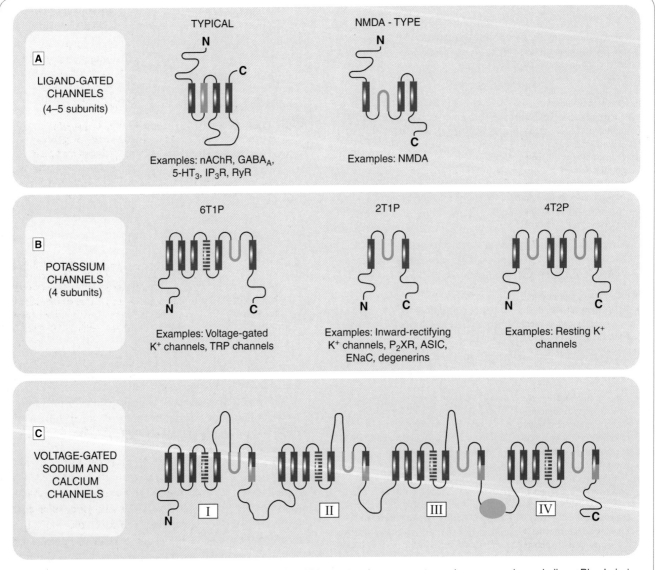

Fig. 3.18 Molecular architecture of ion channels. Red and blue rectangles represent membrane-spanning α helices. Blue hairpins are pore loop (P) domains, present in many channels, blue rectangles being the pore-forming regions of the membrane-spanning α helices. Cross-shaded rectangles represent the voltage-sensing regions of voltage-gated channels. The green symbol represents the inactivating particle of voltage-gated sodium channels. Potassium channel nomenclature is based on the number of transmembrane helices (T) and pore-forming loops (P) in each subunit. Further information on ion channels is given in Chapter 4.
5-HT₃, 5-hydroxytryptamine type 3 receptor; ASIC, acid-sensing ion channel; ENaC, epithelial sodium channel; GABAₐ, GABA type A receptor; IP₃R, inositol trisphosphate receptor; nAChR, nicotinic acetylcholine receptor; P₂ₓR, purine P₂ₓ receptor; RyR, ryanodine receptor.

types of channel, the pore-forming part of the molecule consists of a hairpin loop—the pore (P) loop—between two of the helices.

Voltage-gated channels generally include one transmembrane helix that contains an abundance of basic (i.e. positively charged) amino acids. When the membrane is depolarised, so that the interior of the cell becomes less negative, this region—the voltage sensor—moves slightly towards the outer surface of the membrane, which has the effect of opening the channel. Many voltage-activated channels also show inactivation, which happens when an intracellular appendage of the channel protein moves to plug the channel from the inside. Voltage-gated sodium and calcium channels are remarkable in that the whole structure with four six-helix domains consists of a single huge protein molecule, the domains being linked together by intracellular loops of varying length. Potassium channels comprise the most numerous and heterogeneous class.[13] Voltage-gated potassium channels resemble sodium channels, except that they are made up of four subunits rather than a single long chain. The class of potassium channels known as 'inward rectifier channels' because of their biophysical properties has the two-helix structure shown in Figure 3.18C, whereas others are classed as 'two-pore domain' channels, because each subunit contains two P loops.

The various architectural motifs shown in Figure 3.18 only scrape the surface of the molecular diversity of ion channels. In all cases, the individual subunits come in several molecular varieties, and these can unite in different combinations to form functional channels as hetero-oligomers (as distinct from homo-oligomers built from identical subunits). Furthermore, the channel-forming structures described are usually associated with other membrane proteins, which significantly affect their functional properties. For example, the ATP-gated potassium channel exists in association with the *sulfonylurea receptor (SUR)*, and it is through this linkage that various drugs (including antidiabetic drugs of the sulfonylurea class, see Ch. 26) regulate the channel (see Ashcroft & Gribble, 2000). Good progress is being made in understanding the relation between molecular structure and ion channel function, but we still have only a fragmentary understanding of the physiological role of many of these channels. Many important drugs exert their effects by influencing channel function, either directly or indirectly.

PHARMACOLOGY OF ION CHANNELS

▼ Many drugs and physiological mediators described in this book exert their effects by altering the behaviour of ion channels. Here we outline the general mechanisms as exemplified by the pharmacology of voltage-gated sodium channels (Fig. 3.19). Ion channel pharmacology is likely to be a fertile source of future new drugs (see Clare et al., 2000).

The gating and permeation of both voltage-gated and ligand-gated ion channels is modulated by many factors, including the following.

- *Ligands that bind directly to various sites on the channel protein.* These include many neurotransmitters, and also a variety of drugs and toxins that act in different ways, for example by blocking the channel or by affecting the gating process, thereby either facilitating or inhibiting the opening of the channel.
- *Mediators and drugs that act indirectly, mainly by activation of GPCRs.* The latter produce their effects mainly by affecting the state of phosphorylation of individual amino acids located on the intracellular region of the channel protein. As described above, this modulation involves the production of second messengers that activate protein kinases. The opening of the channel may be facilitated or inhibited, depending on which residues are phosphorylated. Drugs such as opioids (Ch. 41) and β-adrenoceptor agonists (Ch. 11) affect calcium and potassium channel function in this way, producing a wide variety of cellular effects.

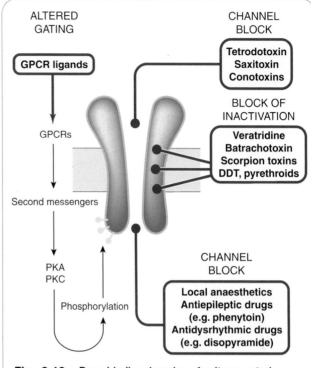

Fig. 3.19 **Drug-binding domains of voltage-gated sodium channels (see Ch. 44).** The multiplicity of different binding sites and effects appears to be typical of many ion channels. DDT, dichlorodiphenyltrichloroethane (dicophane, a well-known insecticide); GPCR, G-protein–coupled receptor; PKA, protein kinase A; PKC, protein kinase C.

- *Intracellular signals, particularly Ca^{2+} and nucleotides such as ATP and GTP (see Ch. 4).* Many ion channels possess binding sites for these intracellular mediators. Increased $[Ca^{2+}]_i$ opens certain types of potassium channels, and inactivates voltage-gated calcium channels. As described in Chapter 4, $[Ca^{2+}]_i$ is itself affected by the function of ion channels and GPCRs. Drugs of the sulfonylurea class (see Ch. 26) act selectively on ATP-gated potassium channels.

Figure 3.19 summarises the main sites and mechanisms by which drugs affect voltage-gated sodium channels, a typical example of this type of drug target.

CONTROL OF RECEPTOR EXPRESSION

Receptor proteins are synthesised by the cells that express them, and the level of expression is itself controlled, via the pathways discussed above, by receptor-mediated events. We can no longer think of the receptors as the fixed elements in cellular control systems, responding to changes in the concentration of ligands, and initiating changes in the components of the signal transduction pathway—they are themselves subject to regulation. Short-term regulation of receptor function generally occurs through desensitisation, as discussed above. Long-term regulation occurs through an increase or decrease of receptor expression. Examples of this type of control (see review by Donaldson et al., 1997) include the proliferation of various postsynaptic receptors after denervation (see Ch. 9), the up-regulation of various G-protein–coupled and cytokine receptors in response to inflammation (see Ch. 13), and

---

[13]The human genome encodes more than 70 distinct potassium channel subtypes–either a nightmare or a golden opportunity for the pharmacologist, depending on one's perspective.

the induction of growth factor receptors by certain tumour viruses (see Ch. 5). Long-term drug treatment invariably induces adaptive responses, which, particularly with drugs that act on the central nervous system, are often the basis for therapeutic efficacy. They may take the form of a very slow onset of the therapeutic effect (e.g. with antidepressant drugs; see Ch. 39), or the development of drug dependence (Ch. 43). Although the details are not yet clear, it is most likely that changes in receptor expression, secondary to the immediate action of the drug, are involved—a kind of 'secondary pharmacology' whose importance is only now becoming clearer. The same principles apply to drug targets other than receptors (ion channels, enzymes, transporters, etc.) where adaptive changes in expression and function follow long-term drug administration, resulting, for example, in resistance to certain anticancer drugs (Ch. 51).

RECEPTORS AND DISEASE

Increasing understanding of receptor function in molecular terms has revealed a number of disease states directly linked to receptor malfunction. The principal mechanisms involved are:

- autoantibodies directed against receptor proteins
- mutations in genes encoding receptors and proteins involved in signal transduction.

An example of the former is *myasthenia gravis* (see Ch. 10), a disease of the neuromuscular junction due to autoantibodies that inactivate nicotinic acetylcholine receptors. Autoantibodies can also mimic the effects of agonists, as in many cases of thyroid hypersecretion, caused by activation of thyrotropin receptors. Activating antibodies have also been discovered in patients with severe hypertension (α-adrenoceptors), cardiomyopathy (β-adrenoceptors), and certain forms of epilepsy and neurodegenerative disorder (glutamate receptors).

Inherited mutations of genes encoding GPCRs account for various disease states (see Spiegel & Weinstein, 2004). Mutated vasopressin and adrenocorticotrophic hormone receptors (see Chs 24 and 28) can result in resistance to these hormones. Receptor mutations can result in activation of effector mechanisms in the absence of agonist. One of these involves the receptor for thyrotropin, producing continuous oversecretion of thyroid hormone; another involves the receptor for luteinising hormone and results in precocious puberty. Adrenoceptor polymorphisms are common in humans, and recent studies suggest that certain mutations of the β_2-adrenoceptor, although they do not directly cause disease, are associated with a reduced efficacy of β-adrenoceptor agonists in treating asthma (Ch. 23) and a poor prognosis in patients with cardiac failure (Ch. 18). Mutations in G-proteins can also cause disease (see Farfel et al., 1999; Spiegel & Weinstein, 2004). For example, mutations of a particular Gα subunit cause one form of hypoparathyroidism, while mutations of a Gβ subunit result in hypertension.

Many cancers are associated with mutations of the genes encoding growth factor receptors, kinases and other proteins involved in signal transduction (see Ch. 5).

REFERENCES AND FURTHER READING

General references

Alexander S P H, Mathie A, Peters J A 2004 Guide to receptors and channels. Br J Pharmacol 141 Supplement 1 (*Comprehensive catalogue of molecular and pharmacological properties of known receptors—also transporters and some enzymes involved in signal transduction*)

Ben-Shlomo I, Hsu S Y, Rauch R et al. 2003 Signalling receptome: a genomic and evolutionary perspective of plasma membrane receptors involved in signal transduction. STKE website: http://www.stke.org

Donaldson L F, Hanley M R, Villablanca A C 1997 Inducible receptors. Trends Pharmacol Sci 18: 171–181 (*Emphasises processes controlling receptor expression*)

IUPHAR receptor database and channel compendium. http://www.iuphar-db.org (*Online catalogue and coding scheme for receptors and channels. Not yet complete, but planned to be updated regularly*)

Laudet V, Adelmant G 1995 Lonesome receptors. Curr Biol 5: 124–127 (*Short review of 'orphan' receptors*)

Walaas S I, Greengard P 1991 Protein phosphorylation and neuronal function. Pharmacol Rev 43: 299–349 (*Excellent general review*)

Receptors
G-protein–coupled receptors

AbdAlla S, Lother H, El Massiery A, Quitterer U 2001 Increased AT$_1$ receptor heterodimers in preeclampsia mediate enhanced angiotensin II responsiveness. Nat Med 7: 1003–1009 (*The first instance of disturbed GPCR heterodimerisation in relation to human disease*)

Angers S, Salahpour A, Bouvier M 2002 Dimerization: an emerging concept for G protein-coupled receptor

ontogeny and function. Annu Rev Pharmacol Toxicol 42: 409–435 (*Review of the unexpected behaviour of GPCRs in linking together as dimers*)

Bockaert J, Pin J P 1999 Molecular tinkering of G protein-coupled receptors: an evolutionary success. EMBO J 18: 1723–1729 (*Short review covering some newer aspects of GPCR function*)

Conigrave A D, Quinn S J, Brown E M 2000 Cooperative multi-modal sensing and therapeutic implications of the extracellular Ca^{2+}-sensing receptor. Trends Pharmacol Sci 21: 401–407 (*Short account of the Ca^{2+}-sensing receptor, an anomalous type of GPCR*)

Costa T, Cotecchia S 2005 Historical review: negative efficacy and the constitutive activity of G-protein – coupled receptors. Trends Pharmacol Sci 26: 618–624 (*A clear and thoughtful review of ideas relating to constitutive receptor activation and inverse agonists*)

Ferguson S S G 2001 Evolving concepts in G protein-coupled receptor endocytosis: the role in receptor desensitization and signaling. Pharmacol Rev 53: 1–24 (*Detailed account of the role of phosphorylation of receptors in fast and slow desensitisation mechanisms*)

Gudermann T, Kalkbrenner F, Schultz G 1996 Diversity and selectivity of receptor–G protein signalling. Annu Rev Pharmacol Toxicol 36: 429–459 (*Discusses how selectivity is achieved between many ligands, receptors and interlinking transduction pathways*)

Hill S J 2006 G-protein-coupled receptors: past, present and future. Br J Pharmacol 147 (Suppl): 27–37 (*Good introductory review*)

Kenakin T 2002 Efficacy at G-protein–coupled receptors. Nat Rev Drug Discov 1: 103–110 (*Mainly theoretical discussion of the implications of agonist trafficking*)

Kilpatrick G, Dautzenberg F M, Martin G R, Eglen R M 1999 7TM receptors: the splicing on the cake. Trends Pharmacol Sci 20: 294–301 (*Review of the importance of mRNA splicing as a source of variation among GPCRs—a salutary reminder that cloning genes is not the last word in defining receptor diversity*)

Koenig J A, Edwardson J M 1997 Endocytosis and recycling of G protein-coupled receptors. Trends Pharmacol Sci 18: 276–287 (*Excellent review of the complex life cycle of a receptor molecule*)

Krupnick J G, Benovic J L 1998 The role of receptor kinases and arrestins in G protein coupled receptor regulation. Annu Rev Pharmacol Toxicol 38: 298–319 (*Review on GPCR phosphorylation, arrestins and desensitisation*)

Liu F, Wan Q, Pristupa Z et al. 2000 Direct protein–protein coupling enables cross-talk between dopamine D$_5$ and γ-aminobutyric acid A receptors. Nature 403: 274–280. (*The first demonstration of direct coupling of a GPCR with an ion channel. Look, no G-protein!*)

Milligan G 1995 Signal sorting by G-protein–linked receptors. Adv Pharmacol 32: 1–29 (*More on the selectivity problem*)

Ossofskaya V S, Bunnett N W 2004 Protease-activated receptors: contribution to physiology and disease. Physiol Rev 84: 579–621 (*Review of current knowledge of pathophysiological role of protease-activated receptors*)

Pierce K L, Premont R T, Lefkowitz R J 2002 Seven-transmembrane receptors. Nat Rev Mol Cell Biol 3: 639–650 (*Useful general review of GPCRs, including desensitisation mechanisms, signal transduction pathways and dimerisation*)

Schwartz T W 1996 Molecular structure of G-protein–coupled receptors. In: Foreman J C, Johanesen T (eds) Textbook of receptor pharmacology. CRC Press, Boca Raton (*Useful account without unnecessary detail*)

Spiegel A M, Weinstein L S 2004 Inherited diseases involving G proteins and G protein-coupled receptors. Annu Rev Med 55: 27–39 (*Short review article*)

Teitler M, Herrick-Davis K, Purohit A 2002 Constitutive activity of G-protein coupled receptors: emphasis on serotonin receptors. Curr Top Med Chem 2: 529–538 (*Review of evidence that spontaneous activity is common among both native and mutated GPCRs*)

Vergnolle N 2004 Modulation of visceral pain and inflammation by protease-activated receptors. Br J Pharmacol 141: 1264–1274 (*Describes properties of PARs, which are likely to be useful therapeutic targets when specific inhibitors are discovered*)

Vergnolle N, Wallace J L, Bunnett N W, Hollenberg M D 2001 Protease-activated receptors in inflammation, neuronal signalling and pain. Trends Pharmacol Sci 22: 146–152 (*Short review article on this recently discovered family of GPCRs*)

Wess J 1998 Molecular basis of receptor/G-protein–coupling selectivity. Pharmacol Ther 80: 231–264 (*Detailed review of molecular biology of GPCRs and G-proteins, emphasising what is known about the thorny question of how selectivity is achieved*)

Kinase-linked receptors

Barbacid M 1996 Neurotrophic factors and their receptors. Curr Biol 7: 148–155 (*Useful review of neural growth factors and their associated tyrosine kinase–linked receptors*)

Cohen P 2002 Protein kinases—the major drug targets of the twenty-first century? Nat Rev Drug Discov 1: 309–315 (*General review on pharmacological aspects of protein kinases*)

Cook D N, Pisetsky D S, Schwartz D A 2004 Toll-like receptors in the pathogenesis of human disease. Nat Immunol 5: 975–979 (*Review emphasising the role of this class of receptor tyrosine kinases in many human disease states*)

Ihle J N 1995 Cytokine receptor signalling. Nature 377: 591–594

Pawson T 2002 Regulation and targets of receptor tyrosine kinases. Eur J Cancer 38: S3–S10 (*Short review of RTK signalling*)

Schenk P W, Snaar-Jakelska B E 1999 Signal perception and transduction: the role of protein kinases. Biochim Biophys Acta 1449: 1–24 (*General review of receptor–protein kinase interactions*)

Nuclear receptors

Bourguet W, Germain P, Gronemeyer H 2000 Nuclear receptor ligand-binding domains: three-dimensional structures, molecular interactions and pharmacological implications. Trends Pharmacol Sci 21: 381–388 (*Review concentrating on distinction between agonist and antagonist effects at the molecular level*)

Chawla A, Repa J J, Evans R M, Mangelsdorf D J 2001 Nuclear receptors and lipid physiology: opening the X-files. Science 294: 1866–1870 (*Accessible review that deals mainly with the role of nuclear receptors in lipid metabolism*)

Falkenstein E, Tillmann H-C, Christ M et al. 2000 Multiple actions of steroid hormones—a focus on rapid, non-genomic effects. Pharmacol Rev 52: 513–553 (*Comprehensive review article describing the non-classical effects of steroids*)

Giguere V 1999 Orphan nuclear receptors: from gene to function. Endocr Rev 20: 689–725 (*Very comprehensive review for the serious reader*)

Kersten S, Desvergne B, Wahli W 2000 Roles of PPARs in health and disease. Nature 405: 421–424 (*General review of an important class of nuclear receptors*)

Murphy G J, Holder J C 2000 PPAR-γ agonists: therapeutic role in diabetes, inflammation and cancer. Trends Pharmacol Sci 21: 469–474 (*Account of the emerging importance of nuclear receptors of the PPAR family as therapeutic targets*)

Novac N, Heinzel T 2004 Nuclear receptors: overview and classification. Curr Drug Targets Inflamm Allergy 3: 335–346 (*Excellent general review*)

Synold TW, Dussault I, Forman BM 2001 The orphan nuclear receptor SXR coordinately regulates drug metabolism and efflux. Nature Med 7: 584–590

Walters MR, Nemere I 2004 Receptors for steroid hormones: membrane-associated and nuclear forms. Cell Mol Life Sci 61: 2309–2321 (*Good discussion about alternative types of steroid hormone receptors*)

Signal transduction

Beavo J A 1995 Cyclic nucleotide phosphodiesterase. Functional implications of multiple isoforms. Physiol Rev 75: 725–748 (*Useful account of the numerous PDE subtypes, selective inhibitors of which have many potential therapeutic applications*)

Bishop A L, Hall R A 2000 Rho–GTPases and their effector proteins. Biochem J 348: 241–255 (*General review article on the Rho/Rho kinase system and the various pathways and functions that it controls*)

Brzostowski J A, Kimmel A R 2001 Signaling at zero G: G-protein–independent functions for 7TM receptors. Trends Biochem Sci 26: 291–297 (*Review of evidence for GPCR signalling that does not involve G-proteins, thus conflicting with the orthodox dogma*)

Chang L, Karin M 2001 Mammalian MAP kinase signalling cascades. Nature 410: 37–40 (*Short and rather dense review article*)

Clapham D, Neer E 1997 G-protein βγ subunits. Annu Rev Pharmacol Toxicol 37: 167–203 (*On the diversity and role in signalling of G-protein βγ subunits—the poor relations of the α subunits*)

Farfel Z, Bourne H R, Iiri T 1999 The expanding spectrum of G protein diseases. New Engl J Med 340: 1012–1020 (*Review of recent work revealing how G-protein mutations lead to disease—useful for reference*)

Garrington T P, Johnson G L 1999 Organization and regulation of mitogen-activated protein kinase signaling pathways. Curr Opin Cell Biol 11: 211–218

Hollinger S, Hepler J R 2002 Cellular regulation of RGS proteins: modulators and integrators of G protein signaling. Physiol Rev 54: 527–559 (*Describes the nature of this family of proteins that bind to α subunits and modulate G-protein signalling in many situations*)

Irvine R F 2001 Does IP_4 run a protection racket? Curr Biol 11: R172–R174 (*Discussion of possible second messenger roles of IP_4*)

Karin M, Yamamoto Y, Wang M 2004 The IKK–NFκB system: a treasure trove for drug development. Nat Rev Drug Discov 3: 17–26 (*Describes the transcription factor NFκB, which plays a key role in inflammation, and its control by kinase cascades*)

Lucas K A, Pitari J M, Kazerounian S et al. 2000 Pharmacol Rev 52: 376–413 (*Detailed review of guanylyl cyclase and its role in signalling. Covers both membrane receptors linked to guanylyl cyclase, and soluble guanylyl cyclases that respond to nitric oxide, etc.*)

Marshall C J 1996 Ras effectors. Curr Opin Cell Biol 8: 197–204 (*Account of one of the most important signal transduction pathways*)

Milligan G, Kostenis E 2006 Heterotrimeric G-proteins: a short history. Br J Pharmacol 147 (Suppl): 46–55

Nahorski S R 2006 Pharmacology of intracellular signalling pathways. Br J Pharmacol 147 (Suppl): 38–45 (*Useful short review*)

Nishizuka Y 1988 The molecular heterogeneity of protein kinase C and its implications for cellular regulation. Nature 334: 661–665 (*As above*)

Offermanns S 2003 G-proteins as transducers in transmembrane signalling. Prog Biophys Mol Biol 83: 101–130 (*Detailed review of G-protein subtypes and their function in signal transduction*)

Simonds W F 1999 G-protein regulation of adenylate cyclase. Trends Pharmacol Sci 20: 66–72. (*Review of mechanisms by which G-proteins affect adenylate cyclase at the level of molecular structure*)

Ion channels

Ashcroft F M 2000 Ion channels and disease. Academic Press, London (*A useful textbook covering all aspects of ion channel physiology and its relevance to disease, with a lot of pharmacological information for good measure*)

Ashcroft F M, Gribble F M 2000 New windows on the mechanism of action of K_{ATP} channel openers. Trends Pharmacol Sci 21: 439–445

Barritt G J 1999 Receptor-activated Ca^{2+} inflow in animal cells: a variety of pathways tailored to meet different intracellular Ca^{2+} signalling requirements. Biochem J 337: 153–169 (*Useful overview of mechanisms involved in Ca^{2+} signalling*)

Catterall W A 2000 From ionic currents to molecular mechanisms: the structure and function of voltage-gated sodium channels. Neuron 26: 13–25 (*General review of sodium channel structure, function and pharmacology*)

Clapham D E 1995 Calcium signaling. Cell 80: 259–268 (*Excellent general review*)

Clare J J, Tate S N, Nobbs M, Romanos M A 2000 Voltage-gated sodium channels as therapeutic targets. Drug Discov Today 5: 506–520 (*Useful review dealing at a basic level with the therapeutic potential of drugs affecting sodium channels*)

Galzi J-L, Changeux J-P 1994 Neurotransmitter-gated ion channels as unconventional allosteric proteins. Curr Opin Struct Biol 4: 554–565 (*Review focusing on molecular mechanisms of channel activation*)

Hille B 2001 Ionic channels of excitable membranes. Sinauer Associates, Sunderland (*A clear and detailed account of the basic principles of ion channels, with emphasis on their biophysical properties*)

Jin R, Banke T, Mayer M et al. 2003 Structural basis for partial agonist action at ionotropic glutamate receptors. Nat Neurosci 6: 803–819 (*Shows that partial agonists for glutamate receptors induce different conductance states of the channel*)

Karlin A 1993 Structure of nicotinic acetylcholine receptors. Curr Opin Neurobiol 3: 299–309 (*Excellent general review*)

Miyazawa A, Fujiyoshi Y, Unwin N 2003 Structure and gating mechanism of the acetylcholine receptor pore. Nature 423: 949–955. (*Description of how the channel is opened by agonists, based on high-resolution crystallography*)

Unwin N 1993 Nicotinic acetylcholine receptor at 9A resolution. J Mol Biol 229: 1101–1124 (*The first structural study of a channel-linked receptor*)

Unwin N 1995 Acetylcholine receptor channel imaged in the open state. Nature 373: 37–43 (*Refinement of 1993 paper, showing for the first time how channel opening occurs—a technical tour de force*)

Wickham K D, Clapham, D E 1995 G-protein regulation of ion channels. Curr Opin Neurobiol 5: 278–285 (*Discusses direct and indirect regulation of ion channels by G-protein–coupled receptors*)

Transporters

Nelson N 1998 The family of Na^+/Cl^- neurotransmitter transporters. J Neurochem 71: 1785–1803 (*Review article describing the molecular characteristics of the different families of neurotransporters*)

4

How drugs act: cellular aspects—excitation, contraction and secretion

- the storage and release of Ca^{2+} by intracellular organelles
- Ca^{2+}-dependent regulation of enzymes, contractile proteins and vesicle proteins.

More detailed coverage of the topics presented in this chapter can be found in Nicholls et al. (2000), Nestler et al. (2001) and Levitan & Kaczmarek (2002).

Because $[Ca^{2+}]_i$ plays such a key role in cell function, a wide variety of drug effects results from interference with one or more of these mechanisms. If love makes the human world go round, $[Ca^{2+}]_i$ does the same for cells. Knowledge of the molecular and cellular details has expanded remarkably in the past decade, and here we focus on the aspects that help to explain drug effects.

OVERVIEW

The link between a drug interacting with a molecular target and its effect at the pathophysiological level, such as a change in blood glucose concentration or the shrinkage of a tumour, involves events at the cellular level. Whatever their specialised physiological function, cells generally share much the same repertoire of signalling mechanisms. In the next two chapters, we describe the parts of this repertoire that are of particular significance in understanding drug action at the cellular level. In this chapter, we describe mechanisms that operate mainly over a short timescale (milliseconds to hours), particularly *excitation, contraction* and *secretion*, which account for many physiological responses; Chapter 5 deals with the slower processes (generally days to months), including *cell division, growth, differentiation* and *cell death*, that determine the body's structure and constitution.

The short-term regulation of cell function depends mainly on the following components and mechanisms, which regulate, or are regulated by, the free concentration of Ca^{2+} in the cytosol, $[Ca^{2+}]_i$:

- ion channels and transporters in the plasma membrane

REGULATION OF INTRACELLULAR CALCIUM LEVELS

Ever since the famous accident by Sidney Ringer's technician, which showed that using tap water rather than distilled water to make up the bathing solution for isolated frog hearts would allow them to carry on contracting, the role of Ca^{2+} as the most important regulator of cell function has never been in question. Many drugs and physiological mechanisms operate, directly or indirectly, by influencing $[Ca^{2+}]_i$. Here we consider the main ways in which it is regulated, and later we describe some of the ways in which $[Ca^{2+}]_i$ controls cell function. Details of the molecular components and drug targets are presented in Chapter 3, and descriptions of drug effects on integrated physiological function are given in later chapters.

The study of Ca^{2+} regulation took a big step forward in the 1970s with the development of fluorescent techniques based on the Ca^{2+}-sensitive photoprotein *aequorin*, and dyes such as Fura-2, which, for the first time, allowed free $[Ca^{2+}]_i$ to be continuously monitored in living cells with a high level of temporal and spatial resolution.

Most of the Ca^{2+} in a resting cell is sequestered in organelles, particularly the endoplasmic or sarcoplasmic reticulum (ER or SR) and the mitochondria, and the free $[Ca^{2+}]_i$ is kept to a low level, about 10^{-7} M. The Ca^{2+} concentration in tissue fluid $[Ca^{2+}]_o$, is about 2.4 mM, so there is a large concentration gradient favouring Ca^{2+} entry. $[Ca^{2+}]_i$ is kept low (a) by the operation of active transport mechanisms that eject cytosolic Ca^{2+} through the plasma membrane and pump it into the ER, and (b) by the normally low Ca^{2+} permeability of the plasma and ER membranes. Regulation of $[Ca^{2+}]_i$ involves three main mechanisms:

- control of Ca^{2+} entry
- control of Ca^{2+} extrusion
- exchange of Ca^{2+} between the cytosol and the intracellular stores.

These mechanisms are described in more detail below and are summarised in Figure 4.1 (see reviews by Berridge et al., 2000, 2003).

CALCIUM ENTRY MECHANISMS

There are four main routes by which Ca^{2+} enters cells across the plasma membrane:

- voltage-gated calcium channels
- ligand-gated calcium channels

- store-operated calcium channels (SOCs)
- Na^+–Ca^{2+} exchange (can operate in either direction; see *Calcium extrusion mechanisms*).

VOLTAGE-GATED CALCIUM CHANNELS

The pioneering work of Hodgkin and Huxley on the ionic basis of the nerve action potential (see below) identified voltage-dependent Na^+ and K^+ conductances as the main participants. It was later found that some invertebrate nerve and muscle cells could produce action potentials that depended on Ca^{2+} rather than Na^+, and improved voltage clamp methods revealed that vertebrate cells also possess voltage-activated calcium channels capable of allowing substantial amounts of Ca^{2+} to enter the cell when the membrane is depolarised. These voltage-gated channels are highly selective for Ca^{2+} (although they also conduct Ba^{2+} ions, which are often used as a substitute in electrophysiological experiments), and do not conduct Na^+ or K^+; they are ubiquitous in excitable cells and allow Ca^{2+} to enter the cell whenever the membrane is depolarised, for example by a conducted action potential.

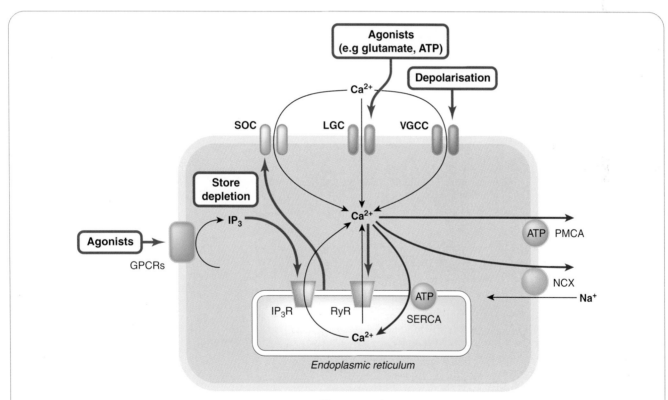

Fig. 4.1   Regulation of intracellular calcium. The main routes of transfer of Ca^{2+} into, and out of, the cytosol and endoplasmic reticulum are shown for a typical cell (see text for details). Black arrows: routes into the cytosol. Blue arrows: routes out of the cytosol. Red arrows: regulatory mechanisms. Most of the channels and transporters have been characterised at the molecular level, but the mechanism by which store-operated calcium channels (SOCs) are linked to the state of the intracellular Ca^{2+} store is uncertain. Normally, $[Ca^{2+}]_i$ is regulated to about 10^{-7} mol/l in a 'resting' cell. Mitochondria (not shown) also function as Ca^{2+} storage organelles but release Ca^{2+} only under pathological conditions, such as ischaemia (see text). There is also evidence for an intracellular store (not shown) activated by the second messenger nicotinic acid dinucleotide phosphate. GPCR, G-protein–coupled receptor; IP_3, inositol trisphosphate; IP_3R, inositol trisphosphate receptor; LGC, ligand-gated cation channel; NCX, Na^+–Ca^{2+} exchange transporter; PMCA, plasma membrane Ca^{2+}–ATPase; RyR, ryanodine receptor; SERCA, sarcoplasmic/endoplasmic reticulum ATPase; VGCC, voltage-gated calcium channel.

A combination of electrophysiological and pharmacological criteria suggests that there are five distinct subtypes of voltage-gated calcium channels: L, T, N, P and R.[1] The subtypes vary with respect to their activation and inactivation kinetics, their voltage threshold for activation, their conductance, and their sensitivity to blocking agents, as summarised in Table 4.1. The molecular basis for this heterogeneity has been worked out in some detail. The main pore-forming subunits (termed $\alpha 1$, see Fig. 3.4) occur in at least 10 molecular subtypes, and they are associated with other subunits (β, γ, δ) that also exist in different forms. Different combinations of these subunits give rise to the different physiological subtypes. In general, L channels are particularly important in regulating contraction of cardiac and smooth muscle (see below), and N channels (and also P/Q) are involved in neurotransmitter and hormone release, while T channels mediate Ca^{2+} entry into neurons and thereby control various Ca^{2+}-dependent functions such as regulation of other channels, enzymes, etc. Clinically used drugs that act directly on these channels include the group of 'Ca^{2+} antagonists' consisting of dihydro-pyridines (e.g. **nifedipine**), **verapamil** and **diltiazem** (used for their cardiovascular effects; see Chs 18 and 19), and also **gabapentin** and **pregabalin** (used to treat epilepsy and pain; see Chs 40, 41). Many drugs affect calcium channels indirectly by acting on G-protein–coupled receptors (see Ch. 3; Triggle, 1999). A number of toxins act selectively on one or other type of calcium channel (Table 4.1), and these are used as experimental tools.

---

[1]A sixth (Q) has also been found, but its properties so closely resemble those of P that they usually get lumped together. The terminology is less than poetic: L stands for long-lasting; T stands for transient; N stands for neither long-lasting nor transient; and P, Q and R carry on alphabetically from N, with O (of course) omitted.

LIGAND-GATED CHANNELS

Most ligand-gated cation channels (see Ch. 3) that are activated by excitatory neurotransmitters are relatively non-selective, and

---

Table 4.1 Types and functions of calcium channels

Gated by:	Main types	Characteristics	Location and function	Drug effects
Voltage	L	High activation threshold. Slow inactivation.	Plasma membrane of many cells. Main Ca^{2+} source for contraction in smooth and cardiac muscle.	Blocked by dihydropyridines, **verapamil, diltiazem**. Activated by **BayK 8644.**
	N	Low activation threshold. Slow inactivation.	Main Ca^{2+} source for transmitter release by nerve terminals.	Blocked by ω-**conotoxin** (component of *Conus* snail venom).
	T	Low threshold. Fast inactivation.	Widely distributed. Important in cardiac pacemaker and atria (role in dysrhythmias).	Blocked by **mibefradil**.
	P/Q	Low activation threshold. Slow inactivation.	Nerve terminals. Transmitter release.	Blocked by ω-**agatoxin** (component of funnel web spider venom).
	R	Low threshold. Fast inactivation.	?	–
Inositol trisphosphate	IP₃ receptor	Ligand-gated channel activated by IP₃.	Located in endoplasmic/sarcoplasmic reticulum. Mediates Ca^{2+} release produced by GPCR activation.	Not directly targeted by drugs. Some experimental blocking agents known (e.g. heparin, injected intracellularly). Responds to GPCR agonists and antagonists in many cells.
Ca^{2+}, sensitised by cyclic ADP ribose	Ryanodine receptor	Directly activated in striated muscle via dihydropyridine receptor of T tubules.	Located in endoplasmic/sarcoplasmic reticulum. Mediates Ca^{2+}-evoked Ca^{2+} release in muscle. Also activated by the second messenger cyclic ADP ribose.	Activated by **caffeine** (high concentrations). Blocked by **ryanodine**. Mutations may lead to drug-induced malignant hyperthermia.
Store depletion	Store-operated channels	Indirectly coupled to endoplasmic/sarcoplasmic reticulum Ca^{2+} stores.	Located in plasma membrane.	Activated indirectly by agents that deplete intracellular stores (e.g. GPCR agonists, **thapsigargin**). Not directly targeted by drugs.
NAADP	–	Activated by NAADP formed as second messenger.	Located in lysosomes. Functional role not clear.	–

GPCR, G-protein–coupled receptor; NAADP, nicotinic acid dinucleotide phosphate.

conduct Ca^{2+} ions as well as other cations. Most important in this respect is the glutamate receptor of the NMDA type (Ch. 33), which has a particularly high permeability to Ca^{2+} and is a major contributor to Ca^{2+} uptake by postsynaptic neurons (and also glial cells) in the central nervous system. Activation of this receptor can readily cause so much Ca^{2+} entry that the cell dies, mainly through activation of Ca^{2+}-dependent proteases but also by triggering apoptosis (see Ch. 5). This mechanism, termed *excitotoxicity*, probably plays a part in various neurodegenerative disorders (see Ch. 35).

For many years, there has been dispute about the existence of 'receptor-operated channels' in smooth muscle, responding directly to mediators such as adrenaline (epinephrine), acetylcholine and histamine. Now it seems (see Kuriyama et al., 1998) that the P_{2X} receptor (see Ch. 3), activated by ATP, is the only example of a true ligand-gated channel in smooth muscle, and this constitutes an important route of entry for Ca^{2+}. Other mediators, acting on G-protein–coupled receptors, affect Ca^{2+} entry indirectly, mainly by regulating voltage-gated calcium channels or potassium channels.

STORE-OPERATED CALCIUM CHANNELS

These are channels that occur in the plasma membrane and open to allow Ca^{2+} entry when the ER stores are depleted. They are distinct from other membrane calcium channels, and belong to the large, recently discovered group of TRP (standing for 'transient receptor potential') channels, which have many different functions (see Clapham, 2003). SOCs remain somewhat mysterious, because it is unclear what kind of linkage couples them to the ER (see Berridge, 1997; Barritt, 1999). Like the ER and SR channels, they can serve to amplify the rise in $[Ca^{2+}]_i$ resulting from Ca^{2+} release from the stores. So far, only experimental compounds are known to block these channels, but efforts are being made to develop specific blocking agents for therapeutic use as relaxants of smooth muscle.

CALCIUM EXTRUSION MECHANISMS

Active transport of Ca^{2+} outwards across the plasma membrane, and inwards across the membranes of the ER or SR, depends on the activity of a Ca^{2+}-dependent ATPase, similar to the Na^+/K^+-dependent ATPase that pumps Na^+ out of the cell in exchange for K^+. Several subtypes of the Ca^{2+}-dependent ATPase have been cloned, but the physiological significance of this heterogeneity remains unclear. They have not been implicated in pharmacological responses, with the exception that **thapsigargin** (derived from a Mediterranean plant, *Thapsia garganica*) specifically blocks the ER pump, causing loss of Ca^{2+} from the ER. It is a useful experimental tool but has no therapeutic significance.

Calcium is also extruded from cells in exchange for Na^+, by Na^+–Ca^{2+} exchange. The transporter that does this has been fully characterised and cloned, and (as you would expect) comes in several molecular subtypes whose functions remain to be worked out. The exchanger transfers three Na^+ ions for one Ca^{2+}, and therefore produces a net depolarising current when it is extruding Ca^{2+}. The energy for Ca^{2+} extrusion comes from the electrochemical gradient for Na^+, not directly from ATP hydrolysis. This means that a reduction in the Na^+ concentration gradient resulting from Na^+ entry will reduce Ca^{2+} extrusion by the exchanger, causing a secondary rise in $[Ca^{2+}]_i$, a mechanism that is particularly important in cardiac muscle (see Ch. 18). The exchanger can actually function in reverse if $[Na^+]_i$ rises excessively, resulting in increased Ca^{2+} entry into the cell (see above). The effect of **digoxin** on cardiac muscle (Ch. 18) is produced in this way.

CALCIUM RELEASE MECHANISMS

There are two main types of calcium channel in the ER and SR membrane, which play an important part in controlling the release of Ca^{2+} from these stores.

- The *inositol trisphosphate receptor* (IP_3R) is activated by inositol trisphosphate (IP_3), a second messenger produced by the action of many ligands on G-protein–coupled receptors (see Ch. 3). IP_3R is a ligand-gated ion channel, although its molecular structure differs from that of ligand-gated channels in the plasma membrane. This is the main mechanism by which activation of G-protein–coupled receptors causes an increase in $[Ca^{2+}]_i$.

- The *ryanodine receptor* (RyR) is so called because it was first identified through the specific blocking action of the plant alkaloid **ryanodine**. It is particularly important in skeletal muscle, where there is direct coupling between the RyRs of the SR and the dihydropyridine receptors of the T-tubules (see below); this coupling results in Ca^{2+} release following the action potential in the muscle fibre. RyRs are also present in other types of cell that lack T tubules; they are activated by a small rise in $[Ca^{2+}]_i$, producing the effect known as *calcium-induced calcium release* (CICR), which serves to amplify the Ca^{2+} signal produced by other mechanisms such as opening of calcium channels in the plasma membrane. CICR means that release tends to be regenerative, because an initial puff of Ca^{2+} releases more, resulting in localised 'sparks' or 'waves' of Ca^{2+} release (see Berridge, 1997).

The functions of IP_3Rs and RyRs are modulated by a variety of other intracellular signals (see Berridge et al., 2003), which affect the magnitude and spatiotemporal patterning of Ca^{2+} signals. Fluorescence imaging techniques have revealed a remarkable level of complexity of Ca^{2+} signals, and much remains to be discovered about the importance of this patterning in relation to physiological and pharmacological mechanisms. The Ca^{2+} sensitivity of RyRs is increased by **caffeine**, causing Ca^{2+} release from the SR even at resting levels of $[Ca^{2+}]_i$. This is used experimentally but rarely happens in humans, because the other pharmacological effects of caffeine (see Ch. 42) occur at much lower doses. The blocking effect of **dantrolene**, a compound related to ryanodine, is used therapeutically to relieve muscle spasm in the rare condition of *malignant hyperthermia* (see Ch. 36), which is associated with inherited abnormalities in the RyR protein. There are as yet few other examples of drugs that directly affect these Ca^{2+} release mechanisms.

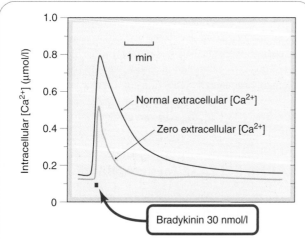

Fig. 4.2 **Increase in intracellular calcium concentration in response to receptor activation.** The records were obtained from a single rat sensory neuron grown in tissue culture. The cells were loaded with the fluorescent Ca^{2+} indicator Fura-2, and the signal from a single cell monitored with a fluorescence microscope. A brief exposure to the peptide bradykinin, which causes excitation of sensory neurons (see Ch. 41), causes a transient increase in $[Ca^{2+}]_i$ from the resting value of about 150 nmol/l. When Ca^{2+} is removed from the extracellular solution, the bradykinin-induced increase in $[Ca^{2+}]_i$ is still present but is smaller and briefer. The response in the absence of extracellular Ca^{2+} represents the release of stored intracellular Ca^{2+} resulting from the intracellular production of inositol trisphosphate. The difference between this and the larger response when Ca^{2+} is present extracellularly is believed to represent Ca^{2+} entry through store-operated ion channels in the cell membrane.
(Figure kindly provided by G M Burgess and A Forbes, Novartis Institute for Medical Research.)

A typical $[Ca^{2+}]_i$ signal resulting from activation of a G-protein–coupled receptor is shown in Figure 4.2. The response produced in the absence of extracellular Ca^{2+} represents release of intracellular Ca^{2+}. The larger and more prolonged response when extracellular Ca^{2+} is present shows the contribution of SOC-mediated Ca^{2+} entry.

OTHER SECOND MESSENGERS

▼ Two intracellular metabolites, *cyclic ADP-ribose* (*cADPR*; see Guse, 2000) and *nicotinic acid dinucleotide phosphate* (NAADP; see Chini & De Toledo, 2002), formed from the ubiquitous coenzymes nicotinamide adenine dinucleotide (NAD) and NAD phosphate, also affect Ca^{2+} signalling. cADPR acts by increasing the sensitivity of RyRs to Ca^{2+}, thus increasing the 'gain' of the CICR effect. NAADP releases Ca^{2+} from lysosomes by activating channels not yet identified but evidently distinct from the IP$_3$R and RyR.

The levels of these messengers in mammalian cells may be regulated mainly in response to changes in the metabolic status of the cell, although the details are not yet clear. Abnormal Ca^{2+} signalling is involved in many pathophysiological conditions, such as ischaemic cell death, endocrine disorders and cardiac dysrhythmias, where the roles of cADPR and NAADP, and their interaction with other mechanisms that regulate $[Ca^{2+}]_I$, are the subject of much current work (see Berridge et al., 2003).

THE ROLE OF MITOCHONDRIA

▼ Under normal conditions, mitochondria accumulate Ca^{2+} passively as a result of the intramitochondrial potential, which is strongly negative with respect to the cytosol. This negativity is maintained by active extrusion of protons, and is lost—thus releasing Ca^{2+} into the cytosol—if the cell runs short of ATP, for example under conditions of hypoxia. This only happens in extremis, and the resulting Ca^{2+} release contributes to the cytotoxicity associated with severe metabolic disturbance. Cell death resulting from brain ischaemia or coronary ischaemia (see Chs 18 and 35) involves this mechanism, along with others that contribute to an excessive rise in $[Ca^{2+}]_i$.

CALMODULIN

Calcium exerts its control over cell functions by virtue of its ability to regulate the activity of many different proteins, including enzymes (particularly kinases and phosphatases), channels, transporters, transcription factors, synaptic vesicle proteins, and many others. In most cases, a Ca^{2+}-binding protein serves as an intermediate between Ca^{2+} and the regulated functional protein, the best known such binding protein being the ubiquitous *calmodulin*. This regulates at least 40 different functional proteins—indeed a powerful fixer. Calmodulin is a dimer, with

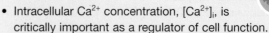

Calcium regulation

- Intracellular Ca^{2+} concentration, $[Ca^{2+}]_i$, is critically important as a regulator of cell function.
- Intracellular Ca^{2+} is determined by (a) Ca^{2+} entry; (b) Ca^{2+} extrusion; and (c) Ca^{2+} exchange between the cytosol, endoplasmic reticulum (ER) and mitochondria.
- Calcium entry occurs by various routes, including voltage- and ligand-gated calcium channels and Na^+–Ca^{2+} exchange.
- Calcium extrusion depends mainly on an ATP-driven Ca^{2+} pump.
- Calcium ions are stored by the ER or sarcoplasmic reticulum (SR), from which they are released in response to various stimuli.
- Calcium ions are released from ER/SR stores by (a) the second messenger inositol trisphosphate acting on inositol trisphosphate receptors; or (b) increased $[Ca^{2+}]_i$ itself acting on ryanodine receptors, a mechanism known as Ca^{2+}-induced Ca^{2+} release.
- Other second messengers, cyclic ADP-ribose and nicotinic acid dinucleotide phosphate, also promote the release of Ca^{2+} from Ca^{2+} stores.
- Depletion of ER/SR Ca^{2+} stores promotes Ca^{2+} entry through the plasma membrane, via store-operated channels.
- Calcium ions affect many aspects of cell function by binding to proteins such as calmodulin, which in turn bind other proteins and regulate their function.

four Ca^{2+}-binding sites. When all are occupied, it undergoes a conformational change, exposing a 'sticky' hydrophobic domain that lures many proteins into association, thereby affecting their functional properties.

EXCITATION

Excitability describes the ability of a cell to show a regenerative all-or-nothing electrical response to depolarisation of its membrane, this membrane response being known as an *action potential*. It is a characteristic of most neurons and muscle cells (including striated, cardiac and smooth muscle), and of many endocrine gland cells. In neurons and muscle cells, the ability of the action potential, once initiated, to propagate to all parts of the cell membrane, and often to spread to neighbouring cells, explains the importance of membrane excitation in intra- and intercellular signalling. In the nervous system, and in striated muscle, action potential propagation is the mechanism responsible for communication over long distances at high speed, indispensable for large, fast-moving creatures. In cardiac and smooth muscle, as well as in some central neurons, spontaneous rhythmic activity occurs. In gland cells, the action potential, where it occurs, serves to amplify the signal that causes the cell to secrete. In each type of tissue, the properties of the excitation process reflect the special characteristics of the ion channels that underlie the process. The molecular nature of ion channels, and their importance as drug targets, is considered in Chapter 3; here we discuss the cellular processes that depend primarily on ion channel function. For more detail, see Hille (2001).

THE 'RESTING' CELL

The resting cell is not resting at all but very busy controlling the state of its interior, and it requires a continuous supply of energy to do so. In relation to the topics discussed in this chapter, the following characteristics are especially important:

- membrane potential
- permeability of the plasma membrane to different ions
- intracellular ion concentrations, especially $[Ca^{2+}]_i$.

Under resting conditions, all cells maintain a negative internal potential between about -30 mV and -80 mV, depending on the cell type. This arises because (a) the membrane is relatively impermeable to Na^+, and (b) Na^+ ions are actively extruded from the cell in exchange for K^+ ions by an energy-dependent transporter, the Na^+ pump (or Na^+–K^+ ATPase). The result is that the intracellular K^+ concentration, $[K^+]_i$, is higher, and $[Na^+]_i$ is lower, than the respective extracellular concentrations. In many cells, other ions, particularly Cl^-, are also actively transported and unequally distributed across the membrane. In many cases (e.g. in neurons), the membrane permeability to K^+ is relatively high, and the membrane potential settles at a value of -60 to -80 mV, close to the equilibrium potential for K^+ (Fig. 4.3). In other cells (e.g. smooth muscle), anions play a larger part, and the membrane potential is generally lower (-30 to -50 mV) and less dependent on K^+.

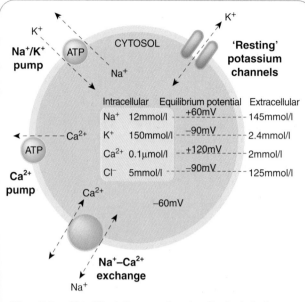

Fig. 4.3   Simplified diagram showing the ionic balance of a typical 'resting' cell. The main transport mechanisms that maintain the ionic gradients across the plasma membrane are the ATP-driven Na^+–K^+ and Ca^{2+} pumps and the Na^+–Ca^{2+} exchange transporter. The membrane is relatively permeable to K^+, because potassium channels are open at rest, but impermeable to other cations. The unequal ion concentrations on either side of the membrane give rise to the 'equilibrium potentials' shown. The resting membrane potential, typically about -60 mV but differing between different cell types, is determined by the equilibrium potentials and the permeabilities of the various ions involved, and by the 'electrogenic' effect of the transporters. For simplicity, anions and other ions, such as protons, are not shown, although these play an important role in many cell types.

Within the figure:

	Intracellular	Equilibrium potential	Extracellular
Na^+	12 mmol/l	$+60$ mV	145 mmol/l
K^+	150 mmol/l	-90 mV	2.4 mmol/l
Ca^{2+}	0.1 µmol/l	$+120$ mV	2 mmol/l
Cl^-	5 mmol/l	-90 mV	125 mmol/l

-60 mV

Na^+/K^+ pump — ATP; Ca^{2+} pump — ATP; Na$^+$–Ca^{2+} exchange; 'Resting' potassium channels; CYTOSOL

ELECTRICAL AND IONIC EVENTS UNDERLYING THE ACTION POTENTIAL

Our present understanding of electrical excitability rests firmly on the work of Hodgkin, Huxley and Katz on squid axons, published in 1949–52. Their experiments (see Katz, 1966) revealed the existence of voltage-gated ion channels (see above) and showed that the action potential is generated by the interplay of two processes:

1. a rapid, transient increase in Na^+ permeability that occurs when the membrane is depolarised beyond about -50 mV
2. a slower, sustained increase in K^+ permeability.

Because of the inequality of Na^+ and K^+ concentrations on the two sides of the membrane, an increase in Na^+ permeability causes an inward current of Na^+ ions, whereas an increase in K^+ permeability causes an outward current. The separate nature of these two currents can be most clearly demonstrated by the use of drugs blocking sodium and potassium channels, as shown in Figure 4.4. During the physiological initiation or propagation of a nerve impulse, the first event is a small depolarisation of the membrane, produced either by transmitter action or by the approach of an action potential passing along the axon. This

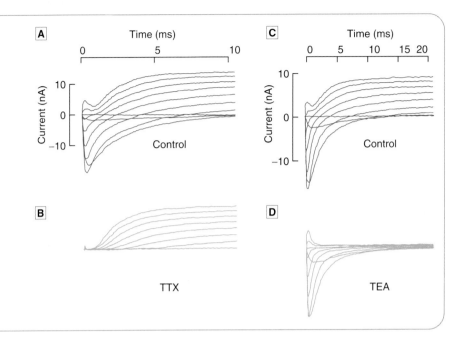

Fig. 4.4 Separation of sodium and potassium currents in the nerve membrane. Voltage clamp records from the node of Ranvier of a single frog nerve fibre. At time 0, the membrane potential was stepped to a depolarised level, ranging from –60 mV (lower trace in each series) to +60 mV (upper trace in each series) in 15-mV steps. A C Control records from two fibres. B Effect of tetrodotoxin (TTX), which abolishes Na^+ currents. D Effect of tetraethylammonium (TEA), which abolishes K^+ currents.
(From Hille B 1970 Prog Biophys 21: 1.)

opens sodium channels, allowing an inward current of Na^+ ions to flow, which depolarises the membrane still further. The process is thus a regenerative one, and the increase in Na^+ permeability is enough to bring the membrane potential close to E_{Na}. The increased Na^+ conductance is transient, because the channels inactivate rapidly and the membrane returns to its resting state.

In many types of cell, including most nerve cells, repolarisation is assisted by the opening of voltage-dependent potassium channels. These function in much the same way as sodium channels, but their activation kinetics are about 10 times slower and they do not inactivate appreciably. This means that the potassium channels open later than the sodium channels, and contribute to the rapid termination of the action potential. The behaviour of the sodium and potassium channels during an action potential is shown in Figure 4.5.

The foregoing account, based on Hodgkin & Huxley's work 50 years ago, involves only Na^+ and potassium channels. Subsequently (see Hille, 2001), voltage-gated calcium channels (see Fig. 4.1) were discovered. These function in basically the same way as sodium channels; they contribute to action potential generation in many cells, particularly cardiac and smooth muscle cells, but also in neurons and secretory cells. Ca^{2+} entry through voltage-gated calcium channels plays a key role in intracellular signalling, as described above.

CHANNEL FUNCTION

The discharge patterns of excitable cells vary greatly. Skeletal muscle fibres are quiescent unless stimulated by the arrival of a nerve impulse at the neuromuscular junction. Cardiac muscle fibres discharge spontaneously at a regular rate (see Ch. 18). Neurons may be normally silent, or they may discharge spontaneously, either regularly or in bursts; smooth muscle cells show a similar variety of firing patterns. The frequency at which

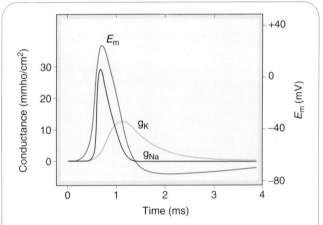

Fig. 4.5 Behaviour of sodium and potassium channels during a conducted action potential. Rapid opening of sodium channels occurs during the action potential upstroke. Delayed opening of potassium channels, and inactivation of sodium channels, causes repolarisation. E_m, membrane potential g_{Na}, g_k, membrane conductance to Na^+, K^+

different cells normally discharge action potentials also varies greatly, from several hundred Hertz for fast-conducting neurons, down to about 1 Hz for cardiac muscle cells. These very pronounced functional variations reflect the different characteristics of the ion channels expressed in different cell types.

Drugs that alter channel characteristics, either by interacting directly with the channel itself or indirectly through second messengers, affect the function of many organ systems, including the nervous, cardiovascular, endocrine, respiratory and reproductive systems, and are a frequent theme in this book. Here we describe some of the key mechanisms involved in the regulation of excitable cells.

In general, action potentials are initiated by membrane currents that cause depolarisation of the cell. These currents may be produced by synaptic activity, by an action potential approaching from another part of the cell, by a sensory stimulus, or by spontaneous *pacemaker* activity. The tendency of such currents to initiate an action potential is governed by the *excitability* of the cell, which depends mainly on the state of (a) the voltage-gated sodium and/or calcium channels, and (b) the potassium channels of the resting membrane. Anything that increases the number of available sodium or calcium channels, or reduces their activation threshold, will tend to increase excitability, whereas increasing the resting K^+ conductance reduces it. Agents that do the reverse, by blocking channels or interfering with their opening, will have the opposite effect. Some examples are shown in Figures 4.6 and 4.7 and in Table 4.1.

USE DEPENDENCE AND VOLTAGE DEPENDENCE

▼ Voltage-gated channels can exist in three functional states (Fig.4.8): *resting* (the closed state that prevails at the normal resting potential), *activated* (the open state favoured by brief depolarisation) and *inactivated* (the blocked state resulting from a trap door–like occlusion of the channel by a floppy intracellular appendage of the channel protein). After the action potential has passed, many sodium channels are in the inactivated state; after the membrane potential returns to its resting value, the inactivated channels revert to the resting state and thus become available for activation once more. In the meantime, the membrane is temporarily *refractory*. Each action potential causes the channels to cycle through these states. The duration of the refractory period, which determines the maximum frequency at which action potentials can occur, depends on the rate of recovery from inactivation. Drugs that block sodium channels, such as local anaesthetics (Ch. 44), antidysrhythmic drugs (Ch. 18) and antiepileptic drugs (Ch. 40), commonly show a selective affinity for one or other of these functional states of the channel, and in their presence the proportion of channels in the high-affinity state is increased. Of particular importance are drugs that bind most strongly to the inactivated state of the channel and thus favour the adoption of this state, thus prolonging the refractory period and reducing the maximum frequency at which action potentials can be generated. This type of block is called *use-dependent*, because the binding of such drugs increases as a function of the rate of action potential discharge, which governs the rate at which inactivated—and therefore drug-sensitive—channels are generated. This is important for some antidysrhythmic drugs (see Ch. 18) and for antiepileptic drugs (Ch. 40), because high-frequency discharges can be inhibited without affecting excitability at normal frequencies. Drugs that readily block sodium channels in their resting state (e.g. local anaesthetics, Ch. 44) prevent excitation at low as well as high frequencies.

Most sodium channel–blocking drugs are cationic at physiological pH and are therefore affected by the voltage gradient across the cell membrane, so that their blocking action is favoured by depolarisation. This phenomenon, known as *voltage dependence*, is also of relevance to the action of antidysrhythmic and antiepileptic drugs, because the cells that are the seat of dysrhythmias or seizure activity are generally somewhat depolarised and therefore more strongly blocked than 'healthy' cells. Similar considerations apply also to drugs that block potassium or calcium channels, but we know less about the importance of use and voltage dependence for these than we do for sodium channels.

SODIUM CHANNELS

In most excitable cells, the regenerative inward current that initiates the action potential results from activation of voltage-gated sodium channels. The early voltage clamp studies by Hodgkin & Huxley on the squid giant axon, described above, revealed the essential functional properties of these channels. Later, advantage was taken of the potent and highly selective blocking action of **tetrodotoxin** (TTX, see Ch.44) to label and purify the channel protein, and subsequently to clone it, revealing the complex structure shown in Figure 3.18, with four similar domains each comprising six membrane-spanning helices (reviewed by Catterall, 2000). One of these helices, S4, contains several basic amino acids and forms the voltage sensor, and moves outwards, thus opening the channel, when the membrane is depolarised. One of the intracellular loops is designed to swing across and block the channel when S4 is displaced, thus inactivating the channel.

It was known from physiological studies that the sodium channels of heart and skeletal muscle differ in various ways from those of neurons. In particular, cardiac sodium channels are relatively insensitive to TTX, and slower in their kinetics (as are those of some sensory neurons), compared with most neuronal sodium channels. Nine distinct molecular subtypes have so far been identified, more than enough to explain the functional diversity.

Various experimental compounds affect sodium channel gating and inactivation, the most important being **tetrodotoxin,** a highly potent and selective blocking agent (Ch.44), and certain substances (e.g. **batrachotoxin** and **veratridine**) that prevent inactivation and therefore cause sodium channels to remain open after activation. Therapeutic agents that act by blocking sodium channels include **local anaesthetic drugs** (Ch.44), antiepileptic drugs (Ch.40) and **antidysrhythmic drugs** (Ch.18). The sodium channel–blocking actions of these drugs were in most cases discovered long after their clinical applications were recognised; many of them lack specificity and produce a variety of unwanted side effects. The use of induced mutations in cloned sodium channels expressed in cell lines is now revealing which regions of the very large channel molecule are involved in the binding of particular agents, and it is hoped that this information will allow more specific drugs to be designed in the future. Certain inherited neurological disorders are associated with sodium channel mutations (see Ashcroft, 2000).

POTASSIUM CHANNELS

In a typical resting cell (see above), the membrane is selectively permeable to K^+, and the membrane potential (about $-60\,mV$) is somewhat positive to the K^+ equilibrium (about $-90\,mV$). This resting permeability comes about because potassium channels are open. If more potassium channels open, the membrane hyperpolarises and the cell is inhibited, whereas the opposite happens if potassium channels close. As well as affecting *excitability* in this way, potassium channels also play an important role in regulating the *duration* of the action potential and the *temporal patterning* of action potential discharges; altogether, these channels play a central role in regulating cell function. As mentioned in Chapter 3, the number and variety of potassium channel subtypes is extraordinary, implying that evolution has been driven by the scope for biological advantage to be gained from subtle variations in the functional properties of these channels. A recent résumé lists over 60 different pore-forming subunits, plus another 20

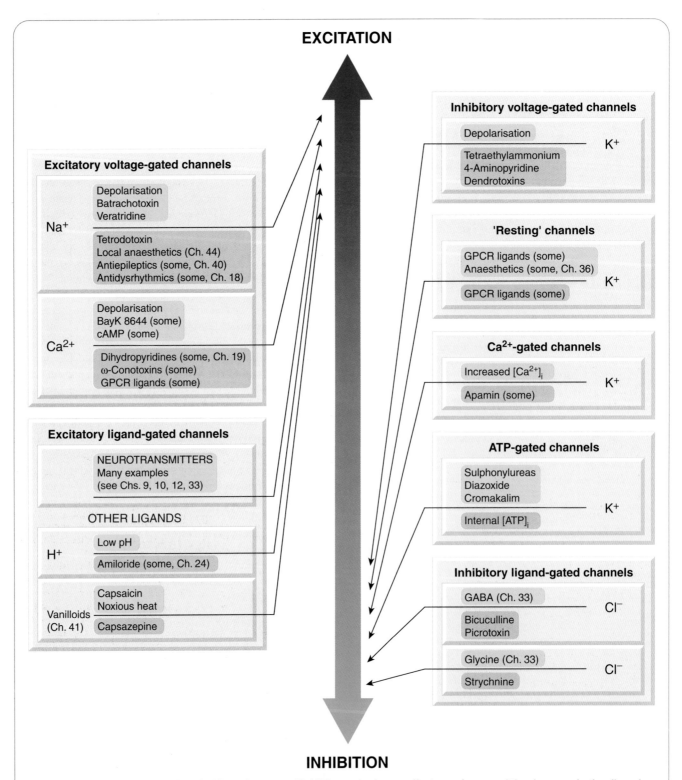

EXCITATION

Excitatory voltage-gated channels

Na+
Depolarisation
Batrachotoxin
Veratridine

Tetrodotoxin
Local anaesthetics (Ch. 44)
Antiepileptics (some, Ch. 40)
Antidysrhythmics (some, Ch. 18)

Ca2+
Depolarisation
BayK 8644 (some)
cAMP (some)

Dihydropyridines (some, Ch. 19)
ω-Conotoxins (some)
GPCR ligands (some)

Excitatory ligand-gated channels

NEUROTRANSMITTERS
Many examples
(see Chs. 9, 10, 12, 33)

OTHER LIGANDS

H+
Low pH
Amiloride (some, Ch. 24)

Vanilloids
(Ch. 41)
Capsaicin
Noxious heat
Capsazepine

Inhibitory voltage-gated channels

Depolarisation

Tetraethylammonium
4-Aminopyridine
Dendrotoxins
K+

'Resting' channels

GPCR ligands (some)
Anaesthetics (some, Ch. 36)

GPCR ligands (some)
K+

Ca2+-gated channels

Increased [Ca2+]i

Apamin (some)
K+

ATP-gated channels

Sulphonylureas
Diazoxide
Cromakalim

Internal [ATP]i
K+

Inhibitory ligand-gated channels

GABA (Ch. 33)

Bicuculline
Picrotoxin
Cl−

Glycine (Ch. 33)

Strychnine
Cl−

INHIBITION

Fig. 4.6   **Ion channels associated with excitatory and inhibitory membrane effects, and some of the drugs and other ligands that affect them.** Channel openers are shown in green boxes, blocking agents and inhibitors in pink boxes. GPCR, G-protein–coupled receptor.

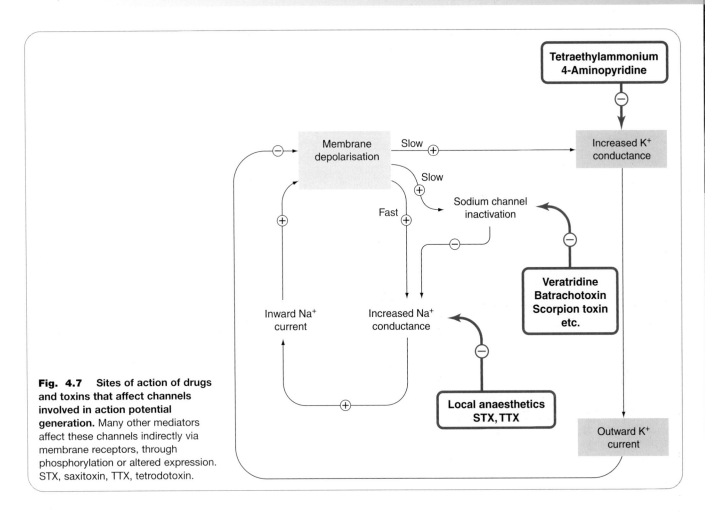

Fig. 4.7 **Sites of action of drugs and toxins that affect channels involved in action potential generation.** Many other mediators affect these channels indirectly via membrane receptors, through phosphorylation or altered expression. STX, saxitoxin, TTX, tetrodotoxin.

or so auxiliary subunits. An impressive evolutionary display, maybe, but hard going for most of us. Here we outline the main types that are known to be important pharmacologically. For more details, and information on potassium channels and the various drugs and toxins that affect them, see Shieh et al. (2000), Gutman et al. (2003) and Jenkinson (2006).

▼ Potassium channels fall into three main classes (Table 4.2),[2] of which the structures are shown in Figure 3.18.

- *Voltage-gated potassium channels*, which possess six membrane-spanning helices, one of which serves as the voltage sensor, causing the channel to open when the membrane is depolarised. Included in this group are channels of the *shaker* family, accounting for most of the voltage-gated K[+] currents familiar to electrophysiologists, and others such as *Ca[2+]-activated potassium channels* and two subtypes that are important in the heart, *HERG* and *LQT channels*. Disturbance of these

channels, either by genetic mutations or by unwanted drug effects, is a major factor in causing cardiac dysrhythmias, which can cause sudden death (see Ch. 18). Many of these channels are blocked by drugs such as **tetraethylammonium** and **4-aminopyridine**.
- *Inwardly rectifying potassium channels*, so called because they allow K[+] to pass inwards much more readily than outwards (see review by Reimann & Ashcroft, 1999). These have two membrane-spanning helices and a single pore-forming loop (P loop). These channels are regulated by interaction with G-proteins (see Ch. 3) and mediate the inhibitory effects of many agonists acting on G-protein–coupled receptors. Certain types are important in the heart, particularly in regulating the duration of the cardiac action potential (Ch. 18); others are the target for the action of **sulfonylureas** (antidiabetic drugs that stimulate insulin secretion by blocking them; see Ch. 26) and smooth muscle relaxant drugs, such as **cromakalim** and **diazoxide**, which open them (see Ch. 19).
- *Two-pore domain potassium channels*, with four helices and two P loops (see review by Goldstein et al., 2001). These show outward rectification and therefore exert a strong repolarising influence, opposing any tendency to excitation. They may contribute to the resting K[+] conductance in many cells, and are susceptible to regulation via G-proteins; certain subtypes have been implicated in the action of volatile anaesthetics such as halothane (Ch. 36).

Inherited abnormalities of potassium channels (*channelopathies*) contribute to a rapidly growing number of cardiac, neurological and other diseases. These include the *long QT syndrome* associated with mutations in cardiac voltage-gated potassium channels, causing episodes of ventricular arrest that can result in sudden death. Certain familial types of deafness and epilepsy are

---

[2]Potassium channel terminology is confusing, to put it mildly. Electrophysiologists have christened K[+] currents prosaically on the basis of their functional properties (I_{KV}, I_{KCa}, I_{KATP}, I_{KIR}, etc.); geneticists have named genes somewhat fancifully according to the phenotypes associated with mutations (shaker, ether-a-go-go, etc.), while molecular biologists have introduced a rational but unmemorable nomenclature on the basis of sequence data (KCNK, KCNQ, etc., with numerical suffixes). The rest of us have to make what we can of the unlovely jargon of labels such as HERG (which—don't blink—stands for Human Ether-a-go-go Related Gene), TWIK, TREK and TASK.

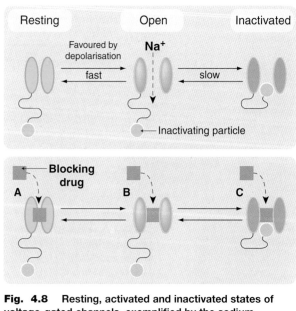

Fig. 4.8 Resting, activated and inactivated states of voltage-gated channels, exemplified by the sodium channel. Membrane depolarisation causes a rapid transition from the resting (closed) state to the open state. The inactivating particle (part of the intracellular domain of the channel protein) is then able to block the channel. Blocking drugs (e.g. local anaesthetics and antiepileptic drugs) often show preference for one of the three channel states, and thus affect the kinetic behaviour of the channels, with implications for their clinical application.

Ion channels and electrical excitability

- Excitable cells generate an all-or-nothing action potential in response to membrane depolarisation. This occurs in most neurons and muscle cells, and also in some gland cells. The ionic basis and time course of the response varies between tissues.
- The regenerative response results from the depolarising current associated with opening of voltage-dependent cation channels (mainly Na+ and Ca^{2+}). It is terminated by spontaneous closure of these channels accompanied by opening of potassium channels.
- The sodium, calcium and potassium channels exist in many molecular varieties, with specific functions in different types of cell.
- The membrane of the 'resting' cell is relatively permeable to K+ but impermeable to Na+ and Ca^{2+}. Drugs or mediators that open potassium channels reduce membrane excitability, and vice versa. Inhibitors of sodium or calcium channel function have the same effect.
- Cardiac muscle cells, some neurons and some smooth muscle cells generate spontaneous action potentials whose amplitude, rate and rhythm is affected by drugs that affect ion channel function.

---

associated with mutations in voltage-gated potassium channels. Other genetic disorders—mostly very rare—involving potassium channels are described by Ashcroft (2000).

MUSCLE CONTRACTION

Effects of drugs on the contractile machinery of smooth muscle are the basis of many therapeutic applications, for smooth muscle is an important component of most physiological systems, including blood vessels and the gastrointestinal and respiratory tracts. For many decades, smooth muscle pharmacology with its trademark technology—the isolated organ bath—held the centre of the pharmacological stage, and neither the subject nor the technology show any sign of flagging, even though the stage has become much more crowded. Cardiac muscle contractility is also the target of important drug effects, whereas striated muscle contractility is only rarely affected by drugs.

Although in each case the basic molecular basis of contraction is similar, namely an interaction between actin and myosin, fuelled by ATP and initiated by an increase in [Ca^{2+}]$_i$, there are differences between these three kinds of muscle that account for their different responsiveness to drugs and chemical mediators.

These differences (Fig. 4.9) involve (a) the linkage between membrane events and increase in [Ca^{2+}]$_i$, and (b) the mechanism by which [Ca^{2+}]$_i$ regulates contraction.

SKELETAL MUSCLE

Skeletal muscle possesses an array of transverse T tubules extending into the cell from the plasma membrane. The action potential of the plasma membrane depends on voltage-gated sodium channels, as in most nerve cells, and propagates rapidly from its site of origin, the motor endplate (see Ch. 10), to the rest of the fibre. The T tubule membrane contains L-type calcium channels, which respond to membrane depolarisation conducted passively along the T tubule when the plasma membrane is invaded by an action potential. These calcium channels are located extremely close to *ryanodine receptors* (see Ch. 3) in the adjacent SR membrane, and activation of these RyRs causes release of Ca^{2+} from the SR. There is evidence of direct coupling between the calcium channels of the T tubule and the RyRs of the SR (as shown in Fig. 4.9); however, Ca^{2+} entry through the T-tubule channels into the restricted zone between these channels and associated RyRs may also contribute. Through this link, depolarisation rapidly activates the RyRs, releasing a short puff of Ca^{2+} from the SR into the sarcoplasm. The Ca^{2+} binds to *troponin*, a protein that normally blocks the interaction between actin and myosin. When Ca^{2+} binds, troponin moves out of the way and allows the contractile machinery to operate. Ca^{2+} release is rapid and brief, and the muscle responds with a short-lasting 'twitch' response. This is a relatively fast and direct mechanism compared with the arrangement in cardiac and smooth muscle

Table 4.2   Types and functions of potassium channels

Structural class[a]	Functional subtypes[b]	Functions	Drug effects	Notes
Voltage-gated (6T, 1P)	Voltage-gated potassium channels	Action potential repolarisation. Limits maximum firing frequency.	Blocked by **tetraethyl-ammonium, 4-aminopyridine.** Certain subtypes blocked by **dendrotoxins** (from mamba snake venom).	Subtypes in the heart include HERG and LQT channels, which are involved in congenital and drug-induced dysrhythmias. Other subtypes may be involved in inherited forms of epilepsy.
	Ca^{2+}-activated potassium channels	Inhibition following stimuli that increase [Ca^{2+}]$_i$	Certain subtypes blocked by **apamin** (from bee venom), and **charybdotoxin** (from scorpion venom).	Important in many excitable tissues to limit repetitive discharges, also in secretory cells.
Inward rectifying (2T, 1P)	G-protein–activated	Mediate effects of many GPCRs that cause inhibition by increasing K$^+$ conductance.	GPCR agonists and antagonists. No important direct interactions.	Other inward-rectifying potassium channels important in kidney.
	ATP-sensitive	Found in many cells. Channels open when [ATP] is low, causing inhibition. Important in control of insulin secretion.	Association of one subtype with the sulfonylurea receptor results in modulation by sulfonylureas (e.g. **glibenclamide**), which close channels, and by potassium channel openers (e.g. **diazoxide, pinacidil**), which relax smooth muscle.	–
Two-pore domain (4T, 2P)	Several subtypes identified (TWIK, TRAAK, TREK, TASK, etc.)	Most are voltage-insensitive; some are normally open and contribute to the 'resting' K$^+$ conductance. Modulated by GPCRs.	Certain subtypes are activated by volatile anaesthetics (e.g. **halothane**). No selective blocking agents. Modulation by GPCR agonists and antagonists.	Recently discovered, so knowledge is fragmentary as yet.

GPCR, G-protein–coupled receptor.

[a]Potassium channel structures (see Fig.3.17) are defined according to the number of transmembrane helices (T) and the number of pore-forming loops (P) in each α subunit. Functional channels contain several subunits (often four), which may be identical or different, and they are often associated with accessory (β) subunits.

[b]Within each functional subtype, several molecular variants have been identified, often restricted to particular cells and tissues. The physiological and pharmacological significance of this heterogeneity is not yet understood.

(see below), and consequently less susceptible to pharmacological modulation. The few examples of drugs that directly affect skeletal muscle contraction are shown in Table 4.1.

CARDIAC MUSCLE

Cardiac muscle (see review by Bers, 2002) differs from skeletal muscle in several important respects. The nature of the cardiac action potential, the ionic mechanisms underlying its inherent rhythmicity, and the effects of drugs on the rate and rhythm of the heart are described in Chapter 18. Cardiac muscle cells lack T tubules, and there is no direct coupling between the plasma membrane and the SR. The cardiac action potential varies in its configuration in different parts of the heart, but commonly shows a 'plateau' lasting several hundred milliseconds following the initial rapid depolarisation. The plasma membrane contains many L-type calcium channels, which open during this plateau and allow Ca^{2+} to enter the cell, although not in sufficient quantities to activate the contractile machinery directly. Instead, this initial Ca^{2+} entry acts on RyRs (a different molecular type from those of skeletal muscle) to release Ca^{2+} from the SR, producing a secondary and much larger wave of Ca^{2+}. Because the RyRs of cardiac muscle are themselves activated by Ca^{2+}, the [Ca^{2+}]$_i$ wave is a regenerative, all-or-nothing event. The initial Ca^{2+} entry that triggers this event is highly dependent on the action potential duration, and on the functioning of the membrane L-type channels. Some of the drugs that affect it are shown in Table 4.1. With minor differences, the mechanism by which Ca^{2+} activates the contractile machinery is the same as in skeletal muscle.

SMOOTH MUSCLE

The properties of smooth muscle vary considerably in different organs, and the link between membrane events and contraction is less direct and less well understood than in other kinds of muscle. The action potential of smooth muscle is generally a

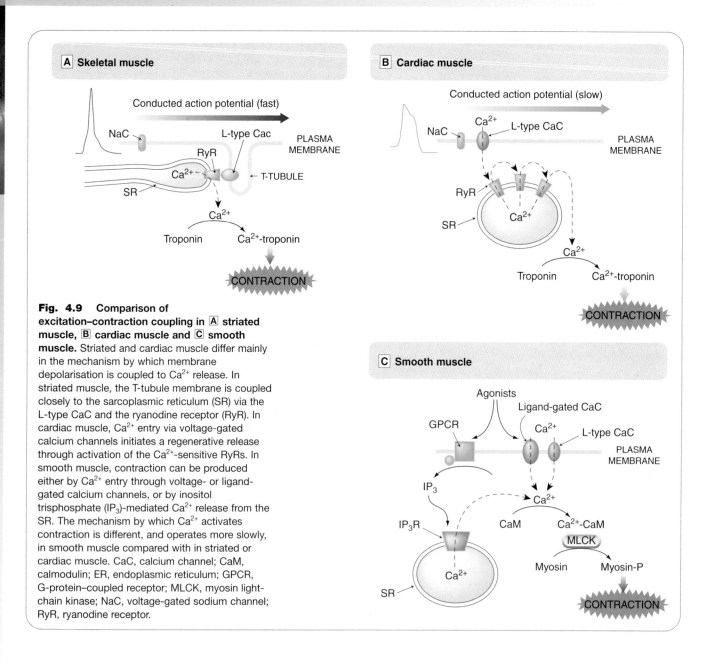

Fig. 4.9 Comparison of excitation–contraction coupling in Ⓐ **striated muscle,** Ⓑ **cardiac muscle and** Ⓒ **smooth muscle.** Striated and cardiac muscle differ mainly in the mechanism by which membrane depolarisation is coupled to Ca^{2+} release. In striated muscle, the T-tubule membrane is coupled closely to the sarcoplasmic reticulum (SR) via the L-type CaC and the ryanodine receptor (RyR). In cardiac muscle, Ca^{2+} entry via voltage-gated calcium channels initiates a regenerative release through activation of the Ca^{2+}-sensitive RyRs. In smooth muscle, contraction can be produced either by Ca^{2+} entry through voltage- or ligand-gated calcium channels, or by inositol trisphosphate (IP_3)-mediated Ca^{2+} release from the SR. The mechanism by which Ca^{2+} activates contraction is different, and operates more slowly, in smooth muscle compared with in striated or cardiac muscle. CaC, calcium channel; CaM, calmodulin; ER, endoplasmic reticulum; GPCR, G-protein–coupled receptor; MLCK, myosin light-chain kinase; NaC, voltage-gated sodium channel; RyR, ryanodine receptor.

rather lazy and vague affair compared with the more military behaviour of skeletal and cardiac muscle, and it propagates through the tissue much more slowly and uncertainly. The action potential is, in most cases, generated by L-type calcium channels rather than by voltage-gated sodium channels, and this is one important route of Ca^{2+} entry. In addition, many smooth muscle cells possess ligand-gated cation channels, which allow Ca^{2+} entry when they respond to transmitters. The best characterised of these are the receptors of the P_{2X} type (see Ch. 12), which respond to ATP released from autonomic nerves. Smooth muscle cells also store Ca^{2+} in the ER, from which it can be released when the IP_3R is activated (see Ch. 3). IP_3 is generated by activation of many types of G-protein–coupled receptor. Thus, in contrast to skeletal and cardiac muscle, Ca^{2+} release and contraction can occur in smooth muscle when such receptors are activated without necessarily involving depolarisation and Ca^{2+} entry through the plasma membrane.

The contractile machinery of smooth muscle is activated when the *myosin light chain* undergoes phosphorylation, causing it to become detached from the actin filaments. This phosphorylation is catalysed by a kinase, *myosin light-chain kinase (MLCK)*, which is activated when it binds to Ca^{2+}–calmodulin (see p. 58). A second enzyme, *myosin phosphatase*, reverses the phosphorylation and causes relaxation. The activity of MLCK and myosin phosphatase thus exerts a balanced effect, promoting contraction and relaxation, respectively. Both enzymes are regulated by cyclic nucleotides (cAMP and cGMP; see Ch. 3), and many drugs that cause smooth muscle contraction or relaxation mediated through G-protein–coupled receptors or through guanylate cyclase–linked receptors act in this way. Figure 4.10 summarises the main mechanisms by which drugs control smooth muscle contraction. The complexity of these control mechanisms and interactions explains why pharmacologists have been entranced for so long by smooth muscle. Many therapeutic

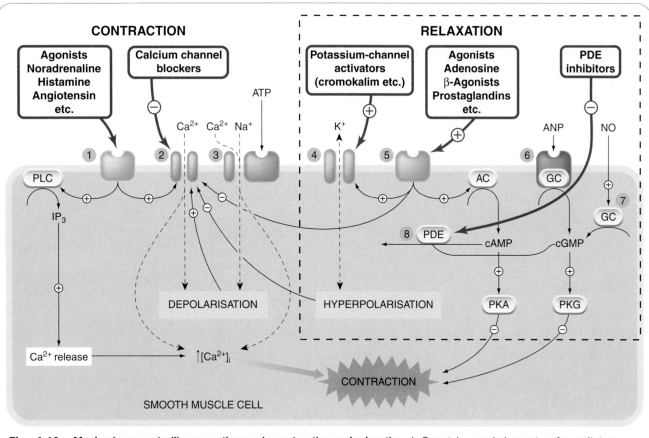

Fig. 4.10 **Mechanisms controlling smooth muscle contraction and relaxation.** 1. G-protein–coupled receptors for excitatory agonists, mainly regulating inositol trisphosphate formation and calcium channel function. 2. Voltage-gated calcium channels. 3. Ligand-gated cation channels (the P_{2X} receptor for ATP is the main example). 4. Potassium channels. 5. G-protein–coupled receptors for inhibitory agonists, mainly regulating cAMP formation and potassium and calcium channel function. 6. Receptor for atrial natriuretic peptide (ANP), coupled directly to guanylate cyclase (GC). 7. Soluble guanylate cyclase, activated by nitric oxide (NO). 8. Phosphodiesterase (PDE), the main route of inactivation of cAMP and cGMP. AC, adenylate cyclase; PKA, protein kinase A; PKG, protein kinase G; PLC, phospholipase C.

drugs work by contracting or relaxing smooth muscle, particularly those affecting the cardiovascular, respiratory and gastrointestinal systems, as discussed in later chapters, where details of specific drugs and their physiological effects are given.

RELEASE OF CHEMICAL MEDIATORS

Much of pharmacology is based on interference with the body's own chemical mediators, particularly neurotransmitters, hormones and inflammatory mediators. Here we discuss some of the common mechanisms involved in the release of such mediators, and it will come as no surprise that Ca^{2+} plays a central role. Drugs and other agents that affect the various control mechanisms that regulate $[Ca^{2+}]_i$ will therefore also affect mediator release, and this accounts for many of the physiological effects that they produce.

Chemical mediators that are released from cells fall into two main groups (Fig. 4.11).

- Mediators that are preformed and packaged in storage vesicles—sometimes called storage granules—from which they are released by *exocytosis*. This large group comprises all the conventional neurotransmitters and neuromodulators (see Chs 9 and 32), and many hormones. It also includes secreted proteins such as cytokines (Ch. 13) and various growth factors (Ch. 16).
- Mediators that are produced on demand and are released by diffusion or by membrane carriers. This group includes nitric oxide (Ch. 17) and many lipid mediators (e.g. prostanoids, Ch. 13, and endocannabinoids, Ch. 15).[3]

Calcium ions play a key role in both cases, because a rise in $[Ca^{2+}]_i$ initiates exocytosis and is also the main activator of the enzymes responsible for the synthesis of diffusible mediators.

In addition to mediators that are released from cells, some are formed from precursors in the plasma, two important examples being *kinins* (Ch. 13) and *angiotensin* (Ch. 19), which are peptides produced by protease-mediated cleavage of circulating proteins.

---

[3]Carrier-mediated release can also occur with neurotransmitters that are stored in vesicles but is quantitatively less significant than exocytosis (see Ch.9).

Muscle contraction

- Muscle contraction occurs in response to a rise in $[Ca^{2+}]_i$.
- In skeletal muscle, depolarisation causes rapid Ca^{2+} release from the sarcoplasmic reticulum (SR); in cardiac muscle, Ca^{2+} enters through voltage-gated channels, and this initial entry triggers further release from the SR; in smooth muscle, the Ca^{2+} signal is due partly to Ca^{2+} entry and partly to inositol trisphosphate (IP_3)-mediated release from the SR.
- In smooth muscle, contraction can occur without action potentials, for example when agonists at G-protein–coupled receptors lead to IP_3 formation.
- Activation of the contractile machinery in smooth muscle involves phosphorylation of the myosin light chain, a mechanism that is regulated by a variety of second messenger systems.

EXOCYTOSIS

Exocytosis, occurring in response to an increase of $[Ca^{2+}]_i$, is the principal mechanism of transmitter release (see Fig. 4.11) in the peripheral and central nervous systems, as well as in endocrine cells and mast cells. The secretion of enzymes and other proteins by gastrointestinal and exocrine glands and by vascular endothelial cells is also basically similar. Exocytosis (see Burgoyne & Morgan, 2002) involves fusion between the membrane of synaptic vesicles and the inner surface of the plasma membrane. The vesicles are preloaded with stored transmitter, and release occurs in discrete packets, or *quanta*, each representing the contents of a single vesicle. The first evidence for this (see Nicholls et al., 2000) came from the work of Katz and his colleagues in the 1950s, who recorded spontaneous 'miniature endplate potentials' at the frog neuromuscular junction, and showed that each resulted from the spontaneous release of a packet of the transmitter, acetylcholine. They also showed that release evoked by nerve stimulation occurred by the synchronous release of several hundred such quanta, and was highly dependent on the presence of Ca^{2+} in the bathing solution. Unequivocal evidence that the quanta represented vesicles releasing their contents by exocytosis came from electron microscopic studies, in which the tissue was rapidly frozen in mid-release, revealing vesicles in the process of extrusion, and from elegant electrophysiological measurements showing that membrane capacitance (reflecting the area of the presynaptic membrane) increased in a stepwise way as each vesicle fused, and then gradually returned as the vesicle membrane was recovered from the surface. There is also biochemical evidence showing that, in addition to the transmitter, other constituents of the vesicles are released at the same time.

In nerve terminals specialised for fast synaptic transmission, Ca^{2+} enters through voltage-gated calcium channels, mainly of the N and P type (see above), and the synaptic vesicles are 'docked' at *active zones*—specialised regions of the presynaptic

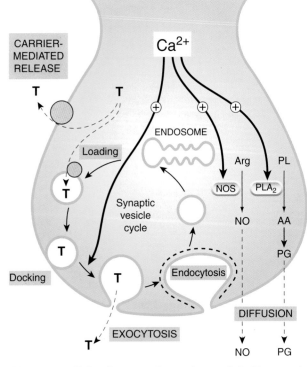

Fig. 4.11 Role of exocytosis, carrier-mediated transport and diffusion in mediator release. The main mechanism of release of monoamine and peptide mediators is Ca^{2+}-mediated exocytosis, but carrier-mediated release from the cytosol also occurs. T represents a typical amine transmitter, such as noradrenaline (norepinephrine) or 5-hydroxytryptamine. Nitric oxide (NO) and prostaglandins (PGs) are released by diffusion as soon as they are formed, from arginine (Arg) and arachidonic acid (AA), respectively, through the action of Ca^{2+}-activated enzymes, nitric oxide synthase (NOS) and phospholipase A_2 (see Chs 16 and 17 for more details).

membrane from which exocytosis occurs, situated close to the relevant calcium channels and opposite receptor-rich zones of the postsynaptic membrane (see Stanley, 1997). Elsewhere, where speed is less critical, Ca^{2+} may come from intracellular stores as described above, and the spatial organisation of active zones is less clear. It is common for secretory cells, including neurons, to release more than one mediator (for example, a 'fast' transmitter such as glutamate and a 'slow' transmitter such as a neuropeptide) from different vesicle pools (see Ch. 9). The fast transmitter vesicles are located close to active zones, while the slow transmitter vesicles are further away. Release of the fast transmitter, because of the tight spatial organisation, occurs as soon as the neighbouring calcium channels open, before the Ca^{2+} has a chance to diffuse throughout the terminal, whereas release of the slow transmitter requires the Ca^{2+} to diffuse more widely. As a result, release of fast transmitters occurs impulse by impulse, even at low stimulation frequencies, whereas release of slow transmitters builds up only at higher stimulation frequencies. The release rates of the two therefore depend critically on the frequency and patterning of firing of the presynaptic neuron (Fig. 4.12). In non-excitable cells (e.g. most exocrine and endocrine glands), the

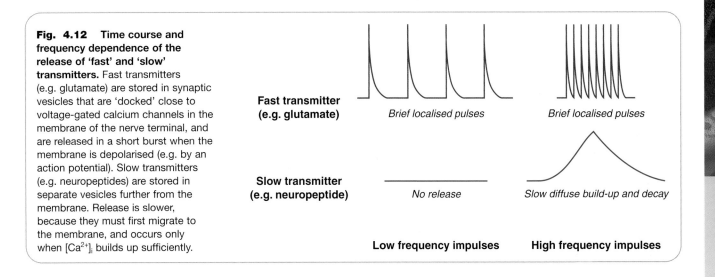

Fig. 4.12 Time course and frequency dependence of the release of 'fast' and 'slow' transmitters. Fast transmitters (e.g. glutamate) are stored in synaptic vesicles that are 'docked' close to voltage-gated calcium channels in the membrane of the nerve terminal, and are released in a short burst when the membrane is depolarised (e.g. by an action potential). Slow transmitters (e.g. neuropeptides) are stored in separate vesicles further from the membrane. Release is slower, because they must first migrate to the membrane, and occurs only when $[Ca^{2+}]_i$ builds up sufficiently.

Fast transmitter (e.g. glutamate)
Brief localised pulses   *Brief localised pulses*

Slow transmitter (e.g. neuropeptide)
No release   *Slow diffuse build-up and decay*

Low frequency impulses   **High frequency impulses**

slow mechanism predominates and is activated mainly by Ca^{2+} release from intracellular stores.

▼ Calcium causes exocytosis by binding to the vesicle-bound protein *synaptotagmin*, and this favours association between a second vesicle-bound protein, *synaptobrevin*, and a related protein, *synaptotaxin*, on the inner surface of the plasma membrane. This association brings the vesicle membrane into close apposition with the plasma membrane, causing membrane fusion. This group of proteins, known collectively as *SNAREs*, play a key role in exocytosis.

Having undergone exocytosis, the empty vesicle[4] is recaptured by endocytosis and returns to the interior of the terminal, where it fuses with the larger endosomal membrane. The endosome buds off new vesicles, which take up transmitter from the cytosol by means of specific transport proteins and are again docked on the presynaptic membrane. This sequence, which typically takes several minutes, is controlled by various trafficking proteins associated with the plasma membrane and the vesicles, as well as cytosolic proteins. Further details about exocytosis and vesicle recycling are given by Calakos & Scheller (1996), Nestler et al. (2001) and Südhof (2004). So far, there are few examples of drugs that affect transmitter release by interacting with synaptic proteins, although the **botulinum neurotoxins** (see Ch. 10) produce their effects by proteolytic cleavage of SNARE proteins.

NON-VESICULAR RELEASE MECHANISMS

If this neat and tidy picture of transmitter packets ready and waiting to pop obediently out of the cell in response to a puff of Ca^{2+} seems a little too good to be true, rest assured that the picture is not quite so simple. Acetylcholine, noradrenaline (norepinephrine) and other mediators can leak out of nerve endings from the cytosolic compartment, independently of vesicle fusion, by utilising carriers in the plasma membrane (Fig. 4.11). Drugs such as amphetamines, which release amines from central and peripheral nerve terminals (see Chs 11 and 32), do so by displacing the endogenous amine from storage vesicles into the cytosol,

whence it escapes via the monoamine transporter in the plasma membrane, a mechanism that does not depend on Ca^{2+}.

Nitric oxide (see Ch. 17) and arachidonic acid metabolites (e.g. prostaglandins; Ch. 19) are two important examples of mediators that are released by diffusion across the membrane or by carrier-mediated extrusion, rather than by exocytosis. The mediators are not stored but escape from the cell as soon as they are synthesised. In both cases, the synthetic enzyme is activated by Ca^{2+}, and the moment-to-moment control of the rate of synthesis depends on $[Ca^{2+}]_i$. This kind of release is necessarily slower than the classic exocytotic mechanism, but in the case of nitric oxide is fast enough for it to function as a true transmitter (see Ch. 17).

> **Mediator release**
>
> • Most chemical mediators are packaged into storage vesicles and released by exocytosis. Some are synthesised on demand and released by diffusion or the operation of membrane carriers.
> • Exocytosis occurs in response to increased $[Ca^{2+}]_i$ as a result of a Ca^{2+}-mediated interaction between proteins of the synaptic vesicle and the plasma membrane, causing the membranes to fuse.
> • After releasing their contents, vesicles are recycled and reloaded with transmitter.
> • Many secretory cells contain more than one type of vesicle, loaded with different mediators and secreted independently.
> • Stored mediators (e.g. neurotransmitters) may be released directly from the cytosol independently of Ca^{2+} and exocytosis by drugs that interact with membrane transport mechanisms.
> • Non-stored mediators, such as prostanoids and nitric oxide, are released by increased $[Ca^{2+}]_i$, which activates the enzymes responsible for their synthesis.

---

[4]The vesicle contents may not always discharge completely. Instead, vesicles may fuse transiently with the cell membrane and release only part of their contents (see Burgoyne & Morgan, 2002) before becoming disconnected (termed *kiss-and run exocytosis*).

EPITHELIAL ION TRANSPORT

Fluid-secreting epithelia include the renal tubule, salivary glands, gastrointestinal tract and airways epithelia. In each case, epithelial cells are arranged in sheets separating the interior (blood-perfused) compartment from the exterior lumen compartment, into which, or from which, secretion takes place. Fluid secretion involves two distinct mechanisms, which often coexist in the same cell and indeed interact with each other. Greger (2000) and Ashcroft (2000) give more detailed accounts. The two mechanisms (Fig. 4.13) are concerned, respectively, with Na^+ transport and Cl^- transport.

In the case of Na^+ transport, secretion occurs because Na^+ enters the cell passively at one end and is pumped out actively at the other, with water following passively. Critical to this mechanism is a class of highly regulated epithelial sodium channels (ENaCs) that allow Na^+ entry.

Epithelial sodium channels (see De la Rosa et al., 2000) are widely expressed, not only in epithelial cells but also in neurons and other excitable cells, where their function is largely unknown. They are regulated mainly by **aldosterone**, a hormone produced by the adrenal cortex that enhances Na^+ reabsorption by the kidney (Ch. 24). Aldosterone, like other steroid hormones, exerts its effects by regulating gene expression (see Ch. 3), and causes an increase in ENaC expression, thereby increasing the rate of Na^+ and fluid transport. This takes a few hours, and aldosterone also affects ENaC function through other more rapid mechanisms, but the details are not well understood. ENaCs are selectively blocked by certain diuretic drugs, notably **amiloride** (see Ch. 24), a compound that is widely used to study the functioning of ENaCs in other situations.

Chloride transport is particularly important in the airways and gastrointestinal tract. In the airways, it is essential for fluid secretion, whereas in the colon it mediates fluid reabsorption, the difference being due to the different arrangement of various transporters and channels with respect to the polarity of the cells. The simplified diagram in Figure 4.13B represents the situation in the pancreas, where secretion depends on Cl^- transport. The key molecule in Cl^- transport is the *cystic fibrosis transmembrane conductance regulator* (*CFTR*; see Hwang & Sheppard, 1999), so named because early studies on the inherited disorder cystic fibrosis showed it to be associated with impaired Cl^- conductance in the membrane of secretory epithelial cells, and the CFTR gene, identified through painstaking genetic linkage studies and isolated in 1989, was found to encode a Cl^- conducting ion channel. Severe physiological consequences follow from the impairment of secretion, particularly in the airways but also in many other systems, such as sweat glands and pancreas. Genetic studies revealed mutations in the CFTR gene; this knowledge has produced a flood of research on the molecular mechanisms involved in Cl^- transport, but as yet no significant therapeutic advance. So far, no drugs are known that interact specifically with CFTRs.

Both Na^+ and Cl^- transport are regulated by intracellular messengers, notably by Ca^{2+} and cAMP, the latter exerting its effects by activating protein kinases and thereby causing

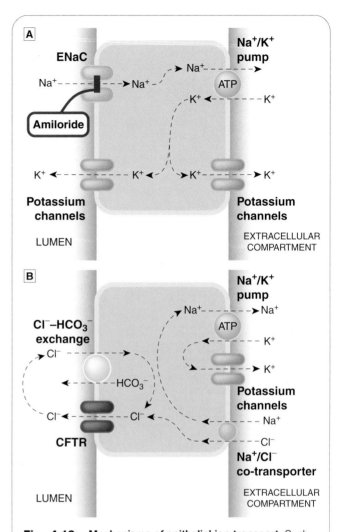

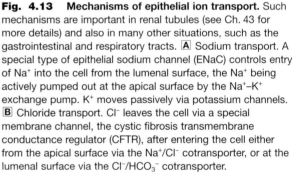

Fig. 4.13 **Mechanisms of epithelial ion transport.** Such mechanisms are important in renal tubules (see Ch. 43 for more details) and also in many other situations, such as the gastrointestinal and respiratory tracts. **A** Sodium transport. A special type of epithelial sodium channel (ENaC) controls entry of Na^+ into the cell from the lumenal surface, the Na^+ being actively pumped out at the apical surface by the Na^+–K^+ exchange pump. K^+ moves passively via potassium channels. **B** Chloride transport. Cl^- leaves the cell via a special membrane channel, the cystic fibrosis transmembrane conductance regulator (CFTR), after entering the cell either from the apical surface via the Na^+/Cl^- cotransporter, or at the lumenal surface via the Cl^-/HCO_3^- cotransporter.

phosphorylation of channels and transporters. CFTR itself is activated by cAMP. In the gastrointestinal tract, increased cAMP formation causes a large increase in the rate of fluid secretion, an effect that leads to the copious diarrhoea produced by cholera infection (see Ch. 3) and also by inflammatory conditions in which prostaglandin formation is increased (see Ch. 13). Activation of G-protein–coupled receptors, which cause release of Ca^{2+}, also stimulates secretion, possibly also by activating CFTR. Many examples of therapeutic drugs that affect epithelial secretion by activating or blocking G-protein–coupled receptors appear in later chapters.

Epithelial ion transport

- Many epithelia (e.g. renal tubules, exocrine glands, and airways) are specialised to transport specific ions.
- This type of transport depends on a class of sodium channels known as epithelial sodium channels, which allow Na^+ entry into the cell at one surface, coupled to active extrusion of Na^+, or exchange for another ion, from the opposite surface.

- Anion transport depends on a specific chloride channel (the cystic fibrosis transmembrane conductance regulator), mutations of which result in cystic fibrosis.
- The activity of channels, pumps and exchange transporters is regulated by various second messengers and nuclear receptors, which control the transport of ions in specific ways.

REFERENCES AND FURTHER READING

General references

Katz B 1966 Nerve, muscle and synapse. McGraw Hill, New York (*A classic account of the ground-breaking electrophysiological experiments that established the basis of nerve and muscle function*)

Levitan I B, Kaczmarek L K 2002 The neuron: cell and molecular biology, 3rd edn. Oxford University Press, New York (*Useful textbook covering ion channels and synaptic mechanisms as well as other aspects of neuronal function*)

Nestler E J, Hyman S E, Malenka R C 2001 Molecular neuropharmacology. McGraw-Hill, New York (*Excellent modern textbook*)

Nicholls J G, Fuchs P A, Martin A R, Wallace B G 2000 From neuron to brain. Sinauer, Sunderland (*Excellent, well-written textbook of neuroscience*)

Second messengers and calcium regulation

Barritt G J 1999 Receptor-activated Ca^{2+} inflow in animal cells: a variety of pathways tailored to meet different intracellular Ca^{2+} signalling requirements. Biochem J 337: 153–169 (*Useful overview of mechanisms involved in Ca^{2+} signalling*)

Berridge M J 1997 Elementary and global aspects of calcium signalling. J Physiol 499: 291–306 (*Review of Ca^{2+} signalling, emphasising the various intracellular mechanisms that produce spatial and temporal patterning—'sparks', 'waves', etc.*)

Berridge M J, Bootman M D, Llewellyn Roderick H 2003 Calcium signalling: dynamics, homeostasis and remodelling. Nat Rev Mol Cell Biol 4: 517–529

Berridge M J, Lipp P, Bootman M D 2000 The versatility and universality of calcium signalling. Nat Rev Cell Mol Biol 1: 11–21

Chini E N, De Toledo F G H 2002 Nicotinic acid adenine dinucleotide phosphate: a new intracellular second messenger. Am J Physiol Cell Physiol 292: C1191–C1198 (*Current state of knowledge of NAADP as a second messenger involved in Ca^{2+} signalling*)

Guse A H 2000 Cyclic ADP-ribose. J Mol Med 78: 26–35 (*Review article describing the role of cADPR, a recently discovered second messenger similar to IP_3*)

Excitation and ion channels

Ashcroft F M 2000 Ion channels and disease. Academic Press, San Diego (*A very useful textbook that describes the physiology of different kinds of ion channels, and relates it to their molecular structure; the book emphasises the importance of 'channelopathies', genetic channel defects associated with disease states*)

Catterall W A 2000 From ionic currents to molecular mechanisms: the structure and function of voltage-gated sodium channels Neuron 26: 13–25 (*Useful review article*)

Clapham D E 2003 TRP channels as cellular sensors. Nature 426: 517–524 (*Review article on the recently discovered multipurpose TRP family of channels*)

De la Rosa D A, Canessa C M, Fyfe G K, Zhang P 2000 Structure and regulation of amiloride-sensitive sodium channels. Annu Rev Physiol 62: 573–594 (*General review on the nature and function of 'epithelial' sodium channels*)

Goldstein S A N, Bockenhauer D, Zilberberg N 2001 Potassium leak channels and the KCNK family of two–P-domain subunits. Nat Rev Neurosci 2: 175–184 (*Review on the current state of knowledge of a recently discovered class of potassium channels*)

Gutman G A et al 2003 IUPHAR compendium of voltage-gated ion channels: potassium channels. Pharmacol Rev 55: 583–586

Hille B 2001 Ionic channels of excitable membranes. Sinauer Associates, Sunderland (*A clear and detailed account of the basic principles of ion channels, with emphasis on their biophysical properties*)

Jenkinson D H 2006 Potassium channels—multiplicity and challenges. Br J Pharmacol 147 (Suppl): 63–71

Reimann F, Ashcroft F M 1999 Inwardly rectifying potassium channels. Curr Opin Cell Biol 11: 503–508 (*Review describing the various mechanisms by which the inwardly rectifying potassium channels are modulated*)

Shieh C-C, Coghlan M, Sullivan J P, Gopalakrishnan M 2000 Potassium channels: molecular defects, diseases and therapeutic opportunities. Pharmacol Rev 52: 557–593 (*Comprehensive review of potassium channel pathophysiology and pharmacology*)

Triggle D J 1999 The pharmacology of ion channels: with particular reference to voltage-gated Ca^{2+} channels. Eur J Pharmacol 375: 311–325 (*Review focusing mainly on various types of calcium channel blockers, many of which are important therapeutically*)

Muscle contraction

Bers D M 2002 Cardiac excitation–contraction coupling. Nature 415: 198–205 (*Short, well-illustrated review article*)

Kuriyama H, Kitamura K, Itoh T, Inoue R 1998 Physiological features of visceral smooth muscle cells, with special reference to receptors and ion channels. Physiol Rev 78: 811–920 (*Comprehensive review article*)

Secretion and exocytosis

Burgoyne R D, Morgan A 2002 Secretory granule exocytosis. Physiol Rev 83: 581–632 (*Comprehensive review of the molecular machinery responsible for secretory exocytosis*)

Calakos N, Scheller R H 1996 Synaptic vesicle biogenesis, docking and fusion: a molecular description. Physiol Rev 76: 1–29 (*Summarises recent advances in the understanding of the mechanism of exocytosis*)

Greger R 2000 The role of CFTR in the colon. Annu Rev Physiol 62: 467–491 (*A useful résumé of information about CFTR and epithelial secretion, more general than its title suggests*)

Hwang T-C, Sheppard D N 1999 Molecular pharmacology of the CFTR channel. Trends Pharmacol Sci 20: 448–453 (*Description of approaches aimed at finding therapeutic drugs aimed at altering the function of the CFTR channel*)

Stanley E E 1997 The calcium channel and the organization of the presynaptic transmitter release face. Trends Neurosci 20: 404–409 (*Discusses the microphysiology of vesicular release*)

Südhof T C 2004 The synaptic vesicle cycle. Annu Rev Neurosci 27: 509–547 (*Summarises recent advances in the understanding of vesicular release at the molecular level*)

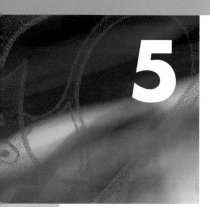

5 Cell proliferation and apoptosis

OVERVIEW

In the postembryonic body, about 10 billion new cells are manufactured daily through division of existing cells—a prodigious output that must be counterbalanced by the elimination of a similar number of cells. A balance between cell generation and cell removal is also critical during embryogenesis and development. This chapter covers the main elements involved in the processes of cell proliferation and cell removal. We consider the changes that occur within an individual cell when, after stimulation by growth factors, it gears up to divide into two daughter cells. We consider the interaction of cells, growth factors and the extracellular matrix in cell proliferation. We consider the phenomenon of apoptosis—a programmed series of events leading to cell death—detailing the changes that occur in a cell preparing to die and describing the intracellular pathways that lead to its demise.

Last, the pathophysiological significance of the events described is considered and their implications for the potential development of clinically useful drugs briefly discussed.

CELL PROLIFERATION

Cell proliferation is involved in many physiological and pathological processes including growth, healing, repair, hypertrophy, hyperplasia and the development of tumours. Angiogenesis (the development of new blood vessels) necessarily occurs during many of these processes.

Proliferating cells go through what is termed the *cell cycle*, during which the cell replicates all its components and then bisects itself into two identical daughter cells. Important components of the signalling pathways in proliferating cells are receptor tyrosine kinases or receptor-linked kinases, and the mitogen-activated kinase cascade (see Ch. 3). In all cases, the pathways eventually lead to transcription of the genes that control the cell cycle.

THE CELL CYCLE

The cell cycle is an ordered series of events consisting of several sequential phases: G_1, S, G_2 and M (see Fig. 5.1).

- M is the phase of m̲itosis
- S is the phase of DNA s̲ynthesis
- G_1 is the gap between the mitosis that gave rise to the cell and the S phase; during G_1, the cell is preparing for DNA synthesis
- G_2 is the gap between S phase and the mitosis that will give rise to two daughter cells; during G_2, the cell is preparing for the mitotic division into two daughter cells.

Cell division requires the controlled timing of two critical events of the cell cycle: S phase (DNA replication) and M phase (mitosis). Entry into each of these phases is carefully regulated, and there are thus two 'check points'[2] (restriction points) in the cycle: one at the start of S and one at the start of M. DNA damage results in the cycle being stopped at one or other of these. The integrity of the check points is critical for the maintenance of genetic stability (explained below), and failure of the check points to stop the cycle when it is appropriate to do so is a hallmark of cancer.

---

[1]In cells that are dividing continuously, G_1, S and G_2 comprise *interphase*—the phase between one mitosis and the next.

[2]Some authorities have challenged the concept of cells simultaneously being arrested at the check points and, on the basis of cell culture studies, favour a continuum model in which arrest does not occur at a defined point in the cycle.

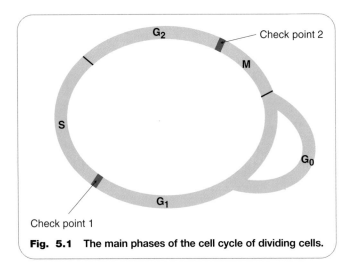

Fig. 5.1 **The main phases of the cell cycle of dividing cells.**

In the adult, most cells are not constantly dividing; most spend a varying amount of time in a quiescent phase outside the cycle as it were, in the phase termed G_0 (Fig. 5.1). (Note that G_0 means 'G nought', not the word 'Go'.) Neurons and skeletal muscle cells spend all their lifetime in G_0; bone marrow cells and the lining cells of the gastrointestinal tract divide daily.

Quiescent cells can be activated into G_1 by chemical stimuli associated with damage; for example, a quiescent skin cell can be stimulated by a wound into dividing and repairing the lesion. The impetus for a cell to start off on the cell cycle (i.e. to move from G_0 into G_1) can be provided by several stimuli, the most important being growth factor action though G-protein–coupled receptors, which can also stimulate cell proliferation. The action of ligands on G-protein–coupled receptors (dealt with in Ch. 4) can also stimulate the cell to embark on the cell cycle (Johnson & Walker, 1999; Cummings et al., 2004).

Growth factors stimulate the production of signal transducers of two types:

- positive regulators of the cell cycle that control the changes necessary for cell division
- negative regulators that control the positive regulators.

The maintenance of normal cell numbers in tissues and organs requires that there be a balance between the positive regulatory forces and the negative regulatory forces. Apoptosis also has a role in the control of cell numbers (see below).

POSITIVE REGULATORS OF THE CELL CYCLE

The cycle is initiated when a growth factor acts on a quiescent cell, provoking it to divide. One of the main actions of a growth factor is to stimulate production of the cell cycle regulators, which are coded for by the delayed response genes (explained below).

The main components of the control system that determines progress through the cycle are two families of proteins: *cyclins*[3] and *cyclin-dependent kinases (cdks)*. Recently, another family of kinases—Polo-like kinases (Plks)—have been shown to play an important role in the cell cycle (see below).

The cdks phosphorylate various proteins (e.g. enzymes)—activating some and inhibiting others—to coordinate their activities.

Sequential functioning of several different cdks activates the processes that promote progress through the phases of the cycle. Each cdk is inactive until it binds to a cyclin, the binding enabling the cdk to phosphorylate the protein(s) necessary for a particular step in the cycle. It is the cyclin that determines which protein(s) are phosphorylated. After the phosphorylation event has taken place, the cyclin is degraded (Fig. 5.2) by the ubiquitin/protease system. This involves several enzymes (E_1, E_2, E_3) acting sequentially to add small molecules of ubiquitin to the cyclin, with the resulting ubiquitin polymer acting as an 'address label' that directs the cyclin to the proteasome where it is degraded.

There are eight main groups of cyclins. Those important in the control of the cell cycle are cyclins A, B, D and E. Each cyclin is associated with and activates particular cdk(s). Cyclin A activates cdks 1 and 2; cyclin B, cdk 1; cyclin D, cdks 4 and 6; and cyclin E, cdk 2. Precise timing of each activity is essential, and many cycle proteins are degraded after they have carried out their functions. The actions of the cyclin/cdk complexes in the cell cycle are depicted in Figure 5.3.

---

[3]The name 'cyclin' comes from the fact that these proteins undergo a cycle of synthesis and breakdown during each cell division.

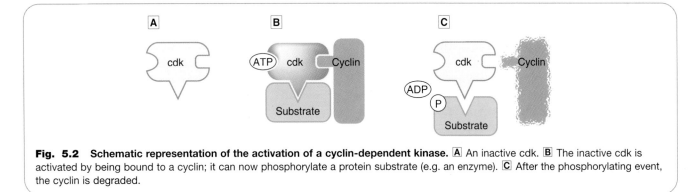

Fig. 5.2 **Schematic representation of the activation of a cyclin-dependent kinase.** **A** An inactive cdk. **B** The inactive cdk is activated by being bound to a cyclin; it can now phosphorylate a protein substrate (e.g. an enzyme). **C** After the phosphorylating event, the cyclin is degraded.

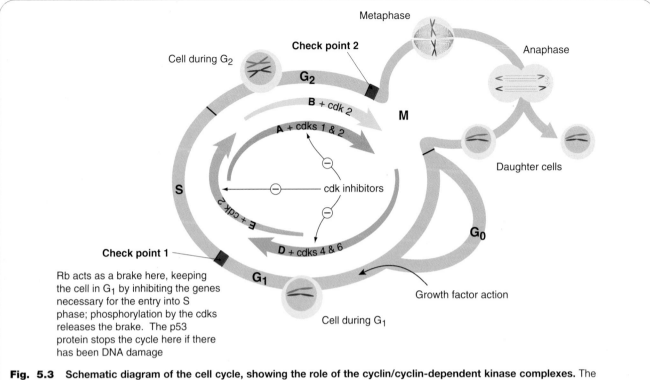

Check point 1 —

Rb acts as a brake here, keeping the cell in G_1 by inhibiting the genes necessary for the entry into S phase; phosphorylation by the cdks releases the brake. The p53 protein stops the cycle here if there has been DNA damage

Fig. 5.3   Schematic diagram of the cell cycle, showing the role of the cyclin/cyclin-dependent kinase complexes. The processes outlined in the cycle occur inside a cell such as the one shown in Figure 5.4. A quiescent cell (in G_0 phase), when stimulated to divide by growth factors, is propelled into G_1 phase and prepares for DNA synthesis. Progress through the cycle is determined by sequential action of the cyclin/cdk complexes—depicted here by coloured arrows, the arrows being given the names of the relevant cyclins: D, E, A and B. The cdks (cyclin-dependent kinases) are given next to the relevant cyclins. The thickness of each arrow represents the intensity of action of the cdk at that point in the cycle. The activity of the cdks is regulated by cdk inhibitors. If there is DNA damage, the products of the tumour suppressor gene *p53* stop the cycle at check point 1, allowing for repair. If repair fails, apoptosis (see Fig. 5.5) is initiated. The state of the chromosomes is shown schematically in each G phase—as a single pair in G_1, and each duplicated and forming two daughter chromatids in G_2. Some changes that occur during mitosis (metaphase, anaphase) are shown in a subsidiary circle. After the mitotic division, the daughter cells may enter G_1 or G_0 phase. Rb, retinoblastoma gene.

The activity of these cyclin/cdk complexes is modulated by various negative regulatory forces (considered below), most of which act at one or other of the two check points.

Cells in G_0

In quiescent G_0 cells, cyclin D is present in low concentration, and an important regulatory protein—the Rb protein[4]—is hypophosphorylated.

Hypophosphorylated Rb holds the cell cycle in check at check point 1 by inhibiting the expression of several proteins critical for cell cycle progression. The Rb protein accomplishes this by binding to the E2F transcription factors, which control the expression of the genes that code for cyclins E and A, for DNA polymerase, for thymidine kinase, for dihydrofolate reductase, etc.—all essential for DNA replication during S phase.

Growth factor action on a cell in G_0 propels it into G_1 phase.

Phase G_1

G_1 is the phase in which the cell is preparing for S phase by synthesising the messenger RNAs and proteins needed for DNA replication. During G_1, the concentration of cyclin D increases and the cyclin D/cdk complex phosphorylates and activates the necessary proteins.

In mid-G_1, the cyclin D/cdk complex phosphorylates the Rb protein, releasing transcription factor E2F; this then activates the genes for the components specified above that are essential for the next phase—DNA synthesis—namely cyclins E and A, DNA polymerase and so on.

The action of the cyclin E/cdk complex is necessary for transition from G_1 to S phase, i.e. past check point 1. Once past check point 1, the processes that have been set in motion cannot be reversed, and the cell is committed to continue with DNA replication and mitosis.

S phase

Cyclin E/cdk and cyclin A/cdk regulate progress through S phase, phosphorylating and thus activating proteins/enzymes involved in DNA synthesis.

---

[4]The Rb protein is coded for by the *Rb* gene. The *Rb* gene is so named because mutations of this gene are associated with retinoblastoma tumours.

G₂ phase

In G₂ phase, the cell, which now has double the number of chromosomes, must duplicate all other cellular components for allocation to the two daughter cells. Synthesis of the necessary messenger RNAs and proteins occurs.

Cyclin A/cdk and cyclin B/cdk complexes are active during G₂ phase and are necessary for entry into M phase, i.e. for passing check point 2. The presence of cyclin B/cdk complexes in the nucleus is required for mitosis to commence.

Unlike cyclins C, D and E, which are short-lived, cyclins A and B remain stable throughout interphase but undergo proteolysis by a ubiquitin-dependent pathway during mitosis.

Mitosis

Mitosis is a continuous process but can be considered to consist of four stages.

- *Prophase.* The duplicated chromosomes (which have up to this point formed a tangled mass filling the nucleus) condense, each now consisting of two daughter chromatids (the original chromosome and a copy). These are released into the cytoplasm as the nuclear membrane disintegrates.
- *Metaphase.* The chromosomes are aligned at the equator (see Fig. 5.3).

- *Anaphase.* A specialised device, the *mitotic apparatus*, captures the chromosomes and draws them to opposite poles of the dividing cell (see Fig. 5.3).
- *Telophase.* A nuclear membrane forms round each set of chromosomes. Finally, the cytoplasm divides between the two forming daughter cells. Each daughter cell will be in G₀ phase and will remain there unless stimulated into G₁ phase as described above.

During metaphase, the cyclin A and B complexes phosphorylate cytoskeletal proteins, histones, and possibly components of the spindle (the microtubules along which the chromatids are pulled during metaphase).

Polo-like kinases

Polo-like kinases (Plks) are a family of kinases that are involved in the regulation of the cell cycle (Dai, 2005). There are four Plks in humans: Plks 1–4. In G₁, they are active in centrosome dynamics and the DNA damage response; their action is important at the point where the cell enters the mitotic phase, they play a part in spindle assembly, their action peaks cyclically during anaphase–telophase, and they have a role in postmitotic function when the cell passes into the G₀ phase.

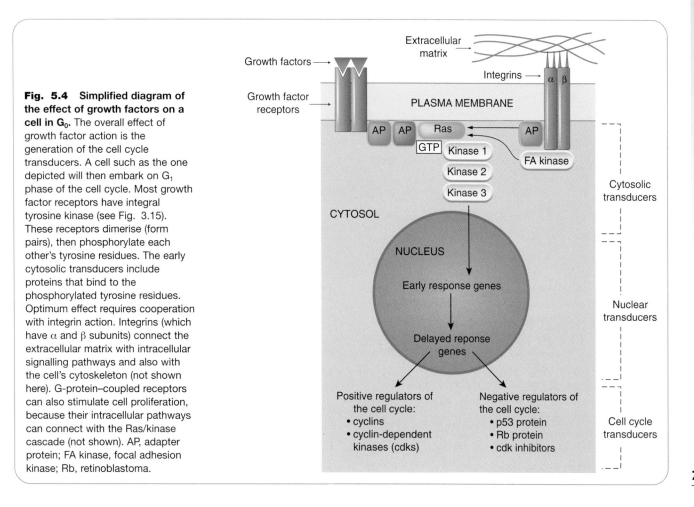

Fig. 5.4 Simplified diagram of the effect of growth factors on a cell in G₀. The overall effect of growth factor action is the generation of the cell cycle transducers. A cell such as the one depicted will then embark on G₁ phase of the cell cycle. Most growth factor receptors have integral tyrosine kinase (see Fig. 3.15). These receptors dimerise (form pairs), then phosphorylate each other's tyrosine residues. The early cytosolic transducers include proteins that bind to the phosphorylated tyrosine residues. Optimum effect requires cooperation with integrin action. Integrins (which have α and β subunits) connect the extracellular matrix with intracellular signalling pathways and also with the cell's cytoskeleton (not shown here). G-protein–coupled receptors can also stimulate cell proliferation, because their intracellular pathways can connect with the Ras/kinase cascade (not shown). AP, adapter protein; FA kinase, focal adhesion kinase; Rb, retinoblastoma.

NEGATIVE REGULATORS OF THE CELL CYCLE

One of the main negative regulators has already been mentioned—the Rb protein that holds the cycle in check while it is hypophosphorylated.

Another negative regulatory mechanism is the action of the inhibitors of the cdks. These bind to and inhibit the action of the complexes, their main action being at check point 1.

There are two families of inhibitors:

- the CIP family (cdk inhibitory proteins, also termed KIP or kinase inhibitory proteins)—p21, p27 and p57
- the Ink family (inhibitors of kinases)—p16, p19, and p15.

The action of p21 (explained below) serves as an example of the role of a cyclin/cdk inhibitor. Protein p21 is under the control of the *p53* gene—a particularly important negative regulator that operates at check point 1.

Inhibition of the cycle at check point 1

The *p53* gene has been called the 'guardian of the genome'. It codes for a protein transcription factor—the *p53 protein*. In normal healthy cells, the steady-state concentration of the p53 protein is low. But when there is DNA damage, the protein accumulates and activates the transcription of several genes, one of which codes for p21. Protein p21 inactivates cyclin/cdk complexes, thus preventing Rb phosphorylation, which means that the cycle is arrested at check point 1. This allows for DNA repair. If the repair is successful, the cycle proceeds past check point 1 into S phase. If the repair is unsuccessful, the p53 gene triggers apoptosis—cell suicide (see below).

Inhibition of the cycle at check point 2

There is evidence that DNA damage can result in the cycle being stopped at check point 2, but the mechanisms involved are less clear than those at check point 1. Inhibition of the accumulation of cyclin B/cdk complex in the nucleus seems to be a factor.

For more detail on the control of the cell cycle, see Swanton (2004).

INTERACTIONS BETWEEN CELLS, GROWTH FACTORS AND THE EXTRACELLULAR MATRIX

During cell proliferation, there is integrated interplay between growth factors, cells, the extracellular matrix, and the matrix metalloproteinases. The extracellular matrix supplies the supporting framework for the cells of the body and is secreted by the cells themselves. It also profoundly influences cell behaviour through the cell's integrins (see below). Matrix expression is regulated by the action on the cell of growth factors and cytokines (see Chang & Werb, 2001; McCawley & Matrisian, 2001). The activation status of some growth factors is, in turn, determined by the matrix, because they are sequestered by inter-action with matrix components and released by enzymes (e.g. metalloproteinases, see below) secreted by the cells.

It is clear that the action of growth factors—which act through receptor tyrosine kinases or receptor-coupled kinases (see Ch. 3)

The cell cycle 🔑

- The term *cell cycle* refers to the sequence of events that take place within a cell as it tools up for division.
- The phases of the cell cycle are:
  G_1—preparation for DNA synthesis
  S—DNA synthesis
  G_2—preparation for division
  mitosis—division into two daughter cells.
- Growth factor action stimulates a quiescent cell—said to be in G_0 (G nought)—to divide, i.e. to start on G_1 phase.
- In G_0 phase, a hypophosphorylated protein, coded for by the *Rb* gene, holds the cycle in check by inhibiting expression of critical factors necessary for DNA replication.
- Progress through the cycle is controlled by specific kinases (cyclin-dependent kinases, cdks) that are activated by binding to proteins termed *cyclins*.
- Four main cyclin/cdk complexes involving cyclins D, E, A and B drive the cycle; the first complex, cyclin D/cdk, releases the Rb protein–mediated inhibition.
- Various families of proteins act as cdk inhibitors. Important is protein p21, which is expressed when DNA damage causes transcription of gene *p53*. The p21 protein stops the cycle at check point 1.

---

initiating the cell cycle (see above)—is a fundamental part of these processes. There are numerous growth factors, important examples being fibroblast growth factor (FGF), epidermal growth factor (EGF), platelet-dependent growth factor (PDGF), vascular endothelial growth factor (VEGF) and transforming growth factor (TGF-β). (But as pointed out above, there is also a role for ligands acting on G-protein–coupled receptors in cell cycle initiation; see also Ch. 3.)

The main components of the extracellular matrix are as follows.

- *Proteoglycans*. These have a growth-regulating role, in part by functioning as a reservoir of sequestrated growth factors (as specified above). Some proteoglycans are associated with the cell surface, where they help to bind cells to the matrix (Kresse & Schönherr, 2001).
- *Collagens*. These are the main proteins of the extracellular matrix.
- *Adhesive proteins* (e.g. fibronectin). These link the various elements of the matrix together, and also form links between the cells and the matrix through integrins on the cells (see below).

THE ROLE OF INTEGRINS

Integrins are transmembrane receptors, with α and β subunits, that on interaction with the extracellular matrix elements outside the cell (e.g. fibronectin) mediate various cell responses, such as cytoskeletal rearrangement (not considered here) and coregulation of growth factor function. Intracellular signalling by both growth factor receptors and integrins is important for optimal cell proliferation (Fig. 5.4). Integrin stimulation activates an intracellular transduction pathway, which, through an adapter protein and an enzyme (focal adhesion kinase), can activate the kinase cascade that forms part of the growth factor signalling pathway (Fig. 5.4). Cross-talk between the integrin and growth factor pathways occurs by several other means as well. Autophosphorylation of growth factor receptors (Ch. 3) is enhanced by integrin activation, and integrin-mediated adhesion to the extracellular matrix (Fig. 5.4) not only suppresses the concentrations of cdk inhibitors p21 and p27 but is required for the expression of cyclins A and D, and therefore for the progression of the cell cycle. Furthermore, integrin action stimulates apoptosis-inhibiting signals (see below), further facilitating growth factor action. See reviews by Schwartz & Baron (1999), Dedhar (2000), Eliceiri (2001), and Schwartz (2001).

THE ROLE OF MATRIX METALLOPROTEINASES

Degradation of the extracellular matrix by metalloproteinases is necessary during the growth, repair and remodelling of tissues. These enzymes are secreted as inactive precursors by local cells. When growth factors stimulate a cell to enter the cell cycle, they also stimulate the secretion of metalloproteinases, which then sculpt the matrix—producing the local changes necessary for the resulting increase in cell numbers. Metalloproteinases in turn play a part in releasing growth factors from the matrix as described above and, in some cases (e.g. interleukin IL-1β), in processing them from precursor to active form.

The action of these enzymes is regulated by TIMPS (tissue inhibitors of metalloproteinases), which are also secreted by local cells.

In addition to the physiological function outlined above, metalloproteinases are involved in the tissue destruction that occurs in various diseases, such as rheumatoid arthritis, osteoarthritis, periodontitis, macular degeneration, and myocardial restenosis. They also have a critical role in the growth, invasion and metastasis of tumours etc. See reviews by Chang & Werb (2001), McCawley & Matrisian (2001), Sternlicht & Werb (2001), Von Adrian & Engelhardt (2003) and Skiles et al. (2004).

ANGIOGENESIS

Angiogenesis, which normally accompanies cell proliferation, is the formation of new capillaries from existing small blood vessels. Angiogenic stimuli, in the context of cell proliferation, include the action of various growth factors and cytokines, in particular VEGF. The sequence of events is as follows.

1. VEGF induces nitric oxide and also the expression of proteases (e.g. metalloproteinases). Nitric oxide (see Ch. 17) causes local vasodilatation; and the proteases degrade the local basement membrane and the local matrix, and they also mobilise further growth factors from the matrix.

> **Interactions between cells, growth factors and the matrix** 🔑
>
> - Cells are embedded in the extracellular matrix (ECM), which is secreted by the cells themselves.
> - The ECM profoundly influences the cells through the cells' integrins; it also forms a store of growth factors by sequestering them.
> - Integrins are transmembrane receptors that on interaction with elements of the ECM, cooperate with growth factor signalling pathways (this is necessary for optimum cell division) and also mediate cytoskeletal adjustments within the cell.
> - On stimulation with growth factors, cells release metalloproteinases that degrade the local matrix in preparation for the increase in cell numbers.
> - Metalloproteinases release growth factors from the ECM and can activate some that are present in precursor form.

2. Endothelial cells migrate out, forming a solid capillary sprout.
3. The endothelial cells behind the leading cells are activated by growth factors and start to divide.
4. A lumen forms in the sprout.
5. Local fibroblasts, activated by growth factors, proliferate and lay down matrix around the capillary sprout.
6. A process of 'maturation' occurs in which there is stabilisation of the endothelial layer through cell to cell binding by adherence proteins and integrin binding of the cells to the matrix.

APOPTOSIS AND CELL REMOVAL

Apoptosis is cell suicide by a built-in self-destruct mechanism consisting of a genetically programmed sequence of biochemical events. It is thus unlike necrosis, which is disorganised disintegration of damaged cells resulting in products that trigger the inflammatory response.

> **Angiogenesis** 🔑
>
> Angiogenesis is the formation of new capillaries from existing blood vessels, an important stimulus being vascular endothelial growth factor (VEGF). The sequence of events is as follows.
> 1. The basement membrane is degraded locally by proteases.
> 2. Endothelial cells migrate out, forming a sprout.
> 3. Endothelial cells following the leading cells proliferate under the influence of VEGF.
> 4. Matrix is laid down around the new capillary.

Apoptosis plays an essential role in embryogenesis, helping to shape organs during development by eliminating cells that have become redundant. It is the mechanism that each day unobtrusively removes 10 billion cells from the human body. It is involved in numerous physiological events: the shedding of the intestinal lining, the death of time-expired neutrophils, and the turnover of tissues as the newborn infant grows to maturity. It is the basis for the development of self-tolerance in the immune system (Ch. 13) and is implicated in the pathophysiology of many conditions—from cancer (Ch. 51), where there is insufficient apoptosis, to conditions in which there is disturbed or increased apoptosis, such as autoimmune diseases (Ch. 13), neurodegenerative conditions (Ch. 35), cardiovascular diseases (Chs 19 and 20), diseases of bone metabolism (Ch. 31), and AIDS (Ch. 47). Apoptosis has a role in the monitoring of cancerous change because it acts as a first-line defence against mutations—purging cells with abnormal DNA that could become malignant.

▼Apoptosis is particularly important in the regulation of the immune response and in the many conditions in which it is an underlying component. There is recent evidence that T cells have a negative regulatory pathway controlled by surface programmed cell death receptors (e.g. the PD-1 receptor), and that there is normally a balance between the stimulatory pathways triggered by antigens and this negative regulatory apoptosis-inducing pathway. The balance is important in the maintenance of peripheral tolerance, in that the receptor is up-regulated on autoreactive T cells (Okazaki et al., 2002). A disturbance of this balance is seen in autoimmune disease, in the 'exhaustion' of T cells in chronic viral diseases such as HIV (see Ch. 47), and possibly in tumour escape from immune destruction (Greenwald et al., 2002; Zha et al., 2004).

It is known that apoptosis is a default response, i.e. that *continuous active signalling* by tissue-specific trophic factors, cytokines, hormones, and cell-to-cell contact factors (adhesion molecules, integrins, etc.) may be required for cell survival and viability, and that the self-destruct mechanism is automatically triggered unless it is actively and continuously inhibited by these antiapoptotic factors. Different cell types require differing sets of survival factors, which function only locally. If a cell strays or is dislodged from the area where its paracrine survival signals operate, it will die.

Withdrawal of these cell survival factors—which has been termed 'death by neglect'—is not the only pathway to apoptosis (see Fig. 5.5). The death machinery can be activated by ligands that stimulate death receptors ('death by design') and by DNA damage. But it is generally accepted that cell proliferation processes and apoptosis are tightly connected (see below).

MORPHOLOGICAL CHANGES IN APOPTOSIS

As the cell dies it rounds up, the chromatin in the nucleus condenses into dense masses and the cytoplasm shrinks. This is followed by blebbing of the plasma membrane, and finally transformation of the cell into a cluster of membrane-bound entities constituting the corpse of the cell; this displays 'eat me' signals—surface exposure of phosphatidylserine and changes in surface sugars. Macrophages recognise these signals and rapidly phagocytose the remains. The fact that the remains are membrane-bound is important, because release of the internal constituents (enzymes, mitochondrial components, DNA fragments, etc.) into the cell's surroundings could trigger an unwanted inflammatory reaction. An additional safeguard against this is that macrophages that are engaged in the clearance of the cell corpses release anti-inflammatory mediators such as TGF-β and IL-10.

THE MAJOR PLAYERS IN APOPTOSIS

The repertoire of reactions in apoptosis is extremely complex and can vary not only between species but between cell types. Yet it could be, as some authorities have suggested, that the pivotal reaction(s) that lead to either cell survival or cell death are controlled by a single gene or combination of genes. If so, the exciting possibility exists that these genes could be attainable targets in the development of drugs for many proliferative diseases.

▼ Only a simple outline of the apoptotic repertoire of reactions can be given here. Intriguingly, an increased understanding of the critical control points of apoptosis has resulted from comparison of the process in mammals with that in the nematode *Caenorhabditis elegans*. This nematode undergoes an unvarying procedure of apoptosis in which 131 cells out of a total of 1090 die during the development of the worm, which thus eventually consists of just 959 cells. It seems that some critical control points for cell death are not all that different in worm and mammal (see Danial & Korsmeyer, 2004.). More recently, an even more interesting and potentially very fruitful approach to dissecting out the detail of the apoptotic pathways has been proposed: the use of gene silencing by RNA interference (RNAi) technology. This permits very efficient and precision silencing of gene expression and is being used to identify antiapoptotic genes (Milner, 2004). For simple overviews of RNA silencing, see Black & Newbury (2004) and Zhang (2004).

The major players are the caspases—a family of cysteine proteases present in the cell in inactive form. They do not perform generalised proteolysis; they undertake delicate protein surgery, selectively cleaving a specific set of target proteins (enzymes, structural components), inactivating some and activating others. A cascade of about nine different caspases take part in bringing about apoptosis, some functioning as *initiators* that transmit the initial apoptotic signals, and some being responsible for the final *effector* phase of cell death (Fig. 5.5).

The caspases are not the only executors of apoptotic change. Various pathways that result in apoptosis without the action of the caspase fraternity have been described. One involves a protein termed AIF (apoptotic initiating factor) that is released from the mitochondria, enters the nucleus and triggers cell suicide.

Note that not all caspases are death-mediating enzymes; some have a role in the processing and activating of cytokines (e.g. caspase 8 is active in processing the inflammatory cytokines IL-1 and IL-18).

PATHWAYS TO APOPTOSIS

There are two main routes to cell death, one involving stimulation of death receptors by external ligands, and one arising within the cell and involving the mitochondria. Both these routes activate initiator caspases and both converge on a final common effector caspase pathway.

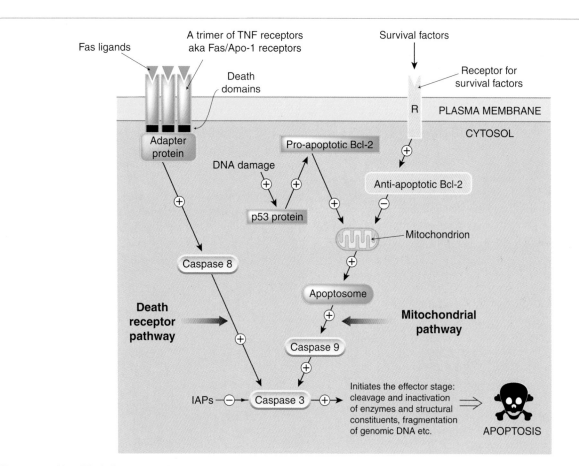

Fig. 5.5 **Simplified diagram of the two main signalling pathways in apoptosis.** The death receptor pathway is activated when death receptors such as members of the tumour necrosis factor (TNF) family are stimulated by specific death ligands. This recruits adapter proteins that activate initiator caspases (e.g. caspase 8), which in turn activate effector caspases such as caspase 3. The mitochondrial pathway is activated by diverse signals, one being DNA damage. In the presence of DNA damage that cannot be repaired, the p53 protein (see text and Figs 5.3 and 5.4) activates a subpathway that results in release of cytochrome *c* from the mitochondrion, with subsequent involvement of the apoptosome and activation of an initiator caspase, caspase 9. The apoptosome is a complex of procaspase 9, cytochrome *c* and apoptotic-activating protease factor-1 (Apaf-1). Both these pathways converge on the effector caspase (e.g. caspase 3), which brings about the demise of the cell. The survival factor subpathway (shown here faded) normally holds apoptosis at bay by inhibiting the mitochondrion pathway through activation of the antiapoptotic factor Bcl-2. The receptor labelled 'R' represents the respective receptors for trophic factors, growth factors, cell-to-cell contact factors (adhesion molecules, integrins), etc. Continuous stimulation of these receptors is necessary for cell survival/proliferation. If this pathway is non-functional (as depicted here by being shown in grey), this antiapoptotic drive is withdrawn. IAP, inhibitor of apoptosis.

THE DEATH RECEPTOR PATHWAY

Lurking in the plasma membrane of most cell types are members of the tumour necrosis factor receptor (TNFR) superfamily, which function as death receptors (Fig. 5.5). Important family members are TNFR-1 and CD95 (aka Fas or Apo-1), but there are many others.[5] Each receptor has a 'death domain' in its cytoplasmic tail. Stimulation of the receptors by an external ligand such as tumour necrosis factor (TNF) itself or TRAIL[6] causes them to get together in threes (trimerise), and recruit an adapter protein that complexes with the trimer by associating with the death domains. The resulting complex activates caspase 8, an initiator caspase that in turn activates the effector caspases (Fig. 5.5).

THE MITOCHONDRIAL PATHWAY

This pathway can be called into action in two principal ways: by DNA damage and by withdrawal of the action of cell survival factors.

DNA damage and the mitochondrial pathway

In the presence of DNA damage that cannot be repaired, the p53 protein activates a subpathway involving the p21 protein (see above) and proapoptotic members of the Bcl-2 protein family—Bid, Bax and Bak. In addition to these proapoptotic

---

[5]There are two gene families, which include 28 receptors and 18 ligands. PD-1 is a death receptor that can be induced on activated T cells, as discussed.

[6]TRAIL is tumour necrosis factor-α–related apoptosis-inducing ligand of course; what else? See Janssen et al. (2005) for discussion of a role of TRAIL. PD-L1, a ligand for the PD-1 receptor, is found on all haemopoietic cells and many other tissues, and on many tumours in mice (Latchman et al., 2004).

Apoptosis

- Apoptosis is programmed cell death, essential in embryogenesis and tissue homeostasis; it is brought about principally by a cascade of proteases—the caspases. Two sets of initiator caspases converge on a set of effector caspases.
- There are two main pathways to activation of the effector caspases: the death receptor pathway and the mitochondrial pathway.
  - The death receptor pathway involves stimulation of members of the tumour necrosis factor receptor family; and the main initiator caspase is caspase 8.
  - The mitochondrial pathway is activated by internal factors such as DNA damage, which results in transcription of gene *p53*. The p53 protein activates a subpathway that results in release from the mitochondrion of cytochrome *c*. This in turn complexes with protein Apaf-1, and together they activate initiator caspase 9.
- In undamaged cells, survival factors (cytokines, hormones, cell-to-cell contact factors) continuously activate antiapoptotic mechanisms. Withdrawal of survival factor stimulation causes cell death through the mitochondrial pathway.
- The effector caspases (e.g. caspase 3) start a pathway that results in cleavage of cell constituents, DNA, cytoskeletal components, enzymes, etc. This reduces the cell to a cluster of membrane-bound entities that are eventually phagocytosed by macrophages.

individuals, this family has antiapoptotic members.[7] They meet at the surface of mitochondria and compete with each other. The proapoptotic branch of the family (e.g. Bax) promotes release of *cytochrome* c from the mitochondria; the antiapoptotic branch inhibits this. The released cytochrome *c* complexes with a protein termed *Apaf-1* (apoptotic protease-activating factor-1), and the two then combine with procaspase 9 and activate it. This latter enzyme orchestrates the effector caspase pathway. The three-party composite of cytochrome *c*, Apaf-1 and procaspase 9 is termed the *apoptosome* (see Fig. 5.5).

Note that nitric oxide (see Ch. 17) is another mediator that can have proapoptotic and antiapoptotic actions (Chung et al., 2001).

---

[7]Another brake on the cell death mechanisms is a family of caspase-inhibiting proteins called, you will not be surprised to learn, IAPs (inhibitors of apoptosis proteins).

Withdrawal of survival factors and the mitochondrial pathway

In normal cells, survival factors (specified above) continuously activate antiapoptotic mechanisms, and the withdrawal of survival factors can cause death in several different ways depending on the cell type. But a common mechanism is a tipping of the balance between Bcl-2 family members leading to loss of the stimulation of antiapoptotic Bcl-2 protein action, with resultant unopposed action of the proapoptotic Bcl-2 proteins (see Fig. 5.5).

Cross-talk between the death receptor pathway and the mitochondrial pathway

The two main pathways to cell death are connected to each other, in that caspase 8 in the death receptor pathway can activate the proapoptotic Bcl-2 and thus activate the mitochondrial pathway.

THE EFFECTOR STAGE CASPASES

The effector stage caspases (e.g. caspase 3) cleave and inactivate cell constituents such as the DNA repair enzymes, protein kinase C, and cytoskeletal components. A DNAase is activated and cuts genomic DNA between the nucleosomes, generating DNA fragments of approximately 180 base pairs.

THE FINAL STAGE: DISPOSAL OF THE REMAINS

When the effector caspases have carried out their functions, the cell is reduced to a cluster of membrane-bound bodies, each containing a variety of organelles. This is the corpse of the cell, which, as described above, is phagocytosed by macrophages.

PATHOPHYSIOLOGICAL IMPLICATIONS

OUTLINE

It has been briefly mentioned above that cell proliferation and apoptosis are involved in many physiological and pathological processes. These are:

- the growth of tissues and organs in the embryo and later during childhood
- the replenishment of lost or time-expired cells such as leucocytes, gut epithelium, and uterine endometrium
- the development of immunological tolerance to host proteins
- repair and healing after injury or inflammation
- the hyperplasia (increase in cell number and in connective tissue) associated with chronic inflammatory, hypersensitivity and autoimmune diseases (Ch. 13)
- the growth, invasion and metastasis of tumours
- regeneration of tissues.

The role of cell proliferation and apoptosis in the first two processes listed is self evident and needs no further comment, and their involvement in immune tolerance is discussed briefly above. But the other processes need further comment.

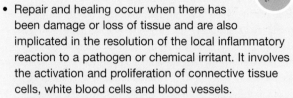

REPAIR AND HEALING

Repair occurs when there has been damage or loss of tissue; it is also implicated in the resolution of the local inflammatory reaction to a pathogen or chemical irritant. In some instances, damage or tissue loss can lead to regeneration, which is quite different to repair and is considered separately below.

In repair and healing, there is an ordered series of events involving cell migration, angiogenesis, proliferation of connective tissue cells, synthesis of extracellular matrix and finally remodelling—all coordinated by the growth factors and cytokines that are relevant for the particular tissue involved. TGF-β is a key cytokine in several of these processes. (There is considerable overlap between the inflammatory reaction and repair in terms of the cells and mechanisms activated.)

HYPERPLASIA

Hyperplasia (cell proliferation and matrix expansion) are hallmarks of chronic inflammatory, hypersensitivity and autoimmune diseases such as rheumatoid arthritis (Ch. 13), psoriasis, chronic ulcers, chronic obstructive lung disease, the processes underlying the bronchial hyperreactivity of chronic asthma (Ch. 23), and glomerular nephritis. The cells that take part and the events themselves are described in more detail in Chapter 13 (p. 205).

Cell proliferation and apoptotic events are also implicated in atherosclerosis, restenosis, and myocardial repair after infarction.

THE GROWTH, INVASION AND METASTASIS OF TUMOURS

One doesn't need to be a rocket scientist to be aware that tumour cells proliferate, but what may not be so obvious is that perturbations in the growth factor signalling pathways, the antiapoptotic pathways, and the function of the cell cycle controllers have an important role in the *pathogenesis* of malignancy. New understanding of this is leading to novel approaches to the treatment of cancer. See below and in Chapter 51 (p. 718).

Regeneration is distinct from the processes above and needs to be considered in more detail.

REGENERATION

Regeneration after damage or tissue loss implies restitution or replacement of the area so that it is identical to what was there before.

Many animals (e.g. amphibians and other lower orders) have an impressive power to regenerate their tissues, even to regrow an organ such as a limb. The essential process is the activation of stem cells—primitive cells that are multipotent, i.e. they have the potential to develop into any or most of the specialised cells in the body. Amphibians have a plentiful supply of these primitive cells in their organs and, furthermore, many of their specialised cells can dedifferentiate to become stem cells. These stem cells then multiply and retrace the pathways that generated the organ (e.g. a limb) during fetal life, proliferating again and again and

> **Repair, healing and regeneration**
>
> - Repair and healing occur when there has been damage or loss of tissue and are also implicated in the resolution of the local inflammatory reaction to a pathogen or chemical irritant. It involves the activation and proliferation of connective tissue cells, white blood cells and blood vessels.
> - Regeneration is the replacement of the tissue or organ that has been damaged or lost. It involves the activation of primitive stem cells that have the potential to develop into any cell in the body. Regeneration of a tissue or organ is rare in mammals. If a mammal is injured or has its tissue removed, *repair processes*—often with subsequent scarring—usually make good the damage.
> - It may be that repair (with rapid closure of the defect after tissue loss) is an evolutionary trade-off in mammals for the lost power of regeneration. But recent work has suggested that it might be possible to activate in mammals the original regenerative pathways—at least to some extent and in some organs.

eventually differentiating into the various cell types needed to replace the missing part.

However, during evolution, mammals in general have lost this ability and now have regenerative capacity in only a few tissues. Blood cells, intestinal epithelium and the outer layers of the skin are replaced continuously throughout life. Of the more discrete organs, there is a low degree of turnover and replacement of cells in such organs as liver, kidney and bone. This is in essence physiological renewal and is effected by local tissue-specific stem cells.

Almost alone, the liver has significant ability to replace itself if much of it is removed. It can regenerate to its original size in a remarkably short time, provided that at least 25% has been left intact.[8] And the mature parenchymal liver cells participate in this process as well as all the other cellular components of the liver.

What underlies the different regenerative abilities of mammals and amphibians is that although stem cells are known to exist in most tissues in adult mammals, they are very sparse in number, the vast majority of cells in most tissues being *irreversibly* differentiated. If a mammal is injured or its tissue is removed, *repair processes*—often with subsequent scarring—usually make good the damage. It seems that rapid closure of the defect after tissue loss (which is much more speedily accomplished by

---

[8]There is an account of liver regeneration in Greek myths. Prometheus stole the secret of fire from Zeus and gave it to mankind. To punish him, Zeus had him shackled to a crag in the Caucasus, and every day an eagle tore at his flesh and devoured much of his liver. But during the night, it regenerated and in the morning was whole again. The legend doesn't say whether the requisite 25% was left after the eagle had had its fill, and the regeneration described is unphysiologically speedy—rat liver takes 2 weeks or more to get back to the original size after 66% hepatectomy.

repair mechanisms) takes priority over regeneration. Until recently, it was assumed that this was an unalterable situation, except for a few examples, some mentioned above.

But recent work has suggested that it might be possible to activate in mammals the original regenerative pathways—at least to some extent and in some organs. Regeneration of a lost limb as happens in amphibians is manifestly not possible in humans, but regeneration of limited areas of a tissue or of a small part of an organ may well be feasible. For this to happen, it would be necessary to encourage some stem cells to proliferate, develop and differentiate at the relevant sites. Or—and this is a rather more remote prospect in humans—to persuade some local specialised cells to dedifferentiate. This can occur in some mammals under special circumstances (see below). However, it may be that repair is the Janus face of regeneration, repair being an evolutionary trade-off in mammals for the lost power of regeneration.

▼ Where are the relevant stem cells that could be responsible for regeneration processes? And what sort of stem cells are they? There are two possibilities:

- some tissues (e.g. bone marrow) in the postembryonic body have a cohort of reserve pluripotent stem cells[9] set aside during fetal life that could seed other tissues and, with the right signals, develop into the requisite tissue-specific cells
- some tissues contain tissue-specific stem cells developed during fetal life.

In the first case, the adult stem cells would have to be continuously self-renewing, with an unusual first mitotic division—one daughter cell maturing to develop into a tissue-specific cell of one sort or another when it reaches a particular tissue,[10] and one daughter cell remaining as a multipotent stem cell. The tissue-specific cells in a particular organ would presumably be one step further along the differentiation pathway and yet still be 'stem cells' undergoing, at intervals, a second unusual mitotic division.

This subject is too complex to cover here, but reviews by Raff (2003) and Rosenthal (2003) each provide a fascinating discussion of this topic. Suffice it to say here that the possibility of making use of the body's own pool of stem cells in the treatment of disease by using pharmacological means (e.g. cytokines) to coax them into regenerative service is being vigorously investigated.

Requisites for replacement of a portion of a tissue or organ

What would need to happen if, after loss, a portion of a tissue such as, for example, the liver or the heart were to regenerate? Replacement of the lost specialised parenchymal cells is a *sine qua non*, and growth factor stimulation of the local tissue-specific stem cells to start them off on the cell cycle and continue to proliferate would be one of the first requirements for this. But other essential processes would be:

- angiogenesis to supply the necessary blood vessels
- activation of matrix metalloproteinases to replace the matrix in which the new cells would need to be embedded

---

[9]Referred to as being *plastic* in their development potential, or having *plasticity*.

[10]Not all authors are convinced that there is plasticity of stem cells, i.e. that any stem cell is pluripotent and can, on being transferred to or homing on a particular organ, give rise to the specific parenchymal cells of that organ.

- interaction between matrix and integrins and fibronectin to link the new elements together.

Concomitant replacement of components of the lost connective tissue (fibroblasts, macrophages, etc.) would also be necessary.

Not all regenerative processes involve replacement of all the elements in a tissue. In the case of regeneration of a peripheral nerve after damage or cutting, the cell bodies in the spinal cord are intact and it is the sensory axons that are replaced. This is associated with the transport of retrograde injury signals from the damage site to the dorsal root ganglion neurons. These signals trigger the expression of genes controlling the regenerative process (Blesch & Tuszynski, 2004).

Is it possible to stimulate regeneration of damaged tissue in humans?

This is an important question, because drugs that could awaken the lost regenerative ability could be of immense value in numerous diseases.

To approach the question of whether it would be possible to stimulate regeneration pharmacologically, we need to consider some of the tissues in which there is little or no regeneration after damage or loss, and consider to what extent the pathways are lost and to what extent they are merely dormant but capable, with the right stimulation, of being reactivated. The central nervous system and the myocardium are taken as examples here, but the regenerative capacity of other tissues and the role of stem cells therein are also under investigation.

The central nervous system

The adult central nervous system, unlike the peripheral nervous system, has virtually no capacity to regenerate. The reasons are not fully understood, although there is some understanding of the lethal events at the site of injury. Apoptosis of cells is certainly implicated. Thus there is evidence that in the spinal cord, injury triggers increased expression of the death receptor CD95/Fas in the neurons and other cells at the damage site, and also up-regulation of the natural ligand for the CD95/Fas—which leads to apoptosis (Barthélémy & Henderson, 2004). Necrosis also occurs.

Regeneration after injury to the central nervous system is hampered by two main obstacles.

- *Inhibition by myelin-derived factors.* Three of these inhibitors have been identified, the receptor for at least one of them has been cloned, and small GTP kinases of the Rho family are believed to be involved in the inhibitory action. (For further discussion, see Ch. 35.)
- *The development of a glial scar by the astrocytes.*

In recent years, work on these aspects in experimental systems has resulted in significant advances in getting axons to regrow. This is discussed further in Chapter 35 (see also Filbin, 2003).

Heart muscle

The usual assumption is that cardiac muscle has no power to regenerate. But in a particular strain of mouse, when part of the heart is damaged by freezing, repair processes do not start up; instead, the area is replaced by regeneration within a few months. The implication of this is that in this mouse strain, the genes that direct the mechanisms for repair of cardiac muscle have been switched off and those that direct regeneration (silent in other mouse strains—and in humans) are activated.

Mice are not the only mammals to be imbued with the ability to replace areas of the myocardium: there is regeneration of heart tissue in dogs after acute heart failure. Mitosis of myocytes is seen in the normal human heart, and cell proliferation of myocytes immediately after infarction has been reported. Indeed, the sequence of events described above (under *Requisites for replacement of a portion of a tissue or organ*) has been shown to occur during the process of remodelling after myocardial infarction in rodents (Nian et al., 2004).

▼ Cytokines such as TNF-α and IL-6 are produced after the ischaemic injury of myocardial infarction and are implicated in the *immediate* events: cell death, recruitment of inflammatory cells, and repair. Their *sustained* presence has a role in remodelling—activation of matrix metalloproteinases, angiogenesis, the regulation of integrins and the recruitment of progenitor cells. TNF-α is able to self-amplify by targeting the transcription factor nuclear factor (NF) κB and initiating a positive feedback loop because NFκB activates the expression of cytoprotective genes that promote cell survival (Nian et al., 2004).

It is not certain whether the myocytes that proliferate after an insult to the heart are derived from local stem cells or from stem cells from other tissues that have homed to the heart (Anversa & Nadal-Ginard, 2002).

Some researchers are of the opinion that the sleeping regenerative pathways in humans could possibly be reawakened. If this were possible, it would be of immense therapeutic benefit because death of heart muscle underlies myocardial infarction and other serious cardiac conditions.

THERAPEUTIC IMPLICATIONS

Considerable effort is being expended on finding compounds that will inhibit or modify the processes described in this chapter, much work being aimed at developing new drugs for cancer therapy. Theoretically, all the processes could constitute targets for new drug development. Here we concentrate on those approaches that are proving or are likely to prove fruitful.

APOPTOTIC MECHANISMS

As outlined above, disrupted apoptosis is a factor in several diseases, and compounds that could modify it are being intensively investigated (Nicholson, 2000; Reed, 2002; Melnikova & Golden, 2004).

Examples of *over-exuberant apoptosis* with increase of cell death (Melnikova & Golden, 2004) include:

- neurodegenerative diseases such as Alzheimer's, multiple sclerosis, and Parkinson's disease (Ch. 35)

- conditions with tissue damage or cell loss, such as myocardial infarction (Ch. 18), stroke, and spinal cord injury (Ch. 35)
- depletion of T cells in HIV infection (Ch. 47)
- osteoarthritis (Ch. 31)
- haematological disease such as aplastic anaemia (Ch. 22).

Examples of *defective apoptosis* (Melnikova & Golden, 2004) include:

- cancer evasion of the immune response and resistance to cancer chemotherapy (Ch. 51)
- autoimmune/inflammatory diseases such as myasthenia gravis, rheumatoid arthritis (Chs 13 and 14), and bronchial asthma (Ch. 23)
- viral infections with ineffective eradication of virus-infected cells (Ch. 47).

Potential apoptosis-modulating compounds are being actively investigated (see Cummings et al., 2004; Melnikova & Golden, 2004). Here we can only outline some of the more important approaches.

Promoters of apoptosis

The Bcl-2 family as a target for new drugs
The Bcl-2 protein is oncogenic because it inhibits apoptosis and increases resistance to cancer chemotherapy; other antiapoptotic members of the Bcl-2 family are Bcl-x_L and Mcl-1. These are all current targets for anticancer drugs.

▼ An antisense compound against Bcl-2 (oblimersen) is in phase III trial for multiple myeloma and leukaemia. Investigations of antisense compounds against Mcl-1 are in progress (Melnikova & Golden, 2004).

Death receptors and their ligands as target for new drugs
Death receptors for ligands such as TRAIL (see above) are expressed on cancer cells and undergo apoptosis when TRAIL binds. Monoclonal antibodies to TRAIL are in phase I trial for cancer chemotherapy (Melnikova & Golden, 2004) and could well become important in conditions in which the immune response might need to be enhanced (Janssen et al., 2005).

▼ Viral infections are controlled largely by the action of cytotoxic T cells (see Fig. 13.3), and the persistence and chronicity of viral infections (such as HIV) is mainly due to exhaustion of T-cell cytolytic activity and cytokine production. A monoclonal antibody has been shown to block the interaction of the apoptosis-inducing PD-1 receptor and its ligand and reverse this exhaustion in mice with chronic lymphocytic choriomeningitis (Barber et al., 2006). This approach—the use of a blocking antibody to the PD-1 receptor and its like—is mooted as being a potentially fruitful new avenue to explore for the treatment of HIV, hepatitis B and hepatitis C infections—three chronic infections that affect > 500 million individuals worldwide—as well as other chronic infections and some cancers that express the ligand for PD-1(Williams & Bevan, 2006).

Indirect promoters of apoptosis
Various compounds that act on the cell survival and proliferation pathways can induce cell death indirectly; see *Cell cycle regulators as targets for new drug development* below.

A new indirect target is the proteasome, which is the part of the cell's machinery for degradation of proteins—including those involved in apoptosis. A new drug, bortemozib, which inhibits the proteasome, is on the market for the treatment of selected cancers. It causes the build-up of Bax, an apoptotic promoter protein of the Bcl-2 family that acts by inhibiting antiapoptotic Bcl-2. Bortemozib is recognised as acting partly by inhibiting NFκB action.[11]

An endogenous caspase inhibitor, *survivin*, occurs in high concentration in certain tumours, its gene being one of the most cancer-specific genes in the genome. The possibility of developing compounds that inhibit this inhibitor (IAPs) is being pursued, the object being to free caspases to induce cancer cell suicide. Drugs based on antisense approaches to survivin inhibition are being considered for clinical trial (Cummings et al., 2004).

Inhibitors of apoptosis

Apoptosis inhibitors such as the caspases are activated by stimuli produced by damaged or diseased tissue. Several **caspase inhibitors** are under investigation for use in the treatment of myocardial infarction, stroke, liver disease, organ transplantation and sepsis. One, still only with a number for its name, is in phase II trial.

ANGIOGENESIS AND METALLOPROTEINASES

As outlined above, metalloproteinases and angiogenesis have critical roles in numerous bodily processes, some physiological (e.g. growth, repair) and some pathological (e.g. tumour growth, chronic inflammatory conditions), and disturbances of these processes are implicated in many diseases. There has been a considerable amount of work done in the attempt to find clinically useful inhibitors, but this has not so far been successful. At present, only one new drug has been approved for use in cancer treatment: the antiangiogenesis compound bevacizumab, a monoclonal antibody that acts against VEGF.

CELL CYCLE REGULATORS AS TARGETS FOR NEW DRUG DEVELOPMENT

The main endogenous positive regulators of the cell cycle are the cdks. During the past decade, these have been cloned and small molecule inhibitors sought (Senderowicz, 2003).

Cyclin-dependent kinases

Several small molecules that target the ATP-binding sites of these kinases have been developed; examples are flavopiridol, roscovitine and UCN-01 (7-hydroxystaurosporine). Flavopiridol inhibits all the cdks, causing arrest of the cell cycle; it also promotes apoptosis, has antiangiogenic ability and can induce differentiation. All three compounds are in early clinical trial (see Senderowicz, 2003; Swanton, 2004).

Some compounds affect upstream pathways for cdk activation. Examples are lovastatin and perifosine.

Proteasome-mediated degradation of cell cycle proteins as a target

Bortezomib, a boronate compound, covalently binds the proteasome. Early results of a phase III trial in melanoma patients have proved promising (Richardson et al., 2005).

The growth factor signalling pathway

Of the various components of the growth factor signalling pathway, receptor tyrosine kinases, the Ras protein and cytoplasmic kinases have been the subjects of most interest, and several new drugs have been developed. Their main use is in cancer therapy, and details are given in Chapter 51 (p. 730) and Figure 51.1.

STEM CELLS AND THE REGENERATION PATHWAYS AS TARGETS FOR NEW DRUGS

The potential use of *embryonic stem cells* in the treatment of human disease is a thorny and emotionally charged topic—and is beyond the remit of this book. But that *endogenous adult stem cells* could have a therapeutic role in regeneration and repair is a possibility for the future (see above). There is some experimental evidence that cytokines and secreted proteins might be able to kick-start regeneration pathways (Bock-Marquette et al., 2004; Liberto et al., 2004). Retinoic acid, a biologically active metabolite of vitamin A, has been shown to induce alveolar regeneration in rats and mice with experimental emphysema or with alveoli disrupted by various noxious treatments (Maden & Hind, 2003).

Many researchers in regenerative medicine are reasonably optimistic that it may eventually become possible to reawaken the lost regenerative pathways at least to some extent and in some organs.

---

[11]Nuclear factor κB is a transcription factor that, among multiple other actions, is involved in the integration of many of the survival-signalling pathways. It also inhibits activation of caspase 8 by up-regulating its inhibitor, FLIP (see Fig. 5.5).

REFERENCES AND FURTHER READING

Apoptosis (general)

Ashkenasi A 2002 Targeting death and decoy receptors of the tumour necrosis receptor superfamily. Nat Rev Cancer 2: 420–429 (*Exemplary review, comprehensive; good diagrams*)

Chung H T, Pae H O, Choi B M et al. 2001 Nitric oxide as a bioregulator of apoptosis. Biochem Biophys Res Commun 282: 1075–1079

Cummings J, Ward T, Ranson M, Dive C 2004 Apoptosis pathway-targeted drugs—from the bench to the clinic.

Biochim Biophys Acta 1705: 53–66 (*Good review discussing—in the context of anticancer drug development—Bcl-2 proteins, IAPs, growth factors, tyrosine kinase inhibitors, and assays for apoptosis-inducing drugs*)

Danial N N, Korsmeyer S J 2004 Cell death: critical control points. Cell 116: 205–219 (*Definitive review of the biology and control of apoptosis; includes evidence from C. elegans, Drosophila and mammals*)

Friedlander R M 2003 Apoptosis and caspases in neurodegenerative disease. N Engl J Med 348: 1365–1375 (*Reviews evidence linking apoptosis to central nervous system diseases; discusses new therapeutic strategies*)

Hipfner D R, Cohen S M 2004 Connecting proliferation and apoptosis in development and disease. Nat Rev Mol Cell Biol 5: 805–811 (*Extensive, detailed review*)

Melnikova A, Golden J 2004 Apoptosis-targeting therapies. Nat Rev Drug Discov 3: 905–906 (*Crisp overview*)

Milner J 2004 Death without stress: the stiletto approach against disease. Biochemist October: 16–18 (*Pithy article; when new gene targets for anticancer therapy are identified, RNAi provides the means for their selective therapeutic silencing*) Also in the journal are related articles that provide helpful reading: Zhang (pp. 20–23) and Black & Newbury (pp. 7–10) (*Both give an overview of RNAi*)

Nicholson D W 2000 From bench to clinic with apoptosis-based therapeutic agents. Nature 407: 810–816 (*Useful review that covers the potential of apoptosis modulation for the treatment of human disease*)

Reed J C 2002 Apoptosis-based therapies. Nat Rev Drug Discov 1: 111–121 (*Excellent coverage, useful tables, good diagrams*)

Riedl S J, Shi Y 2004 Molecular mechanisms of caspase regulation during apoptosis. Nat Rev Mol Cell Biol 5: 897–905 (*Systematic review*)

Salvesen G S, Duckett C S 2002 IAP proteins: blocking the road to death's door. Nat Rev Mol Cell Biol 3: 401–410 (*Review covering the molecular biology of IAPs—inhibitors of apoptosis proteins—and their functions*)

The apoptosis-inducing surface receptor PD-1

Barber D L, Wherry E J, Masopust D et al. 2006 Restoring function in exhausted CD8 T cells during chronic viral infection. Nature 439: 682–687 (*Antibody that blocks the interaction between the PD-1 receptor and its ligand reverses T-cell exhaustion in a chronic viral infection*)

Greenwald R J, Latchman Y E, Sharpe A H 2002 Negative co-receptors on lymphocytes. Curr Opin Immunol 14: 391–396

Janssen E M, Droin N M, Lemmens E E 2005 CD4+ T-cell-help controls CD4+ T cell memory via TRAIL-mediated activation-induced cell death. Nature 434: 88–92 (*Control of TRAIL expression could explain the role of CD4+ T cells in CD8+ T-cell help*)

Latchman Y E, Liang S C, Wu Y et al. 2004 PD-L1–deficient mice show that PD-L1 on T cells, antigen-presenting cells, and host tissues negatively regulates T cells. Proc Natl Acad Sci USA 101: 10691–10696 (*Covers down-regulation of T-cell activity by the interaction of PD-1 ligand in peripheral tissues with the apoptosis-inducing PD-1 receptor on T cells*)

Okazaki T, Iwai Y, Honjo T 2002 New regulatory co-receptors: inducible co-stimulator and PD-1. Curr Opin Immunol 14: 779–782 (*Coreceptor signalling has a pivotal role in the control of autoreactive lymphocytes*)

Rodig N, Ryan T, Allen J A et al. 2003 Endothelial expression of PD-L1 and PD-L2 down-regulates CD8+ T-cell activation and cytolysis. Eur J Immunol 33: 3117–3126 (*The PD-1 receptor ligand on endothelium can activate apoptosis of cytotoxic T cells*)

Williams M A, Bevan M J 2006 Exhausted T cells perk up. Nature 439: 669–670 (*Succinct article assesses the work on reversing T-cell exhaustion*)

Zha Y, Blank C, Gajewski T F 2004 Negative regulation of T-cell function by PD-1. Crit Rev Immunol 24: 229–237 (*Article on the balance between stimulatory and inhibitory signalling and its relevance to self tolerance and the pathogenesis of autoimmune diseases*)

Growth factor signalling and the cell cycle

Blume-Jensen P, Hunter T 2001 Oncogenic kinase signalling. Nature 411: 355–365 (*Excellent article, which emphasises oncogenic receptor tyrosine kinases and cytoplasmic tyrosine kinases; useful figures and tables. Note that there are eight other relevant articles in the same issue of Nature*)

Dai W 2005 Polo-like kinases, an introduction. Oncogene 24: 214–216 (*Short overview of the role of Plks in the control of cell proliferation; useful diagram*)

Dispenzieri A 2005 Bortezomib for myeloma—much ado about something. N Engl Med J 352: 2546–2548 (*Assesses the role of bortezomib in the treatment of myeloma*)

English J M, Cobb M H 2002 Pharmacological inhibitors of MAPK pathways. Trends Pharmacol Sci 23: 40–45 (*Lists mitogen-activated protein kinases (MAPKs) and discusses small molecule inhibitors under investigation*)

Favoni R E, de Cupis A 2000 The role of polypeptide growth factors in human carcinomas: new targets for a novel pharmacological approach. Pharmacol Rev 52: 179–206 (*Thorough coverage; outlines growth factor signalling; describes 14 growth factor families and their possible role in cancer; discusses possible drug action on signalling pathways*)

Johnson D G, Walker C L 1999 Cyclins and cell cycle checkpoints. Annu Rev Pharmacol Toxicol 39: 295–312 (*Admirably clear description of the cell cycle, detailing the progression from G_0 through the cycle, the inhibitors of cdks, the alterations seen in cancer, and therapeutic targets*)

Li J M, Brooks G 1999 Cell cycle regulatory molecules (cyclins, cyclin-dependent kinases and cyclin-dependent kinase inhibitors) and the cardiovascular system: potential targets for therapy. Eur Heart J 20: 406–420 (*Adroit overview of the cell cycle; considers cycle control in vascular disease and potential therapeutic manipulation*)

Richardson P G, Sommeveld P et al. 2005 Bortezomib or high-dose dexamethasone for relapsed multiple myeloma. N Engl Med J 352: 2487–2498 (*Results of clinical trial*)

Senderowicz A M 2003 Novel small molecule cyclin-dependent kinase modulators in human clinical trials. Cancer Biol Ther 2(suppl 1): S84–S95 (*Review*)

Swanton C 2004 Cell-cycle targeted therapies. Lancet 5: 27–36 (*Definitive review of the protein families controlling the cell cycle and their alterations in malignancy as targets for new drugs*)

Talapatra S, Thompson C B 2001 Growth factor signaling in cell survival: implications for cancer treatment. J Pharmacol Exp Ther 298: 873–878 (*Succinct overview of death receptor–induced apoptosis, the role of growth factors in preventing it, and potential drugs*)

Integrins, extracellular matrix, metalloproteinases, and angiogenesis

Carmeliet P, Jain R K 2000 Angiogenesis in cancer and other diseases. Nature 407: 249–257 (*Gives details of mechanisms involved in angiogenesis; lists biological activators and inhibitors, and agents in clinical trials; excellent figures*)

Chang C, Werb Z 2001 The many faces of metalloproteinases: cell growth, invasion, angiogenesis and metastasis. Trends Cell Biol 11: S37–S43 (*Covers the role of matrix metalloproteinases in cell proliferation, the release of growth regulators, and angiogenesis*)

Dedhar S 2000 Cell–substrate interactions and signaling through ILK. Curr Opin Cell Biol 12: 250–256 (*Discusses the role of integrin-linked kinase in the cross-talk between integrin and growth factor signalling for cell cycle progression and cell growth*)

Dimmler S 2005 Platelet-derived growth factor CC—a clinically useful angiogenic factor at last? N Engl J Med 352: 1815–1816 (*Pithy article; clear diagram*)

Eliceiri B P 2001 Integrin and growth factor receptor cross-talk. Circ Res 89: 1104–1110 (*Gives experimental evidence for cooperation between integrins and growth factors in cell growth and angiogenesis*)

Ferrara N, Hillan K J, Gerber H P, Novotny W 2004 Discovery and development of bevacizumab, an anti-VEGF antibody for treating cancer. Nat Rev Drug Discov 3: 391–400 (*Comprehensive coverage of the discovery and development of bevacizumab, an angiogenesis inhibitor*)

Griffioen A, Molema G 2000 Angiogenesis: potentials for pharmacologic intervention in the treatment of cancer, cardiovascular diseases and chronic inflammation. Pharmacol Rev 52: 237–268 (*Comprehensive review covering virtually all aspects of angiogenesis and the potential methods of modifying it*)

Kresse H, Schönherr E 2001 Proteoglycans of the extracellular matrix and growth control. J Cell Physiol 189: 266–274 (*Describes how proteoglycans can affect cell growth directly and through modulation of growth factor activities*)

McCawley L J, Matrisian L M 2001 Matrix metalloproteinases: they're not just for matrix anymore. Curr Opin Cell Biol 13: 534–540 (*Succinct coverage; discusses matrix and non-matrix metalloproteinase substrates involved in cell growth, apoptosis or tumour progression*)

Schwartz M A 2001 Integrin signalling revisited. Trends Cell Biol 11: 466–470 (*Good readable review*)

Schwartz M A, Baron V 1999 Interactions between mitogenic stimuli, or a thousand and one connections. Curr Opin Cell Biol 11: 197–202 (*Discusses cross-talk between integrins, G-protein–coupled receptors and tyrosine kinase receptors in cell proliferation*)

Skiles J W, Gonnella N C, Jeng A Y 2004 The design, structure and clinical update of small molecular weight matrix metalloproteinase inhibitors. Curr Med Chem 11: 2911–2977 (*Results of trials with early matrix metalloproteinases were disappointing; the authors discuss the proposed usefulness of matrix metalloproteinase inhibitors and review newly patented drugs*)

Sternlicht M D, Werb Z 2001 How matrix metalloproteinases regulate cell behaviour. Annu Rev Cell Dev Biol 17: 463–516 (*Comprehensive review of the regulation of metalloproteinases, their regulation of cell signalling, and their role in development and disease*)

Von Adrian U H, Engelhardt B 2003 α_4 Integrins as therapeutic targets in autoimmune disease. N Engl J Med 348: 68–72 (*Describes physiological and pathological functions of α_4 integrins (with good diagram), and a recombinant antibody against α_4 integrins in clinical trial for multiple sclerosis and Crohn's disease*)

Regeneration and repair

Anversa P, Nadal-Ginard B 2002 Myocyte renewal and ventricular remodeling. Nature 415: 240–243 (*Discusses promising results of animal experiments*)

Barthélémy C, Henderson C 2004 Spinal cord alive and kicking. Nat Med 10: 229–340 (*Discusses the significance for axonal regeneration of blocking a death receptor; lucid précis of a more detailed article in the same journal*)

Blesch A, Tuszynski M H 2004 Nucleus hears the axon's pain. Nat Med 10: 236–237 (*Brief discussion of importins—proteins that transport injury signals from axon to nucleus—in the context of enhancing regeneration in the central nervous system*)

Bock-Marquette I, Saxena A et al. 2004 Thymosin β₄ activates integrin-linked kinase and promotes cardiac cell migration, survival and cardiac repair. Nature 432: 466–472. (*After obstruction of the coronary artery in mice, injection of the secreted protein thymosin β₄ reduces myocyte death, scarring and heart dysfunction*)

Curt A, Schwab M E, Dietz V 2004 Providing the clinical basis for new interventional therapies: refine diagnosis and assessment of recovery after spinal cord injury. Spinal Cord 42: 1–6 (*Concise review*)

David S, Lacroix S 2003 Molecular approaches to spinal cord repair. Annu Rev Neurosci 26: 411–440 (*Endogenous axon growth inhibitors can now be neutralised; this could be the basis of new approaches to stimulate regeneration after spinal cord injury*)

Eickelberg O 2001 Endless healing: TGF-β, SMADS, and fibrosis. FEBS Lett 506: 11–14

Filbin M T 2003 Myelin-associated inhibitors of axonal regeneration in the adult mammalian CNS. Nat Rev Neurosci 4: 703–713 (*Excellent review*)

Lee D H S, Strittmatter S M, Sah D W Y 2003 Targeting the Nogo receptor to treat central nervous system injuries. Nat Rev Drug Discov 2: 872–879 (*Discusses the Nogo receptor as target for potential regenerative drugs*)

Liberto C M, Albrecht P J et al. 2004 Pro-regenerative properties of cytokine-activated astrocytes. J Neurochem 89: 1092–1100 (*Review of studies that support the view that cytokines elicit potent neuroprotective and regenerative responses from astrocytes*)

Maden M, Hind M 2003 Retinoic acid, a regeneration-inducing molecule. Dev Dyn 226: 237–244

Nat Rev Drug Discovery August 2006 vol 5 has a series of articles on nerve regeneration (*The articles 'highlight recent progress in knowledge of the molecular, cellular and circuitry, level responses to injuries to the adult mammalian CNS, with a view to understanding the underlying mechanism that will enable the development of appropriate therapeutic strategies'.*)

Nian M, Lee P, Khaper N, Liu P 2004 Inflammatory cytokines and postmyocardial infarction remodeling. Circ Res 94: 1543–1553 (*Excellent, forward-looking article on the possibility of using cytokines to improve healing and cardiac remodeling*)

Varus T J, Wickenhauser C, Kvasnicka H M et al. 2004 Regeneration of heart muscle tissue: quantification of chimeric cardiomyocytes and endothelial cells following transplantation Histol Histopathol 19: 201–209

Wilson C 2003 The regeneration game. New Scientist 179: 2414–2427 (*Very readable article on the possibility of regeneration of mammalian tissues and organs*)

Woolf C J 2001 Turbocharging neurons for growth: accelerating regeneration in the adult CNS. Nat Neurosci 4: 7–9 (*Succinct overview*)

Stem cells

Dorkin K 2002 Multilineage development from adult bone marrow stem cells. Nat Immunol 3: 311–313 (*Crisp review*)

Raff M 2003 Adult stem cell plasticity: fact or artifact? Annu Rev Cell Biol 19: 1–22 (*Outstanding review; considers a question the answer of which is important for possible regenerative therapy*)

Rosenthal N 2003 Prometheus's vulture and the stem-cell promise. N Engl J Med 349: 267–286 (*Excellent article, entrancingly written; discusses the problem of regeneration of tissues and organs*)

Sylvester K G, Longmaker M T 2004 Stem cells: review and update. Arch Surg 139: 93–99 (*Concise review*)

Method and measurement in pharmacology

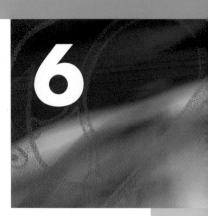

6

OVERVIEW

We emphasised in Chapters 2 and 3 that drugs, being molecules, produce their effects by interacting with other molecules. This interaction can lead to effects at all levels of biological organisation, from molecules to human populations (Fig. 6.1).[1]

In this chapter, we cover the principles of metrication at the various organisational levels, ranging from laboratory methods to clinical trials. Assessment of drug action at the population level is the concern of *pharmacoepidemiology* and *pharmacoeconomics* (see Ch. 1), disciplines that are beyond the scope of this book.

We consider first the general principles of bioassay, and its extension to studies in human beings; we describe the development of animal models to bridge the predictive gap between animal physiology and human disease; we next discuss aspects of clinical trials used to evaluate therapeutic efficacy in a clinical setting; finally, we consider the principles of balancing benefit and risk. Experimental design and statistical analysis are central to the interpretation of all types of pharmacological data. Kirkwood & Sterne (2003) provide an excellent introduction.

BIOASSAY

Methods for measuring drug effects are needed in order that we may compare the properties of different substances, or the same substance under different circumstances, requirements that are met by the techniques of *bioassay*, defined as the estimation of the concentration or potency of a substance by measurement of the biological response that it produces.

USES OF BIOASSAY

The uses of bioassay are:

- to measure the pharmacological activity of new or chemically undefined substances
- to investigate the function of endogenous mediators
- to measure drug toxicity and unwanted effects.

▼ Bioassay plays a key role in the development of new drugs, discussed in Chapter 56.

In the past, bioassay was often used to measure the *concentration* of drugs and other active substances in the blood or other body fluids, an application now superseded by analytical chemistry techniques.

Bioassay is useful in the study of new hormonal or other chemically mediated control systems. Mediators in such systems are often first recognised by the biological effects that they produce. The first clue may be the finding that a tissue extract or some other biological sample produces an effect on an assay system. For example, the ability of extracts of the posterior lobe of the pituitary to produce a rise in blood pressure and a contraction of the uterus was observed at the beginning of the 20th century. These actions were developed as quantitative assay procedures, and a standard preparation of the extract was established by international agreement in 1935. By use of these assays, it was shown that two distinct peptides—*vasopressin* and *oxytocin*—were responsible, and they were eventually identified and synthesised in 1953. Biological assay had already revealed much about the synthesis, storage and release of the hormones, and was essential for their purification and identification. Nowadays, it does not take 50 years of laborious bioassays to identify new hormones before they are chemically characterised,[2] but bioassay still plays a key role.

---

[1]Consider the effect of cocaine on organised crime, of organophosphate 'nerve gases' on the stability of dictatorships, or of anaesthetics on the feasibility of surgical procedures for examples of molecular interactions that affect the behaviour of populations and societies.

---

[2]In 1988, a Japanese group (Yanagisawa et al., 1988) described in a single remarkable paper the bioassay, purification, chemical analysis and synthesis, and DNA cloning of a new vascular peptide, endothelin (see Ch. 19).

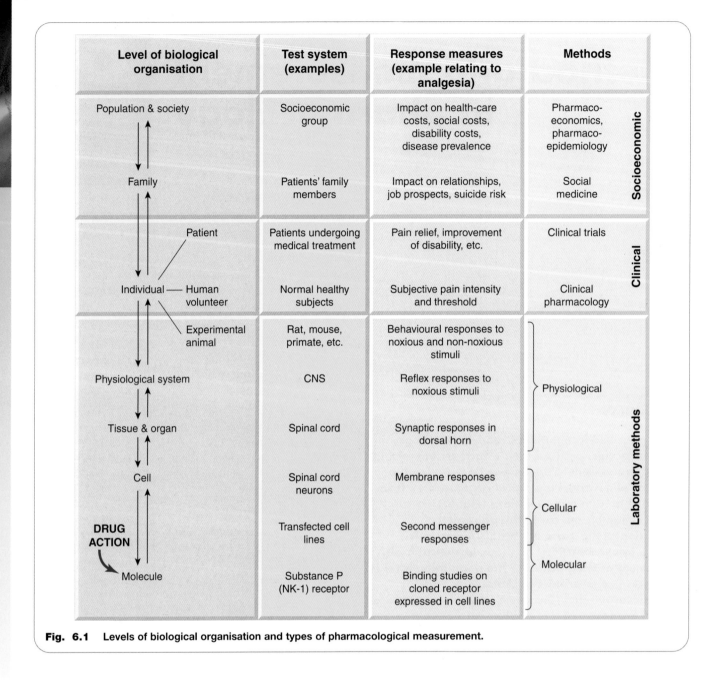

Level of biological organisation	Test system (examples)	Response measures (example relating to analgesia)	Methods	
Population & society	Socioeconomic group	Impact on health-care costs, social costs, disability costs, disease prevalence	Pharmaco-economics, pharmaco-epidemiology	Socioeconomic
Family	Patients' family members	Impact on relationships, job prospects, suicide risk	Social medicine	Socioeconomic
Patient	Patients undergoing medical treatment	Pain relief, improvement of disability, etc.	Clinical trials	Clinical
Individual — Human volunteer	Normal healthy subjects	Subjective pain intensity and threshold	Clinical pharmacology	Clinical
Experimental animal	Rat, mouse, primate, etc.	Behavioural responses to noxious and non-noxious stimuli	Physiological	Laboratory methods
Physiological system	CNS	Reflex responses to noxious stimuli	Physiological	Laboratory methods
Tissue & organ	Spinal cord	Synaptic responses in dorsal horn	Physiological	Laboratory methods
Cell	Spinal cord neurons	Membrane responses	Cellular	Laboratory methods
DRUG ACTION	Transfected cell lines	Second messenger responses	Cellular	Laboratory methods
Molecule	Substance P (NK-1) receptor	Binding studies on cloned receptor expressed in cell lines	Molecular	Laboratory methods

Fig. 6.1   Levels of biological organisation and types of pharmacological measurement.

BIOLOGICAL TEST SYSTEMS

Nowadays, an important use of bioassay is to provide information that will predict the effect of the drug in the clinical situation (where the aim is to improve function in patients suffering from the effects of disease). The choice of laboratory test systems (in vitro and in vivo 'models') that provide this predictive link is an important aspect of quantitative pharmacology. As our understanding of drug action at the molecular level advances (Ch. 3), this knowledge, and the technologies underlying it, have greatly extended the range of models that are available for measuring drug effects. By the 1960s, pharmacologists had become adept at using isolated organs and laboratory animals (usually under anaesthesia) for quantitative experiments, and had developed the

principles of bioassay to allow reliable measurements to be made with these sometimes difficult and unpredictable test systems.

Bioassays on different test systems may be run in parallel to reveal the profile of activity of an unknown mediator. This was developed to an almost baroque splendour in the work of Vane and his colleagues, who studied the generation and destruction of endogenous active substances such as prostanoids (see Ch. 13) by the technique of *cascade superfusion* (Fig. 6.2). In this technique, the sample is run sequentially over a series of test preparations chosen to differentiate between different active constituents of the sample. The pattern of responses produced identifies the active material, and the use of such assay systems for 'on line' analysis of biological samples has been invaluable in studying

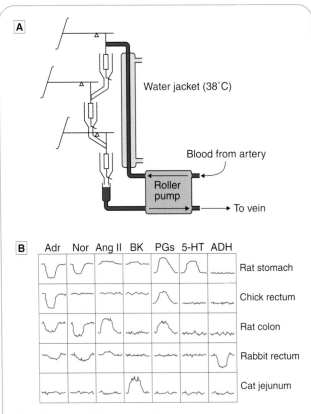

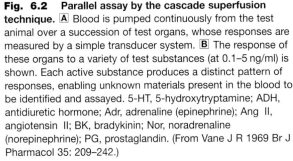

Fig. 6.2 **Parallel assay by the cascade superfusion technique.** **A** Blood is pumped continuously from the test animal over a succession of test organs, whose responses are measured by a simple transducer system. **B** The response of these organs to a variety of test substances (at 0.1–5 ng/ml) is shown. Each active substance produces a distinct pattern of responses, enabling unknown materials present in the blood to be identified and assayed. 5-HT, 5-hydroxytryptamine; ADH, antidiuretic hormone; Adr, adrenaline (epinephrine); Ang II, angiotensin II; BK, bradykinin; Nor, noradrenaline (norepinephrine); PG, prostaglandin. (From Vane J R 1969 Br J Pharmacol 35: 209–242.)

the production and fate of short-lived mediators such as prostanoids and the endothelium-derived relaxing factor (Ch. 14).

These 'traditional' assay systems address drug action at the physiological level—roughly, the mid-range of the organisational hierarchy shown in Fig. 6.1. Subsequent developments have extended the range of available models in both directions, towards the molecular and towards the clinical. The introduction of binding assays (Ch. 3) in the 1970s was a significant step towards analysis at the molecular level. More recently, the use of cell lines engineered to express specific human receptor subtypes has become widespread as a screening tool for drug discovery (see Ch. 56). Indeed, the range of techniques for analysing drug effects at the molecular and cellular levels is now very impressive. Bridging the gap between effects at the physiological and the therapeutic levels has, however, proved much more difficult, because human illness cannot, in many cases, be accurately reproduced in experimental animals. The use of transgenic animals to model human disease represents a real advance, and is discussed in more detail below.

GENERAL PRINCIPLES OF BIOASSAY

THE USE OF STANDARDS

J H Burn wrote in 1950: 'Pharmacologists today strain at the king's arm, but they swallow the frog, rat and mouse, not to mention the guinea pig and the pigeon.' He was referring to the fact that the 'king's arm' had been long since abandoned as a standard measure of length, whereas drug activity continued to be defined in terms of dose needed to cause, say, vomiting of a pigeon or cardiac arrest in a mouse. A plethora of 'pigeon units', 'mouse units' and the like, which no two laboratories could agree on, contaminated the literature.[3] Even if two laboratories cannot agree—because their pigeons differ—on the activity in pigeon units of the same sample of an active substance, they should nonetheless be able to agree that preparation X is, say, 3.5 times as active as standard preparation Y on the pigeon test. Biological assays are therefore designed to measure the *relative* potency of two preparations, usually a standard and an unknown. The best kind of standard is, of course, the pure substance, but it may be necessary to establish standard preparations of various hormones, natural products and antisera against which laboratory samples can be calibrated, even though the standard preparations are not chemically pure.

THE DESIGN OF BIOASSAYS

Given the aim of comparing the activity of two preparations, a standard (S) and an unknown (U) on a particular preparation, a bioassay must provide an estimate of the dose or concentration of U that will produce the same biological effect as that of a known dose or concentration of S. As Figure 6.3 shows, provided that the log dose–effect curves for S and U are parallel, the ratio, M, of equiactive doses will not depend on the magnitude of response chosen. Thus M provides an estimate of the potency ratio of the two preparations. A comparison of the magnitude of the effects produced by equal doses of S and U does not provide an estimate of M (see Fig. 6.3).

The main problem with all types of bioassay is that of biological variation, and the design of bioassays is aimed at:

- minimising variation
- avoiding systematic errors resulting from variation
- estimation of the limits of error of the assay result.

▼ Many different experimental designs have been proposed to maximise the efficiency and reliability of bioassays (see Laska & Meisner, 1987). Commonly, comparisons are based on analysis of dose–response curves, from which the matching doses of S and U are calculated. This analysis is much simpler if the dose–response curves are linear, which can often be achieved by using a logarithmic dose scale and restricting observations

---

[3]More picturesque examples of absolute units of the kind that Burn would have frowned on are the PHI and the mHelen. PHI, cited by Colquhoun (1971), stands for 'purity in heart index' and measures the ability of a virgin pure-in-heart to transform, under appropriate conditions, a he-goat into a youth of surpassing beauty. The mHelen is a unit of beauty, 1 mHelen being sufficient to launch 1 ship.

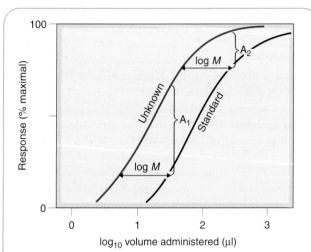

Fig. 6.3   Comparison of the potency of unknown and standard by bioassay. Note that comparing the magnitude of responses produced by the same dose (i.e. volume) of standard and unknown gives no quantitative estimate of their relative potency. (The differences, A_1 and A_2, depend on the dose chosen.) Comparison of equieffective doses of standard and unknown gives a valid measure of their relative potencies. Because the lines are parallel, the magnitude of the effect chosen for the comparison is immaterial; i.e. log M is the same at all points on the curves.

to the middle region of the $\log_{10}$ dose–effect curve, which is usually close to a straight line (see Ch. 2). The use of a logarithmic dose scale means that the curves for S and U will normally be parallel, and the potency ratio (M) is estimated from the horizontal distance between the two curves (Fig. 6.3). Assays of this type are known as *parallel line assays*, the minimal design being the 2 + 2 assay, in which two doses of standard (S_1 and S_2) and two of unknown (U_1 and U_2) are used. The doses are chosen to give responses lying on the linear part of the $\log_{10}$ dose–response curve, and are given repeatedly in randomised order, providing an inherent measure of the variability of the test system, which can be used, by means of straightforward statistical analysis, to estimate the *confidence limits* of the final result.

In practice, most bioassays will give results whose 5% confidence limits lie within ± 20%, and many will do better than this.

The 2 + 2 assay also detects whether or not the two log dose–effect lines deviate significantly from parallelism. If the lines are not parallel, which may be the case if the assay is used to compare two drugs whose mechanism of action is not the same, it is not possible to define the relative potencies of S and U unambiguously in terms of a simple ratio. The experimenter must then face up to the fact that there are qualitative as well as quantitative differences between the two, so that comparison requires measurement of more than a single dimension of potency. An example of this kind of difficulty is met when diuretic drugs (Ch. 24) are compared. Some ('low ceiling') diuretics are capable of producing only a small diuretic effect, no matter how much is given; others ('high ceiling') can produce a very intense diuresis (described as 'torrential' by authors with vivid imaginations). A comparison of two such drugs requires not only a measure of the doses needed to produce an equal low-level diuretic effect, but also a measure of the relative heights of the ceilings. More generally, full and partial agonists at the same receptor (see Ch. 2) will generate non-parallel log dose–response curves, so the difference between them cannot be expressed simply in terms of a potency ratio.

QUANTAL AND GRADED RESPONSES

▼ An assay may be based on a *graded response* (e.g. change in blood glucose concentration, contraction of a strip of smooth muscle, change in the time taken for a rat to run a maze), or on *all-or-nothing responses* (e.g. death, loss of righting reflex, success in maze running within a stipulated time). With the latter, sometimes known as a *discontinuous* or *quantal response*, the proportion of animals responding will increase with dose. The shape and slope of such a curve is governed by the individual variation between animals—the more uniform the population, the steeper the curve and the more precise the assay. With graded responses, the steepness of the dose–response curve is a property of the test system and has nothing to do with biological variation. Quantal responses can be used in essentially the same way as graded responses for the purposes of bioassay, although the appropriate statistical procedures are slightly different.

BIOASSAYS IN HUMANS

Studies involving human subjects fall into two distinct categories. The first, *human pharmacology*, focuses on using human subjects (either healthy volunteers or patients) essentially as experimental animals, for example to check whether mechanisms that operate in other species also apply to humans, or to take advantage of the much broader response capabilities of a person compared with a rat. The scientific principles underlying such measurements are the same, but the ethical and safety issues are paramount, and ethical committees associated with all medical research centres tightly control the type of experiment that can be done.

▼ An example of an experiment to compare two analgesic drugs (see Ch. 41) in humans is shown in Figure 6.4. Although many animal tests have been devised (e.g. measuring the effect of an analgesic drug on the

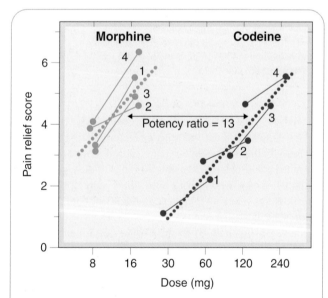

Fig. 6.4   Assay of morphine and codeine as analgesics in humans. Each of four patients (numbered 1–4) was given, on successive occasions in random order, four different treatments (high and low morphine, and high and low codeine) by intramuscular injection, and the subjective pain relief score calculated for each. The calculated regression lines gave a potency ratio estimate of 13 for the two drugs. (After Houde R W et al. 1965 In: Analgetics. Academic Press, New York.)

mean time taken for groups of mice to jump off a surface heated to a mildly painful temperature), they often fail to predict accurately the subjective relief of pain in humans. Figure 6.4 shows a comparison of morphine and codeine in humans, based on a modified 2 + 2 design. Each of the four doses was given on different occasions to each of the four subjects, the order being randomised and both subject and observer being unaware of the dose given. Subjective pain relief was assessed by a trained observer, and the results showed morphine to be 13 times as potent as codeine. This, of course, does not prove its superiority, but merely shows that a smaller dose is needed to produce the same effect. Such a measurement is, however, an essential preliminary to assessing the relative therapeutic merits of the two drugs, for any comparison of other factors, such as side effects, duration of action, tolerance or dependence, needs to be done on the basis of doses that are equiactive as analgesics.

The second type of human assay, the *clinical trial*, is designed to measure therapeutic effectiveness, an important and highly specialised form of biological assay. The need to use patients for experimental purposes imposes many restrictions. Below, we discuss some of the basic principles involved in clinical trials; the role of such trials in the course of drug development is described in Chapter 56.

ANIMAL MODELS OF DISEASE

There are many examples where simple intuitive models predict with fair accuracy therapeutic efficacy in humans. Ferrets, when housed in swaying cages, respond by vomiting, and drugs that prevent this are also found to relieve motion sickness and other types of nausea in humans. Irritant chemicals injected into rats' paws cause them to become swollen and tender, and this test predicts very well the efficacy of drugs used for symptomatic relief in inflammatory conditions such as rheumatoid arthritis in humans. As discussed elsewhere in this book, models for many important disorders, such as epilepsy, diabetes, hypertension, and gastric ulceration, based on knowledge of the physiology of the condition, are available, and have been used successfully to produce new drugs, even though their success in predicting therapeutic efficacy is far from perfect.[4]

Generalising, we can say that an animal model should ideally resemble the human disease in the following ways:

1. similar pathophysiological phenotype (sometimes called *face validity*)
2. similar causation (sometimes called *construct validity*)
3. similar response to treatment (sometimes called *predictive validity*).

In practice, there are many difficulties, and the shortcomings of animal models are one of the main roadblocks on the route from basic medical science to improvements in therapy. The difficulties include the following.

- Many diseases, particularly in psychiatry, are defined by phenomena in humans that are difficult or impossible to observe in animals, which rules out criterion 1. As far as we know, mania or delusions have no counterpart in rats, nor can we recognise in them anything resembling a migraine attack or suicidal behaviour. Pathophysiological similarity is also inapplicable to conditions such as depression or anxiety disorders, where no clear brain pathology has been defined.
- The 'cause' (criterion 2) of many human diseases is complex or unknown. For many degenerative diseases (e.g. Alzheimer's disease, osteoarthritis, Parkinson's disease), we need to model the upstream (causative) factors rather than the downstream (symptomatic) features of the disease, although the latter are the basis of most of the simple physiological models used hitherto.
- Relying on response to treatment (criterion 3) as a test of validity carries the risk that drugs acting by novel mechanisms could be missed, because the model will have been selected on the basis of its responsiveness to known drugs. With schizophrenia (Ch. 38) for example, it is clear that dopamine antagonists are effective, and many of the models used are designed to reflect dopamine function in the brain, rather than other potential mechanisms that need to be identified if drug discovery is to move on.

Bioassay

- Bioassay is the measurement of potency of a drug or unknown mediator from the magnitude of the biological effect that it produces.
- Bioassay normally involves comparison of the unknown preparation with a standard. Estimates that are not based on comparison with standards are usually unreliable and vary from laboratory to laboratory.
- Comparisons are best made on the basis of dose–response curves, which allow estimates of the equiactive concentrations of unknown and standard to be used as a basis for the potency comparison. Parallel line assays follow this principle.
- The biological response may be quantal (the proportion of tests in which a given all-or-nothing effect is produced) or graded. Different statistical procedures are appropriate in each case.
- Different approaches to metrication apply according to the level of biological organisation at which the drug effect needs to be measured. Approaches range through molecular and chemical techniques, in vitro and in vivo animal studies, and clinical studies on volunteers and patients, to measurement of effects at the socioeconomic level.

---

[4]There have been many examples of drugs that were highly effective in experimental animals (e.g. in reducing brain damage following cerebral ischaemia) but ineffective in humans (stroke victims). Similarly, recent work on substance P antagonists (Ch. 16) showed them to be very effective in animal tests for analgesia, but they proved inactive in humans. How many errors in the opposite direction may have occurred we shall never know, because such drugs will not have been tested in humans.

GENETIC AND TRANSGENIC ANIMAL MODELS

Nowadays, genetic approaches are increasingly used as an adjunct to conventional physiological and pharmacological approaches to disease modelling.

By selective breeding, it is possible to obtain pure animal strains with characteristics closely resembling certain human diseases. Genetic models of this kind include spontaneously hypertensive rats, genetically obese mice, epilepsy-prone dogs and mice, rats with deficient vasopressin secretion, and many other examples. In most cases, the genes responsible have not been identified.

More recently, deliberate genetic manipulation of the germline is increasingly used to generate *transgenic animals* as a means of replicating human disease states in experimental animals, and thereby providing animal models that are expected to be more predictive of therapeutic drug effects in humans (see reviews by Rudolph & Moehler, 1999; Törnell & Snaith, 2002). This versatile technology, first reported in 1980, can be used in many different ways, for example:

- to inactivate individual genes, or mutate them to pathological forms
- to introduce new (e.g. human) genes
- to overexpress genes by inserting additional copies
- to allow gene expression to be controlled by the experimenter.[5]

Currently, most transgenic technologies are applicable in mice but much more difficult in other mammals.[6]

Examples of such models include transgenic mice that overexpress mutated forms of the *amyloid precursor protein* or *presenilins* (see Yamada & Nabeshima, 2000), which are important in the pathogenesis of Alzheimer's disease (see Ch. 35). When they are a few months old, these mice develop pathological lesions and cognitive changes resembling Alzheimer's disease, and provide very useful models with which to test possible new therapeutic approaches to the disease. Another neurodegenerative condition, Parkinson's disease (Ch. 35) has been modelled in transgenic mice that overexpress *synuclein*, a protein found in the brain inclusions that are characteristic of the disease (see Beal, 2001). Transgenic mice with mutations in tumour suppressor genes and oncogenes (see Ch. 5) are widely used as models for human cancers. Mice in which the gene for a particular adenosine receptor subtype has been inactivated show distinct behavioural and cardiovascular abnormalities, such as increased aggression, reduced response to noxious stimuli, and raised blood pressure (Ledent et al., 1997). These findings serve to pinpoint the physiological role of this receptor, whose function was hitherto unknown, and to suggest new ways in which agonists or antagonists for these receptors might be developed for therapeutic use (e.g. to reduce aggressive behaviour or to treat hypertension). Transgenic mice can, however, be misleading in relation to human disease. For example, the gene defect responsible for causing cystic fibrosis (a disease affecting mainly the lungs in humans), when reproduced in mice causes a disorder that mainly affects the intestine.

The use of transgenic animals in pharmacological research is increasing rapidly as the technology improves. For more detailed information, see Offermanns & Hein (2004).

CLINICAL TRIALS

A clinical trial is a method for comparing objectively, by a prospective study, the results of two or more therapeutic procedures. For new drugs, this is carried out during phase III of clinical development (Ch. 56). It is important to realise that, until about 30 years ago, methods of treatment were chosen on the basis of clinical impression and personal experience rather than objective testing.[7] Although many drugs, with undoubted effectiveness, remain in use without ever having been subjected to a controlled clinical trial, any new drug is now required to have been tested in this way before being licensed for general clinical use.[8]

On the other hand, *digitalis* (see Ch. 18) was used for 200 years to treat cardiac failure before a controlled trial showed it to be of very limited value except in a particular type of patient.

A good account of the principles and organisation of clinical trials is given by Friedman et al. (1996). A clinical trial aims to compare the response of a test group of patients receiving a new treatment (A) with that of a control group receiving an existing 'standard' treatment (B). Treatment A might be a new drug or a new combination of existing drugs, or any other kind of therapeutic intervention, such as a surgical operation, a diet, physiotherapy

---

[5]With conventional transgenic technology, the genetic abnormality is expressed throughout development, sometimes proving lethal or causing major developmental abnormalities. Conditional transgenesis is now possible, allowing the mutation to remain silent until triggered by the administration of a chemical promoter (e.g. the tetracycline analogue, doxycycline, in the most widely used Cre-Lox conditional system). This avoids the complications of developmental effects and long-term adaptations, and may allow adult disease to be modelled more accurately.

[6]On the other hand, nematodes, fruit flies and zebra fish—fast-multiplying species whose genetics has been extensively studied, are very amenable to transgenic approaches and, unlike mice, can be used in automated high-throughput drug-screening assays (see Ch. 56).

[7]Not exclusively. James Lind conducted a controlled trial in 1753 on 12 mariners, which showed that oranges and lemons offered protection against scurvy. However, 40 years passed before the British Navy acted on his advice, and a further century before the US Navy did.

[8]It is fashionable in some quarters to argue that to require evidence of efficacy of therapeutic procedures in the form of a controlled trial runs counter to the doctrines of 'holistic' medicine. This is a fundamentally antiscientific view, for science advances only by generating predictions from hypotheses and by subjecting the predictions to experimental test. Very few 'alternative' or 'complementary' medical procedures, such as homeopathy, aromatherapy, acupuncture or 'detox', have been so tested. Standing up for the scientific approach is the evidence-based medicine movement (see Sackett et al., 1996), which sets out strict criteria for assessing therapeutic efficacy, based on randomised, controlled clinical trials, and urges scepticism about therapeutic doctrines whose efficacy have not been so demonstrated.

and so on. The standard against which it is judged (treatment B) might be a currently used drug treatment or (if there is no currently available effective treatment) a placebo or no treatment at all.

The use of *controls* is crucial in clinical trials. Claims of therapeutic efficacy based on reports that, for example, 16 out of 20 patients receiving drug X got better within 2 weeks are of no value without a knowledge of how 20 patients receiving no treatment, or a different treatment, would have fared. Usually, the controls are provided by a separate group of patients from those receiving the test treatment, but sometimes a cross-over design is possible in which the same patients are switched from test to control treatment or vice versa, and the results compared. *Randomisation* is essential to avoid bias in assigning individual patients to test or control groups. Hence, the *randomised controlled clinical trial* is now regarded as the essential tool for assessing clinical efficacy of new drugs.

Concern inevitably arises over the ethics of assigning patients at random to an untreated control group when the doctor in charge believes the test treatment to have advantages. However, the reason for setting up a trial is that doubt exists in the minds of many doctors that the treatment is efficacious, so for these doctors there is no ethical dilemma. If individual doctors are personally convinced that the treatment is beneficial, they should clearly avoid participating in a controlled trial. All would agree on the principle of informed consent,[9] whereby each patient must be told the nature and risks of the trial, and agree to participate on the basis that he or she will be randomly and unknowingly assigned to either the test or the control group.

Unlike the kind of bioassay discussed earlier, the clinical trial does not normally give any information about potency or the form of the dose–response curve, but merely compares the response produced by two stipulated therapeutic regimens. Additional questions may be posed, such as the prevalence and severity of side effects, or whether the treatment works better or worse in particular classes of patient, but only at the expense of added complexity and numbers of patients, and most trials are kept as simple as possible. The investigator must decide in advance what dose to use and how often to give it, and the trial will reveal only whether the chosen regimen performed better or worse than the control treatment. It will not say whether increasing or decreasing the dose would have improved the response; another trial would be needed to ascertain that. The basic question posed by a clinical trial is thus simpler than that addressed by most conventional bioassays. However, the organisation of clinical trials, with the problem of avoiding bias, is immeasurably more complicated, time-consuming and expensive than that of any laboratory-based assay.

---

[9]Even this can be contentious, because patients who are unconscious, demented or mentally ill are unable to give such consent, yet no one would want to preclude trials that might offer improved therapies to these needy patients. Clinical trials in children are particularly problematic but are necessary if the treatment of childhood diseases is to be placed on the same evidence base as is judged appropriate for adults. There are many examples where experience has shown that children respond differently from adults, and there is now increasing pressure on pharmaceutical companies to perform trials in children, despite the difficulties of carrying out such studies. The same concerns apply to trials in elderly patients.

> **Animal models**
>
> - Animal models of disease are important for the discovery of new therapeutic agents. Animal models generally reproduce imperfectly only certain aspects of human disease states. Models of psychiatric illness are particularly problematic.
> - Transgenic animals are produced by introducing mutations into the germ cells of animals (usually mice), which allow new genes to be introduced ('knock-ins') or existing genes to be inactivated ('knockouts') or mutated in the animals in a breeding colony.
> - Insertion or deletion of certain genes sometimes results in phenotypic changes resembling human disease, and is an approach increasingly used to develop disease models for drug testing. Many such models are now available.
> - The induced mutation operates throughout the development and lifetime of the animal, and may be lethal. The new technique of conditional mutagenesis is an advance that allows the abnormal gene to be switched on or off at a chosen time.

AVOIDANCE OF BIAS

There are two main strategies that aim to minimise bias in clinical trials, namely:

- randomisation
- the double-blind technique.

If two treatments, A and B, are being compared on a series of selected patients, the simplest form of randomisation is to allocate each patient to A or B by reference to a series of random numbers. One difficulty with simple randomisation, particularly if the groups are small, is that the two groups may turn out to be ill-matched with respect to characteristics such as age, sex, or disease severity. *Stratified randomisation* is often used to avoid the difficulty. Thus the subjects might be divided into age categories, random allocation to A or B being used within each category. It is possible to treat two or more characteristics of the trial population in this way, but the number of strata can quickly become large, and the process is self-defeating when the number of subjects in each becomes too small. As well as avoiding error resulting from imbalance of groups assigned to A and B, stratification can also allow more sophisticated conclusions to be reached. B might, for example, prove to be better than A in a particular group of patients even if it is not significantly better overall.

The *double-blind technique*, which means that neither subject nor investigator is aware at the time of the assessment which treatment is being used, is intended to minimise subjective bias. It has been repeatedly shown that, with the best will in the world, subjects and investigators both contribute to bias if they know which treatment is which, so the use of a double-blind technique is an important safeguard. It is not always possible, however. A dietary regimen or a surgical operation, for example, can seldom be disguised, and even with drugs, pharmacological effects may reveal to patients what they are taking and predispose them to report accordingly.[10] In general, however, the use of a double-blind procedure, with precautions if necessary to disguise such clues as the taste or appearance of the two drugs, is an important principle.

Maintaining the blind can be problematic. In an attempt to determine whether melatonin is effective in countering jet lag, a pharmacologist selected a group of fellow pharmacologists attending a congress in Australia, providing them with unlabelled capsules of melatonin or placebo, with a jet lag questionnaire to fill in when they arrived. Many of them (one of the authors included), with analytical resources easily to hand, opened the capsules and consigned them to the bin on finding that they contained placebo. Pharmacologists are only human.

THE SIZE OF THE SAMPLE

Both ethical and financial considerations dictate that the trial should involve the minimum number of subjects, and much statistical thought has gone into the problem of deciding in advance how many subjects will be required to produce a useful result. The results of a trial cannot, by their nature, be absolutely conclusive. This is because it is based on a sample of patients, and there is always a chance that the sample was atypical of the population from which it came. Two types of erroneous conclusion are possible, referred to as *type I* and *type II errors*. A type I error occurs if a difference is found between A and B when none actually exists (false positive). A type II error occurs if no difference is found although A and B do actually differ (false negative). A major factor that determines the size of sample needed is the degree of certainty the investigator seeks in avoiding either type of error. The probability of incurring a type I error is expressed as the *significance* of the result. To say that A and B are different at the 0.05 level of significance means that the probability of obtaining a false positive result (i.e. incurring a type I error) is less than 1 in 20. For most purposes, this level of significance is considered acceptable as a basis for drawing conclusions.

The probability of avoiding a type II error (i.e. failing to detect a real difference between A and B) is termed the *power* of the trial. We tend to regard type II errors more leniently than type I errors, and trials are often designed with a power of 0.8–0.9. To increase the significance and the power of a trial requires more patients. The second factor that determines the sample size required is the magnitude of difference between A and B that is

regarded as clinically significant. For example, to detect that a given treatment reduces the mortality in a certain condition by at least 10 percentage points, say from 50% (in the control group) to 40% (in the treated group), would require 850 subjects, assuming that we wanted to achieve a 0.05 level of significance and a power of 0.9. If we were content only to reveal a reduction by 20 percentage points (and very likely miss a reduction by 10 points), only 210 subjects would be needed. In this example, missing a real 10-point reduction in mortality could result in abandonment of a treatment that would save 100 lives for every 1000 patients treated—an extremely serious mistake from society's point of view. This simple example emphasises the need to assess clinical benefit (which is often difficult to quantify) in parallel with statistical considerations (which are fairly straightforward) in planning trials.

▼ A trial may give a significant result before the planned number of patients have been enrolled, so it is common for interim analyses to be carried out (by an independent team so that the trial team remains unaware of the results). If this analysis gives a conclusive result, or if it shows that continuation is unlikely to give a conclusive result, the trial can be terminated, thus reducing the number of subjects tested. In one such large-scale trial (Beta-blocker Heart Attack Trial Research Group, 1982) of the value of long-term treatment with the β-adrenoceptor–blocking drug propranolol (Ch. 18) following heart attacks, the interim results showed a significant reduction in mortality, which led to the early termination of the trial. In *sequential trials*, the results are computed case by case (each case being paired with a control) as the trial proceeds, and the trial stopped as soon as a result (at a predetermined level of significance) is achieved.

Various 'hybrid' trial designs, which have the advantage of sequential trials in minimising the number of patients needed but do not require strict pairing of subjects, have been devised (see Friedman et al. (1996).

CLINICAL OUTCOME MEASURES

The measurement of clinical outcome can be a complicated business, and is becoming increasingly so as society becomes more preoccupied with assessing the efficacy of therapeutic procedures in terms of improved quality of life, societal and economic benefit, rather than in terms of objective clinical effects, such as lowering of blood pressure, improved airways conductance or increased life expectancy. Various scales for assessing 'health-related quality of life' have been devised and tested (see Drummond et al., 1997; Walley & Haycocks, 1997), and the tendency is to combine these with measures of life expectancy to arrive at the measure 'quality-adjusted life years' (QALYs) as an overall measure of therapeutic efficacy, which attempts to combine both survival time and relief from suffering in assessing overall benefit.[11] In

---

[10]The distinction between a true pharmacological response and a beneficial clinical effect produced by the knowledge (based on the pharmacological effects that the drug produces) that an active drug is being administered is not easy to draw, and we should not expect a mere clinical trial to resolve such a fine semantic issue.

[11]As may be imagined, trading off duration and quality of life raises issues about which many of us feel decidedly squeamish. Not so economists, however. They approach the problem by asking such questions as: 'How many years of life would you be prepared to sacrifice in order to live the rest of your life free of the disability you are currently experiencing?' Or, even more disturbingly: 'If you could gamble on surviving free of disability for your normal lifespan, or (if you lose the gamble) dying immediately, what odds would you accept?' Imagine being asked this by your doctor. 'But I only wanted something for my sore throat' you protest weakly.

planning clinical trials, it is necessary to decide the purpose of the trial in advance, and to define the outcome measures accordingly.

FREQUENTIST AND BAYESIAN APPROACHES

▼ The conventional approach to analysis of scientific data (including clinical trials data) is known as 'frequentist' and is based on a null hypothesis, for example of the form *treatment A is no more effective than treatment B*. Rejection of the hypothesis implies that A is more effective than B. Suppose that a trial shows, on average, that patients treated with A live longer than patients treated with B. Conventional frequentist statistics addresses the question: *If A were actually no more effective than B, what is the probability (P) of obtaining the results that were actually obtained in the trial?* In other words, given that treatment A is no better than B, how often, had we repeated the trial many times, would we have obtained results suggesting that A is better? If this probability is low (say less than 0.05), we reject the null hypothesis and conclude that A is most likely better. If *P* is larger, the results could quite easily have been obtained without there being any true difference between A and B, and we cannot reject the null hypothesis.

If we have no prior reason for thinking that A will be better than B, the frequentist approach is perfectly appropriate, and it is the usual principle on which trials of unknown drugs are based. But often, in real life, there will be good reason, based on previous trials or clinical experience, to believe that A is actually better than B. Using a Bayesian approach allows this to be taken into account formally and explicitly by defining a *prior probability* for the effect of A. The data from the new trial, which can be smaller than a conventional trial, are then statistically superimposed on the prior probability curve to produce a *posterior probability* curve, in effect an update of the prior probability curve that takes account of the new data. The Bayesian approach is controversial, depending as it does on expressing the often subjective prior assumption in explicit mathematical terms, and the statistical analysis is complex. Nevertheless, it can be argued that to ignore altogether prior knowledge and experience when interpreting new data is unjustified, and even unethical, and the Bayesian approach is consequently gaining acceptance, although most trials are still based on frequentist principles.

The principles underlying Bayesian approaches, which are being increasingly applied to clinical trials, are described by Spiegelhalter et al. (1999) and Lilford & Braunholtz (2000).

PLACEBOS

▼ A placebo is a dummy medicine containing no active ingredient (or alternatively, a dummy surgical procedure, diet, or other kind of therapeutic intervention), which the patient believes is (or could be, in the context of a controlled trial) the real thing. The 'placebo response' is widely believed to be a powerful therapeutic effect, producing a significant beneficial effect in about one-third of patients. While many clinical trials include a placebo group that shows improvement, only a small minority have compared this group with untreated controls. A recent survey of these trial results (Hróbjartsson & Grøtsche, 2001) showed that the placebo effect was generally insignificant, except in the case of pain relief, where it was small but significant. They concluded that the popular belief in the strength of the placebo effect is misplaced, and probably reflects in part the tendency of many symptoms to improve spontaneously and in part the reporting bias of patients who want to please their doctors. The ethical case for using placebos as therapy, which has been the subject of much public discussion, may therefore be weaker than has been argued. The risks of placebo therapies should not be underestimated. The use of active medicines may be delayed. The necessary element of deception risks undermining the confidence of patients in the integrity of doctors. A state of 'therapy dependence' may be produced in people who are not ill, because there is no way of assessing whether a patient still 'needs' the placebo.

META-ANALYSIS

▼ It is possible, by the use of statistical techniques, to combine the data obtained in several individual trials (provided each has been conducted according to a randomised design) in order to gain greater power and significance. This procedure, known as *meta-analysis or overview analysis*, can be very useful in arriving at a conclusion on the basis of several published trials, of which some claimed superiority of the test treatment over the control while others did not. As an objective procedure, it is certainly preferable to the 'take your pick' approach to conclusion forming adopted by most human beings when confronted with contradictory data. It has several drawbacks, however (see Naylor, 1997), the main one being 'publication bias', because negative studies are generally considered less interesting, and are therefore less likely to be published, than positive studies. Double counting, caused by the same data being incorporated into more than one trial report, is another problem.

THE ORGANISATION OF CLINICAL TRIALS

The organisation of large-scale clinical trials involving hundreds or thousands of patients at many different centres is a massive and expensive undertaking that makes up one of the major costs of developing a new drug, and can easily go wrong.

One large trial (Anturane Reinfarction Trial Research Group, 1978) involved 1620 patients at 26 research centres in the USA and Canada, 98 collaborating researchers, and a formidable list of organising committees, including two independent audit committees to check that the work was being carried out in conformity with the strict protocols established. The conclusion was that the drug under test (sulfinpyrazone) reduced by almost one-half the mortality from repeat heart attacks in the 8-month period after a first attack, and could save many lives. The US Food and Drug Administration, however, refused to grant a licence for the use of the drug, criticising the trial as unreliable and biased in several respects. Their independent analysis of the data showed the beneficial effect of the drug to be slight and insignificant. Further analysis and further trials, however, supported the original conclusion, but by then the efficacy of aspirin in this condition had been established, so the use of sulfinpyrazone never found favour.

BALANCING BENEFIT AND RISK

THERAPEUTIC INDEX

Ehrlich recognised that a drug must be judged not only by its useful properties, but also by its toxic effects, and he expressed the *therapeutic index* of a drug in terms of the ratio between the average minimum effective dose and the average maximum tolerated dose in a group of subjects, i.e.

$$\text{Therapeutic index} = \frac{\text{Maximum non-toxic dose}}{\text{Minimum effective dose}}$$

Unfortunately, the variability between individuals is not taken into account in this definition. Even if for a particular subject there is a large margin between the maximum tolerated dose and minimum effective dose, individuals may vary widely in their sensitivity, so it is quite possible that the effective dose in some individuals will be toxic to others.

An often-quoted definition that aims to take into account individual variation is:

$$\text{Therapeutic index} = LD_{50}/ED_{50}$$

where LD_{50} is the dose that is lethal in 50% of the population, and ED_{50} is the dose that is 'effective' in 50%.

Thus defined, therapeutic index is intended to indicate the *margin of safety* in use of a drug, by drawing attention to the relationship between the effective and toxic doses, but it has obvious limitations and is therefore very rarely quoted as a number. For many reasons, it is not a useful guide to the safety of a drug in clinical use.

- LD_{50} does not reflect toxicity in the therapeutic setting, which produces unwanted effects but rarely death.
- ED_{50} is often not definable, because it depends on what measure of effectiveness is used. For example, the ED_{50} for aspirin used for a mild headache is much lower than for aspirin as an antirheumatic drug.
- Some very important forms of toxicity are *idiosyncratic* (i.e. only a small proportion of individuals are susceptible; see Ch. 53). In other cases, toxicity depends greatly on the clinical state of the patient. Thus propranolol is dangerous to an asthmatic patient in doses that are harmless to a normal individual. More generally, we can say that wide individual variation (see Ch. 52) in either the effective dose or the toxic dose of a drug makes it inherently less predictable, and therefore less safe, although this is not reflected in the therapeutic index.

In conclusion, therapeutic index is of little value as a measure of the clinical usefulness of a drug, It may have some relevance as a measure of the impunity with which an overdose may be given. Thus one reason why the benzodiazepines replaced barbiturates as hypnotic drugs (see Ch. 37) is that their therapeutic index is much greater, and they are much less likely to kill when taken in accidental or deliberate overdose. Ironically, though, thalidomide —probably the most harmful drug ever marketed—was promoted specifically on the basis of its exceptionally high therapeutic index.

Although therapeutic index expresses a valid general concept by emphasising the balance between risk and benefit, its pseudo-quantitative precision is misleading, and it provides no measure of the usefulness of a drug.

OTHER MEASURES OF BENEFIT AND RISK

Alternative ways of quantifying the benefits and risks of drugs in clinical use have received much attention. One useful approach is to estimate from clinical trial data the proportion of test and control patients who will experience (a) a defined level of clinical benefit (e.g. survival beyond 2 years, pain relief to a certain predetermined level, slowing of cognitive decline by a given amount), and (b) adverse effects of defined degree. These estimates of proportions of patients showing beneficial or harmful reactions can be expressed as *number needed to treat* (*NNT*; i.e. the number of patients who need to be treated in order for one to show the given effect, whether beneficial or adverse). For example, in a recent study of pain relief by antidepressant drugs compared with placebo, the findings were: for benefit (a defined level of pain relief), NNT = 3; for minor unwanted effects, NNT = 3; for major adverse effects, NNT = 22. Thus of 100 patients treated with the drug, on average 33 will experience pain relief, 33 will experience minor unwanted effects, and 4 or 5 will experience major adverse effects, information that is helpful in guiding therapeutic choices. One advantage of this type of analysis is that it can take into account the underlying disease severity in quantifying benefit. Thus if drug A halves the mortality of an often fatal disease (reducing it from 50% to 25%, say), the NNT to save one life is 4; if drug B halves the mortality of a rarely fatal disease (reducing it from 5% to 2.5%, say), the NNT to save one life is 40. Notwithstanding other considerations, drug A is judged to be more valuable than drug B, even though both reduce mortality by a half. Furthermore, the clinician must realise that to save one life with drug B, 40 patients must be exposed to a risk of adverse effects, whereas only 4 are exposed for each life saved with drug A.

REFERENCES AND FURTHER READING

General references

Colquhoun D 1971 Lectures on biostatistics. Oxford University Press, Oxford (*Standard textbook*)

Drummond M F, O'Brien B, Stoddart G I, Torrance G W 1997 Methods for the economic evaluation of health care programmes. Oxford University Press, Oxford (*Includes good explanation of the principles of pharmacoeconomics*)

Kirkwood B R, Sterne J A C 2003 Medical statistics, 2nd edn. Blackwell, Malden (*Clear introductory textbook covering statistical principles and methods*)

Lilford R J, Braunholtz D 2000 Who's afraid of Thomas Bayes? J Epidemiol Community Health 54: 731–739 (*Explains the principles of Bayesian analysis in a non-mathematical way*)

Walley T, Haycocks A 1997 Pharmacoeconomics: basic concepts and terminology. Br J Clin Pharmacol 43: 343–348 (*Useful introduction to analytical principles that are becoming increasingly important for therapeutic policy makers*).

Yanagisawa M, Kurihara H, Kimura S et al. 1988 A novel potent vasoconstrictor peptide produced by vascular endothelial cells. Nature 332: 411–415 (*The first paper describing endothelin—a remarkably full characterisation of an important new mediator*)

Bioassay

Laska E M, Meisner M J 1987 Statistical methods and the applications of bioassay. Annu Rev Pharmacol 27: 385–397 (*Useful references for those concerned with statistical principles of assay design and analysis*)

Animal models

Beal M F 2001 Experimental models of Parkinson's disease. Nat Rev Neurosci 2: 325–332 (*Review of the various approaches to producing valid models for Parkinson's disease, including transgenics; although

the focus is on one disorder, the principles apply generally*)

Ledent C, Veaugois J-M, Schiffmann S N et al. 1997 Aggressiveness, hypoalgesia and high blood pressure in mice lacking the adenosine A_{2a} receptor. Nature 388: 674–676 (*Examples of the use of a transgenic model to study receptor function*)

Maerki U, Haerri A 1996 Transgenic technology: principles. Int J Exp Pathol 77: 247–250 (*Short review article*)

Offermanns S, Hein L (eds) 2004 Transgenic models in pharmacology. Handb Exp Pharmacol 159 (*A comprehensive series of review articles describing transgenic mouse models used to study different pharmacological mechanisms and disease states*)

Plueck A 1996 Conditional mutagenesis in mice: the Cre/loxP recombination system. Int J Exp Pathol 77: 269–278 (*An emerging technology for allowing genes to be switched on or off during the lifetime of an animal*)

Polites H G 1996 Transgenic model applications to drug discovery. Int J Exp Pathol 77: 257–262 (*Useful general review*)

Rudolph U, Moehler H 1999 Genetically modified animals in pharmacological research: future trends. Eur J Pharmacol 375: 327–337 (*Good review of uses of transgenic animals in pharmacological research, including application to disease models*)

Törnell J, Snaith M 2002 Transgenic systems in drug discovery: from target identification to humanized mice. Drug Discov Today 7: 463–470

Yamada K, Nabeshima T 2000 Animal models of Alzheimer's disease and evaluation of anti-dementia drugs. Pharmacol Ther 88: 93–113 (*Good review of models of Alzheimer's disease, including transgenics*)

Clinical trials

Anturane Reinfarction Trial Research Group 1978 Sulfinpyrazone in the prevention of cardiac death after myocardial infarction. N Engl J Med 298: 289–295 (*Example of a large-scale clinical trial*)

Beta-blocker Heart Attack Trial Research Group 1982 A randomised trial of propranolol in patients with acute myocardial infarction. 1. Mortality results. JAMA 247: 1707–1714 (*A trial that was terminated early when clear evidence of benefit emerged*)

Friedman L M, Furberg C D, DeMets D L 1996 Fundamentals of clinical trials, 3rd edn. Mosby, St Louis (*Standard textbook*)

Hróbjartsson A, Grøtsche P C 2001 Is the placebo powerless? An analysis of clinical trials comparing placebo with no treatment. N Engl J Med 344: 1594–1601 (*An important survey of clinical trial data, which shows, contrary to common belief, that placebos in general have no significant effect on clinical outcome, except—to a small degree—in pain relief trials*)

Naylor C D 1997 Meta-analysis and the meta-epidemiology of clinical research. Br Med J 315: 617–619 (*Thoughtful review on the strengths and weaknesses of meta-analysis*)

Sackett D L, Rosenburg W M C, Muir-Gray J A et al. 1996 Evidence-based medicine: what it is and what it isn't. Br Med J 312: 71–72 (*Balanced account of the value of evidence-based medicine—an important recent trend in medical thinking*)

Spiegelhalter D J, Myles J P, Jones D R, Abrams K R 1999 An introduction to Bayesian methods in health technology assessment. Br Med J 319: 508–512 (*Short non-mathematical explanation of the Bayesian approach to data analysis*)

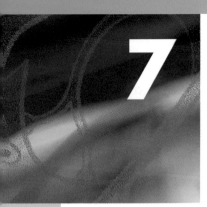

7 Absorption and distribution of drugs

OVERVIEW

In order to work, drugs need to achieve an adequate concentration in their target tissues. The two fundamental processes that determine the concentration of a drug at any moment and in any region of the body are:

- translocation of drug molecules
- chemical transformation.

In this chapter, we discuss drug translocation and the factors that determine absorption and distribution. These are critically important for choosing appropriate routes of administration, and this aspect is emphasised. Chemical transformation by drug metabolism and other processes involved in drug elimination are described in Chapter 8.

TRANSLOCATION OF DRUG MOLECULES

Drug molecules move around the body in two ways:

- bulk flow (i.e. in the bloodstream)
- diffusion (i.e. molecule by molecule, over short distances).

The chemical nature of a drug makes no difference to its transfer by bulk flow. The cardiovascular system provides a rapid long-distance distribution system. In contrast, diffusional characteristics differ markedly between different drugs. In particular, ability to cross hydrophobic diffusion barriers is strongly influenced by lipid solubility. Aqueous diffusion is also part of the overall mechanism of drug transport, because it is this process that delivers drug molecules to and from the non-aqueous barriers. The rate of diffusion of a substance depends mainly on its molecular size, the diffusion coefficient for small molecules being inversely proportional to the square root of molecular weight. Consequently, while large molecules diffuse more slowly than small ones, the variation with molecular weight is modest. Many drugs fall within the molecular weight range 200–1000, and variations in aqueous diffusion rate have only a small effect on their overall pharmacokinetic behaviour. For most purposes, we can regard the body as a series of interconnected well-stirred compartments within each of which the drug concentration is uniform. It is movement between compartments, generally involving penetration of non-aqueous diffusion barriers, that determines where, and for how long, a drug will be present in the body after it has been administered. The analysis of drug movements with the help of a simple compartmental model is discussed in Chapter 8.

THE MOVEMENT OF DRUG MOLECULES ACROSS CELL BARRIERS

Cell membranes form the barriers between aqueous compartments in the body. A single layer of membrane separates the intracellular from the extracellular compartments. An epithelial barrier, such as the gastrointestinal mucosa or renal tubule, consists of a layer of cells tightly connected to each other so that molecules must traverse at least two cell membranes (inner and outer) to pass from one side to the other. Vascular endothelium is more complicated, its anatomical disposition and permeability varying from one tissue to another. Gaps between endothelial cells are packed with a loose matrix of proteins that act as filters, retaining large molecules and letting smaller ones through. The cut-off of molecular size is not exact: water transfers rapidly whereas molecules of 80 000–100 000 Da transfer very slowly. In some organs, especially the central nervous system (CNS) and the placenta, there are tight junctions between the cells, and the endothelium is encased in an impermeable layer of periendothelial cells (*pericytes*). These features prevent potentially harmful molecules from leaking from the blood into these organs and have major pharmacokinetic consequences for drug distribution.[1]

In other organs (e.g. the liver and spleen) endothelium is discontinuous, allowing free passage between cells. In the liver, hepatocytes form the barrier between intra- and extravascular compartments and take on several endothelial cell functions. Fenestrated endothelium occurs in endocrine glands, facilitating transfer to the bloodstream of hormones or other molecules through pores in the endothelium. Angiogenesis of fenestrated endothelium is controlled by a specific endocrine gland–derived vascular endothelial growth factor (dubbed EG-VEGF). Endothelial cells lining postcapillary venules have specialised functions relating to leucocyte migration and inflammation: the sophistication of the intercellular junction can be appreciated from the observation that leucocyte migration can occur without any detectable leak of water or small ions (see Ch. 13).

There are four main ways by which small molecules cross cell membranes (Fig. 7.1):

- by diffusing directly through the lipid
- by diffusing through aqueous pores formed by special proteins ('aquaporins') that traverse the lipid
- by combination with a transmembrane carrier protein that binds a molecule on one side of the membrane then changes conformation and releases it on the other
- by pinocytosis.

Of these routes, *diffusion through lipid* and *carrier-mediated transport* are particularly important in relation to pharmacokinetic mechanisms. Diffusion through *aquaporins* (membrane glycoproteins that can be blocked by mercurial reagents such as *para-chloromercurobenzene sulfonate*) is probably important in the transfer of gases such as carbon dioxide, but the pores are too small in diameter (about 0.4 nm) to allow most drug molecules (which usually exceed 1 nm in diameter) to pass through. Consequently, drug distribution is not notably abnormal in patients with genetic diseases affecting aquaporins. *Pinocytosis* involves invagination of part of the cell membrane and the trapping within the cell of a small vesicle containing extracellular constituents. The vesicle contents can then be released within the cell, or extruded from its other side. This mechanism appears to be important for the transport of some macromolecules (e.g. insulin, which crosses the blood–brain barrier by this process), but not for small molecules. Diffusion through lipid and carrier-mediated transport will now be discussed in more detail.

DIFFUSION THROUGH LIPID

Non-polar molecules (in which electrons are uniformly distributed) dissolve freely in membrane lipids (which are liquid at body

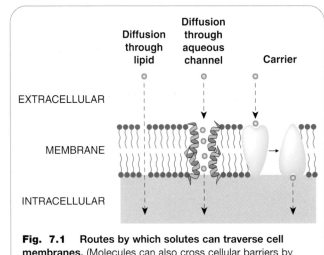

Fig. 7.1   Routes by which solutes can traverse cell membranes. (Molecules can also cross cellular barriers by pinocytosis.)

temperature), and consequently diffuse readily across cell membranes. The number of molecules crossing the membrane per unit area in unit time is determined by the permeability coefficient, P, and the concentration difference across the membrane. Permeant molecules must be present within the membrane in sufficient numbers and must be mobile within the membrane if rapid permeation is to occur. Thus two physicochemical factors contribute to P, namely solubility in the membrane (which can be expressed as a partition coefficient for the substance distributed between the membrane phase and the aqueous environment) and diffusivity, which is a measure of the mobility of molecules within the lipid and is expressed as a diffusion coefficient. Among different drug molecules, the diffusion coefficient varies only slightly, as noted above, so the most important variable is the partition coefficient (Fig. 7.2). Consequently, there is a close correlation between lipid solubility and the permeability of the cell membrane to different substances. For this reason, lipid solubility is one of the most important determinants of the pharmacokinetic characteristics of a drug, and many properties—such as rate of absorption from the gut, penetration into the brain and other tissues, and the extent of renal elimination—can be predicted from knowledge of a drug's lipid solubility.

pH and ionisation

One important complicating factor in relation to membrane permeation is that many drugs are weak acids or bases, and therefore exist in both unionised and ionised form, the ratio of the two forms varying with pH. For a weak base, the ionisation reaction is

$$BH^+ \; \overset{K_a}{\rightleftharpoons} \; B \; + \; H^+$$

and the dissociation constant pK_a is given by the Henderson–Hasselbalch equation

$$pK_a \; = \; pH \; + \; \log_{10} \frac{[BH^+]}{[B]}$$

---

[1]This is illustrated by strain and species differences. For example, collie dogs lack the multidrug resistance gene (*mdr1*) and a P-glycoprotein that contributes importantly to the blood–brain barrier (see p. 102), with important consequences for veterinary medicine because ivermectin (an anthelminthic drug, Ch. 50, p. 715) is consequently severely neurotoxic in the many breeds with collie ancestry (see Mealey et al., 2001; Neff et al., 2004).

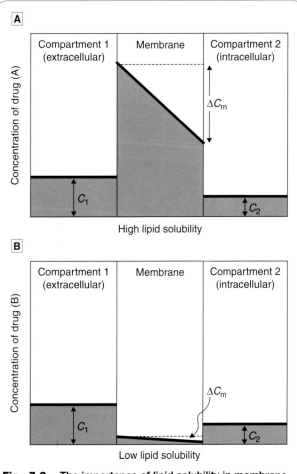

Fig. 7.2   The importance of lipid solubility in membrane permeation. $\boxed{A}$ and $\boxed{B}$ Figures show the concentration profile in a lipid membrane separating two aqueous compartments. A lipid-soluble drug (A) is subject to a much larger transmembrane concentration gradient (ΔC_m) than a lipid-insoluble drug (B). It therefore diffuses more rapidly, even though the aqueous concentration gradient (C_1–C_2) is the same in both cases.

For a weak acid:

$$AH \underset{}{\overset{K_a}{\rightleftharpoons}} A^- + H^+$$

$$pK_a = pH + \log_{10} \frac{[AH]}{[A^-]}$$

In either case, the ionised species, BH^+ or A^-, has very low lipid solubility and is virtually unable to permeate membranes except where a specific transport mechanism exists. The lipid solubility of the uncharged species, B or AH, depends on the chemical nature of the drug; for many drugs, the uncharged species is sufficiently lipid-soluble to permit rapid membrane permeation, although there are exceptions (e.g. aminoglycoside antibiotics; see Ch. 46) where even the uncharged molecule is insufficiently lipid-soluble to cross membranes appreciably. This is usually because of the occurrence of hydrogen-bonding groups (such as hydroxyl in sugar moieties in aminoglycosides) that render the uncharged molecule hydrophilic.

pH partition and ion trapping

Ionisation affects not only the rate at which drugs permeate membranes but also the steady-state distribution of drug molecules between aqueous compartments, if a pH difference exists between them. Figure 7.3 shows how a weak acid (e.g. aspirin, pK_a 3.5); and a weak base (e.g. *pethidine*, pK_a 8.6) would be distributed at equilibrium between three body compartments, namely plasma (pH 7.4), alkaline urine (pH 8) and gastric juice (pH 3). Within each compartment, the ratio of ionised to unionised drug is governed by the pK_a of the drug and the pH of that compartment. It is assumed that the unionised species can cross the membrane, and therefore reaches an equal concentration in each compartment. The ionised species is assumed not to cross at all. The result is that, at equilibrium, the total (ionised + unionised) concentration of the drug will be different in the two compartments, with an acidic drug being concentrated in the compartment with high pH ('ion trapping'), and vice versa. The concentration gradients produced by ion trapping can theoretically be very large if there is a large pH difference between compartments. Thus aspirin would be concentrated more than fourfold with respect to plasma in an alkaline renal tubule, and about 6000-fold in plasma with respect to the acidic gastric contents. Such large gradients are, however, unlikely to be achieved in reality for two main reasons. First, the attribution of total impermeability to the charged species is not realistic, and even a small permeability will considerably attenuate the concentration difference that can be reached. Second, body compartments rarely approach equilibrium. Neither the gastric contents nor the renal tubular fluid stands still, and the resulting flux of drug molecules reduces the concentration gradients well below the theoretical equilibrium conditions. The pH partition mechanism nonetheless correctly explains some of the qualitative effects of pH changes in different body compartments on the pharmacokinetics of weakly acidic or basic drugs, particularly in relation to renal excretion and to penetration of the blood–brain barrier.

pH partition is not the main determinant of the site of absorption of drugs from the gastrointestinal tract. This is because the enormous absorptive surface area of the villi and microvilli in the ileum compared with the much smaller surface area in the stomach is of overriding importance. Thus absorption of an acidic drug such as **aspirin** is promoted by drugs that accelerate gastric emptying (e.g. **metoclopramide**; see pp. 392-393) and retarded by drugs that slow gastric emptying (e.g. **propantheline**; see p. 395), despite the fact that the acidic pH of the stomach contents favours absorption of weak acids. Values of pK_a for some common drugs are shown in Figure 7.4.

There are several important consequences of pH partition.

- Urinary acidification accelerates excretion of weak bases and retards that of weak acids.
- Urinary alkalinisation has the opposite effects: it reduces excretion of weak bases and increases excretion of weak acids.
- Increasing plasma pH (e.g. by administration of sodium bicarbonate) causes weakly acidic drugs to be extracted from the CNS into the plasma. Conversely, reducing plasma pH (e.g. by administration of a carbonic anhydrase inhibitor such as **acetazolamide**; see p. 375) causes weakly acidic drugs to

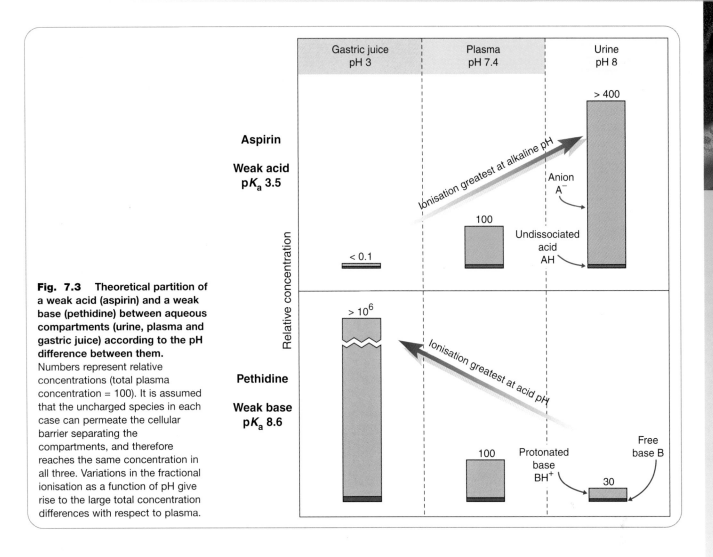

Fig. 7.3 Theoretical partition of a weak acid (aspirin) and a weak base (pethidine) between aqueous compartments (urine, plasma and gastric juice) according to the pH difference between them. Numbers represent relative concentrations (total plasma concentration = 100). It is assumed that the uncharged species in each case can permeate the cellular barrier separating the compartments, and therefore reaches the same concentration in all three. Variations in the fractional ionisation as a function of pH give rise to the large total concentration differences with respect to plasma.

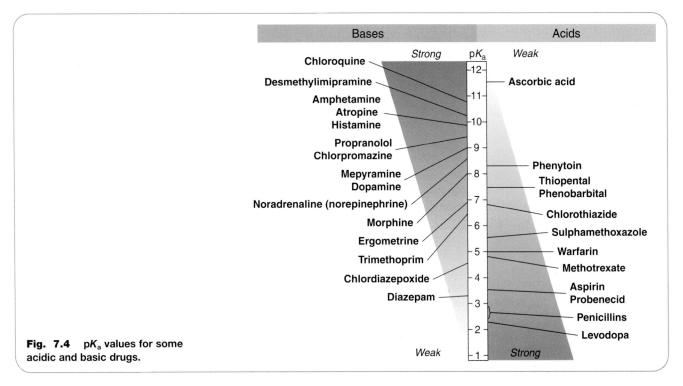

Fig. 7.4 pK_a values for some acidic and basic drugs.

become concentrated in the CNS, increasing their neurotoxicity. This has practical consequences in choosing a means to alkalinise urine in treating aspirin overdose (see p. 119): bicarbonate and acetazolamide each increase urine pH and hence increase salicylate elimination, but bicarbonate reduces whereas acetazolamide increases distribution of salicylate to the CNS.

CARRIER-MEDIATED TRANSPORT

Many cell membranes possess specialised transport mechanisms that regulate entry and exit of physiologically important molecules, such as sugars, amino acids, neurotransmitters and metal ions. Generally, such transport systems involve a carrier molecule, i.e. a transmembrane protein that binds one or more molecules or ions, changes conformation, and releases them on the other side of the membrane. Such systems may operate purely passively, without any energy source; in this case, they merely facilitate the process of transmembrane equilibration of the transported species in the direction of its electrochemical gradient, and the mechanism is called *facilitated diffusion*. Alternatively, they may be coupled to the electrochemical gradient of Na^+; in this case, transport can occur against an electrochemical gradient and is called *active transport*. Carrier-mediated transport, because it involves a binding step, shows the characteristic of saturation. With simple diffusion, the rate of transport increases directly in proportion to the concentration gradient, whereas with carrier-mediated transport the carrier sites become saturated at high ligand concentrations and the rate of transport does not increase beyond this point. Furthermore, competitive inhibition of transport can occur in the presence of a second ligand that binds the carrier.

Carriers of this type are ubiquitous, and many pharmacological effects are the result of interference with them. Thus nerve terminals have transport mechanisms for accumulating specific neurotransmitters, and there are many examples of drugs that act by inhibiting these transport mechanisms (see Chs 10, 11 and 32). From a general pharmacokinetic point of view, however, there are only a few sites where carrier-mediated drug transport is important, the main ones being:

- the blood–brain barrier
- the gastrointestinal tract
- the renal tubule
- the biliary tract
- the placenta.

P-glycoprotein (the drug transporter responsible for multidrug resistance in neoplastic cells; p. 731) is present in renal tubular brush border membranes, in bile canaliculi, in astrocyte foot processes in brain microvessels, and in the gastrointestinal tract. It plays an important part in absorption, distribution and elimination of many drugs. The characteristics of transport systems are discussed later, when patterns of distribution and elimination in the body as a whole are considered more fully.

In addition to the processes so far described, which govern the transport of drug molecules across the barriers between different aqueous compartments, two additional factors have a major influence on drug distribution and elimination. These are:

- binding to plasma proteins
- partition into body fat and other tissues.

BINDING OF DRUGS TO PLASMA PROTEINS

At therapeutic concentrations in plasma, many drugs exist mainly in bound form. The fraction of drug that is free in aqueous solution can be as low as 1%, the remainder being associated with plasma protein. It is the unbound drug that is pharmacologically active. The most important plasma protein in relation to drug binding is *albumin*, which binds many acidic drugs (e.g. **warfarin** [see p. 338], non-steroidal anti-inflammatory drugs, sulfonamides) and a smaller number of basic drugs (e.g. tricyclic antidepressants and **chlorpromazine**; see p. 551). Other plasma proteins, including β-globulin and an acid glycoprotein that increases in inflammatory disease, have also been implicated in the binding of certain basic drugs, such as **quinine** (see p. 706).

The amount of a drug that is bound to protein depends on three factors:

- the concentration of free drug
- its affinity for the binding sites
- the concentration of protein.

As a first approximation, the binding reaction can be regarded as a simple association of the drug molecules with a finite population of binding sites, exactly analogous to drug–receptor binding (see Ch. 2).

Movement of drugs across cellular barriers

- To traverse cellular barriers (e.g. gastrointestinal mucosa, renal tubule, blood–brain barrier, placenta), drugs have to cross lipid membranes.
- Drugs cross lipid membranes mainly (a) by passive diffusional transfer and (b) by carrier-mediated transfer.
- The main factor that determines the rate of passive diffusional transfer across membranes is a drug's lipid solubility. Molecular weight is less important.
- Many drugs are weak acids or weak bases; their state of ionisation varies with pH according to the Henderson–Hasselbalch equation.
- With weak acids or bases, only the uncharged species (the protonated form for a weak acid, the unprotonated form for a weak base) can diffuse across lipid membranes; this gives rise to pH partition.
- pH partition means that weak acids tend to accumulate in compartments of relatively high pH, whereas weak bases do the reverse.
- Carrier-mediated transport (e.g. in the renal tubule, blood–brain barrier, gastrointestinal epithelium) is important for some drugs that are chemically related to endogenous substances.

$$D + S \rightleftharpoons DS$$
free   binding   complex
drug   site

The usual concentration of albumin in plasma is about 0.6 mmol/l (4 g/100 ml). With two sites per albumin molecule, the drug-binding capacity of plasma albumin would therefore be about 1.2 mmol/l. For most drugs, the total plasma concentration required for a clinical effect is much less than 1.2 mmol/l, so with usual therapeutic doses the binding sites are far from saturated, and the concentration bound [DS] varies nearly in direct proportion to the free concentration [D]. Under these conditions, the fraction bound, [DS]/([D] + [DS]), is independent of the drug concentration. However, some drugs, for example **tolbutamide** (Ch. 26) and some sulfonamides (Ch. 46), work at plasma concentrations at which the binding to protein is approaching saturation (i.e. on the flat part of the binding curve). This means that adding more drug to the plasma increases its free concentration disproportionately. Doubling the dose of such a drug can therefore more than double the free (pharmacologically active) concentration. This is illustrated in Figure 7.5.

Binding sites on plasma albumin bind many different drugs, so competition can occur between them. If two drugs (A and B) compete in this way, administration of drug B can reduce the protein binding, and hence increase the free plasma concentration, of drug A. To do this, drug B needs to occupy an appreciable fraction of the binding sites. Few therapeutic drugs affect the binding of other drugs because they occupy, at therapeutic plasma concentrations, only a tiny fraction of the available sites. Sulfonamides (Ch. 46) are an exception, because they occupy about 50% of the binding sites at therapeutic concentrations and

so can cause harmful effects by displacing other drugs or, in premature babies, *bilirubin* (Ch. 52, p. 747). Much has been made of binding interactions of this kind as a source of untoward drug interactions in clinical medicine, but this type of competition is less important than was once thought (see Ch. 52).

PARTITION INTO BODY FAT AND OTHER TISSUES

Fat represents a large, non-polar compartment. In practice, this is important for only a few drugs, mainly because the effective fat:water partition coefficient is relatively low for most drugs. **Morphine** (see p. 596), for example, although quite lipid-soluble enough to cross the blood–brain barrier, has a lipid:water partition coefficient of only 0.4, so sequestration of the drug by body fat is of little importance. **Thiopental** (p. 532), by comparison (fat:water partition coefficient approximately 10), accumulates substantially in body fat. This has important consequences that limit its usefulness as an intravenous anaesthetic to short-term initiation ('induction') of anaesthesia (Ch. 36).

The second factor that limits the accumulation of drugs in body fat is its low blood supply—less than 2% of the cardiac output. Consequently, drugs are delivered to body fat rather slowly, and the theoretical equilibrium distribution between fat and body water is approached slowly. For practical purposes, therefore, partition into body fat when drugs are given acutely is important only for a few highly lipid-soluble drugs (e.g. general anaesthetics; Ch. 36). When lipid-soluble drugs are given chronically, however, accumulation in body fat is often significant (e.g. benzodiazepines; Ch. 37). Furthermore, there are some environmental contaminants ('xenobiotics'), such as insecticides, that are poorly metabolised. If ingested regularly, such xenobiotics accumulate slowly but progressively in body fat.

Body fat is not the only tissue in which drugs can accumulate. **Chloroquine**—an antimalarial drug (Ch. 49) used additionally to treat rheumatoid arthritis (Ch. 14)—has a high affinity for melanin and is taken up by tissues such as retina that are rich in melanin granules, which may account for the retinopathy that can occur

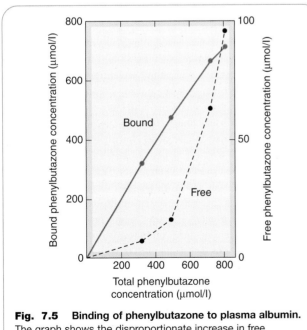

Fig. 7.5 Binding of phenylbutazone to plasma albumin. The graph shows the disproportionate increase in free concentration as the total concentration increases, owing to the binding sites approaching saturation. (Data from Brodie B, Hogben C A M 1957 J Pharm Pharmacol 9: 345.)

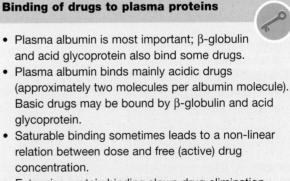

Binding of drugs to plasma proteins

- Plasma albumin is most important; β-globulin and acid glycoprotein also bind some drugs.
- Plasma albumin binds mainly acidic drugs (approximately two molecules per albumin molecule). Basic drugs may be bound by β-globulin and acid glycoprotein.
- Saturable binding sometimes leads to a non-linear relation between dose and free (active) drug concentration.
- Extensive protein binding slows drug elimination (metabolism and/or glomerular filtration).
- Competition between drugs for protein binding can lead, rarely, to clinically important drug interactions.

during prolonged treatment of patients with rheumatoid disease. Tetracyclines (Ch. 46) accumulate slowly in bones and teeth, because they have a high affinity for calcium, and should not be used in children for this reason. Very high concentrations of **amiodarone** (an antidysrhythmic drug; Ch. 18) accumulate in liver and lung, where they can cause adverse effects of (respectively) hepatitis and interstitial fibrosis.

DRUG DISPOSITION

We will now consider how the physical processes described above—diffusion, penetration of membranes, binding to plasma protein, and partition into fat and other tissues—influence the overall disposition of drug molecules in the body. Drug disposition is divided into four stages:

- absorption from the site of administration
- distribution within the body
- metabolism
- excretion.

Absorption and distribution are considered here, metabolism and excretion in Chapter 8. The main routes of drug administration and elimination are shown schematically in Figure 7.6.

DRUG ABSORPTION
ROUTES OF ADMINISTRATION

Absorption is defined as the passage of a drug from its site of administration into the plasma. It is therefore important for all routes of administration, except intravenous injection. There are instances, such as inhalation of a bronchodilator aerosol to treat asthma (Ch. 23), where absorption as just defined is not required for the drug to act, but in most cases the drug must enter plasma before reaching its site of action.

The main routes of administration are:

- oral
- sublingual
- rectal
- application to other epithelial surfaces (e.g. skin, cornea, vagina and nasal mucosa)
- inhalation
- injection
  —subcutaneous
  —intramuscular
  —intravenous
  —intrathecal.

ORAL ADMINISTRATION

Most drugs are taken by mouth and swallowed. Little absorption occurs until the drug enters the small intestine.

Drug absorption from the intestine

The mechanism of drug absorption is the same as for other epithelial barriers, namely passive transfer at a rate determined by the ionisation and lipid solubility of the drug molecules. Figure 7.7 shows the absorption of a series of weak acids and bases as a function of pK_a. As expected, strong bases of pK_a 10 or higher are poorly absorbed, as are strong acids of pK_a less than 3, because they are fully ionised. The arrow poison curare used by South American Indians contained quaternary ammonium compounds that block neuromuscular transmission (Ch. 10). These strong bases are poorly absorbed from the gastrointestinal tract, so the meat from animals killed in this way was safe to eat.

There are a few instances where intestinal absorption depends on carrier-mediated transport rather than simple lipid diffusion. Examples include **levodopa**, used in treating Parkinson's disease (see Ch. 35), which is taken up by the carrier that normally transports phenylalanine, and **fluorouracil** (Ch. 51), a cytotoxic drug that is transported by the system that carries natural pyrimidines (thymine and uracil). Iron is absorbed via specific carriers in the surface membranes of jejunal mucosa, and calcium is absorbed by means of a vitamin D-dependent carrier system.

Factors affecting gastrointestinal absorption

Typically, about 75% of a drug given orally is absorbed in 1–3 hours, but numerous factors alter this, some physiological and some to do with the formulation of the drug. The main factors are:

- gastrointestinal motility
- splanchnic blood flow
- particle size and formulation
- physicochemical factors.

Gastrointestinal motility has a large effect. Many disorders (e.g. migraine, diabetic neuropathy) cause gastric stasis and slow drug absorption. Drug treatment can also affect motility, either reducing (e.g. drugs that block muscarinic receptors; see Ch. 10) or increasing it (e.g. **metoclopramide**, an antiemetic used in migraine to facilitate absorption of analgesic). Excessively rapid movement of gut contents (e.g. in some forms of diarrhoea) can impair absorption. Conversely, a drug taken after a meal is often more slowly absorbed because its progress to the small intestine is delayed. There are exceptions, however, and several drugs (e.g. **propranolol**; see p. 16) reach a higher plasma concentration if they are taken after a meal, probably because food increases splanchnic blood flow. Conversely, splanchnic blood flow is greatly reduced by hypovolaemia or heart failure, with a resultant reduction of drug absorption.

Particle size and formulation have major effects on absorption. In 1971, patients in a New York hospital were found to require unusually large maintenance doses of **digoxin** (Ch. 18). In a study on normal volunteers, it was found that standard digoxin tablets from different manufacturers resulted in grossly different plasma concentrations (Fig. 7.8), even though the digoxin content of the tablets was the same, because of differences in particle size. Because digoxin is rather poorly absorbed, small differences in the pharmaceutical formulation can make a large difference to the extent of absorption.

Therapeutic drugs are formulated pharmaceutically to produce desired absorption characteristics. Capsules may be designed to remain intact for some hours after ingestion in order to delay absorption, or tablets may have a resistant coating to give the

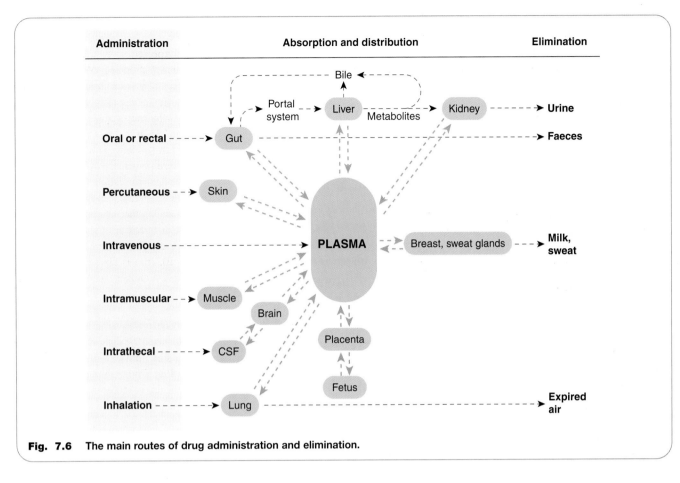

Fig. 7.6 **The main routes of drug administration and elimination.**

same effect. In some cases, a mixture of slow- and fast-release particles is included in a capsule to produce rapid but sustained absorption. More elaborate pharmaceutical systems include various modified-release preparations (e.g. a long-acting form of **nifedipine**, see pp. 295-296, that permits once-daily use). Such preparations

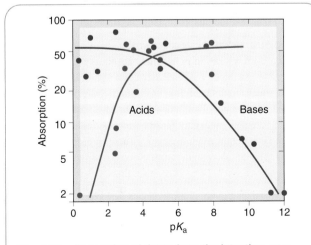

Fig. 7.7 **Absorption of drugs from the intestine, as a function of pK_a, for acids and bases.** Weak acids and bases are well absorbed; strong acids and bases are poorly absorbed. (Redrawn from Schanker L S et al. 1957 J Pharmacol 120: 528.)

not only increase the dose interval but also reduce adverse effects related to high peak plasma concentrations following administration of a conventional formulation (e.g. flushing following regular nifedipine). Osmotically driven 'minipumps' can be implanted experimentally, and some oral extended-release preparations that are used clinically use the same principle, the tablet containing an osmotically active core and being bound by an impermeable membrane with a precisely engineered pore to allow drug to exit in solution, delivering drug at an approximately constant rate into the bowel lumen. Such preparations may, however, cause problems related to high local concentrations of drug in the intestine (an osmotically released preparation of the anti-inflammatory drug **indometacin**, Ch. 14, had to be withdrawn because it caused small bowel perforation), and are subject to variations in small bowel transit time that occur during ageing and with disease.

Physicochemical factors (including some drug interactions; Ch. 52) affect drug absorption. **Tetracycline** binds strongly to Ca^{2+}, and calcium-rich foods (especially milk) prevent its absorption (Ch. 46). Bile acid–binding resins such as **colestyramine** (used to treat diarrhoea caused by bile acids) bind several drugs, for example **warfarin** (Ch. 21) and **thyroxine** (Ch. 29).

When drugs are administered by mouth, the intention is usually that they should be absorbed and cause a systemic effect, but there are exceptions. **Vancomycin** (p. 674) is very poorly absorbed, and is administered orally to eradicate toxin-forming *Clostridium difficile* from the gut lumen in patients with

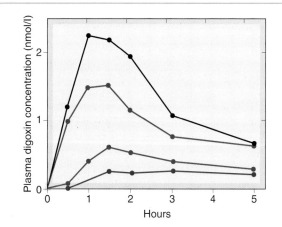

Fig. 7.8 **Variation in oral absorption among different formulations of digoxin.** The four curves show the mean plasma concentrations attained for the four preparations, each of which was given on separate occasions to four subjects. The large variation has caused the formulation of digoxin tablets to be standardised since this study was published. (From Lindenbaum J et al. 1971 N Engl J Med 285: 1344.)

pseudomembranous colitis (an adverse effect of broad-spectrum antibiotics caused by appearance of this organism in the bowel). **Mesalazine** (p. 395) is a formulation of 5-aminosalicylic acid in a pH-dependent acrylic coat that degrades in the terminal ileum and proximal colon, and is used to treat inflammatory bowel disease affecting this part of the gut. **Olsalazine** (p. 395) is a prodrug consisting of a dimer of two molecules of 5-aminosalicylic acid that is cleaved by colonic bacteria in the distal bowel and is used to treat patients with distal colitis.

Bioavailability

To get from the lumen of the small intestine into the systemic circulation, a drug must not only penetrate the intestinal mucosa, it must also run the gauntlet of enzymes that may inactivate it in gut wall and liver. The term *bioavailability* (*F*) is used to indicate the fraction of an orally administered dose that reaches the systemic circulation as intact drug, taking into account both absorption and local metabolic degradation. *F* is measured by determining the plasma drug concentration versus time curves in a group of subjects following oral and (on separate occasions) intravenous administration (the fraction absorbed following an intravenous dose is 1 by definition). The areas under the plasma concentration time curves (AUC) are used to estimate *F* as $AUC_{oral}/AUC_{intravenous}$. AUC is estimated using the 'trapezoidal rule', by calculating the area under each pair of data points as a trapezoid (i.e. a rectangle with a triangle on top). The areas of all the trapezoids are summed, and the area from the last point to infinite time is estimated as C_{last}/k, where C_{last} is the last measured concentration and k is the elimination rate constant of the slowest elimination phase. Bioavailability is not a characteristic solely of the drug preparation: variations in enzyme activity of gut wall or liver, in gastric pH or intestinal motility all affect it. Because of this, one cannot speak strictly of the bioavailability of a particular preparation, but only of that preparation in a given

individual on a particular occasion, and *F* determined in a group of healthy volunteer subjects may differ substantially from the value determined in patients with diseases of gastrointestinal or circulatory systems.

Even with these caveats, the concept is of limited use because it relates only to the total proportion of the drug that reaches the systemic circulation and neglects the *rate* of absorption. If a drug is completely absorbed in 30 minutes, it will reach a much higher peak plasma concentration (and have a more dramatic effect) than if it were absorbed more slowly. For these reasons, regulatory authorities—which have to make decisions about the licensing of products that are 'generic equivalents' of patented products—lay importance on evidence of *bioequivalence*, i.e. evidence that the new product behaves sufficiently similarly to the existing one to be substituted for it without causing clinical problems.

SUBLINGUAL ADMINISTRATION

Absorption directly from the oral cavity is sometimes useful (provided the drug does not taste too horrible) when a rapid response is required, particularly when the drug is either unstable at gastric pH or rapidly metabolised by the liver. **Glyceryl trinitrate** is an example of a drug that is often given sublingually (Ch. 18). Drugs absorbed from the mouth pass directly into the systemic circulation without entering the portal system, and so escape first-pass metabolism by enzymes in the gut wall and liver.

RECTAL ADMINISTRATION

Rectal administration is used for drugs that are required either to produce a local effect (e.g. anti-inflammatory drugs for use in ulcerative colitis) or to produce systemic effects. Absorption following rectal administration is often unreliable, but this route can be useful in patients who are vomiting or are unable to take medication by mouth (e.g. postoperatively). It is used to administer **diazepam** to children who are in status epilepticus (Ch. 40), in whom it is difficult to establish intravenous access.

APPLICATION TO EPITHELIAL SURFACES

Cutaneous administration

Cutaneous administration is used when a local effect on the skin is required (e.g. topically applied steroids). Appreciable absorption may nonetheless occur and lead to systemic effects.

Most drugs are absorbed very poorly through unbroken skin. However, a number of organophosphate insecticides (see Ch. 10), which need to penetrate an insect's cuticle in order to work, are absorbed through skin, and accidental poisoning occurs in farm workers.

▼ A case is recounted of a 35-year-old florist in 1932. 'While engaged in doing a light electrical repair job at a work bench he sat down in a chair on the seat of which some "Nico-Fume liquid" (a 40% solution of free nicotine) had been spilled. He felt the solution wet through his clothes to the skin over the left buttock, an area about the size of the palm of his hand. He thought nothing further of it and continued at his work for about 15 minutes, when he was suddenly seized with nausea and faintness ... and found himself in a drenching sweat. On the way to hospital he lost consciousness.' He survived, just, and then 4 days later: 'On discharge from the hospital he was given the same clothes that he had worn when he was brought in. The clothes had been kept in a paper bag and were still damp where they had been wet with the nicotine solution.' The sequel was predictable. He survived again but felt thereafter 'unable to enter a greenhouse where nicotine was being sprayed'. Transdermal dosage forms of nicotine are now used to reduce the withdrawal symptoms that accompany stopping smoking (Ch. 54).

Transdermal dosage forms, in which the drug is incorporated in a stick-on patch applied to the skin, are used increasingly, and several drugs—for example **oestrogen** for hormone replacement (Ch. 30)—are available in this form. Such patches produce a steady rate of drug delivery and avoid presystemic metabolism. However, the method is suitable only for lipid-soluble drugs and is relatively expensive.

Nasal sprays

Some peptide hormone analogues, for example of antidiuretic hormone (Ch. 24) and of gonadotrophin-releasing hormone (see Ch. 30), are given as nasal sprays, as is **calcitonin** (Ch. 31). Absorption is believed to take place through mucosa overlying nasal-associated lymphoid tissue. This is similar to mucosa overlying Peyer's patches in the small intestine, which is also unusually permeable.

Eye drops

Many drugs are applied as eye drops, relying on absorption through the epithelium of the conjunctival sac to produce their effects. Desirable local effects within the eye can be achieved without causing systemic side effects; for example, **dorzolamide** is a carbonic anhydrase inhibitor that is given as eye drops to lower ocular pressure in patients with glaucoma. It achieves this without affecting the kidney (see Ch. 24), thus avoiding the acidosis that is caused by oral administration of **acetazolamide**. Some systemic absorption from the eye occurs, however, and can result in unwanted effects (e.g. bronchospasm in asthmatic patients using **timolol** eye drops; see Table 10.4 on p. 153, for glaucoma).

Administration by inhalation

Inhalation is the route used for volatile and gaseous anaesthetics (see Ch. 36), the lung serving as the route of both administration and elimination. The rapid exchange resulting from the large surface area and blood flow makes it possible to achieve rapid adjustments of plasma concentration. The pharmacokinetic behaviour of inhalation anaesthetics is discussed more fully in Chapter 36. Recently, the potential of the lung as a site of absorption of peptides and proteins has been appreciated, and inhaled human insulin is now available for use in diabetes mellitus (see Ch. 26).

Drugs used for their effects on the lung are also given by inhalation, usually as an aerosol. Glucocorticoids (e.g. **beclometasone dipropionate**) and bronchodilators (e.g. **salbutamol**; Ch. 23) are given in this way to achieve high local concentrations in the lung while minimising systemic side effects. However, drugs given by inhalation in this way are usually partly absorbed into the circulation, and systemic side effects (e.g. tremor following salbutamol) can occur. Chemical modification of a drug may minimise such absorption. For example, **ipratropium**, a muscarinic receptor antagonist (Chs 10 and 23), is a quaternary ammonium ion analogue of **atropine**. It is used as an inhaled bronchodilator because its poor absorption minimises systemic adverse effects.

ADMINISTRATION BY INJECTION

Intravenous injection is the fastest and most certain route of drug administration. Bolus injection produces a very high concentration of drug, first in the right heart and lungs and then in the systemic circulation. The peak concentration reaching the tissues depends critically on the rate of injection. Administration by steady intravenous infusion avoids the uncertainties of absorption from other sites, while avoiding high peak plasma concentrations caused by bolus injection. Drugs given intravenously include several antibiotics, anaesthetics such as **propofol** (Ch. 36), and **diazepam** for patients with status epilepticus (Ch. 40).

Subcutaneous or intramuscular injection of drugs usually produces a faster effect than oral administration, but the rate of absorption depends greatly on the site of injection and on local blood flow. The rate-limiting factors in absorption from the injection site are:

- diffusion through the tissue
- removal by local blood flow.

Absorption from a site of injection is increased by increased blood flow. *Hyaluronidase* (an enzyme that breaks down the intercellular matrix, thereby increasing diffusion) also increases drug absorption from the site of injection. Conversely, absorption is reduced in patients with circulatory failure ('shock') in whom tissue perfusion is reduced (Ch. 19).

Methods for delaying absorption

It may be desirable to delay absorption, either to produce a local effect or to prolong systemic action. For example, addition of **adrenaline (epinephrine)**—see p. 177—to a local anaesthetic reduces absorption of the anaesthetic into the general circulation, usefully prolonging the anaesthetic effect. Formulation of **insulin** with protamine or zinc produces a long-acting form (see Ch. 26, p. 404). **Procaine penicillin** (Ch. 46) is a poorly soluble salt of penicillin; when injected as an aqueous suspension, it is slowly absorbed and exerts a prolonged action. Esterification of steroid hormones (e.g. **medroxyprogesterone acetate, testosterone propionate**; see Ch. 30) and antipsychotic drugs (e.g. **fluphenazine decanoate**; Ch. 38) increases their solubility in oil and slows their rate of absorption when they are injected in an oily solution.

Another method used to achieve slow and continuous absorption of certain steroid hormones (e.g. **estradiol**; Ch. 30) is the subcutaneous implantation of solid pellets. The rate of absorption is proportional to the surface area of the implant.

Intrathecal injection

Injection of a drug into the subarachnoid space via a lumbar puncture needle is used for some specialised purposes. **Methotrexate** (Ch. 51) is administered in this way in the treatment of certain childhood leukaemias to prevent relapse in the CNS. Regional anaesthesia can be produced by intrathecal administration of a local anaesthetic such as **bupivacaine** (see Ch. 44); opiate analgesics can also be used in this way (Ch. 41). **Baclofen** (a GABA analogue; Ch. 33) is used to treat disabling muscle spasms. It has been administered intrathecally to minimise its adverse effects. Some antibiotics (e.g. aminoglycosides) cross the blood–brain barrier very slowly, and in rare clinical situations where they are essential (e.g. nervous system infections with bacteria resistant to other antibiotics) can be given intrathecally or directly into the cerebral ventricles via a reservoir.

DISTRIBUTION OF DRUGS IN THE BODY

BODY FLUID COMPARTMENTS

Body water is distributed into four main compartments, as shown in Figure 7.9. The total body water as a percentage of body weight varies from 50 to 70%, being rather less in women than in men.

Extracellular fluid comprises the blood plasma (about 4.5% of body weight), interstitial fluid (16%) and lymph (1.2%). Intracellular fluid (30–40%) is the sum of the fluid contents of all cells in the body. Transcellular fluid (2.5%) includes the cerebrospinal, intraocular, peritoneal, pleural and synovial fluids, and digestive secretions. The fetus may also be regarded as a special type of transcellular compartment. Within each of these aqueous compartments, drug molecules usually exist both in free solution and in bound form; furthermore, drugs that are weak acids or bases will exist as an equilibrium mixture of the charged and uncharged forms, the position of the equilibrium depending on the pH (see pp. 99-100).

The equilibrium pattern of distribution between the various compartments will therefore depend on:

- permeability across tissue barriers
- binding within compartments

> **Drug absorption and bioavailability**
>
> - Drugs of very low lipid solubility, including those that are strong acids or bases, are generally poorly absorbed from the gut.
> - A few drugs (e.g. levodopa) are absorbed by carrier-mediated transfer.
> - Absorption from the gut depends on many factors, including:
>   - gastrointestinal motility
>   - gastrointestinal pH
>   - particle size
>   - physicochemical interaction with gut contents (e.g. chemical interaction between calcium and tetracycline antibiotics).
> - Bioavailability is the fraction of an ingested dose of a drug that gains access to the systemic circulation. It may be low because absorption is incomplete, or because the drug is metabolised in the gut wall or liver before reaching the systemic circulation.
> - Bioequivalence implies that if one formulation of a drug is substituted for another, no clinically untoward consequences will ensue.

- pH partition
- fat:water partition.

To enter the transcellular compartments from the extracellular compartment, a drug must cross a cellular barrier, a particularly important example in the context of pharmacokinetics being the blood–brain barrier.

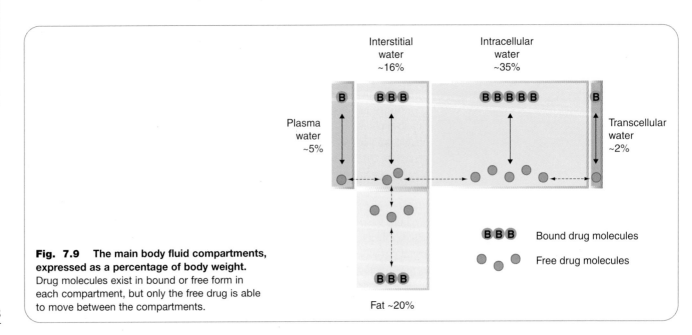

Fig. 7.9 The main body fluid compartments, expressed as a percentage of body weight. Drug molecules exist in bound or free form in each compartment, but only the free drug is able to move between the compartments.

Interstitial water ~16%

Intracellular water ~35%

Plasma water ~5%

Transcellular water ~2%

Ⓑ Ⓑ Ⓑ Bound drug molecules

⬤ ⬤ ⬤ Free drug molecules

Fat ~20%

THE BLOOD–BRAIN BARRIER

The concept of the blood–brain barrier was introduced by Paul Ehrlich to explain his observation that intravenously injected dye stained most tissues yet the brain remained unstained. The barrier consists of a continuous layer of endothelial cells joined by tight junctions and surrounded by pericytes. The brain is consequently inaccessible to many drugs, including many anticancer drugs and some antibiotics such as the aminoglycosides, with a lipid solubility that is insufficient to allow penetration of the blood–brain barrier. However, inflammation can disrupt the integrity of the blood –brain barrier, allowing normally impermeant substances to enter the brain (Fig. 7.10); consequently, **penicillin** (Ch. 46) can be given intravenously (rather than intrathecally) to treat bacterial meningitis (which is accompanied by intense inflammation).

Furthermore, in some parts of the CNS, including the chemoreceptor trigger zone, the barrier is leaky. This enables **domperidone**, an antiemetic dopamine receptor antagonist (Ch. 25) that does not penetrate the blood–brain barrier but does access the chemoreceptor trigger zone, to be used to prevent the nausea caused by dopamine agonists such as **apomorphine** (see p. 547) when these are used to treat advanced Parkinson's disease. This is achieved without loss of efficacy, because dopamine receptors in the basal ganglia are accessible only to drugs that have traversed the blood–brain barrier.

An opioid antagonist (*ADL 8-2698*) with extremely limited gastrointestinal absorption has been developed to prevent ileus, the transient reduction in bowel motility that often complicates abdominal surgery. It does not cross the blood–brain barrier. When given by mouth postoperatively, it speeds recovery of bowel function without impairing the pain relief provided by opioid analgesics.

Several peptides, including *bradykinin* and *enkephalins*, increase blood–brain barrier permeability. There is interest in exploiting this to improve penetration of chemotherapy during treatment of brain tumours. In addition, extreme stress renders the blood–brain barrier permeable to drugs such as pyridostigmine (Ch. 10), which normally act peripherally.[2]

VOLUME OF DISTRIBUTION

The apparent volume of distribution, V_d, is defined as the volume of fluid required to contain the total amount, Q, of drug in the body at the same concentration as that present in the plasma, C_p.

$$V_d = \frac{Q}{C_p}$$

Values of V_d[3] have been measured for many drugs (Table 7.1). Some general patterns can be distinguished, but it is important to avoid identifying a given range of V_d too closely with a particular anatomical compartment. For example, **insulin** has a measured V_d similar to the volume of plasma water but exerts its effects on muscle, fat and liver via receptors that are exposed to interstitial fluid but not to plasma (Ch. 26).

Drugs confined to the plasma compartment

The plasma volume is about 0.05 l/kg body weight. A few drugs, such as heparin (Ch. 21), are confined to plasma because the molecule is too large to cross the capillary wall easily. More often, retention of a drug in the plasma following a single dose reflects strong binding to plasma protein. It is, nevertheless, the free drug in the interstitial fluid that exerts a pharmacological effect. Following repeated dosing, equilibration occurs and measured V_d increases. Some dyes, such as Evans blue, bind so strongly to plasma albumin that its V_d is used experimentally to measure plasma volume.

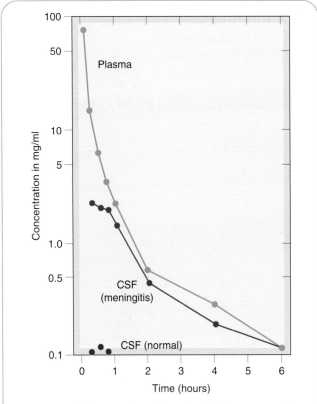

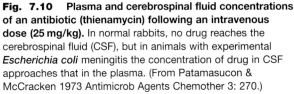

Fig. 7.10 Plasma and cerebrospinal fluid concentrations of an antibiotic (thienamycin) following an intravenous dose (25 mg/kg). In normal rabbits, no drug reaches the cerebrospinal fluid (CSF), but in animals with experimental *Escherichia coli* meningitis the concentration of drug in CSF approaches that in the plasma. (From Patamasucon & McCracken 1973 Antimicrob Agents Chemother 3: 270.)

---

[2]This has been invoked to explain the central symptoms of cholinesterase inhibition experienced by some soldiers during the Gulf War. These soldiers may have been exposed to cholinesterase inhibitors (developed as chemical weapons and also, somewhat bizarrely, used externally during the conflict to prevent insect infestation) in the context of the stress of warfare.

[3]The experimental measurement of V_d is complicated by the fact that Q does not stay constant (because of metabolism and excretion of the drug) during the time that it takes for it to be distributed among the various body compartments that contribute to the overall V_d. It therefore has to be calculated indirectly from a series of measurements of plasma concentrations as a function of time (see Fig. 8.6, p. 121).

Drug distribution

- The major compartments are:
  - plasma (5% of body weight)
  - interstitial fluid (16%)
  - intracellular fluid (35%)
  - transcellular fluid (2%)
  - fat (20%).
- Volume of distribution (V_d) is defined as the volume of plasma that would contain the total body content of the drug at a concentration equal to that in the plasma.
- Lipid-insoluble drugs are mainly confined to plasma and interstitial fluids; most do not enter the brain following acute dosing.
- Lipid-soluble drugs reach all compartments and may accumulate in fat.
- For drugs that accumulate outside the plasma compartment (e.g. in fat or by being bound to tissues), V_d may exceed total body volume.

Drugs distributed in the extracellular compartment

The total extracellular volume is about 0.2 l/kg, and this is the approximate V_d for many polar compounds, such as **vecuronium** (Ch. 10), **gentamicin** and **carbenicillin** (Ch. 46). These drugs cannot easily enter cells because of their low lipid solubility, and they do not traverse the blood–brain or placental barriers freely.

Distribution throughout the body water

Total body water represents about 0.55 l/kg. This approximates the distribution of relatively lipid-soluble drugs that readily cross cell membranes, such as **phenytoin** (Ch. 40) and **ethanol** (Ch. 43). Binding of drug outside the plasma compartment, or partitioning into body fat, increases V_d beyond total body water. Consequently, there are many drugs with V_d greater than the total body volume, such as **morphine** (Ch. 41), tricyclic antidepressants (Ch. 39) and **haloperidol** (Ch. 38). Such drugs are not efficiently removed from the body by haemodialysis, which is therefore unhelpful in managing overdose with such agents.

SPECIAL DRUG DELIVERY SYSTEMS

Several approaches are being explored in an attempt to improve drug delivery. They include:

- biologically erodable microspheres
- prodrugs
- antibody–drug conjugates
- packaging in liposomes
- coating implantable devices.

Biologically erodable microspheres

Microspheres of biologically erodable polymers (see Varde & Pack, 2004) can be engineered to adhere to mucosal epithelium in the

Table 7.1 Distribution volumes for some drugs compared with volume of body fluid compartments

Volume (l/kg body weight)	Compartment	Volume of distribution (V_d; l/kg body weight)	Drug(s)
0.05	Plasma	0.05–0.1	Heparin Insulin
		0.1–0.2	Warfarin Sulfamethoxazole Glibenclamide Atenolol
0.2	Extracellular fluid	0.2–0.4	Tubocurarine
		0.4–0.7	Theophylline
0.55	Total body water		Ethanol Neostigmine Phenytoin
		1–2	Methotrexate Indomethacin Paracetamol Diazepam Lidocaine (lignocaine)
		2–5	Glyceryl trinitrate Morphine Propranolol Digoxin Chlorpromazine
		> 10	Nortriptyline Imipramine

gut. Such microspheres can be loaded with drugs, including high-molecular-weight substances, as a means of improving absorption, which occurs both through mucosal absorptive epithelium and also through epithelium overlying Peyer's patches. This approach has yet to be used clinically, but microspheres made from polyanhydride copolymers of fumaric and sebacic acids by a technique known as phase inversion nanoencapsulation have been used to produce systemic absorption of insulin and of plasmid DNA following oral administration in rats. Because drug delivery is a critical problem in gene therapy (Ch.55), this is potentially momentous!

Prodrugs

Prodrugs are inactive precursors that are metabolised to active metabolites; they are described in Chapter 8. Some of the examples in clinical use confer no obvious benefits and have been found to be prodrugs only retrospectively, not having been designed with this in mind. However, some do have advantages. For example, the cytotoxic drug **cyclophosphamide** (see Ch. 51) becomes active only after it has been metabolised in the liver; it can therefore be taken orally without causing serious damage to the gastrointestinal epithelium. **Levodopa** is absorbed from the gastrointestinal tract and crosses the blood–brain barrier via an amino acid transport mechanism before conversion to active dopamine in nerve terminals in the basal ganglia (Ch. 35). **Zidovudine** is phosphorylated to its active trisphosphate metabolite only in cells containing appropriate reverse transcriptase, hence conferring selective toxicity towards cells infected with HIV (Ch. 47). **Valaciclovir** and **famciclovir** are each ester prodrugs of prodrugs; respectively, of **aciclovir** and of **penciclovir**. Their bioavailability is greater than that of aciclovir and penciclovir, each of which is converted into active metabolites in virally infected cells (Ch. 47).

Other problems could theoretically be overcome by the use of suitable prodrugs; for example, instability of drugs at gastric pH, direct gastric irritation (**aspirin** was synthesised in the 19th century in a deliberate attempt to produce a prodrug of salicylic acid that would be tolerable when taken by mouth), failure of drug to cross the blood–brain barrier and so on. Progress with this approach remains slow, however, and the optimistic prodrug designer was warned as long ago as 1965: 'he will have to bear in mind that an organism's normal reaction to a foreign substance is to burn it up for food'.

Antibody–drug conjugates

One of the aims of cancer chemotherapy is to improve the selectivity of cytotoxic drugs (see Ch. 51). One interesting possibility is to attach the drug to an antibody directed against a tumour-specific antigen, which will bind selectively to tumour cells. Such approaches look promising in experimental animals, but it is still too early to say whether they will succeed in humans.

Packaging in liposomes

Liposomes are minute vesicles produced by sonication of an aqueous suspension of phospholipids. They can be filled with non–lipid-soluble drugs or nucleic acids (Ch. 55), which are retained until the liposome is disrupted. Liposomes are taken up by reticuloendothelial cells, especially in the liver. They are also concentrated in malignant tumours, and there is a possibility of achieving selective delivery of drugs in this way. **Amphotericin**, an antifungal drug used to treat systemic mycoses (Ch. 48), is available in a liposomal formulation that is less nephrotoxic and better tolerated than the conventional form, albeit considerably more expensive. In the future, it may be possible to direct drugs or genes selectively to a specific target by incorporating antibody molecules into liposomal membrane surfaces.

Coated implantable devices

Impregnated coatings have been developed that permit localised drug delivery from implants. Examples include hormonal delivery to the endometrium from intrauterine devices, and delivery of antithrombotic and antiproliferative agents (drugs or radiopharmaceuticals) to the coronary arteries from stents (devices inserted via a catheter after a diseased coronary artery has been dilated with a balloon). Stents reduce the occurrence of restenosis, but this can still occur at the margin of the device. Coating stents with drugs such as **sirolimus** (a potent immunosuppressant; see Ch. 14) embedded in a surface polymer prevents this important clinical problem.

REFERENCES AND FURTHER READING

Drug distribution (including blood–brain barrier)
Abbott N J 2002 Astrocyte–endothelial interactions and blood–brain barrier permeability. J Anat 200: 629–638 (*'The BBB phenotype develops under the influence of ... astrocytic glia, and consists of more complex tight junctions than in other capillary endothelia, and a number of specific transport and enzyme systems which regulate molecular traffic across the endothelial cells. Transporters characteristic of the BBB phenotype include both uptake mechanisms (e.g. GLUT-1 glucose carrier, L1 amino acid transporter) and efflux transporters (e.g. P-glycoprotein) ... endothelial cells are involved in both long- and short-term chemical communication with neighbouring cells, with the perivascular end feet of astrocytes being of particular importance.'*)

Bauer B, Hartz A M S, Fricker G, Miller D S 2005 Modulation of P-glycoprotein transport function at the blood–brain barrier. Exp Biol Med 230: 118–127 (*Reviews mechanisms by which P-glycoprotein activity can be modulated, including direct inhibition by specific competitors, and functional and transcriptional modulation*)
Cooper G J, Boron W F 1998 Effect of pCMBS on the CO_2 permeability of *Xenopus* oocytes expressing aquaporin 1 or its C189S mutant. Am J Physiol 275: C1481–C1486 (*Carbon dioxide acidification depends on transfer via a channel called aquaporin 1, rather than free diffusion as thought previously*)
de Boer A G, van der Sandt I C J, Gaillard P J 2003 The role of drug transporters at the blood–brain barrier. Ann Rev Pharmacol Toxicol 43: 629–656 (*Reviews the*

role of carrier- and receptor-mediated transport systems in the blood–brain barrier; these include P-glycoprotein, multidrug-resistance proteins 17, nucleoside transporters, organic anion transporters, and large amino acid transporters, the transferrin-1 and -2 receptors, and the scavenger receptors SB-AI and SB-BI)
Doan K M M, Humphreys J E, Webster L O et al. 2002 Passive permeability and P-glycoprotein–mediated efflux differentiate central nervous system (CNS) and non-CNS marketed drugs. J PET 303: 1029–1037 (*Study on 48 CNS and 45 non-CNS drugs, comparing permeability and P-glycoprotein–mediated efflux between compounds; concludes that for CNS delivery, a drug should ideally have an in vitro passive permeability > 150 nm/s and not be a good P-glycoprotein substrate*)

Eraly S A, Bush K T, Sampogna R V et al. 2004 The molecular pharmacology of organic anion transporters: from DNA to FDA? Mol Pharmacol 65: 479–487 (*Reviews aspects of the molecular biology and pharmacology of the organic anion transporters, and discusses their structural biology, paired genomic organisation, developmental regulation, toxicology, and pharmacogenetics*)

Friedman A, Kaufer D, Shemer J et al. 1996 Pyridostigmine brain penetration under stress enhances neuronal excitability and induces early immediate transcriptional response. Nat Med 2: 1382–1385 (*Peripherally acting drugs administered during severe stress may unexpectedly penetrate the blood–brain barrier; see also accompanying comment: Hanin I The Gulf War, stress and a leaky blood brain barrier, pp. 1307–1308*)

Koepsell H 2004 Polyspecific organic cation transporters: their functions and interactions with drugs. Trends Pharmacol Sci 25: 375–381 (*Reviews organic cation transporters [OCT]1–3, which are expressed in gut, liver, kidney, heart, placenta, lung and brain and facilitate diffusion of structurally diverse organic cations including monoamine neurotransmitters and many drugs; studies in knockout mice implicate OCT1 in the hepatic uptake and biliary excretion of cationic drugs, and OCT1 and 2 in renal proximal tubules participate in secreting cationic drugs into urine*)

McNamara P J, Abbassi M 2004 Neonatal exposure to drugs in breast milk. Pharm Res 21: 555–566 (*Review*)

Mealey K L, Bentjen S A, Gay J M, Cantor G H 2001 Ivermectin sensitivity in collies is associated with a deletion mutation of the mdr1 gene. Pharmacogenetics 11: 727–733 (*Reports a deletion mutation of the mdr1 gene that is associated with ivermectin sensitivity. The deletion results in premature termination of P-glycoprotein synthesis. Dogs that are homozygous for the mutation are exquisitely sensitive to ivermectin, while those that are homozygous normal or heterozygous are not.*)

Neff M W, Robertson K R, Wong A K et al. 2004 Breed distribution and history of canine mdr1-1 delta, a pharmacogenetic mutation that marks the emergence of breeds from the collie lineage. Proc Natl Acad Sci USA 101: 11725–11730 (*The breed distribution and frequency of mdr1-1δ have applications in veterinary medicine, whereas the allele's history recounts the emergence of formally recognised breeds from an admixed population of working sheepdogs*)

Ritter C A, Jedlitschky G, Schwabedissen H M Z et al. 2005 Cellular export of drugs and signaling molecules by the ATP-binding cassette transporters MRP4 (ABCC4) and MRP5 (ABCC5). Drug Metab Rev 37: 253–278 (*Members of the multidrug resistance–associated protein [MRP] subfamily of ATP-binding cassette transporters, MRP4 and 5 are organic anion transporters; they transport nucleotides and nucleotide analogues, and also cyclic nucleotides,*

so are implicated in signal transduction. MRP4 also transports conjugated steroids, prostaglandins, and glutathione.)

Sasaki M, Suzuki H, Aoki J et al. 2004 Prediction of in vivo biliary clearance from the in vitro transcellular transport of organic anions across a double-transfected Madin–Darby canine kidney II monolayer expressing both rat organic anion transporting polypeptide 4 and multidrug resistance associated protein 2. Mol Pharmacol 66: 450–459 (*Double-transfected Madin–Darby canine kidney cell monolayer may be useful in analysing hepatic transport of organic anions and in predicting in vivo biliary clearance*)

van Montfoort J E, Hagenbuch B, Groothuis G M M et al. 2003 Drug uptake systems in liver and kidney. Curr Drug Metab 4: 185–211 (*Reviews the tissue distribution, substrate specificity, transport and regulation of the organic anion–transporting polypeptide superfamily [solute carrier family SLC21A] and the SLC22A family–containing transporters for organic cations and organic anions*)

Zhang Y, Schuetz J D, Elmquist W F et al. 2004 Plasma membrane localization of multidrug resistance-associated protein homologs in brain capillary endothelial cells. J PET 311: 449–455 (*Predominantly apical plasma membrane distribution for MRP1 and MRP5, and an almost equal distribution of MRP4 on the apical and basolateral plasma membrane of bovine brain microvessel endothelial cells; MRPs in the endothelial cells forming the blood–brain barrier is different from that observed in polarised epithelial cells, and may contribute to the reduced entry and enhanced elimination of organic anions and nucleotides in the brain*)

Drug delivery

Blanc E, Bonnafous C, Merida P et al. 2004 Peptide-vector strategy bypasses P-glycoprotein efflux, and enhances brain transport and solubility of paclitaxel. Anti-Cancer Drugs 15: 947–954 (*Paclitaxel coupled to a peptide vector enhances the solubility of paclitaxel and its brain uptake in mice. In wild-type mice, vectorised paclitaxel bypasses P-glycoprotein present at the lumenal side of the blood–brain barrier—cf. P-glycoprotein–deficient mice. The effect of vectorised paclitaxel on cancer cells was similar to that of free paclitaxel. 'Vectorization of paclitaxel may have significant potential for the treatment of brain tumors.'*)

Cornford E M, Cornford M E 2002 New systems for delivery of drugs to the brain in neurological disease. Lancet Neurol 1: 306–315 (*Reviews augmentation of pinocytosis to deliver drugs to the brain. Macromolecules can be conjugated to peptidomimetic ligands that bind peptide receptors, and are then internalised and transported in small vesicles across the cytoplasmic brain–capillary barrier. Such conjugates can remain effective in animal models of neurological disease.*)

Goldberg M, Gomez-Orellana I 2003 Challenges for the oral delivery of macromolecules. Nat Rev Drug Discov 2: 289–295 (*Reviews the current status and future prospects of oral macromolecular drug delivery*)

Le Couter J et al. 2001 Identification of an angiogenic mitogen selective for endocrine gland endothelium. Nature 412: 877–884 (*See also accompanying editorial comment: Carmeliet P Creating unique blood vessels, pp. 868–869*)

Mahato R I, Narang A S, Thoma L, Miller D D 2003 Emerging trends in oral delivery of peptide and protein drugs. Crit Rev Ther Drug Carrier Syst 20: 153–214 (*Various strategies currently under investigation include amino acid backbone modifications; formulation approaches; chemical conjugation of hydrophobic or targeting ligand; and use of enzyme inhibitors, mucoadhesive polymers, and absorption enhancers*)

Mathiovitz E, Jacob J S, Jong Y S et al. 1997 Biologically erodable microspheres as potential oral drug delivery systems. Nature 386: 410–414 (*Oral delivery of three model substances of different molecular size: dicoumarol, insulin and plasmid DNA*)

Medina O P, Zhu Y, Kairemo K 2004 Targeted liposomal drug delivery in cancer. Curr Pharm Des 10: 2981–2989 (*Reviews in vivo trafficking of liposomes visualised by positron emission tomography and discusses the characteristics of liposomes that affect the targeting of drugs in vivo*)

Mizuno N, Niwa T, Yotsumoto Y, Sugiyama Y 2003 Impact of drug transporter studies on drug discovery and development. Pharmacol Rev 55: 425–461 (*Reviews drug transport in intestine, liver, kidney and brain, and its roles in absorption, distribution and excretion*)

Schinkel A H, Jonker J W 2003 Mammalian drug efflux transporters of the ATP binding cassette (ABC) family: an overview. Adv Drug Deliv Rev 55: 3–29 (*Overviews mammalian ATP-binding cassette (ABC) transporters known to transport clinically important drugs*)

Skyler J S, Cefalu W T, Kourides I A et al. 2001 Efficacy of inhaled human insulin in type 1 diabetes mellitus: a randomized proof-of-concept study. Lancet 357: 324–325 (*Preprandial inhaled insulin is a less invasive alternative to injection*)

Taguchi A, Sharma N, Saleem R M 2001 Selective postoperative inhibition of gastrointestinal opioid receptors. N Engl J Med 345: 935–940 (*Speeds recovery of bowel function and shortens hospitalisation: notionally 'poor' absorption is used to advantage by providing a selective action on the gut*)

Varde N K, Pack D W 2004 Microspheres for controlled release drug delivery. Exp Opin Biol Ther 4: 35–51 (*Describes methods of microparticle fabrication and factors controlling the release rates of encapsulated drugs; recent advances for delivery of single-shot vaccines, plasmid DNA and therapeutic proteins are discussed*)

Drug elimination and pharmacokinetics

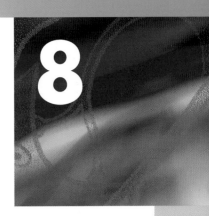

8

OVERVIEW

In the first part of this chapter, we describe the main pathways of drug metabolism, factors that influence drug elimination by the kidney, and biliary excretion and enterohepatic recirculation of drugs. The second part presents a simple approach to quantitative pharmacokinetics, explaining how drug clearance determines the steady-state plasma concentration during constant-rate drug administration and how the characteristics of absorption and distribution (considered in Ch. 7), plus metabolism and excretion, determine the time course of drug concentration in the blood before and after steady state and how these vary with different dosing regimens.

INTRODUCTION

Drug elimination is the irreversible loss of drug from the body. It occurs by two processes: metabolism and excretion. Metabolism involves enzymic conversion of one chemical entity to another within the body, whereas excretion consists of elimination from the body of chemically unchanged drug or its metabolites. The main routes by which drugs and their metabolites leave the body are:

- the kidneys
- the hepatobiliary system
- the lungs (important for volatile/gaseous anaesthetics).

Most drugs leave the body in the urine, either unchanged or as polar metabolites. Some drugs are secreted into bile via the liver, but most of these are then reabsorbed from the intestine. There are, however, instances (e.g. **rifampicin**; see Ch. 46, p. 675) where faecal loss accounts for the elimination of a substantial fraction of unchanged drug in healthy individuals, and faecal elimination of drugs such as **digoxin** that are normally excreted in urine (Ch. 18, p. 292) becomes progressively more important in patients with advancing renal failure. Excretion via the lungs occurs only with highly volatile or gaseous agents (e.g. general anaesthetics; Ch. 36). Small amounts of some drugs are also excreted in secretions such as milk or sweat. Elimination by these routes is quantitatively negligible compared with renal excretion, although excretion into milk can sometimes be important because of effects on the baby (e.g. see McNamara & Abbassi, 2004).

Lipophilic substances are not eliminated efficiently by the kidney (see p. 119). Consequently, most lipophilic drugs are metabolised to more polar products, which are then excreted in urine. Drug metabolism occurs predominantly in the liver, especially by the *cytochrome P450* (*CYP*) system. Some P450 enzymes are extrahepatic and play an important part in the biosynthesis of steroid hormones (Ch. 28) and eicosanoids (Ch. 13), but here we are concerned with catabolism of drugs by the hepatic P450 system.

DRUG METABOLISM

Animals have evolved complex systems that detoxify foreign chemicals, including carcinogens and toxins present in poisonous plants. Drugs are a special case of such foreign chemicals and, like plant alkaloids, they often exhibit distinct chirality (i.e. there is more than one stereoisomer), which affects their overall metabolism. Drug metabolism involves two kinds of reaction, known as *phase I* and *phase II*. These often, although not invariably, occur sequentially.

Phase I reactions are catabolic (e.g. oxidation, reduction or hydrolysis), and the products are often more chemically reactive and hence, paradoxically, sometimes more toxic or carcinogenic than the parent drug. Phase II reactions are synthetic ('anabolic') and involve conjugation, which usually results in inactive products (although there are exceptions, e.g. the active sulfate metabolite of **minoxidil**, a potassium channel activator used to treat severe hypertension; Ch. 19). Phase I reactions often introduce a reactive group, such as hydroxyl, into the molecule, a process known as 'functionalisation'. This group then serves as the point of attack for the conjugating system to attach a substituent such as glucuronide (Fig. 8.1), explaining why phase I reactions so often precede phase II reactions. Both phases decrease lipid solubility, thus increasing renal elimination.

Phase I and phase II reactions take place mainly in the liver, although some drugs are metabolised in plasma (e.g. hydrolysis of **suxamethonium** by plasma cholinesterase; see Ch. 10), lung (e.g. various prostanoids; see Ch. 13) or gut (e.g. **tyramine**, **salbutamol**; Chs 9 and 23). Many hepatic drug-metabolising enzymes, including CYP enzymes, are embedded in the smooth endoplasmic reticulum. They are often called 'microsomal' enzymes because, on homogenisation and differential centrifugation, the endoplasmic reticulum is broken into very small fragments that sediment only after prolonged high-speed centrifugation in the microsomal fraction. To reach these metabolising enzymes in life, a drug must cross the plasma membrane. Polar molecules do this less readily than non-polar molecules except where there are specific transport mechanisms (Ch. 7), so intracellular metabolism is in general less important for polar drugs than for lipid-soluble drugs, and the former tend to be excreted unchanged in the urine. Conversely, non-polar drugs can readily access intracellular enzymes, but are eliminated very inefficiently by the kidneys because of passive tubular reabsorption (see p. 119).

Stereoselectivity

Many clinically important drugs, such as **sotalol** (Ch. 18), **warfarin** (Ch. 21) and **cyclophosphamide** (Ch. 51), are mixtures of stereoisomers, the components of which differ not only in their pharmacological effects but also in their metabolism, which may follow completely distinct pathways. Several clinically important drug interactions involve stereospecific inhibition of metabolism of one drug by another (Ch. 52). In some cases, drug toxicity is mainly linked to one of the stereoisomers, not necessarily the pharmacologically active one. Where practicable, regulatory authorities urge that new drugs should consist of pure stereoisomers to avoid these complications.[1]

PHASE I REACTIONS

THE P450 MONOOXYGENASE SYSTEM

Nature, classification and mechanism of P450 enzymes

Cytochrome P450 enzymes are haem proteins, comprising a large family ('superfamily') of related but distinct enzymes (each referred to as CYP followed by a defining set of numbers and a letter). These enzymes differ from one another in amino acid sequence, in sensitivity to inhibitors and inducing agents, and in the specificity of the reactions that they catalyse (see Coon, 2005, for a review). Different members of the family have distinct, but often overlapping, substrate specificities, with some enzymes acting on the same substrates as each other but at different rates. Purification of P450 enzymes and complementary DNA cloning form the basis of the current classification, which is based on

---

[1]No doubt a good idea; less happily, some in the industry have perceived a commercial opportunity, and 'novel' entities that are actually just the active isomers of well-established and safe racemates have been licensed and aggressively marketed.

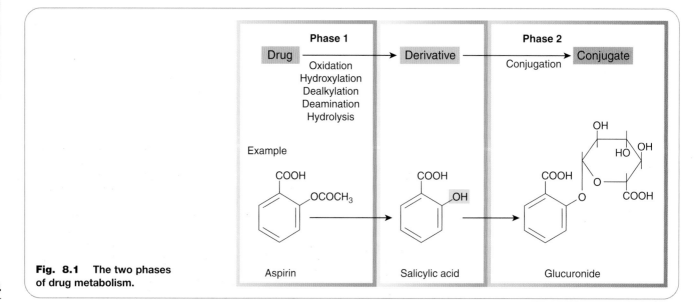

Fig. 8.1 The two phases of drug metabolism.

amino acid sequence similarities. Seventy-four CYP gene families have been described, of which three main ones (CYP1, CYP2 and CYP3) are involved in drug metabolism in human liver. Examples of therapeutic drugs that are substrates for some important P450 isoenzymes are shown in Table 8.1. Drug oxidation by the monooxygenase P450 system requires drug (substrate, 'DH'), P450 enzyme, molecular oxygen, NADPH and a flavoprotein (NADPH–P450 reductase). The mechanism involves a complex cycle (Fig. 8.2), but the overall net effect of the reaction is quite simple, namely the addition of one atom of oxygen (from molecular oxygen) to the drug to form a hydroxyl group (product, 'DOH'), the other atom of oxygen being converted to water.

▼ The P450 enzymes have unique spectral properties, and the reduced forms combine with carbon monoxide to form a pink compound (hence 'P') with absorption peaks near 450 nm (range 447–452 nm). The first clue that there are multiple forms of CYP came from the observation that treatment of rats with 3-methylcholanthrene, an inducing agent (see below), causes a shift in the absorption maximum from 450 to 448 nm.

Cytochrome P450 enzymes have unique redox properties that are fundamental to their diverse functions. These relate to the variable spin state (high/low) of the haem iron, which lies in an octahedral complex with six ligands and within which it can adopt either a penta- or hexacoordinate configuration. NADPH–P450 reductase supplies one or both electrons needed for the oxidation, and restores the redox state of the P450. Cyclic oxidation/reduction of haem iron occurs in conjunction with substrate binding and oxygen activation. The ferric iron (Fe^{3+}) in free P450 is mainly in a low-spin form. After binding DH, a conformational change converts the ferric Fe^{3+} iron to the high-spin state, making it easier to reduce. Reduction from Fe^{3+} to Fe^{2+} is achieved by a single electron, which is relayed from NADPH (electron donor) to P450 via the flavoprotein NADPH–P450 reductase. Molecular oxygen binds the reduced $Fe^{2+}·DH$ complex to form a $Fe^{2+}O_2$–DH complex. This then accepts a second electron from NADPH–P450 reductase (or alternatively from cytochrome b_5) and a proton, to yield a peroxide complex: $Fe^{2+}OOH$–DH. Addition of a second proton cleaves the $Fe^{2+}OOH$–DH complex to yield water and a ferric oxene $(FeO)^{3+}$ drug complex: $(FeO)^{3+}$–DH. $(FeO)^{3+}$ extracts a hydrogen atom from DH to form a pair of transient free radicals: D• and $Fe^{2+}OH$•. D• acquires the bound OH• radical to form hydroxylated drug (DOH), which is released from the complex with regeneration of P450 in its initial state.

P450 and biological variation

There are important variations in the expression and regulation of P450 enzymes between species. For instance, the activation pathways of certain dietary heterocyclic amines (formed when meat is cooked) to genotoxic products involves one member of the P450 superfamily (CYP1A2) that is constitutively present in humans and rats (which develop colon tumours after treatment with such amines) but not in cynomolgus monkeys (which do not). Such species differences have crucial implications for the choice of species to be used for toxicity and carcinogenicity testing during the development of new drugs for use in humans.

Within human populations, there are major sources of interindividual variation in P450 enzymes that are of great importance in therapeutics. These include genetic polymorphisms: for example, one variant of the gene *CYP2D6* leads to poor or extensive hydroxylation of **debrisoquine**. Environmental factors (Ch. 52) are also important. Enzyme inhibitors and inducers are present in the diet and environment. For example, a component of grapefruit juice inhibits drug metabolism (leading to potentially

Table 8.1 Examples of drugs that are substrates for P450 isoenzymes

Isoenzyme P450	Drug(s)
CYP1A2	Caffeine, paracetamol (→ NAPQI; see p. XXX), tacrine, theophylline
CYP2B6	Cyclophosphamide, methadone
CYP2C8	Paclitaxel, repaglinide
CYP2C19	Omeprazole, phenytoin
CYP2C9	Ibuprofen, tolbutamide, warfarin
CYP2D6	Codeine, debrisoquine, *S*-metoprolol
CYP2E1	Alcohol, paracetamol
CYP3A4, 5, 7	Ciclosporin, nifedipine, indinavir, simvastatin

(Adapted from http://medicine.iupui.edu/flockhart/table.htm.)

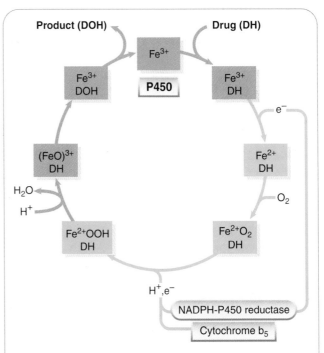

Fig. 8.2 The monooxygenase P450 cycle. P450 containing ferric iron (Fe^{3+}) combines with a molecule of drug ('DH'); receives an electron from NADPH–P450 reductase, which reduces the iron to Fe^{2+}; combines with molecular oxygen, a proton and a second electron (either from NADPH–P450 reductase or from cytochrome b_5) to form an $Fe^{2+}OOH$–DH complex. This combines with another proton to yield water and a ferric oxene $(FeO)^{3+}$–DH complex. $(FeO)^{3+}$ extracts a hydrogen atom from DH, with the formation of a pair of short-lived free radicals (see text), liberation from the complex of oxidised drug ('DOH'), and regeneration of P450 enzyme.

disastrous consequences, including cardiac dysrhythmias; Ch. 52, p. 748), whereas Brussels sprouts and cigarette smoke induce P450 enzymes. Components of St John's wort (used to treat depression in 'alternative' medicine) induce CYP450 isoenzymes and *P-glycoprotein*, which is important in drug distribution and excretion (see below, and Henderson et al., 2002).

Inhibition of P450

Inhibitors of P450 differ in their selectivity towards different isoforms of the enzyme, and are classified by their mechanism of action. Some drugs compete for the active site but are not themselves substrates (e.g. **quinidine** is a potent competitive inhibitor of CYP2D6 but is not a substrate for it). Non-competitive inhibitors include drugs such as **ketoconazole**, which forms a tight complex with the Fe^{3+} form of the haem iron of CYP3A4, causing reversible non-competitive inhibition. So-called mechanism-based inhibitors require oxidation by a P450 enzyme. Examples include **gestodene** (CYP3A4) and **diethylcarbamazine** (CYP2E1)—see p. 450 and p. 715, respectively. An oxidation product (e.g. a postulated epoxide intermediate of gestodene) binds covalently to the enzyme, which then destroys itself ('suicide inhibition'). Many clinically important interactions between drugs are the result of inhibition of P450 enzymes (see Ch. 52, p. 742).

OTHER PHASE I REACTIONS

Not all drug oxidation reactions involve the P450 system. For example, **ethanol** is metabolised by a soluble cytoplasmic enzyme, *alcohol dehydrogenase*, in addition to CYP2E1. Other P450-independent enzymes involved in drug oxidation include *xanthine oxidase*, which inactivates **6-mercaptopurine** (Ch. 51), and *monoamine oxidase*, which inactivates many biologically active amines (e.g. noradrenaline [norepinephrine], tyramine, 5-hydroxytryptamine; see Chs 11 and 12).

Reductive reactions are much less common than oxidations, but some are important. For example, **warfarin** (Ch. 21) is inactivated by conversion of a ketone to a hydroxyl group by CYP2A6.

Hydrolytic reactions (e.g. of **aspirin**, Fig. 8.1; see Ch. 14) do not involve hepatic microsomal enzymes but occur in plasma and in many tissues. Both ester and (less readily) amide bonds are susceptible to hydrolysis.

PHASE II REACTIONS

If a drug molecule has a suitable 'handle' (e.g. a hydroxyl, thiol or amino group), either in the parent molecule or in a product resulting from phase I metabolism, it is susceptible to conjugation, i.e. attachment of a substituent group. This synthetic step is called a phase II reaction. The resulting conjugate is almost always pharmacologically inactive and less lipid-soluble than its precursor, and is excreted in urine or bile.

The groups most often involved are glucuronyl (Fig. 8.3), sulfate, methyl, acetyl and glycyl. The tripeptide glutathione can conjugate drug metabolites via its sulfhydryl group, as in the detoxification of **paracetamol** (see Fig. 53.1, p. 755). Glucuronide formation involves the formation of a high-energy phosphate compound, uridine diphosphate (UDP) glucuronic acid (UDPGA),

from which glucuronic acid is transferred to an electron-rich atom (N, O or S) on the substrate, forming an amide, ester or thiol bond. UDP glucuronyl transferase, which catalyses these reactions, has very broad substrate specificity embracing many drugs and other foreign molecules. Several important endogenous substances, including bilirubin and adrenal corticosteroids, are conjugated by the same system.

Acetylation and *methylation* reactions occur with acetyl-CoA and *S*-adenosyl methionine, respectively, acting as the donor compounds. Many of these conjugation reactions occur in the liver, but other tissues, such as lung and kidney, are also involved.

INDUCTION OF MICROSOMAL ENZYMES

A number of drugs, such as **rifampicin** (Ch. 46), **ethanol** (Ch. 43) and **carbamazepine** (Ch. 40), increase the activity of microsomal oxidase and conjugating systems when administered repeatedly. Many carcinogenic chemicals (e.g. benzpyrene, 3-methyl-cholanthrene) also have this effect, which can be substantial; Figure 8.4 shows a nearly 10-fold increase in the rate of benzpyrene metabolism 2 days after a single dose. The effect is referred to as induction, and is the result of increased synthesis and/or reduced breakdown of microsomal enzymes—see recent reviews, for example Park et al. (1996) and Dickins (2004), for more detail.

Enzyme induction can *increase* drug toxicity and carcinogenicity (Park et al., 2005), because several phase I metabolites are toxic or carcinogenic: **paracetamol** is an important example of a drug with a highly toxic metabolite (see Ch. 53).

The mechanism of induction is incompletely understood but is similar to that involved in the action of steroid and other hormones that bind to nuclear receptors (see Ch. 3). The most thoroughly studied inducing agents are polycyclic aromatic hydrocarbons. These bind to the ligand-binding domain of a soluble protein, termed the *aromatic hydrocarbon* (*Ah*) receptor. This complex is transported to the nucleus by an Ah receptor nuclear translocator and binds Ah receptor response elements in the DNA, thereby promoting transcription of the gene *CYP1A1*. In addition to enhanced transcription, some inducing agents (e.g. ethanol, which induces CYP2E1 in humans) also stabilise mRNA or P450 protein.

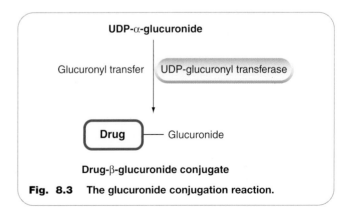

Fig. 8.3 The glucuronide conjugation reaction.

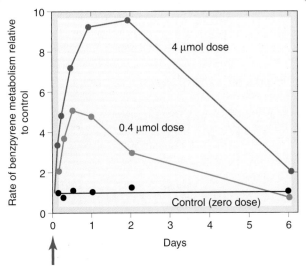

Fig. 8.4   Stimulation of hepatic metabolism of benzpyrene. Young rats were given benzpyrene (intraperitoneally) in the doses shown, and the benzpyrene-metabolising activity of liver homogenates was measured at times up to 6 days. (From Conney A H et al. 1957 J Biol Chem 228: 753.)

Table 8.2   Examples of drugs that undergo substantial first-pass elimination

Aspirin	Metoprolol
Glyceryl trinitrate	Morphine
Isosorbide dinitrate	Propranolol
Levodopa	Salbutamol
Lidocaine	Verapamil

FIRST-PASS (PRESYSTEMIC) METABOLISM

Some drugs are extracted so efficiently by the liver or gut wall that the amount reaching the systemic circulation is considerably less than the amount absorbed. This is known as *first-pass* or *presystemic* metabolism and reduces bioavailability (Ch. 7, p. 106) even when a drug is well absorbed from the gut. Presystemic metabolism is important for many therapeutic drugs (Table 8.2 shows some examples), and is a problem because:

- a much larger dose of the drug is needed when it is given orally than when it is given by other routes
- marked individual variations occur in the extent of first-pass metabolism of a given drug (see Ch. 52), resulting in unpredictability when such drugs are taken orally.

PHARMACOLOGICALLY ACTIVE DRUG METABOLITES

In some cases (see Table 8.3), a drug becomes pharmacologically active only after it has been metabolised. For example, **azathioprine**, an immunosuppressant drug (Ch. 14), is metabolised to **mercaptopurine**; and **enalapril**, an angiotensin-converting enzyme inhibitor (Ch. 19), is hydrolysed to its active form **enalaprilat**. Such drugs, in which the parent compound lacks activity of its own, are known as *prodrugs*. These are sometimes designed deliberately to overcome problems of drug delivery (Ch. 7). Metabolism can alter the pharmacological actions of a drug qualitatively. **Aspirin** inhibits some platelet functions and has anti-inflammatory activity (Ch 21, pp. 341-342; Ch. 14, pp. 234-235). It is hydrolysed to salicylic acid (Fig. 8.1), which has anti-inflammatory but not antiplatelet activity. In other instances, metabolites have pharmacological actions similar to those of the parent compound (e.g. benzodiazepines, many of which form long-lived active metabolites that cause sedation to persist after the parent drug has disappeared; Ch. 37). There are also cases in which metabolites are responsible for toxicity. Hepatotoxicity of **paracetamol** is one example (see Ch. 53), and bladder toxicity of **cyclophosphamide**, which is caused by its toxic metabolite *acrolein* (Ch. 51, p. 724), is another. Methanol and ethylene glycol both exert their toxic effects via metabolites formed by alcohol dehydrogenase. Poisoning with these agents is treated with ethanol (or with a more potent inhibitor), which competes for the active site of the enzyme. **Terfenadine**, a non-sedating antihistamine (p. 237-238), can, rarely, cause serious cardiac dysrhythmias by blocking cardiac potassium channels. Its pharmacologically active metabolite (**fexofenadine**) blocks histamine H_1 receptors but not cardiac potassium channels, and has now largely replaced terfenadine in therapeutic use for this

---

Drug metabolism

- Phase I reactions involve oxidation, reduction and hydrolysis. They:
  - usually form more chemically reactive products, which can be pharmacologically active, toxic or carcinogenic
  - often involve a monooxygenase system in which cytochrome P450 plays a key role.
- Phase II reactions involve conjugation (e.g. glucuronidation) of a reactive group (often inserted during phase I reaction) and usually lead to inactive and polar products that are readily excreted.
- Some conjugated products are excreted via bile, are reactivated in the intestine and then reabsorbed ('enterohepatic circulation').
- Induction of P450 enzymes can greatly accelerate hepatic drug metabolism. It can increase the toxicity of drugs with toxic metabolites.
- Presystemic metabolism in liver or gut wall reduces the bioavailability of several drugs when they are administered by mouth.

Table 8.3 Some drugs that produce active or toxic metabolites

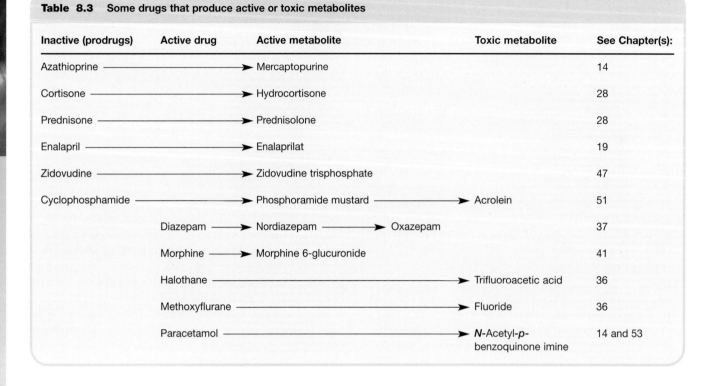

Inactive (prodrugs)	Active drug	Active metabolite	Toxic metabolite	See Chapter(s):
Azathioprine		→ Mercaptopurine		14
Cortisone		→ Hydrocortisone		28
Prednisone		→ Prednisolone		28
Enalapril		→ Enalaprilat		19
Zidovudine		→ Zidovudine trisphosphate		47
Cyclophosphamide		→ Phosphoramide mustard	→ Acrolein	51
	Diazepam →	Nordiazepam → Oxazepam		37
	Morphine →	Morphine 6-glucuronide		41
Halothane			→ Trifluoroacetic acid	36
Methoxyflurane			→ Fluoride	36
Paracetamol			→ *N*-Acetyl-*p*-benzoquinone imine	14 and 53

reason. Hepatic necrosis is a rare but sometimes fatal complication of **halothane** anaesthesia. It is caused by immune sensitisation to new antigens formed by trifluoroacetylation of liver protein (Ch. 53, p. 763). **Disulfiram** (see pp. 632-633) inhibits CYP2E1 and reduces substantially the formation of trifluoroacetic acid during halothane anaesthesia, raising the intriguing possibility that it could prevent halothane hepatitis (Kharasch et al., 1996).

BILIARY EXCRETION AND ENTEROHEPATIC CIRCULATION

Liver cells transfer various substances, including drugs, from plasma to bile by means of transport systems similar to those of the renal tubule and that involve P-glycoprotein (see Ch. 7). Various hydrophilic drug conjugates (particularly glucuronides) are concentrated in bile and delivered to the intestine, where the glucuronide is usually hydrolysed, releasing active drug once more; free drug can then be reabsorbed and the cycle repeated (enterohepatic circulation). The effect of this is to create a 'reservoir' of recirculating drug that can amount to about 20% of total drug in the body and prolongs drug action. Examples where this is important include **morphine** (Ch. 41) and **ethinylestradiol** (Ch. 30). Several drugs are excreted to an appreciable extent in bile. **Vecuronium** (a non-depolarising muscle relaxant; Ch. 10) is an example of a drug that is excreted mainly unchanged in bile. **Rifampicin** (Ch. 46) is absorbed from the gut and slowly deacetylated, retaining its biological activity. Both forms are secreted in the bile, but the deacetylated form is not reabsorbed,

so eventually most of the drug leaves the body in this form in the faeces.

RENAL EXCRETION OF DRUGS AND DRUG METABOLITES

Drugs differ greatly in the rate at which they are excreted by the kidney, ranging from **penicillin** (Ch. 46), which is cleared from the blood almost completely on a single transit through the kidney, to **diazepam** (Ch. 37), which is cleared extremely slowly. Most drugs fall between these extremes, and metabolites are nearly always cleared more quickly than the parent drug. Three fundamental processes account for renal drug excretion:

- glomerular filtration
- active tubular secretion
- passive diffusion across tubular epithelium.

GLOMERULAR FILTRATION

Glomerular capillaries allow drug molecules of molecular weight below about 20 000 to diffuse into the glomerular filtrate. Plasma albumin (molecular weight approximately 68 000) is almost completely impermeable, but most drugs—with the exception of macromolecules such as **heparin** (Ch. 21)—cross the barrier freely. If a drug binds appreciably to plasma albumin, its concentration in the filtrate will be less than the total plasma concentration. If, like **warfarin** (Ch. 21), a drug is approximately 98% bound to albumin, the concentration in the filtrate is only 2% of that in plasma, and clearance by filtration is correspondingly reduced.

TUBULAR SECRETION

Up to 20% of renal plasma flow is filtered through the glomerulus, leaving at least 80% of delivered drug to pass on to the peritubular capillaries of the proximal tubule. Here, drug molecules are transferred to the tubular lumen by two independent and relatively non-selective carrier systems. One of these transports acidic drugs (as well as various endogenous acids, such as uric acid), while the other handles organic bases. Some of the more important drugs that are transported by these two carrier systems are shown in Table 8.4. The carriers can transport drug molecules against an electrochemical gradient, and can therefore reduce the plasma concentration nearly to zero. Because at least 80% of the drug delivered to the kidney is presented to the carrier, tubular secretion is potentially the most effective mechanism of renal drug elimination. Unlike glomerular filtration, carrier-mediated transport can achieve maximal drug clearance even when most of the drug is bound to plasma protein.[2] **Penicillin** (Ch. 46), for example, although about 80% protein-bound and therefore cleared only slowly by filtration, is almost completely removed by proximal tubular secretion, and its overall rate of elimination is very high.

Many drugs compete for the same transport system (Table 8.4), leading to drug interactions. For example, **probenecid** (see p. 239) was developed originally to prolong the action of penicillin by retarding its tubular secretion.

DIFFUSION ACROSS THE RENAL TUBULE

Water is reabsorbed as fluid traverses the tubule, the volume of urine emerging being only about 1% of that of the glomerular filtrate. If the tubule is freely permeable to drug molecules, some 99% of the filtered drug will be reabsorbed passively. Lipid-soluble drugs are therefore excreted poorly, whereas polar drugs of low tubular permeability remain in the lumen and become progressively concentrated as water is reabsorbed. Drugs handled in this way include **digoxin** (p. 292) and aminoglycoside antibiotics. These exemplify a relatively small but important group of drugs (Table 8.5) that are not inactivated by metabolism, the rate of renal elimination being the main factor that determines their duration of action. These drugs have to be used with special care in individuals whose renal function may be impaired, including the elderly and patients with renal disease or any severe acute illness (Ch. 52, pp. 740-745).

---

[2]Because filtration involves isosmotic movement of both water and solutes, it does not affect the free concentration of drug in the plasma. Thus the equilibrium between free and bound drug is not disturbed, and there is no tendency for bound drug to dissociate as blood traverses the glomerular capillary. The rate of clearance of a drug by filtration is therefore reduced directly in proportion to the fraction that is bound. In the case of active tubular secretion, this is not so; secretion may be retarded very little even though the drug is mostly bound. This is because the carrier transports drug molecules unaccompanied by water. As free drug molecules are taken from the plasma, therefore, the free plasma concentration falls, causing dissociation of bound drug from plasma albumin. Consequently, effectively 100% of the drug, bound and free, is available to the carrier.

Table 8.4 Important drugs and related substances actively secreted into the proximal renal tubule

Acids	Bases
p-Aminohippuric acid	Amiloride
Furosemide (frusemide)	Dopamine
Glucuronic acid conjugates	Histamine
Glycine conjugates	Mepacrine
Indometacin	Morphine
Methotrexate	Pethidine
Penicillin	Quaternary ammonium probenecid compounds
Sulfate conjugates	Quinine
Thiazide diuretics	5-Hydroxytryptamine (serotonin)
Uric acid	Triamterene

Many drugs, being weak acids or weak bases, change their ionisation with pH (see pp. 99-100), and this can markedly affect renal excretion. The ion-trapping effect means that a basic drug is more rapidly excreted in an acid urine, because the low pH within the tubule favours ionisation and thus inhibits reabsorption. Conversely, acidic drugs are most rapidly excreted if the urine is alkaline (Fig. 8.5). Urinary alkalinisation is used to accelerate the excretion of salicylate in treating selected cases of **aspirin** overdose (p. 100).

RENAL CLEARANCE

Elimination of drugs by the kidneys is best quantified by the renal clearance (CL_r). This is defined as the volume of plasma

Elimination of drugs by the kidney

- Most drugs, unless highly bound to plasma protein, cross the glomerular filter freely.
- Many drugs, especially weak acids and weak bases, are actively secreted into the renal tubule and thus more rapidly excreted.
- Lipid-soluble drugs are passively reabsorbed by diffusion across the tubule, so are not efficiently excreted in the urine.
- Because of pH partition, weak acids are more rapidly excreted in alkaline urine, and vice versa.
- Several important drugs are removed predominantly by renal excretion, and are liable to cause toxicity in elderly persons and patients with renal disease.

Table 8.5 Examples of drugs that are excreted largely unchanged in the urine

Percentage	Drugs excreted
100–75	Furosemide (frusemide), gentamicin, methotrexate, atenolol, digoxin
75–50	Benzylpenicillin, cimetidine, oxytetracycline, neostigmine
~50	Propantheline, tubocurarine

containing the amount of substance that is removed by the kidney in unit time. It is calculated from the plasma concentration, C_p, the urinary concentration, C_u, and the rate of flow of urine, V_u, by the equation:

$$CL_r = \frac{C_u \times V_u}{C_p} \qquad (8.1)$$

CL_r varies greatly for different drugs, from less than 1 ml/min to the theoretical maximum set by the renal plasma flow, which is approximately 700 ml/min, measured by p-aminohippuric acid (PAH) clearance (renal extraction of PAH approaches 100%).

PHARMACOKINETICS

Definition and uses of pharmacokinetics

The relationship between the time course of drug concentrations attained in different regions of the body during and after dosing is termed *pharmacokinetics* ('what the body does to the drug'), to distinguish it from *pharmacodynamics* ('what the drug does to the body', i.e. events consequent on interaction of the drug with its receptor or other primary site of action). The distinction is useful, although the words cause dismay to etymological purists.

Knowledge of pharmacokinetics is crucial for drug development, both to make sense of preclinical toxicity testing and of whole animal pharmacology,[3] and to decide on an appropriate dosing regimen for pivotal phase III studies of efficacy. Understanding the general principles of pharmacokinetics is also important for clinicians, who need to understand how dosage recommendations in the product information provided with licensed drugs have been arrived at if they are to use the drug optimally and understand its limitations. In particular, clinicians dealing with a severely ill patient often need to individualise the dose regimen depending on how rapidly a therapeutic plasma concentration is required, and whether the clearance of the drug is impaired because of renal or liver disease.

Scope

In this section, we explain how the total clearance of a drug determines its steady-state plasma concentration during continuous administration. We then present a simple model in which the body is represented as a single well-stirred compartment, of volume V_d, that describes the situation before steady state is reached in terms of elimination half life ($t_{1/2}$). Three dosing situations are

---

[3]For example, doses used in experimental animals often need to be much greater than those in humans (on a 'per unit body weight' basis), because drug metabolism is commonly much more rapid in rodents.

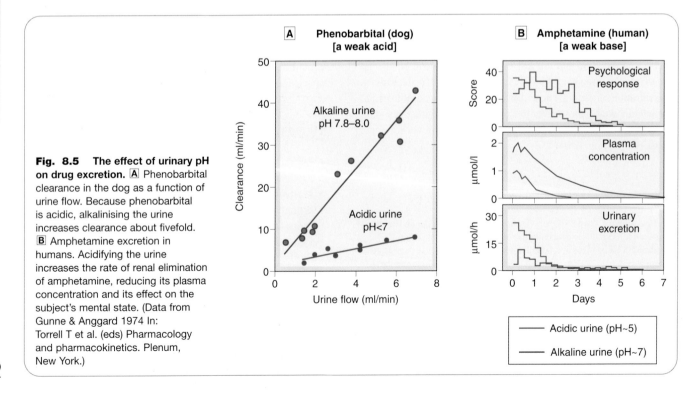

Fig. 8.5 **The effect of urinary pH on drug excretion.** A Phenobarbital clearance in the dog as a function of urine flow. Because phenobarbital is acidic, alkalinising the urine increases clearance about fivefold. B Amphetamine excretion in humans. Acidifying the urine increases the rate of renal elimination of amphetamine, reducing its plasma concentration and its effect on the subject's mental state. (Data from Gunne & Anggard 1974 In: Torrell T et al. (eds) Pharmacology and pharmacokinetics. Plenum, New York.)

considered: continuous intravenous infusion, bolus dose administration and repeated administration. Finally, we consider some situations where the simple model is inadequate, and either a two-compartment model or a model where clearance varies with drug concentration ('non-linear kinetics') is needed. More detailed accounts are provided by Rowland & Tozer (1995) and Birkett (2002); Atkinson et al. (2002) describe an alternative approach.

DRUG ELIMINATION EXPRESSED AS CLEARANCE

The overall clearance of a drug (CL) is the volume of plasma containing the total amount of drug that is removed from the body in unit time. It is the fundamental pharmacokinetic parameter that relates the rate of elimination of a drug to its plasma concentration (C):

$$\text{Rate of drug elimination} = C \times CL \qquad (8.2)$$

Drug clearance can be determined in an individual subject by measuring the plasma concentration of the drug (in units of, say, mg/l) at intervals during a constant-rate intravenous infusion (say X mg/h), until a steady state is approximated (Fig. 8.6A). At steady state, the rate of input to the body is equal to the rate of elimination, so:

$$X = C_{SS} \times CL \qquad (8.3)$$

Rearranging this,

$$CL = \frac{X}{C_{SS}} \qquad (8.4)$$

where C_{SS} is the plasma concentration at steady state, and CL is in units of volume/time (l/h in the example given).

For many drugs, the clearance in an individual subject is the same at different doses (at least within the range of doses used therapeutically—but see the *Saturation kinetics* section below, pp. 124–126, for exceptions), so knowing CL enables one to calculate the dose rate needed to achieve a desired steady-state plasma concentration from equation 8.3.

CL can also be estimated by measuring plasma concentrations at intervals following a single intravenous bolus dose of, say, Q mg (Fig. 8.6B).

$$CL = \frac{Q}{\text{AUC}} \qquad (8.5)$$

where AUC is the area under the curve relating C to time (see Ch. 7, p. 106, and Birkett, 2002, for a fuller account of AUC and how it is estimated).

SINGLE-COMPARTMENT MODEL

Consider a highly simplified model of a human being, which consists of a single well-stirred compartment, of volume V_d (distribution volume), into which a quantity of drug Q is introduced rapidly by intravenous injection, and from which it can escape either by being metabolised or by being excreted (Fig. 8.7). For most drugs, V_d is an apparent volume rather than the volume of an anatomical compartment. It links the total amount of drug in

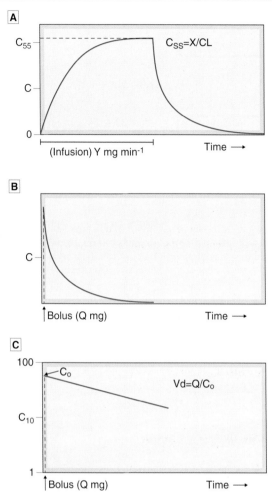

Fig. 8.6 Plasma drug concentration–time curves.
A During a constant intravenous infusion at rate X mg/min, indicated by the horizontal bar, the plasma concentration (**C**) increases from zero to a steady-state value (**C**$_{SS}$); when the infusion is stopped, **C** declines to zero. **B** Following an intravenous bolus dose (Q mg), the plasma concentration rises abruptly and then declines towards zero. **C** If the data from panel B are plotted with **C** on a logarithmic scale, there is a linear portion during which the concentration declines approximately exponentially. Extrapolation of this portion of the curve back to the ordinate at zero time gives an estimate of **C**$_0$, the concentration at zero time, and hence of **V**$_d$, the volume of distribution.

the body to its concentration in plasma (see Ch. 7, p. 109). The quantity of drug in the body when it is administered as a single bolus is equal to the administered dose Q. The initial concentration, C_0, will therefore be given by:

$$C_0 = \frac{Q}{V_d} \qquad (8.6)$$

In practice, C_0 is estimated by extrapolating the linear portion of a semilogarithmic plot of C against time back to its intercept at time 0 (Fig. 8.6C). The concentration C_t at a later time t will depend on the rate of elimination of the drug (i.e. on its total clearance, CL). Many drugs exhibit first-order kinetics where the

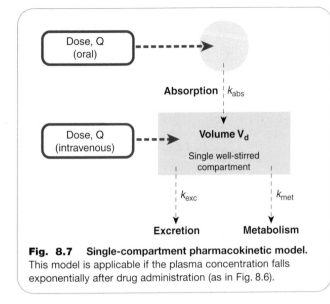

Fig. 8.7   **Single-compartment pharmacokinetic model.** This model is applicable if the plasma concentration falls exponentially after drug administration (as in Fig. 8.6).

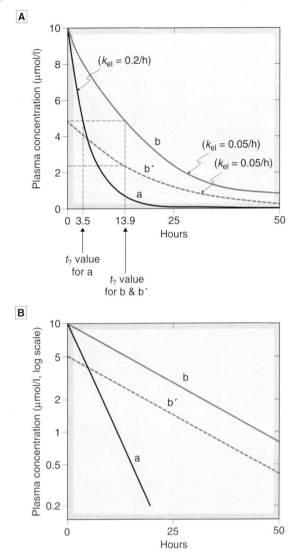

Fig. 8.8   **Predicted behaviour of single-compartment model following intravenous drug administration at time 0.** Drugs a and b differ only in their elimination rate constant, k_{el}. Curve b shows the plasma concentration time course for a smaller dose of b. Note that the half-life ($t_{1/2}$) (indicated by broken lines) does not depend on the dose. **A** Linear concentration scale. **B** Logarithmic concentration scale.

rate of elimination is directly proportional to drug concentration. Drug concentration then decays exponentially (Fig. 8.8), being described by the equation:

$$C(t) = C_{(0)}\exp\frac{-CL_s}{V_d}t \qquad (8.7)$$

Taking logarithms:

$$\ln C(t) = \ln C_{(0)} - \frac{-CL_s}{V_d}t \qquad (8.8)$$

Plotting C_t on a logarithmic scale against t (on a linear scale) yields a straight line with slope CL_s/V_d. The inverse of this slope (CL_s/V_d) is the elimination rate constant k_{el}. The elimination half-life, $t_{1/2}$, is an easily conceptualised parameter inversely related to k_{el}. It is the time taken for C_t to decrease by 50%, and is equal to $\ln2/k_{el}$ ($0.693/k_{el}$). The plasma half-life is therefore determined by V_d and CL_s.

When the single-compartment model is applicable, the drug concentration in plasma approaches the steady-state value approximately exponentially during a constant infusion (Fig. 8.6A). When the infusion is discontinued, the concentration falls exponentially towards zero: after one half-life, the concentration will have fallen to half the initial concentration; after two half-lives, it will have fallen to one-quarter the initial concentration; after three half-lives, to one eighth; and so on. It is intuitively obvious that the longer the half-life, the longer the drug will persist in the body after dosing is discontinued. It is less obvious, but nonetheless true, that during chronic drug administration the longer the half-life the longer it will take for the drug to accumulate to its steady-state level: one half-life to reach 50% of the steady-state value, two to reach 75%, three to reach 87.5%, and so on. This is extremely helpful to a clinician deciding how to start treatment. If the drug in question has a half-life of approximately 24 hours, for example, it will take 3–5 days to approximate the steady-state concentration during a constant-rate infusion. If this is too slow in the face of the prevailing clinical situation, a

loading dose may be used (see below). The size of such a dose is determined by the volume of distribution (equation 8.6).

EFFECT OF REPEATED DOSAGE

Drugs are usually given as repeated doses rather than single injections or a constant infusion. Repeated injections (each of dose Q) give a more complicated pattern than the smooth exponential rise during intravenous infusion, but the principle is the same (Fig. 8.9). The concentration will rise to a mean steady-state concentration with an approximately exponential time course, but will oscillate (through a range Q/V_d). The smaller and more

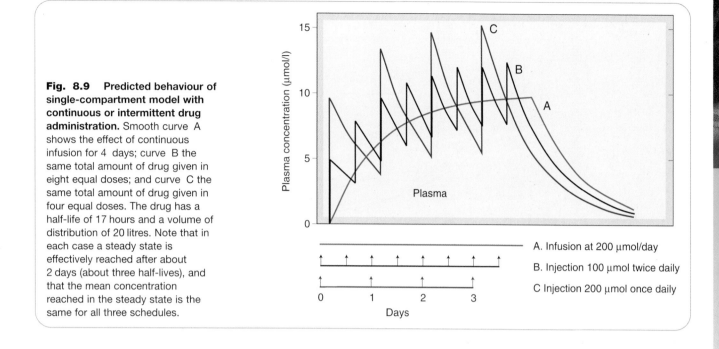

Fig. 8.9 Predicted behaviour of single-compartment model with continuous or intermittent drug administration. Smooth curve A shows the effect of continuous infusion for 4 days; curve B the same total amount of drug given in eight equal doses; and curve C the same total amount of drug given in four equal doses. The drug has a half-life of 17 hours and a volume of distribution of 20 litres. Note that in each case a steady state is effectively reached after about 2 days (about three half-lives), and that the mean concentration reached in the steady state is the same for all three schedules.

A. Infusion at 200 µmol/day

B. Injection 100 µmol twice daily

C Injection 200 µmol once daily

frequent the doses, the more closely the situation approaches that of a continuous infusion, and the smaller the swings in concentration. The exact dosage schedule, however, does not affect the mean steady-state concentration, nor the rate at which it is approached. In practice, a steady state is effectively achieved after three to five half-lives. Speedier attainment of the steady state can be achieved by starting with a larger dose, as explained above. Such a loading dose is sometimes used when starting treatment with a drug with a half-life that is long in the context of the urgency of the clinical situation, as may be the case when treating cardiac dysrhythmias with drugs such as **amiodarone** or **digoxin** (Ch. 18).

EFFECT OF VARIATION IN RATE OF ABSORPTION

If a drug is absorbed slowly from the gut or from an injection site into the plasma, it is (in terms of a compartmental model) as though it were being injected slowly into the bloodstream. For the purpose of kinetic modelling, the transfer of drug from the site of administration to the central compartment can be represented approximately by a rate constant, k_{abs} (see Fig. 8.7). This assumes that the rate of absorption is directly proportional, at any moment, to the amount of drug still unabsorbed, which is at best a rough approximation to reality. The effect of slow absorption on the time course of the rise and fall of the plasma concentration is shown in Figure 8.10. The curves show the effect of spreading out the absorption of the same total amount of drug over different times. In each case, the drug is absorbed completely, but the peak concentration appears later and is lower and less sharp if absorption is slow. In the limiting case, a dosage form that releases drug at a constant rate as it traverses the ileum (Ch. 7,

p. 100) approximates a constant-rate infusion. Once absorption is complete, the plasma concentration declines with the same half-time, irrespective of the rate of absorption.

▼ For the kind of pharmacokinetic model discussed here, the area under the plasma concentration–time curve (AUC) is directly proportional to the total amount of drug introduced into the plasma compartment, irrespective of the rate at which it enters. Incomplete absorption, or destruction by first-pass metabolism before the drug reaches the plasma compartment, reduces AUC after oral administration (see Ch. 7, p. 106). Changes in the *rate* of absorption, however, do not affect AUC. Again, it is worth noting that provided absorption is complete, the relation between the rate of administration and the steady-state plasma concentration (equation 8.4) is unaffected by k_{abs}, although the size of the oscillation of plasma concentration with each dose is reduced if absorption is slow.

MORE COMPLICATED KINETIC MODELS

So far, we have considered a single-compartment pharmacokinetic model in which the rates of absorption, metabolism and excretion are all assumed to be directly proportional to the concentration of drug in the compartment from which transfer is occurring. This is a useful way to illustrate some basic principles but is clearly a physiological oversimplification. The characteristics of different parts of the body, such as brain, body fat and muscle, are quite different in terms of their blood supply, partition coefficient for drugs, and the permeability of their capillaries to drugs. These differences, which the single-compartment model ignores, can markedly affect the time courses of drug distribution and action, and much theoretical work has gone into the mathematical analysis of more complex models (see Rowland & Tozer, 1995; Atkinson et al., 2002). They are beyond the scope of this book, and perhaps also beyond the limit of what is actually useful, for the experimental data on pharmacokinetic properties of drugs are

123

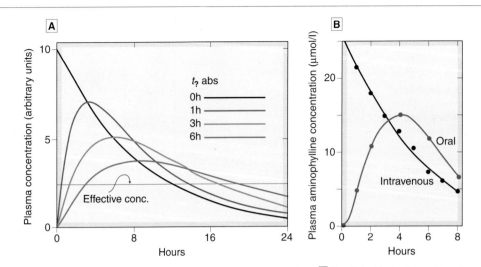

Fig. 8.10   The effect of slow drug absorption on plasma drug concentration. $\boxed{A}$ Predicted behaviour of single-compartment model with drug absorbed at different rates from the gut or an injection site. The elimination half-time is 6 hours. The absorption half-times ($t_{1/2}$ abs) are marked on the diagram. (Zero indicates instantaneous absorption, corresponding to intravenous administration.) Note that the peak plasma concentration is reduced and delayed by slow absorption, and the duration of action is somewhat increased. $\boxed{B}$ Measurements of plasma aminophylline concentration in humans following equal oral and intravenous doses. (Data from Swintowsky J V 1956 J Am Pharm Assoc 49: 395.)

seldom accurate or reproducible enough to enable complex models to be tested critically.

The two-compartment model, which introduces a separate 'peripheral' compartment to represent the tissues, in communication with the 'central' plasma compartment, more closely resembles the real situation without involving excessive complications.

TWO-COMPARTMENT MODEL

The two-compartment model is a widely used approximation in which the tissues are lumped together as a peripheral compartment. Drug molecules can enter and leave the peripheral compartment only via the central compartment (Fig. 8.11), which usually represents the plasma (or plasma plus some extravascular space

in the case of a few drugs that distribute especially rapidly). The effect of adding a second compartment to the model is to introduce a second exponential component into the predicted time course of the plasma concentration, so that it comprises a fast and a slow phase. This pattern is often found experimentally, and is most clearly revealed when the concentration data are plotted semilogarithmically (Fig. 8.12). If, as is often the case, the transfer of drug between the central and peripheral compartments is relatively fast compared with the rate of elimination, then the fast phase (often called the α phase) can be taken to represent the redistribution of the drug (i.e. drug molecules passing from plasma to tissues, thereby rapidly lowering the plasma concentration). The plasma concentration reached when the fast phase is complete, but before any elimination has occurred, allows a measure of the combined distribution volumes of the two compartments; the half-time for the slow phase (the β phase) provides an estimate of k_{el}. If a drug is rapidly metabolised, the α and β phases are not well separated, and the calculation of V_d and k_{el} is not straightforward. Problems also arise with drugs (e.g. very fat-soluble drugs) for which it is unrealistic to lump all the peripheral tissues together.

SATURATION KINETICS

In a few cases, such as **ethanol**, **phenytoin** and **salicylate**, the time course of disappearance of drug from the plasma does not follow the exponential or biexponential patterns shown in Figures 8.8 and 8.12 but is initially linear (i.e. drug is removed at a constant rate that is independent of plasma concentration). This is often called *zero-order kinetics* to distinguish it from the usual *first-order kinetics* that we have considered so far (these terms have their origin in chemical kinetic theory). *Saturation kinetics* is a better term. Figure 8.13 shows the example of ethanol. It can

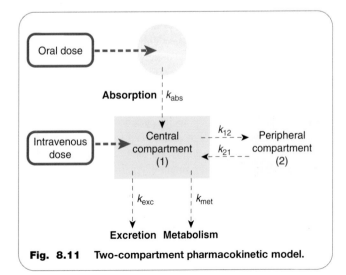

Fig. 8.11   Two-compartment pharmacokinetic model.

Pharmacokinetics

- Total clearance (*CL*) of a drug is the fundamental parameter describing its elimination: the rate of elimination equals *CL* times plasma concentration.
- *CL* determines steady-state plasma concentration (C_{ss}): C_{ss} = rate of drug administration/*CL*.
- For many drugs, disappearance from the plasma follows an approximately exponential time course. Such drugs can be described by a model where the body is treated as a single well-stirred compartment of volume V_d. V_d is an apparent volume linking the amount of drug in the body at any time to the plasma concentration.
- Elimination half-life ($t_{1/2}$) is directly proportional to V_d and inversely proportional to *CL*.
- With repeated dosage or sustained delivery of a drug, the plasma concentration approaches a steady value within three to five plasma half-lives.
- In urgent situations, a loading dose may be needed to achieve therapeutic concentration rapidly.
- The loading dose needed to achieve a desired initial plasma concentration is determined by V_d.
- A two-compartment model is often needed. In this case, the kinetics are biexponential. The two components roughly represent the processes of transfer between plasma and tissues (α phase) and elimination from the plasma (β phase).
- Some drugs show non-exponential 'saturation' kinetics, with important clinical consequences, especially a disproportionate increase in steady-state plasma concentration when daily dose is increased.

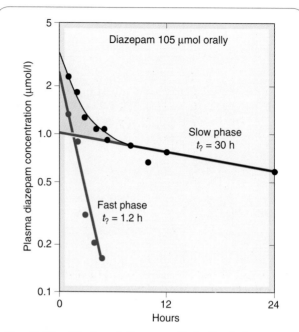

Fig. 8.12 Kinetics of diazepam elimination in humans following a single oral dose. The graph shows a semilogarithmic plot of plasma concentration versus time. The experimental data (black symbols) follow a curve that becomes linear after about 8 hours (slow phase). Plotting the deviation of the early points (pink shaded area) from this line on the same coordinates (red symbols) reveals the fast phase. This type of two-component decay is consistent with the two-compartment model (Fig. 8.11) and is obtained with many drugs. (Data from Curry S H 1980 Drug disposition and pharmacokinetics. Blackwell, Oxford.)

be seen that the rate of disappearance of ethanol from the plasma is constant at about 4 mmol/l per hour, irrespective of its plasma concentration. The explanation for this is that the rate of oxidation by the enzyme alcohol dehydrogenase reaches a maximum at low ethanol concentrations, because of limited availability of the cofactor NAD^+ (see Ch. 43, p. 632, Fig. 43.6).

Saturation kinetics has several important consequences (see Fig. 8.14). One is that the duration of action is more strongly dependent on dose than is the case with drugs that do not show metabolic saturation. Another consequence is that the relationship between dose and steady-state plasma concentration is steep and unpredictable, and it does not obey the proportionality rule implicit in equation 8.4 for non-saturating drugs. The maximum rate of metabolism sets a limit to the rate at which the drug can be administered; if this rate is exceeded, the amount of drug in the body will, in principle, increase indefinitely and never reach a steady state (Fig. 8.14). This does not actually happen, because there is always some dependence of the rate of elimination on the plasma concentration (usually because other, non-saturating metabolic pathways or renal excretion contribute significantly at

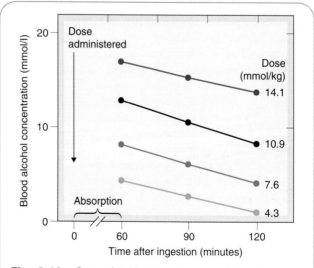
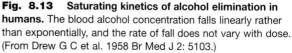

Fig. 8.13 Saturating kinetics of alcohol elimination in humans. The blood alcohol concentration falls linearly rather than exponentially, and the rate of fall does not vary with dose. (From Drew G C et al. 1958 Br Med J 2: 5103.)

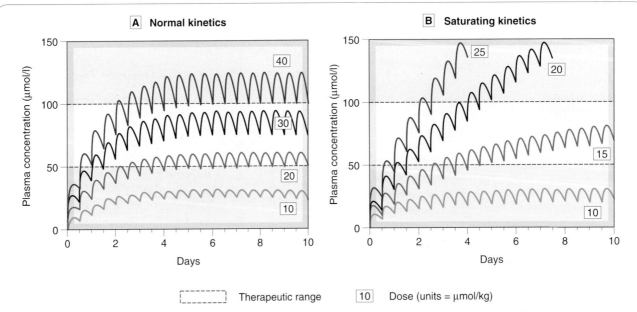

Fig. 8.14 **Comparison of non-saturating and saturating kinetics for drugs given orally every 12 hours.** The curves show an imaginary drug, similar to the antiepileptic drug phenytoin at the lowest dose, but with linear kinetics. The curves for saturating kinetics are calculated from the known pharmacokinetic parameters of phenytoin (see Ch. 40). Note A that no steady state is reached with higher doses of phenytoin, and B that a small increment in dose results after a time in a disproportionately large effect on plasma concentration. With linear kinetics, the steady-state plasma concentration is directly proportional to dose. (Curves were calculated with the Sympak pharmacokinetic modelling program written by Dr J G Blackman, University of Otago.)

high concentrations). Nevertheless, steady-state plasma concentrations of drugs of this kind vary widely and unpredictably with dose. Similarly, variations in the rate of metabolism (e.g. through enzyme induction) cause disproportionately large changes in the plasma concentration. These problems are well recognised for drugs such as **phenytoin**, an anticonvulsant for which plasma concentration needs to be closely controlled to achieve an optimal clinical effect (see Ch. 40, p. 582, Fig. 40.3).

Clinical applications of pharmacokinetics are summarised in the clinical box.

Pharmacokinetics

- Pharmacokinetic studies performed during drug development underpin the standard dose regimens approved by regulatory agencies.
- Clinicians sometimes need to individualise dose regimens to account for individual variation in a particular patient (e.g. a neonate, a patient with impaired and changing renal function, or a patient taking drugs that interfere with drug metabolism; see Ch. 52).
- Drug effect (*pharmacodynamics*) is often used for such individualisation, but there are drugs (including some anticonvulsants, antidysrhythmics and antineoplastics) where a therapeutic range of plasma concentrations has been defined, and for which it is useful to adjust the dose to achieve a concentration in this range.
- Knowledge of kinetics enables rational dose adjustment. For example:
  - the dose interval of a drug such as gentamicin eliminated by renal excretion may need to be

markedly increased in a patient with renal failure (Ch. 46, pp. 670-671)
  - the dose increment needed to achieve a target plasma concentration range of a drug such as **phenytoin** with saturation kinetics (Ch. 40, p. 582, Fig. 40.3) is much less than for a drug with linear kinetics.
- Knowing the approximate $t_{1/2}$ of a drug can be very useful, even if a therapeutic concentration is not known:
  - in correctly interpreting adverse events that occur some considerable time after starting regular treatment (e.g. benzodiazepines; see Ch. 37, pp. 541-542)
  - in deciding on the need or otherwise for an initial loading dose when starting treatment with drugs such as **digoxin** and **amiodarone** (Ch. 18, pp. 290 and 292).
- The volume of distribution (V_d) of a drug determines the size of loading dose needed. If V_d is large (as for many tricyclic antidepressants), haemodialysis will not be an effective way of increasing the rate of elimination in treating overdose.

REFERENCES AND FURTHER READING

Pharmacogenetics

Bertilsson L, Dahl M L, Dalen P, Al-Shurbaji A 2002 Molecular genetics of CYP2D6: clinical relevance with focus on psychotropic drugs. Br J Clin Pharmacol 53: 111–122 (*Reviews the influence of genetic variability in CYP2D6 on the clinical pharmacokinetics and therapeutic effects/adverse effects of psychotropic drugs*)

Walker D K 2004 The use of pharmacokinetic and pharmacodynamic data in the assessment of drug safety in early drug development. Br J Clin Pharmacol 58: 601–608 (*A factor in the assessment of safety during early drug development is the pharmacokinetic profile of the compound, which allows safety data such as QT interval to be considered in the light of systemic drug exposure before human exposure. CYP2D6 genotype can result in widely differing systemic drug exposure in the patient population due to polymorphic expression.*)

Drug metabolism

Dickins M 2004 Induction of cytochromes P450. Curr Top Med Chem 4: 1745–1766 (*Recent advances*)

Gonzalez F J, Korzekwa K R 1995 Cytochromes P450 expression systems. Annu Rev Pharmacol Toxicol 35: 369–390 (*Catalytically active P450 enzymes can be expressed in bacterial, yeast or mammalian cells*)

Gooderham N J, Murray S, Lynch A M et al. 1996 Heterocyclic amines: evaluation of their role in diet associated human cancer. Br J Clin Pharmacol 42: 91–98 (*Heterocyclic amines are formed during cooking; they are absorbed after eating meat and converted into genotoxic hydroxylamines by CYP1A2 in human liver, and they are both mutagenic and carcinogenic in bioassays.*)

Hutt A J, Tan S C 1996 Drug chirality and its clinical significance. Drugs 52: 1–12 (*Short review*)

Kharasch E D, Hankins D, Mautz D, Thummel K E 1996 Identification of the enzyme responsible for oxidative halothane metabolism: implications for prevention of halothane hepatitis. Lancet 347: 1367–1371 (*Evidence that CYP2E1 is important in human oxidative halothane metabolism: 'single dose disulfiram may prove effective prophylaxis against halothane hepatitis'*)

Kim D, Guengerich F P 2005 Cytochrome P450 activation of arylamines and heterocyclic amines. Annu Rev Pharmacol Toxicol 45: 27–49 (*Arylamines are of particular interest as carcinogens; the activation of these, and also some arylamine drugs, involves N-hydroxylation, usually by CYP 1A2*)

Kinirons M T, O'Mahony M S 2004 Drug metabolism and ageing. Br J Clin Pharmacol 57: 540–544 (*Reviews age-related changes in drug metabolism*)

Park B K, Kitteringham N R, Maggs J L et al. 2005 The role of metabolic activation in drug-induced hepatotoxicity. Annu Rev Pharmacol Toxicol 45: 177–202 (*Reviews the evidence for reactive metabolite formation from hepatotoxic drugs, including paracetamol, tamoxifen, diclofenac, and troglitazone, and the current hypotheses of how this leads to liver injury*)

P450 enzyme induction and inhibition

Halpert J R 1995 Structural basis of selective cytochrome P450 inhibition. Annu Rev Pharmacol Toxicol 35: 29–53 (*Complementary properties of isoform-selective P450 inhibitors and their target enzymes determine inhibitor selectivity*)

Henderson L et al. 2002 St John's wort (*Hypericum perforatum*): drug interactions and clinical outcomes. Br J Clin Pharmacol 54: 349–356 (*Reviews the induction of CYP450 isoenzymes and of P-glycoprotein by constituents in this herbal remedy*)

Lin J H, Lu A Y 2001 Interindividual variability in inhibition and induction of cytochrome P450 enzymes. Annu Rev Pharmacol Toxicol 41: 535–567

Park B K, Kitteringham N R, Pirmohamed M, Tucker G T 1996 Relevance of induction of human drug-metabolizing enzymes: pharmacological and toxicological implications. Br J Clin Pharmacol 41: 477–491 (*Reviews the mechanism and biological importance of enzyme induction, including implications for toxicity/carcinogenicity testing of new drugs*)

Sueyoshi T, Negishi M 2001 Phenobarbital response elements of cytochrome P450 genes and nuclear receptors. Annu Rev Pharmacol Toxicol 41: 123–143

Drug elimination

Keppler D, Konig J 2000 Hepatic secretion of conjugated drugs and endogenous substances. Semin Liver Dis 20: 265–272 (*'Conjugate export pumps of the multidrug resistance protein—MRP—family mediate ATP-dependent secretion of anionic conjugates across the canalicular and the basolateral hepatocyte membrane into bile and sinusoidal blood, respectively. Xenobiotic and endogenous lipophilic substances may be conjugated with glutathione, glucuronate, sulfate, or other negatively charged groups and thus become substrates for export pumps of the MRP family'*)

McNamara P J, Abbassi M 2004 Neonatal exposure to drugs in breast milk. Pharm Res 21: 555–566

Others

Atkinson A J, Daniels C E, Dedrick R L et al. (eds) 2002 Principles of clinical pharmacology. Academic Press, London (*Section on pharmacokinetics includes the application of Laplace transformations, effects of disease, compartmental versus non-compartmental approaches, population pharmacokinetics, drug metabolism and transport*)

Birkett D J 2002 Pharmacokinetics made easy (revised), 2nd edn. McGraw-Hill Australia, Sydney (*Excellent slim volume that lives up to the promise of its title*)

Coon M J 2005 Cytochrome P450: nature's most versatile biological catalyst. Annu Rev Pharmacol Toxicol 45: 1–25 (*Summarises the individual steps in the P450 and reductase reaction cycles*)

Mangoni A A, Jackson S H D 2004 Age-related changes in pharmacokinetics and pharmacodynamics: basic principles and practical applications. Br J Clin Pharmacol 57: 6–14 (*Reviews the main age-related physiological changes affecting different organ systems, and their implications for pharmacokinetics and pharmacodynamics*)

Rowland M, Tozer T N 1995 Clinical pharmacokinetics: concepts and applications, 3rd edn. Williams & Wilkins, Baltimore (*Excellent text, over-modestly described by its authors as a 'primer'; emphasises clinical applications*)

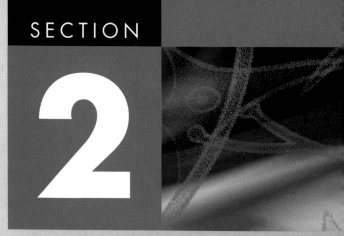

CHEMICAL MEDIATORS

Chemical mediators and the autonomic nervous system

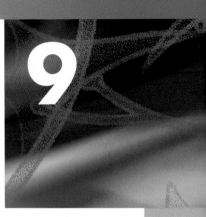

9

OVERVIEW

The network of chemical signals and associated receptors by which cells in the body communicate with one another provides many targets for drug action, and has always been a focus of attention for pharmacologists. Chemical transmission in the peripheral nervous system, and the various ways in which the process can be pharmacologically subverted, are discussed in this chapter. In addition to neurotransmission, we also consider briefly the less clearly defined processes, collectively termed *neuromodulation,* **by which many mediators and drugs exert control over the function of the nervous system. The relative anatomical and physiological simplicity of the peripheral nervous system has made it the proving ground for most of the important discoveries about chemical transmission, and the same general principles apply to the central nervous system (see Ch. 32). For more detail than is given here, see Broadley (1996), Brading (1999), and Cooper et al. (2004).**

HISTORICAL ASPECTS

▼ Studies initiated on the peripheral nervous system have been central to the understanding and classification of many major types of drug action, so it is worth recounting a little history. Excellent accounts are given by Bacq (1975) and Valenstein (2005).

Experimental physiology became established as an approach to the understanding of the function of living organisms in the middle of the 19th century. The peripheral nervous system, and particularly the autonomic nervous system, received a great deal of attention. The fact that electrical stimulation of nerves could elicit a whole variety of physiological effects —from blanching of the skin to arrest of the heart—presented a real challenge to comprehension, particularly of the way in which the signal was passed from the nerve to the effector tissue. In 1877, Du Bois-Reymond was the first to put the alternatives clearly: 'Of known natural processes that might pass on excitation, only two are, in my opinion, worth talking about—either there exists at the boundary of the contractile substance a stimulatory secretion ... or the phenomenon is electrical in nature'. The latter view was generally favoured. In 1869, it had been shown that an exogenous substance, **muscarine**, could mimic the effects of stimulating the vagus nerve, and that **atropine** could inhibit the actions both of muscarine and of nerve stimulation. In 1905, Langley showed the same for **nicotine** and **curare** acting at the neuromuscular junction. Most physiologists interpreted these phenomena as stimulation and inhibition of the nerve endings, respectively, rather than as evidence for chemical transmission. Hence the suggestion of T R Elliott, in 1904, that **adrenaline (epinephrine)** might act as a chemical transmitter mediating the actions of the sympathetic nervous system was coolly received, until Langley, the Professor of Physiology at Cambridge and a powerful figure at that time, suggested, a year later, that transmission to skeletal muscle involved the secretion by the nerve terminals of a substance related to nicotine.

One of the key observations for Elliott was that degeneration of sympathetic nerve terminals did not abolish the sensitivity of smooth muscle preparations to adrenaline (which the electrical theory predicted) but actually enhanced it. The hypothesis of chemical transmission was put to direct test in 1907 by Dixon, who tried to show that vagus nerve stimulation released from a dog's heart into the blood a substance capable of inhibiting another heart. The experiment failed, and the atmosphere of scepticism prevailed.

It was not until 1921, in Germany, that Loewi showed that stimulation of the vagosympathetic trunk connected to an isolated and cannulated frog's heart could cause the release into the cannula of a substance ('Vagusstoff') that, if the cannula fluid was transferred from the first heart to a second, would inhibit the second heart. This is a classic and much-quoted experiment that proved extremely difficult for even Loewi to perform reproducibly. In an autobiographical sketch, Loewi tells us that the idea of chemical transmission arose in a discussion that he had in 1903, but no way of testing it experimentally occurred to him until he dreamed of the appropriate experiment one night in 1920. He wrote some notes of this very important dream in the middle of the night, but

131

in the morning could not read them. The dream obligingly returned the next night and, taking no chances, he went to the laboratory at 3 a.m. and carried out the experiment successfully. Loewi's experiment may be, and was, criticised on numerous grounds (it could, for example, have been potassium rather than a neurotransmitter that was acting on the recipient heart), but a series of further experiments proved him to be right. His findings can be summarised as follow.

- Stimulation of the vagus caused the appearance in the perfusate of the frog heart of a substance capable of producing, in a second heart, an inhibitory effect resembling vagus stimulation.
- Stimulation of the sympathetic nervous system caused the appearance of a substance capable of accelerating a second heart. By fluorescence measurements, Loewi concluded later that this substance was adrenaline.
- Atropine prevented the inhibitory action of the vagus on the heart but did not prevent release of Vagusstoff. Atropine thus prevented the effects, rather than the release, of the transmitter.
- When Vagusstoff was incubated with ground-up heart muscle, it became inactivated. This effect is now known to be due to enzymatic destruction of acetylcholine by cholinesterase.
- **Physostigmine (eserine)**, which potentiated the effect of vagus stimulation on the heart, prevented destruction of Vagusstoff by heart muscle, providing evidence that the potentiation is due to inhibition of cholinesterase, which normally destroys the transmitter substance acetylcholine.

A few years later, in the early 1930s, Dale showed convincingly that acetylcholine was also the transmitter substance at the neuromuscular junction of striated muscle and at autonomic ganglia. One of the keys to Dale's success lay in the use of very highly sensitive bioassays, especially the leech dorsal muscle, for measuring acetylcholine release. Chemical transmission at sympathetic nerve terminals was demonstrated at about the same time as cholinergic transmission and by very similar methods. Cannon and his colleagues at Harvard first showed unequivocally the phenomenon of chemical transmission at sympathetic nerve endings, by experiments in vivo in which tissues made supersensitive to adrenaline by prior sympathetic denervation were shown to respond, after a delay, to the transmitter released by stimulation of the sympathetic nerves to other parts of the body. The chemical identity of the transmitter, tantalisingly like adrenaline but not identical to it, caused confusion for many years, until in 1946 von Euler showed it to be the non-methylated derivative **noradrenaline (norepinephrine)**.

THE PERIPHERAL NERVOUS SYSTEM

The peripheral nervous system consists of the following principal elements:

- autonomic nervous system, which includes the enteric nervous system
- somatic efferent nerves, innervating skeletal muscle
- somatic and visceral afferent nerves.

In this chapter, we focus on the autonomic nervous system, which for a long time occupied centre stage in the pharmacology of chemical transmission. Aspects of the somatic efferent system are considered in Chapter 10. Afferent nerves (particularly the non-myelinated nerves subserving nociceptive and other functions; see Ch. 41) also have important effector functions in the periphery, mediated mainly by neuropeptides (Ch. 16). Many afferent fibres are present in autonomic nerves and are anatomically part of the autonomic nervous system, but it is the efferent pathways that are the main concern of this chapter.

BASIC ANATOMY AND PHYSIOLOGY OF THE AUTONOMIC NERVOUS SYSTEM

The autonomic nervous system (see Appenzeller & Oribe, 1997) consists of three main anatomical divisions: *sympathetic* and *parasympathetic* (see Fig. 9.1), and the *enteric* nervous system, consisting of the intrinsic nerve plexuses of the gastrointestinal tract, which are closely interconnected with the sympathetic and parasympathetic systems.

The autonomic nervous system conveys all the outputs from the central nervous system to the rest of the body, except for the motor innervation of skeletal muscle. The enteric nervous system has sufficient integrative capabilities to allow it to function independently of the central nervous system, but the sympathetic and parasympathetic systems are agents of the central nervous system and cannot function without it. The autonomic nervous system is largely outside the influence of voluntary control. The main processes that it regulates are:

- contraction and relaxation of vascular and visceral smooth muscle
- all exocrine and certain endocrine secretions
- the heartbeat
- energy metabolism, particularly in liver and skeletal muscle.

A degree of autonomic control also affects many other systems, including the kidney, immune system and somatosensory system. The main difference between the autonomic and the somatic efferent pathways is that the former consists of two neurons arranged in series, whereas in the latter a single motor neuron connects the central nervous system to the skeletal muscle fibre (Fig. 9.2). The two neurons in the autonomic pathway are known, respectively, as *preganglionic* and *postganglionic*. In the sympathetic nervous system, the intervening synapses lie in *autonomic ganglia*, which are outside the central nervous system, and contain the nerve endings of preganglionic fibres and the cell bodies of postganglionic neurons. In parasympathetic pathways, the postganglionic cells are mainly found in the target organs, discrete parasympathetic ganglia (e.g. the ciliary ganglion) being found only in the head and neck.

The cell bodies of the sympathetic preganglionic neurons lie in the lateral horn of the grey matter of the thoracic and lumbar segments of the spinal cord, and the fibres leave the spinal cord in the spinal nerves as the *thoracolumbar sympathetic outflow*. The preganglionic fibres synapse in the *paravertebral chains* of sympathetic ganglia, lying on either side of the spinal column. These ganglia contain the cell bodies of the postganglionic sympathetic neurons, the axons of which rejoin the spinal nerve. Many of the postganglionic sympathetic fibres reach their peripheral destinations via the branches of the spinal nerves. Others, destined for abdominal and pelvic viscera, have their cell bodies in a group of unpaired *prevertebral ganglia* in the abdominal cavity. The only exception to the two-neuron arrangement is the innervation of the adrenal medulla. The catecholamine-secreting cells of the adrenal medulla are, in effect, modified postganglionic sympathetic neurons, and the nerves supplying the gland are equivalent to preganglionic fibres.

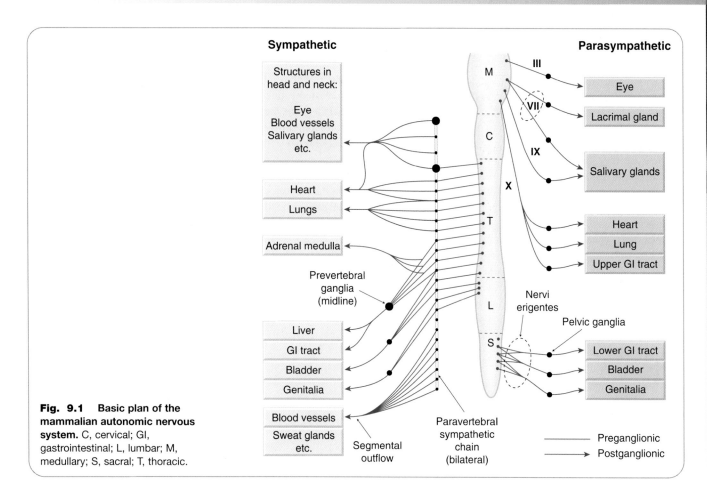

Fig. 9.1   Basic plan of the mammalian autonomic nervous system. C, cervical; GI, gastrointestinal; L, lumbar; M, medullary; S, sacral; T, thoracic.

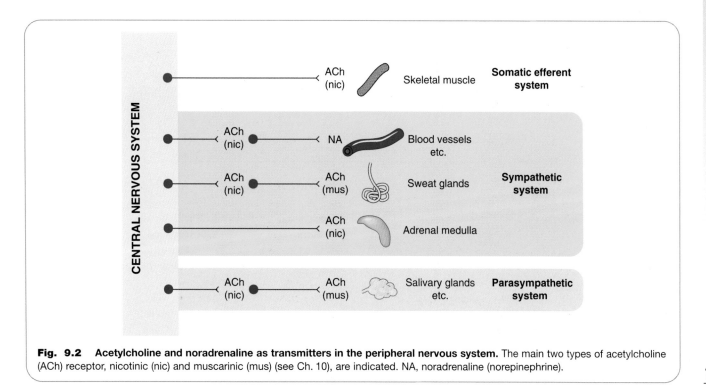

Fig. 9.2   Acetylcholine and noradrenaline as transmitters in the peripheral nervous system. The main two types of acetylcholine (ACh) receptor, nicotinic (nic) and muscarinic (mus) (see Ch. 10), are indicated. NA, noradrenaline (norepinephrine).

The parasympathetic nerves emerge from two separate regions of the central nervous system. The *cranial outflow* consists of preganglionic fibres in certain cranial nerves, namely the oculomotor nerve (carrying parasympathetic fibres destined for the eye), the facial and glossopharyngeal nerves (carrying fibres to the salivary glands and the nasopharynx), and the vagus nerve (carrying fibres to the thoracic and abdominal viscera). The ganglia lie scattered in close relation to the target organs; the postganglionic neurons are very short compared with those of the sympathetic system. Parasympathetic fibres destined for the pelvic and abdominal viscera emerge as the *sacral outflow* from the spinal cord in a bundle of nerves known as the *nervi erigentes* (because stimulation of these nerves evokes genital erection—a fact of some importance to those responsible for artificial insemination of livestock). These fibres synapse in a group of scattered pelvic ganglia, whence the short postganglionic fibres run to target tissues such as the bladder, rectum and genitalia. The pelvic ganglia carry both sympathetic and parasympathetic fibres, and the two divisions are not anatomically distinct in this region.

The *enteric nervous system* (reviewed by Goyal & Hirano, 1996) consists of the neurons whose cell bodies lie in the intramural plexuses in the wall of the intestine. It is estimated that there are more cells in this system than in the spinal cord, and functionally they do not fit simply into the sympathetic/parasympathetic classification. Incoming nerves from both the sympathetic and the parasympathetic systems terminate on enteric neurons, as well as running directly to smooth muscle, glands and blood vessels. Some enteric neurons function as mechanoreceptors or chemoreceptors, providing local reflex pathways that can control gastrointestinal function without external inputs. The enteric nervous system is pharmacologically more complex than the sympathetic or parasympathetic systems, involving many neuropeptide and other transmitters (such as 5-hydroxytryptamine, nitric oxide and ATP).

In some places (e.g. in the visceral smooth muscle of the gut and bladder, and in the heart), the sympathetic and the parasympathetic systems produce opposite effects, but there are others where only one division of the autonomic system operates. The sweat glands and most blood vessels, for example, have only a sympathetic innervation, whereas the ciliary muscle of the eye has only a parasympathetic innervation. Bronchial smooth muscle has only a parasympathetic (constrictor) innervation (although its tone is highly sensitive to circulating adrenaline—acting probably to inhibit the constrictor innervation rather than on the smooth muscle directly). Resistance arteries (see Ch. 19) have a sympathetic vasoconstrictor innervation but no parasympathetic innervation; instead, the constrictor tone is opposed by a background release of nitric oxide from the endothelial cells (see Ch. 17). There are other examples, such as the salivary glands, where the two systems produce similar, rather than opposing, effects.

It is therefore a mistake to think of the sympathetic and parasympathetic systems simply as physiological opponents. Each serves its own physiological function and can be more or less active in a particular organ or tissue according to the need of the moment. Cannon rightly emphasised the general role of the sympathetic system in evoking 'fight or flight' reactions in an emergency, but emergencies are rare for most animals. In everyday life, the autonomic nervous system functions continuously to control specific local functions, such as adjustments to postural changes, exercise or ambient temperature (see Jänig & McLachlan, 1992). The popular concept of a continuum from the extreme 'rest and digest' state (parasympathetic active, sympathetic quiescent) to the extreme emergency fight or flight state (sympathetic active, parasympathetic quiescent) is an oversimplification.

Table 9.1 lists some of the more important autonomic responses in humans.

Table 9.1   The main effects of the autonomic nervous system

Organ	Sympathetic effect	Adrenergic receptor type[a]	Parasympathetic effect	Cholinergic receptor type[a]
Heart				
Sinoatrial node	Rate ↑	β_1	Rate ↓	M_2
Atrial muscle	Force ↑	β_1	Force ↓	M_2
Atrioventricular node	Automaticity ↑	β_1	Conduction velocity ↓	M_2
			Atrioventricular block	M_2
Ventricular muscle	Automaticity ↑ Force ↑	β_1	No effect	M_2
Blood vessels				
Arterioles				
Coronary	Constriction	α	No effect	–
Muscle	Dilatation	β_2	No effect	–
Viscera, skin, brain	Constriction	α	No effect	–
Erectile tissue	Constriction	α	Dilatation	$M_3{}^{b}$
Salivary gland	Constriction	α	Dilatation	$M_3{}^{b}$

Table 9.1 (cont'd)   The main effects of the autonomic nervous system

Organ	Sympathetic effect	Adrenergic receptor type[a]	Parasympathetic effect	Cholinergic receptor type[a]
Veins	Constriction	α	No effect	–
	Dilatation	β_2	No effect	–
Viscera				
Bronchi				
Smooth muscle	No sympathetic innervation, but dilated by circulating adrenaline (epinephrine)	β_2	Constriction	M_3
Glands	No effect	–	Secretion	M_3
Gastrointestinal tract				
Smooth muscle	Motility ↓	$\alpha_1, \alpha_2, \beta_2$	Motility ↑	M_3
Sphincters	Constriction	α_2, β_2	Dilatation	M_3
Glands	No effect	–	Secretion	M_3
			Gastric acid secretion	M_1
Bladder	Relaxation	β_2	Contraction	M_3
	Sphincter contraction	α_1	Sphincter relaxation	M_3
Uterus				
Pregnant	Contraction	α	Variable	–
Non-pregnant	Relaxation	β_2		
Male sex organs	Ejaculation	α	Erection	M_3
Eye				
Pupil	Dilatation	α	Constriction	M_3
Ciliary muscle	Relaxation (slight)	β	Contraction	M_3
Skin				
Sweat glands	Secretion (mainly cholinergic via M_3 receptors)	–	No effect	
Pilomotor	Piloerection	α	No effect	–
Salivary glands	Secretion	α, β	Secretion	M_3
Lacrimal glands	No effect	–	Secretion	M_3
Kidney	Renin secretion	β_1	No effect	–
Liver	Glycogenolysis Gluconeogenesis	α, β_2	No effect	

[a]The adrenergic and cholinergic receptor types shown are described more fully in Chapters 7 and 8. Transmitters other than acetylcholine and noradrenaline (norepinephrine) contribute to many of these responses (see Table 9.2).
[b]Vasodilator effects of M_3 receptors are due to nitric oxide release from endothelial cells (see Ch. 15).

TRANSMITTERS IN THE AUTONOMIC NERVOUS SYSTEM

The two main neurotransmitters that operate in the autonomic system are **acetylcholine** and **noradrenaline**, whose sites of action are shown diagrammatically in Figure 9.2. This diagram also shows the type of postsynaptic receptor with which the transmitters interact at the different sites (discussed more fully in Chs 10 and 11). Some general rules apply.

- All motor nerve fibres leaving the central nervous system release acetylcholine, which acts on nicotinic receptors (although in autonomic ganglia a minor component of excitation is due to activation of muscarinic receptors; see Ch. 10).
- All postganglionic parasympathetic fibres release acetylcholine, which acts on muscarinic receptors.
- All postganglionic sympathetic fibres (with one important exception) release noradrenaline, which may act on either α- or β-adrenoceptors (see Ch. 11). The exception is the

Basic anatomy of the autonomic nervous system

- The autonomic nervous system comprises three divisions: sympathetic, parasympathetic and enteric.
- The basic (two-neuron) pattern of the sympathetic and parasympathetic systems consists of a preganglionic neuron with a cell body in the central nervous system (CNS) and a postganglionic neuron with cell body in an autonomic ganglion.
- The parasympathetic system is connected to the CNS via:
  - cranial nerve outflow (III, VII, IX, X)
  - sacral outflow.
- Parasympathetic ganglia usually lie close to or within the target organ.
- Sympathetic outflow leaves the CNS in thoracic and lumbar spinal roots. Sympathetic ganglia form two paravertebral chains, plus some midline ganglia.
- The enteric nervous system consists of neurons lying in the intramural plexuses of the gastrointestinal tract. It receives inputs from sympathetic and parasympathetic systems, but can act on its own to control the motor and secretory functions of the intestine.

Physiology of the autonomic nervous system

- The autonomic system controls smooth muscle (visceral and vascular), exocrine (and some endocrine) secretions, rate and force of the heart, and certain metabolic processes (e.g. glucose utilisation).
- Sympathetic and parasympathetic systems have opposing actions in some situations (e.g. control of heart rate, gastrointestinal smooth muscle), but not in others (e.g. salivary glands, ciliary muscle).
- Sympathetic activity increases in stress ('fight or flight' response), whereas parasympathetic activity predominates during satiation and repose. Both systems exert a continuous physiological control of specific organs under normal conditions, when the body is at neither extreme.

sympathetic innervation of sweat glands, where transmission is due to acetylcholine acting on muscarinic receptors. In some species, but not humans, vasodilatation in skeletal muscle is produced by cholinergic sympathetic nerve fibres.

Acetylcholine and noradrenaline are the grandees among autonomic transmitters, and are central to understanding autonomic pharmacology. However, many other chemical mediators are also released by autonomic neurons (see below), and their functional significance is gradually becoming clearer.

SOME GENERAL PRINCIPLES OF CHEMICAL TRANSMISSION

The essential processes in chemical transmission—the release of mediators, and their interaction with receptors on target cells—are described in Chapters 4 and 3, respectively. Here we consider some general characteristics of chemical transmission of particular relevance to pharmacology. Many of these principles apply also to the central nervous system and are taken up again in Chapter 32.

DALE'S PRINCIPLE

▼ Dale's principle, advanced in 1934, states, in its modern form: 'A mature neuron releases the same transmitter (or transmitters) at all of its synapses'. Dale considered it unlikely that a single neuron could store and release different transmitters at different nerve terminals, and his view was supported by physiological and neurochemical evidence. It is known, for example, that the axons of motor neurons have branches that synapse on interneurons in the spinal cord, in addition to the main branch that innervates skeletal muscle fibres in the periphery. The transmitter at both the central and the peripheral nerve endings is acetylcholine, in accordance with Dale's principle. Recent work, however, suggests that there are situations where different transmitters are released from different terminals of the same neuron. Further, we now know that most neurons release more than one transmitter (see *Cotransmission*, below) and may change their transmitter repertoire, for example during development or in response to injury. Moreover (see Fig. 4.12), the balance of the cocktail of mediators released by a nerve terminal can vary with stimulus conditions, and in response to presynaptic modulators. Dale's principle was, of course, framed long before these complexities were discovered, and it has probably now outlived its usefulness, although purists seem curiously reluctant to let it go.

DENERVATION SUPERSENSITIVITY

It is known, mainly from the work of Cannon on the sympathetic system, that if a nerve is cut and its terminals allowed to degenerate, the structure supplied by it becomes supersensitive to the transmitter substance released by the terminals. Thus skeletal muscle, which normally responds to injected acetylcholine only if a large dose is given directly into the arterial blood supply, will, after denervation, respond by contracture to much smaller amounts. Other organs, such as salivary glands and blood vessels, show similar supersensitivity to acetylcholine and noradrenaline when the postganglionic nerves degenerate, and there is evidence that pathways in the central nervous system show the same phenomenon.

▼ Several mechanisms contribute to denervation supersensitivity, and the extent and mechanism of the phenomenon varies from organ to organ. Reported mechanisms include the following.

- *Proliferation of receptors.* This is particularly marked in skeletal muscle, in which the number of acetylcholine receptors increases 20-fold or more after denervation; the receptors, normally localised to the endplate region of the fibres, spread over the whole surface. Elsewhere, much smaller increases in receptor number (about twofold) have often been reported, but there are examples where no change occurs.
- *Loss of mechanisms for transmitter removal.* At noradrenergic synapses, the loss of neuronal uptake of noradrenaline (see Ch. 11) contributes substantially to denervation supersensitivity. At cholinergic synapses, a partial loss of cholinesterase occurs (see Ch. 10).
- *Increased postjunctional responsiveness.* In some cases, the postsynaptic cells become supersensitive without a corresponding increase in the

number of receptors. Thus smooth muscle cells become partly depolarised and hyperexcitable, and this phenomenon contributes appreciably to their supersensitivity. The mechanism of this change and its importance for other synapses is not known.

Supersensitivity can occur, but is less marked, when transmission is interrupted by processes other than nerve section. Pharmacological block of ganglionic transmission, for example, if sustained for a few days, causes some degree of supersensitivity of the target organs, and long-term blockade of postsynaptic receptors also causes receptors to proliferate, leaving the cell supersensitive when the blocking agent is removed. Phenomena such as this are of importance in the central nervous system, where such supersensitivity can cause 'rebound' effects when drugs that impair synaptic transmission are given for some time and then stopped.

PRESYNAPTIC MODULATION

The presynaptic terminals that synthesise and release transmitter in response to electrical activity in the nerve fibre are often themselves sensitive to transmitter substances and to other substances that may be produced locally in tissues (for reviews see Starke et al., 1989; Fuder & Muscholl, 1995). Such presynaptic effects most commonly act to inhibit transmitter release, but may enhance it. Figure 9.3 shows the inhibitory effect of adrenaline on the release of acetylcholine (evoked by electrical stimulation) from the postganglionic parasympathetic nerve terminals of the intestine. The release of noradrenaline from nearby sympathetic nerve terminals can also inhibit release of acetylcholine. Noradrenergic and cholinergic nerve terminals often lie close together in the myenteric plexus, so the opposing effects of the sympathetic and parasympathetic systems result not only from the opposite effects of the two transmitters on the smooth muscle cells, but also from the inhibition of acetylcholine release by

noradrenaline acting on the parasympathetic nerve terminals. A similar situation of mutual presynaptic inhibition exists in the heart, where noradrenaline inhibits acetylcholine release, as in the myenteric plexus, and acetylcholine also inhibits noradrenaline release. These are examples of *heterotropic* interactions, where one neurotransmitter affects the release of another. *Homotropic* interactions also occur, where the transmitter, by binding to presynaptic autoreceptors, affects the nerve terminals from which it is being released. This type of autoinhibitory feedback acts powerfully at noradrenergic nerve terminals (see Starke et al., 1989). One of the strongest pieces of evidence is that the amount of noradrenaline released from tissues in response to repetitive stimulation of sympathetic nerves is increased 10-fold or more in the presence of an antagonist that blocks the presynaptic noradrenaline receptors (see Ch. 11). This suggests that the released noradrenaline can inhibit further release by at least 90%. In the brain, acetylcholine release is modulated by a similar autoinhibitory feedback involving presynaptic muscarinic acetylcholine receptors.

In both the noradrenergic and cholinergic systems, the presynaptic autoreceptors are pharmacologically distinct from the postsynaptic receptors (see Chs 10 and 11), and there are drugs that act selectively, as agonists or antagonists, on the pre- or postsynaptic receptors.

Cholinergic and noradrenergic nerve terminals respond not only to acetylcholine and noradrenaline, as described above, but also to other substances that are released as cotransmitters, such as **ATP** and **neuropeptide Y** (**NPY**), or derived from other sources, including **nitric oxide**, **prostaglandins**, **adenosine**, **dopamine**, **5-hydroxytryptamine**, **GABA**, **opioid peptides**, **endocannabinoids** and many other substances. The physiological role and pharmacological significance of these various interactions is still unclear (see review by Vizi, 2001), but the description of the autonomic nervous system represented in Figure 9.2 is undoubtedly oversimplified. Figure 9.4 shows some of the main presynaptic interactions between autonomic neurons, and summarises the many chemical influences that regulate transmitter release from noradrenergic neurons.

Presynaptic receptors regulate transmitter release mainly by affecting Ca^{2+} entry into the nerve terminal (see Ch. 4). Most presynaptic receptors are of the G-protein–coupled type (see Ch. 3), which control the function of calcium channels and potassium channels either through second messengers that regulate the state of phosphorylation of the channel proteins, or by a direct interaction of G-proteins with the channels. Transmitter release is inhibited when calcium channel opening is inhibited, or when potassium channel opening is increased (see Ch. 4); in many cases, both mechanisms operate simultaneously. Presynaptic regulation by receptors linked directly to ion channels (ionotropic receptors; see Ch. 3) rather than to G-proteins also occurs (see MacDermott et al., 1999). Nicotinic acetylcholine receptors (nAChRs) are particularly important in this respect. They facilitate the release of other transmitters, such as glutamate (see Ch. 33), and most of the nAChRs expressed in the central nervous system are located presynaptically. Another example is the GABA$_A$ receptor, whose action is to inhibit transmitter release (see Chs 4 and 33). Other ionotropic receptors, such as those activated by ATP and 5-hydroxytryptamine (Ch. 12), may have similar effects on transmitter release.

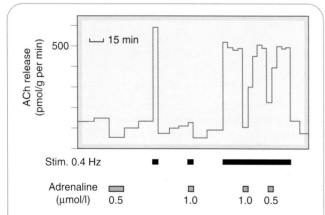

Fig. 9.3 **Inhibitory effect of adrenaline on acetylcholine (ACh) release from postganglionic parasympathetic nerves in the guinea pig ileum.** The intramural nerves were stimulated electrically where indicated, and the ACh released into the bathing fluid determined by bioassay. Adrenaline strongly inhibits ACh release. (From Vizi E S 1979 Prog Neurobiol 12: 181.)

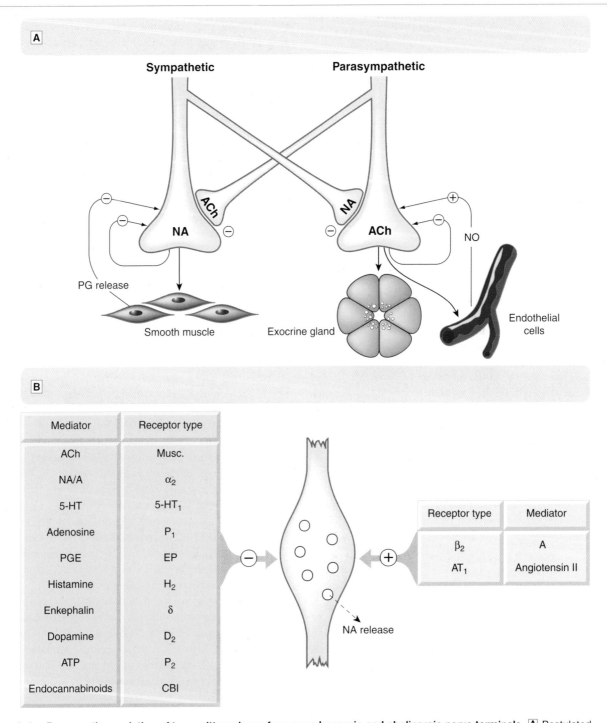

Fig. 9.4 Presynaptic regulation of transmitter release from noradrenergic and cholinergic nerve terminals. [A] Postulated homotropic and heterotropic interactions between sympathetic and parasympathetic nerves. [B] Some of the known inhibitory and facilitatory influences on noradrenaline release from sympathetic nerve endings. 5-HT, 5-hydroxytryptamine; A, adrenaline; ACh, acetylcholine; NA, noradrenaline; NO, nitric oxide; NPY, neuropeptide Y; PG, prostaglandin; PGE, prostaglandin E.

POSTSYNAPTIC MODULATION

Chemical mediators often act on postsynaptic structures, including neurons, smooth muscle cells, cardiac muscle cells, etc., in such a way that their excitability or spontaneous firing pattern is altered. In many cases, as with presynaptic modulation, this is caused by changes in calcium and/or potassium channel function mediated by a second messenger. We give only a few examples here.

- The slow excitatory effect produced by various mediators, including acetylcholine and peptides such as substance P (see Ch. 41), on many peripheral and central neurons results mainly from a decrease in K⁺ permeability. Conversely, the inhibitory effect of various opiates is mainly due to increased K⁺ permeability.

- **Benzodiazepine** tranquillisers (Ch. 37) act directly on receptors for GABA (see Ch. 33) to facilitate their inhibitory effect. There is some evidence that drugs such as **galantamine** act similarly on nAChRs to facilitate the excitatory effect of acetylcholine in the brain, which may have relevance for the use of such drugs to treat dementia (see Ch. 35).
- Neuropeptide Y, which is released as a cotransmitter with noradrenaline at many sympathetic nerve endings and enhances the vasoconstrictor effect of noradrenaline, thus greatly facilitating transmission (Fig. 9.5); the mechanism is not known.

The pre- and postsynaptic effects described above are often described as *neuromodulation*, because the mediator acts to increase or decrease the efficacy of synaptic transmission without participating directly as a transmitter. Many neuropeptides, for example, affect membrane ion channels in such a way as to increase or decrease excitability and thus control the firing pattern of the cell. Neuromodulation is loosely defined but, in general, involves slower processes (taking seconds to days) than

neurotransmission (which occurs in milliseconds), and operates through cascades of intracellular messengers (Ch. 3) rather than directly on ligand-gated ion channels. Some aspects of this problem of terminology are discussed in Chapter 16.

TRANSMITTERS OTHER THAN ACETYLCHOLINE AND NORADRENALINE

As mentioned above, acetylcholine or noradrenaline are not the only autonomic transmitters. The rather grudging realisation that this was so dawned many years ago when it was noticed that autonomic transmission in many organs could not be completely blocked by drugs that abolish responses to these transmitters. The dismal but tenacious term *non-adrenergic non-cholinergic (NANC)* transmission was coined. Later, fluorescence and immunocytochemical methods showed that neurons, including autonomic neurons, contain many potential transmitters, often several in the same cell. Compounds believed to function as NANC transmitters include ATP, vasoactive intestinal peptide (VIP), NPY and nitric oxide (see Fig. 9.6 and Table 9.2), which function at postganglionic nerve terminals, as well as substance P, 5-hydroxytryptamine, GABA and dopamine, which play a

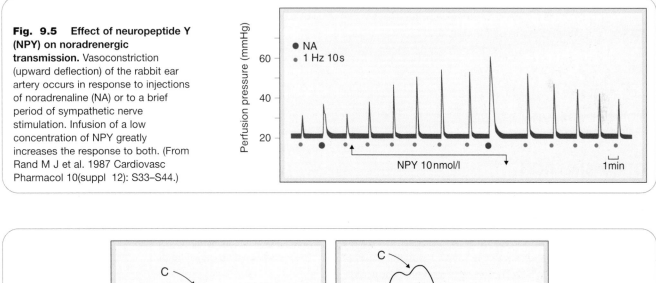

Fig. 9.5 Effect of neuropeptide Y (NPY) on noradrenergic transmission. Vasoconstriction (upward deflection) of the rabbit ear artery occurs in response to injections of noradrenaline (NA) or to a brief period of sympathetic nerve stimulation. Infusion of a low concentration of NPY greatly increases the response to both. (From Rand M J et al. 1987 Cardiovasc Pharmacol 10(suppl 12): S33–S44.)

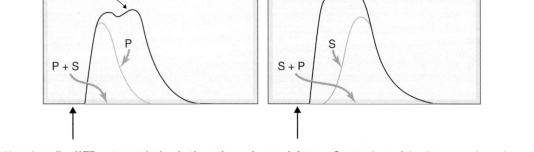

Fig. 9.6 Noradrenaline/ATP cotransmission in the guinea pig vas deferens. Contractions of the tissue are shown in response to a single electrical stimulus causing excitation of sympathetic nerve endings. With no blocking drugs present, a twin-peaked response is produced (C). The early peak is selectively abolished by the ATP antagonist suramin (S), while the late peak is blocked by the α₁-adrenoceptor antagonist prazosin (P). The response is completely eliminated when both drugs are present. (Reproduced with permission from von Kugelglen & Starke 1991 Trends Pharmacol Sci 12: 319–324.)

Table 9.2 Examples of non-noradrenergic non-cholinergic transmitters and cotransmitters in the peripheral nervous system

Transmitter	Location	Function
Non-peptides		
ATP	Postganglionic sympathetic neurons (e.g. blood vessels, vas deferens)	Fast depolarisation/contraction of smooth muscle cells
GABA, 5-hydroxytryptamine	Enteric neurons	Peristaltic reflex
Dopamine	Some sympathetic neurons (e.g. kidney)	Vasodilatation
Nitric oxide	Pelvic nerves Gastric nerves	Erection Gastric emptying
Peptides		
Neuropeptide Y	Postganglionic sympathetic neurons (e.g. blood vessels)	Facilitates constrictor action of noradrenaline; inhibits noradrenaline release
Vasoactive intestinal peptide	Parasympathetic nerves to salivary glands NANC innervation of airways smooth muscle	Vasodilatation; cotransmitter with acetylcholine Bronchodilatation
Gonadotrophin-releasing hormone	Sympathetic ganglia	Slow depolarisation; cotransmitter with acetylcholine
Substance P	Sympathetic ganglia Enteric neurons	Slow depolarisation Cotransmitter with acetylcholine
Calcitonin gene–related peptide	Non-myelinated sensory neurons	Vasodilatation; vascular leakage; neurogenic inflammation

NANC, non-noradrenergic non-cholinergic.

role in ganglionic transmission (see Lundberg, 1996, for a comprehensive review).

COTRANSMISSION

It is probably the rule rather than the exception that neurons release more than one transmitter or modulator (see Lundberg, 1996), each of which interacts with specific receptors and produces effects, often both pre- and postsynaptically. We are only just beginning to understand the functional implications of this (see Kupfermann, 1991). The example of noradrenaline/ATP cotransmission at the sympathetic nerve endings is shown in Figure 9.6, and the best-studied examples and mechanisms are summarised in Table 9.2 and Figures 9.7 and 9.8.

What, one might well ask, could be the functional advantage of cotransmission, compared with a single transmitter acting on various different receptors? The possible advantages include the following.

- One constituent of the cocktail (e.g. a peptide) may be removed or inactivated more slowly than the other (e.g. a monoamine), and therefore reach targets further from the site of release and produce longer-lasting effects. This appears to be the case, for example, with acetylcholine and gonadotrophin-releasing hormone in sympathetic ganglia (Jan & Jan, 1983).

- The balance of the transmitters released may vary under different conditions. At sympathetic nerve terminals, for example, where noradrenaline and NPY are stored in separate vesicles, NPY is preferentially released at high stimulation frequencies (see Stjärne, 1989), so that differential release of one or other mediator may result from varying impulse patterns. Differential effects of presynaptic modulators are also possible; for example, activation of β-adrenoceptors inhibits ATP release while enhancing noradrenaline release from sympathetic nerve terminals (Gonçalves et al., 1996).

TERMINATION OF TRANSMITTER ACTION

Chemically transmitting synapses other than the peptidergic variety (Ch. 16) invariably incorporate a mechanism for disposing rapidly of the released transmitter, so that its action remains brief and localised. At cholinergic synapses (Ch. 10), the released acetylcholine is inactivated very rapidly in the synaptic cleft by acetylcholinesterase. In most other cases (see Fig. 9.9), transmitter action is terminated by active reuptake into the presynaptic nerve, or into supporting cells such as glia. Such reuptake depends on transporter proteins, each being specific for a particular transmitter (see Nelson, 1998; Torres et al., 2003). They belong to a distinct family of membrane proteins, each possessing 12 transmembrane helices. Different members of the family show selectivity for

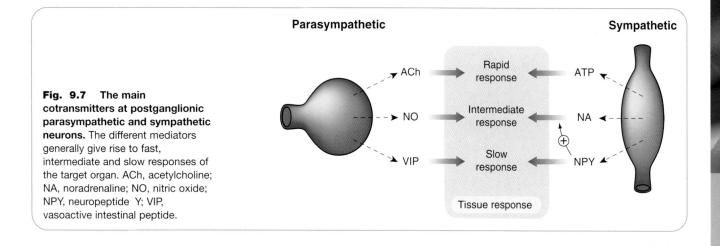

Fig. 9.7 **The main cotransmitters at postganglionic parasympathetic and sympathetic neurons.** The different mediators generally give rise to fast, intermediate and slow responses of the target organ. ACh, acetylcholine; NA, noradrenaline; NO, nitric oxide; NPY, neuropeptide Y; VIP, vasoactive intestinal peptide.

each of the main monoamine transmitters (e.g. the *norepinephrine transporter*, *NET*, which transports noradrenaline; the *serotonin transporter*, *SERT*, which transports 5-hydroxytryptamine); transporters for glutamate and GABA show greater diversity, several subtypes of each having been described. *Vesicular transporters* (Ch. 4), which load synaptic vesicles with transmitter molecules, are closely related to the membrane transporters. Membrane transporters usually act as cotransporters of Na^+, Cl^- and transmitter molecules, and it is the inwardly directed 'downhill' gradient for Na^+ that provides the energy for the inward 'uphill' movement of the transmitter. The simultaneous transport of ions along with the transmitter means that the process generates a net

current across the membrane, which can be measured directly and used to monitor the transport process. Very similar mechanisms are responsible for other physiological transport processes, such as glucose uptake (Ch. 26) and renal tubular transport of amino acids. Because it is the electrochemical gradient for Na^+ that drives the inward transport of transmitter molecules, a reduction of this gradient can reduce or even reverse the flow of transmitter. This is probably not important under normal conditions, but when the nerve terminals are depolarised or abnormally loaded with sodium (e.g. in ischaemic conditions) the resulting non-vesicular release of transmitter (and inhibition of the normal synaptic reuptake mechanism) may play a significant role in the effects of ischaemia on tissues such as heart and brain (see Chs 18 and 35). Studies with transgenic 'knockout' mice (see Torres et al., 2003) show that the store of releasable transmitter is substantially depleted in animals lacking the membrane transporter, showing that synthesis is unable to maintain the store if the recapture mechanism is disabled.

As we shall see in subsequent chapters, both membrane and vesicular transporters are targets for various drug effects, and defining the physiological role and pharmacological properties of these molecules is the focus of much current research.

BASIC STEPS IN NEUROCHEMICAL TRANSMISSION: SITES OF DRUG ACTION

Figure 9.9 summarises the main processes that occur in a classical chemically transmitting synapse, and provides a useful basis for understanding the actions of the many different classes of drug, discussed in later chapters, that act by facilitating or blocking neurochemical transmission.

All the steps shown in Figure 9.9 (except for transmitter diffusion, step 8) can be influenced by drugs. For example, the enzymes involved in synthesis or inactivation of the transmitter can be inhibited, as can the transport systems responsible for the neuronal and vesicular uptake of the transmitter or its precursor. The actions of the great majority of drugs that act on the peripheral nervous system (Chs 10 and 11) and the central nervous system fit into this general scheme.

Transmitters of the autonomic nervous system 🔑

- The principal transmitters are acetylcholine (ACh) and noradrenaline.
- Preganglionic neurons are cholinergic, and ganglionic transmission occurs via nicotinic ACh receptors (although excitatory muscarinic ACh receptors are also present on postganglionic cells).
- Postganglionic parasympathetic neurons are cholinergic, acting on muscarinic receptors in target organs.
- Postganglionic sympathetic neurons are mainly noradrenergic, although a few are cholinergic (e.g. sweat glands).
- Transmitters other than noradrenaline and acetylcholine (NANC transmitters) are also used extensively in the autonomic nervous system. The main ones are nitric oxide and vasoactive intestinal peptide (parasympathetic), ATP and neuropeptide Y (sympathetic). Others, such as 5-hydroxytryptamine, GABA and dopamine, also play a role.
- Cotransmission is a general phenomenon.

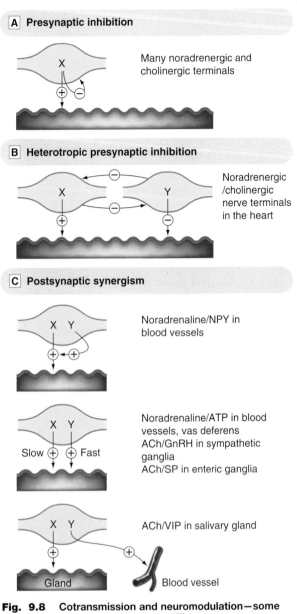

A Presynaptic inhibition

Many noradrenergic and cholinergic terminals

B Heterotropic presynaptic inhibition

Noradrenergic /cholinergic nerve terminals in the heart

C Postsynaptic synergism

Noradrenaline/NPY in blood vessels

Noradrenaline/ATP in blood vessels, vas deferens
ACh/GnRH in sympathetic ganglia
ACh/SP in enteric ganglia

ACh/VIP in salivary gland

Gland   Blood vessel

Fig. 9.8   Cotransmission and neuromodulation—some examples. Ⓐ Presynaptic inhibition. Ⓑ Heterotropic presynaptic inhibition. Ⓒ Postsynaptic synergism. ACh, acetylcholine; GnRH, gonadotrophin-releasing hormone (luteinising hormone–releasing hormone); NPY, neuropeptide Y; SP, substance P; VIP, vasoactive intestinal peptide.

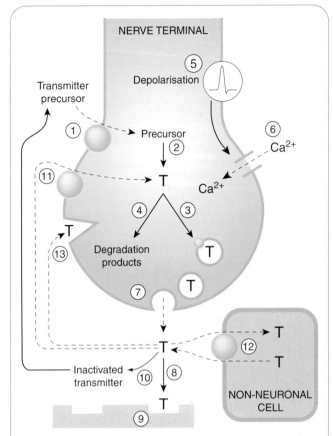

Fig. 9.9   The main processes involved in synthesis, storage and release of amine and amino acid transmitters. 1, Uptake of precursors; 2, synthesis of transmitter; 3, uptake/transport of transmitter into vesicles; 4, degradation of surplus transmitter; 5, depolarisation by propagated action potential; 6, influx of Ca^{2+} in response to depolarisation; 7, release of transmitter by exocytosis; 8, diffusion to postsynaptic membrane; 9, interaction with postsynaptic receptors; 10, inactivation of transmitter; 11, reuptake of transmitter or degradation products by nerve terminals; 12, uptake of transmitter by non-neuronal cells; and 13, interaction with presynaptic receptors. The transporters (11 and 12) can release transmitter under certain conditions by working in reverse. These processes are well characterised for many transmitters (e.g. acetylcholine, monoamines, amino acids, ATP). Peptide mediators (see Ch. 16) differ in that they may be synthesised and packaged in the cell body rather than the terminals.

Neuromodulation and presynaptic interactions

- As well as functioning directly as neurotransmitters, chemical mediators may regulate:
  - presynaptic transmitter release
  - neuronal excitability.
- Both are examples of neuromodulation and generally involve second messenger regulation of membrane ion channels.
- Presynaptic receptors may inhibit or increase transmitter release, the former being more important.
- Inhibitory presynaptic autoreceptors occur on noradrenergic and cholinergic neurons, causing each transmitter to inhibit its own release (autoinhibitory feedback).
- Many endogenous mediators (e.g. GABA, prostaglandins, opioid and other peptides), as well as the transmitters themselves, exert presynaptic control (mainly inhibitory) over autonomic transmitter release.

REFERENCES AND FURTHER READING

General references

Appenzeller O, Oribe E 1997 The autonomic nervous system: an introduction to basic and clinical concepts, 5th edn. Elsevier, New York (*Comprehensive textbook*)

Bacq Z M 1975 Chemical transmission of nerve impulses: a historical sketch. Pergamon Press, Oxford (*Lively account of the history of the discovery of chemical transmission*)

Brading A F 1999 The autonomic nervous system and its effectors. Blackwell, Oxford

Broadley K J 1996 Autonomic pharmacology. Taylor & Francis, London (*Comprehensive textbook*)

Cooper J C, Bloom F E, Roth R H 2004 The biochemical basis of neuropharmacology, 8th edn. Oxford University Press, New York (*Excellent general account covering a broad area of neuropharmacology*)

Goyal R K, Hirano I 1996 The enteric nervous system. N Engl J Med 334: 1106–1115 (*Excellent review article*)

Jänig W, McLachlan E M 1992 Characteristics of function-specific pathways in the sympathetic nervous system. Trends Neurosci 15: 475–481 (*Short article emphasising that the sympathetic system is far from being an all-or-none alarm system*)

Nestler E J, Hyman S E, Malenka R C 2001 Molecular neuropharmacology. McGraw-Hill, New York (*A very good advanced textbook covering the actions of mediators and neuroactive drugs at the molecular and cellular level*)

Valenstein E S 2005 The war of the soups and the sparks. Columbia university Press, New York

(*Readable and informative account of origins of the theory of chemical transmission*)

Presynaptic modulation

Fuder H, Muscholl E 1995 Heteroreceptor-mediated modulation of noradrenaline and acetylcholine release from peripheral nerves. Rev Physiol Biochem Pharmacol 126: 263–412 (*Comprehensive review of presynaptic modulation*)

Gonçalves J, Bueltmann R, Driessen B 1996 Opposite modulation of cotransmitter release in guinea-pig vas deferens: increase of noradrenaline and decrease of ATP release by activation of prejunctional β-receptors. Naunyn-Schmiedeberg's Arch Pharmacol 353: 184–192 (*Shows that presynaptic regulation can affect specific transmitters in different ways*)

MacDermott A B, Role L W, Siegelbaum S A 1999 Presynaptic ionotropic receptors and the control of transmitter release. Annu Rev Pharmacol 22: 442–485 (*Detailed review of presynaptic ionotropic receptor mechanisms—as distinct from the more familiar G-protein–coupled receptors—controlling transmitter release*)

Starke K, Gothert M, Kilbinger H 1989 Modulation of neurotransmitter release by presynaptic autoreceptors. Physiol Rev 69: 864–989 (*Comprehensive review article*)

Cotransmission

Jan Y N, Jan L Y 1983 A LHRH-like peptidergic neurotransmitter capable of 'action at a distance' in autonomic ganglia. Trends Neurosci 6: 320–325 (*Electrophysiological analysis of cotransmission*)

Kupfermann I 1991 Functional studies of cotransmission. Physiol Rev 71: 683–732 (*Good review article*)

Lundberg J M 1996 Pharmacology of co-transmission in the autonomic nervous system: integrative aspects on amines, neuropeptides, adenosine triphosphate, amino acids and nitric oxide. Pharmacol Rev 48: 114–192 (*Detailed and informative review article*)

Stjarne L 1989 Basic mechanisms and local modulation of nerve impulse–induced secretion of neurotransmitters from individual sympathetic nerve varicosities. Rev Physiol Biochem Pharmacol 112: 1–137 (*Excellent review on presynaptic regulation*)

Transporters

Nelson N 1998 The family of Na$^+$/Cl$^-$ neurotransmitter transporters. J Neurochem 71: 1785–1803 (*Review article describing the molecular characteristics of the different families of neurotransporters*)

Torres G E, Gainetdinov R R, Caron M G 2003 Plasma membrane monoamine transporters: structure, regulation and function. Nat Rev Neurosci 4: 13–25 (*Describes molecular, physiological, and pharmacological aspects of transporters*)

Vizi E S 2001 Role of high-affinity receptors and membrane transporters in non-synaptic communication and drug action in the central nervous system. Pharmacol Rev 52: 63–89 (*Comprehensive review on pharmacological relevance of presynaptic receptors and transporters; useful for reference*)

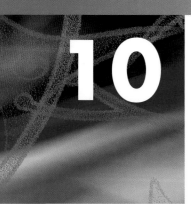

10

Cholinergic transmission

OVERVIEW

This chapter is concerned mainly with cholinergic transmission in the periphery, and the ways in which drugs affect it. Here we describe the different types of acetylcholine (ACh) receptors and their functions, as well as the synthesis and release of ACh. Drugs that act on ACh receptors, many of which have clinical uses, are described in this chapter. Cholinergic mechanisms in the central nervous system (CNS) and their relevance to dementia are discussed in Chapters 32 and 35.

MUSCARINIC AND NICOTINIC ACTIONS OF ACETYLCHOLINE

▼ The discovery of the pharmacological action of ACh came, paradoxically, from work on adrenal glands, extracts of which were known to produce a rise in blood pressure owing to their content of adrenaline (epinephrine). In 1900, Reid Hunt found that after adrenaline had been removed from such extracts, they produced a fall in blood pressure instead of a rise. He attributed the fall to the presence of choline, but later concluded that a more potent derivative of choline must be responsible. With Taveau, he tested a number of choline derivatives and discovered that ACh was some

100 000 times more active than choline in lowering the rabbit's blood pressure. The physiological role of ACh was not apparent at that time, and it remained a pharmacological curiosity until Loewi and Dale and their colleagues discovered its transmitter role in the 1930s.

Analysing the pharmacological actions of ACh in 1914, Dale distinguished two types of activity, which he designated as *muscarinic* and *nicotinic*. The muscarinic actions of ACh are those that can be reproduced by the injection of **muscarine**, the active principle of the poisonous mushroom *Amanita muscaria*, and can be abolished by small doses of **atropine**. Muscarinic actions closely resemble the effects of parasympathetic stimulation, as shown in Table 9.1. After the muscarinic effects have been blocked by atropine, larger doses of ACh produce another set of effects, closely similar to those of **nicotine**. They include:

- stimulation of all autonomic ganglia
- stimulation of voluntary muscle
- secretion of adrenaline from the adrenal medulla.

The muscarinic and nicotinic actions of ACh are demonstrated in Figure 10.1. Small and medium doses of ACh produce a transient fall in blood pressure due to arteriolar vasodilatation and slowing of the heart—muscarinic effects that are abolished by atropine. A large dose of ACh given after atropine produces nicotinic effects: an initial rise in blood pressure due to a stimulation of sympathetic ganglia and consequent vasoconstriction, and a secondary rise resulting from secretion of adrenaline.

Dale's pharmacological classification corresponds closely to the main physiological functions of ACh in the body. The muscarinic actions correspond to those of ACh released at postganglionic parasympathetic nerve endings, with two significant exceptions:

- Acetylcholine causes generalised vasodilatation, even though most blood vessels have no parasympathetic innervation. This is an indirect effect: ACh (like many other mediators) acts on vascular endothelial cells to release nitric oxide (see Ch. 17), which relaxes smooth muscle. The physiological function of this is uncertain, because ACh is not normally present in circulating blood.
- Acetylcholine evokes secretion from sweat glands, which are innervated by cholinergic fibres of the sympathetic nervous system (see Table 9.1).

The nicotinic actions correspond to those of ACh acting on autonomic ganglia of the sympathetic and parasympathetic systems, the motor endplate of voluntary muscle, and the secretory cells of the adrenal medulla.

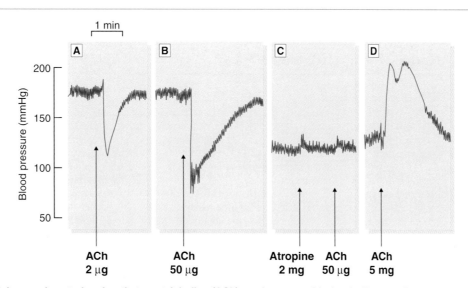

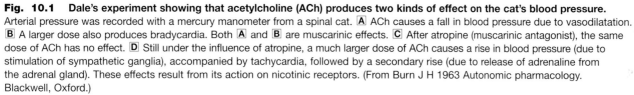

Fig. 10.1 Dale's experiment showing that acetylcholine (ACh) produces two kinds of effect on the cat's blood pressure. Arterial pressure was recorded with a mercury manometer from a spinal cat. **A** ACh causes a fall in blood pressure due to vasodilatation. **B** A larger dose also produces bradycardia. Both **A** and **B** are muscarinic effects. **C** After atropine (muscarinic antagonist), the same dose of ACh has no effect. **D** Still under the influence of atropine, a much larger dose of ACh causes a rise in blood pressure (due to stimulation of sympathetic ganglia), accompanied by tachycardia, followed by a secondary rise (due to release of adrenaline from the adrenal gland). These effects result from its action on nicotinic receptors. (From Burn J H 1963 Autonomic pharmacology. Blackwell, Oxford.)

ACETYLCHOLINE RECEPTORS

Although Dale himself dismissed the concept of receptors as sophistry rather than science, his classification provided the basis for distinguishing the two major classes of ACh receptor (see Ch. 3).

NICOTINIC RECEPTORS

Nicotinic ACh receptors (nAChRs) fall into three main classes, the muscle, ganglionic and CNS types, whose subunit composition is summarised in Table 10.1. Muscle receptors are confined to the skeletal neuromuscular junction; ganglionic receptors are responsible for transmission at sympathetic and parasympathetic ganglia; and CNS-type receptors are widespread in the brain, and are heterogeneous with respect to their molecular composition and location (see Ch. 35).

▼ All nAChRs are pentameric structures that function as ligand-gated ion channels (see Ch. 3). The five subunits that form the receptor–channel complex are similar in structure, and so far 16 different members of the family have been identified and cloned, designated α (nine types), β (four types), γ, δ and ε (one of each). The five subunits each possess four membrane-spanning helical domains, and one of these helices (M_2) from each subunit defines the central pore (see Ch. 3). nAChR subtypes generally contain both α and β subunits, the exception being the homomeric $(\alpha7)_5$ subtype found mainly in the brain (Ch. 35). The adult muscle receptor has the composition $(\alpha1)_2/\beta1\gamma\varepsilon$, while the main ganglionic subtype is $(\alpha3)_2(\beta4)_3$. The two binding sites for ACh (both of which need to be occupied to cause the channel to open) reside at the interface between the extracellular domain of each of the α subunits and its neighbour. The diversity of the nAChR family (see Hogg et al., 2003, for details), which emerged from cloning studies in the 1980s, took pharmacologists somewhat by surprise. Although they knew that the neuromuscular and ganglionic synapses differed pharmacologically, and suspected that

cholinergic synapses in the CNS might be different again, the diversity goes far beyond this, and its functional significance is not yet clear (for reviews see McGehee & Role, 1995; Cordero-Erauskin et al., 2000).

The different action of agonists and antagonists on ganglionic and neuromuscular synapses is of practical importance and mainly reflects the differences between the muscle and neuronal nAChRs (Table 10.1).

MUSCARINIC RECEPTORS

Muscarinic receptors (mAChRs) are typical G-protein–coupled receptors (see Ch. 3), and five molecular subtypes (M_1–M_5) are known (see Wess, 1996). The odd-numbered members of the group (M_1, M_3, M_5) couple with G_q to activate the inositol phosphate pathway (Ch. 3), while the even-numbered receptors (M_2, M_4) act through G_i to inhibit adenylyl cyclase and thus reduce intracellular cAMP (see Goyal, 1989).

Three of these (M_1, M_2, M_3) are well characterised (Table 10.2). M_1 receptors ('neural') are found mainly on CNS and peripheral neurons and on gastric parietal cells. They mediate excitatory effects, for example the slow muscarinic excitation mediated by ACh in sympathetic ganglia (Ch. 9) and central neurons. This excitation is produced by a decrease in K^+ conductance, which causes membrane depolarisation. Deficiency of this kind of ACh-mediated effect in the brain is possibly associated with dementia (see Ch. 35), although transgenic M_1 receptor knockout mice show only slight cognitive impairment (see Wess, 2004). M_1 receptors are also involved in the increase of gastric acid secretion following vagal stimulation (see Ch. 25).

M_2 receptors ('cardiac') occur in the heart, and also on the presynaptic terminals of peripheral and central neurons. They

Table 10.1 Nicotinic receptor subtypes[a]

	Muscle type	Ganglion type	CNS type		Notes
Main molecular form	$(\alpha1)_2\beta1\delta\epsilon$ (adult form)	$(\alpha3)_2(\beta4)_3$	$(\alpha4)_2(\beta2)_3$	$(\alpha7)_5$	–
Main synaptic location	Skeletal neuromuscular junction: mainly postsynaptic	Autonomic ganglia: mainly postsynaptic	Many brain regions: pre- and postsynaptic	Many brain regions: pre- and postsynaptic	– –
Membrane response	Excitatory Increased cation permeability (mainly Na^+, K^+)	Excitatory Increased cation permeability (mainly Na^+, K^+)	Pre- and postsynaptic excitation Increased cation permeability (mainly Na^+, K^+)	Pre- and postsynaptic excitation Increased Ca^{2+} permeability	$(\alpha7)_5$ receptor produces large Ca^{2+} entry, evoking transmitter release
Agonists	Acetylcholine Carbachol Succinylcholine	Acetylcholine Carbachol Nicotine Epibatidine Dimethylphenyl-piperazinium	Nicotine Epibatidine Acetylcholine Cytosine	Epibatidine Dimethylphenyl-piperazinium	$(\alpha4)_2(\beta2)_3$ is brain 'nicotine receptor' (see Ch. 34)
Antagonists	Tubocurarine Pancuronium Atracurium Vecuronium α-Bungarotoxin α-Conotoxin	Mecamylamine Trimetaphan Hexamethonium α-Conotoxin	Mecamylamine Methylaconitine	α-Bungarotoxin α-Conotoxin Methylaconitine	

[a]This table shows only the main subtypes expressed in mammalian tissues. Several other subtypes are expressed in selected brain regions, and also in the peripheral nervous system and in non-neuronal tissues. For further details, see Chapter 34 and reviews by Lindstrom (2000), Cordero-Erausquin et al. (2000) and Dajas-Bailador & Wonnacott (2004).

exert inhibitory effects, mainly by increasing K^+ conductance and by inhibiting calcium channels (see Ch. 4). M_2 receptor activation is responsible for cholinergic inhibition of the heart, as well as presynaptic inhibition in the CNS and periphery (Ch. 9). They are also coexpressed with M_3 receptors in visceral smooth muscle, and contribute to the smooth-muscle–stimulating effect of muscarinic agonists in several organs.

M_3 receptors ('glandular/smooth muscle') produce mainly excitatory effects, i.e. stimulation of glandular secretions (salivary, bronchial, sweat, etc.) and contraction of visceral smooth muscle. M_3 receptors also mediate relaxation of smooth muscle (mainly vascular), which results from the release of nitric oxide from neighbouring endothelial cells (Ch. 17). M_1, M_2 and M_3 receptors occur also in specific locations in the CNS (see Ch. 34). M_4 and M_5 receptors are largely confined to the CNS, and their functional role is not well understood, although mice lacking these receptors do show behavioural changes (Wess, 2004).

The pharmacological classification of these receptor types relies on the limited selectivity of certain agonists and antagonists that can distinguish between them. Most agonists are non-selective, but two experimental compounds, **McNA343** and **oxotremorine**, are selective for M_1 receptors; **carbachol** is relatively inactive on these receptors. Other M_1-selective agonists (e.g. **xanomeline**) have recently been discovered and are in development as possible

treatments for dementia. There is more selectivity among antagonists. Although most of the classic muscarinic antagonists (e.g. **atropine**, **scopolamine**) are non-selective, **pirenzepine** is selective for M_1 receptors, and **darifenacin** for M_3 receptors. **Gallamine**, better known as a neuromuscular-blocking drug (see p. 157), is also a selective, although weak, M_2 receptor antagonist. Recently, toxins from the venom of the green mamba have been discovered to be highly selective mAChR antagonists (see Table 10.2), as well as various synthetic compounds with some degree of selectivity (see Eglen et al., 1999, for more details). Compounds that have recently been approved for clinical use are described below (p. 152).

PHYSIOLOGY OF CHOLINERGIC TRANSMISSION

The physiology of cholinergic transmission is described in detail by Nicholls et al. (2001). The main ways in which drugs can affect cholinergic transmission are shown in Figure 10.2.

▼ Acetylcholine is synthesised and stored in many tissues that lack cholinergic innervation, such as the placenta and cornea. Despite speculation about possible regulatory and trophic functions (see review by Wessle et al., 1998), the role of non-neuronal acetylcholine is uncertain.

Table 10.2 Muscarinic receptor subtypes[a]

	M₁ ('neural')	M₂ ('cardiac')	M₃ ('glandular/ smooth muscle')	M₄	M₅
Main locations	Autonomic ganglia Glands: gastric, salivary, etc. Cerebral cortex	Heart: atria CNS: widely distributed	Exocrine glands: gastric, salivary, etc. Smooth muscle: gastrointestinal tract, eye, airways, bladder Blood vessels: endothelium CNS	CNS	CNS: very localised expression in substantia nigra Salivary glands Iris/ciliary muscle
Cellular response	↑ IP₃, DAG Depolarisation Excitation (slow epsp) ↓ K+ conductance	↓ cAMP Inhibition ↓ Ca²⁺ conductance ↑ K⁺ conductance	↑ IP₃ Stimulation ↑ [Ca²⁺]ᵢ	↓ cAMP Inhibition	↑ IP₃ Excitation
Functional response	CNS excitation (?memory) Gastric secretion	Cardiac inhibition Neural inhibition Central muscarinic effects (e.g. tremor, hypothermia)	Gastric, salivary secretion Gastrointestinal smooth muscle contraction Ocular accommodation Vasodilatation	Enhanced locomotion	Not known
Agonists (non-selective, except those in italics) See also Table 10.3	Acetylcholine Carbachol Oxotremorine *McNA343* *Talsaclidine*	As M₁	As M₁	As M₁	As M₁
Antagonists (non-selective, except those in italics) See also Table 10.5	Atropine Dicycloverine Tolterodine Oxybutynin Ipratropium *Pirenzepine* *Mamba toxin MT7*	Atropine Dicycloverine Tolterodine Oxybutynin Ipratropium Gallamine	Atropine Dicycloverine Tolterodine Oxybutynin Ipratropium *Darifenacin*	Atropine Dicycloverine Tolterodine Oxybutynin *Ipratropium* *Mamba toxin MT3*	Atropine Dicycloverine Tolterodine Oxybutynin Ipratropium

CNS, central nervous system; DAG, diacylglycerol; epsp, excitatory postsynaptic potential; IP3, inositol trisphosphate.
[a]This table shows only the predominant subtypes expressed in mammalian tissues. For further details, see Chapter 34 and reviews by Caulfield & Birdsall (1998) and Wess (2004).

ACETYLCHOLINE SYNTHESIS AND RELEASE

Acetylcholine metabolism is well reviewed by Parsons et al. (1993). ACh is synthesised within the nerve terminal from choline, which is taken up into the nerve terminal by a specific carrier (Ch. 9), similar to that which operates for many transmitters. The difference is that it transports the precursor, choline, not ACh, so it is not important in terminating the action of the transmitter. The concentration of choline in the blood and body fluids is normally about 10 μmol/l, but in the immediate vicinity of cholinergic nerve terminals it increases, probably to about 1 mmol/l, when the released ACh is hydrolysed, and more than 50% of this choline is normally recaptured by the nerve terminals. Free choline within the nerve terminal is acetylated by a cytosolic enzyme, *choline acetyltransferase (CAT)*, which transfers the acetyl group from acetyl coenzyme A. The rate-limiting process in ACh synthesis appears to be choline transport, the activity of which is regulated according to the rate at which ACh is being released. Cholinesterase

is present in the presynaptic nerve terminals, and ACh is continually being hydrolysed and resynthesised. Inhibition of the nerve terminal cholinesterase causes the accumulation of 'surplus' ACh in the cytosol, which is not available for release by nerve impulses (although it is able to leak out via the choline carrier). Most of the ACh synthesised, however, is packaged into synaptic vesicles, in which its concentration is very high (about 100 mmol/1), and from which release occurs by exocytosis triggered by Ca²⁺ entry into the nerve terminal (see Ch. 4).

Cholinergic vesicles accumulate ACh actively, by means of a specific transporter (see Usdin et al., 1995; Liu & Edwards, 1997) belonging to the family of amine transporters described in Chapter 9. Accumulation of ACh is coupled to the large electrochemical gradient for protons that exists between intracellular organelles and the cytosol; it is blocked selectively by the experimental drug **vesamicol** (see Parsons et al., 1993). Following its release, the ACh diffuses across the synaptic cleft to combine with receptors on the postsynaptic cell. Some of it succumbs on the way to hydrolysis

Acetylcholine receptors

- Main subdivision is into nicotinic (nAChR) and muscarinic (mAChR) subtypes.
- nAChRs are directly coupled to cation channels, and mediate fast excitatory synaptic transmission at the neuromuscular junction, autonomic ganglia, and various sites in the central nervous system (CNS). Muscle and neuronal nAChRs differ in their molecular structure and pharmacology.
- mAChRs and nAChRs occur presynaptically as well as postsynaptically, and function to regulate transmitter release.
- mAChRs are G-protein–coupled receptors causing:
  - activation of phospholipase C (hence formation of inositol trisphosphate and diacylglycerol as second messengers)
  - inhibition of adenylyl cyclase
  - activation of potassium channels or inhibition of calcium channels.
- mAChRs mediate acetylcholine effects at postganglionic parasympathetic synapses (mainly heart, smooth muscle, glands), and contribute to ganglionic excitation. They occur in many parts of the CNS.
- Three main types of mAChR occur.
  - M_1 receptors ('neural') producing slow excitation of ganglia. They are selectively blocked by pirenzepine.
  - M_2 receptors ('cardiac') causing decrease in cardiac rate and force of contraction (mainly of atria). They are selectively blocked by gallamine. M_2 receptors also mediate presynaptic inhibition.
  - M_3 receptors ('glandular') causing secretion, contraction of visceral smooth muscle, vascular relaxation.
- Two further molecular mAChR subtypes, M_4 and M_5, occur mainly in the CNS.
- All mAChRs are activated by acetylcholine and blocked by atropine. There are also subtype-selective agonists and antagonists.

by acetylcholinesterase (AChE), an enzyme that is bound to the basement membrane, which lies between the pre- and postsynaptic membranes. At fast cholinergic synapses (e.g. the neuromuscular and ganglionic synapses), but not at slow ones (smooth muscle, gland cells, heart, etc.), the released ACh is hydrolysed very rapidly (within 1 ms), so that it acts only very briefly.

▼ At the neuromuscular junction, which is a highly specialised synapse, a single nerve impulse releases about 300 synaptic vesicles (altogether about three million ACh molecules) from the nerve terminals supplying a single muscle fibre, which contain altogether about three million synaptic vesicles. Approximately two million ACh molecules combine with receptors, of which there are about 30 million on each muscle fibre, the rest being hydrolysed without reaching a receptor. The ACh molecules remain bound to receptors for, on average, about 2 ms, and are quickly hydrolysed after dissociating, so that they cannot combine with

a second receptor. The result is that transmitter action is very rapid and very brief, which is important for a synapse that has to initiate speedy muscular responses, and that may have to transmit signals faithfully at high frequency. Muscle cells are much larger than neurons and require much more synaptic current to generate an action potential. Thus all the chemical events happen on a larger scale than at a neuronal synapse; the number of transmitter molecules in a quantum, the number of quanta released, and the number of receptors activated by each quantum are all 10–100 times greater. Our brains would be huge, but not very clever, if their synapses were built on the industrial scale of the neuromuscular junction.

PRESYNAPTIC MODULATION

Acetylcholine release is regulated by mediators, including ACh itself, acting on presynaptic receptors, as discussed in Chapter 9. At postganglionic parasympathetic nerve endings, inhibitory M_2 receptors participate in autoinhibition of ACh release; other mediators, such as noradrenaline, also inhibit the release of ACh (see Ch. 9). At the neuromuscular junction, on the other hand, presynaptic nAChRs are believed to facilitate ACh release (see Prior et al., 1995), a mechanism that may allow the synapse to function reliably during prolonged high-frequency activity. In the brain (see review by Dajas-Bailador & Wonnacott, 2004), most of the nAChRs are located presynaptically and serve to facilitate transmission by other mediators, such as glutamate and dopamine.

ELECTRICAL EVENTS IN TRANSMISSION AT FAST CHOLINERGIC SYNAPSES

Acetylcholine, acting on the postsynaptic membrane of a nicotinic (neuromuscular or ganglionic) synapse, causes a large increase in its permeability to cations, particularly to Na^+ and K^+, and to a lesser extent Ca^{2+}. The resulting inflow of Na^+ depolarises the postsynaptic membrane. This transmitter-mediated depolarisation is called an *endplate potential* (*epp*) in a skeletal muscle fibre, or a *fast excitatory postsynaptic potential* (*fast epsp*) at the ganglionic synapse. In a muscle fibre, the localised epp spreads to adjacent, electrically excitable parts of the muscle fibre; if its amplitude reaches the threshold for excitation, an action potential is initiated, which propagates to the rest of the fibre and evokes a contraction (Ch. 4).

In a nerve cell, depolarisation of the soma or a dendrite by the fast epsp causes a local current to flow. This depolarises the axon hillock region of the cell, where, if the epsp is large enough, an action potential is initiated. Figure 10.3 shows that **tubocurarine**, a drug that blocks postsynaptic ACh receptors (see p. 158), reduces the amplitude of the fast epsp until it no longer initiates an action potential, although the cell is still capable of responding when it is stimulated antidromically. Most ganglion cells are supplied by several presynaptic axons, and it requires simultaneous activity in more than one to make the postganglionic cell fire. At the neuromuscular junction, only one nerve fibre supplies each muscle fibre. Nevertheless, the amplitude of the epp is normally more than enough to initiate an action potential—indeed, transmission still occurs when the epp is reduced by 70–80%, and is said to show a large *margin of safety* so that fluctuations in transmitter release (e.g. during repetitive stimulation) do not affect transmission.

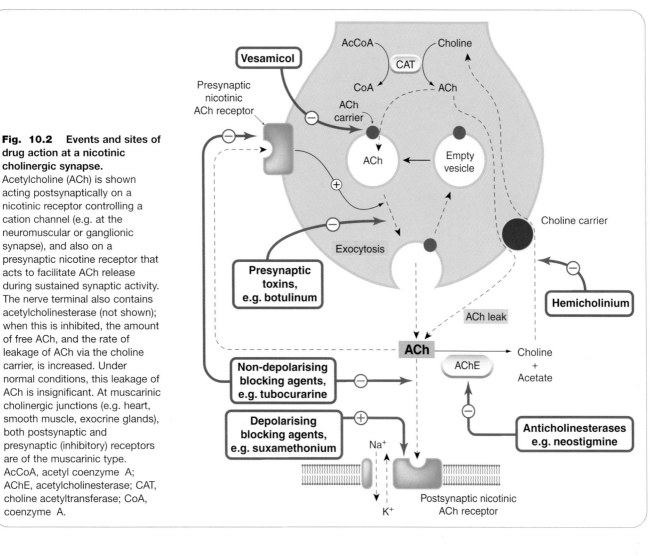

Fig. 10.2 Events and sites of drug action at a nicotinic cholinergic synapse.
Acetylcholine (ACh) is shown acting postsynaptically on a nicotinic receptor controlling a cation channel (e.g. at the neuromuscular or ganglionic synapse), and also on a presynaptic nicotine receptor that acts to facilitate ACh release during sustained synaptic activity. The nerve terminal also contains acetylcholinesterase (not shown); when this is inhibited, the amount of free ACh, and the rate of leakage of ACh via the choline carrier, is increased. Under normal conditions, this leakage of ACh is insignificant. At muscarinic cholinergic junctions (e.g. heart, smooth muscle, exocrine glands), both postsynaptic and presynaptic (inhibitory) receptors are of the muscarinic type. AcCoA, acetyl coenzyme A; AChE, acetylcholinesterase; CAT, choline acetyltransferase; CoA, coenzyme A.

▼ Transmission at the ganglionic synapse is more complex than at the neuromuscular junction. Although the primary event at both is the epp or fast epsp produced by ACh acting on nAChRs, this is followed in the ganglion by a succession of much slower postsynaptic responses, comprising the following.

- *A slow inhibitory (hyperpolarising) postsynaptic potential (slow ipsp) lasting 2–5 seconds.* This mainly reflects a muscarinic (M_2) receptor –mediated increase in K^+ conductance, but other transmitters, such as dopamine and adenosine, also contribute.
- *A slow epsp, which lasts for about 10 seconds.* This is produced by ACh acting on M_1 receptors, which close potassium channels.
- *A late slow epsp, lasting for 1–2 minutes.* This is thought to be mediated by a peptide cotransmitter, which may be substance P in some ganglia, and a gonadotrophin-releasing hormone–like peptide in others (see Ch. 9). Like the slow epsp, it is produced by a decrease in K^+ conductance.

DEPOLARISATION BLOCK

Depolarisation block occurs at cholinergic synapses when the excitatory nAChRs are persistently activated, and it results from a decrease in the electrical excitability of the postsynaptic cell. This is shown in Figure 10.4. Application of nicotine to a sympathetic ganglion causes a depolarisation of the cell, which at first initiates action potential discharge. After a few seconds, this discharge ceases and transmission is blocked. The loss of electrical excitability at this time is shown by the fact that antidromic stimuli also fail to produce an action potential. The main reason for the loss of electrical excitability during a period of maintained depolarisation is that the voltage-sensitive sodium channels (see Ch. 4) become inactivated (i.e. refractory) and no longer able to open in response to a brief depolarising stimulus.

▼ A second type of effect is also seen in the experiment shown in Figure 10.4. After nicotine has acted for several minutes, the cell partially repolarises and its electrical excitability returns but, despite this, transmission remains blocked. This type of secondary, non-depolarising block occurs also at the neuromuscular junction if repeated doses of the depolarising drug **succinylcholine** (see below) are used. The main factor responsible for the secondary block (known clinically as phase II block) appears to be receptor desensitisation (see Ch. 2). This causes the depolarising action of the blocking drug to subside, but transmission remains blocked because the receptors are desensitised to ACh.

EFFECTS OF DRUGS ON CHOLINERGIC TRANSMISSION

As shown in Figure 10.2, drugs can influence cholinergic transmission either by acting on postsynaptic ACh receptors as

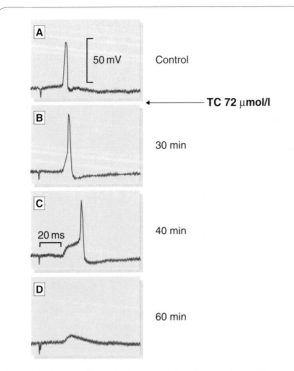

Fig. 10.3 Cholinergic transmission in an autonomic ganglion cell. Records were obtained with an intracellular microelectrode from a guinea pig parasympathetic ganglion cell. The artefact at the beginning of each trace shows the moment of stimulation of the preganglionic nerve. Tubocurarine (TC), an acetylcholine antagonist, causes the epsp to become smaller. In record C, it only just succeeds in triggering the action potential, and in D it has fallen below the threshold. Following complete block, antidromic stimulation (not shown) will still produce an action potential (cf. depolarisation block, Fig. 10.4). (From Blackman J G et al. 1969 J Physiol 201: 723.)

Cholinergic transmission

- Acetylcholine (ACh) synthesis:
  - requires choline, which enters the neuron via carrier-mediated transport
  - requires acetylation of choline, utilising acetyl coenzyme A as source of acetyl groups, and involves choline acetyl transferase, a cytosolic enzyme found only in cholinergic neurons.
- ACh is packaged into synaptic vesicles at high concentration by carrier-mediated transport.
- ACh release occurs by Ca^{2+}-mediated exocytosis. At the neuromuscular junction, one presynaptic nerve impulse releases 100–500 vesicles.
- At the neuromuscular junction, ACh acts on nicotinic receptors to open cation channels, producing a rapid depolarisation (endplate potential), which normally initiates an action potential in the muscle fibre. Transmission at other 'fast' cholinergic synapses (e.g. ganglionic) is similar.
- At 'fast' cholinergic synapses, ACh is hydrolysed within about 1 ms by acetylcholinesterase, so a presynaptic action potential produces only one postsynaptic action potential.
- Transmission mediated by muscarinic receptors is much slower in its time course, and synaptic structures are less clearly defined. In many situations, ACh functions as a modulator rather than as a direct transmitter.
- Main mechanisms of pharmacological block: inhibition of choline uptake, inhibition of ACh release, block of postsynaptic receptors or ion channels, persistent postsynaptic depolarisation.

agonists or antagonists (Tables 10.1 and 10.2), or by affecting the release or destruction of endogenous ACh.

In the rest of this chapter, we describe the following groups of drugs, subdivided according to their physiological site of action:

- muscarinic agonists
- muscarinic antagonists
- ganglion-stimulating drugs
- ganglion-blocking drugs
- neuromuscular-blocking drugs
- anticholinesterases and other drugs that enhance cholinergic transmission.

DRUGS AFFECTING MUSCARINIC RECEPTORS

MUSCARINIC AGONISTS

Structure–activity relationships

Muscarinic agonists, as a group, are often referred to as *parasympathomimetic*, because the main effects that they produce in the whole animal resemble those of parasympathetic stimulation. The structures of the most important compounds are

given in Table 10.3. ACh itself and related choline esters are agonists at both mAChRs and nAChRs, but act more potently on mAChRs (see Fig. 10.1). Only **bethanechol** and **pilocarpine** are now used clinically.

The key features of the ACh molecule that are important for its activity are the quaternary ammonium group, which bears a positive charge, and the ester group, which bears a partial negative charge and is susceptible to rapid hydrolysis by cholinesterase. Variants of the choline ester structure (Table 10.3) have the effect of reducing the susceptibility of the compound to hydrolysis by cholinesterase, and altering the relative activity on mAChRs and nAChRs.

Carbachol and **methacholine** are used as experimental tools. Bethanechol, which is a hybrid of these two molecules, is stable to hydrolysis and selective for mAChRs, and is occasionally used clinically. Pilocarpine is a partial agonist and shows some selectivity in stimulating secretion from sweat, salivary, lacrimal and bronchial glands, and contracting iris smooth muscle (see below), with weak effects on gastrointestinal smooth muscle and the heart.

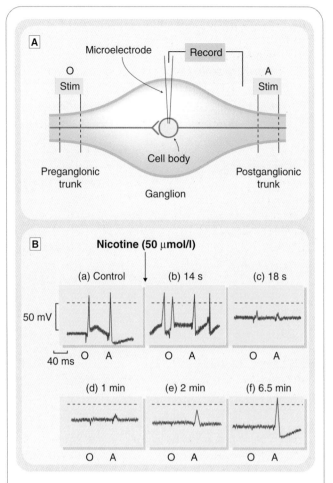

Fig. 10.4 Depolarisation block of ganglionic transmission by nicotine. A System used for intracellular recording from sympathetic ganglion cells of the frog, showing the location of orthodromic (O) and antidromic (A) stimulating (stim) electrodes. Stimulation at O excites the cell via the cholinergic synapse, whereas stimulation at A excites it by electrical propagation of the action potential. B The effect of nicotine: (a) Control records. The membrane potential is −55 mV (dotted line = 0 mV), and the cell responds to both O and A. (b) Shortly after adding nicotine, the cell is slightly depolarised and spontaneously active, but still responsive to O and A. (c and d) The cell is further depolarised, to −25 mV, and produces only a vestigial action potential. The fact that it does not respond to A shows that it is electrically inexcitable. (e and f) In the continued presence of nicotine, the cell repolarises and regains its responsiveness to A, but it is still unresponsive to O because the ACh receptors are desensitised by nicotine. (From Ginsborg B L, Guerrero S 1964 J Physiol 172: 189.)

Effects of muscarinic agonists

The main actions of muscarinic agonists are readily understood in terms of the parasympathetic nervous system.

Cardiovascular effects. These include cardiac slowing and a decrease in cardiac output. The latter action is due mainly to a decreased force of contraction of the atria, because the ventricles have only a sparse parasympathetic innervation and a low sensitivity to muscarinic agonists. Generalised vasodilatation also occurs

(a nitric oxide–mediated effect; see Ch. 17), and these two effects combine to produce a sharp fall in arterial pressure (Fig. 10.1). The mechanism of action of muscarinic agonists on the heart is discussed in Chapter 18.

Smooth muscle. Smooth muscle other than vascular smooth muscle contracts in response to muscarinic agonists. Peristaltic activity of the gastrointestinal tract is increased, which can cause colicky pain, and the bladder and bronchial smooth muscle also contract.

Sweating, lacrimation, salivation and bronchial secretion. These result from stimulation of exocrine glands. The combined effect of bronchial secretion and constriction can interfere with breathing.

Effects on the eye. Such effects are of some importance. The parasympathetic nerves to the eye supply the *constrictor pupillae* muscle, which runs circumferentially in the iris, and the *ciliary muscle*, which adjusts the curvature of the lens (Fig. 10.5). Contraction of the ciliary muscle in response to activation of mAChRs pulls the ciliary body forwards and inwards, thus relaxing the tension on the suspensory ligament of the lens, allowing the lens to bulge more and reducing its focal length. This parasympathetic reflex is thus necessary to accommodate the eye for near vision. The constrictor pupillae is important not only for adjusting the pupil in response to changes in light intensity, but also in regulating the intraocular pressure. Aqueous humour is secreted slowly and continuously by the cells of the epithelium covering the ciliary body, and it drains into the canal of Schlemm (Fig. 10.5), which runs around the eye close to the outer margin of the iris. The intraocular pressure is normally 10–15 mmHg above atmospheric, which keeps the eye slightly distended. Abnormally raised intraocular pressure (associated with glaucoma) damages the eye and is one of the commonest preventable causes of blindness. In acute glaucoma, drainage of aqueous humour becomes impeded when the pupil is dilated, because folding of the iris tissue occludes the drainage angle, causing the intraocular pressure to rise. Activation of the constrictor pupillae muscle by muscarinic agonists in these circumstances lowers the intraocular pressure, although in a normal individual it has little effect. The increased tension in the ciliary muscle produced by these drugs may also play a part in improving drainage by realigning the connective tissue trabeculae through which the canal of Schlemm passes.

▼ In addition to these peripheral effects, muscarinic agonists that are able to penetrate the blood–brain barrier produce marked central effects due to activation mainly of M_1 receptors in the brain. These include tremor, hypothermia and increased locomotor activity, as well as improved cognition (see Ch. 34). M_1-selective agonists (e.g. **taclifensine**) are being investigated for possible use in treating dementia (see Eglen et al., 1999; Ch. 35).

Clinical use

The main use of muscarinic agonists is in treating glaucoma, by local instillation in the form of eye drops. Pilocarpine is the most effective as, being a tertiary amine, it can cross the conjunctival membrane. It is a stable compound whose action lasts for about 1 day. A variety of drugs with different mechanisms of action are now available for the treatment of glaucoma, and are summarised in Table 10.4.

Table 10.3 Muscarinic agonists

Drug	Structure	Receptor specificity		Hydrolysis by acetylcholinesterase	Clinical uses
		Muscarinic	Nicotinic		
Acetylcholine		+++	+++	+++	None
Carbachol		++	+++	–	None
Methacholine		+++	+	++	None
Bethanechol		+++	–	–	Bladder[a] and gastrointestinal hypotonia
Muscarine		+++	–	–	None[b]
Pilocarpine		++	–	–	Glaucoma
Oxotremorine		++	–	–	None

[a]Necessary first to ensure that bladder neck is not obstructed.
[b]Cause of mushroom poisoning.

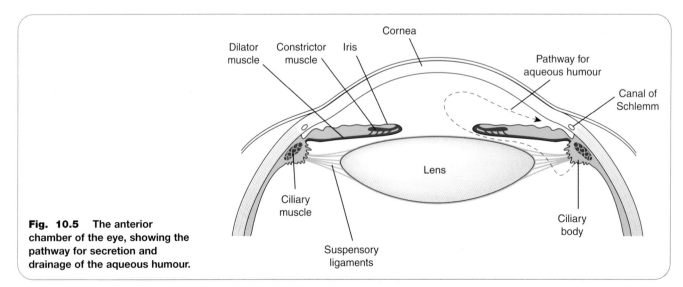

Fig. 10.5   The anterior chamber of the eye, showing the pathway for secretion and drainage of the aqueous humour.

Table 10.4 Drugs that lower intraocular pressure

Drug[a]	Mechanism	Notes	Reference
Pilocarpine	Muscarinic agonist	Widely used as eye drops	This chapter
Ecothiopate	Anticholinesterase	Widely used as eye drops. Can cause muscle spasm and systemic effects.	This chapter
Timolol, carteolol	β-Adrenoceptor antagonist	Given as eye drops but may still cause systemic side effects: bradycardia, bronchoconstriction.	Chapter 11
Acetazolamide, dorzolamide	Carbonic anhydrase inhibitor	Acetazolamide is given systemically. Side effects include diuresis, loss of appetite, tingling, neutropenia. Dorzolamide is used as eye drops. Side effects include bitter taste and burning sensation.	Chapter 24
Clonidine, apraclonidine	α_2-Adrenoceptor agonist	Used as eye drops	Chapter 11
Latanoprost	Prostaglandin analogue	Can cause ocular pigmentation	Chapter 13

[a]The most important drugs are shown in bold type.

Bethanechol is very occasionally used to assist bladder emptying or to stimulate gastrointestinal motility (see Table 10.3). It acts mainly on M_3 receptors and has little effect on the heart. In principle, a selective M_2 agonist would be useful for treating cardiac dysrhythmias, but such drugs remain to be discovered.

MUSCARINIC ANTAGONISTS

Muscarinic receptor antagonists (*parasympatholytic* drugs; Table 10.5) are competitive antagonists whose chemical structures usually contain ester and basic groups in the same relationship as ACh, but they have a bulky aromatic group in place of the acetyl group. The two naturally occurring compounds, **atropine** and **hyoscine** (scopolamine) are alkaloids found in solanaceous plants. The deadly nightshade (*Atropa belladonna*) contains mainly atropine, whereas the thorn apple (*Datura stramonium*) contains mainly hyoscine. These are tertiary ammonium compounds that are sufficiently lipid-soluble to be readily absorbed from the gut or conjunctival sac and, importantly, to penetrate the blood–brain barrier. The quaternary derivative of atropine, **atropine methonitrate,** has peripheral actions very similar to those of atropine but, because of its exclusion from the brain, lacks central actions. **Tiotropium** and **ipratropium** are also quaternary derivatives that are poorly absorbed from the lung. Given by inhalation, they act on airways smooth muscle and are used to treat asthma and chronic obstructive pulmonary disease. **Cyclopentolate** and **tropicamide** are tertiary amines developed for ophthalmic use and administered as eye drops. **Pirenzepine** is a relatively selective M_1 receptor antagonist. **Oxybutynin, tolterodine and darifenacin (M_3-selective)** are new drugs that act on the bladder to inhibit micturition, and are used for treating urinary incontinence. They produce unwanted effects typical of muscarinic antagonists, such as dry mouth, constipation and blurred vision, but these are less severe than with earlier drugs.

Effects of muscarinic antagonists

All the muscarinic antagonists produce basically similar peripheral effects, although some show a degree of selectivity, for example for the heart or the gastrointestinal tract, reflecting heterogeneity among mAChRs (see p. 145).

The main effects of atropine are as follow.

Inhibition of secretions. Salivary, lacrimal, bronchial and sweat glands are inhibited by very low doses of atropine, producing an uncomfortably dry mouth and skin. Gastric secretion is only slightly reduced. Mucociliary clearance in the bronchi is inhibited, so that residual secretions tend to accumulate in the lungs. Ipratropium lacks this effect.

Effects on heart rate. Atropine causes tachycardia through block of cardiac mAChRs. The tachycardia is modest, up to 80–90 beats/min in humans. This is because there is no effect on the sympathetic system, but only inhibition of the existing parasympathetic tone. Tachycardia is most pronounced in young people, in whom vagal tone at rest is highest; it is often absent in the elderly. At very low doses, atropine causes a paradoxical bradycardia, possibly due to a central action. The response of the heart to exercise is unaffected. Arterial blood pressure is unaffected, because most resistance vessels have no cholinergic innervation.

Effects on the eye. The pupil is dilated (*mydriasis*) by atropine administration, and becomes unresponsive to light. Relaxation of the ciliary muscle causes paralysis of accommodation (*cycloplegia*), so that near vision is impaired. Intraocular pressure may rise; although this is unimportant in normal individuals, it can be dangerous in patients suffering from narrow-angle glaucoma.

Effects on the gastrointestinal tract. Gastrointestinal motility is inhibited by atropine, although this requires larger doses than the other effects listed, and is not complete. This is because excitatory transmitters other than ACh are important in normal function of the myenteric plexus (see Ch. 9). Atropine is used in pathological conditions in which there is increased gastrointestinal motility; agents selective for M_3 receptors, which are being developed, may be preferable. Pirenzepine, owing to its selectivity for M_1 receptors, inhibits gastric acid secretion in doses that do not affect other systems.

Table 10.5   Muscarinic antagonists[a]

Compound	Pharmacological properties	Clinical uses	Notes
Atropine	Non-selective antagonist Well absorbed orally CNS stimulant	Adjunct for anaesthesia (reduced secretions, bronchodilatation) Anticholinesterase poisoning Bradycardia Gastrointestinal hypermotility (antispasmodic)	Belladonna alkaloid Main side effects: urinary retention, dry mouth, blurred vision Dicycloverine (dicyclomine) is similar and used mainly as antispasmodic agent
Hyoscine	Similar to atropine CNS depressant	As atropine Motion sickness	Belladonna alkaloid (also known as scopolamine) Causes sedation; other side effects as atropine
Atropine methonitrate	Similar to atropine but poorly absorbed and lacks CNS effects Significant ganglion-blocking activity	Mainly for gastrointestinal hypermotility	Quaternary ammonium derivative Similar drugs include methscopolamine, propantheline
Tiotropium	Similar to atropine methonitrate Does not inhibit mucociliary clearance from bronchi	By inhalation for asthma, bronchitis	Quaternary ammonium compound Ipratropium similar
Tropicamide	Similar to atropine May raise intraocular pressure	Ophthalmic use to produce mydriasis and cycloplegia (as eye drops) Short acting	–
Cyclopentolate	Similar to tropicamide	As tropicamide (long acting)	–
Pirenzepine	Selective for M_1 receptors Inhibits gastric secretion by action on ganglion cells Little effect on smooth muscle or CNS	Peptic ulcer	Fewer side effects than other muscarinic antagonists Largely superseded by other antiulcer drugs (see Ch. 25)
Darifenacin	Selective for M_3 receptors	Urinary incontinence	Few side effects

[a]For chemical structures, see Hardman J G, Limbird L E, Gilman A G, Goodman-Gilman A et al. 2001 Goodman and Gilman's pharmacological basis of therapeutics, 10th edn. McGraw-Hill, New York.

Effects on other smooth muscle. Bronchial, biliary and urinary tract smooth muscle are all relaxed by atropine. Reflex bronchoconstriction (e.g. during anaesthesia) is prevented by atropine, whereas bronchoconstriction caused by local mediators, such as **histamine** and **leukotrienes** (e.g. in asthma; Ch. 23) is unaffected. Biliary and urinary tract smooth muscle are only slightly affected, probably because transmitters other than ACh (see Ch. 6) are important in these organs; nevertheless, atropine and similar drugs commonly precipitate urinary retention in elderly men with prostatic enlargement.

Effects on the CNS. Atropine produces mainly excitatory effects on the CNS. At low doses, this causes mild restlessness; higher doses cause agitation and disorientation. In atropine poisoning, which occurs mainly in young children who eat deadly nightshade berries, marked excitement and irritability result in hyperactivity and a considerable rise in body temperature, which is accentuated by the loss of sweating. These central effects are the result of blocking mAChRs in

the brain, and they are opposed by anticholinesterase drugs such as **physostigmine**, which is an effective antidote to atropine poisoning. Scopolamine in low doses causes marked sedation, but has similar effects in high dosage. Scopolamine also has a useful antiemetic effect and is used in treating motion sickness. Muscarinic antagonists also affect the extrapyramidal system, reducing the involuntary movement and rigidity of patients with Parkinson's disease (Ch. 35) and counteracting the extrapyramidal side effects of many antipsychotic drugs (Ch. 38).

Clinical use

The main uses of muscarinic antagonists are shown in Table 10.5 and the clinical box (p. 156). Apart from pirenzepine (M_1-selective), currently used muscarinic antagonists show little subtype selectivity. M_3-selective antagonists, which may be useful as smooth muscle relaxants, are in development, but none has so far been approved for clinical use.

DRUGS AFFECTING AUTONOMIC GANGLIA
GANGLION STIMULANTS

Most nAChR agonists affect both ganglionic and motor endplate receptors, but **nicotine**, **lobeline** and **dimethylphenylpiperazinium** (**DMPP**) affect ganglia preferentially (Table 10.6).

Nicotine and lobeline are tertiary amines found in the leaves of tobacco and lobelia plants, respectively. Nicotine belongs in pharmacological folklore, as it was the substance on the tip of Langley's paintbrush causing stimulation of muscle fibres when applied to the endplate region, leading him to postulate in 1905 the existence of a 'receptive substance' on the surface of the fibres (Ch. 9). DMPP is a synthetic compound that is selective for ganglionic receptors.

Only nicotine is used clinically (to help people to stop smoking; see Ch. 43); otherwise these drugs are used only as experimental tools. They cause complex peripheral responses associated with generalised stimulation of autonomic ganglia. The effects of nicotine on the gastrointestinal tract and sweat glands are familiar to neophyte smokers (see Ch. 43), although usually insufficient to act as an effective deterrent.

GANGLION-BLOCKING DRUGS

Ganglion block is often used in experimental studies on the autonomic nervous system but is of little clinical importance. It can occur by several mechanisms.

- By interference with ACh release, as at the neuromuscular junction (see p. 161 and Ch. 9). **Botulinum toxin** and **hemicholinium** work in this way.
- By prolonged depolarisation. Nicotine (see Fig. 10.4) can block ganglia, after initial stimulation, in this way, as can ACh itself if cholinesterase is inhibited so that it can exert a continuing action on the postsynaptic membrane.
- By interference with the postsynaptic action of ACh. The few ganglion-blocking drugs of practical importance act by blocking neuronal nAChRs or the associated ion channels.

▼ Fifty years ago, Paton and Zaimis investigated a series of linear bisquaternary compounds. Compounds with five or six carbon atoms (**hexamethonium**; Table 10.6) in the methylene chain linking the two quaternary groups produced ganglionic block, whereas compounds with nine or ten carbon atoms (decamethonium) produced neuromuscular block.[1]

Hexamethonium, although no longer used, deserves recognition as the first effective antihypertensive agent (see Ch. 19). The only ganglion-blocking drug currently in clinical use is **trimetaphan** (Table 10.6; see below).

---

[1]Based on their structural similarity to ACh, these compounds were originally believed to act as competitive antagonists. However, they are now known to act mainly by blocking the ion channel rather than the receptor site itself.

Table 10.6 Nicotine receptor agonists and antagonists

Drug(s)	Main site	Type of action	Notes
Agonists			
Nicotine	Autonomic ganglia	Stimulation then block	See Chapter 43
	CNS	Stimulation	For CNS effects, see Chapter 43
Lobeline	Autonomic ganglia	Stimulation	–
	Sensory nerve terminals	Stimulation	–
Epibatidine	Autonomic ganglia, CNS	Stimulation	Isolated from frog skin; Highly potent; No clinical uses
Suxamethonium	Neuromuscular junction	Depolarisation block	Used clinically as muscle relaxant
Decamethonium	Neuromuscular junction	Depolarisation block	No clinical use
Antagonists			
Hexamethonium	Autonomic ganglia	Transmission block	No clinical use
Trimetaphan	Autonomic ganglia	Transmission block	Blood pressure–lowering in surgery (rarely used)
Tubocurarine	Neuromuscular junction	Transmission block	Now rarely used
Pancuronium Atracurium Vecuronium	Neuromuscular junction	Transmission block	Widely used as muscle relaxants in anaesthesia

Clinical uses of muscarinic antagonists

Cardiovascular
- Treatment of *sinus bradycardia* (e.g. after myocardial infarction; see Ch. 18): **atropine**.

Ophthalmic
- To *dilate the pupil*: for example **tropicamide** or **cyclopentolate** eye drops.

Neurological
- Prevention of *motion sickness*: for example **hyoscine** (orally or transdermally).
- *Parkinsonism* (see Ch. 35), especially to counteract movement disorders caused by antipsychotic drugs (see Ch. 38): for example **benzhexol, benztropine**.

Respiratory
- *Asthma* and *chronic obstructive pulmonary disease* (see Ch. 23, clinical boxes): **ipratropium** or **tiotropium** by inhalation.

Anaesthetic premedication
- To dry secretions: for example **atropine, hyoscine**. (Current anaesthetics are relatively non-irritant, see Ch. 36, so this use is now less important.)

Gastrointestinal
- To facilitate endoscopy and gastrointestinal radiology by relaxing gastrointestinal smooth muscle (*antispasmodic* action; see Ch. 25): for example **hyoscine**.
- As an antispasmodic in irritable bowel syndrome or colonic diverticular disease: for example **dicycloverine** (dicyclomine).
- To treat peptic ulcer disease by suppressing gastric acid secretion (see Ch. 25): for example **pirenzepine** (M_1-selective antagonist). This is used less since the introduction of histamine H_2 antagonists and proton pump inhibitors.

Drugs acting on muscarinic receptors

Muscarinic agonists
- Important compounds include acetylcholine, carbachol, methacholine, muscarine and pilocarpine. They vary in muscarinic/nicotinic selectivity, and in susceptibility to cholinesterase.
- Main effects are bradycardia and vasodilatation (endothelium-dependent), leading to fall in blood pressure; contraction of visceral smooth muscle (gut, bladder, bronchi, etc.); exocrine secretions, pupillary constriction and ciliary muscle contraction, leading to decrease of intraocular pressure.
- Main use is in treatment of glaucoma (especially pilocarpine).
- Most agonists show little receptor subtype selectivity, but more selective compounds are in development.

Muscarinic antagonists
- Most important compounds are atropine, scopolamine, ipratropium and pirenzepine.
- Main effects are inhibition of secretions; tachycardia, pupillary dilatation and paralysis of accommodation; relaxation of smooth muscle (gut, bronchi, biliary tract, bladder); inhibition of gastric acid secretion (especially pirenzepine); central nervous system effects (mainly excitatory with atropine; depressant, including amnesia, with scopolamine), including antiemetic effect and antiparkinsonian effect.

Effects of ganglion-blocking drugs

The effects of ganglion-blocking drugs are numerous and complex, as would be expected, because both divisions of the autonomic nervous system are blocked indiscriminately. The description by Paton of 'hexamethonium man' cannot be bettered:

▼He is a pink-complexioned person, except when he has stood in a queue for a long time, when he may get pale and faint. His handshake is warm and dry. He is a placid and relaxed companion; for instance he may laugh but he can't cry because the tears cannot come. Your rudest story will not make him blush, and the most unpleasant circumstances will fail to make him turn pale. His collars and socks stay very clean and sweet. He wears corsets and may, if you meet him out, be rather fidgety (corsets to compress his splanchnic vascular pool, fidgety to keep the venous return going from his legs). He dislikes speaking much unless helped with something to moisten his dry mouth and throat. He is long-sighted and easily blinded by bright light. The redness of his eyeballs may suggest irregular habits and in fact his head is rather weak. But he always behaves like a gentleman and never belches or hiccups. He tends to get cold and keeps well wrapped up. But his health is good; he does not have chilblains and those diseases of modern civilization, hypertension and peptic ulcer, pass him by. He gets thin because his appetite is modest; he never feels hunger pains and his stomach never rumbles. He gets rather constipated so that his intake of liquid paraffin is high. As old age comes on, he will suffer from retention of urine and impotence, but frequency, precipitancy and strangury will not worry him. One is uncertain how he will end, but perhaps if he is not careful, by eating less and less and getting colder and colder, he will sink into a symptomless, hypoglycaemic coma and die, as was proposed for the universe, a sort of entropy death.

(From Paton W D M 1954 The principles of ganglion block. Lectures on the scientific basis of medicine, vol. 2.)

In practice, the important effects are on the cardiovascular system. A marked fall in arterial blood pressure results mainly from block of sympathetic ganglia, which causes arteriolar vasodilatation. Most cardiovascular reflexes are blocked. In particular, the venoconstriction, which occurs normally when a subject stands up, and which is necessary to prevent the central venous pressure from falling sharply, is reduced. Standing thus causes a sudden fall in cardiac output and arterial pressure (postural hypotension) that can cause fainting. Similarly, the vasodilatation of skeletal muscle during exercise is normally accompanied by vasoconstriction elsewhere (e.g. splanchnic area) produced by sympathetic activity. If this adjustment is prevented, the overall peripheral resistance falls and the blood pressure also falls (postexercise hypotension).

Clinical use

Ganglion-blocking drugs, because of their many side effects, are clinically obsolete, with the exception of **trimetaphan**, a very short-acting drug that can be administered as an intravenous infusion for certain types of anaesthetic procedure. Tilting of the operating table results in controlled hypotension, used to minimise bleeding during certain kinds of surgery. Trimetaphan can also be used to lower blood pressure as an emergency procedure.

NEUROMUSCULAR-BLOCKING DRUGS

The pharmacology of neuromuscular function is well reviewed by Bowman (1990). Drugs can block neuromuscular transmission either by acting presynaptically to inhibit ACh synthesis or release, or by acting postsynaptically, the latter being the site of action of all the clinically important drugs (except for botulinum toxin; see below).

Clinically, neuromuscular block is used only as an adjunct to anaesthesia, when artificial ventilation is available; it is not a therapeutic intervention. The drugs that are used all work by interfering with the postsynaptic action of ACh. They fall into two categories:

- non-depolarising blocking agents (the majority), which act by blocking ACh receptors (and, in some cases, also by blocking ion channels)
- depolarising blocking agents, which are agonists at ACh receptors.

NON-DEPOLARISING BLOCKING AGENTS

In 1856, Claude Bernard, in a famous experiment, showed that 'curare' causes paralysis by blocking neuromuscular transmission, rather than by abolishing nerve conduction or muscle contractility. Curare is a mixture of naturally occurring alkaloids found in various South American plants and used as arrow poisons by South American Indians. The most important component is **tubocurarine**, the structure of which was elucidated in 1935. Tubocurarine is now rarely used in clinical medicine, being superseded by synthetic drugs with improved properties. The most important are **pancuronium**, **vecuronium** and **atracurium** (Table 10.7), which differ mainly in their duration of action. **Gallamine** was the first useful synthetic successor to tubocurarine, but has been replaced by compounds with fewer side effects. These substances are all quaternary ammonium compounds, which means that they are poorly absorbed and generally rapidly excreted. They also fail to cross the placenta, which is important in relation to their use in obstetric anaesthesia. The low oral absorption of tubocurarine allowed it to be used safely in the hunting of animals for food.

Mechanism of action

Non-depolarising blocking agents all act as competitive antagonists (see Ch. 2) at the ACh receptors of the endplate. The amount of ACh released by a nerve impulse normally exceeds by several-fold what is needed to elicit an action potential in the muscle fibre. It is therefore necessary to block 70–80% of the receptor sites before transmission actually fails. When this happens, it is still possible to record a subthreshold epp in the muscle fibre (Fig. 10.6). In any individual muscle fibre, transmission is all or nothing, so graded degrees of block represent a varying proportion of muscle fibres failing to respond. In this situation, where the amplitude of epp in all the fibres is close to threshold (just above in some, just below in others), small variations in the amount of transmitter released, or in the rate at which it is destroyed, will have a large effect on the proportion of fibres contracting, so the degree of block is liable to vary according to various physiological circumstances (e.g. stimulation frequency, temperature, and cholinesterase inhibition), which normally have relatively little effect on the efficiency of transmission.

Some non-depolarising blocking agents also appear to block presynaptic autoreceptors, and thus inhibit the release of ACh during repetitive stimulation of the motor nerve (see Prior et al., 1995). This may play a part in causing the 'tetanic fade' seen with these drugs (see p. 160).

Drugs acting on autonomic ganglia

Ganglion-stimulating drugs
- Compounds include nicotine, dimethylphenylpiperazinium (DMPP).
- Both sympathetic and parasympathetic ganglia are stimulated, so effects are complex, including tachycardia and increase of blood pressure; variable effects on gastrointestinal motility and secretions; increased bronchial, salivary and sweat secretions. Additional effects result from stimulation of other neuronal structures, including sensory and noradrenergic nerve terminals.
- Ganglion stimulation may be followed by depolarisation block.
- Nicotine also has important central nervous system effects.
- No therapeutic uses, except for nicotine to assist giving up smoking.

Ganglion-blocking drugs
- Compounds include hexamethonium, trimetaphan, tubocurarine (also nicotine; see above).
- Block all autonomic ganglia and enteric ganglia. Main effects: hypotension and loss of cardiovascular reflexes, inhibition of secretions, gastrointestinal paralysis, impaired micturition.
- Clinically obsolete, except for occasional use of trimetaphan to produce controlled hypotension in anaesthesia.

Table 10.7 Characteristics of neuromuscular-blocking drugs[a]

Drug	Speed of onset	Duration of action	Main side effects	Notes
Tubocurarine	Slow (> 5 min)	Long (1–2 h)	Hypotension (ganglion block plus histamine release) Bronchoconstriction (histamine release)	Plant alkaloid, now rarely used **Alcuronium** is a semisynthetic derivative with similar properties but fewer side effects
Pancuronium	Intermediate (2–3 min)	Long	Slight tachycardia No hypotension	The first steroid-based compound Better side effect profile than tubocurarine Widely used **Pipecuronium** is similar
Vecuronium	Intermediate	Intermediate (30–40 min)	Few side effects	Widely used Occasionally causes prolonged paralysis, probably owing to active metabolite **Rocuronium** is similar, with faster onset
Atracurium	Intermediate	Intermediate (< 30 min)	Transient hypotension (histamine release)	Unusual mechanism of elimination (spontaneous non-enzymic chemical degradation in plasma); degradation slowed by acidosis Widely used **Doxacurium** is chemically similar but stable in plasma, giving it long duration of action **Cisatracurium** is the pure isomeric constituent of atracurium, similar but with less histamine release
Mivacurium	Fast (~2 min)	Short (~15 min)	Transient hypotension (histamine release)	New drug, chemically similar to atracurium but rapidly inactivated by plasma cholinesterase (therefore longer acting in patients with liver disease or with genetic cholinesterase deficiency (see p. 160)
Suxamethonium	Fast	Short (~10 min)	Bradycardia (muscarinic agonist effect) Cardiac dysrhythmias (increased plasma K+ concentration—avoid in patients with burns or severe trauma) Raised intraocular pressure (nicotinic agonist effect on extraocular muscles) Postoperative muscle pain	Acts by depolarisation of endplate (nicotinic agonist effect)—the only drug of this type still in use Paralysis is preceded by transient muscle fasciculations Short duration of action owing to hydrolysis by plasma cholinesterase (prolonged action in patients with liver disease or genetic deficiency of plasma cholinesterase) Used for brief procedures (e.g. tracheal intubation, electroconvulsive shock therapy) Rocuronium has similar speed of onset and recovery, with fewer unwanted effects

[a]For chemical structures, see Hardman J G, Limbird L E, Gilman A G, Goodman-Gilman A et al. 2001 Goodman and Gilman's pharmacological basis of therapeutics, 10th edn. McGraw-Hill, New York.

Effects of non-depolarising blocking drugs

The effects of non-depolarising neuromuscular-blocking agents are mainly due to motor paralysis, although some of the drugs also produce clinically significant autonomic effects. The first muscles to be affected are the extrinsic eye muscles (causing double vision) and the small muscles of the face, limbs and pharynx (causing difficulty in swallowing). Respiratory muscles are the last to be affected and the first to recover. An experiment in 1947 in which a heroic volunteer was fully curarised under artificial ventilation established this orderly paralytic march, and showed that consciousness and awareness of pain were quite normal even when paralysis was complete. The special characteristics of non-depolarising block, and the ways in which it differs from depolarisation block, are described on page 160.

Unwanted effects

The main side effect of tubocurarine is a fall in arterial pressure, chiefly due to ganglion block. An additional cause is the release

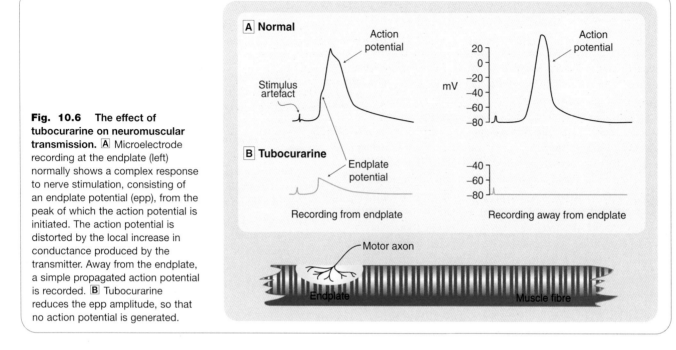

Fig. 10.6 The effect of tubocurarine on neuromuscular transmission. **A** Microelectrode recording at the endplate (left) normally shows a complex response to nerve stimulation, consisting of an endplate potential (epp), from the peak of which the action potential is initiated. The action potential is distorted by the local increase in conductance produced by the transmitter. Away from the endplate, a simple propagated action potential is recorded. **B** Tubocurarine reduces the epp amplitude, so that no action potential is generated.

of histamine from mast cells (see Ch. 13), which can also give rise to bronchospasm in sensitive individuals. This is unrelated to nAChRs but also occurs with atracurium and mivacurium (as well as with some unrelated drugs such as morphine, Ch. 41). The other non-depolarising blocking drugs lack these side effects, and hence cause less hypotension. Gallamine, and to a lesser extent pancuronium, block mAChRs, particularly in the heart, which results in tachycardia.

Pharmacokinetic aspects

Neuromuscular-blocking agents are used mainly in anaesthesia to produce muscle relaxation. They are given intravenously but differ in their rates of onset and recovery (Fig. 10.7 and Table 10.7).

Most of the non-depolarising blocking agents are metabolised by the liver or excreted unchanged in the urine, exceptions being **atracurium**, which hydrolyses spontaneously in plasma, and **mivacurium**, which, like **succinylcholine**, is hydrolysed by plasma cholinesterase. Their duration of action varies between about 15 minutes and 1–2 hours (Table 10.7), by which time the patient regains enough strength to cough and breathe properly, although residual weakness may persist for much longer. The route of elimination is important, because many patients undergoing anaesthesia have impaired renal or hepatic function, which, depending on the drug used, can enhance or prolong the paralysis to an important degree.

Atracurium was designed to be chemically unstable at physiological pH (splitting into two inactive fragments by cleavage at one of the quaternary nitrogen atoms), although indefinitely stable when stored at an acid pH. It has a short duration of action, which is unaffected by renal or hepatic function. Because of the marked pH dependence of its degradation, however, its action becomes considerably briefer during respiratory alkalosis caused by hyperventilation.

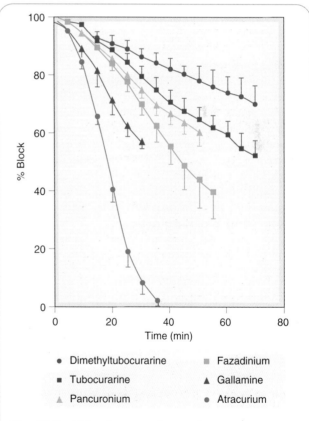

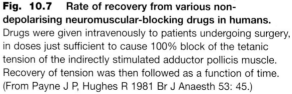

Fig. 10.7 Rate of recovery from various non-depolarising neuromuscular-blocking drugs in humans. Drugs were given intravenously to patients undergoing surgery, in doses just sufficient to cause 100% block of the tetanic tension of the indirectly stimulated adductor pollicis muscle. Recovery of tension was then followed as a function of time. (From Payne J P, Hughes R 1981 Br J Anaesth 53: 45.)

DEPOLARISING BLOCKING AGENTS

This class of neuromuscular-blocking drugs was discovered by Paton and Zaimis in their study of the effects of symmetrical bisquaternary ammonium compounds. One of these, **decamethonium**, was found to cause paralysis without appreciable ganglion-blocking activity. Several features of its action showed it to be different from competitive blocking drugs such as tubocurarine. In particular, it was found to produce a transient twitching of skeletal muscle (fasciculation) before causing block, and when it was injected into chicks it caused a powerful extensor spasm,[2] whereas tubocurarine simply caused flaccid paralysis. In 1951, Burns and Paton showed that its action was to cause a maintained depolarisation at the endplate region of the muscle fibre, which led to a loss of electrical excitability (see p. 149), and they coined the term *depolarisation block*. Fasciculation occurs because the developing endplate depolarisation initially causes a discharge of action potentials in the muscle fibre. This subsides after a few seconds as the electrical excitability of the endplate region of the fibre is lost.

Decamethonium itself was used clinically but has the disadvantage of too long a duration of action. Suxamethonium (Table 10.7) is closely related in structure to both decamethonium and ACh (consisting of two ACh molecules linked by their acetyl groups). Its action is shorter than that of decamethonium, because it is quickly hydrolysed by plasma cholinesterase. Suxamethonium and decamethonium act—like ACh—as agonists on the receptors of the motor endplate. However, when given as drugs, they diffuse relatively slowly to the endplate and remain there for long enough that the depolarisation causes loss of electrical excitability. ACh, in contrast, when released from the nerve, reaches the endplate in very brief spurts and is rapidly hydrolysed in situ, so it never causes sufficiently prolonged depolarisation to result in block. If cholinesterase is inhibited, however (see p. 164), it is possible for the circulating ACh concentration to reach a level sufficient to cause depolarisation block.

Comparison of non-depolarising and depolarising blocking drugs

There are several differences in the pattern of neuromuscular block produced by depolarising and non-depolarising mechanisms.

- Anticholinesterase drugs are very effective in overcoming the blocking action of competitive agents. This is because the released ACh, protected from hydrolysis, can diffuse further within the synaptic cleft, and so gains access to a wider area of postsynaptic membrane than it normally would. The chances of an ACh molecule finding an unoccupied receptor before being hydrolysed are thus increased. This diffusional effect seems to be of more importance than a truly competitive

interaction, for it is unlikely that appreciable dissociation of the antagonist can occur in the short time for which the ACh is present. In contrast, depolarisation block is unaffected, or even increased, by anticholinesterase drugs.

- The fasciculations seen with suxamethonium (see Table 10.7) as a prelude to paralysis do not occur with competitive drugs. There appears to be a correlation between the amount of fasciculation and the severity of the postoperative muscle pain that is often produced by succinylcholine.
- *Tetanic fade* (a term used to describe the failure of muscle tension to be maintained during a brief period of nerve stimulation at a frequency high enough to produce a fused tetanus) is increased by non-depolarising blocking drugs, compared with normal muscle. This is probably due mainly to the block of presynaptic nAChRs, which normally serve to sustain transmitter release during a tetanus (see Prior et al., 1995), and it does not occur with depolarisation block. This forms the basis of a simple test used by anaesthetists to discover which type of block is present. Electrodes are applied to the skin over a peripheral nerve, such as the ulnar nerve, and muscle contraction is observed during a short period of tetanic stimulation.

Unwanted effects and dangers of depolarising drugs

Suxamethonium, the only drug of this type in clinical use, can produce a number of important adverse effects (see Table 10.7).

Bradycardia. This is preventable by atropine and is probably due to a direct muscarinic action.

Potassium release. The increase in cation permeability of the motor endplates causes a net loss of K^+ from muscle, and thus a small rise in plasma K^+ concentration. In normal individuals, this is not important, but in cases of trauma, especially burns or injuries causing muscle denervation, it may be (Fig. 10.8). This is because denervation causes ACh receptors to spread to regions of the muscle fibre away from the endplates (see Ch. 9), so that a much larger area of membrane is sensitive to succinylcholine. The resulting hyperkalaemia can be enough to cause ventricular dysrhythmia or even cardiac arrest.

Increased intraocular pressure. This results from contracture of extraocular muscles applying pressure to the eyeball. It is particularly important to avoid this if the eyeball has been injured.

Prolonged paralysis. The action of succinylcholine given intravenously normally lasts for less than 5 minutes, because the drug is hydrolysed by plasma cholinesterase. Its action is prolonged by various factors that reduce the activity of this enzyme:

- Genetic variants in which plasma cholinesterase is abnormal (see Ch. 52). Severe deficiency, enough to increase the duration of action to 2 hours or more, occurs in only about 1 in 2000 individuals. Very rarely, the enzyme is completely absent and the paralysis lasts for many hours.
- Anticholinesterase drugs. The use of organophosphates to treat glaucoma (see Table 10.4) can inhibit plasma cholinesterase and prolong the action of succinylcholine. Competing substrates for plasma cholinesterase (e.g. procaine, propanidid) can also have this effect.

---

[2]Birds possess a special type of skeletal muscle, rare in mammals, that has many endplates scattered over the surface of each muscle fibre. A drug that causes endplate depolarisation produces a widespread depolarisation in such muscles, resulting in a maintained contracture. In normal skeletal muscle, with only one endplate per fibre, endplate depolarisation is too localised to cause contracture on its own.

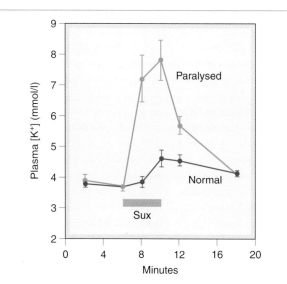

Fig. 10.8   Effect of succinylcholine (Sux) on plasma potassium concentration in humans. Blood was collected from veins draining paralysed and non-paralysed limbs of seven injured patients undergoing surgery. The injuries had resulted in motor nerve degeneration, and hence denervation supersensitivity of the affected muscles. (From Tobey R E et al. 1972 Anaesthesiology 37: 322.)

- Neonates and patients with liver disease may have low plasma cholinesterase activity and show prolonged paralysis with succinylcholine.

Malignant hyperthermia. This is a rare inherited condition, due to a mutation of the Ca^{2+} release channel of the sarcoplasmic reticulum (the ryanodine receptor, see Ch. 4), which results in intense muscle spasm and a dramatic rise in body temperature when certain drugs are given (see Ch. 51). The most commonly implicated drugs are **suxamethonium** and **halothane**, although it can be precipitated by a variety of other drugs. The condition carries a very high mortality (about 65%) and is treated by administration of **dantrolene**, a drug that inhibits muscle contraction by preventing Ca^{2+} release from the sarcoplasmic reticulum.

DRUGS THAT ACT PRESYNAPTICALLY

DRUGS THAT INHIBIT ACETYLCHOLINE SYNTHESIS

The steps in the synthesis of ACh in the presynaptic nerve terminals are shown in Figure 10.2. The rate-limiting process appears to be the transport of choline into the nerve terminal. **Hemicholinium** blocks this transport and thereby inhibits ACh synthesis. It is useful as an experimental tool but has no clinical applications. Its blocking effect on transmission develops slowly, as the existing stores of ACh become depleted. **Vesamicol**, which acts by blocking ACh transport into synaptic vesicles, has a similar effect.

Neuromuscular-blocking drugs

- Substances that block choline uptake: for example hemicholinium (not used clinically).
- Substances that block acetylcholine release: aminoglycoside antibiotics, botulinum toxin.
- Drugs used to cause paralysis during anaesthesia are as follows.
  - Non-depolarising neuromuscular-blocking agents: tubocurarine, pancuronium, atracurium, vecuronium. These act as competitive antagonists at nicotinic acetylcholine receptors and differ mainly in duration of action.
  - Depolarising neuromuscular-blocking agents: suxamethonium.
- Important characteristics of non-depolarising and depolarising blocking drugs:
  - non-depolarising block is reversible by anticholinesterase drugs, depolarising block is not
  - depolarising block produces initial fasciculations and often postoperative muscle pain
  - suxamethonium is hydrolysed by plasma cholinesterase and is normally very short-acting, but may cause long-lasting paralysis in a small group of congenitally cholinesterase-deficient individuals.
- Main side effects: tubocurarine causes ganglion block, histamine release, hence hypotension, bronchoconstriction; newer non-depolarising blocking drugs have fewer side effects; suxamethonium may cause bradycardia, cardiac dysrhythmias due to K^+ release (especially in burned or injured patients), increased intraocular pressure, malignant hyperthermia (rare).

DRUGS THAT INHIBIT ACETYLCHOLINE RELEASE

Acetylcholine release by a nerve impulse involves the entry of Ca^{2+} into the nerve terminal; the increase in $[Ca^{2+}]_i$ stimulates exocytosis and increases the rate of quantal release (Fig. 10.2). Agents that inhibit Ca^{2+} entry include Mg^{2+} and various aminoglycoside antibiotics (e.g. **streptomycin** and **neomycin**; see Ch. 46), which occasionally produce muscle paralysis as an unwanted side effect when used clinically.

Two potent neurotoxins, namely **botulinum toxin** and **β-bungarotoxin**, act specifically to inhibit ACh release. Botulinum toxin is a protein produced by the anaerobic bacillus *Clostridium botulinum*, an organism that can multiply in preserved food and can cause botulism, an extremely serious type of food poisoning. The potency of botulinum toxin is extraordinary, the minimum lethal dose in a mouse being less than 10^{-12} g—only a few million molecules. It belongs to the group of potent bacterial exotoxins that includes tetanus and diphtheria toxins. They possess two subunits, one of which binds to a membrane receptor and is responsible for cellular specificity. By this means, the toxin enters the cell, where the other subunit produces the toxic effect (see Montecucco & Schiavo, 1995). Botulinum toxin contains several components (A–G). They are peptidases that cleave specific proteins involved in exocytosis (*synaptobrevins*, *syntaxins*, etc.—see Ch. 9), thereby producing a long-lasting block of synaptic function. Each toxin component inactivates a different functional protein—a remarkably coordinated attack by a humble bacterium on a vital component of mammalian physiology.

Botulinum poisoning causes progressive parasympathetic and motor paralysis, with dry mouth, blurred vision and difficulty in swallowing, followed by progressive respiratory paralysis. Treatment with antitoxin is effective only if given before symptoms appear, for once the toxin is bound its action cannot be reversed. Mortality is high, and recovery takes several weeks. Anticholinesterases and drugs that increase transmitter release (see p. 163) are ineffective in restoring transmission. Among the more spectacular outbreaks of botulinum poisoning was an incident on Loch Maree in Scotland in 1922, when all eight members of a fishing party died after eating duck pâté for their lunch. Their ghillies, consuming humbler fare no doubt, survived. The innkeeper committed suicide.

Botulinum toxin, injected locally into muscles, is used to treat a form of persistent and disabling eyelid spasm (blepharospasm) as well as other types of local muscle spasm, for example in spasticity (see Tsui, 1996). Botox is also fashionable as a wrinkle remover, removing frown lines by paralysing the superficial muscles that pucker the skin. Injections must be repeated every few months to sustain the effect. For the same agent to figure as a beauty treatment as well as a weapon of biological warfare reflects strangely on the modern world.

▼ **β-Bungarotoxin** is a protein contained in the venom of various snakes of the cobra family, and has a similar action to botulinum toxin, although its active component is a phospholipase rather than a peptidase. The same venoms also contain **α-bungarotoxin** (see p. 27), which blocks postsynaptic ACh receptors, so these snakes evidently cover all eventualities as far as causing paralysis of their victims is concerned.

DRUGS THAT ENHANCE CHOLINERGIC TRANSMISSION

Drugs that enhance cholinergic transmission act either by inhibiting cholinesterase (the main group) or by increasing ACh release. In this chapter, we focus on the peripheral actions of such drugs; drugs affecting cholinergic transmission in the CNS, used to treat senile dementia, are discussed in Chapter 35.

DISTRIBUTION AND FUNCTION OF CHOLINESTERASE

There are two distinct types of cholinesterase, namely *acetylcholinesterase* and *butyrylcholinesterase* (*BuChE*), closely related in molecular structure but differing in their distribution, substrate specificity and functions (see Chatonnet & Lockridge, 1989). Both consist of globular catalytic subunits, which constitute the soluble forms found in plasma (BuChE) and cerebrospinal

fluid (AChE). Elsewhere, the catalytic units are linked to collagen-like proteins or to glycolipids, through which they are tethered, like a bunch of balloons, to the cell membrane or the basement membrane at various sites, including cholinergic synapses (and also, oddly, the erythrocyte membrane, where the function of the enzyme is unknown).

The bound AChE at cholinergic synapses serves to hydrolyse the released transmitter and terminate its action rapidly. Soluble AChE is also present in cholinergic nerve terminals, where it seems to have a role in regulating the free ACh concentration, and from which it may be secreted; the function of the secreted enzyme is so far unclear. AChE is quite specific for ACh and closely related esters such as methacholine. Certain neuropeptides, such as substance P (Ch. 16) are inactivated by AChE, but it is not known whether this is of physiological significance. Overall, there is poor correspondence between the distribution of cholinergic synapses and that of AChE, both in the brain and in the periphery, and AChE most probably has functions other than disposal of ACh, although the details remain unclear (see review by Soreq & Seidman, 2001).

Butyrylcholinesterase (or pseudocholinesterase) has a widespread distribution, being found in tissues such as liver, skin, brain and gastrointestinal smooth muscle, as well as in soluble form in the plasma. It is not particularly associated with cholinergic synapses, and its physiological function is unclear. It has a broader substrate specificity than AChE. It hydrolyses the synthetic substrate butyrylcholine more rapidly than ACh, as well as other esters, such as **procaine**, **succinylcholine** and **propanidid** (a short-acting anaesthetic agent; see Ch. 36). The plasma enzyme is important in relation to the inactivation of the drugs listed above. Genetic variants of BuChE occur (see Ch. 52), and these partly account for the variability in the duration of action of these drugs. The very short duration of action of ACh given intravenously (see Fig. 10.1) results from its rapid hydrolysis in the plasma. Normally, AChE and BuChE between them keep the plasma ACh at an undetectably low level, so ACh (unlike noradrenaline) is strictly a neurotransmitter and not a hormone.

Both AChE and BuChE belong to the class of serine hydrolases, which includes many proteases, such as trypsin. The active site of AChE comprises two distinct regions: an *anionic site* (glutamate residue), which binds the basic (choline) moiety of ACh; and an *esteratic site* (histidine + serine). As with other serine hydrolases, the acidic (acetyl) group of the substrate is transferred to the serine hydroxyl group, leaving (transiently) an acetylated enzyme molecule and a molecule of free choline. Spontaneous hydrolysis of the serine acetyl group occurs rapidly, and the overall turnover number of AChE is extremely high (over 10 000 molecules of ACh hydrolysed per second by a single active site).

DRUGS THAT INHIBIT CHOLINESTERASE

Peripherally acting anticholinesterase drugs fall into three main groups according to the nature of their interaction with the active site, which determines their duration of action. Most of them inhibit AChE and BuChE about equally. Centrally acting anticholinesterases, developed for the treatment of dementia, are discussed in Chapter 35.

Short-acting anticholinesterases

The only important drug among the short-acting anticholinesterases is **edrophonium** (Table 10.8), a quaternary ammonium compound that binds to the anionic site of the enzyme only. The ionic bond formed is readily reversible, and the action of the drug is very brief. It is used mainly for diagnostic purposes, because improvement of muscle strength by an anticholinesterase is characteristic of myasthenia gravis (see p. 165) but does not occur when muscle weakness is due to other causes.

Medium-duration anticholinesterases

The medium-duration anticholinesterases (Table 10.8) include **neostigmine** and **pyridostigmine**, which are quaternary ammonium compounds of clinical importance, and **physostigmine** (eserine), a tertiary amine, which occurs naturally in the Calabar bean.[3]

These drugs are all carbamyl, as opposed to acetyl, esters, and all possess basic groups that bind to the anionic site. Transfer of the carbamyl group to the serine hydroxyl group of the esteratic site occurs as with ACh, but the carbamylated enzyme is very much slower to hydrolyse (Fig. 10.9), taking minutes rather than microseconds. The anticholinesterase drug is therefore hydrolysed,

---

[3]Otherwise known as the ordeal bean. In the Middle Ages, extracts of these beans were used to determine the guilt or innocence of those accused of crime or heresy. Death implied guilt.

Table 10.8 Anticholinesterase drugs

Drug	Structure	Duration of action	Main site of action	Notes
Edrophonium	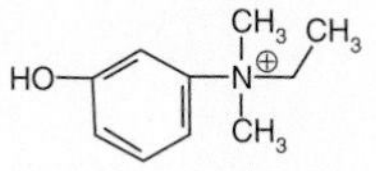	Short	NMJ	Used mainly in diagnosis of myasthenia gravis Too short acting for therapeutic use
Neostigmine	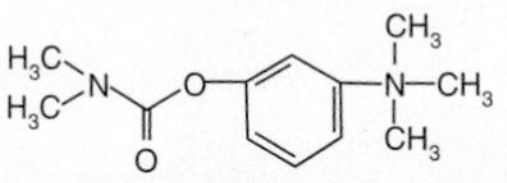	Medium	NMJ	Used intravenously to reverse competitive neuromuscular block Used orally in treatment of myasthenia gravis Visceral side effects
Physostigmine	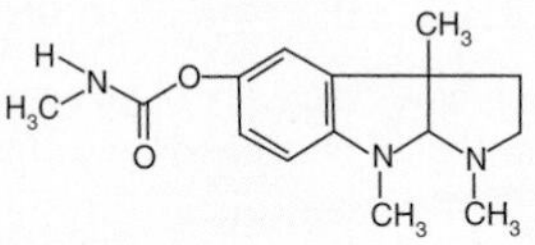	Medium	P	Used as eye drops in treatment of glaucoma
Pyridostigmine	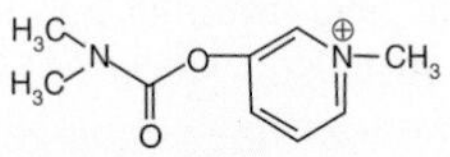	Medium	NMJ	Used orally in treatment of myasthenia gravis Better absorbed than neostigmine and has longer duration of action
Dyflos	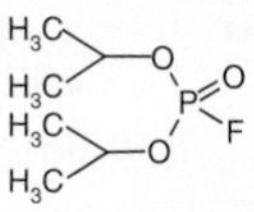	Long	P	Highly toxic organophosphate, with very prolonged action Has been used as eye drops for glaucoma
Ecothiopate	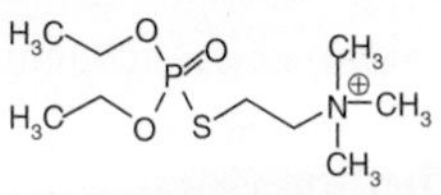	Long	P	Used as eye drops in treatment of glaucoma Prolonged action; may cause systemic effects
Parathion	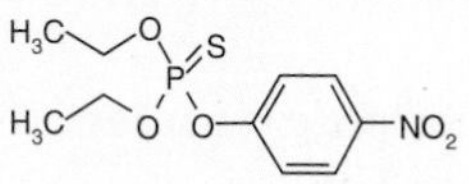	Long	–	Converted to active metabolite by replacement of sulfur by oxygen Used as insecticide but commonly causes poisoning in humans

NMJ, neuromuscular junction; P, postganglionic parasympathetic junction.

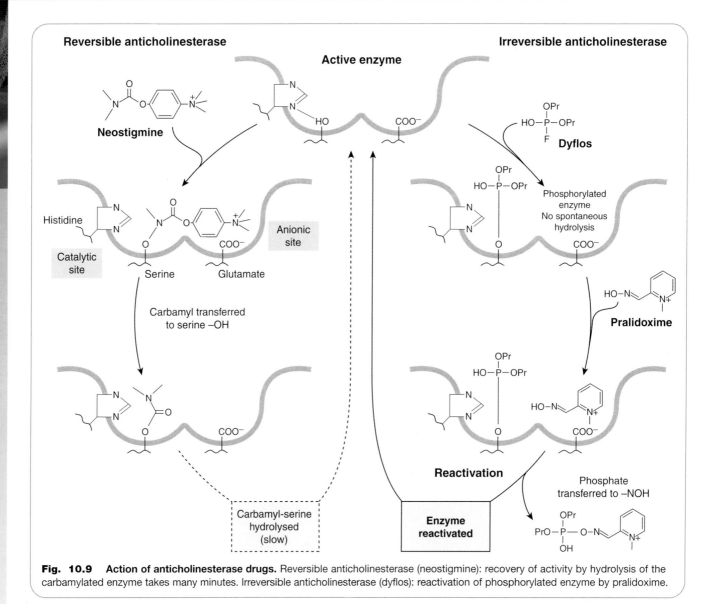

Fig. 10.9 **Action of anticholinesterase drugs.** Reversible anticholinesterase (neostigmine): recovery of activity by hydrolysis of the carbamylated enzyme takes many minutes. Irreversible anticholinesterase (dyflos): reactivation of phosphorylated enzyme by pralidoxime.

but at a negligible rate compared with ACh, and the slow recovery of the carbamylated enzyme means that the action of these drugs is quite long-lasting.

Irreversible anticholinesterases

Irreversible anticholinesterases (Table 10.8) are pentavalent phosphorus compounds containing a labile group such as fluoride (in **dyflos**) or an organic group (in **parathion** and **ecothiopate**). This group is released, leaving the serine hydroxyl group of the enzyme phosphorylated (Fig. 10.9). Most of these organophosphate compounds, of which there are many, developed as war gases and pesticides as well as for clinical use; they interact only with the esteratic site of the enzyme and have no cationic group. Ecothiopate is an exception in having a quaternary nitrogen group designed to bind also to the anionic site.

The inactive phosphorylated enzyme is usually very stable. With drugs such as dyflos, no appreciable hydrolysis occurs, and recovery of enzymic activity depends on the synthesis of new enzyme molecules, a process that may take weeks. With other

drugs, such as ecothiopate, slow hydrolysis occurs over the course of a few days, so that their action is not strictly irreversible. Dyflos and parathion are volatile non-polar substances of very high lipid solubility, and are rapidly absorbed through mucous membranes and even through unbroken skin and insect cuticles; the use of these agents as war gases or insecticides relies on this property. The lack of a specificity-conferring quaternary group means that most of these drugs block other serine hydrolases (e.g. trypsin, thrombin), although their pharmacological effects result mainly from cholinesterase inhibition.

Effects of anticholinesterase drugs

Cholinesterase inhibitors affect peripheral as well as central cholinergic synapses.

Some organophosphate compounds can produce, in addition, a severe form of neurotoxicity.

Effects on autonomic cholinergic synapses. These mainly reflect enhancement of ACh activity at parasympathetic postganglionic synapses (i.e. increased secretions from salivary, lacrimal, bronchial and gastrointestinal glands; increased peristaltic activity; broncho-constriction; bradycardia and hypotension; pupillary constriction; fixation of accommodation for near vision; fall in intraocular pressure). Large doses can stimulate, and later block, autonomic ganglia, producing complex autonomic effects. The block, if it occurs, is a depolarisation block and is associated with a build-up of ACh in the plasma and body fluids. Neostigmine and pyridostigmine tend to affect neuromuscular transmission more than the autonomic system, whereas physostigmine and organo-phosphates show the reverse pattern. The reason is not clear, but therapeutic usage takes advantage of this partial selectivity.

Acute anticholinesterase poisoning (e.g. from contact with insecticides or war gases) causes severe bradycardia, hypotension and difficulty in breathing. Combined with a depolarising neuro-muscular block, and central effects (see below), the result may be fatal.

Effects on the neuromuscular junction. The twitch tension of a muscle stimulated via its motor nerve is increased by anticholinesterases, owing to repetitive firing in the muscle fibre associated with prolongation of the epp. Normally, the ACh is hydrolysed so quickly that each stimulus initiates only one action potential in the muscle fibre, but when AChE is inhibited this is converted to a short train of action potentials in the muscle fibre, and hence greater tension. Much more important is the effect produced when transmission has been blocked by a competitive blocking agent such as tubocurarine. In this case, addition of an anticholinesterase can dramatically restore transmission. If a large proportion of the receptors are blocked, the majority of ACh molecules will normally encounter, and be destroyed by, an AChE molecule before reaching a vacant receptor; inhibiting AChE gives the ACh molecules a greater chance of finding a vacant receptor before being destroyed, and thus increase the epp so that it reaches threshold. In myasthenia gravis (see below), transmission fails because there are too few ACh receptors, and cholinesterase inhibition improves transmission just as it does in curarised muscle.

In large doses, such as can occur in poisoning, anticholinesterases initially cause twitching of muscles. This is because spontaneous ACh release can give rise to epps that reach the firing threshold. Later, paralysis may occur due to depolarisation block, which is associated with the build-up of ACh in the plasma and tissue fluids.

Effects on the CNS. Tertiary compounds, such as physostigmine, and the non-polar organophosphates penetrate the blood–brain barrier freely and affect the brain. The result is an initial excitation, which can result in convulsions, followed by depression, which can cause unconsciousness and respiratory failure. These central effects result mainly from the activation of mAChRs, and are antagonised by atropine. The use of anticholinesterases to treat senile dementia is discussed in Chapter 35.

Neurotoxicity of organophosphates. Many organophosphates can cause a severe type of peripheral nerve demyelination, leading to progressive weakness and sensory loss. This is not a problem with clinically used anticholinesterases but occasionally occurs with accidental poisoning with insecticides. In 1931, an estimated 20 000 Americans were affected, some fatally, by contamination of fruit juice with an organophosphate insecticide, and other similar outbreaks have been recorded. The mechanism of this reaction is only partly understood, but it seems to result from inhibition of an esterase (not cholinesterase itself) specific to myelin.

The main uses of anticholinesterases are summarised in the clinical box.

CHOLINESTERASE REACTIVATION

Spontaneous hydrolysis of phosphorylated cholinesterase is extremely slow, a fact that makes poisoning with organophosphates very dangerous. **Pralidoxime** (Figs 10.9 and 10.10) reactivates the enzyme by bringing an oxime group into close proximity with the phosphorylated esteratic site. This group is a strong nucleophile and lures the phosphate group away from the serine hydroxyl group of the enzyme. The effectiveness of pralidoxime in reactivating plasma cholinesterase activity in a poisoned subject is shown in Figure 10.10. The main drawback to its use as an antidote to organophosphate poisoning is that, within a few hours, the phosphorylated enzyme undergoes a chemical change ('ageing') that renders it no longer susceptible to reactivation, so that

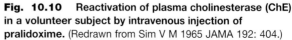

Clinical uses of anticholinesterase drugs

- To reverse the action of non-depolarising neuromuscular-blocking drugs at the end of an operation (**neostigmine**).
- To treat *myasthenia gravis* (**neostigmine** or **pyridostigmine**).
- As a test for myasthenia gravis and to distinguish weakness caused by anticholinesterase overdosage ('cholinergic crisis') from the weakness of myasthenia itself ('myasthenic crisis'): **edrophonium**, a short-acting drug given intravenously.
- *Alzheimer's dieases* (e.g. **donepezil**; see Ch. 35).
- *Glaucoma* (**ecothiopate** eye drops).

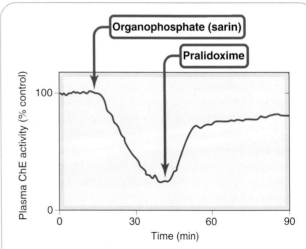

Fig. 10.10 **Reactivation of plasma cholinesterase (ChE) in a volunteer subject by intravenous injection of pralidoxime.** (Redrawn from Sim V M 1965 JAMA 192: 404.)

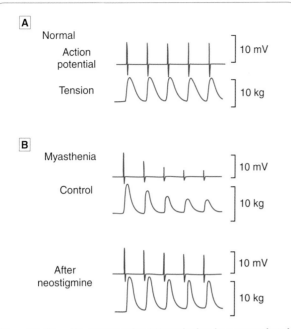

Fig. 10.11 Neuromuscular transmission in a normal and a myasthenic human subject. Electrical activity was recorded with a needle electrode in the adductor pollicis muscle, in response to ulnar nerve stimulation (3 Hz) at the wrist. **A** In a normal subject, electrical and mechanical response is well sustained. **B** In a myasthenic patient, transmission fails rapidly when nerve is stimulated. Treatment with neostigmine improves transmission. (From Desmedt J E 1962 Bull Acad Roy Med Belg VII 2: 213.)

affects it (see Lindstrom, 2000). This disease affects about 1 in 2000 individuals, who show muscle weakness and increased fatiguability resulting from a failure of neuromuscular transmission. The tendency for transmission to fail during repetitive activity can be seen in Figure 10.11. Functionally, it results in the inability of muscles to produce sustained contractions, of which the characteristic drooping eyelids of myasthenic patients are a sign. The effectiveness of anticholinesterase drugs in improving muscle strength in myasthenia was discovered in 1931, long before the cause of the disease was known.

The cause of the transmission failure is an autoimmune response that causes a loss of nAChRs from the neuromuscular junction, first revealed in studies showing that the number of bungarotoxin-binding sites at the endplates of myasthenic patients was reduced by about 70% compared with normal. It had been suspected that myasthenia had an immunological basis, because removal of the thymus gland was frequently of benefit. Immunisation of rabbits with purified ACh receptor causes, after a delay, symptoms very similar to those of human myasthenia gravis. The presence of antibody directed against the ACh receptor protein can be detected in the serum of myasthenic patients, but the reason for the development of the autoimmune response in humans is still unknown (see Lindstrom, 2000).

The improvement of neuromuscular function by anticholinesterase treatment (shown in Fig. 10.11) can be dramatic, but if the disease progresses too far, the number of receptors remaining may become too few to produce an adequate epp, and anticholinesterase drugs will then cease to be effective.

Alternative approaches to the treatment of myasthenia are to remove circulating antibody by plasma exchange, which is transiently effective, or, for a more prolonged effect, to inhibit antibody production with steroids (e.g. **prednisolone**) or immunosuppressant drugs (e.g. **azathioprine**; see Ch. 14).

OTHER DRUGS THAT ENHANCE CHOLINERGIC TRANSMISSION

▼ It was observed many years ago that **tetraethylammonium**, better known as a ganglion-blocking drug, could reverse the neuromuscular-blocking action of tubocurarine, and this was shown to be because it increases the release of transmitter evoked by nerve stimulation. Subsequently, **aminopyridines**, which block potassium channels (see Ch. 4), and thus prolong the action potential in the presynaptic nerve terminal, were found to act similarly and to be considerably more potent and selective in their actions than tetraethylammonium. These drugs are not selective for cholinergic nerves but increase the evoked release of many different transmitters, so have too many unwanted effects to be useful in treating neuromuscular disorders.

pralidoxime must be given early in order to work. Pralidoxime does not enter the brain, but related compounds have been developed to treat the central effects of organophosphate poisoning.

Myasthenia gravis

▼ The neuromuscular junction is a robust structure that very rarely fails, myasthenia gravis being one of the very few disorders that specifically

---

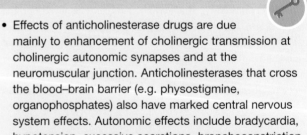

Cholinesterase and anticholinesterase drugs

- There are two main forms of cholinesterase: acetylcholinesterase (AChE), which is mainly membrane-bound, relatively specific for acetylcholine, and responsible for rapid acetylcholine hydrolysis at cholinergic synapses; and butyrylcholinesterase (BuChE) or pseudocholinesterase, which is relatively non-selective and occurs in plasma and many tissues. Both enzymes belong to the family of serine hydrolases.

- Anticholinesterase drugs are of three main types: short-acting (edrophonium); medium-acting (neostigmine, physostigmine); irreversible (organophosphates, dyflos, ecothiopate). They differ in the nature of their chemical interaction with the active site of cholinesterase.

- Effects of anticholinesterase drugs are due mainly to enhancement of cholinergic transmission at cholinergic autonomic synapses and at the neuromuscular junction. Anticholinesterases that cross the blood–brain barrier (e.g. physostigmine, organophosphates) also have marked central nervous system effects. Autonomic effects include bradycardia, hypotension, excessive secretions, bronchoconstriction, gastrointestinal hypermotility, decrease of intraocular pressure. Neuromuscular action causes muscle fasciculation and increased twitch tension, and can produce depolarisation block.

- Anticholinesterase poisoning may occur from exposure to insecticides or nerve gases.

REFERENCES AND FURTHER READING

General references

Nicholls J G, Martin A R, Wallace B G, Fuchs P 2001 From neuron to brain. Sinauer, Sunderland (*Excellent general textbook*)

Wessle I, Kilpatrick C J, Racke K 1998 Non-neuronal acetylcholine, a locally-acting molecule, widely distributed in biological systems: expression and function in humans. Pharmacol Ther 77: 59–79 (*Speculative review describing possible roles of non-neuronal ACh*)

Acetylcholine receptors

Caulfield M P, Birdsall N J 1998 International Union of Pharmacology. XVII. Classification of muscarinic acetylcholine receptors. Pharmacol Rev 50: 279–290 (*The accepted definitions and characteristics of mAChRs*)

Cordero-Erauskin M, Marubio L M, Clink R, Changeux J-P 2000 Nicotinic receptor function: new perspectives from knockout mice. Trends Pharmacol Sci 21: 211–217

Dajas-Bailador F, Wonnacott S 2004 Nicotinic acetylcholine receptors and the regulation of neuronal signalling. Trends Pharmacol Sci 25: 217–324 (*Short review article focusing on the presynaptic actions of nAChRs in the CNS and periphery*)

Eglen R M, Choppin A, Dillon M P, Hedge S 1999 Muscarinic receptor ligands and their therapeutic potential. Curr Opin Chem Biol 3: 426–432 (*Review of the future development of muscarinic agonists and antagonists for different indications*)

Goyal R K 1989 Muscarinic receptor subtypes: physiology and clinical implications. New Engl J Med 321: 1022–1029 (*Good general review*)

Hogg R C, Raggenbass M, Bertrand D 2003 Nicotinic acetylcholine receptors: from structure to brain function. Rev Physiol Biochem Pharmacol 147: 1–46 (*Comprehensive review covering all aspects of nAChR structure and function*)

McGehee D S, Role L W 1995 Physiological diversity of nicotinic acetylcholine receptors expressed by vertebrate neurons. Annu Rev Physiol 57: 521–546 (*Summarises molecular and physiological diversity among neuronal receptors in the CNS and periphery*)

Wess J 1996 Molecular biology of muscarinic acetylcholine receptors. Crit Rev Neurobiol 10: 69–99 (*Describes receptor subtypes in detail*)

Wess J 2004 Muscarinic acetylcholine receptor knockout mice: novel phenotypes and clinical implications. Annu Rev Pharmacol Toxicol 44: 423–450 (*Progress in assigning function to different receptor subtypes by studying gene knockouts*)

Cholinergic transmission

Lindstrom J M 2000 Acetylcholine receptors and myasthenia. Muscle Nerve 23: 453–477 (*Good review article on nAChR subtypes and current views on the pathophysiology of myasthenia gravis and related neuromuscular disorders*)

Liu Y, Edwards R H 1997 The role of vesicular transport proteins in synaptic transmission and neural degeneration. Annu Rev Neurosci 20: 125–156 (*Review of recent ideas about the functional role of transporters*)

Parsons S M, Prior C, Marshall I G 1993 Acetylcholine transport, storage and release. Int Rev Neurobiol 35: 279–390 (*Useful review of the local metabolism of ACh*)

Usdin T B, Eiden L E, Bonner T I, Erickson J D 1995 Molecular biology of the vesicular ACh transporter. Trends Neurosci 18: 218–224 (*Short review article*)

Drugs affecting the neuromuscular junction

Bowman W C 1990 Pharmacology of neuromuscular function. Wright, Bristol (*Detailed textbook*)

Montecucco C, Schiavo G 1995 Structure and function of botulinum neurotoxins. Q Rev Biophys 28: 423–472 (*Discusses the mode of action of an important group of presynaptic neurotoxins*)

Prior C, Tian L, Dempster J, Marshall I G 1995 Prejunctional actions of muscle relaxants: synaptic vesicles and transmitter mobilization as sites of action. Gen Pharmacol 26: 659–666 (*Emphasises the role of presynaptic inhibition in the action of neuromuscular-blocking drugs*)

Tsui J K C 1996 Botulinum toxin as a therapeutic agent. Pharmacol Ther 72: 13–24 (*A lethal toxin can be useful in therapeutics*)

Cholinesterase

Chatonnet A, Lockridge O 1989 Comparison of butyrylcholinesterase and acetylcholinesterase. Biochem J 260: 625–634 (*Short review on the nature and functions of cholinesterases*)

Soreq H, Sediman S 2001 Acetycholinesterase—new roles for an old actor. Nat Rev Neurosci 2 294–302 (*Speculative review of evidence suggesting functions for AChE other than ACh hydrolysis*)

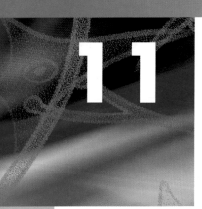

Noradrenergic transmission

OVERVIEW

The peripheral noradrenergic neuron is an important target for drug action, both as an object for investigation in its own right and as a point of attack for many clinically useful drugs. In this chapter, we describe the physiology and function of noradrenergic neurons and the properties of adrenoceptors, and discuss the various classes of drugs that affect them. For convenience, much of the pharmacological information is summarised later in the chapter.

CATECHOLAMINES

Catecholamines are compounds containing a catechol moiety (a benzene ring with two adjacent hydroxyl groups) and an amine side-chain (Fig. 11.1). Pharmacologically, the most important ones are:

- **Noradrenaline (norepinephrine[1])**, a transmitter released by sympathetic nerve terminals

- **Adrenaline (epinephrine)**, a hormone secreted by the adrenal medulla
- **Dopamine**, the metabolic precursor of noradrenaline and adrenaline, also a transmitter/neuromodulator in the central nervous system
- **Isoproterenol** (previously **isoprenaline**), a synthetic derivative of noradrenaline, not present in the body.

CLASSIFICATION OF ADRENOCEPTORS

In 1896, Oliver and Schafer demonstrated that injection of extracts of adrenal gland caused a rise in arterial pressure. Following the subsequent isolation of **adrenaline** as the active principle, it was shown by Dale in 1913 that adrenaline causes two distinct kinds of effect, namely vasoconstriction in certain vascular beds (which normally predominates and, together with its actions on the heart —see below—causes the rise in arterial pressure) and vasodilatation in others. Dale showed that the vasoconstrictor component disappeared if the animal was first injected with an ergot derivative[2] (see p. 193), and noticed that adrenaline then caused a fall, instead of a rise, in arterial pressure. This result paralleled Dale's demonstration of the separate muscarinic and nicotinic components of the action of acetylcholine (see Ch. 10). He avoided interpreting it in terms of different types of receptor, but later pharmacological work, beginning with that of Ahlquist in 1948, showed clearly the existence of several subclasses of adrenoceptor. Ahlquist found that the rank order of the potencies of various catecholamines, including **adrenaline**, **noradrenaline** and **isoproterenol**, fell into two distinct patterns, depending on what response was being measured. He postulated the existence of two kinds of receptor, α and β, defined in terms of agonist potencies as follows:

α: noradrenaline > adrenaline > isoproterenol
β: isoproterenol > adrenaline > noradrenaline.

---

[1]The conventional British names (e.g. adrenaline, noradrenaline) are used, although the recommended international non-proprietary names (rINNs) are now epinephrine and norepinephrine.

[2]Dale was a new recruit in the laboratories of the Wellcome pharmaceutical company, given the job of checking the potency of batches of adrenaline coming from the factory. He tested one batch at the end of a day's experimentation on a cat that he had earlier injected with an ergot preparation. Because it produced a fall in blood pressure rather than the expected rise, he had advised that the whole expensive consignment should be rejected. Unknown to him, he was given the same sample to test a few days later, and reported it to be normal. How he explained this to Wellcome's management is not recorded.

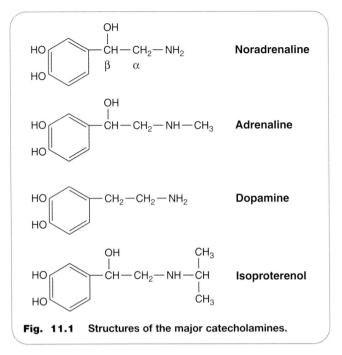

Fig. 11.1   Structures of the major catecholamines.

It was then recognised that certain ergot alkaloids, which Dale had studied, act as selective α-receptor antagonists, and that Dale's adrenaline reversal experiment reflected the unmasking of the β effects of adrenaline by α-receptor blockade. Selective β-receptor antagonists were not developed until 1955, when their effects fully confirmed Ahlquist's original classification and also suggested the existence of further subdivisions of both α and β receptors. Subsequent studies with agonists and antagonists have confirmed the existence of two main α-receptor subtypes (α_1 and α_2) and three β-receptor subtypes (β_1, β_2 and β_3; Table 11.1).

All are typical G-protein–coupled receptors, and cloning has revealed that α_1 and α_2 receptors each comprise three further sub-classes, which are expressed in different locations but whose functions are, for the most part, still unclear (Bylund, 1994; Insel, 1996).

Each of these receptor classes is associated with a specific second messenger system (Table 11.1). Thus α_1 receptors are coupled to phospholipase C and produce their effects mainly by the release of intracellular Ca^{2+}; α_2 receptors are negatively coupled to adenylyl cyclase, and reduce cAMP formation as well as inhibiting calcium channels; and all three types of β-receptor act by stimulation of adenylyl cyclase. The major effects that are

Table 11.1   Characteristics of adrenoceptors

	α_1	α_2	β_1	β_2	β_3
Tissues and effects					
Smooth muscle					
Blood vessels	Constrict	Constrict/dilate	–	Dilate	–
Bronchi	Constrict	–	–	Dilate	–
Gastrointestinal tract	Relax	Relax (presynaptic effect)	–	Relax	–
Gastrointestinal sphincters	Contract	–	–	–	–
Uterus	Contract	–	–	Relax	–
Bladder detrusor	–	–	–	Relax	–
Bladder sphincter	Contract	–	–	–	–
Seminal tract	Contract	–	–	Relax	–
Iris (radial muscle)	Contract	–	–	–	–
Ciliary muscle	–	–	–	Relax	–
Heart					
Rate	–	–	Increase	Increase[a]	
Force of contraction	–	–	Increase	Increase[a]	–
Skeletal muscle	–	–	–	Tremor Increased muscle mass and speed of contraction Glycogenolysis	Thermogenesis
Liver	Glycogenolysis	–	–	Glycogenolysis	–
Fat	–	–	–	–	Lipolysis Thermogenesis
Pancreatic islets	–	Decrease insulin secretion	–	–	–
Nerve terminals					
Adrenergic	–	Decrease release	–	Increase release	–
Cholinergic	–	Decrease release	–	–	–

Table 11.1 (cont'd) Characteristics of adrenoceptors

	α_1	α_2	β_1	β_2	β_3
Salivary gland	K⁺ release	–	Amylase secretion	–	–
Platelets	–	Aggregation	–	–	–
Mast cells	–	–	–	Inhibition of histamine release	–
Brain stem	–	Inhibits sympathetic outflow	–	–	–
Second messengers and effectors	Phospholipase C activation ↑ inositol trisphosphate ↑ diacylglycerol ↑ Ca²⁺	↓ cAMP ↓ Calcium channels ↑ Potassium channels	↑ cAMP	↑ cAMP	↑ cAMP
Agonist potency order	NA ≥ A >> ISO	A > NA >> ISO	ISO > NA > A	ISO > A > NA	ISO > NA = A
Selective agonists	Phenylephrine, methoxamine	Clonidine	Dobutamine, xamoterol	Salbutamol, terbutaline, salmeterol, formoterol clenbuterol	BRL 37344
Selective antagonists	Prazosin, doxazosin	Yohimbine, idazoxan	Atenolol, metoprolol	Butoxamine	–

A, adrenaline; ISO, isoproterenol; NA, noradrenaline.
ªMinor component normally but may increase in heart rise.

produced by these receptors, and the main drugs that act on them, are shown in Table 11.1.

The distinction between β_1- and β_2-receptors is an important one, for β_1-receptors are found mainly in the heart, where they are responsible for the positive inotropic and chronotropic effects of catecholamines (see Ch. 18). β_2-receptors, on the other hand, are responsible for causing smooth muscle relaxation in many organs. The latter is often a useful therapeutic effect, while the former is more often harmful; consequently, considerable efforts have been made to find selective β_2 agonists, which would relax smooth muscle without affecting the heart, and selective β_1 antagonists, which would exert a useful blocking effect on the heart without at the same time blocking β_2-receptors in bronchial smooth muscle (see Table 11.1). It is important to realise that the selectivity of these drugs is relative rather than absolute. Thus compounds used as selective β_1-antagonists invariably have some action on β_2-receptors as well, which can cause unwanted effects such as bronchoconstriction.

In relation to vascular control, it is broadly true that α_1- and β_2-receptors act mainly on the smooth muscle cells themselves, while α_2-receptors act on presynaptic terminals, but different vascular beds deviate from this general rule. Both α- and β-receptor subtypes are expressed in smooth muscle cells, nerve terminals and endothelial cells, and their role in physiological regulation

and pharmacological responses of the cardiovascular system is only partly understood (see Guimaraes & Moura, 2001).

Partial agonist effects

▼ Several drugs that act on adrenoceptors have the characteristics of partial agonists (see Ch. 2), i.e. they block receptors and thus antagonise the actions of full agonists, but also have a weak agonist effect of their own. Examples include **ergotamine** (α_1-receptors) and clonidine (α_2-receptors). Some β-adrenoceptor–blocking drugs (e.g. **alprenolol, oxprenolol**) cause, under resting conditions, an increase of heart rate while at the same time opposing the tachycardia produced by sympathetic stimulation. This has been interpreted as a partial agonist effect, although there is evidence that mechanisms other than β-receptor activation may contribute to the tachycardia.

There are several additional factors that make β-adrenoceptor pharmacology more complicated than it appears at first sight, and may have implications for the clinical use of β-adrenoceptor antagonists:

- The high degree of receptor specificity found for some compounds in laboratory animals is seldom found in humans
- As well as β_1-receptors, β_2-receptors contribute to the cardiostimulant effects of catecholamines. Normally, the β_1 contribution predominates, but in failing hearts (see Ch. 18) β_2-receptors become more important.
- There is evidence that β-adrenoceptor agonists and partial agonists may act not only through cAMP formation, but also through other signal transduction pathways (e.g. the mitogen-activated protein kinase pathway; see Ch. 3), and that the relative contribution of these signals

Classification of adrenoceptors

- Main pharmacological classification into α and β subtypes, based originally on order of potency among agonists, later on selective antagonists.
- Adrenoceptor subtypes:
  — two main α-receptor subtypes, α_1 and α_2, each divided into three further subtypes
  — three β-adrenoceptor subtypes (β_1, β_2, β_3)
  — all belong to the superfamily of G-protein–coupled receptors.
- Second messengers:
  — α_1-receptors activate phospholipase C, producing inositol trisphosphate and diacylglycerol as second messengers
  — α_2-receptors inhibit adenylate cyclase, decreasing cAMP formation
  — all types of β-receptor stimulate adenylyl cyclase.
- The main effects of receptor activation are as follows.
  — α_1-receptors: vasoconstriction, relaxation of gastrointestinal smooth muscle, salivary secretion and hepatic glycogenolysis
  — α_2-receptors: inhibition of transmitter release (including noradrenaline and acetylcholine release from autonomic nerves), platelet aggregation, contraction of vascular smooth muscle, inhibition of insulin release
  — β_1-receptors: increased cardiac rate and force
  — β_2-receptors: bronchodilatation, vasodilatation, relaxation of visceral smooth muscle, hepatic glycogenolysis and muscle tremor
  — β_3-receptors: lipolysis.

differs for different drugs. Furthermore, the pathways show different levels of constitutive activation, which is reduced by ligands that function as inverse agonists. Clinically used β-adrenoceptor antagonists differ in respect of these properties, and drugs classified as partial agonists may actually activate one pathway while blocking the other (see Baker et al., 2003).

The possible clinical significance of antagonists, partial agonists and inverse agonists is discussed under the headings of individual drugs later in this chapter. The pharmacology of ergot derivatives is discussed in Chapter 12.

PHYSIOLOGY OF NORADRENERGIC TRANSMISSION

THE NORADRENERGIC NEURON

Noradrenergic neurons in the periphery are postganglionic sympathetic neurons whose cell bodies lie in sympathetic ganglia. They generally have long axons that end in a series of varicosities strung along the branching terminal network. These varicosities contain numerous synaptic vesicles, which are the sites of synthesis and release of noradrenaline and of coreleased mediators such as

ATP and neuropeptide Y (see Ch. 12). Fluorescence histochemistry, in which formaldehyde treatment is used to convert catecholamines to fluorescent quinone derivatives, shows that noradrenaline is present at high concentration in these varicosities, where it is stored in large dense-core vesicles, and released by exocytosis. In most peripheral tissues, the tissue content of noradrenaline closely parallels the density of the sympathetic innervation. With the exception of the adrenal medulla, sympathetic nerve terminals account for all the noradrenaline content of peripheral tissues. Organs such as the heart, spleen, vas deferens and some blood vessels are particularly rich in noradrenaline (5–50 nmol/g of tissue) and have been widely used for studies of noradrenergic transmission. For detailed information on noradrenergic neurons, see Trendelenburg & Weiner (1988) and Cooper et al. (1996).

NORADRENALINE SYNTHESIS

The biosynthetic pathway for noradrenaline synthesis is shown in Figure 11.2. The metabolic precursor for noradrenaline is L-tyrosine, an aromatic amino acid that is present in the body fluids, and is taken up by adrenergic neurons. *Tyrosine hydroxylase*, a cytosolic

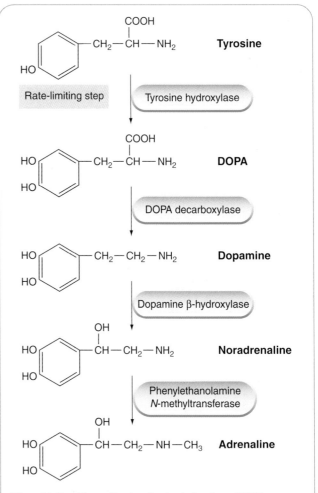

Fig. 11.2 Biosynthesis of catecholamines. DOPA, dihydroxyphenylalanine.

enzyme that catalyses the conversion of tyrosine to dihydroxy-phenylalanine (dopa) is found only in catecholamine-containing cells. It is a rather selective enzyme; unlike other enzymes involved in catecholamine metabolism, it does not accept indole derivatives as substrates, and so is not involved in 5-hydroxytryptamine (5-HT) metabolism. This first hydroxylation step is the main control point for noradrenaline synthesis. Tyrosine hydroxylase is inhibited by the end-product of the biosynthetic pathway, noradrenaline, and this provides the mechanism for the moment-to-moment regulation of the rate of synthesis; much slower regulation, taking hours or days, occurs by changes in the rate of production of the enzyme.

The tyrosine analogue α-**methyltyrosine** strongly inhibits tyrosine hydroxylase and may be used experimentally to block noradrenaline synthesis.

The next step, conversion of dopa to dopamine, is catalysed by *dopa decarboxylase*, a cytosolic enzyme that is by no means confined to catecholamine-synthesising cells. It is a relatively non-specific enzyme, and catalyses the decarboxylation of various other L-aromatic amino acids, such as L-histidine and L-tryptophan, which are precursors in the synthesis of histamine (Ch. 13) and 5-HT (Ch. 12), respectively. Dopa decarboxylase activity is not rate-limiting for noradrenaline synthesis. Although various factors, including certain drugs, affect the enzyme, it is not an effective means of regulating noradrenaline synthesis.

Dopamine-β-hydroxylase (*DBH*) is also a relatively non-specific enzyme, but is restricted to catecholamine-synthesising cells. It is located in synaptic vesicles, mainly in membrane-bound form. A small amount of the enzyme is released from adrenergic nerve terminals in company with noradrenaline, representing the small proportion in a soluble form within the vesicle. Unlike noradrenaline, the released DBH is not subject to rapid degradation or uptake, so its concentration in plasma and body fluids can be used as an index of overall sympathetic nerve activity.

Many drugs inhibit DBH, including copper-chelating agents and **disulfiram** (a drug used mainly for its effect on ethanol metabolism; see Chs 8 and 54). Such drugs can cause a partial depletion of noradrenaline stores and interference with sympathetic transmission.

Phenylethanolamine N-*methyl transferase* (*PNMT*) catalyses the N-methylation of noradrenaline to adrenaline. The main location of this enzyme is in the adrenal medulla, which contains a population of adrenaline-releasing (A) cells separate from the smaller proportion of noradrenaline-releasing (N) cells. The A cells, which appear only after birth, lie adjacent to the adrenal cortex, and the production of PNMT is induced by an action of the steroid hormones secreted by the adrenal cortex (see Ch. 28). PNMT is also found in certain parts of the brain, where adrenaline may function as a transmitter, but little is known about its role.

Noradrenaline turnover can be measured under steady-state conditions by measuring the rate at which labelled noradrenaline accumulates when a labelled precursor, such as tyrosine or dopa, is administered. The turnover time is defined as the time taken for an amount of noradrenaline equal to the total tissue content to be degraded and resynthesised. In peripheral tissues, the turnover time is generally about 5–15 hours, but it becomes much shorter if sympathetic nerve activity is increased. Under normal circumstances, the rate of synthesis closely matches the rate of release,

so that the noradrenaline content of tissues is constant regardless of how fast it is being released.

NORADRENALINE STORAGE

Most of the noradrenaline in nerve terminals or chromaffin cells is contained in vesicles; only a little is free in the cytoplasm under normal circumstances. The concentration in the vesicles is very high (0.3–1.0 mol/l) and is maintained by the *vesicular monoamine transporter*, which is similar to the amine transporter responsible for noradrenaline uptake into the nerve terminal, but uses the transvesicular proton gradient as its driving force (see Liu & Edwards, 1997). Certain drugs, such as **reserpine** (see below; Table 11.2) block this transport and cause nerve terminals to become depleted of their noradrenaline stores. The vesicles contain two major constituents besides noradrenaline, namely ATP (about four molecules per molecule of noradrenaline) and a protein called *chromogranin A*. These substances are released along with noradrenaline, and it is generally assumed that a reversible complex, depending partly on the opposite charges on the molecules of noradrenaline and ATP, is formed within the vesicle. This would serve both to reduce the osmolarity of the vesicle contents and also to reduce the tendency of noradrenaline to leak out of the vesicles within the nerve terminal.

ATP itself has a transmitter function at adrenergic synapses (see Lundberg 1996; Ch. 12), being responsible for the fast excitatory synaptic potential and the rapid phase of contraction produced by sympathetic nerve activity in many smooth muscle tissues.

NORADRENALINE RELEASE

The processes linking the arrival of a nerve impulse at a noradrenergic nerve terminal to the release of noradrenaline are basically the same as those at other chemically transmitting synapses (see Ch. 4). Depolarisation of the nerve terminal membrane opens calcium channels in the nerve terminal membrane, and the resulting entry of Ca^{2+} promotes the fusion and discharge of synaptic vesicles. A surprising feature of the release mechanism at the varicosities of noradrenergic nerves is that the probability of release, even of a single vesicle, when a nerve impulse arrives at a varicosity, is very low (less than 1 in 50; see Cunnane, 1984). A single neuron possesses many thousand varicosities, so one impulse leads to the discharge of a few hundred vesicles, scattered over a wide area. This contrasts sharply with the neuromuscular junction (Ch. 10), where the release probability at a single terminal is high, and release of acetylcholine is sharply localised.

Regulation of noradrenaline release

Noradrenaline release is affected by a variety of substances that act on presynaptic receptors (see Ch. 9). Many different types of nerve terminal (cholinergic, noradrenergic, dopaminergic, 5-HT-ergic, etc.) are subject to this type of control, and many different mediators (e.g. acetylcholine acting through muscarinic receptors, catecholamines acting through α- and β-receptors, angiotensin II, prostaglandins, purine nucleotides, neuropeptides, etc.) can act on presynaptic terminals. Presynaptic modulation represents

Table 11.2 Characteristics of noradrenaline (norepinephrine) transport systems

	Uptake 1[a]	Uptake 2	Vesicular[a]
Transport of NA (rat heart) V_{max} (nmol/g per min)	1.2	100	–
K_m (μmol/l)	0.3	250	~0.2
Specificity	NA > A > ISO	A > NA > ISO	NA = A = ISO
Location	Neuronal membrane	Non-neuronal cell membrane (smooth muscle, cardiac muscle, endothelium)	Synaptic vesicle membrane
Other substrates	Methylnoradrenaline Tyramine Adrenergic neuron–blocking drugs (e.g. guanethidine)	(+)-Noradrenaline Dopamine 5-Hydroxytryptamine Histamine	Dopamine 5-Hydroxytryptamine Guanethidine MPP+ (see Ch. 35)
Inhibitors	Cocaine Tricyclic antidepressants (e.g. desipramine) Phenoxybenzamine Amphetamine	Normetanephrine Steroid hormones (e.g. corticosterone) Phenoxybenzamine	Reserpine Tetrabenazine

A, adrenaline; ISO, isoprenaline; NA, noradrenaline.
[a]Transporters corresponding to uptake 1 and vesicular transporter have been cloned and termed *noradrenaline transporter* and *vesicular monoamine transporter*, respectively (see review by Nelson 1998 J Neurochem 71: 1785–1803). The uptake 2 transporter has not yet been identified.

an important physiological control mechanism throughout the nervous system.

Furthermore, noradrenaline, by acting on presynaptic receptors, can regulate its own release, and also that of coreleased ATP (see Ch. 9). This is believed to occur physiologically, so that released noradrenaline exerts a local inhibitory effect on the terminals from which it came—the so-called *autoinhibitory feedback* mechanism (Fig. 11.3; see Starke et al., 1989). Agonists or antagonists affecting these presynaptic receptors can have large effects on sympathetic transmission. The physiological significance of presynaptic autoinhibition in the sympathetic nervous system is still somewhat contentious, and there is evidence that, in most tissues, it is less influential than biochemical measurements of transmitter overflow would imply. Thus, although blocking autoreceptors causes large changes in noradrenaline *overflow*—the amount of noradrenaline released into the bathing solution or the bloodstream when sympathetic nerves are stimulated—the associated changes in the tissue response are often rather small. This suggests that what is measured in overflow experiments may not be the physiologically important component of transmitter release.

The inhibitory feedback mechanism operates through α_2 receptors, which inhibit adenylate cyclase and prevent the opening of calcium channels. Sympathetic nerve terminals also possess β_2-receptors, coupled to activation of adenylyl cyclase, which cause an increased noradrenaline release. Whether they have any physiological function is not yet clear.

UPTAKE AND DEGRADATION OF CATECHOLAMINES

The action of released noradrenaline is terminated mainly by reuptake of the transmitter into noradrenergic nerve terminals. Some is also sequestered by other cells in the vicinity. Circulating adrenaline and noradrenaline are degraded enzymically, but much more slowly than acetylcholine (see Ch. 10), where synaptically located acetylcholinesterase inactivates the transmitter in milliseconds. The two main catecholamine-metabolising enzymes are located intracellularly, so uptake into cells necessarily precedes metabolic degradation.

Uptake of catecholamines

Radioactive noradrenaline injected into the bloodstream is rapidly taken up into tissues. Part of this uptake is by sympathetic neurons (for it disappears when sympathetic nerves are caused to degenerate), from which it can be released again by sympathetic nerve stimulation. In a study of noradrenaline uptake by isolated rat hearts, Iversen identified two distinct uptake mechanisms, each having the characteristics of a saturable active transport system capable of accumulating catecholamines against a large concentration gradient. These two mechanisms, called **uptake 1** and **uptake 2**, correspond to neuronal and extraneuronal uptake, respectively. About 75% of the noradrenaline released by sympathetic neurons is recycled via uptake 1, the remainder being captured by other cells in the vicinity via uptake 2. Thus uptake 1

Noradrenergic transmission

- Transmitter synthesis involves the following.
  - L-tyrosine is converted to dihydroxyphenylalanine (dopa) by tyrosine hydroxylase (rate-limiting step). Tyrosine hydroxylase occurs only in catecholaminergic neurons.
  - Dopa is converted to dopamine by dopa decarboxylase.
  - Dopamine is converted to noradrenaline by dopamine β-hydroxylase (DBH), located in synaptic vesicles.
  - In the adrenal medulla, noradrenaline is converted to adrenaline by phenylethanolamine *N*-methyl transferase.
- Transmitter storage: noradrenaline is stored at high concentration in synaptic vesicles, together with ATP, chromogranin and DBH, all of which are released by exocytosis. Transport of noradrenaline into vesicles occurs by a **reserpine**-sensitive transporter. Noradrenaline content of cytosol is normally low due to monoamine oxidase in nerve terminals.
- Transmitter release occurs normally by Ca^{2+}-mediated exocytosis from varicosities on the terminal network. Non-exocytotic release occurs in response to indirectly acting sympathomimetic drugs (e.g. **amphetamine**), which displace noradrenaline from vesicles. Noradrenaline escapes via uptake 1 (reverse transport).
- Transmitter action is terminated mainly by transporter-mediated reuptake of noradrenaline into nerve terminals (uptake 1). Uptake 1 is blocked by **tricyclic antidepressant drugs** and **cocaine**.
- Noradrenaline release is controlled by autoinhibitory feedback mediated by α_2 receptors.
- Cotransmission occurs at many noradrenergic nerve terminals, ATP and neuropeptide Y being frequently coreleased with NA. ATP mediates the early phase of smooth muscle contraction in response to sympathetic nerve activity.

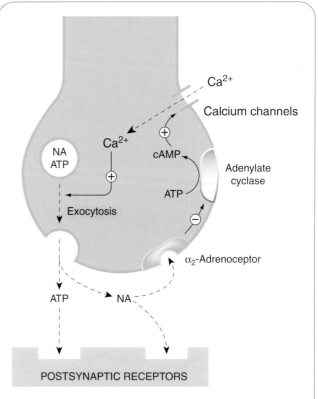

Fig. 11.3 **Feedback control of noradrenaline release.** The presynaptic α_2 receptor inhibits adenylate cyclase, thereby reducing intracellular cAMP. cAMP acts to promote Ca^{2+} influx in response to membrane depolarisation, and hence to promote the release of noradrenaline and ATP.

serves to cut short the action of the transmitter, and to recycle it, whereas uptake 2 serves mainly to limit its spread. Uptakes 1 and 2 are associated with distinct transporter molecules, which have different kinetic properties as well as different substrate and inhibitor specificity, as summarised in Table 11.2. Uptake 1 is a high-affinity system, relatively selective for noradrenaline, with a low maximum rate of uptake, and it is important in maintaining releasable stores of noradrenaline. Uptake 2 has low affinity, and transports adrenaline and isoproterenol as well as noradrenaline, at a much higher maximum rate than uptake 1. The effects of several important drugs that act on noradrenergic neurons depend on their ability either to inhibit uptake 1 or to enter the nerve terminal with it shelp (see Table 11.2).

Noradrenaline transporters belong to the family of neurotransmitter transporter proteins (NET, DAT, SERT, etc.) specific for different amine transmitters, described in Chapter 9; these act as cotransporters of Na^+, Cl^- and the amine in question, using the electrochemical gradient for Na^+ as a driving force. Changes in this gradient can alter, or even reverse, the operation of uptake 1, with marked effects on the availability of the released transmitter at postsynaptic receptors. Uptake of noradrenaline from the cytosol into the synaptic vessel is carried out by a different transporter, the *vesicular monoamine transporter* (VMAT).

Metabolic degradation of catecholamines

Endogenous and exogenous catecholamines are metabolised mainly by two enzymes: *monoamine oxidase (MAO)* and *catechol-O-methyl transferase (COMT)*. MAO occurs within cells, bound to the surface membrane of mitochondria. It is abundant in noradrenergic nerve terminals but is also present in many other places, such as liver and intestinal epithelium. MAO converts catecholamines to their corresponding aldehydes, which, in the periphery, are rapidly metabolised by aldehyde dehydrogenase to the corresponding carboxylic acid (3,4-dihydroxyphenylglycol being formed from noradrenaline; Fig. 11.4). MAO can also oxidise other monoamines, important ones being dopamine and 5-HT. It is inhibited by various drugs (see Table 11.3), which are used mainly for their effects on the central nervous system, where these three amines all have transmitter functions (see Ch. 34). These drugs have important side effects that are related to disturbances of peripheral adrenergic transmission. Within sympathetic neurons, MAO controls the content of dopamine and noradrenaline, and the releasable store of noradrenaline increases if the enzyme is inhibited. MAO and its inhibitors are discussed in more detail in Chapter 39.

The second major pathway for catecholamine metabolism involves methylation of one of the catechol hydroxyl groups to give a methoxy derivative. COMT is absent from noradrenergic neurons but present in the adrenal medulla and many other cells and tissues. The final product formed by the sequential action of MAO and COMT is *3-hydroxy-4-methoxyphenylglycol* (*MHPG*; see Fig. 11.4). This is partly conjugated to sulfate or glucuronide derivatives, which are excreted in the urine, but most of it is converted to *vanillylmandelic acid* (*VMA*; Fig. 11.4) and excreted in the urine in this form.[3] In patients with tumours of chromaffin

tissue that secrete these amines (a rare cause of high blood pressure), the urinary excretion of VMA is markedly increased, this being used as a diagnostic test for this condition.

In the periphery, neither MAO nor COMT is primarily responsible for the termination of transmitter action, most of the released noradrenaline being quickly recaptured by uptake 1. Circulating catecholamines are usually inactivated by a combination of uptake 1, uptake 2 and COMT, the relative importance of these processes varying according to the agent concerned. Thus circulating noradrenaline is removed mainly by uptake 1, whereas adrenaline is more dependent on uptake 2. Isoproterenol, on the other hand, is not a substrate for uptake 1, and is removed by a combination of uptake 2 and COMT.

In the central nervous system (see Ch. 32), MAO is more important as a means of terminating transmitter action than it is in the periphery, and MAO knockout mice show a greater enhancement of noradrenergic transmission in the brain than do NET knockouts, in which neuronal stores of noradrenaline are much depleted (see Gainetdinov & Caron, 2003). The main excretory product of noradrenaline released in the brain is MHPG.

---

[3]The amounts of MHPG and VMA excreted are often taken to reflect noradrenaline release from sympathetic neurons and central nervous system neurons, respectively, but this is now believed to be unreliable (see Eisenhofer et al., 2004).

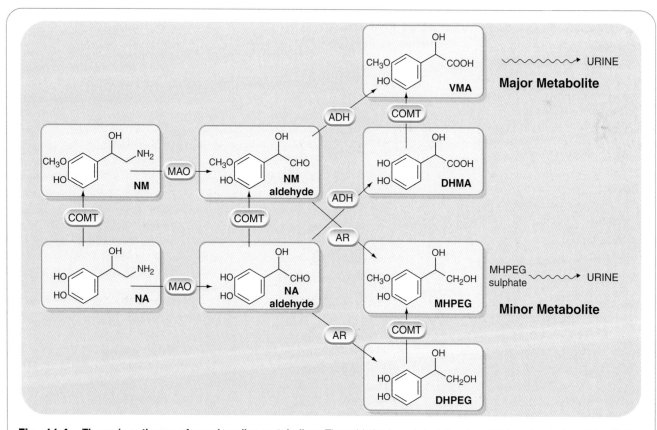

Fig. 11.4 **The main pathways of noradrenaline metabolism.** The oxidative branch (catalysed by ADH) predominates, giving VMA as the main urinary metabolite. The reductive branch (catalysed by AR) produces the less abundant metabolite, MHPEG, which is conjugated to MHPEG sulfate before being excreted. ADH, aldehyde dehydrogenase; AR, aldehyde reductase; CNS, central nervous system; COMT, catechol-O-methyl transferase; DHMA, 3,4-dihydroxymandelic acid; DHPEG, 3,4-dihydroxyphenylglycol; MAO, monoamine oxidase; MHPEG, 3-methoxy, 4-hydroxyphenylglycol; NA, noradrenaline; NM, normetanephrine; VMA, vanillylmandelic acid.

DRUGS ACTING ON NORADRENERGIC TRANSMISSION

Many clinically important drugs, particularly those used to treat cardiovascular, respiratory and psychiatric disorders (see Chs 18, 19, 23 and 39) act by affecting noradrenergic neuron function. The main drug targets are:

* adrenoceptors
* monoamine transporters
* catecholamine-metabolising enzymes.

The properties of the most important drugs that act on adrenergic transmission are summarised in Table 11.3.

DRUGS ACTING ON ADRENOCEPTORS

The overall activity of these drugs is governed by their affinity, efficacy and selectivity with respect to different types of adrenoceptor, and intensive research has been devoted to developing drugs with the right properties for specific clinical indications. As a result, the pharmacopoeia is awash with adrenoceptor ligands. Many clinical needs are met, it turns out, by drugs that relax smooth muscle in different organs of the body;[4] on the other hand, cardiac stimulation is generally undesirable. Broadly speaking, β-adrenoceptor agonists are useful as bronchodilators, while β-adrenoceptor antagonists (often called β-blockers) and α-adrenoceptor antagonists are used mainly in cardiovascular indications, by virtue of their respective cardiodepressant and vasodilator effects.

ADRENOCEPTOR AGONISTS

Examples of the main types of adrenoceptor agonist are given in Table 11.1, and the characteristics of individual drugs are summarised in Table 11.3.

Actions

The major physiological effects mediated by different types of adrenoceptor are summarised in Table 11.1.

Smooth muscle

All types of smooth muscle, except that of the gastrointestinal tract, contract in response to stimulation of α_1-adrenoceptors, through activation of the signal transduction mechanism described in Chapter 4.

When α agonists are given systemically to experimental animals or humans, the most important action is on vascular smooth muscle, particularly in the skin and splanchnic vascular beds, which are strongly constricted. Large arteries and veins, as well as arterioles, are also constricted, resulting in decreased vascular compliance, increased central venous pressure and increased peripheral resistance, all of which contribute to an increase in systolic and diastolic arterial pressure and increased cardiac work. Some vascular beds (e.g. cerebral, coronary and pulmonary) are relatively little affected.

In the whole animal, baroreceptor reflexes are activated by the rise in arterial pressure produced by α agonists, causing reflex bradycardia and inhibition of respiration.

Smooth muscle in the vas deferens, spleen capsule and eyelid retractor muscles (or nictitating membrane, in some species) is also stimulated by α agonists, and these organs are often used for pharmacological studies.

The α-receptors involved in smooth muscle contraction are mainly α_1 in type, although vascular smooth muscle possesses both α_1 and α_2-receptors. It appears that α_1-receptors lie close to the sites of release (and are mainly responsible for neurally mediated vasoconstriction), while α_2-receptors lie elsewhere on the muscle fibre surface and are activated by circulating catecholamines.

Stimulation of β-receptors causes relaxation of most kinds of smooth muscle by increasing cAMP formation (see Ch. 4). Additionally, β-receptor activation enhances Ca^{2+} extrusion and intracellular Ca^{2+} binding, both effects acting to reduce intracellular Ca^{2+} concentration.

Relaxation is usually produced by β_2-receptors, although the receptor that is responsible for this effect in gastrointestinal smooth muscle is not clearly β_1 or β_2. In the vascular system, β_2-mediated vasodilatation is (particularly in humans) mainly endothelium-dependent and mediated by nitric oxide release (see Ch. 17). It occurs in many vascular beds and is especially marked in skeletal muscle.

The powerful inhibitory effect of the sympathetic system on gastrointestinal smooth muscle is produced by both α and β-receptors, this tissue being unusual in that α-receptors cause relaxation in most regions. Part of the effect is due to stimulation of presynaptic α_2-receptors (see below), which inhibit the release of excitatory transmitters (e.g. acetylcholine) from intramural nerves, but there are also α-receptors on the muscle cells, stimulation of which hyperpolarises the cell (by increasing the membrane permeability to K^+) and inhibits action potential discharge. The sphincters of the gastrointestinal tract are contracted by α-receptor activation.

Bronchial smooth muscle is strongly dilated by activation of β_2-adrenoceptors, and selective β_2 agonists are important in the treatment of asthma (see Ch. 23). Uterine smooth muscle responds similarly, and these drugs are also used to delay premature labour (Ch. 30).

α-Adrenoceptors also mediate a long-lasting trophic response, stimulating smooth muscle proliferation in various tissues, for example in blood vessels and in the prostate gland, which is of pathological importance. Benign prostatic hyperplasia (see Ch. 30) is commonly treated with α-adrenoceptor antagonists (see the clinical box on p. 179). 'Cross-talk' between the α_1-adrenoceptor and the growth factor signalling pathways (see Ch. 3) probably accounts for this effect.

Nerve terminals

Presynaptic adrenoceptors are present on both cholinergic and noradrenergic nerve terminals (see Chs 4 and 9). The main effect

---

[4]And conversely, contracting smooth muscle is usually bad news. This bald statement must not be pressed too far, but the exceptions (such as nasal decongestants and drugs acting on the eye) are surprisingly few.

(α_2-mediated) is inhibitory, but a weaker facilitatory action of β-receptors on adrenergic nerve terminals has also been described.

Heart

Catecholamines, acting on β_1-receptors, exert a powerful stimulant effect on the heart (see Ch. 18). Both the heart rate (*chronotropic effect*) and the force of contraction (*inotropic effect*) are increased, resulting in a markedly increased cardiac output and cardiac oxygen consumption. The cardiac efficiency (see Ch. 18) is reduced. Catecholamines can also cause disturbance of the cardiac rhythm, culminating in ventricular fibrillation. (Paradoxically, but importantly, adrenaline is also used to treat ventricular fibrillation arrest as well as other forms of cardiac arrest—Ch. 18, Table 18.1.) In normal hearts, the dose required to cause marked dysrhythmia is greater than that which produces the chronotropic and inotropic effects, but in ischaemic conditions dysrhythmias are produced much more readily. Figure 11.5 shows the overall pattern of cardiovascular responses to catecholamine infusions in humans, reflecting their actions on both the heart and vascular system.

Cardiac hypertrophy occurs in response to activation of α_1-receptors, probably by a mechanism similar to the hypertrophy of vascular and prostatic smooth muscle. This may be important in the pathophysiology of hypertension and cardiac failure (see Ch. 18).

Metabolism

Catecholamines encourage the conversion of energy stores (glycogen and fat) to freely available fuels (glucose and free fatty acids), and cause an increase in the plasma concentration of the latter substances. The detailed biochemical mechanisms (see review by Nonogaki, 2000) vary from species to species, but in most cases the effects on carbohydrate metabolism of liver and muscle (Fig. 11.6) are mediated through β_1-receptors (although hepatic glucose release can also be produced by α agonists), and the stimulation of lipolysis is produced by β_3-receptors (see Table 11.1). Insulin secretion is through α_2-receptors, an effect that further contributes to the hyperglycaemia. Additionally, the production of **leptin** by adipose tissue (see Ch. 27) is inhibited. Adrenaline-induced hyperglycaemia in humans is blocked completely by a combination of α and β antagonists but not by either on its own. Selective β_3-receptor agonists (e.g. BRL 37344) have been developed as possible treatments for obesity, but their action is too transient for them to be clinically useful.

Other effects

Skeletal muscle is affected by adrenaline, acting on β_2-receptors, although the effect is far less dramatic than that on the heart. The twitch tension of fast-contracting fibres (white muscle) is increased by adrenaline, particularly if the muscle is fatigued, whereas the twitch of slow (red) muscle is reduced. These effects depend on an action on the contractile proteins, rather than on the membrane, and the mechanism is poorly understood. In humans, adrenaline and other β_2 agonists cause a marked tremor, the shakiness that accompanies fear, excitement or the excessive use of β_2 agonists (e.g. salbutamol) in the treatment of asthma being examples of this. It probably results from an increase in muscle spindle discharge, coupled with an effect on the contraction kinetics of the fibres, these effects combining to produce an instability in the reflex control of muscle length. β-Receptor antagonists are sometimes used to control pathological tremor. The β_2 agonists also cause long-term changes in the expression of sarcoplasmic reticulum proteins that control contraction kinetics, and thereby increase the rate and force of contraction of skeletal muscle (see Zhang et al., 1996). **Clenbuterol**, an 'anabolic' drug used illicitly by athletes to improve performance (see Ch. 54), is a β_2 agonist that acts in this way.

Histamine release by human and guinea pig lung tissue in response to anaphylactic challenge (see Ch. 13) is inhibited by catecholamines, acting apparently on β_2-receptors.

Lymphocytes and other cells of the immune system also express adrenoceptors (mainly β-adrenoceptors). Lymphocyte proliferation, lymphocyte-mediated cell killing, and production of many cytokines are inhibited by β-adrenoceptor agonists. The physiological and clinical importance of these effects has not yet been established. For a review of the effects of the sympathetic nervous system on immune function, see Elenkov et al., 2000.

Clinical use

The main clinical uses of adrenoceptor agonists are summarised in the clinical box (p. 179).

ADRENOCEPTOR ANTAGONISTS

The main drugs are listed in Table 11.1, and further information is given in Table 11.3. In contrast to the situation with agonists, most adrenoceptor antagonists are selective for α or β-receptors, and many are also subtype-selective.

Adrenoceptor agonists

- **Noradrenaline** and **adrenaline** show relatively little receptor selectivity.
- Selective α_1 agonists include **phenylephrine** and **oxymetazoline**.
- Selective α_2 agonists include **clonidine** and α-**methylnoradrenaline**. They cause a fall in blood pressure, partly by inhibition of noradrenaline release and partly by a central action. Methylnoradrenaline is formed as a false transmitter from **methyldopa**, developed as a hypotensive drug (now largely obsolete).
- Selective β_1 agonists include **dobutamine**. Increased cardiac contractility may be useful clinically, but all β_1 agonists can cause cardiac dysrhythmias.
- Selective β_2 agonists include **salbutamol, terbutaline** and **salmeterol**, used mainly for their bronchodilator action in asthma.
- Selective β_3 agonists may be developed for the control of obesity.

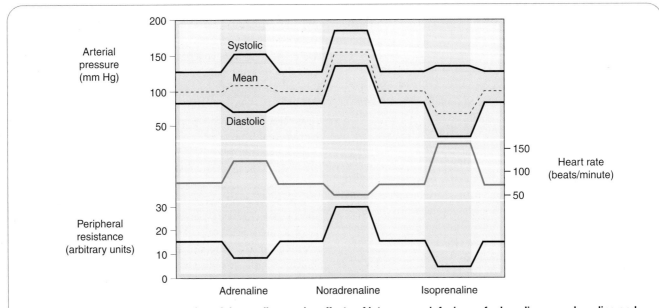

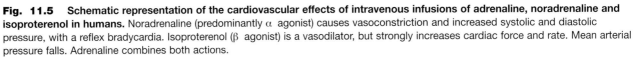

Fig. 11.5 Schematic representation of the cardiovascular effects of intravenous infusions of adrenaline, noradrenaline and isoproterenol in humans. Noradrenaline (predominantly α agonist) causes vasoconstriction and increased systolic and diastolic pressure, with a reflex bradycardia. Isoproterenol (β agonist) is a vasodilator, but strongly increases cardiac force and rate. Mean arterial pressure falls. Adrenaline combines both actions.

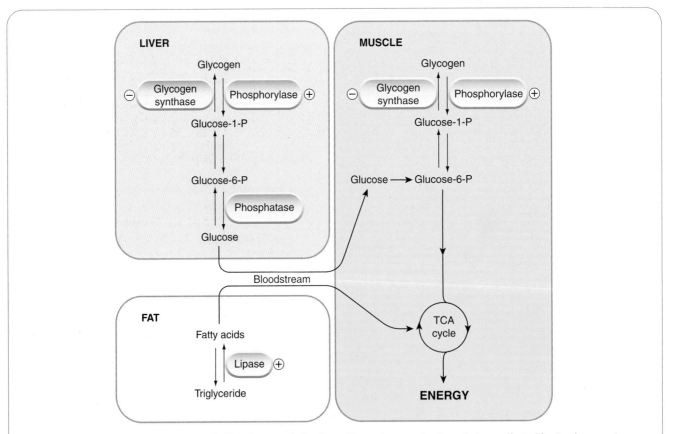

Fig. 11.6 Regulation of energy metabolism by catecholamines. The main enzymic steps that are affected by β-adrenoceptor activation are indicated by + and – signs, denoting stimulation and inhibition, respectively. The overall effect is to mobilise glycogen and fat stores to meet energy demands.

α-Adrenoceptor antagonists

The main groups of α-adrenoceptor antagonists are:

- non-selective α-receptor antagonists (e.g. **phenoxybenzamine, phentolamine**)
- α_1-selective antagonists (e.g. **prazosin, doxazosin, terazosin**)
- α_2-selective antagonists (e.g. **yohimbine, idazoxan**)
- ergot derivatives (e.g. **ergotamine, dihydroergotamine**). This group of compounds has many actions in addition to α-receptor block, and is discussed in Chapter 12. Their action on α-adrenoceptors is of pharmacological interest (see p. 168) but not used therapeutically.

Non-selective α-adrenoceptor antagonists

Phenoxybenzamine is not specific for α-receptors, and also antagonises the actions of acetylcholine, histamine and 5-HT. It is long-lasting because it binds covalently to the receptor. **Phentolamine** is more selective, but it binds reversibly and its action is short-lasting. In humans, these drugs cause a fall in arterial pressure (because of block of α-receptor–mediated vasoconstriction) and postural hypotension. The cardiac output and heart rate are increased. This is a reflex response to the fall in arterial pressure, mediated through β-receptors. The concomitant block of α_2-receptors tends to increase noradrenaline release, which has the effect of enhancing the reflex tachycardia that occurs with any blood pressure–lowering agent. Phenoxybenzamine retains a niche (but vital) use in preparing patients with phaeochromocytoma for surgery; its irreversible antagonism and the resultant depression in the maximum of the agonist dose–response curve (cf. Ch 2, Fig. 2.10) are desirable in a situation where surgical manipulation of the tumour may release a large bolus of pressor amine into the circulation.

Labetalol and **carvedilol** are mixed α and β-receptor–blocking drugs, although clinically they act predominantly on β-receptors. Much has been made of the fact that they combine both activities in one molecule. To a pharmacologist, accustomed to putting specificity of action high on the list of pharmacological saintly virtues, this may seem like a step backwards rather than forwards. Carvedilol is used mainly to treat hypertension and heart failure (see Chs 18 and 19); labetalol is used to treat hypertension in pregnancy.

Selective α_1 antagonists

Prazosin was the first α_1-selective antagonist. Similar drugs with longer half-lives (e.g. **doxazosin, terazosin**), which have the advantage of allowing once-daily dosing, are now available. They are highly selective for α_1-adrenoceptors and cause vasodilatation and fall in arterial pressure, but less tachycardia than occurs with non-selective α-receptor antagonists, presumably because they do not increase noradrenaline release from sympathetic nerve terminals. Some postural hypotension may occur.

The α_1-receptor antagonists cause relaxation of the smooth muscle of the bladder neck and prostate capsule, and inhibit hypertrophy of these tissues, and are therefore useful in treating urinary retention associated with benign prostatic hypertrophy. **Tamsulosin**, an α_{1A}-receptor antagonist, shows some selectivity

> **Clinical uses of α-adrenoceptor antagonists**
>
> - *Severe hypertension* (see Ch. 19): α_1-selective antagonists (e.g. **doxazosin**) in combination with other drugs.
> - *Benign prostatic hypertrophy* (e.g. **tamsulosin**, a selective α_{1A}-receptor antagonist).
> - *Phaeochromocytoma*: **phenoxybenzamine** (irreversible antagonist) in preparation for surgery.

> **Clinical uses of adrenoceptor agonists**
>
> - Cardiovascular system:
>   - *cardiac arrest*: **adrenaline**
>   - *cardiogenic shock* (see Ch. 19): **dobutamine** (β_1 agonist)
> - *Anaphylaxis* (acute hypersensitivity, see Ch. 13, and Ch. 23): **adrenaline**.
> - Respiratory system:
>   - *asthma* (Ch. 23): selective β_2-receptor agonists (**salbutamol, terbutaline, salmeterol, formoterol**)
>   - *nasal decongestion*: drops containing **xylometazoline** or **ephedrine** for short-term use.
> - Miscellaneous indications:
>   - **adrenaline**: with local anaesthetics to prolong their action (see Ch. 44)
>   - *premature labour* (**salbutamol**; see Ch. 30)
>   - α_2 agonists (e.g. **clonidine**): to lower blood pressure (Ch. 19) and intraocular pressure; as an adjunct during drug withdrawal in addicts (Ch. 43; Table 43.2); to reduce menopausal flushing; and to reduce frequency of migraine attacks (Ch. 12).

> **α-Adrenoceptor antagonists**
>
> - Drugs that block α_1 and α_2 adrenoceptors (e.g. **phenoxybenzamine** and **phentolamine**) were once used to produce vasodilatation in the treatment of peripheral vascular disease, but this use is now largely obsolete.
> - Selective α_1 antagonists (e.g. **prazosin, doxazosin, terazosin**) are used in treating hypertension. Postural hypotension and impotence are unwanted effects.
> - Yohimbine is a selective α_2 antagonist. It is not used clinically.
> - **Tamsulosin** is α_{1A}-selective and acts mainly on the urogenital tract.
> - Some drugs (e.g. **labetalol, carvedilol**) block both α and β adrenoceptors.

for the bladder, and causes less hypotension than drugs such as prazosin, which act on α_{1B}-receptors to control vascular tone.

It is believed that α_{1A}-receptors play a part in the pathological hypertrophy not only of prostatic and vascular smooth muscle, but also in the cardiac hypertrophy that occurs in hypertension, and the use of selective α_{1A}-receptor antagonists to treat these chronic conditions is under investigation.

Selective α_2 antagonists

Yohimbine is a naturally occurring alkaloid; various synthetic analogues have been made, such as **idazoxan**. These drugs are used experimentally to analyse α-receptor subtypes, and yohimbine, probably by virtue of its vasodilator effect, historically enjoyed notoriety as an aphrodisiac, but they are not used therapeutically.

General clinical uses and unwanted effects of α-adrenoceptor antagonists

The main uses of α-adrenoceptor antagonists are related to their cardiovascular actions, and are summarised in the clinical box (below). They have been tried for many purposes, but have only limited therapeutic applications. In hypertension, non-selective α-blocking drugs are unsatisfactory, because of their tendency to produce tachycardia and cardiac dysrhythmias, and increased gastrointestinal activity. Selective α_1-receptor antagonists (especially the longer-acting compounds doxazosin and terazosin) are, however, useful. They do not affect cardiac function appreciably, and postural hypotension is less troublesome than with prazosin or non-selective α-receptor antagonists. They have a place in treating severe hypertension, where they are added to treatment with first- and second-line drugs, but are not used as first-line agents (see Ch. 19). Unlike other antihypertensive drugs, they cause a modest decrease in low-density lipoprotein, and an increase in high-density lipoprotein cholesterol (see Ch. 20), although the clinical importance of these ostensibly beneficial effects is uncertain. They are also used to control urinary retention in patients with benign prostatic hypertrophy.

Phaeochromocytoma is a catecholamine-secreting tumour of chromaffin tissue, which causes episodes of severe hypertension. A combination of α- and β-receptor antagonists is the most effective way of controlling the blood pressure. The tumour may be surgically removable, and it is essential to block α- and β-receptors before surgery is begun, to avoid the effects of a sudden release of catecholamines when the tumour is disturbed. A combination of **phenoxybenzamine** and **atenolol** is effective for this purpose.

β-Adrenoceptor antagonists

The β-adrenoceptor antagonists are an important group of drugs. They were first discovered in 1958, 10 years after Ahlquist had postulated the existence of β-adrenoceptors. The first compound, **dichloroisoproterenol**, had fairly low potency and was a partial agonist. Further development led to **propranolol**, which is much more potent and a pure antagonist that blocks β_1- and β_2-receptors equally. The potential clinical advantages of drugs with some partial agonist activity, and/or with selectivity for β_1-receptors, led to the development of **practolol** (selective for β_1-receptors but withdrawn because of its toxicity), **oxprenolol** and **alprenolol** (non-selective with considerable partial agonist activity), and **atenolol** (β_1-selective with no agonist activity). Two newer drugs are **carvedilol** (a non-selective β-adrenoceptor antagonist with additional α_1-blocking activity) and **nebivolol** (a β_1-selective

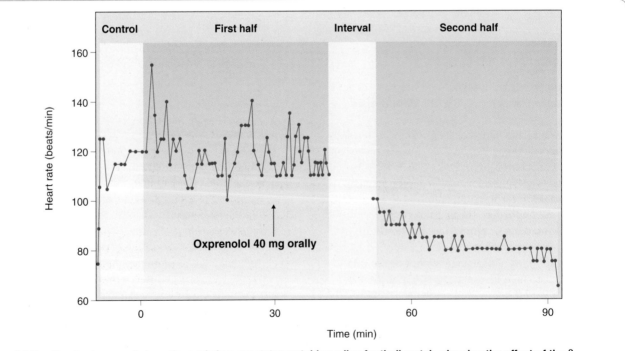

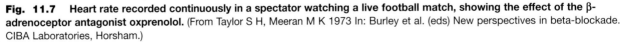

Fig. 11.7 Heart rate recorded continuously in a spectator watching a live football match, showing the effect of the β-adrenoceptor antagonist oxprenolol. (From Taylor S H, Meeran M K 1973 In: Burley et al. (eds) New perspectives in beta-blockade. CIBA Laboratories, Horsham.)

antagonist that also causes vasodilatation through an endothelium-dependent mechanism). Both of these drugs have proven more effective than conventional β-adrenoceptor antagonists in treating heart failure (see Ch. 18). The characteristics of the most important compounds are set out in Table 11.3. Most β-receptor antagonists are inactive on β_3-receptors so do not affect lipolysis.

Actions

The pharmacological actions of β-receptor antagonists can be deduced from Table 11.1. The effects produced in humans depend on the degree of sympathetic activity and are slight in subjects at rest. The most important effects are on the cardiovascular system and on bronchial smooth muscle (see Chs 19 and 23).

In a subject at rest, propranolol causes little change in heart rate, cardiac output or arterial pressure, but reduces the effect of exercise or excitement on these variables (Fig. 11.7). Drugs with partial agonist activity, such as oxprenolol, increase the heart rate at rest but reduce it during exercise. Maximum exercise tolerance is considerably reduced in normal subjects, partly because of the limitation of the cardiac response, and partly because the β-mediated vasodilatation in skeletal muscle is reduced. Coronary flow is reduced, but relatively less than the myocardial oxygen consumption, so oxygenation of the myocardium is improved, an effect of importance in the treatment of angina pectoris (see Ch. 18). In normal subjects, the reduction of the force of contraction of the heart is of no importance, but it may have serious consequences for patients with heart disease (see below).

An important, and somewhat unexpected, effect of β-receptor antagonists is their antihypertensive action (see Ch. 19). Patients with hypertension (although not normotensive subjects) show a gradual fall in arterial pressure that takes several days to develop fully. The mechanism is complex and involves the following:

- reduction in cardiac output
- reduction of renin release from the juxtaglomerular cells of the kidney
- a central action, reducing sympathetic activity.

Carvedilol and nebivolol (see above) are particularly effective in lowering blood pressure, because of their additional vasodilator properties.

Blockade of the facilitatory effect of presynaptic β-receptors on noradrenaline release (see Table 11.1) may also contribute to the antihypertensive effect. The antihypertensive effect of β-receptor antagonists is clinically very useful. Because reflex vasoconstriction is preserved, postural and exercise-induced hypotension (see Ch. 19) are less troublesome than with many other antihypertensive drugs.

Many β-receptor antagonists have an antidysrhythmic effect on the heart, which is of clinical importance (see Ch. 18).

Airways resistance in normal subjects is only slightly increased by β-receptor antagonists, and this is of no consequence. In asthmatic subjects, however, non-selective β-receptor antagonists (such as propranolol) can cause severe bronchoconstriction, which does not, of course, respond to the usual doses of drugs such as salbutamol or adrenaline. This danger is less with β_1-selective antagonists, but none are so selective that this danger can be ignored.

Despite the involvement of β-receptors in the hyperglycaemic actions of adrenaline, β-receptor antagonists cause only minor metabolic changes in normal subjects. They do not affect the onset of hypoglycaemia following an injection of insulin, but somewhat delay the recovery of blood glucose concentration. In diabetic patients, the use of β-receptor antagonists increases the likelihood of exercise-induced hypoglycaemia, because the normal adrenaline-induced release of glucose from the liver is diminished.

Clinical use

The main uses of β-receptor antagonists are connected with their effects on the cardiovascular system, and are discussed in Chapters 18 and 19. They are as summarised in the clinical box (p. 182).

The use of β-receptor antagonists in cardiac failure deserves special mention, as clinical opinion has undergone a U-turn in recent years. Patients with heart disease may rely on a degree of sympathetic drive to the heart to maintain an adequate cardiac output, and removal of this by blocking β receptors can exacerbate cardiac failure, so using these drugs in patients with cardiac failure was considered ill-advised. In theory, drugs with partial agonist activity (e.g. oxprenolol, alprenolol) offer an advantage because they can, by their own action, maintain a degree of β_1-receptor activation, while at the same time blunting the cardiac response to increased sympathetic nerve activity or to circulating adrenaline. Clinical trials, however, have not shown a clear advantage of these drugs measurable as a reduced incidence of cardiac failure.

Paradoxically, β-receptor antagonists are increasingly being used in low doses to *treat* cardiac failure, although at the outset there is a danger of exacerbating the problem. Several mechanisms may contribute, including inhibition of central sympathetic outflow, direct vasodilator effects (see review by Pfeffer & Stevenson, 1996), and prevention of cardiac hypertrophy by interference with signalling pathways other than the major cAMP pathway—a phenomenon still poorly understood. **Carvedilol** is often used for this purpose.

Unwanted effects

The main side effects of β-receptor antagonists result from their receptor-blocking action.

Bronchoconstriction. This is of little importance in the absence of airways disease, but in asthmatic patients the effect can be dramatic and life-threatening. It is also of clinical importance in patients with other forms of obstructive lung disease (e.g. chronic bronchitis, emphysema).

Cardiac depression. Cardiac depression can occur, leading to signs of heart failure, particularly in elderly people. Patients suffering from heart failure who are treated with β-receptor antagonists (see above) often deteriorate in the first few weeks before the beneficial effect develops.

Bradycardia. This side effect can lead to life-threatening heart block and can occur in patients with coronary disease, particularly if they are being treated with antiarrhythmic drugs that impair cardiac conduction (see Ch. 18).

Hypoglycaemia. Glucose release in response to adrenaline is a safety device that may be important to diabetic patients and to

Clinical uses of β-adrenoceptor antagonists

- Cardiovascular (see Chs 18 and 19):
  - *angina pectoris*
  - *myocardial infarction*
  - *dysrhythmias*
  - *heart failure*
  - *hypertension* (no longer first choice; Ch. 19)
- Other uses:
  - *glaucoma* (e.g. **timolol** eye drops)
  - *thyrotoxicosis* (Ch. 29), as adjunct to definitive treatment (e.g. preoperatively)
  - *anxiety* (Ch. 37), to control somatic symptoms (e.g. palpitations, tremor)
  - *migraine* prophylaxis (Ch. 12)
  - *benign essential tremor* (a familial disorder).

β-Adrenoceptor antagonists

- Non-selective between β₁ and β₂ adrenoceptors: **propranolol, alprenolol, oxprenolol**.
- β₁-selective: atenolol, nebivolol.
- **Alprenolol** and **oxprenolol** have partial agonist activity.
- Many clinical uses (see clinical box).
- Important hazards are bronchoconstriction, and bradycardia and cardiac failure (possibly less with partial agonists).
- Side effects include cold extremities, insomnia, depression, fatigue.
- Some show rapid first-pass metabolism, hence poor bioavailability.

other individuals prone to hypoglycaemic attacks. The sympathetic response to hypoglycaemia produces symptoms (especially tachycardia) that warn patients of the urgent need for carbohydrate (usually in the form of a sugary drink). β-Receptor antagonists reduce these symptoms, so incipient hypoglycaemia is more likely to go unnoticed by the patient. The use of β-receptor antagonists is generally to be avoided in patients with poorly controlled diabetes. There is a theoretical advantage in using β₁-selective agents, because glucose release from the liver is controlled by β₂-receptors.

Fatigue. This is probably due to reduced cardiac output and reduced muscle perfusion in exercise. It is a frequent complaint of patients taking β receptor–blocking drugs.

Cold extremities. These are presumably due to a loss of β-receptor–mediated vasodilatation in cutaneous vessels, and are a common side effect. Theoretically, β₁-selective drugs are less likely to produce this effect, but it is not clear that this is so in practice.

Other side effects associated with β-receptor antagonists are not obviously the result of β-receptor blockade. One is the occurrence of bad dreams, which occur mainly with highly lipid-soluble drugs such as propranolol, which enter the brain easily.

DRUGS THAT AFFECT NORADRENERGIC NEURONS

Emphasis in this chapter is placed on peripheral sympathetic transmission. The same principles, however, are applicable to the central nervous system (see Ch. 34), where many of the drugs mentioned here also act.

DRUGS THAT AFFECT NORADRENALINE SYNTHESIS

Only a few clinically important drugs affect noradrenaline synthesis directly. Examples are **α-methyltyrosine**, which inhibits tyrosine hydroxylase (used rarely to treat phaeochromacytoma), and **carbidopa**, a hydrazine derivative of dopa, which inhibits dopa decarboxylase and is used in the treatment of parkinsonism (see Ch. 35).

Methyldopa, a drug still used in the treatment of hypertension during pregnancy (see Ch. 19) is taken up by noradrenergic neurons, where it is converted to the false transmitter α-methylnoradrenaline. This substance is not deaminated within the neuron by MAO, so it accumulates and displaces noradrenaline from the synaptic vesicles. α-Methylnoradrenaline is released in the same way as noradrenaline, but is less active than noradrenaline on α₁-receptors and thus is less effective in causing vasoconstriction. On the other hand, it is more active on presynaptic (α₂) receptors, so the autoinhibitory feedback mechanism operates more strongly than normal, thus reducing transmitter release below the normal levels. Both of these effects (as well as a central effect, probably caused by the same cellular mechanism) contribute to the hypotensive action. It produces side effects typical of centrally acting antiadrenergic drugs (e.g. sedation), as well as carrying a risk of immune haemolytic reactions and liver toxicity, so it is now little used, except for hypertension in late pregnancy.

6-Hydroxydopamine (identical with dopamine except that it possesses an extra ring hydroxyl group) is a neurotoxin of the Trojan horse kind. It is taken up selectively by noradrenergic nerve terminals, where it is converted to a reactive quinone, which destroys the nerve terminal, producing a 'chemical sympathectomy'. The cell bodies survive, and eventually the sympathetic innervation recovers. The drug is useful for experimental purposes but has no clinical uses. If injected directly into the brain, it selectively destroys those nerve terminals (i.e. dopaminergic, noradrenergic and adrenergic) that take it up, but it does not reach the brain if given systemically. **MPTP** (1-methyl-4-phenyl-1,2,3,5-tetrahydropyridine; see Ch. 35) is a rather similar selective neurotoxin.

DRUGS THAT AFFECT NORADRENALINE STORAGE

Reserpine is an alkaloid from the shrub *Rauwolfia*, which has been used in India for centuries for the treatment of mental disorders. Reserpine, at very low concentration, blocks the transport of noradrenaline and other amines into synaptic vesicles, by blocking the vesicular monoamine transporter. Noradrenaline accumulates instead in the cytoplasm, where it is degraded by MAO. The noradrenaline content of tissues drops to a low level, and sympathetic transmission is blocked. Reserpine also causes depletion of 5-HT and dopamine from neurons in the brain, in which these amines are transmitters (see Ch. 34). Reserpine is now used only experimentally, but was at one time used as an antihypertensive drug. Its central effects, especially depression, which probably result from impairment of noradrenergic and 5-HT–mediated transmission in the brain (see Ch. 39) are a serious disadvantage.

DRUGS THAT AFFECT NORADRENALINE RELEASE

Drugs can affect noradrenaline release in four main ways:

- by directly blocking release (noradrenergic neuron–blocking drugs)
- by evoking noradrenaline release in the absence of nerve terminal depolarisation (indirectly acting sympathomimetic drugs)
- by interacting with presynaptic receptors that indirectly inhibit or enhance depolarisation-evoked release (e.g. α_2 agonists, angiotensin II, dopamine, and prostaglandins). Effects mediated through α_2-adrenoceptors are discussed elsewhere in this chapter; the other mechanisms are probably more important in the central than in the peripheral nervous system.
- by increasing or decreasing available stores of noradrenaline (e.g. reserpine, see above; MAO inhibitors, see Chapter 39).

NORADRENERGIC NEURON–BLOCKING DRUGS

Noradrenergic neuron–blocking drugs (e.g. **guanethidine**) were first discovered in the mid-1950s when alternatives to ganglion-blocking drugs, for use in the treatment of hypertension, were being sought. The main effect of guanethidine is to inhibit the release of noradrenaline from sympathetic nerve terminals. It has little effect on the adrenal medulla, and none on nerve terminals that release transmitters other than noradrenaline. Drugs very similar to it include **bretylium**, **bethanidine**, and **debrisoquin** (which is of interest mainly as a tool for studying drug metabolism; see Ch. 8).

Actions

Drugs of this class reduce or abolish the response of tissues to sympathetic nerve stimulation, but do not affect (or may potentiate) the effects of circulating noradrenaline.

The action of guanethidine on noradrenergic transmission is complex (see Broadley, 1996). It is selectively accumulated by noradrenergic nerve terminals, being a substrate for uptake 1. Its initial blocking activity is due to block of impulse conduction in the nerve terminals that selectively accumulate the drug. Its action is prevented by drugs, such as tricyclic antidepressants (see Ch. 39), which block uptake 1.

Guanethidine is also concentrated in synaptic vesicles by means of the vesicular transporter, possibly interfering with their ability

to undergo exocytosis, and also displacing noradrenaline. In this way, it causes a gradual and long-lasting depletion of noradrenaline in sympathetic nerve endings, similar to the effect of reserpine.

Given in large doses, guanethidine causes structural damage to noradrenergic neurons, which is probably due to the fact that the terminals accumulate the drug in high concentration. It can therefore be used experimentally as a selective neurotoxin.

Guanethidine, bethanidine and debrisoquin are no longer used clinically, now that better antihypertensive drugs are available. Although extremely effective in lowering blood pressure, they produce severe side effects associated with the loss of sympathetic reflexes. The most troublesome are postural hypotension, diarrhoea, nasal congestion and failure of ejaculation.

INDIRECTLY ACTING SYMPATHOMIMETIC AMINES

Mechanism of action and structure–activity relationships

The most important drugs in the indirectly acting sympathomimetic amine category are **tyramine**, **amphetamine** and **ephedrine**, which are structurally related to noradrenaline. Drugs that act similarly and are used for their central effects (see Ch. 42) include **methylphenidate** and **atomoxetine**.

These drugs have only weak actions on adrenoceptors, but sufficiently resemble noradrenaline to be transported into nerve terminals by uptake 1. Once inside the nerve terminals, they are taken up into the vesicles by the vesicular monoamine transporter, in exchange for noradrenaline, which escapes into the cytosol. Some of the cytosolic noradrenaline is degraded by MAO, while the rest escapes via uptake 1, in exchange for the foreign monoamine, to act on postsynaptic receptors (Fig. 11.8). Exocytosis is not involved in the release process, so their actions do not require the presence of Ca^{2+}. They are not completely specific in their actions, and act partly by a direct effect on adrenoceptors, partly by inhibiting uptake 1 (thereby enhancing the effect of the released noradrenaline), and partly by inhibiting MAO.

As would be expected, the effects of these drugs are strongly influenced by other drugs that modify noradrenergic transmission. Thus reserpine or 6-hydroxydopamine abolishes their effects by depleting the terminals of noradrenaline. MAO inhibitors, on the other hand, strongly potentiate their effects by preventing inactivation, within the terminals, of the transmitter displaced from the vesicles. MAO inhibition particularly enhances the action of **tyramine**, because this substance is itself a substrate for MAO. Normally, dietary tyramine is destroyed by MAO in the gut wall and liver before reaching the systemic circulation. When MAO is inhibited this is prevented, and ingestion of tyramine-rich foods such as fermented cheese (e.g. ripe Brie) can then provoke a sudden and dangerous rise in blood pressure. Inhibitors of uptake 1, such as **imipramine** (see below), interfere with the effects of indirectly acting sympathomimetic amines by preventing their uptake into the nerve terminals.

These drugs, especially amphetamine, have important effects on the central nervous system (see Ch. 39) that depend on their ability to release not only noradrenaline, but also 5-HT and dopamine from nerve terminals in the brain. An important

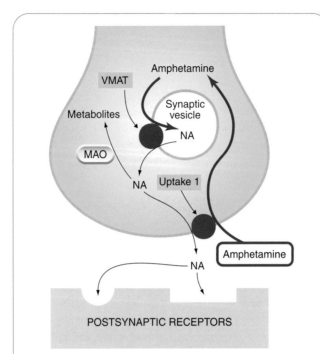

Fig. 11.8   The mode of action of amphetamine, an indirectly acting sympathomimetic amine. Amphetamine enters the nerve terminal via the noradrenaline (NA) transporter (uptake 1) and enters synaptic vesicles via the vesicular monoamine transporter (VMAT), in exchange for NA, which accumulates in the cytosol. Some of the NA is degraded by monoamine oxidase (MAO) within the nerve terminal and some escapes, in exchange for amphetamine via the noradrenaline transporter, to act on postsynaptic receptors. Amphetamine also reduces NA reuptake via the transporter, so enhancing the action of the released NA.

characteristic of the effects of indirectly acting sympathomimetic amines is that marked tolerance develops. Repeated doses of amphetamine or tyramine, for example, produce progressively smaller pressor responses. This is probably caused by a depletion of the releasable store of noradrenaline. A similar tolerance to the central effects also develops with repeated administration, which partly accounts for the liability of amphetamine and related drugs to cause dependence.

Actions

The peripheral actions of the indirectly acting sympathomimetic amines include bronchodilatation, raised arterial pressure, peripheral vasoconstriction, increased heart rate and force of myocardial contraction, and inhibition of gut motility. They have important central actions, which account for their significant abuse potential and for their limited therapeutic applications (see Chs 43 and 54). Apart from ephedrine, which is still sometimes used as a nasal decongestant because it has much less central action, these drugs are no longer used for their peripheral sympathomimetic effects.

> **Drugs acting on noradrenergic nerve terminals**
>
> - Drugs that inhibit noradrenaline synthesis include:
>   — **α-methyltyrosine**: blocks tyrosine hydroxylase; not used clinically
>   — **carbidopa**: blocks dopa decarboxylase and is used in treatment of parkinsonism (see Ch. 35); not much effect on noradrenaline synthesis.
> - **Methyldopa** gives rise to false transmitter (methylnoradrenaline), which is a potent α_2 agonist, thus causing powerful presynaptic inhibitory feedback (also central actions). Rarely used as antihypertensive agent.
> - **Reserpine** blocks carrier-mediated noradrenaline accumulation in vesicles, thus depleting noradrenaline stores and blocking transmission. Effective in hypertension but may cause severe depression. Clinically obsolete.
> - Noradrenergic neuron–blocking drugs (e.g. **guanethidine, bethanidine**) are selectively concentrated in terminals (uptake 1) and in vesicles (vesicular transporter), and block transmitter release, partly by local anaesthetic action. Effective in hypertension but cause severe side effects (postural hypotension, diarrhoea, nasal congestion, etc.), so now little used.
> - **6-Hydroxydopamine** is selectively neurotoxic for noradrenergic neurons, because it is taken up and converted to a toxic metabolite. Used experimentally to eliminate noradrenergic neurons, not clinically.
> - Indirectly acting sympathomimetic amines (e.g. **amphetamine, ephedrine, tyramine**) are accumulated by uptake 1 and displace noradrenaline from vesicles, allowing it to escape. Effect is much enhanced by monoamine oxidase (MAO) inhibition, which can lead to severe hypertension following ingestion of tyramine-rich foods by patients treated with MAO inhibitors.
> - Indirectly acting sympathomimetic agents are central nervous system stimulants. **Methylphenidate** and **atomoxetine** are used to treat attention deficit–hyperactivity disorder.
> - Drugs that inhibit uptake 1 include **cocaine** and **tricyclic antidepressant drugs**. Sympathetic effects are enhanced by such drugs.

INHIBITORS OF NORADRENALINE UPTAKE

Neuronal reuptake of released noradrenaline (uptake 1) is the most important mechanism by which its action is brought to an end. Many drugs inhibit this transport, and thereby enhance the effects of both sympathetic nerve activity and circulating noradrenaline.

Uptake 1 is not responsible for clearing circulating adrenaline, so these drugs do not affect responses to this amine.

The main class of drugs whose primary action is inhibition of uptake 1 are the **tricyclic antidepressants** (see Ch. 39), for example **desipramine**. These drugs have their major effect on the central nervous system but also cause tachycardia and cardiac dysrhythmias, reflecting their peripheral effect on sympathetic transmission. **Cocaine**, known mainly for its abuse liability (Ch. 43) and local anaesthetic activity (Ch. 44), enhances sympathetic transmission, causing tachycardia and increased arterial pressure. Its central effects of euphoria and excitement (Ch. 42) are probably a manifestation of the same mechanism acting in the brain. It strongly potentiates the actions of noradrenaline in experimental animals or in isolated tissues provided the sympathetic nerve terminals are intact.

Many drugs that act mainly on other steps in sympathetic transmission also inhibit uptake 1 to some extent, presumably because the carrier molecule has structural features in common with other noradrenaline recognition sites, such as receptors and degradative enzymes.

Extraneuronal uptake (uptake 2), which is important in clearing circulating adrenaline from the bloodstream, is not affected by most of the drugs that block uptake 1. It is inhibited by phenoxybenzamine, however, and also by various **corticosteroids** (see Ch. 14). This action of corticosteroids may have some relevance to their therapeutic effect in conditions such as asthma, but is probably of minor importance.

The main sites of action of drugs that affect adrenergic transmission are summarised in Figure 11.9.

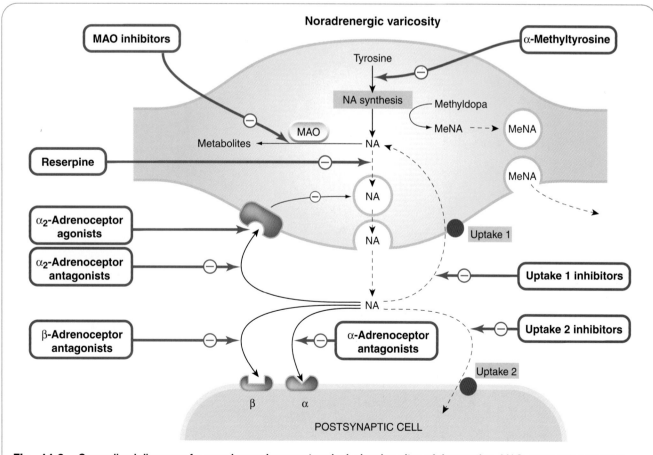

Fig. 11.9 Generalised diagram of a noradrenergic nerve terminal, showing sites of drug action. MAO, monoamine oxidase; MeNA, methylnoradrenaline; NA, noradrenaline.

Table 11.3 Summary of drugs that affect noradrenergic transmission

Type	Drug[a]	Main action	Uses/function	Unwanted effects	Pharmacokinetic aspects	Notes
Sympathomimetic (directly acting)	Norepinephrine[b]	α/β Agonist	Not used clinically Transmitter at postganglionic sympathetic neurons, and in CNS Hormone of adrenal medulla	Hypertension, vasoconstriction, tachycardia (or reflex bradycardia), ventricular dysrhythmias	Poorly absorbed by mouth Rapid removal by tissues Metabolised by MAO and COMT Plasma $t_{1/2}$ ~2 min	–
	Epinephrine[b]	α/β Agonist	Asthma (emergency treatment), anaphylactic shock, cardiac arrest Added to local anaesthetic solutions Main hormone of adrenal medulla	As norepinephrine	As norepinephrine Given i.m. or s.c.	See Chapter 23
	Isoproterenol	β Agonist (non-selective)	Asthma (obsolete) Not an endogenous substance	Tachycardia, dysrhythmias	Some tissue uptake, followed by inactivation (COMT) Plasma $t_{1/2}$ ~2 h	Now replaced by salbutamol in treatment of asthma (see Ch. 23)
	Dobutamine	β_1 Agonist (non-selective)	Cardiogenic shock	Dysrhythmias	Plasma $t_{1/2}$ ~2 min Given i.v.	Chapter 18
	Salbutamol	β_2 Agonist	Asthma, premature labour	Tachycardia, dysrhythmias, tremor, peripheral vasodilatation	Given orally or by aerosol Mainly excreted unchanged Plasma $t_{1/2}$ ~4 h	Chapter 23
	Salmeterol	β_2 Agonist	Asthma	As salbutamol	Given by aerosol Long acting	Formoterol is similar
	Terbutaline	β_2 Agonist	Asthma Delay of parturition	As salbutamol	Poorly absorbed orally Given by aerosol Mainly excreted unchanged Plasma $t_{1/2}$ ~4 h	Chapter 23
	Clenbuterol	β_2 Agonist	'Anabolic' action to increase muscle strength	As salbutamol	Active orally Long acting	Illicit use in sport
	Ritodrine	β_2 Agonist	Delay of parturition	As salbutamol	Poorly absorbed by mouth; given i.v.	Rarely used
	Phenylephrine	α_1 Agonist	Nasal decongestion	Hypertension, reflex bradycardia	Given intranasally Metabolised by MAO Short plasma $t_{1/2}$	–
	Methoxamine	α Agonist (non-selective)	Nasal decongestion	As phenylephrine	Given intranasally Plasma $t_{1/2}$ ~1 h	–
	Clonidine	α_2 Partial agonist	Hypertension, migraine	Drowsiness, orthostatic hypotension, oedema and weight gain, rebound hypertension	Well absorbed orally Excreted unchanged and as conjugate Plasma $t_{1/2}$ ~12 h	See Chapter 18
Sympathomimetic (indirectly acting)	Tyramine	NA release	No clinical uses Present in various foods	As norepinephrine	Normally destroyed by MAO in gut Does not enter brain	Chapter 39
	Amphetamine	NA release, MAO inhibitor, uptake 1 inhibitor, CNS stimulant	Used as CNS stimulant in narcolepsy, also (paradoxically) in hyperactive children Appetite suppressant Drug of abuse	Hypertension, tachycardia, insomnia Acute psychosis with overdose Dependence	Well absorbed orally Penetrates freely into brain Excreted unchanged in urine Plasma $t_{1/2}$ ~12 h, depending on urine flow and pH	Chapter 42 Methylphenidate and atomoxetine are similar (used for CNS effects; see Ch. 42)
	Ephedrine	NA release, β agonist, weak CNS stimulant	Nasal decongestion	As amphetamine but less pronounced	Similar to amphetamine	Contraindicated if MAO inhibitors are given

Table 11.3 (cont'd) Summary of drugs that affect noradrenergic transmission

Type	Drug[a]	Main action	Uses/function	Unwanted effects	Pharmacokinetic aspects	Notes
Adrenoceptor antagonists	Phenoxybenzamine	α Antagonist (non-selective, irreversible) Uptake 1 inhibitor	Phaeochromocytoma	Hypotension, flushing, tachycardia, nasal congestion, impotence	Absorbed orally Plasma $t_{1/2}$ ~12 h	Action outlasts presence of drug in plasma, because of covalent binding to receptor
	Phentolamine	α Antagonist (non-selective), vasodilator	Rarely used	As phenoxybenzamine	Usually given i.v. Metabolised by liver Plasma $t_{1/2}$ ~2 h	Tolazoline is similar
	Prazosin	α_1 Antagonist	Hypertension	As phenoxybenzamine	Absorbed orally Metabolised by liver Plasma $t_{1/2}$ ~4 h	Doxazosin, terazosin are similar but longer acting See Chapter 19
	Tamsulosin	α_1 Antagonist ('uroselective')	Prostatic hyperplasia	Failure of ejaculation	Absorbed orally Plasma $t_{1/2}$ ~5 h	Selective for α_{1A} adrenoceptor
	Yohimbine	α_2 Antagonist	Not used clinically Claimed to be aphrodisiac	Excitement, hypertension	Absorbed orally Metabolised by liver Plasma $t_{1/2}$ ~4 h	Idazoxan is similar
	Propranolol	β Antagonist (non-selective)	Angina, hypertension, cardiac dysrhythmias, anxiety tremor, glaucoma	Bronchoconstriction, cardiac failure, cold extremities, fatigue and depression, hypoglycaemia	Absorbed orally Extensive first-pass metabolism About 90% bound to plasma protein Plasma $t_{1/2}$ ~4 h	Timolol is similar and used mainly to treat glaucoma See Chapter 18
	Alprenolol	β Antagonist (non-selective) (partial agonist)	As propranolol	As propranolol	Absorbed orally Metabolised by liver Plasma $t_{1/2}$ ~4 h	Oxprenolol and pindolol are similar See Chapter 18
	Practolol	β_1 Antagonist	Hypertension, angina, dysrhythmias	As propranolol, also oculomucocutaneous syndrome	Absorbed orally Excreted unchanged in urine Plasma $t_{1/2}$ ~4 h	Withdrawn from clinical use
	Metoprolol	β_1 Antagonist	Angina, hypertension, dysrhythmias	As propranolol, less risk of bronchoconstriction	Absorbed orally Mainly metabolised in liver Plasma $t_{1/2}$ ~3 h	Atenolol is similar, with a longer half-life See Chapter 18
	Nebivolol	β_1 Antagonist Enhances nitric oxide–mediated transmission	Hypertension	Fatigue, headache	Absorbed orally $t_{1/2}$ ~10 h	–
	Butoxamine	β_2 Antagonist, weak α agonist	No clinical uses	–	–	–
	Labetalol	α/β Antagonist	Hypertension in pregnancy	Postural hypotension, brochoconstriction	Absorbed orally Conjugated in liver Plasma $t_{1/2}$ ~4 h	Chapters 18 and 19
	Carvedilol	α/β Antagonist	Heart failure	As for other β-blockers Initial exacerbation of heart failure Renal failure	Absorbed orally $t_{1/2}$ ~10 h	Additional actions may contribute to clinical benefit (Ch. 18)
Drugs affecting NA synthesis	α-Methyl-p-tyrosine	Inhibits tyrosine hydroxylase	Occasionally used in phaeochromocytoma	Hypotension, sedation	–	–
	Carbidopa	Inhibits dopa decarboxylase	Used as adjunct to levodopa to prevent peripheral effects	–	Absorbed orally Does not enter brain	Chapter 35
	Methyldopa	False transmitter precursor	Hypertension in pregnancy	Hypotension, drowsiness, diarrhoea, impotence, hypersensitivity reactions	Absorbed slowly by mouth Excreted unchanged or as conjugate Plasma $t_{1/2}$ ~6 h	Chapter 19

Table 11.3 (cont'd) Summary of drugs that affect noradrenergic transmission

Type	Drug[a]	Main action	Uses/function	Unwanted effects	Pharmacokinetic aspects	Notes
Drugs affecting NA release	Reserpine	Depletes NA stores by inhibiting vesicular uptake of NA	Hypertension (obsolete)	As methyldopa Also depression, parkinsonism, gynaecomastia	Poorly absorbed orally Slowly metabolised Plasma $t_{1/2}$ ~100 h Excreted in milk	Antihypertensive effect develops slowly and persists when drug is stopped
	Guanethidine	Inhibits NA release Also causes NA depletion and can damage NA neurons irreversibly	Hypertension (obsolete)	As methyldopa Hypertension on first administration	Poorly absorbed orally Mainly excreted unchanged in urine Plasma $t_{1/2}$ ~100 h	Action prevented by uptake 1 inhibitors Bethanidine and debrisoquin are similar
Drugs affecting NA uptake	Imipramine	Blocks uptake 1 Also has atropine-like action	Depression	Atropine-like side effects Cardiac dysrhythmias in overdose	Well absorbed orally 95% bound to plasma protein Converted to active metabolite (desmethylimipramine) Plasma $t_{1/2}$ ~4 h	Desipramine and amitriptyline are similar See Chapter 39
	Cocaine	Local anaesthetic; blocks uptake 1 CNS stimulant	Rarely used local anaesthetic Major drug of abuse	Hypertension, excitement, convulsions, dependence	Well absorbed orally or intranasally	See Chapters 42 and 53

COMT, catechol-*O*-methyltransferase; MAO, monoamine oxidase; NA, noradrenaline.

[a]For chemical structures, see Hardman J G, Limbird L E, Gilman A G, Goodman-Gilman A et al. 2001 Goodman and Gilman's pharmacological basis of therapeutics, 10th edn. McGraw-Hill, New York.

[b]Note that norepinephrine and epinephrine are the recommended drug names for noradrenaline and adrenaline, respectively.

REFERENCES AND FURTHER READING

General

Broadley K J 1996 Autonomic pharmacology. Taylor & Francis, London (*Detailed textbook*)

Cooper J R, Bloom F E, Roth R H 1996 The biochemical basis of neuropharmacology. Oxford University Press, New York (*Excellent standard textbook*)

Trendelenburg U, Weiner N 1988 Catecholamines. Handbook of experimental pharmacology, vol 90, parts 1 and 2. Springer-Verlag, Berlin (*Massive compilation of knowledge to date*)

Adrenoceptors

Baker J G, Hall I P, Hill S J 2003 Agonist and inverse agonist actions of β-blockers at the human β2-adrenoceptor provide evidence for agonist-directed signalling. Mol Pharmacol 64: 1357–1369 (*Recent studies showing that β-blockers differ in their ability to activate and block cAMP and mitogen-activated protein kinase pathways, possibly explaining why some are better than others in treating heart disease*)

Guimaraes S, Moura D 2001 Vascular adrenoceptors: an update. Pharmacol Rev 53: 319–356 (*Review describing the complex roles of different adrenoceptors in blood vessels*)

Insel P A 1996 Adrenergic receptors—evolving concepts and clinical implications. New Engl J Med 334: 580–585 (*Excellent review focusing on applications*)

Noradrenergic neurons

Bylund D B 1994 Nomenclature of adrenoceptors. Pharmacol Rev 46: 121–136 (*Rationalisation of the taxonomy of adrenoceptors*)

Cunnane T C 1984 The mechanism of neurotransmitter release from sympathetic nerves. Trends Neurosci 7: 248–253 (*Points out important differences between adrenergic and cholinergic neurons*)

Elenkov I J, Wilder R L, Chrousos G P, Vizi E S 2000 The sympathetic nerve—an integrative interface between two supersystems: the brain and the immune system. Pharmacol Rev 52: 595–638 (*Detailed catalogue of effects of catecholamines and the sympathetic nervous system on the immune system*)

Gainetdinov R R, Caron M G 2003 Monoamine transporters: from genes to behaviour. Annu Rev Pharmacol Toxicol 43: 261–284 (*Review article focusing on the characteristics of transgenic mice lacking specific monoamine transporters*)

Liu Y, Edwards R H 1997 The role of vesicular transport proteins in synaptic transmission and neural degeneration. Annu Rev Neurosci 20: 125–156 (*Review of recent ideas about the functional role of transporters*)

Lundberg J M 1996 Pharmacology of co-transmission in the autonomic nervous system: integrative aspects on amines, neuropeptides, adenosine triphosphate, amino acids and nitric oxide. Pharmacol Rev 48: 114–192 (*Comprehensive and informative review*)

Starke K, Göthert M, Kilbinger H 1989 Modulation of transmitter release by presynaptic autoreceptors. Physiol Rev 69: 864–989 (*Comprehensive review*)

Miscellaneous topics

Eisenhofer G, Kopin I J, Goldstein D S 2004 Catecholamine metabolism: a contemporary view with implications for physiology and medicine. Pharmacol Rev 56: 331–349 (*Review that dismisses a number of fallacies concerning the routes by which catecholamines from different sources are metabolised and excreted*)

Nonogaki K 2000 New insights into sympathetic regulation of glucose and fat metabolism. Diabetologia 43: 533–549 (*Review of the complex adrenoceptor-mediated effects on the metabolism of liver muscle and adipose tissue; up to date, but not a particularly easy read*)

Pfeffer M A, Stevenson L W 1996 β-adrenergic blockers and survival in heart failure. New Engl J Med 334: 1396–1397 (*Shows that β-adrenergic blockers in low doses can be beneficial in heart failure*)

Zhang K-M, Hu P, Wang S-W et al. 1996 Salbutamol changes the molecular and mechanical properties of canine skeletal muscle. J Physiol 496: 211–220 (*Surprising finding that salbutamol affects muscle function by non-receptor mechanisms*)

Other peripheral mediators: 5-hydroxytryptamine and purines

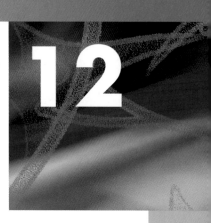

12

OVERVIEW

In this chapter, we discuss two types of mediator, both of which play a role as neurotransmitters in the brain and periphery and also function as local hormones. 5-Hydroxytryptamine (5-HT) has a longer pharmacological history than purines (nucleosides and nucleotides), and numerous drugs in current use act wholly or partly on 5-HT receptors, of which no fewer than 15 subtypes have been identified. Purine pharmacology is currently a less well-exploited area, but this is changing and there is increasing interest in the potential role of purinergic agents in the treatment of thrombotic and respiratory disorders. In the case of both mediators, the physiological significance— and hence therapeutic relevance—of the various receptor subtypes is still being unravelled. In our discussion, therefore, we will focus on the more secure hypotheses, recognising that the overall picture is far from complete. Useful reviews include Burnstock (2002) and Gershon (2004).

5-HYDROXYTRYPTAMINE

Serotonin was the name given to an unknown vasoconstrictor substance found in the serum after blood had clotted. It was identified chemically as 5-hydroxytryptamine in 1948 and shown to originate from platelets. It was subsequently found in the gastrointestinal tract and central nervous system (CNS), and shown to function both as a neurotransmitter and as a local hormone in the peripheral vascular system. This chapter deals with the metabolism, distribution and possible physiological roles of 5-HT in the periphery, and with the different types of 5-HT receptor and the drugs that act on them. Further information on the role of 5-HT in the brain, and its relationship to psychiatric disorders and the actions of psychotropic drugs, is presented in Chapters 32, 38 and 39. The use of drugs that modulate 5-HT in the gut is dealt with in Chapter 25.

DISTRIBUTION, BIOSYNTHESIS AND DEGRADATION

5-Hydroxytryptamine occurs in the highest concentrations in three organs.

- *In the wall of the intestine.* Over 90% of the total amount in the body is present in the *enterochromaffin* cells in the gut (endocrine cells with distinctive staining properties). These are cells derived from the neural crest and resemble those of the adrenal medulla. They are interspersed with mucosal cells, mainly in the stomach and small intestine. Some 5-HT also occurs in nerve cells of the myenteric plexus, where it functions as an excitatory neurotransmitter (see Chs 9 and 25).
- *In blood.* 5-HT is present in high concentrations in platelets, which accumulate it from the plasma by an active transport system and release it when they aggregate at sites of tissue damage (see Ch. 21).
- *In the CNS.* 5-HT is a transmitter in the CNS and is present in high concentrations in localised regions of the midbrain. Its functional role is discussed in Chapter 34.

Although 5-HT is present in the diet, most of this is metabolised before entering the bloodstream. Endogenous 5-HT arises from a biosynthetic pathway similar to that which generates noradrenaline (norepinephrine; see Ch. 11), except that the precursor amino acid is *tryptophan* instead of tyrosine (Fig. 12.1). Tryptophan is converted to 5-hydroxytryptophan (in chromaffin cells and neurons, but not in platelets) by the action of *tryptophan hydroxylase*, an enzyme confined to 5-HT–producing cells. The 5-hydroxytryptophan is then decarboxylated to 5-HT by a ubiquitous *amino acid decarboxylase* that also participates in the synthesis of catecholamines (Ch. 11) and histamine (Ch. 13).

Platelets (and neurons) possess a high-affinity 5-HT uptake mechanism, and platelets become loaded with 5-HT as they pass through the intestinal circulation, where the local concentration is relatively high. The mechanisms of synthesis, storage, release and reuptake of 5-HT are very similar to those of noradrenaline. Many drugs affect both processes indiscriminately (see Ch. 11), but selective serotonin reuptake inhibitors have been developed and are important therapeutically as antidepressants (Ch. 39). 5-HT is often stored in neurons and chromaffin cells as a cotransmitter together with various peptide hormones, such as *somatostatin*, *substance P* or *vasoactive intestinal polypeptide*.

Degradation of 5-HT (Fig. 12.1) occurs mainly through oxidative deamination, catalysed by *monoamine oxidase*, followed by oxidation to *5-hydroxyindoleacetic acid (5-HIAA)*, the pathway being the same as that of noradrenaline catabolism. 5-HIAA is excreted in the urine and serves as an indicator of 5-HT production in the body. This is used, for example, in the diagnosis of *carcinoid syndrome* (see below).

PHARMACOLOGICAL EFFECTS

The actions of 5-HT are numerous and complex, and there is considerable species variation. This complexity reflects a profusion of 5-HT receptor subtypes, which has been revealed in recent years (see below). The main sites of action are as follows.

Gastrointestinal tract. 5-HT subserves complex and important roles in the regulation of gastrointestinal function (see Gershon, 2004). Only about 10% of 5-HT in the intestine is located in neurons, where it acts as a neurotransmitter, while the remainder is located in the enterochromaffin cells, which act as sensors to transduce information about the state of the gut. The 5-HT is released from enterochromaffin cells into the *lamina propria*, where it stimulates receptors located on enteric neurons. Acting at 5-HT$_{1B}$ receptors, 5-HT initiates secretory and peristaltic reflexes. Stimulation of presynaptic 5-HT$_4$ receptors amplifies neurotransmission in some enteric neurons, resulting in increased

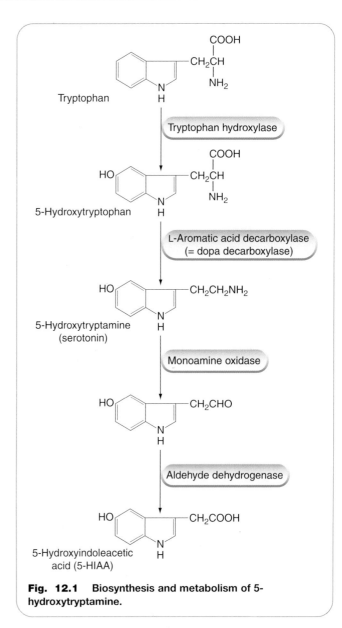

Fig. 12.1 Biosynthesis and metabolism of 5-hydroxytryptamine.

Distribution, biosynthesis and degradation of 5-hydroxytryptamine

- Tissues rich in 5-HT are:
  - gastrointestinal tract (chromaffin cells and enteric neurons)
  - platelets
  - central nervous system.
- Metabolism closely parallels that of noradrenaline.
- 5-HT is formed from dietary tryptophan, which is converted to 5-hydroxytryptophan by tryptophan hydroxylase, then to 5-HT by a non-specific decarboxylase.
- 5-HT is transported into cells by a specific transport system.
- Degradation occurs mainly by monoamine oxidase, forming 5-hydroxyindoleacetic acid (5-HIAA), which is excreted in urine.

prokinetic activity in the gut, and may also play a part in the regulation of colonic motility. Stimulation of 5-HT$_3$ receptors slows motility and mediates the neurotransmission involved in sensory perception of the gut by the CNS.

The importance of 5-HT in the gut is underlined by the widespread distribution of the *serotonin uptake transporter*, which rapidly and efficiently removes released 5-HT, limiting its action. Back-up transporters have also been identified. Interestingly, there is evidence for defects in this reuptake system in irritable bowel syndrome (Ch. 25), which might explain the rather bewildering symptoms of the disease.

Smooth muscle. In many species (although only to a minor extent in humans), smooth muscle (e.g. uterus and bronchial tree) is contracted by 5-HT.

Blood vessels. The effect of 5-HT on blood vessels depends on various factors, including the size of the vessel, the species and the prevailing sympathetic activity. Large vessels, both arteries and veins, are usually constricted by 5-HT, although the sensitivity varies greatly. This is a direct action on vascular smooth muscle cells, mediated through 5-HT$_{2A}$ receptors (see below). Activation of 5-HT$_1$ receptors causes constriction of large intracranial vessels, dilatation of which contributes to headache (see below). 5-HT can also cause vasodilatation, partly by acting on endothelial cells to release nitric oxide (see Ch. 17) and partly by inhibiting noradrenaline release from sympathetic nerve terminals. If 5-HT is injected intravenously, the blood pressure usually first rises, owing to the constriction of large vessels, and then falls, owing to arteriolar dilatation.

Platelets. 5-HT causes platelet aggregation (see Ch. 21) by acting on 5-HT$_{2A}$ receptors, and the platelets that collect in the vessel release further 5-HT. If the endothelium is intact, 5-HT release from adherent platelets causes vasodilatation, which helps to sustain blood flow; if it is damaged (e.g. by atherosclerosis), 5-HT causes constriction and impairs blood flow further. These effects of platelet-derived 5-HT are thought to be important in vascular disease.

Nerve endings. 5-HT stimulates nociceptive (pain-mediating) sensory nerve endings, an effect mediated mainly by 5-HT$_3$ receptors. If injected into the skin, 5-HT causes pain; when given systemically, it elicits a variety of autonomic reflexes through stimulation of afferent fibres in the heart and lungs, which further complicate the cardiovascular response. Nettle stings contain 5-HT among other mediators. 5-HT also inhibits transmitter release from adrenergic neurons in the periphery.

Central nervous system. 5-HT excites some neurons and inhibits others; it may also act presynaptically to inhibit transmitter release from nerve terminals. Different receptor subtypes and different membrane mechanisms mediate these effects (see Table 12.1; Barnes & Sharp, 1999; Branchek & Blackburn, 2000). The role of 5-HT in the CNS is discussed in Chapter 34.

CLASSIFICATION OF 5-HT RECEPTORS

▼ It was long ago realised that the actions of 5-HT are not all mediated by receptors of the same type, and various pharmacological classifications have come and gone. The current system (Hoyer et al., 1994) was agreed after long deliberation at a summit meeting of 5-HT aficionados and delivered, with puffs of white smoke and much celebration, in 1992. It is summarised in Table 12.1. This classification takes into account sequence data derived from cloning, signal transduction mechanisms and pharmacological specificity. Their diversity is astonishing. Currently, there are 15 known receptor subtypes (see Kroeze et al., 2002). These are divided into seven classes (5-HT$_{1-7}$), one of which (5-HT$_3$) is a ligand-gated ion channel and the remainder G-protein–coupled receptors (GPCRs; see Ch. 3). The six GPCR families are further subdivided into 13 receptor types based on their sequence and pharmacology. Most subtypes are found in all species so far examined, but there are some exceptions (5-HT$_{5B}$ is found in mouse but probably does not exist in humans) and the GPCR structures are highly conserved. The most common second messenger appears to be cAMP produced by activation of adenylate cyclase, but some members (the 5-HT$_2$ subtype) activate phospholipase C to generate phospholipid-derived second messengers (see Ch. 3).

Transgenic mice lacking some functional members of this receptor family have been produced (see for example Bonasera & Tecott, 2000). The functional deficits in such animals are generally quite subtle, suggesting that these receptors may serve to tune, rather than to enable, physiological

responses. Table 12.1 gives an overview of the most important receptors. Some of the more significant drug targets include the following.

5-HT$_1$ receptors. These occur mainly in the brain, the subtypes being distinguished on the basis of their regional distribution and their pharmacological specificity. They function mainly as inhibitory presynaptic receptors and are linked to inhibition of adenylate cyclase. The 5-HT$_{1A}$ subtype is particularly important in the brain, in relation to mood and behaviour (see Chs 37–39). The 5-HT$_{1D}$ subtype, which is expressed in cerebral blood vessels, is believed to be important in migraine (see below) and is the target for **sumatriptan**, an agonist used to treat acute attacks. The cerebral vessels are unusual in that vasoconstriction is mediated by 5-HT$_1$ receptors; in most vessels, 5-HT$_2$ receptors are responsible. The hapless '5-HT$_{1C}$' receptor—actually the first to be cloned —has been officially declared non-existent, having been ignominiously reclassified as the 5-HT$_{2C}$ receptor when it was found to be linked to inositol trisphosphate production rather than adenylate cyclase.

5-HT$_2$ receptors. These are particularly important in the periphery. The effects of 5-HT on smooth muscle and platelets, which have been known for many years, are mediated by the 5-HT$_{2A}$ receptor, as are some of the behavioural effects of agents such as *lysergic acid diethylamide* (LSD; see Table 12.1 and Ch. 42). 5-HT$_2$ receptors are linked to phospholipase C and thus stimulate inositol trisphosphate formation. The 5-HT$_{2A}$ subtype is functionally the most important, the others having a much more limited distribution and functional role. The role of 5-HT$_2$ receptors in normal physiological processes is probably a minor one, but it becomes more prominent in pathological conditions such as asthma and vascular thrombosis (see Chs 21–23).

Actions and functions of 5-hydroxytryptamine

- Important actions are:
  - increased gastrointestinal motility (direct excitation of smooth muscle and indirect action via enteric neurons)
  - contraction of other smooth muscle (bronchi, uterus)
  - mixture of vascular constriction (direct and via sympathetic innervation) and dilatation (endothelium-dependent)
  - platelet aggregation
  - stimulation of peripheral nociceptive nerve endings
  - excitation/inhibition of central nervous system neurons.
- Postulated physiological and pathophysiological roles include:
  - in periphery: peristalsis, vomiting, platelet aggregation and haemostasis, inflammatory mediator, sensitisation of nociceptors and microvascular control
  - in CNS: many postulated functions, including control of appetite, sleep, mood, hallucinations, stereotyped behaviour, pain perception and vomiting.
- Clinical conditions associated with disturbed 5-hydroxytryptamine function include migraine, carcinoid syndrome, mood disorders and anxiety.

Table 12.1   The main 5-HT receptor subtypes[a]

Receptor	Location	Main effects	Second messenger	Agonists	Antagonists
1A	CNS	Neuronal inhibition Behavioural effects: sleep, feeding, thermoregulation, anxiety	↓ cAMP	5-CT 8-OH-DPAT Buspirone (PA)	Spiperone Methiothepin Ergotamine (PA)
1B	CNS Vascular smooth muscle	Presynaptic inhibition Behavioural effects Pulmonary vasoconstriction	↓ cAMP	5-CT Ergotamine (PA)	Methiothepin
1D	CNS Blood vessels	Cerebral vasoconstriction Behavioural effects: locomotion	↓ cAMP	5-CT Sumatriptan	Methiothepin Ergotamine (PA)
2A	CNS PNS Smooth muscle Platelets	Neuronal excitation Behavioural effects Smooth muscle contraction (gut, bronchi, etc.) Platelet aggregation Vasoconstriction/vasodilatation	↑ IP$_3$/DAG	α-Me-5-HT LSD (CNS) LSD (periphery)	Ketanserin Cyproheptadine Pizotifen (non-selective) Methysergide
2B	Gastric fundus	Contraction	↑ IP$_3$/DAG	α-Me-5-HT	–
2C	CNS Choroid plexus	Cerebrospinal fluid secretion	↑ IP$_3$/DAG	α-Me-5-HT LSD	Methysergide
3	PNS CNS	Neuronal excitation (autonomic, nociceptive neurons) Emesis Behavioural effects: anxiety	None—ligand-gated cation channel	2-Me-5-HT Chlorophenyl-biguanide	Ondansetron Tropisetron Granisetron
4	PNS (GI tract) CNS	Neuronal excitation GI motility	↑ cAMP	5-Methoxy-tryptamine Metoclopramide Tegaserod	Various experimental compounds (e.g. GR113808, SB207266)
5	CNS	Not known	Not known	Not known	Not known
6	CNS	Not known	Not known	Not known	Not known
7	CNS GI tract Blood vessels	Not known	↑ cAMP	5-CT LSD No selective agonists	Various 5-HT$_2$ antagonists No selective antagonists

2-Me-5-HT, 2-methyl-5-hydroxytrypamine; 5-CT, 5-carboxamidotryptamine; 8-OH-DPAT, 8-hydroxy-2-(di-*n*-propylamino) tetraline; CNS, central nervous system; DAG, diacylglycerol; GI, gastrointestinal; IP$_3$, inositol trisphosphate; LSD, lysergic acid diethylamide; PA, partial agonist; PNS, peripheral nervous system; α-Me-5-HT, α-methyl 5-hydroxytrypamine.
[a]For further details, see Hoyer et al. (1994). The list of agonists and antagonists includes only the better known compounds. Many new selective 5-HT receptor ligands, known only by code numbers, are being developed.

5-HT$_3$ receptors. These occur mainly in the peripheral nervous system, particularly on nociceptive sensory neurons (see Ch. 41) and on autonomic and enteric neurons, where 5-HT exerts a strong excitatory effect. 5-HT itself evokes pain when injected locally; when given intravenously, it elicits a fine display of autonomic reflexes, which result from excitation of many types of vascular, pulmonary and cardiac sensory nerve fibres. 5-HT$_3$ receptors also occur in the brain, particularly in the *area postrema*, a region of the medulla involved in the vomiting reflex, and selective 5-HT$_3$ antagonists are used as antiemetic drugs (see Ch. 25). 5-HT$_3$ receptors are exceptional in being directly linked to membrane ion channels (Ch. 3) and cause excitation directly, without involvement of any second messenger.

5-HT$_4$ receptors. These occur in the brain, as well as in peripheral organs such as the gastrointestinal tract, bladder and heart. Their main physiological role appears to be in the gastrointestinal tract, where they produce neuronal excitation and mediate the effect of 5-HT in stimulating peristalsis.

DRUGS ACTING ON 5-HT RECEPTORS

Table 12.1 lists some of the agonists and antagonists for the different receptor types. Many are only partly selective. The improved understanding of the location and function of the different

5-Hydroxytryptamine receptors

- There are seven types ($5\text{-}HT_{1-7}$), with further subtypes of $5\text{-}HT_1$ (A–F) and $5\text{-}HT_2$ (A–C). All are G-protein–coupled receptors, except $5\text{-}HT_3$, which is a ligand-gated cation channel.
- *$5\text{-}HT_1$ receptors* occur mainly in central nervous system (CNS) (all subtypes) and some blood vessels ($5\text{-}HT_{1D}$ subtype). Effects, mediated through inhibition of adenylate cyclase, are neural inhibition and vasoconstriction. Specific agonists include sumatriptan (used in migraine therapy) and buspirone (used in anxiety). Ergotamine is a partial agonist. Specific antagonists include spiperone and methiothepin.
- *$5\text{-}HT_2$ receptors* occur in CNS and many peripheral sites (especially blood vessels, platelets, autonomic neurons). Neuronal and smooth muscle effects are excitatory. Some blood vessels dilated as a result of nitric oxide release from endothelial cells. $5\text{-}HT_2$ receptors act through the phospholipase C/inositol trisphosphate pathway. Specific ligands include lysergic acid diethylamide (LSD; agonist in CNS, antagonist in periphery). Specific antagonists are ketanserin, methysergide and cyproheptadine.
- *$5\text{-}HT_3$ receptors* occur in peripheral nervous system, especially nociceptive afferent neurons and enteric neurons, and in CNS. Effects are excitatory, mediated through direct receptor-coupled ion channels. Specific agonist is 2-methyl-5-HT. Specific antagonists include ondansetron and tropisetron. Antagonists are used mainly as antiemetic drugs but may also be anxiolytic.
- *$5\text{-}HT_4$ receptors* occur mainly in the enteric nervous system (also in CNS). Effects are excitatory, through stimulation of adenylate cyclase, causing increased gastrointestinal motility. Specific agonists include metoclopramide (used to stimulate gastric emptying).
- Little is known so far about the function and pharmacology of *$5\text{-}HT_{5-7}$ receptors*.

receptor subtypes has, however, caused an upsurge of interest in developing compounds with improved receptor selectivity, and useful new drugs are likely to appear in the near future.

Important drugs that act on 5-HT receptors in the periphery include the following.

- Selective $5\text{-}HT_{1A}$ agonists, such as 8-hydroxy-2-(di-*n*-propylamino) tetralin (Table 12.1), are potent hypotensive agents, acting by a central mechanism, but are not used clinically.
- $5\text{-}HT_{1D}$ receptor agonists (e.g. sumatriptan) used for treating migraine (see below).
- $5\text{-}HT_2$ receptor antagonists (e.g. **dihydroergotamine, methysergide, cyproheptadine, ketanserin, ketotifen,**

pizotifen) act mainly on $5\text{-}HT_2$ receptors but also block other 5-HT receptors, as well as α adrenoceptors and histamine receptors (Ch. 14). Dihydroergotamine and methysergide belong to the ergot family (see below) and are used mainly for migraine prophylaxis. Other $5\text{-}HT_2$ antagonists are used to control the symptoms of carcinoid tumours.
- $5\text{-}HT_3$ receptor antagonists (e.g. **ondansetron, granisetron, tropisetron**) are used as antiemetic drugs (see Chs 25 and 51), particularly for controlling the severe nausea and vomiting that occurs with many forms of cancer chemotherapy.
- $5\text{-}HT_4$ receptor agonists, which stimulate coordinated peristaltic activity (known as a 'prokinetic action'), are used for treating gastrointestinal disorders (see Ch. 25). **Metoclopramide** acts in this way, although it also affects dopamine receptors. The new drug **tegaserod** is more selective and is used to treat irritable bowel syndrome.

5-HT is also important as a neurotransmitter in the CNS, and several important antipsychotic and antidepressant drugs owe their actions to effects on these pathways (see Chs 34, 38 and 39). LSD is a relatively non-selective 5-HT receptor agonist or partial agonist, which acts centrally as a potent hallucinogen (see Ch. 42).

ERGOT ALKALOIDS

Ergot alkaloids constitute a hard-to-classify group of drugs that have preoccupied pharmacologists for more than a century. Many of them act on 5-HT receptors, but not selectively, and their actions are complex and diverse.

▼ Ergot contains many active substances, and it was the study of their pharmacological properties that led Dale to many important discoveries concerning acetylcholine, histamine and catecholamines. Ergot alkaloids occur naturally in a fungus (*Claviceps purpurea*) that infests cereal crops. Epidemics of ergot poisoning have occurred, and still occur, when contaminated grain is used for food. The symptoms produced include mental disturbances and intensely painful peripheral vasoconstriction leading to gangrene. This came to be known in the Middle Ages as *St Anthony's fire*, because it was believed that it could be cured by a visit to the Shrine of St Anthony (which happened to be in an ergot-free region of France).

Ergot alkaloids are complex molecules based on lysergic acid (a naturally occurring tetracyclic alkaloid). The important members of the group (Table 12.2) include various naturally occurring and synthetic derivatives with different substituent groups arranged around a basic nucleus. These compounds display many different types of pharmacological action, and it is difficult to discern any clear relationship between chemical structure and pharmacological properties.

Actions

Most of the effects of ergot alkaloids appear to be mediated through adrenoceptors, 5-HT or dopamine receptors (Table 12.2), although some effects may be produced through other mechanisms. All alkaloids stimulate smooth muscle, some being relatively selective for vascular smooth muscle while others act mainly on the uterus. **Ergotamine** and dihydroergotamine are, respectively, a partial agonist and an antagonist at α adrenoceptors. **Bromocriptine** is an agonist on dopamine receptors,

Table 12.2 Properties of ergot alkaloids

Drug	5-HT receptor	α Adrenoceptor	Dopamine receptor	Uterine contraction	Main uses	Side effects etc.
Ergotamine	Antagonist/partial agonist (5-HT$_1$)	Partial agonist (blood vessels) Antagonist (other sites)	Inactive	++	Migraine	Emesis Vasoconstriction (avoid in peripheral vascular disease) Avoid in pregnancy
Dihydroergotamine	Antagonist/partial agonist (5-HT$_1$)	Antagonist	Inactive	+	Migraine (largely obsolete)	Less emesis than with ergotamine
Ergometrine	Antagonist/partial agonist (5-HT$_1$) (weak)	Weak antagonist/ partial agonist	Weak	+++	Prevention of postpartum haemorrhage	–
Bromocriptine	Inactive	Weak antagonist	Agonist/partial agonist	–	Parkinson's disease (Ch. 35) Endocrine disorders (Ch. 28)	Emesis
Methylsergide	Antagonist/partial agonist (5-HT$_2$)	–	–	–	Carcinoid syndrome Migraine (prophylaxis)	Retroperitoneal and mediastinal fibrosis Emesis

particularly in the CNS (Ch. 28), and methysergide is an antagonist at 5-HT$_2$ receptors.

The main pharmacological actions and uses of these drugs are summarised in Table 12.2. As one would expect of drugs with so many actions, their physiological effects are complex and rather poorly understood. Ergotamine, dihydroergotamine and methysergide are discussed here; further information on **ergometrine** and bromocriptine is given in Chapters 28, 30 and 35.

Vascular effects. When injected into an anaesthetised animal, ergotamine activates α adrenoceptors, causing vasoconstriction and a sustained rise in blood pressure. At the same time, ergotamine reverses the pressor effect of **adrenaline** (**epinephrine**; see Ch. 9). The vasoconstrictor effect of ergotamine is responsible for the peripheral gangrene of St Anthony's fire, and probably also for some of the effects of **ergot** on the CNS. Methysergide and dihydroergotamine have much less vasoconstrictor effect. Methysergide is a potent 5-HT$_2$ receptor antagonist, whereas ergotamine and dihydroergotamine act selectively on 5-HT$_1$ receptors. Although generally classified as antagonists, they show partial agonist activity in some tissues, and this may account for their activity in treating migraine attacks (see below).

Clinical use. The only use of ergotamine is in the treatment of attacks of migraine unresponsive to simple analgesics (see below). Methysergide is occasionally used for migraine prophylaxis, but its main use is in treating the symptoms of carcinoid tumours (see below). All these drugs can be used orally or by injection.

Unwanted effects. Ergotamine often causes nausea and vomiting, and it must be avoided in patients with peripheral vascular disease because of its vasoconstrictor action. Methysergide also causes nausea and vomiting, but its most serious side effect,

which considerably restricts its clinical usefulness, is retroperitoneal and mediastinal fibrosis, which impairs the functioning of the gastrointestinal tract, kidneys, heart and lungs. The mechanism of this is unknown, but it is noteworthy that similar fibrotic reactions also occur in carcinoid syndrome (see below) in which there is a high circulating level of 5-HT.

Ergot alkaloids

- These active substances are produced by a fungus that infects cereal crops; it is responsible for occasional poisoning incidents. The most important compounds are:
  — ergotamine, dihydroergotamine, used in migraine
  — ergometrine, used in obstetrics to prevent postpartum haemorrhage
  — methysergide, used to treat carcinoid syndrome, and occasionally for migraine prophylaxis
  — bromocriptine, used in parkinsonism and endocrine disorders.
- Main sites of action are 5-HT receptors, dopamine receptors and adrenoceptors (mixed agonist, antagonist and partial agonist effects).
- Unwanted effects include nausea and vomiting, vasoconstriction (ergot alkaloids are contraindicated in patients with peripheral vascular disease).

CLINICAL CONDITIONS IN WHICH 5-HT PLAYS A ROLE

In this section, we discuss two situations in which the peripheral actions of 5-HT are believed to be important, namely migraine and carcinoid syndrome. Further information may be found in Houston & Vanhoutte (1986). The use of 5-HT$_3$ antagonists in treating drug-induced emesis are discussed in Chapter 25. Modulation of 5-HT-mediated transmission in the CNS is an important mechanism of action of antidepressant and antipsychotic drugs (see Chs 34, 38 and 39).

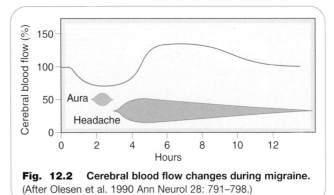

Fig. 12.2 **Cerebral blood flow changes during migraine.** (After Olesen et al. 1990 Ann Neurol 28: 791–798.)

MIGRAINE AND ANTIMIGRAINE DRUGS

Migraine is a common and debilitating condition affecting 10–15% of people, although the causes are not well understood (see Moskowitz, 1992; Edvinsson, 1999; Villalon et al., 2003). A 'textbook' migraine attack consists of an initial visual disturbance (the *aura*), in which a flickering pattern, followed by a blind spot (a 'scintillating scotoma'), progresses gradually across an area of the visual field. This visual disturbance is followed, about 30 minutes later, by a severe throbbing headache, starting unilaterally, often accompanied by photophobia, nausea, vomiting and prostration, which lasts for several hours. In fact, the visual aura occurs only in about 20% of migraine sufferers, although many experience other kinds of premonitory sensation. Sometimes attacks are precipitated by particular foods or by visual stimuli, but more often they occur without obvious cause.

Pathophysiology

Although controversy abounds and opinions vary, there are three fundamental views of the physiological mechanisms underlying migraine, linking it to primary events in blood vessels, the brain or sensory nerves.

The classic *'vascular' theory*, first proposed around 50 years ago by Wolff, implicated an initial humorally mediated intracerebral vasoconstriction causing the aura, followed by an extracerebral vasodilatation causing the headache. This venerable hypothesis has not, however, been generally supported by more recent blood flow studies involving non-invasive monitoring techniques in patients with migraine (see review by Friberg, 1999). In episodes of migraine with aura, there is indeed a biphasic change in cerebral blood flow (Fig. 12.2), with a reduction of 20–30% preceding the premonitory aura, followed by a highly variable increase of similar magnitude. However, the headache usually begins during the initial vasoconstrictor phase, and blood flow changes of similar magnitude caused by other factors do not produce symptoms. The vasoconstriction starts posteriorly and gradually spreads forwards over the hemisphere, implying a neural rather than a humoral cause. These changes occur only in association with an aura and do not occur in the remaining 80% of migraine sufferers. No consistent blood flow changes are associated with the headache phase itself.

The headache originates not in the brain itself, but in extracerebral structures lying within the cranial cavity innervated by nociceptive sensory nerve fibres of the trigeminal pathway, such as the meninges and large arteries. The vascular theory attributes the headache to dilatation in these large arteries. While some studies have shown a unilateral widening of the middle cerebral artery on the same side as the headache sensation, others have shown no clear change. Overall, the evidence for arterial dilatation as a cause of the headache is controversial (see Thomsen, 1997).

The *'brain' hypothesis* (see Lauritzen, 1987) links migraine to the phenomenon of cortical spreading depression. This is a dramatic although poorly understood phenomenon, triggered in experimental animals by local application of K$^+$ to the cortex and thought to occur in concussion. This causes an advancing wave of profound neural inhibition, which progresses slowly over the cortical surface at a rate of about 2 mm/min. In the depressed area, the ionic balance is grossly disturbed, with an extremely high extracellular K$^+$ concentration, and the blood flow is reduced. There is strong evidence to suggest that the aura phase of a migraine attack is associated with a wave of spreading depression, although what initiates it remains obscure. However, spreading depression triggered in animal models does not lead to activation or sensitisation of trigeminal afferents (Ebersberger et al., 2001). It is now believed that the aura is associated with spreading depression, but that this is not a necessary step in the pathogenesis of the migraine attack itself.

The *'sensory nerve' hypothesis* (see Moskowitz, 1992) proposes that activation of trigeminal nerve terminals in the meninges and extracranial vessels is the primary event in a migraine attack. This would cause pain directly and will also induce inflammatory changes through the release of neuropeptides from the sensory nerve terminals (neurogenic inflammation; see Chs 16 and 41). This theory is supported by experiments showing that one such peptide (calcitonin gene–related peptide; see Ch. 16) is released into the meningeal circulation during a migraine attack.

These theories are summarised in Figure 12.3. Many variants of these mechanisms have been proposed, but it is noteworthy that none can explain at the biochemical level what initiates a migraine attack or define the underlying abnormality that predisposes particular individuals to suffer such attacks. In some rare types of familial migraine, inherited mutations affecting calcium channels and Na$^+$-K$^+$ ATPase have been found, suggesting that abnormal membrane function may be responsible, but in most forms of migraine there is no clear genetic cause. Whether one inclines to the view that migraine is a vascular disorder, a type of spontaneous concussion, an inflammatory disease or just

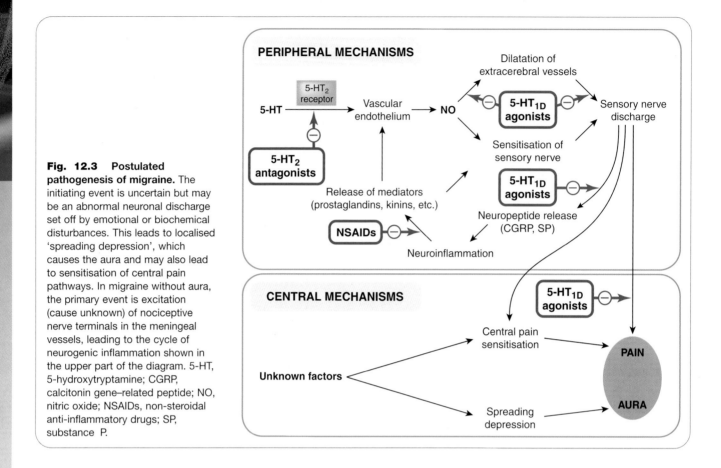

Fig. 12.3 Postulated pathogenesis of migraine. The initiating event is uncertain but may be an abnormal neuronal discharge set off by emotional or biochemical disturbances. This leads to localised 'spreading depression', which causes the aura and may also lead to sensitisation of central pain pathways. In migraine without aura, the primary event is excitation (cause unknown) of nociceptive nerve terminals in the meningeal vessels, leading to the cycle of neurogenic inflammation shown in the upper part of the diagram. 5-HT, 5-hydroxytryptamine; CGRP, calcitonin gene–related peptide; NO, nitric oxide; NSAIDs, non-steroidal anti-inflammatory drugs; SP, substance P.

a bad headache, there are two important factors that implicate 5-HT in its pathogenesis.

- There is a sharp increase in the urinary excretion of the main 5-HT metabolite, 5-HIAA, during the attack. The blood concentration of 5-HT falls, probably because of depletion of platelet 5-HT.
- Many of the drugs that are effective in treating migraine are 5-HT receptor agonists or antagonists. See Figure 12.3 and the clinical box for further information.

Antimigraine drugs

The main drugs used to treat migraine are summarised in Table 12.3, and their postulated sites of action are shown in Figure 12.3. It is important to distinguish between drugs used therapeutically to treat acute attacks of migraine (appropriate when the attacks are fairly infrequent) and drugs that are used for prophylaxis. Apart from 5-HT$_2$ receptor antagonists, the drugs used prophylactically are a mixed bag, and their mechanism of action is poorly understood.

CARCINOID SYNDROME

Carcinoid syndrome (see Creutzfeld & Stockmann, 1987) is a rare disorder associated with malignant tumours of enterochromaffin cells, which usually arise in the small intestine and metastasise to the liver. These tumours secrete a variety of chemical mediators:

Drugs used for migraine

Acute attack
- Simple analgesics (e.g. **aspirin**, **paracetamol**; Ch. 14) with or without metoclopramide (Ch. 25) to hasten absorption.
- **Ergotamine** (5-HT$_{1D}$ receptor partial agonist).
- **Sumatriptan, zolmitriptan** (5-HT$_{1D}$ agonists).

Prophylaxis
- β-Adrenoceptor antagonists (e.g. **propanolol**, **metoprolol**; see Ch. 11).
- **Pizotifen** (5-HT$_2$ receptor antagonist).
- Other 5-HT$_2$ receptor antagonists:
  - **cyproheptadine**: also has antihistamine actions
  - **methysergide**: rarely used because of risk of retroperitoneal fibrosis.
- Tricyclic antidepressants (e.g. **amitriptyline**; Ch. 39).
- **Clonidine**, an α$_2$-adrenoceptor agonist (see Ch. 11).
- Calcium antagonists (e.g. dihydropyridines, **verapamil**; see Ch. 18): headache is a side effect of these drugs but, paradoxically, they may reduce frequency of migraine attacks.

Table 12.3   Antimigraine drugs

Use	Drug(s)	Mode of action	Side effects	Pharmacokinetic aspects	Notes
Acute	Sumatriptan	5-HT_{1D} receptor agonist Constricts large arteries, inhibits trigeminal nerve transmission	Coronary vasoconstriction, dysrhythmias	Poorly absorbed by mouth, hence delayed response Can be given subcutaneously Does not cross blood–brain barrier Plasma half-life 1.5 h	Effective in ~70% of migraine attacks, but short duration of action is a drawback Contraindicated in patients with coronary disease
	Almotriptan Eletriptan Frovatriptan Naratriptan Rizatriptan Zolmitriptan	As sumatriptan, with additional actions on central nervous system	Side effects less than with sumatriptan	Improved bioavailability and duration of action compared with sumatriptan Able to cross blood–brain barrier	Basically sumatriptan lookalikes, with improved pharmacokinetics and reduced cardiac side effects
Acute	Ergotamine	5-HT_1 receptor partial agonist; also affects α adrenoceptors Vasoconstrictor Blocks trigeminal nerve transmission	Peripheral vasoconstriction, including coronary vessels Nausea, vomiting Contracts uterus and may cause fetal damage	Poorly absorbed Sometimes given by suppository, inhalation, etc. Duration of action 12–24 h	Effective, but use limited by side effects
Prophylaxis	Methysergide	5-HT_2 receptor antagonist/partial agonist	Nausea, vomiting, diarrhoea Rarely, but seriously, retroperitoneal or mediastinal fibrosis	Used orally	Effective, but rarely used owing to side effects and insidious toxicity
Prophylaxis	Pizotifen	5-HT_2 receptor antagonist Also muscarinic acetylcholine antagonist	Weight gain Antimuscarinic side effects	Used orally	–
Prophylaxis	Cyproheptadine	5-HT_2 receptor antagonist Also blocks histamine receptors and calcium channels	Sedation, weight gain	Used orally	Rarely used
Prophylaxis	Propranolol and similar drugs (e.g. metoprolol)	β-adrenoceptor antagonists Mechanism of antimigraine effect not clear	Fatigue Bronchoconstriction	Used orally	Effective and widely used for migraine

Notes:
1. Aspirin-like or opiate analgesic drugs (see Ch. 41) are often used to treat acute migraine attacks.
2. Other drugs used for migraine prophylaxis include calcium channel blockers (e.g. nifedipine, see Ch. 19), antidepressants (e.g. amitriptyline, see Ch. 39), valproate (see Ch. 40) and clonidine (Ch. 11). Their efficacy is limited.

5-HT is the most important, but neuropeptides, such as substance P (Ch. 16), and other agents, such as prostaglandins and bradykinin (Ch. 13), are also produced. The release of these substances into the bloodstream results in several unpleasant symptoms, including flushing, diarrhoea, bronchoconstriction and hypotension, which may cause dizziness or fainting. Stenosis of heart valves, which can result in cardiac failure, also occurs. It is reminiscent of retroperitoneal and mediastinal fibrosis, which are adverse effects of methysergide (see above, p. 194), and hence is probably related to an unknown action of 5-HT.

The syndrome is readily diagnosed by measuring the urinary excretion of the main metabolite of 5-HT, 5-HIAA. Excretion in the disease may increase 20-fold and is raised even during periods when the tumour is asymptomatic. 5-HT_2 antagonists, such as cyproheptadine, are effective in controlling some of the symptoms of carcinoid syndrome. A complementary therapeutic approach is to use **octreotide** (a long-acting analogue of somatostatin), which suppresses hormone secretion from neuroendocrine, including carcinoid, cells (see Ch. 28).

PURINES

Nucleosides (especially adenosine) and nucleotides (especially ADP and ATP) produce a wide range of pharmacological effects that are unrelated to their role in energy metabolism. It was shown in 1929 that adenosine injected into anaesthetised animals causes bradycardia, hypotension, vasodilatation and inhibition of intestinal movements. Since then, it has become clear that purines participate in many physiological control mechanisms, including the regulation of coronary flow and myocardial function (Chs 18 and 19), platelet aggregation and immune responses (Chs 13 and 21), and neurotransmission in both the central and peripheral nervous system (Chs 9 and 34; for reviews, see Illes et al., 2000; Cunha, 2001). Figure 12.4 summarises the mechanisms by which purines are released and interconverted, and the main receptor types on which they act.

The full complexity of purinergic control systems, and their importance in many pathophysiological mechanisms, is only now emerging, and there is no doubt that therapeutic agents affecting these systems will assume growing significance.

ATP AS A NEUROTRANSMITTER

The idea that such a workaday metabolite as ATP might be a member of the neurotransmitter elite was resisted for a long time,

but it is now firmly established. ATP is a transmitter in the periphery, both as a primary mediator and as a cotransmitter in noradrenergic nerve terminals (see Burnstock, 1985; Lundberg, 1996; Khakh, 2001). The nucleotide is contained in synaptic vesicles of both adrenergic and cholinergic neurons, and it accounts for many of the actions produced by stimulation of autonomic nerves that are not caused by acetylcholine or noradrenaline (see Ch. 9). These effects include the relaxation of intestinal smooth muscle evoked by sympathetic stimulation, and contraction of the bladder produced by parasympathetic nerves. Burnstock and his colleagues have shown that ATP is released on nerve stimulation in a Ca^{2+}-dependent fashion, and that exogenous ATP, in general, mimics the effects of nerve stimulation in various preparations. Furthermore, the ATP receptor antagonist **suramin** (a drug developed many years ago for treating trypanosome infections) blocks these synaptic responses. Recent work has also shown ATP to function as a conventional 'fast' transmitter in the CNS and in autonomic ganglia (see Khakh, 2001). ATP is present in all cells in millimolar concentrations and is released, independently of exocytosis, if the cells are damaged (e.g. by ischaemia). ATP released from cells is rapidly dephosphorylated by a range of tissue-specific nucleotidases, producing ADP and adenosine (Fig. 12.4), both of which produce a wide variety of receptor-mediated effects. Adenosine, produced following hydrolysis of ATP, exerts presynaptic inhibitory effects on the release of excitatory transmitters in the CNS and periphery.

The role of intracellular ATP in controlling membrane potassium channels, which is important in the control of vascular smooth muscle (Ch. 19) and of insulin secretion (Ch. 26), is quite distinct from its transmitter function.

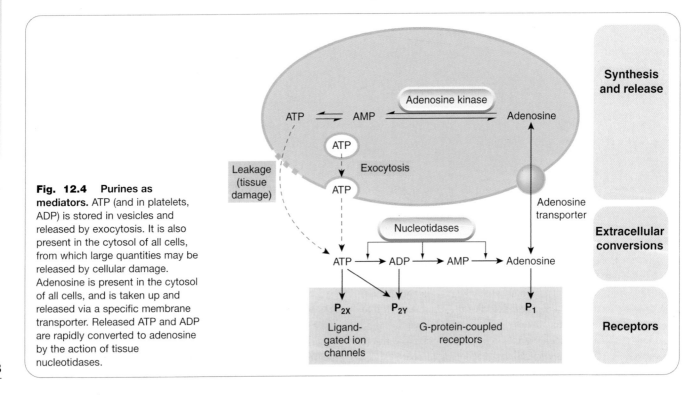

Fig. 12.4 Purines as mediators. ATP (and in platelets, ADP) is stored in vesicles and released by exocytosis. It is also present in the cytosol of all cells, from which large quantities may be released by cellular damage. Adenosine is present in the cytosol of all cells, and is taken up and released via a specific membrane transporter. Released ATP and ADP are rapidly converted to adenosine by the action of tissue nucleotidases.

ADP AND PLATELETS

The secretory vesicles of blood platelets store both ATP and ADP in high concentrations, and release them when the platelets are activated (see Chs 20 and 21). One of the many effects of ADP is to promote platelet aggregation, so this system provides positive feedback—an important mechanism for controlling this process, as attested by the therapeutic effectiveness of **clopidogrel**, which works via antagonism of platelet ADP receptors (Ch. 21, p. 342).

ADENOSINE AS A MEDIATOR

Adenosine differs from ATP in that it is not stored by, and released from, secretory vesicles. Rather, it exists free in the cytosol of all cells and is transported in and out of cells mainly using a membrane transporter. Not much is known about the way in which this is controlled. Adenosine in tissues comes partly from this source and partly from extracellular hydrolysis of released ATP or ADP (Fig. 12.4).

Adenosine produces many pharmacological effects, both in the periphery and in the CNS (see Brundege & Dunwiddie, 1997; Cunha, 2001). Based on its ability to inhibit cell function and thus minimise the metabolic requirements of cells, one of its functions may be as a protective agent released when tissue integrity is threatened (e.g. by coronary or cerebral ischaemia; see Chs 18 and 35). Under less extreme conditions, variations in adenosine release may play a role in controlling blood flow and (through effects on the carotid bodies) respiration, matching them to the metabolic needs of the tissues.

Adenosine is destroyed or taken up within a few seconds of intravenous administration (as in the treatment of supraventricular tachycardias; see Ch. 18), but longer-lasting analogues have been discovered that also show greater receptor selectivity. Adenosine uptake is blocked by **dipyridamole**, a vasodilator and antiplatelet drug (see Ch. 21).

Another area of growing interest is asthma (see Adriaensen and Timmermans, 2004). Adenosine has been identified as a potential mediator of cytokine release from mast cells, of hyper-reactivity of vagal and other airway neurons, and other actions that may directly or indirectly contribute to the disease.

PURINE RECEPTORS

Receptors for purines, like those for other mediators, have undergone classification and reclassification several times, but a rational scheme has now been agreed. There are two main types (see Fredholm et al., 1994).

- *P₁ receptors* (subtypes A_1, A_2 and A_3). These are GPCRs that respond to adenosine and are present in many different tissues. They are linked to stimulation or inhibition of adenylate cyclase.
- *P₂ receptors* (subtypes P_{2X} and P_{2Y}, each with several further subdivisions). These respond to ATP and/or ADP. P_{2X} receptors are multimeric ionotropic receptors (see Ch. 3), whereas P_{2Y} receptors are GPCRs coupled to adenylate cyclase or phosphoinositide metabolism.

These subtypes are distinguished on the basis of their agonist and antagonist selectivity, as well as molecular structure (for recent reviews, see von Kügelgen & Wetter, 2000; Fredholm et al., 2001; Khakh, 2001). Although there are many experimental compounds with varying degrees of receptor selectivity, there are so far few therapeutic agents that act on these receptors, and we will confine this account to some functional aspects that may give rise to therapeutic drugs in the future.

FUNCTIONAL ASPECTS

Adenosine receptors

The main effects of adenosine, and the receptors involved, are as follow.

- Vasodilatation, including coronary vessels (A_2), except in the kidney, where A_1 receptors produce vasoconstriction. Adenosine infusion causes a fall in blood pressure.
- Inhibition of platelet aggregation (A_2).
- Block of cardiac atrioventricular conduction (A_1) and reduction of force of contraction.
- Bronchoconstriction, especially in asthmatic subjects (A_1); the antiasthmatic effect of **methylxanthines** may partly reflect A_1 receptor antagonism.
- Release of mediators from mast cells (A_3): this contributes to bronchoconstriction.
- Stimulation of nociceptive afferent neurons, especially in the heart (A_2): adenosine release in response to ischaemia has been suggested as a mechanism of anginal pain (Ch. 18). Carotid body afferents are also stimulated, causing reflex hyperventilation.
- Inhibition of transmitter release at many peripheral and central synapses (A_1). In the CNS, adenosine generally exerts a pre- and postsynaptic depressant action, reducing motor activity, depressing respiration, inducing sleep and reducing anxiety, all of which effects are the opposite of those produced by methylxanthines (Ch. 42).
- Neuroprotection, in cerebral ischaemia, probably through inhibition of glutamate release through A_1 receptors.

In general, the A_1 receptor has been characterised as a 'homeostatic' receptor with protective functions in many tissues, whereas the A_2 receptor has more specific regulatory functions, especially in the brain, where it is widely expressed.

P₂ receptors and actions

P_2 receptors respond to various adenine nucleotides, generally preferring ATP over ADP or AMP. The role of ATP as a fast transmitter (see above) involves P_{2X} receptors, of which seven subtypes have been identified. These occur as a variety of mixed (heteromeric) assemblies (see Khakh, 2001). Not all their functions are clear, but the following actions are generally agreed.

- P_{2X1} receptors are expressed on various smooth muscle cells. ATP is a cotransmitter released by sympathetic nerves (Ch. 11), and P_{2X1} receptors are responsible for the initial contraction.
- P_{2X2} receptors are expressed in many brain regions and mediate 'fast' transmission by ATP in the brain.

- P_{2X3} receptors occur in nociceptive afferent neurons and may participate in pain associated with ATP released through tissue injury.
- P_{2X7} receptors are unusual in that activation causes a large and non-selective increase in membrane permeability. They are expressed mainly by cells of the immune system, and they control the release of certain cytokines.

The other actions of ATP in mammals are mediated through some eight subtypes of P_{2Y} receptors. These are GPCRs and are linked to various second messenger systems. They occur in many tissues, and the lack of selective antagonists makes it difficult to define their functions individually, although the actions of ADP on platelets and vascular endothelial cells are ascribed to the P_{2Y1} subtype. Drugs acting selectively on P_2 receptors have not yet been developed for clinical purposes.

PHARMACOLOGICAL ASPECTS

Uses of adenosine

Because of its inhibitory effect on cardiac conduction, adenosine may be used as an intravenous bolus injection to terminate supraventricular tachycardia (Ch. 18). It is safer than alternative drugs such as β-adrenoceptor antagonists or **verapamil**, because of its short duration of action. Otherwise, adenosine is not used therapeutically, although longer-lasting A_1 receptor agonists might prove useful in various conditions (e.g. hypertension, ischaemic heart disease and stroke). Selective adenosine receptor antagonists could also have advantages over **theophylline** in the treatment of asthma (see Ch. 23).

Drugs acting on purine receptors

Methylxanthines, especially analogues of theophylline (Ch. 23), are A_1/A_2 receptor antagonists; however, they also increase cAMP by inhibiting phosphodiesterase, which contributes to their pharmacological actions independently of adenosine receptor antagonism. CNS stimulation by methylxanthines such as **caffeine** (see Ch. 42) is partly a result of block of inhibitory A_1/A_2 receptors. Certain derivatives of theophylline are claimed to show greater selectivity for adenosine receptors over phosphodiesterase. P_2 receptors are blocked by suramin and the experimental compound PPADS.

Intensive efforts are underway to develop drugs with improved receptor selectivity for therapeutic purposes. There are many potential applications for such compounds in different indications, including heart disease, stroke, pain and immunological disorders. Probably, their time will come.

Purines as mediators

- *ATP* functions as a neurotransmitter (or cotransmitter) at peripheral neuroeffector junctions and central synapses.
- ATP is stored in vesicles and released by exocytosis. Cytoplasmic ATP may be released when cells are damaged. It also functions as an intracellular mediator, inhibiting the opening of membrane potassium channels.
- ATP acts on two types of *purinoceptor* (P_2), one of which (P_{2X}) is a ligand-gated ion channel responsible for fast synaptic responses. The other (P_{2Y}) is coupled to various second messengers. Suramin blocks the P_{2X} receptor.
- Released ATP is rapidly converted to ADP and adenosine.
- ADP acts on platelets, causing aggregation. This is important in thrombosis. It also acts on vascular and other types of smooth muscle, as well as having effects in the central nervous system (CNS).

- *Adenosine* affects many cells and tissues, including smooth muscle and nerve cells. It is not a conventional transmitter but may be important as a local hormone and 'homeostatic modulator'.
- Adenosine acts through A_1, A_2 and A_3 receptors, coupled to inhibition or stimulation of adenylate cyclase. A_1 and A_2 receptors are blocked by xanthines such as theophylline. The main effects of adenosine are:
  - hypotension (A_2) and cardiac depression (A_1)
  - inhibition of atrioventricular conduction (antidysrhythmic effect, A_1)
  - inhibition of platelet aggregation (A_2)
  - bronchoconstriction (probably secondary to mast cell activation, A_3)
  - presynaptic inhibition in CNS (responsible for neuroprotective effect, A_1).
- Adenosine is very short acting and is sometimes used for its antidysrhythmic effect.
- New adenosine agonists and antagonists are in development, mainly for treatment of ischaemic heart disease and stroke.

REFERENCES AND FURTHER READING

5-hydroxytryptamine

Barnes N M, Sharp T 1999 A review of central 5-HT receptors and their function. Neuropharmacology 38: 1083–1152 (*Useful general review focusing on CNS*)

Bonasera S J, Tecott L H 2000 Mouse models of serotonin receptor function: towards a genetic dissection of serotonin systems. Pharmacol Ther 88: 133–142 (*Review of studies on transgenic mice lacking 5-HT$_1$ or 5-HT$_2$ receptors; shows how difficult it can be to interpret such experiments*)

Branchek T A, Blackburn T P 2000 5-HT$_6$ receptors as emerging targets for drug discovery. Annu Rev Pharmacol Toxicol 40: 319–334 (*Summary of what is known about 5-HT$_6$ receptors, with emphasis on future therapeutic opportunities*)

Gershon M D 2004 Review article: serotonin receptors and transporters—roles in normal and abnormal gastrointestinal motility. Aliment Pharmacol Ther 20 (suppl 7): 3–14

Houston D S, Vanhoutte P M 1986 Serotonin and the vascular system: role in health and disease, and implications for therapy. Drugs 31: 149–163

Hoyer D, Clarke D E, Fozard J R et al. 1994 VII International Union of Pharmacology classification of receptors for 5-hydroxytryptamine. Pharmacol Rev 46: 157–203 (*The official view on 5-HT receptor classification*)

Kroeze W K, Kristiansen K, Roth B L 2002 Molecular biology of serotonin receptors structure and function at the molecular level. Curr Top Med Chem 2: 507–528

Taniyama K et al. 2000 Functions of peripheral 5-hydroxytryptamine receptors, especially 5-HT$_4$ receptor, in gastrointestinal motility. J Gastroenterol 35: 575–582 (*Review describing the role of various 5-HT receptors in the gastrointestinal tract*)

Purines

Adriaensen D, Timmermans J P 2004 Purinergic signalling in the lung: important in asthma and COPD? Curr Opin Pharmacol 4: 207–214

Brundege J M, Dunwiddie T V 1997 Role of adenosine as a modulator of synaptic activity in the central nervous system. Adv Pharmacol 39: 353–391 (*Good review article*)

Burnstock G 1985 Purinergic mechanisms broaden their sphere of influence. Trends Neurosci 8: 5–6 (*Ideas about the functional role of purinergic transmission by the scientist who did much to establish this concept*)

Burnstock G 2002 Potential therapeutic targets in the rapidly expanding field of purinergic signalling. Clin Med 2(1): 45–53

Cunha R A 2001 Adenosine as a neuromodulator and as a homeostatic regulator in the nervous system: different roles, different sources and different receptors. Neurochem Int 38: 107–125 (*Speculative review on the functions of adenosine in the nervous system*)

Fredholm B B, Abbrachio M B, Burnstock G et al. 1994 Nomenclature and classification of purinoceptors. Pharmacol Rev 46: 143–156 (*Useful review*)

Fredholm B B, Arslan G, Halldner L et al. 2001 Structure and function of adenosine receptors and their genes. Naunyn-Schmiedeberg's Arch Pharmacol 362: 364–374 (*General review article*)

Gourine A V, Dale N, Gourine V N, Spyer K M 2004 Fever in systemic inflammation: roles of purines. Front Biosci 9: 1011–1022

Illes P, Klotz K-N, Lohse M J 2000 Signalling by extracellular nucleotides and nucleosides. Naunyn-Schmiedeberg's Arch Pharmacol 362: 295–298 (*Introductory article in a series of useful reviews on purinergic mechanisms in the same issue*)

Khakh B S 2001 Molecular physiology of P$_{2X}$ receptors and signalling at synapses. Nat Rev Neurosci 2: 165–174 (*Summarises data on ATP-mediated synaptic transmission*)

Klotz K-N 2000 Adenosine receptors and their ligands. Naunyn-Schmiedeberg's Arch Pharmacol 362: 382–391 (*Account of known agonists and antagonists at adenosine receptors*)

Liu X J, Salter M W 2005 Purines and pain mechanisms: recent developments. Curr Opin Investig Drugs 6: 65–75

Lundberg J M 1996 Pharmacology of co-transmission in the autonomic nervous system: integrative aspects on amines, neuropeptides, adenosine triphosphate, amino acids and nitric oxide. Pharmacol Rev 48: 114–192 (*Comprehensive and informative review*)

North R A, Barnard E A 1997 Nucleotide receptors. Curr Opin Neurobiol 7: 346–357 (*Review of purinergic receptors*)

Stone T W 2002 Purines and neuroprotection. Adv Exp Med Biol 513: 249–280

von Kügelglen I, Wetter A 2000 Molecular pharmacology of P$_{2Y}$ receptors. Naunyn-Schmiedeberg's Arch Pharmacol 362: 310–323

Migraine and other pathologies

Creutzfeld W, Stockmann F 1987 Carcinoids and carcinoid syndrome. Am J Med 82(suppl 58): 4–16

Ebersberger A, Schaible H-G, Averbeck B, Richter F 2001 Is there a correlation between spreading depression, neurogenic inflammation, and nociception that might cause migraine pain? Ann Neurol 49: 7–13 (*Their conclusion is that there is no connection— spreading depression does not produce inflammation or affect sensory neurons*)

Edvinsson L (ed) 1999 Migraine and headache pathophysiology. Martin Dunitz, London (*Collected articles summarising current, and often conflicting, views on the mechanism of migraine*)

Friberg L 1999 Migraine pathophysiology, its relation to cerebral haemodynamic changes. In: Edvinsson L (ed) Migraine and headache pathophysiology. Martin Dunitz, London (*Useful summary of findings in a controversial area*)

Goadsby P J 2005 Can we develop neurally acting drugs for the treatment of migraine? Nat Rev Drug Discov 4: 741–750 (*Up-to-date review of the causes and treatments of migraine*)

Lauritzen M 1987 Cerebral blood flow in migraine and cortical spreading depression. Acta Neurol Scand Suppl 113: 140 (*Review of clinical measurements of cerebral blood flow in migraine, which overturn earlier hypotheses*)

Moskowitz M A 1992 Neurogenic versus vascular mechanisms of sumatriptan and ergot alkaloids in migraine. Trends Pharmacol Sci 13: 307–311 (*Discussion of controversies about the pathophysiology of migraine*)

Rudolphi K A, Schubert P, Parkinson F E, Fredholm B B 1992 Neuroprotective role of adenosine in cerebral ischaemia. Trends Pharmacol Sci 13: 439–445 (*Argues that adenosine protects neurons against ischaemic damage—important therapeutic implications*)

Thomsen L L 1997 Investigations into the role of nitric oxide and the large intracranial arteries in migraine headache. Cephalalgia 17: 873–895 (*Revisits the old vascular theory of migraine in the light of recent advances in the nitric oxide field*)

Villalon C M, Centurion D, Valdivia L F et al. 2003 Migraine: pathophysiology, pharmacology, treatment and future trends. Curr Vasc Pharmacol 1: 71–84

Books

Cooper J R, Bloom F E, Roth R H 1996 The biochemical basis of neuropharmacology. Oxford University Press, New York (*Excellent general textbook*)

Green A R (ed) 1985 Neuropharmacology of serotonin. Oxford University Press, Oxford (*Useful compilation of articles on 5-HT pharmacology*)

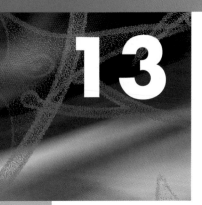

13 Local hormones, inflammation and immune reactions

response acts to protect us, but occasionally it goes awry, leading to a spectrum of inflammatory diseases, and it is under these circumstances that we need to resort to drug therapy to dampen or abolish the inflammatory response.

This chapter deals with this inflammatory response and its regulation. We outline the principal features of the twin pillars of the inflammatory reaction—the innate and the adaptive components—and provide a detailed description of the pathways involved in their activation. We then describe the main chemical mediators that control the responses, emphasising their role in disease. This chapter should be read in conjunction with the next, which explains in more detail how anti-inflammatory drugs themselves actually act.

Unfortunately for the reader, the inflammation literature is rife with acronyms and abbreviations. For this reason, a glossary is provided on p. 224.

OVERVIEW

All living creatures are born into a universe that poses a constant challenge to their physical well-being and survival. Evolution, which has equipped us with homeostatic systems that maintain a stable internal environment in the face of changing external temperatures and fluctuating supplies of food and water, has also provided us with mechanisms for combating the ever-present threat of infection and for promoting healing and restoration to normal function in the event of injury. In mammals, this vital function is subserved by the *innate* and *acquired* (or *adaptive*) immune responses, working together with a variety of mediators and mechanisms that give rise to what we collectively term *inflammation*. Generally this

INTRODUCTION

When facing invasion by disease-causing organisms (pathogens), mammals can call on a daunting arsenal of defensive responses, the deployment of which constitutes the acute inflammatory/immune reaction. When these defences are defective (as for example in AIDS) or are suppressed by drugs, organisms that are not normally pathogenic can cause opportunistic infections, sometimes with fatal consequences. Under other circumstances, these defensive responses may be deployed inappropriately in response to other sorts of injury, such as that caused by chemicals, ultraviolet light or heat, against innocuous foreign substances (e.g. pollen) or against the tissues of the body itself (in autoimmune conditions). When this happens, the inflammation itself inflicts damage and may be responsible for the major symptoms of the disease—either acutely in (for example) anaphylaxis, or chronically in (for example) asthma, rheumatoid arthritis or atherosclerosis. These 'defensive responses' are initiated and regulated by an array of different mediators released from different cell types, and an understanding of the effects, mechanisms of action and clinical use of drugs that affect the inflammatory and the immune responses depends on an appreciation of the way in which these cells and their mediators act and interact.

THE COMPONENTS OF THE ACUTE INFLAMMATORY REACTION

The acute inflammatory reaction has two components:

- an *innate*, non-adaptive response, thought to have been developed early in evolution and present in some form or other in most multicellular organisms
- the *adaptive* immune response.

Some aspects of the *innate response* are non-immunological, for example the histamine-induced vascular changes to ultraviolet damage, and some reactions of the neutrophil polymorphs. Other aspects, particularly those that occur in response to an invading organism, form part of the overall immune response and are referred to as the *innate immune response*. The innate response is activated immediately[1] after infection or injury. A number of multipurpose defences are automatically put in place, and the adaptive immune response is alerted. The innate response also has a role in preventing the adaptive response from targeting and damaging host cells.

The *adaptive immune response* starts up only after a pathogen has been recognised by the innate system. It comprises a range of exquisitely pathogen-specific responses, as well as boosting the actions of the cells and mediators of the innate response. Several 'back-up' systems exist, such that a pathogen can be neutralised or killed in several ways.

In the discussion that follows, we concentrate on the local manifestations of the acute reaction to an invading organism. The outline given will, of necessity, be a very general one, but because everyone has experienced the inflammatory response to a greater or lesser degree during their lifetime, all will be broadly familiar with the *redness*, *swelling*, *heat* and *pain* that are called the *four cardinal signs of inflammation* (there is a fifth too: *loss of function*). The changes occurring within the tissues at this time can be divided into cellular and vascular events. Mediators are generated both from plasma and from cells, and these, in turn, modify and regulate the vascular and cellular reactions.

THE INNATE IMMUNE RESPONSE

The innate immune response has usually been rather airily dismissed by most immunologists as being an ancient throwback that merely provides a temporary holding operation until the more effective specific adaptive immune response gets going. In fact, the innate response has a much more significant role in host defence. An important initiating event in the innate immune response is the recognition by *pattern recognition*, or *Toll*,[2]

---

[1]One immunologist referred to the innate response as the organism's 'knee jerk' response to infection. It is a good description.

[2]These transmembrane receptors were first identified in *Drosophila* and believed to be involved in spatial organisation of the developing embryo. Later, it was appreciated that the receptor was also crucial to host defence. The name, which loosely translates from German as 'Great!' or 'Eureka!', has remained firmly attached to the family.

The acute inflammatory reaction

- The 'acute inflammatory reaction' occurs in tissues in response to a pathogen or other noxious substance.
- It usually has two components: an *innate* non-adaptive response and an *adaptive* (acquired or specific) immunological response.
- These reactions are generally protective, but if inappropriately deployed they are deleterious.
- The normal outcome of the response is healing with or without scarring; alternatively, if injurious agent persists, *chronic* inflammation.
- Many of the diseases that require drug treatment involve inflammation. Understanding the action and use of anti-inflammatory and immunosuppressive drugs necessitates understanding the inflammatory reaction.

receptors on tissue macrophages of specific *pathogen-associated molecular patterns* (PAMPs) on the microorganism (see Medzhitov & Janeway, 2000; Brown, 2001). PAMPs are highly conserved components that are common to entire classes of pathogen (bacteria, viruses and fungi). They are usually crucial structural components of the pathogen that are critical for its survival and virulence.

Examples of bacterial PAMPs are:

- *peptidoglycan*, a constituent of the cell wall common to virtually all bacteria (see Ch. 45)
- *bacterial lipopolysaccharide*, a constituent of the outer membrane of all Gram-negative bacteria.

Unlike the antigen receptors on T and B cells that are generated somatically as the T and B cells develop, endowing each lymphocyte clone with a structurally unique receptor, Toll receptors (TLRs) are encoded in the host DNA and are expressed on the surface of 'professional' antigen-presenting cells (APCs), the dendritic cells and macrophages. Interaction of a PAMP with TLRs triggers the dendritic cell or macrophage to respond immediately; intracellular signal pathways activate the production of the main proinflammatory cytokines (see below) tumour necrosis factor (TNF)-α and interleukin (IL)-1, as well as other mediators (such as prostaglandins and histamine) that act on the vascular endothelial cells of the postcapillary venules, causing expression of adhesion molecules on the intimal surface and an increase in vascular permeability. This allows exudation, into the extravascular space, of fluid containing the components of enzyme cascades (Fig. 13.1) that give rise to more inflammatory mediators (e.g. the chemotaxin C5a).

White blood cells adhere to the endothelial cells through interactions between their cell surface integrins (see below) and adhesion molecules on endothelial cells. This enables them to migrate out of the vessels, attracted by *chemotaxins* generated by the micro-organisms or as a result of their interaction with tissues (see Fig. 13.2). Chemokines released during TLR activation play

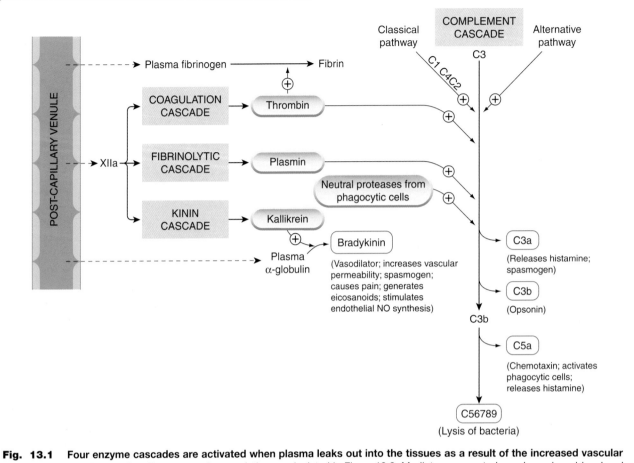

Fig. 13.1 **Four enzyme cascades are activated when plasma leaks out into the tissues as a result of the increased vascular permeability of inflammation.** Factors causing exudation are depicted in Figure 13.2. Mediators generated are shown in red-bordered boxes. Complement components are indicated by C1, C2, etc. When plasmin is formed, it tends to increase kinin formation and decrease the coagulation cascade. (Adapted from Dale et al., 1994.)

an important part in this. (Cytokines and chemokines are considered on pp. 222-223.)

VASCULAR EVENTS AND THE MEDIATORS DERIVED FROM PLASMA

The initial vascular events include dilatation of the small arterioles, resulting in increased blood flow. This is followed by a slowing and eventually stasis of blood, and an increase in the permeability of the postcapillary venules with exudation of fluid. The vasodilatation is brought about by mediators including histamine, prostaglandin (PG) E_2 and PGI_2 (prostacyclin) produced by the interaction of the microorganism with tissue, some of which act together with cytokines to increase vascular permeability.

The fluid exudate contains the components for four proteolytic enzyme cascades: the complement system, the coagulation system, the fibrinolytic system, and the kinin system (see Fig. 13.1). The components of these cascades are proteases that are inactive in their native form but that are activated by proteolytic cleavage, each activated component then activating the next. The exudate is carried by lymphatics to local lymph glands or lymphoid

tissue, where the products of the invading microorganism trigger the adaptive phase of the response.

The complement system comprises nine major components, designated C1 to C9. Activation of the cascade is initiated by substances derived from microorganisms, such as yeast cell walls or endotoxins. This pathway of activation is termed the *alternative pathway* (Fig. 13.1) as opposed to the classic pathway that is dealt with later. One of the main events is the enzymatic splitting of C3, giving rise to various peptides, one of which, *C3a* (termed an *anaphylatoxin*) stimulates mast cells to secrete further chemical mediators and can also directly stimulate smooth muscle, while *C3b* (termed an *opsonin*) attaches to the surface of a microorganism, facilitating ingestion by white blood cells. *C5a*, generated enzymatically from C5, also releases mediators from mast cells and is a powerfully chemotactic attractant and activator of white blood cells.

The final components in the sequence, complement-derived mediators (C5 to C9), attach to certain bacterial membranes, leading to lysis. Complement can therefore mediate the destruction of invading bacteria or damage multicellular parasites; however, it may sometimes cause injury to the host. The principal enzymes

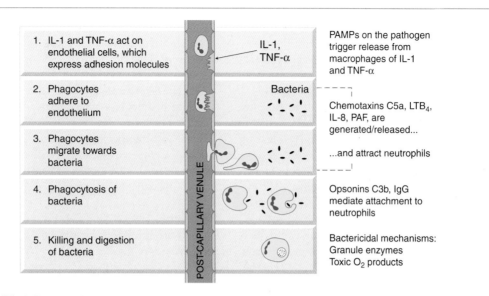

1. IL-1 and TNF-α act on endothelial cells, which express adhesion molecules	IL-1, TNF-α / PAMPs on the pathogen trigger release from macrophages of IL-1 and TNF-α
2. Phagocytes adhere to endothelium	Bacteria / Chemotaxins C5a, LTB$_4$, IL-8, PAF, are generated/released...
3. Phagocytes migrate towards bacteria	...and attract neutrophils
4. Phagocytosis of bacteria	Opsonins C3b, IgG mediate attachment to neutrophils
5. Killing and digestion of bacteria	Bactericidal mechanisms: Granule enzymes Toxic O$_2$ products

POST-CAPILLARY VENULE

Fig. 13.2 **Simplified diagram of the initial events in a local acute inflammatory reaction.** Recognition by tissue macrophages of pathogen-associated molecular patterns (PAMPs) on the pathogen triggers release, from tissue macrophages, of the proinflammatory cytokines interleukin (IL)-1 and tumour necrosis factor-α (TNF-α). These act on the endothelial cells of postcapillary venules, causing exudation of fluid and expression of adhesion factors (e.g. selectins, integrins) to which counter-ligands on blood-borne neutrophils adhere. Subsequent steps are listed in the figure. C5a and C3b, complement components; IgG, immunoglobulin G; LTB$_4$, leukotriene B$_4$; PAF, platelet-activating factor.

of the coagulation and fibrinolytic cascades, thrombin and plasmin, can also activate the cascade by hydrolysing C3, as can enzymes released from white blood cells.

The coagulation system and the *fibrinolytic system* are described in Chapter 21. Factor XII is activated to XIIa (e.g. by collagen), and the end product, fibrin, laid down during a host–pathogen interaction may serve to limit the extent of the infection. Thrombin is additionally involved in the activation of the kinin (Fig. 13.1) and, indirectly, the fibrinolytic systems (see Ch. 21).

The *kinin system* is another enzyme cascade relevant to inflammation. It yields several mediators, in particular *bradykinin* (Fig. 13.1 and see below).

CELLULAR EVENTS

Of the cells involved in inflammation, some (vascular endothelial cells, mast cells and tissue macrophages) are normally present in tissues, while others (platelets and leucocytes) gain access from the blood. The leucocytes are actively motile cells and are of two classes.

- *Polymorphonuclear cells* (cells with multilobed nuclei, also called *granulocytes*), which are further subdivided into *neutrophils*, *eosinophils* and *basophils* according to the staining properties of granules in their cytoplasm. Some use the term to refer exclusively to neutrophils.
- *Mononuclear cells* (or cells with single-lobed nuclei), which are subdivided into *monocytes* and *lymphocytes*.

Mast cells

The mast cell membrane has receptors both for a special class of antibody, immunoglobulin (Ig)E, as well as for the complement

components C3a and C5a. Ligands acting at these receptors trigger mediator release, as does direct physical damage. One of the main substances released is histamine; others include heparin, leukotrienes, PGD$_2$, platelet-activating factor (PAF), nerve growth factor and some interleukins.

Polymorphonuclear leucocytes

Neutrophil polymorphs are the 'shock troops' of inflammation, and are the first of the blood leucocytes to enter an inflamed area (Fig. 13.2). The whole process is cleverly choreographed: under direct observation, the neutrophils may be seen first to *roll* along the activated endothelium, then *adhere* and finally *migrate* out of the blood vessel and into the extravascular space. This process is regulated by the successive activation of different families of adhesion molecules (*selectins*, *intercellular adhesion molecule* [*ICAM*] and *integrins*) on the inflamed endothelium that engage corresponding *counter-ligands* on the neutrophil, capturing it as it rolls along the surface, stabilising its interaction with the endothelial cells, and enabling it to migrate out of the vessel (using a further adhesion molecule termed *PECAM*, platelet endothelium adhesion molecule). The neutrophil is attracted to the invading pathogen by chemicals termed *chemotaxins*, some of which (such as the tripeptide formyl-Met-Leu-Phe) are released by the microorganism, whereas others, such as C5a, are produced locally or by local cells such as macrophages (e.g. chemokines such as IL-8).

Neutrophils can engulf, kill and digest microorganisms. Together with eosinophils, they have surface receptors for C3b, which acts as an *opsonin* that forms a link between neutrophil and invading bacterium. (An even more effective link may be made by antibody; see below.) Neutrophils kill microorganisms by generating toxic oxygen products and other mechanisms, and enzymatic digestion then follows. If the neutrophil is inappropriately activated, the toxic oxygen products and proteolytic enzymes can cause damage to the host's own tissues. When neutrophils have released their toxic chemicals, they undergo apoptosis and must be cleared by macrophages. It is the live and apoptotic neutrophils that constitute 'pus'.

Eosinophils have similar capacities to neutrophils but are also 'armed' with a battery of substances stored in their granules, which, when released, kill multicellular parasites (e.g. helminths). These include *eosinophil cationic protein*, a *peroxidase*, the *eosinophil major basic protein* and a *neurotoxin*. The eosinophil is considered by many to be of primary importance in the pathogenesis of the late phase of asthma where, it is suggested, granule proteins cause damage to bronchiolar epithelium (Fig. 23.3). *Basophils* are very similar in many respects to mast cells. The basophil content of the tissues is negligible—except in certain parasitic infections and hypersensitivity reactions—and in health they form only 0.5% of circulating white blood cells.

Monocytes/macrophages

Monocytes arrive in inflammatory lesions several hours after the polymorphs. Adhesion to endothelium and migration into the tissue follow a pattern similar to that of the neutrophils (see above), although monocyte chemotaxis utilises additional chemokines, such as MCP-1[3] (which, reasonably enough, stands for monocyte chemoattractant protein-1) and RANTES (which very *unreasonably* stands for regulated on activation normal T-cell expressed and secreted—immunological nomenclature has excelled itself here!).

Once in tissues, blood monocytes differentiate into macrophages (literally 'big eaters', compared with neutrophils, originally called microphages or 'little eaters'). The resultant cell has a remarkable range of abilities, being not only a jack of all trades but also master of many (see below). During innate reactions, macrophages bind lipopolysaccharide and other PAMPs using specific cell surface receptors. This stimulates the generation and release of cytokines and chemokines that act on vascular endothelial cells, attract other leucocytes to the area, and give rise to systemic manifestations of the inflammatory response such as fever. Macrophages engulf tissue debris and dead cells, as well as phagocytosing and killing most (but unfortunately not all) microorganisms. When stimulated by glucocorticoids, they secrete annexin-1 (a potent anti-inflammatory polypeptide; see Ch. 28).

Vascular endothelial cells

Vascular endothelial cells (see also Chs 19 and 21), originally considered as passive lining cells, are now known to play an active part in inflammation. Small arteriole endothelial cells secrete nitric oxide (NO), causing relaxation of the underlying smooth muscle (see Ch. 17), vasodilatation, and increased delivery of plasma and blood cells to the inflamed area. The endothelial cells of the postcapillary venules regulate plasma exudation and thus the delivery of plasma-derived mediators (see Fig. 13.1). Vascular endothelial cells express several adhesion molecules (the ICAM and selectin families; see Fig. 13.2), as well as a variety of receptors including those for histamine, acetylcholine and IL-1. In addition to NO, the cells can synthesise and release the vasodilator agent PGI_2, the vasoconstrictor agent endothelin, plasminogen activator, PAF and several cytokines. Endothelial cells also participate in the angiogenesis that occurs during inflammatory resolution, chronic inflammation and cancer (see Chs 5 and 51).

Platelets

Platelets are involved primarily in coagulation and thrombotic phenomena (see Ch. 21) but also play a part in inflammation. They have low-affinity receptors for IgE, and are believed to contribute to the first phase of asthma (Fig. 23.3). In addition to generating thromboxane (TX) A_2 and PAF, they can generate free radicals and proinflammatory cationic proteins. Platelet-derived growth factor contributes to the repair processes that follow inflammatory responses or damage to blood vessels.

Neurons

In addition to relaying impulses to the central nervous system (CNS), some sensory neurons release inflammatory neuropeptides when appropriately stimulated. These neurons are fine afferents (capsaicin-sensitive C and Aδ fibres) with specific receptors at their peripheral terminals. Kinins, 5-hydroxytryptamine and other chemical mediators generated during inflammation act on these receptors, stimulating the release of neuropeptides such as the tachykinins (neurokinin A, substance P) and calcitonin gene-related peptide (CGRP). The neuropeptides are considered further in Chapter 16.

Natural killer cells

Natural killer (NK) cells are a specialised type of lymphocyte. In an unusual twist to the receptor concept, NK cells kill targets (e.g. virus-infected or tumour cells) that *lack* ligands for *inhibitory* receptors on the NK cells themselves. The ligands in question are the *major histocompatibility complex* (*MHC*) molecules, and any cells lacking these become a target for NK-cell attack, a strategy sometimes called the 'mother turkey strategy'.[4] MHC proteins are expressed on the surface of most host cells and, in simple terms, are specific for that individual, enabling the NK cells to avoid damaging host cells. NK cells have other functions: they are equipped with Fc receptors and, in the presence of antibody directed against a target cell, they can kill the cell by *antibody-dependent cellular cytotoxicity*.

---

[3]Human immunodeficiency virus-1 binds to the surface CD4 glycoprotein on monocyte/macrophages but is able to penetrate the cell only after binding also to MCP-1 and RANTES receptors.

[4]Richard Dawkins in *River out of Eden*, citing the zoologist Schliedt, explains that the 'rule ot thumb a mother turkey uses to recognise nest robbers is a dismayingly brusque one; in the vicinity of the nest, attack anything that moves unless it makes a noise like a baby turkey' (quoted by Kärre & Welsh, 1997).

MEDIATORS DERIVED FROM CELLS

When inflammatory cells are stimulated or damaged, another major mediator family, the *eicosanoids*, are called into play. Many anti-inflammatory drugs act, at least in part, by interfering with synthesis of eicosanoids. Other important inflammatory mediators derived from cells are histamine, PAF, NO, neuropeptides and the cytokines.

THE ADAPTIVE IMMUNE RESPONSE

The adaptive immunological response is an immeasurably more efficient defensive manoeuvre and highly specific for the invading pathogen. A simplified version will be given here, stressing only those aspects that are relevant for an understanding of drug action; for more detailed coverage, see Janeway et al. (2004).

The key cells are the *lymphocytes*, of which there are three main groups (see Fig. 13.3):

- *B cells*, responsible for antibody production, i.e. the *humoral* immune response
- *T cells*, which are important in the induction phase of the immune response and in cell-mediated immune reactions
- *NK* cells, which are specialised lymphoid cells that are active in the non-immunological, innate response.

Miraculously, T and B lymphocytes harbour antigen-specific receptors that recognise and react with virtually all foreign proteins and polysaccharides that we are likely to encounter during our lifetime. The specific immune response occurs in two phases:

1. During the *induction phase*, antigen is *presented* to T cells by large *dendritic cells*, and this is followed by complex interactions of those T cells with B cells and other T cells. On first contact with an antigen (foreign protein or polysaccharide), the lymphocytes that have 'recognised' it (by means of surface receptors specific for that antigen) undergo *clonal expansion*, giving rise to a mass of cells that all have the capacity to recognise and respond to that particular antigen. These cells are eventually responsible for the effector phase of the response.
2. During the *effector phase*, these cells differentiate either into *plasma cells* or into *memory cells*. The plasma cells produce antibodies (if they are B cells), or are involved in cell-mediated immune responses such as activating macrophages or killing virus-infected host cells (if they are T cells). Other cells form an increased population of antigen-sensitive memory cells. Any subsequent exposure to the antigen calls forth a greatly enhanced response.

The receptor repertoire on T and B cells is generated randomly and would recognise 'self' proteins as well as foreign antigens if it were not that *tolerance* to self antigens is acquired during fetal life by apoptotic deletion of T-cell clones that recognise the host's own tissues. Dendritic cells and macrophages involved in the innate response also have a role in preventing harmful immune reactions against the host's own cells (see below). A simplified

---

The innate immune response

- The innate response occurs immediately on injury or infection. It comprises vascular and cellular elements. Mediators generated by cells or from plasma modify and regulate the magnitude of the response.
- Tissue macrophages, bearing Toll receptors, recognise specific pathogen-associated molecular patterns on the microorganism and release cytokines, particularly interleukin (IL)-1 and tumour necrosis factor (TNF)-α, as well as various chemokines.
- IL-1 and TNF-α act on local postcapillary venular endothelial cells, causing:
  - vasodilatation and fluid exudation
  - expression of adhesion molecules on the cell surfaces.
- Exudate contains enzyme cascades that generate bradykinin (from kininogen), and C5a and C3a (from complement). Complement activation lyses bacteria.
- C5a and C3a stimulate mast cells to release histamine, which dilates local arterioles.
- Tissue damage and cytokines release prostaglandin (PG) I_2 and PGE_2 (vasodilators) and leukotriene (LT) B_4 (chemotaxin).
- Cytokines stimulate synthesis of vasodilator nitric oxide, which increases vascular permeability.
- Using adhesion molecules, leucocytes roll on, adhere to and finally migrate through vascular endothelium towards the pathogen (attracted by chemokines, IL-8, C5a, and LTB_4), where phagocytosis and killing takes place.

---

outline of the main interactions between cells and mediators is given in Figure 13.3.

THE INDUCTION PHASE

Antigenic molecules reach the local lymph nodes through the lymphatics. APCs ingest and process the antigen and present it on their surface to:

- uncommitted (naive) CD4[+] T-helper lymphocytes, termed Th cells, or T-helper precursor (Thp) cells, in association with class II MHC molecules (see Fig. 13.4) and/or
- naive CD8[+] T lymphocytes in association with class I MHC molecules.[5]

---

[5]The main reason that is difficult to transplant organs such as kidneys from one person to another is that their respective MHC molecules are different. Lymphocytes in the recipient will react to non-self (allogeneic) MHC molecules in the donor tissue, which is then likely to be rejected by a rapid and powerful immunological reaction.

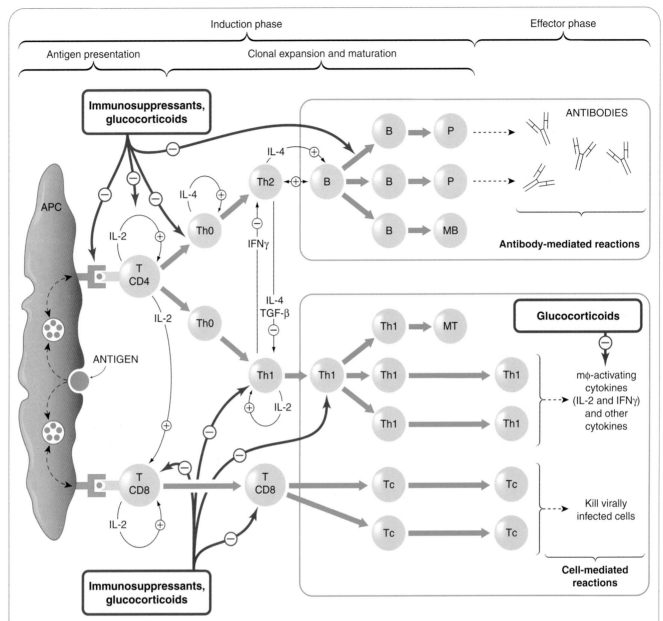

Fig. 13.3 **Simplified diagram of the induction and effector phases of lymphocyte activation with the sites of action of immunosuppressants.** Antigen-presenting cells (APCs) ingest and process antigen (•) and present fragments (•) to naive, uncommitted CD4 T cells in conjunction with major histocompatibility complex (MHC) class II molecules, or to naive CD8 T cells in conjunction with MHC class I molecules (•), thus 'arming' them. The armed CD4⁺ T cells synthesise and express interleukin (IL)-2 receptors and release this cytokine, which stimulates the cells by autocrine action, causing generation and proliferation of T-helper zero (Th0) cells. Autocrine cytokines (e.g. IL-4) cause proliferation of some Th0 cells to give Th2 cells, which are responsible for the development of antibody-mediated immune responses. These Th2 cells cooperate with and activate B cells to proliferate and give rise eventually to memory B cells (MB) and plasma cells (P), which secrete antibodies. Other autocrine cytokines (e.g. IL-2) cause proliferation of Th0 cells to give Th1 cells, which secrete cytokines that activate macrophages (responsible for some cell-mediated immune reactions). The armed CD8⁺ T cells also synthesise and express IL-2 receptors and release IL-2, which stimulates the cells by autocrine action to proliferate and give rise to cytotoxic T cells. These can kill virally infected cells. IL-2 secreted by CD4⁺ cells also plays a part in stimulating CD8⁺ cells to proliferate. Note that the 'effector phase' depicted above relates to the 'protective' action of the immune response. When the response is inappropriately deployed—as in chronic inflammatory conditions such as rheumatoid arthritis—the Th1 component of the immune response is dominant and the activated macrophages (mφ) release IL-1 and tumour necrosis factor-α, which in turn trigger the release of the chemokines and inflammatory cytokines that play a major role in the pathology of the disease.

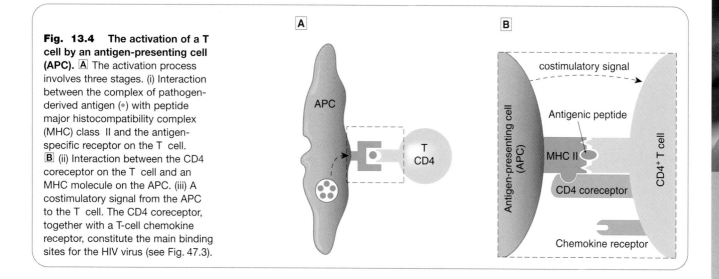

Fig. 13.4 The activation of a T cell by an antigen-presenting cell (APC). **A** The activation process involves three stages. (i) Interaction between the complex of pathogen-derived antigen (●) with peptide major histocompatibility complex (MHC) class II and the antigen-specific receptor on the T cell. **B** (ii) Interaction between the CD4 coreceptor on the T cell and an MHC molecule on the APC. (iii) A costimulatory signal from the APC to the T cell. The CD4 coreceptor, together with a T-cell chemokine receptor, constitute the main binding sites for the HIV virus (see Fig. 47.3).

CD4 and CD8 are *coreceptors* on T lymphocytes that cooperate with the main antigen-specific receptors in antigen recognition. Macrophages also carry surface CD4 proteins.

Activation of a T cell by an APC requires that several signals pass between the two cells (Fig. 13.4; see Medzhitov & Janeway, 2000). Researching the interaction between the APC and the T cell may enable us to exploit these pathways in the treatment of HIV infection and the therapy of immunologically mediated disease.

After activation, the T cells acquire IL-2 receptors and generate IL-2 itself. This cytokine has an autocrine action, causing proliferation and giving rise to a clone of T cells termed *Th0 cells*, which, in turn, give rise to two different subsets of armed helper cells termed *Th1* and *Th2* cells. The action of specific interleukins determines whether Th1 or Th2 cells develop; IL-12 favours progress down the Th1, and IL-4 the Th2, pathway. Each subset of Th cells then produces its own profile of cytokines, which control a unique subset of immune responses. The Th1 pathway mainly controls macrophage-initiated cell-mediated responses, and the Th2 pathway antibody-mediated responses. The cytokines serve as autocrine growth factors for their own subset of T cells and have cross-regulatory actions on the development of the other subset.

The relationship of Th1 and Th2 responses to disease

The T-cell subsets are emphasised here because the balance between the functions of the two subsets is important in immunopathology. Diseases in which Th1 responses are dominant include insulin-dependent diabetes mellitus (Ch. 26), multiple sclerosis, *Helicobacter pylori*–induced peptic ulcer (Ch. 25), aplastic anaemia (Ch. 22) and rheumatoid arthritis (see Ch. 14). Th1 responses are also implicated in allograft rejection (i.e. rejection of grafts between individuals of the same species), although, interestingly, conversion of these Th1 responses to Th2 responses at the maternal/fetal interface prevents rejection of the fetus, which is a sort of foreign 'allograft'.

Th2 responses predominate in allergic conditions such as asthma (Ch. 23). AIDS progression is associated with loss of Th1

cells and is facilitated by Th2 responses. Progression of some diseases is associated with changes in the Th1/Th2 balance; for example, in *tuberculoid leprosy*, Th1 responses predominate, in *lepromatous leprosy* Th2 responses predominate.

Understanding the relationship between T-cell subsets, their respective cytokine profiles and pathological conditions is expected to highlight ways to manipulate the immune responses for disease prevention and treatment. There are already many experimental models in which modulation of the Th1/Th2 balance with recombinant cytokines or cytokine antagonists alters the outcome of the disease.

Th1 cells and cell-mediated events

Th1 cells produce cytokines (IL-2, TNF-β and interferon [IFN]-γ), which:

- *activate macrophages* such that they phagocytose and kill microorganisms (such as mycobacteria) that might otherwise survive and grow intracellularly
- *stimulate CD8+ lymphocytes* to release IL-2 that drives proliferation and the subsequent maturation of the clone into cytotoxic cells that kill virally infected host cells (Fig. 13.3)
- *inhibit Th2 cell functions* (by IFN-γ action).

Th2 cells and antibody-mediated events

Th2 cells produce cytokines (IL-4, transforming growth factor [TGF]-β, IL-10), which:

- *stimulate B cells* to proliferate and mature into plasma cells producing antibodies, particularly IgE, the antibody that fixes to mast cells and, in the lung, to eosinophils
- *stimulate differentiation and activation of eosinophils*
- *inhibit Th1-cell functions*, i.e. the activation of inflammatory cells and the cell-mediated reactions produced by Th1 cytokines. For this reason, these cytokines are often thought of as anti-inflammatory.

The induction of antibody-mediated responses varies with the type of antigen. With most antigens, a cooperative process between

Th2 cells and B cells is necessary to produce a response. B cells can also present antigen to T cells that then release cytokines that act on the B cell. The anti-inflammatory glucocorticoids (see Chs 14 and 28) and the immunosuppressive drug **ciclosporin** (see Ch. 14) affect the events at the stage of induction. The cytotoxic immunosuppressive drugs (see Ch. 14) inhibit the proliferation of both B and T cells. Eicosanoids are believed to play a part in controlling these processes. For example, prostaglandins of the E series inhibit lymphocyte proliferation, probably by inhibiting the release of IL-2.

THE EFFECTOR PHASE

The *effector phase* may be antibody- or cell-mediated. The antibody-mediated (humoral) response is effective in the extracellular fluid, but antibodies cannot neutralise pathogens within cells. Cell-mediated immune mechanisms have evolved to deal with this problem.

The antibody-mediated (humoral) response

There are five classes of antibody—IgG, IgM, IgE, IgA and IgD—which differ from each other in certain structural respects (see Janeway et al., 2004). All are γ-globulins (immunoglobulins) and generally have two functions:

- to recognise and interact specifically with antigens, i.e. proteins or polysaccharides foreign to the host
- to activate one or more further components of the host's defence systems.

The antigen may form part of an invading organism (e.g. the coat of a bacterium) or be released by such an organism (e.g. a bacterial toxin), or it may be a substance introduced experimentally in the laboratory to study the immune response (e.g. the injection of egg albumin into the guinea pig). An antibody is a Y-shaped protein molecule in which the arms of the Y (the *Fab* portions) are the recognition sites for specific antigens, and the stem of the Y (the *Fc* portion) activates host defences. The B cells that are responsible for antibody production recognise foreign molecules by means of surface receptors that are essentially the immunoglobulin that that B-cell clone will eventually produce. Mammals possess a vast number of B-cell clones that produce different antibodies with recognition sites for different antigens.

As you might guess, the ability to make antibodies has huge survival value; children born without this ability suffer repeated infections such as pneumonia, skin infections and tonsillitis. Before the days of antibiotics, they died in early childhood, and even today they require regular replacement therapy with immunoglobulin. Apart from their ability to neutralise pathogens, antibodies can boost the effectiveness and specificity of the host's defence reaction in several ways.

Antibodies and the complement sequence

Formation of the antigen–antibody complex exposes a binding site for complement on the Fc domain. This activates the complement sequence and sets in train its attendant biological effects (see Fig. 13.1). This route to C3 activation (the classic pathway) provides an especially selective way of activating complement in

response to a particular pathogen, because the antigen–antibody reaction that initiates it is not only a highly specific recognition event but also occurs in close association with the pathogen. The lytic property of complement can be used therapeutically: monoclonal antibodies (mAbs) and complement together can be used to clean bone marrow of cancer cells as an adjunct to chemotherapy or radiotherapy (see Ch. 51). Complement lysis is also implicated in the action of antilymphocyte immunoglobulin.

Antibodies and the phagocytosis of bacteria

When antibodies are attached to their antigens on micro-organisms by their Fab portions, the Fc domain is exposed. Phagocytic cells (neutrophils and macrophages) have receptors on their membranes for these projecting Fc portions. Antibodies thus form a very specific link between microorganism and phagocyte that is more effective than C3b as an opsonin in facilitating phagocytosis (see Fig. 13.2).

Antibodies and cellular cytotoxicity

In some cases, for example with parasitic worms, the invader may be too large to be ingested by phagocytes. Antibody molecules can form a link between parasite and the host's white cells (in this case, eosinophils), which are then able to damage or kill the parasite by surface or extracellular actions. NK cells in conjunction with Fc receptors can also kill antibody-coated target cells (an example of antibody-dependent cell-mediated cytoxicity).

Antibodies and mast cells or basophils

Mast cells and basophils have receptors for IgE, a particular form of antibody that can attach ('fix') to their cell membranes. When antigen reacts with this cell-fixed antibody, a whole panoply of pharmacologically active mediators is secreted. This very complex reaction is found widely throughout the animal kingdom and is unlikely to have been developed and retained during evolution unless it offered clear survival value to the host. Having said that, its precise biological significance is not entirely clear, although it may be of importance in association with eosinophil activity as a defence against parasitic worms. When inappropriately triggered by substances not inherently damaging to the host, it is implicated in certain types of allergic reaction (see below) and apparently contributes more to illness than to survival in the modern world.

The cell-mediated immune response

Both cytotoxic T cells (derived from CD8$^+$ cells) and inflammatory (cytokine-releasing) Th1 cells are involved in cell-mediated responses (see Fig. 13.3). They enter inflammatory lesions in a similar manner to neutrophils and macrophages, namely by interaction between adhesion molecules on the endothelial cell and the lymphocyte and attraction to the inflammatory site by chemokines.

Cytotoxic T cells

Armed cytotoxic T cells kill *intracellular* micro-organisms such as viruses. When a virus infects a mammalian cell, there are two aspects to the resulting defensive response. The first step is the expression on the cell surface of peptides derived from the pathogen in association with MHC molecules. The second step is the recognition of the peptide–MHC complex by specific receptors on cytotoxic (CD8$^+$) T cells (Fig. 13.4 shows a similar process for a CD4$^+$ T cell). The cytotoxic T cells then destroy virus-infected cells by programming them to undergo apoptosis. Cooperation with macrophages may be required for killing to occur.

Macrophage-activating CD4$^+$ Th1 cells

Some pathogens (e.g. *mycobacteria*, *listeria*) have evolved strategies for surviving and multiplying within macrophages after ingestion. Armed CD4$^+$ Th1 cells release cytokines that activate macrophages to kill these intracellular pathogens. Th1 cells also recruit macrophages by releasing cytokines that act on vascular endothelial cells (e.g. TNF-α) and chemokines (e.g. macrophage chemotactic factor-1) that attract the macrophages to the sites of infection.

A complex of microorganism–derived peptides plus MHC molecules is expressed on the macrophage surface and is recognised by cytokine-releasing Th1 cells, which then generate cytokines that enable the macrophage to deploy its killing mechanisms. Activated macrophages (with or without intracellular pathogens) are factories for the production of chemical mediators, and can generate and secrete not only many cytokines but also toxic oxygen metabolites and neutral proteases that kill extracellular organisms (e.g. *Pneumocystis carinii* and helminths), complement components, eicosanoids, NO, a fibroblast-stimulating factor, pyrogens and the 'tissue factor' that initiates the extrinsic pathway of the coagulation cascade (Ch. 21), as well as various other coagulation factors. They are also important in the repair processes that must occur for inflammation to 'resolve'. Among the cytokines secreted is IL-12, which has a positive feedback effect, driving the development of further Th1 cells. It is primarily the cell-mediated reaction that is responsible for allograft rejection.

The specific cell-mediated or humoral immunological response is superimposed on the non-specific vascular and cellular reactions described previously, making them not only markedly more effective but much more selective for particular pathogens. An important aspect of the specific immunological response is that the clone of lymphocytes that are programmed to respond to an antigen is greatly expanded after the first contact with the organism and now contains *memory cells*. These changes cause a greatly accelerated and more effective response to subsequent antigen exposure. In some cases, the response is so rapid and efficient that, after one exposure, the pathogen can never gain a foothold again. Immunisation procedures make use of this fact.

The general events of the inflammatory and hypersensitivity reactions specified above vary in some tissues. For example, in the airway inflammation of asthma, eosinophils and neuropeptides play a particularly significant role (see Ch. 23). In CNS inflammation, there is less neutrophil infiltration and monocyte influx is delayed, possibly because of lack of adhesion molecule expression on CNS vascular endothelium and deficient generation of chemotaxins. It has long been known that some tissues—the CNS parenchyma, the anterior chamber of the eye, and the testis—are *privileged sites*, in that a foreign antigen introduced directly does not provoke an immune reaction. However, introduction elsewhere of an antigen already in the CNS parenchyma will trigger the development of immune/inflammatory responses in the CNS.

The adaptive response

- The adaptive (specific, acquired) immunological response boosts the effectiveness of the innate responses. It has two phases, the induction phase and the effector phase, the latter consisting of (i) antibody-mediated and (ii) cell-mediated components.
- During the *induction phase*, naive T cells bearing either the CD4 or the CD8 coreceptors are presented with antigen, triggering proliferation:
  — CD8-bearing T cells develop into cytotoxic T cells that can kill virally infected cells
  — CD4-bearing Th cells are stimulated by cytokines to develop into Th1 or Th2 cells
  — Th2 cells control antibody-mediated responses by stimulating B cells to proliferate, giving rise to antibody-secreting plasma cells and memory cells
  — Th1 cells develop into cells that release cytokines that activate macrophages; these cells, along with cytotoxic T cells, control cell-mediated responses.
- The *effector phase* depends on antibody- and cell-mediated responses.
- Antibodies provide:
  — more selective complement activation
  — more effective pathogen phagocytosis
  — more effective attachment to multicellular parasites, facilitating their destruction
  — direct neutralisation of some viruses and of some bacterial toxins.
- Cell-mediated reactions involve:
  — CD8$^+$ cytotoxic T cells that kill virus-infected cells
  — cytokine-releasing CD4$^+$ T cells that enable macrophages to kill intracellular pathogens such as the tubercle bacillus
  — memory cells primed to react rapidly to a known antigen.
- Inappropriately deployed immune reactions are termed *hypersensitivity reactions*.
- Anti-inflammatory and immunosuppressive drugs are used when the normally protective inflammatory and/or immune responses escape control.

SYSTEMIC RESPONSES IN INFLAMMATION

In addition to the local changes in an inflammatory area, there are often general systemic manifestations of inflammatory disease, including fever, an increase in blood leucocytes termed *leucocytosis* (or *neutrophilia* if the increase is in the neutrophils only), and the release from the liver of *acute-phase proteins*. These include C-reactive protein, α_2-macroglobulin, fibrinogen, α_1-antitrypsin and some complement components. While the function of many of these components is still a matter of conjecture, they all seem to have antimicrobial actions. C-reactive protein, for example, binds to some microorganisms, and the resulting complex activates complement. Other proteins scavenge iron (an essential nutrient for invading organisms) or block proteases, perhaps protecting the host against the worst excesses of the inflammatory response. Cortisol is also increased and exerts an important counter-regulatory effect on the inflammatory response (see Chs 14 and 28).

UNWANTED INFLAMMATORY AND IMMUNE RESPONSES

The immune response has to strike a delicate balance. According to one school of thought, an infection-proof immune system would be a possibility but would come at a serious cost to the host. With approximately 1 trillion potential antigenic sites in the host, such a 'superimmune' system would be some 1000 times more likely to attack the host itself, triggering *autoimmune* disease. In practice, therefore, it is not uncommon to find that innocuous substances such as pollen, or the host's own tissues, sometimes inadvertently activate the immune system; when this occurs, anti-inflammatory or immunosuppressive therapy may be required. Unwanted immune responses, termed *allergic* or *hypersensitivity* reactions, have been classified into four types (Janeway et al., 2004).

Type I: immediate or anaphylactic hypersensitivity

Type I hypersensitivity (often known simply as 'allergy') occurs in individuals who predominantly exhibit a Th2 rather than a Th1 response to antigen. In these individuals, substances that are not inherently noxious (such as grass pollen, house dust mites, certain foodstuffs or drugs, animal fur and so on) provoke the production of antibodies of the IgE type. These fix on mast cells, in the lung, and also to eosinophils. Subsequent contact with the material causes the release of histamine, PAF, eicosanoids and cytokines. The effects may be localised to the nose (hay fever), the bronchial tree (the initial phase of asthma), the skin (urticaria) or the gastrointestinal tract. In some cases, the reaction is more generalised and produces anaphylactic shock, which can be severe and life-threatening. Some important unwanted effects of drugs include *anaphylactic hypersensitivity* responses (see Ch. 53).

Type II: antibody-dependent cytotoxic hypersensitivity

Type II hypersensitivity occurs when the mechanisms outlined above are directed against *cells* within the host that are (or appear to be) foreign. For example, host cells altered by drugs are sometimes mistaken by the immune system for foreign proteins and evoke antibody formation. The antigen–antibody reaction triggers complement activation (and its sequelae) and may promote attack by NK cells. Examples include alteration by drugs of neutrophils, leading to *agranulocytosis* (see Ch. 53), or of platelets, leading to *thrombocytopenic purpura* (Ch. 21). These class II reactions are also implicated in some types of autoimmune thyroiditis (e.g. Hashimoto's disease; see Ch. 29).

Type III: complex-mediated hypersensitivity

Type III hypersensitivity occurs when antibodies react with soluble antigens. The antigen–antibody complexes can activate complement or attach to mast cells and stimulate the release of mediators.

▼An experimental example of this is the *Arthus reaction* that occurs if a foreign protein is injected subcutaneously into a rabbit or guinea pig with high circulating concentrations of antibody. Within 3–8 hours, the area becomes red and swollen because the antigen–antibody complexes precipitate in small blood vessels and activate complement. Neutrophils are attracted and activated (by C5a) to generate toxic oxygen species and to secrete enzymes.

Mast cells are also stimulated by C3a to release mediators. Damage caused by this process is involved in *serum sickness*, caused when antigen persists in the blood after sensitisation causing a severe reaction, as in the response to mouldy hay (known as *farmer's lung*), and in certain types of autoimmune kidney and arterial disease. Type III hypersensitivity is also implicated in *lupus erythematosus* (a chronic, autoimmune inflammatory disease).

Type IV: cell-mediated hypersensitivity

The prototype of *type IV hypersensitivity* (also known as delayed hypersensitivity) is the *tuberculin reaction*, a local inflammatory response seen when proteins derived from cultures of the tubercle bacillus are injected into the skin of a person who has been sensitised by a previous infection or immunisation. An 'inappropriate' cell-mediated immune response is stimulated, accompanied by infiltration of mononuclear cells and the release of various cytokines. Cell-mediated hypersensitivity is also the basis of the reaction seen in some other infections (e.g. mumps and measles), as well as with mosquito and tick bites. It is also important in the skin reactions to drugs or industrial chemicals (see Ch. 53), where the chemical (termed a *hapten*) combines with proteins in the skin to form the 'foreign' substance that evokes the cell-mediated immune response (Fig. 13.3). Other examples of cell-mediated hypersensitivity are rheumatoid arthritis (Ch. 14), multiple sclerosis and type 1 (insulin-dependent) diabetes (Ch. 26).

In essence, inappropriately deployed T-cell activity underlies all types of hypersensitivity, initiating types I, II and III, and being involved in both the initiation and the effector phase in type IV. These reactions are the basis of the clinically important group of autoimmune diseases. Immunosuppressive drugs (Ch. 14) and/or glucocorticoids (Ch. 28) are routinely employed to treat such disorders.

THE OUTCOME OF THE INFLAMMATORY RESPONSE

After outlining the specific immune response, we need to return to a consideration of the local acute inflammatory response that occurs at the site of the host–pathogen interaction. It should now be clear that this comprises an innate, immunologically non-specific component together with a variable involvement of the specific immunological response (either humoral or cell-mediated). The degree to which the latter is implicated depends on several factors, such as the nature of the pathogen and the infected organ or tissue.

It is important not to lose sight of the fact that the inflammatory response is a defence mechanism and not, *ipso facto*, a disease. Its role is to restore normal structure and function to the infected or damaged tissue and, in the vast majority of cases, this is what happens. The healing and resolution phase of the inflammatory response is an active process and does not simply 'happen' in the absence of further inflammation. This is an area that we are just beginning to understand, but it is clear that it utilises its own unique palette of mediators and cytokines (including various growth factors, annexin-A1, lipoxin and IL-10) to terminate residual inflammation and to promote remodelling and repair of damaged tissue.

In some cases, healing will be complete, but if there has been damage (death of cells, pus formation, ulceration) repair is usually necessary and may result in scarring. If the pathogen persists, the acute response is likely to transform into a *chronic* inflammatory response. This is a slow, smouldering reaction that can continue indefinitely, destroying tissue and promoting local proliferation of cells and connective tissue. The principal cell types found in areas of chronic inflammation are mononuclear cells and abnormal macrophage-derived cells. During healing or chronic inflammation, growth factors trigger angiogenesis and cause fibroblasts to lay down fibrous tissue. Infection by some microorganisms, such as syphilis, tuberculosis and leprosy, bears the characteristic hallmarks of chronic inflammation from the start. The cellular and mediator components of this type of inflammation are also seen in many, if not most, chronic autoimmune and hypersensitivity diseases, and are important targets for drug action.

MEDIATORS OF INFLAMMATION AND IMMUNE REACTIONS

Soluble mediators, many of which may be regarded as local hormones, play a key (if sometimes mysterious) role in the orchestration of the inflammatory response. A 'mediator' is operationally defined as a substance that fulfils a set of criteria generally modelled on the original suggestions of Sir Henry Dale in 1933. A modified version, more applicable to the field today, was considered by Dale (1994). The principal mediators of pharmacological significance will be described below.

HISTAMINE

In a classic study, Sir Henry Dale and his colleagues demonstrated that a local anaphylactic reaction (a type I or 'immediate hypersensitivity reaction'; see above) was caused by antigen–antibody reactions in sensitised tissue, and found that histamine mimicked this effect both in vitro and in vivo. The first generation of antihistamine drugs was discovered by Bovet and colleagues, but careful quantitative studies by Schild suggested that there were in fact two types of histamine receptor in the body. Contemporary antihistamines affected only one type, the H_1 *receptors*, and were without action on the second group of H_2 *receptors*, which were important in gastric acid secretion. Utilising Schild's classification, Black and his colleagues developed the second generation of antihistamine drugs, the H_2 *receptor antagonists*. A third subtype of histamine receptor, the H_3 receptor, was cloned in 1999, and the H_4 receptor in 2001 (Zhu et al., 2001).

Synthesis and storage of histamine

Histamine is a basic amine formed from histidine by *histidine decarboxylase*. It is found in most tissues but is present in high concentrations in the lungs and the skin, and in particularly high concentrations in the gastrointestinal tract. At the cellular level, it is found largely in mast cells (approximately 0.1–0.2 pmol/cell) and basophils (0.01 pmol/cell), but non–mast cell histamine occurs in 'histaminocytes' in the stomach and in *histaminergic neurons* in the brain (see Ch. 34). In mast cells and basophils, histamine is complexed in intracellular granules with an acidic protein and a high-molecular-weight heparin termed *macroheparin*.

Histamine release

Histamine is released from mast cells by exocytosis during inflammatory or allergic reactions. Stimuli include C3a and C5a that interact with specific surface receptors, and the combination of antigen with cell-fixed IgE antibodies. In common with many secretory processes (Ch. 4), histamine release is initiated by a rise in cytosolic Ca^{2+}. Various basic drugs, such as **morphine** and **tubocurarine**, release histamine through a non–receptor action. Agents that increase cAMP formation (e.g. β-adrenoceptor agonists; see Ch. 11) inhibit histamine secretion. Replenishment of secreted histamine by mast cells or basophils is a slow process, which may take days or weeks, whereas turnover of histamine in the gastric histaminocyte is very rapid. Histamine is metabolised by *histaminase* and/or by the methylating enzyme *imidazole N-methyltransferase*.

Actions

Histamine acts on specific receptors that may be distinguished by means of selective antagonist drugs. Some details relating to the four main types of histamine receptor, all of which are implicated in the inflammatory response (see Gutzmer et al., 2005, for a review), are given in Tables 13.1 and 13.2. Selective *antagonists* at H_1, H_2 and H_3 receptors include **mepyramine**, **cimetidine** and **thioperamide**, respectively. Selective *agonists* for H_2 and H_3 receptors are, respectively, dimaprit and (*R*)-methylhistamine. Histamine H_1 antagonists are the principal antihistamines used in the treatment of inflammation (notably rhinitis). Other clinical uses of subtype antagonists may be found in Chapters 14, 25 and 34.

Gastric secretion

Histamine stimulates the secretion of gastric acid by action on H_2 receptors. In clinical terms, this is the most important action of histamine, because it is implicated in the pathogenesis of peptic ulcer. It is considered in detail in Chapter 25.

Smooth muscle effects

Histamine, acting on H_1 receptors, contracts the smooth muscle of the ileum, bronchi, bronchioles and uterus. The effect on the ileum is not as marked in humans as it is in the guinea pig (this tissue remains the de facto standard preparation for histamine bioassay). Histamine reduces air flow in the first phase of bronchial asthma (see Ch. 23 and Fig. 23.3).

Cardiovascular effects

Histamine dilates human blood vessels by an action on H_1 receptors, the effect being partly endothelium-dependent in some

Table 13.1   Details of some agonist drugs used to define the three types of histamine receptor

Drug	Relative activity in vitro		
	H_1 receptors (ileum contraction)	H_2 receptors (stimulation of atrial rate)	H_3 receptors (histamine release from brain tissue)
Histamine	100	100	100
Dimaprit	< 0.0001	71	0.0008
(R)-α-Methylhistamine	0.49	1.02	1550

(Data derived from Black J W et al. 1972 Nature 236: 385–390; Ganellin C R 1982 In: Ganellin C R, Parson M E [eds] Pharmacology of histamine receptors. Wright, Bristol, pp.11–102; Arrang J M et al. 1987 Nature 327: 117–123; van der Werf J F, Timmerman H 1989 Trends Pharmacol Sci 10: 159–162.)

Table 13.2   Details of some antagonist drugs used to define the three types of histamine receptor

Drug	Binding constant (K_B; mol/l)		
	H_1	H_2	H_3
Mepyramine	0.4×10^9	–	$> 3 \times 10^6$
Cimetidine	4.5×10^4	0.8×10^6	3.3×10^5
Thioperamide	$> 10^4$	$> 10^5$	4.3×10^9

(Data derived from Black J W et al. 1972 Nature 236: 385–390; Ganellin C R 1982 In: Ganellin C R, Parson M E [eds] Pharmacology of histamine receptors. Wright, Bristol, pp. 11–102; Arrang J M et al. 1987 Nature 327: 117–123; van der Werf J F, Timmerman H 1989 Trends Pharmacol Sci 10: 159–162.)

Histamine

- Histamine is a basic amine, stored in mast cell and basophil granules, and secreted when C3a and C5a interact with specific membrane receptors or when antigen interacts with cell-fixed immunoglobulin E.
- Histamine produces effects by acting on H_1, H_2 or H_3 (and possibly H_4) receptors on target cells.
- The main actions in humans are:
  — stimulation of gastric secretion (H_2)
  — contraction of most smooth muscle, except blood vessels (H_1)
  — cardiac stimulation (H_2)
  — vasodilatation (H_1)
  — increased vascular permeability (H_1).
- Injected intradermally, histamine causes the 'triple response': *reddening* (local vasodilatation), *weal* (direct action on blood vessels) and *flare* (from an 'axon' reflex in sensory nerves releasing a peptide mediator).
- The main pathophysiological roles of histamine are:
  — as a stimulant of gastric acid secretion (treated with H_2-receptor antagonists)
  — as a mediator of type I hypersensitivity reactions such as urticaria and hay fever (treated with H_1-receptor antagonists).
- H_3 receptors occur at presynaptic sites and inhibit the release of a variety of neurotransmitters.

vascular beds. It also increases the rate and the output of the heart by action on cardiac H_2 receptors.

When injected intradermally, histamine causes a reddening of the skin, accompanied by a weal with a surrounding flare. This is the *triple response* described by Sir Thomas Lewis over 50 years ago. The reddening reflects vasodilatation of the small arterioles and precapillary sphincters, and the weal the increased permeability of the postcapillary venules. These effects are mainly mediated through activation of H_1 receptors. The flare is an *axon reflex*: stimulation of sensory nerve fibres evokes antidromic impulses through neighbouring branches of the same nerve, releasing vasodilators such as CGRP (see Chs 14 and 16).

Itching
Itching occurs if histamine is injected into the skin or applied to a blister base, because it stimulates sensory nerve endings by an H_1-dependent mechanism.

Central nervous system effects
Histamine is a transmitter in the CNS (Ch. 34).

Despite the fact that histamine release is evidently capable of producing many of the inflammatory signs and symptoms, histamine H_1 antagonists do not have much clinical utility in the acute inflammatory response per se, because other mediators are more important. Histamine is, however, significant in type I hypersensitivity reactions such as allergic rhinitis and urticaria. The use of H_1 antagonists in these and other conditions is dealt with in Chapter 14.

EICOSANOIDS

Unlike histamine, *eicosanoids* are not preformed in cells but are generated from phospholipid precursors on demand. They are implicated in the control of many physiological processes, and are among the most important mediators and modulators of the inflammatory reaction (Fig. 13.5).

Interest in eicosanoids arose in the 1930s after reports that semen contained a lipid substance that contracted uterine smooth muscle. The substance was believed to originate in the prostate, and was saddled with the misnomer *prostaglandin*. Later, it became clear that prostaglandin was not a single substance but a whole family of compounds that could be generated from 20-carbon unsaturated fatty acids by virtually all cells.

Structure and biosynthesis

In mammals, the main eicosanoid precursor is *arachidonic acid* (5,8,11,14-eicosatetraenoic acid), a 20-carbon unsaturated fatty acid containing four double bonds (hence *eicosa*, referring to the 20 carbon atoms, and *tetraenoic*, referring to the four double bonds). In most cell types, arachidonic acid is esterified in the phospholipid pool, and the concentration of the free acid is low. The principal eicosanoids are the *prostaglandins*, the *thromboxanes* and the *leukotrienes*, although other derivatives of arachidonate,

for example the *lipoxins*, are also produced. (The term *prostanoid* will be used here to encompass both prostaglandins and thromboxanes.)

In most instances, the initial and rate-limiting step in eicosanoid synthesis is the liberation of arachidonate, either in a one-step process (Fig. 13.6) or a two-step process (Fig. 13.7), from phospholipids by the enzyme *phospholipase A₂* (PLA_2). Several species exist, but the most important is probably the highly regulated *cytosolic PLA₂*. This enzyme generates not only arachidonic acid (and thus eicosanoids) but also *lysoglyceryl-phosphorylcholine* (*lyso-PAF*), the precursor of *platelet activating factor*, another inflammatory mediator (see Figs 13.5 and 13.10).

Cytosolic PLA₂ is activated (and hence arachidonic acid liberated) by phosphorylation. This occurs in response to signal transduction events triggered by many stimuli, such as thrombin action on platelets, C5a on neutrophils, bradykinin on fibroblasts, and antigen–antibody reactions on mast cells. General cell damage also triggers the activation process. The free arachidonic acid is metabolised by several pathways, including the following.

- *Fatty acid cyclo-oxygenase (COX)*. Two main isoform forms, COX-1 and COX-2, transform arachidonic acid to prostaglandins and thromboxanes.

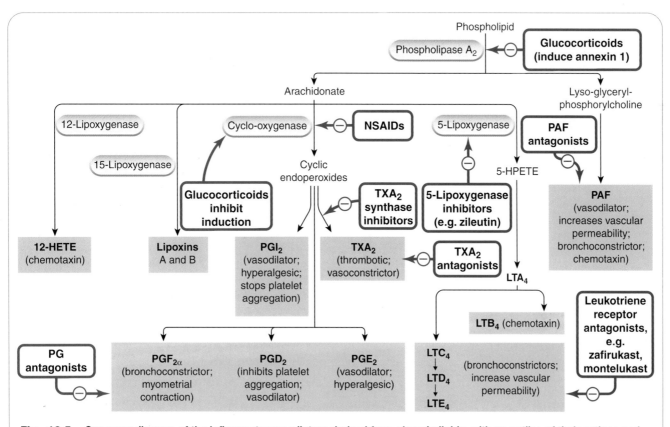

Fig. 13.5 **Summary diagram of the inflammatory mediators derived from phospholipids, with an outline of their actions and the sites of action of anti-inflammatory drugs.** The arachidonate metabolites are *eicosanoids*. The glucocorticoids inhibit transcription of the gene for cyclo-oxygenase-2, induced in inflammatory cells by inflammatory mediators. The effects of prostaglandin (PG) E₂ depend on which of the three receptors for this prostanoid are activated. HETE, hydroxyeicosatetraenoic acid; HPETE, hydroperoxyeicosatetraenoic acid; LT, leukotriene; NSAID, non-steroidal anti-inflammatory drug; PAF, platelet-activating factor; PGI₂, prostacyclin; TX, thromboxane.

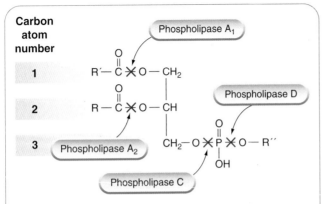

Fig. 13.6 **The structure of phospholipids and the sites of action of phospholipases.** Generally speaking, unsaturated fatty acids such as arachidonic acid are esterified at the C2 position, from which it can be removed by phospholipase A$_2$, but other metabolic routes are known (see Fig. 13.7). The numbering of the carbon atoms in the glycerol 'backbone' is given on the left. This figure shows O-acyl residues on carbon atoms 1 and 2, but O-alkyl residues can occur (see Fig. 13.10). Different bases are found at C3. R' is choline, ethanolamine, serine, inositol or hydrogen.

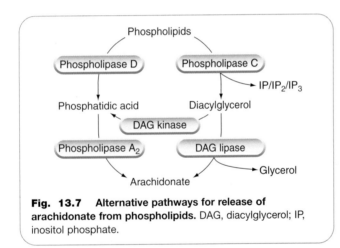

Fig. 13.7 **Alternative pathways for release of arachidonate from phospholipids.** DAG, diacylglycerol; IP, inositol phosphate.

- *Lipoxygenases.* Several subtypes synthesise leukotrienes, lipoxins or other compounds (Figs 13.5 and 13.8).

Chapter 14 deals in detail with the way inhibitors of these pathways (including non-steroidal anti-inflammatory drugs [NSAIDs] and glucocorticoids) produce anti-inflammatory effects.

PROSTANOIDS

Cyclo-oxygenase-1 is present in most cells as a constitutive enzyme that produces prostanoids that act as homeostatic regulators (e.g. modulating vascular responses), whereas COX-2 is not normally present but it is strongly induced by inflammatory stimuli and therefore believed to be more relevant to inflammation therapy (see next chapter for a full discussion of this point). Both enzymes catalyse the incorporation of two molecules of oxygen

into every arachidonate molecule, forming the highly unstable endoperoxides *PGG$_2$* and *PGH$_2$*. These are rapidly transformed by *isomerase* or *synthase* enzymes to PGE$_2$, PGI$_2$, PGD$_2$, PGF$_{2\alpha}$ and TXA$_2$, which are the principal bioactive end products of this reaction. The mix of eicosanoids thus produced varies between cell types depending on the particular endoperoxide isomerases or synthases present. In platelets, for example, TXA$_2$ predominates, whereas in vascular endothelium PGI$_2$ is the main product. Macrophages, neutrophils and mast cells synthesise a mixture of products. If *eicosatrienoic acid* (three double bonds) rather than arachidonic acid is the substrate, the resulting prostanoids have only a single double bond, for example PGE$_1$, while *eicosapentaenoic acid*, which contains five double bonds, yields PGE$_3$. The latter substrate is significant because it is present in abundance in some fish oils and may, if present in sufficient amounts in the diet, come to represent a significant fraction of cellular fatty acids. When this occurs, the production of the proinflammatory PGE$_2$ is diminished and, more significantly, the generation of TXA$_2$ as well. This may underlie the beneficial anti-inflammatory and cardiovascular actions that are ascribed to diets rich in this type of marine product.

Catabolism of the prostanoids

This is a multistep process. After carrier-mediated uptake, most prostaglandins are rapidly inactivated by 'prostaglandin-specific' enzymes, and the inactive products are further degraded by general fatty acid–oxidising enzymes. The prostaglandin-specific enzymes are present in high concentration in the lung, and 95% of infused PGE$_2$, PGE$_1$ or PGF$_{2\alpha}$ is inactivated on first passage. The half-life of most prostaglandins in the circulation is less than 1 minute.

Prostaglandin I$_2$ and TXA$_2$ are slightly different. Both are inherently unstable and decay rapidly (5 minutes and 30 seconds, respectively) in biological fluids into inactive 6-keto-PGF$_{1\alpha}$ and TXB$_2$. Further metabolism occurs, but it is not really relevant to us here.

Prostanoid receptors

There are five main classes of prostanoid receptors (Coleman et al., 1993), all of which are typical G-protein–coupled receptors. They are termed *DP, FP, IP, EP* and *TP receptors*, respectively, depending on whether their ligands are PGD$_2$, PGF$_{2\alpha}$, PGI$_2$, PGE$_2$ or TXA$_2$. Some have further subtypes; for example, the EP receptors are subdivided into three subgroups.

Actions of the prostanoids

The prostanoids affect most tissues and exert a bewildering variety of effects.

- *PGD$_2$* causes vasodilatation, inhibition of platelet aggregation, relaxation of gastrointestinal and uterine muscle, and modification of release of hypothalamic/pituitary hormones. It has a bronchoconstrictor effect through an action on TP receptors.
- *PGF$_{2\alpha}$* causes myometrial contraction in humans (see Ch. 30), luteolysis in some species (e.g. cattle) and bronchoconstriction in other species (cats and dogs).

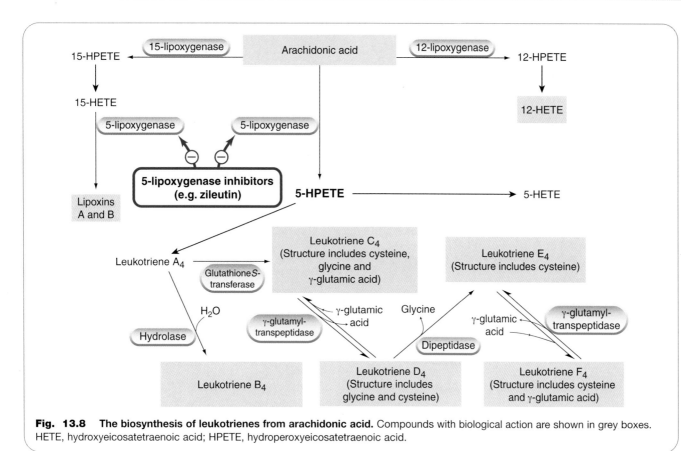

Fig. 13.8 **The biosynthesis of leukotrienes from arachidonic acid.** Compounds with biological action are shown in grey boxes. HETE, hydroxyeicosatetraenoic acid; HPETE, hydroperoxyeicosatetraenoic acid.

- *PGI₂* causes vasodilatation, inhibition of platelet aggregation (see Ch. 21), renin release and natriuresis through effects on tubular reabsorption of Na⁺.
- *TXA₂* causes vasoconstriction, platelet aggregation (see Ch. 21) and bronchoconstriction (more marked in guinea pig than in humans).
- *PGE₂* has the following actions:
  —on EP₁ receptors, it causes contraction of bronchial and gastrointestinal smooth muscle
  —on EP₂ receptors, it causes bronchodilatation, vasodilatation, stimulation of intestinal fluid secretion, and relaxation of gastrointestinal smooth muscle
  —on EP₃ receptors, it causes contraction of intestinal smooth muscle, inhibition of gastric acid secretion (see Ch. 25), increased gastric mucus secretion, inhibition of lipolysis, inhibition of autonomic neurotransmitter release, and stimulation of contraction of the pregnant human uterus (Ch. 30).

The role of the prostanoids in inflammation

The inflammatory response is inevitably accompanied by the release of prostanoids. PGE₂ predominates, although PGI₂ is also important. In areas of acute inflammation, PGE₂ and PGI₂ are generated by the local tissues and blood vessels, while mast cells release mainly PGD₂. In chronic inflammation, cells of the monocyte/macrophage series also release PGE₂ and TXA₂. Together, the prostanoids exert a sort of yin–yang effect in

> **Mediators derived from phospholipids**
>
> - The main phospholipid-derived mediators are the eicosanoids (prostanoids and leukotrienes) and platelet-activating factor (PAF).
> - The eicosanoids are synthesised from arachidonic acid released directly from phospholipids by phospholipase A₂, or by a two-step process involving phospholipase C and diacylglycerol lipase.
> - Arachidonate is metabolised by cyclo-oxygenase (COX)-1 or COX-2 to prostanoids, or by 5-lipoxygenase to leukotrienes.
> - PAF is derived from phospholipid precursors by phospholipase A₂, giving rise to lyso-PAF, which is then acetylated to give PAF.

inflammation, stimulating some responses and decreasing others. The most striking effects are as follow.

In their own right, PGE₂, PGI₂ and PGD₂ are powerful vasodilators and synergise with other inflammatory vasodilators such as histamine and bradykinin. It is this combined dilator action on precapillary arterioles that contributes to the redness and increased blood flow in areas of acute inflammation. Prostanoids do not directly increase the permeability of the postcapillary venules, but potentiate this effect of histamine and bradykinin. Similarly,

Prostanoids

- The term *prostanoids* encompasses the prostaglandins and the thromboxanes.
- Cyclo-oxygenases (COXs) oxidise arachidonate, producing the unstable intermediates prostaglandin (PG) G_2 and PGH_2.
- There are two main COX isoforms: COX-1, a constitutive enzyme, and COX-2, which is often induced by inflammatory stimuli.
- PGI_2 (prostacyclin), predominantly from vascular endothelium, acts on IP receptors, producing vasodilatation and inhibition of platelet aggregation.
- Thromboxane (TX) A_2, predominantly from platelets, acts on TP receptors, causing platelet aggregation and vasoconstriction.
- PGE_2 is prominent in inflammatory responses and is a mediator of fever. Main effects are:
  - EP_1 receptors: contraction of bronchial and gastrointestinal tract (GIT) smooth muscle
  - EP_2 receptors: relaxation of bronchial, vascular and GIT smooth muscle
  - EP_3 receptors: inhibition of gastric acid secretion, increased gastric mucus secretion, contraction of pregnant uterus and of GIT smooth muscle, inhibition of lipolysis and of autonomic neurotransmitter release.
- $PGF_{2\alpha}$ acts on FP receptors, found in uterine (and other) smooth muscle, and corpus luteum, producing contraction of the uterus and luteolysis (in some species).
- PGD_2 is derived particularly from mast cells and acts on DP receptors, causing vasodilatation and inhibition of platelet aggregation.

Clinical uses of prostanoids

- Gynaecological and obstetric (see Ch. 30)
  - termination of pregnancy: **gemeprost** or **misoprostol** (a metabolically stable prostaglandin (PG) E analogue)
  - induction of labour: **dinoprostone** or **misoprostol**
  - postpartum haemorrhage: **carboprost**.
- Gastrointestinal
  - to prevent ulcers associated with non-steroidal anti-inflammatory drug use: **misoprostol** (see Ch. 25).
- Cardiovascular
  - to maintain the patency of the ductus arteriosus until surgical correction of the defect in babies with certain congenital heart malformations: **alprostadil** (PGE_1)
  - to inhibit platelet aggregation (e.g. during haemodialysis): **epoprostenol** (PGI_2), especially if heparin is contraindicated
  - primary pulmonary hypertension: **epoprostenol** (Ch. 19).
- Ophthalmic
  - open-angle glaucoma: **latanoprost** eye drops.

they do not themselves produce pain, but potentiate the effect of bradykinin by sensitising afferent C fibres (see Ch. 41) to the effects of other noxious stimuli. The anti-inflammatory effects of the NSAIDs stem largely from their ability to block these actions of the prostaglandins.

Prostaglandins of the E series are also pyrogenic (i.e. they induce fever). High concentrations are found in cerebrospinal fluid during infection, and there is evidence that the increase in temperature (attributed to cytokines) is actually finally mediated by the release of PGE_2. NSAIDs exert antipyretic actions (Ch. 14) by inhibiting PGE_2 synthesis in the hypothalamus.

However, some prostaglandins have *anti-inflammatory* effects under some circumstances. For example, PGE_2 decreases lysosomal enzyme release and the generation of toxic oxygen metabolites from neutrophils, as well as the release of histamine from mast cells. Several prostanoids are available for clinical use (see clinical box).

LEUKOTRIENES

Leukotrienes (*leuko* because they are made by white cells, and *trienes* because they contain a conjugated triene system of double bonds) are synthesised from arachidonic acid by lipoxygenase-catalysed pathways. These soluble cytosolic enzymes are found in lung, platelets, mast cells and white blood cells. The main enzyme in this group is *5-lipoxygenase*. On cell activation, this enzyme translocates to the nuclear membrane, where it associates with a crucial accessory protein affectionately termed *FLAP* (*five-lipoxygenase activating protein*). The 5-lipoxygenase incorporates a hydroperoxy group at C5 in arachidonic acid (Fig. 13.8), leading to the production of the unstable compound *leukotriene (LT) A_4*. This may be converted enzymically to LTB_4 and is also the precursor of the cysteinyl-containing leukotrienes LTC_4, LTD_4, LTE_4 and LTF_4 (also referred to as the *sulfidopeptide leukotrienes*). Mixtures of these cysteinyl adducts constitute the *slow-reacting substance of anaphylaxis (SRS-A)*, a substance shown many years ago to be generated in guinea pig lung during anaphylaxis, and believed to be important in asthma. LTB_4 is produced mainly by neutrophils, and the cysteinyl-leukotrienes mainly by eosinophils, mast cells, basophils and macrophages. *Lipoxins* and other active products, some of which have anti-inflammatory properties, are also produced from arachidonate by this pathway (Fig. 13.8).

Leukotriene B_4 is metabolised by a unique membrane-bound P450 enzyme in neutrophils, and then further oxidised to 20-carboxy-LTB_4. LTC_4 and LTD_4 are metabolised to LTE_4, which is excreted in the urine.

Actions and receptors of the leukotrienes

Receptors for the leukotrienes are termed *leukotriene receptors*: *BLT* if the ligand is LTB_4, and *CysLT* if the cysteinyl-leukotrienes. LTB_4 acts on specific LTB_4 receptors as defined by selective agonists and antagonists. The transduction mechanism utilises inositol trisphosphate and increased cytosolic Ca^{2+}. LTB_4 is a potent chemotactic agent for neutrophils and macrophages (see Fig. 13.2). On neutrophils, it also up-regulates membrane adhesion molecule expression, and increases the production of toxic oxygen products and the release of granule enzymes. On macrophages and lymphocytes, it stimulates proliferation and cytokine release.

Cysteinyl-leukotrienes have important actions on the respiratory and cardiovascular systems, and specific receptors for LTD_4 have been defined on the basis of numerous selective antagonists.

- *The respiratory system.* Cysteinyl-leukotrienes are potent spasmogens, causing dose-related contraction of human bronchiolar muscle in vitro. LTE_4 is less potent than LTC_4 and LTD_4, but its effect is much longer lasting. All cause an increase in mucus secretion. Given by aerosol to human volunteers, they reduce specific airway conductance and maximum expiratory flow rate, the effect being more protracted than that produced by histamine (Fig. 13.9).
- *The cardiovascular system.* Small amounts of LTC_4 or LTD_4 given intravenously cause a rapid, short-lived fall in blood pressure, and significant constriction of small coronary resistance vessels. Given subcutaneously, they are equipotent with histamine in causing weal and flare. Given topically in the nose, LTD_4 increases nasal blood flow and increases local vascular permeability.

The role of leukotrienes in inflammation

Leukotriene B_4 is found in inflammatory exudates and tissues in many inflammatory conditions, including rheumatoid arthritis, psoriasis and ulcerative colitis. The cysteinyl-leukotrienes are present in the sputum of chronic bronchitis in amounts that are biologically active. On antigen challenge, they are released from samples of human asthmatic lung in vitro, and into nasal lavage fluid in subjects with allergic rhinitis. There is evidence that they contribute to the underlying bronchial hyperreactivity in asthmatics, and it is thought that they are among the main mediators of both the early and late phases of asthma (Fig. 23.2).

The CysLT-receptor antagonists **zafirlukast** and **montelukast** are now in use in the treatment of asthma (see Ch. 23). Cysteinyl-leukotrienes may mediate the cardiovascular changes of acute anaphylaxis. Agents that inhibit 5-lipoxygenase are under development as antiasthmatic agents (see Ch. 23) and anti-inflammatory agents. One such drug, **zileuton**, is available in some parts of the world but has not won a definite place in therapy yet (see Larsson et al., 2006).

LIPOXINS

Recent work has indicated that products of the 15-lipoxygenase enzyme termed *lipoxins* (Fig. 13.8) act on specific receptors on polymorphonuclear leucocytes to oppose the action of LTB_4, supplying what might be called 'stop signals' to inflammation. Oddly, aspirin stimulates the synthesis of these substances, perhaps contributing to its other anti-inflammatory effects (see Gilroy & Perretti, 2005; Serhan, 2005). Lipoxins utilise the same formyl peptide G-protein–coupled receptor system as the anti-inflammatory protein annexin-A1.

PLATELET-ACTIVATING FACTOR

Platelet-activating factor, also variously termed *PAF-acether* and *AGEPC (acetyl-glyceryl-ether-phosphorylcholine)*, is a biologically active lipid that can produce effects at exceedingly low concen-

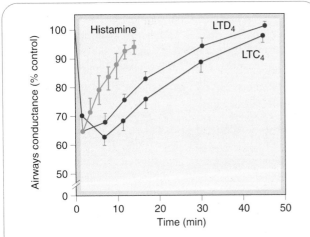

Fig. 13.9 **The time course of action on specific airways conductance of the cysteinyl-leukotrienes and histamine, in six normal subjects.** Specific airways conductance was measured in a constant volume whole-body plethysmograph, and the drugs were given by inhalation. (From Barnes P J, Piper P J, Costello J K 1984 Thorax 39: 500.)

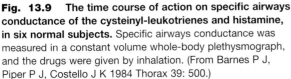

Leukotrienes

- 5-Lipoxygenase oxidises arachidonate to give 5-hydroperoxyeicosatetraenoic acid (5-HPETE), which is converted to leukotriene (LT) A_4. This, in turn, can be converted to either LTB_4 or to a series of glutathione adducts, the cysteinyl-leukotrienes LTC_4, LTD_4 and LTE_4.
- LTB_4, acting on specific receptors, causes adherence, chemotaxis and activation of polymorphs and monocytes, and stimulates proliferation and cytokine production from macrophages and lymphocytes.
- The cysteinyl-leukotrienes cause:
  — contraction of bronchial muscle
  — vasodilatation in most vessels, but coronary vasoconstriction.
- LTB_4 is an important mediator in all types of inflammation; the cysteinyl-leukotrienes are of particular importance in asthma.

trations (less than 10^{-10} mol/l). The name is somewhat misleading, because PAF has actions on a variety of different target cells, and is believed to be an important mediator in both acute and chronic allergic and inflammatory phenomena. PAF is biosynthesised from acyl-PAF in a two-step process (Fig. 13.10). The action of PLA_2 on acyl-PAF produces lyso-PAF, which is then acetylated to give PAF. PAF, in turn, can be deacetylated to the inactive lyso-PAF (Fig. 13.11).

Sources of platelet-activating factor

Platelets stimulated with thrombin and most inflammatory cells can release PAF under the right circumstances.

Actions and role in inflammation

By acting on specific receptors, PAF is capable of producing many of the signs and symptoms of inflammation. Injected locally, it produces vasodilatation (and thus erythema), increased vascular permeability and weal formation. Higher doses produce hyperalgesia. It is a potent chemotaxin for neutrophils and monocytes, and recruits eosinophils into the bronchial mucosa in the late phase of asthma (Fig. 23.3). It can activate PLA_2 and initiates eicosanoid synthesis.

On platelets, PAF triggers arachidonate turnover and TXA_2 generation, producing shape change and the release of the granule contents. This is important in haemostasis and thrombosis (see Ch. 21). PAF has spasmogenic effects on both bronchial and ileal smooth muscle.

The anti-inflammatory actions of the glucocorticoids may be caused, at least in part, by inhibition of PAF synthesis (Fig. 13.5). Competitive antagonists of PAF and/or specific inhibitors of lyso-PAF acetyltransferase could well be useful anti-inflammatory drugs and/or antiasthmatic agents. The PAF antagonist **lexipafant** is in clinical trial in the treatment of acute pancreatitis (see Leveau et al., 2005).

BRADYKININ

Bradykinin and lysyl bradykinin (*kallidin*) are active peptides formed by proteolytic cleavage of circulating proteins termed *kininogens* through a protease cascade pathway (Fig. 13.1).

Source and formation of bradykinin

An outline of the formation of bradykinin from high-molecular-weight kininogen in plasma by the serine protease *kallikrein* is given in Figure 13.12. Kininogen is a plasma α-globulin that exists in both high (M_r 110 000) and low (M_r 70 000) molecular weight forms. Kallikrein is derived from the inactive precursor *prekallikrein* by the action of *Hageman factor* (factor XII; see Ch. 21 and Fig. 13.1). Hageman factor is activated by contact with negatively charged surfaces such as collagen, basement membrane, bacterial lipopolysaccharides, urate crystals and so on. Hageman factor, prekallikrein and the kininogens leak out of the vessels during inflammation because of increased vascular permeability, and exposure to negatively charged surfaces promotes the interaction of Hageman factor with prekallikrein. The activated enzyme then 'clips' bradykinin from its kininogen precursor (Fig. 13.13). Kallikrein can also activate the complement system and can convert plasminogen to plasmin (see Fig. 13.1 and Ch. 21).

In addition to plasma kallikrein, there are other kinin-generating isoenzymes found in pancreas, salivary glands, colon and skin. These *tissue kallikreins* act on both high- and low-

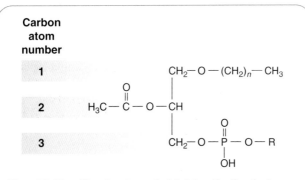

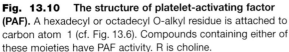

Fig. 13.10 The structure of platelet-activating factor (PAF). A hexadecyl or octadecyl O-alkyl residue is attached to carbon atom 1 (cf. Fig. 13.6). Compounds containing either of these moieties have PAF activity. R is choline.

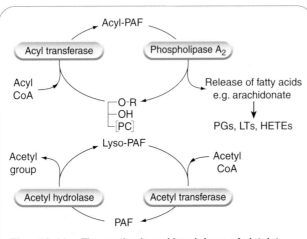

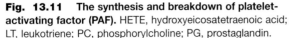

Fig. 13.11 The synthesis and breakdown of platelet-activating factor (PAF). HETE, hydroxyeicosatetraenoic acid; LT, leukotriene; PC, phosphorylcholine; PG, prostaglandin.

Platelet-activating factor

- PAF is released from activated inflammatory cells by phospholipase A_2 and acts on specific receptors in target cells.
- Pharmacological actions include vasodilatation, increased vascular permeability, chemotaxis and activation of leucocytes (especially eosinophils), activation and aggregation of platelets, and smooth muscle contraction.
- PAF is implicated in bronchial hyperresponsiveness and in the delayed phase of asthma.

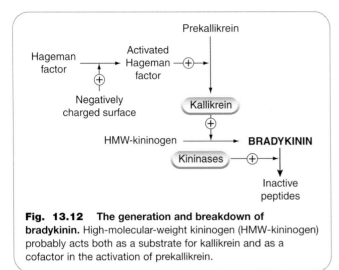

Fig. 13.12 **The generation and breakdown of bradykinin.** High-molecular-weight kininogen (HMW-kininogen) probably acts both as a substrate for kallikrein and as a cofactor in the activation of prekallikrein.

II. Thus kininase II inactivates a vasodilator and activates a vasoconstrictor. Potentiation of bradykinin actions by ACE inhibitors may contribute to some side effects of these drugs (e.g. cough; p. 309). Kinins are also metabolised by various less specific peptidases, including a serum carboxypeptidase that removes the C-terminal arginine, generating *des-Arg⁹-bradykinin*, a specific agonist at one of the two main classes of bradykinin receptor (see below).

Actions and role of bradykinin in inflammation

Bradykinin causes vasodilatation and increased vascular permeability. Its vasodilator action is partly a result of generation of PGI_2 (Fig. 13.5) and release of NO. It is a potent pain-producing agent, and its action is potentiated by the prostaglandins. Bradykinin also has spasmogenic actions on intestinal, uterine and bronchial smooth muscle (in some species). The contraction is slow and sustained in comparison with that produced by histamine (hence *brady*, which means 'slow').

Although bradykinin reproduces many inflammatory signs and symptoms, its role in inflammation and allergy has not been clearly defined, partly because its effects are often part of a complex cascade of events triggered by other mediators. However, excessive bradykinin production contributes to the diarrhoea of gastrointestinal disorders, and in allergic rhinitis it stimulates nasopharyngeal secretion. Bradykinin also contributes to the clinical picture in pancreatitis. Physiologically, the release of bradykinin by tissue kallikrein may regulate blood flow to certain exocrine glands, and influence secretions. It also stimulates ion transport and fluid secretion by some epithelia, including intestine, airways and gall bladder.

molecular-weight kininogens and generate mainly kallidin, a peptide with actions similar to those of bradykinin.

Metabolism and inactivation of bradykinin

Specific enzymes that inactivate bradykinin and related kinins are called *kininases* (Figs 13.12 and 13.13). One of these, *kininase II*, is a peptidyl dipeptidase that inactivates kinins by removing the two C-terminal amino acids. This enzyme, which is bound to the luminal surface of endothelial cells, is identical to *angiotensin-converting enzyme* (ACE; see Ch. 19), which cleaves the two C-terminal residues from the inactive peptide angiotensin I, converting it to the active vasoconstrictor peptide angiotensin

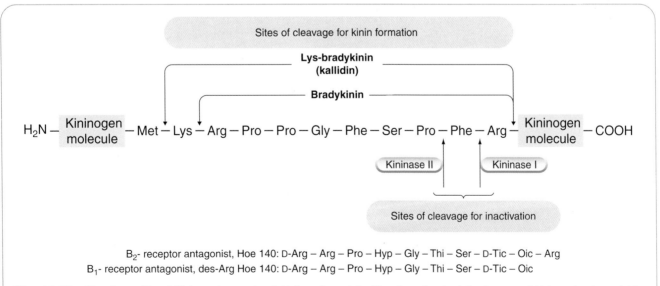

Fig. 13.13 **Structure of bradykinin and some bradykinin antagonists.** The sites of proteolytic cleavage of high-molecular-weight kininogen by kallikrein kallidin involved in the formation of bradykinin are shown in the upper half of the figure; the sites of cleavage associated with bradykinin inactivation are shown in the lower half. The B_2-receptor antagonist icatibant (Hoe 140) has a pA_2 of 9, and the competitive B_1-receptor antagonist des-Arg Hoe 140 has a pA_2 of 8. The Hoe compounds contain unnatural amino acids: Thi, d-Tic and Oic, which are analogues of phenylalanine and proline.

Bradykinin receptors

There are two bradykinin receptors, designated B_1 and B_2. Both are G-protein–coupled receptors and mediate very similar effects. B_1 receptors are normally expressed at very low levels but are strongly induced in inflamed or damaged tissues by cytokines such as IL-1. B_1 receptors respond to des-Arg^9-bradykinin but not to bradykinin itself. A number of selective peptide antagonists are known. It is likely that B_1 receptors play a significant role in inflammation and hyperalgesia, and there is recent interest in developing antagonists for use in cough and neurological disorders (see Chung, 2005; Rodi et al., 2005).

B_2 receptors are constitutively present in many normal cells and are activated by bradykinin and kallidin, but not by des-Arg^9-bradykinin. Peptide and non-peptide antagonists have been developed, the best known being **icatibant**. None are yet available for clinical use.

NITRIC OXIDE

Chapter 17 discusses NO in detail, and here we will consider only its role in inflammation. Inducible NO synthase (iNOS) is the chief isoform relevant to inflammation, and virtually all inflammatory cells express the enzyme in response to cytokine stimulation. iNOS is also present in the bronchial epithelium of asthmatic subjects, in the mucosa of the colon in patients with ulcerative colitis, and in synoviocytes in inflammatory joint disease. NO probably has a net proinflammatory effect: it increases vascular permeability and prostaglandin production, and is a potent vasodilator. Some other properties may be seen as anti-inflammatory; for example, endothelial NO inhibits adhesion of neutrophils and platelets, and platelet aggregation. NO, or

compounds derived from it, also has cytotoxic actions, killing bacteria, fungi, viruses and metazoan parasites, so in this respect NO enhances local defence mechanisms. However, produced in excess, it may also harm host cells.

Inhibitors of iNOS are under investigation for treatment of inflammatory conditions. Patients with septic shock have benefited from inhibitors of iNOS, and in experimental arthritis iNOS inhibitors reduce disease activity. NSAIDs coupled with NO-releasing groups have fewer side effects than conventional NSAIDs and greater anti-inflammatory efficacy (see Ch. 14).

NEUROPEPTIDES

Neuropeptides released from sensory neurons cause *neurogenic inflammation* (Maggi, 1996). The main peptides involved are substance P, neurokinin A and CGRP (see Ch. 16). Substance P and neurokinin A (members of the tachykinin family) act on mast cells, releasing histamine and other mediators, and producing smooth muscle contraction and mucus secretion, whereas CGRP is a potent vasodilator. Neurogenic inflammation is implicated in the pathogenesis of several inflammatory conditions, including the delayed phase of asthma, allergic rhinitis, inflammatory bowel disease and some types of arthritis.

CYTOKINES

Cytokine is an all-purpose functional term that is applied to protein or polypeptide mediators synthesised and released by cells of the immune system during inflammation. More than 100 cytokines have been identified, and the superfamily is generally regarded as comprising:

- interleukins
- chemokines
- interferons
- colony-stimulating factors
- growth factors and TNFs.

Cytokines act locally by autocrine or paracrine mechanisms. On the target cell, they bind to and activate specific, high-affinity receptors that, in most cases, are up-regulated during inflammation. Except for chemokines, which act on G-protein–coupled receptors, most cytokines act on kinase-linked receptors, regulating phosphorylation cascades that affect gene expression, such as the Jak/Stat pathway (Ch. 3).

In addition to their own direct actions on cells, some cytokines amplify inflammation by inducing formation of other inflammatory mediators. Others can induce receptors for other cytokines on their target cell, or engage in synergistic or antagonistic interactions with other cytokines. Cytokines have been likened to a complex signalling language, with the final response of a particular cell involved being determined by the strength and number of different messages received concurrently at the cell surface.

Various systems for classifying cytokines can be found in the literature, as can a multitude of diagrams depicting complex networks of cytokines interacting with each other and with a range of target cells. The cytokine aficionado can find classification tables in Casciari et al. (1996) and Janeway et al. (2004),

---

Bradykinin

- BK is a nonapeptide 'clipped' from a plasma α-globulin, *kininogen*, by *kallikrein*.
- It is converted by *kininase I* to an octapeptide, BK_{1-8} (des-Arg^9-BK), and inactivated by *kininase II* (angiotensin-converting enzyme) in the lung.
- Pharmacological actions:
  - vasodilatation (largely dependent on endothelial cell nitric oxide and prostaglandin I_2)
  - increased vascular permeability
  - stimulation of pain nerve endings
  - stimulation of epithelial ion transport and fluid secretion in airways and gastrointestinal tract
  - contraction of intestinal and uterine smooth muscle.
- There are two main subtypes of BK receptors: B_2, which is constitutively present, and B_1, which is induced in inflammation.
- There are selective competitive antagonists for both B_1 receptors (des-Arg Hoe 140; pA_2:8) and B_2 receptors (icatibant, pA_2:9).

or by using the web links listed at the end of the chapter. A comprehensive coverage of this area is beyond the scope of this book but, for the purposes of this chapter, it is useful to divide cytokines into two main groups:

- those involved in the *induction* of the immune response, described above and outlined in Figure 13.5
- those proinflammatory and anti-inflammatory cytokines involved in the *effector* phase of the immune/inflammatory response, which we will consider below.

Proinflammatory cytokines. These cytokines participate in acute and chronic inflammatory reactions as well as repair and resolution. The primary proinflammatory cytokines are TNF-α and IL-1; see above (Fig. 13.2). The latter cytokine actually comprises a family of three cytokines consisting of two agonists, IL-1α, IL-1β, and, surprisingly, an endogenous IL-1-receptor *antagonist* (IL-1ra). Mixtures of these are released from macrophages and many other cells during inflammation and can initiate the synthesis and release of a cascade of secondary cytokines, among which are the *chemokines* (see below). Various cytokine growth factors (e.g. platelet-derived growth factor, fibroblast growth factor, vascular endothelial growth factor) are crucial to the repair processes and are implicated in chronic inflammation (see Ch. 5).

The anti-inflammatory cytokines. These comprise those that inhibit aspects of the inflammatory reaction, including TGF-β, IL-4, IL-10 and IL-13. They inhibit chemokine production, and the anti-inflammatory interleukins can inhibit responses driven by Th1 cells, whose inappropriate activation is involved in the pathogenesis of several diseases.

CHEMOKINES

Chemokines are defined as *chemoattractant cytokines* that control the migration of leucocytes, functioning as traffic coordinators during immune and inflammatory reactions. The nomenclature (and the classification) is a little confusing here, because some non-cytokine mediators also control leucocyte movement (C5a, LTB₄, f-Met-Leu-Phe, etc.; see Fig. 13.2). Furthermore, many chemokines have other actions, for example causing mast cell degranulation or promoting angiogenesis.

More than 40 chemokines have been identified, and for those of us who are not professional chemokinologists they can be conveniently distinguished by considering whether key cysteine residues in the polypeptide chain are adjacent (*C-C* chemokines) or separated by another residue (*C-X-C* chemokines).

The C-X-C chemokines (main example IL-8; see Fig. 13.2) act on neutrophils and are predominantly involved in *acute* inflammatory responses. The C-C chemokines (main examples MCP-1 and RANTES) act on monocytes, eosinophils and other cells, and are involved predominantly in *chronic* inflammatory responses.

Chemokines act through G-protein–coupled receptors, and alteration or inappropriate expression of these is implicated in multiple sclerosis, cancer, rheumatoid arthritis and some cardiovascular diseases (Gerard & Rollins, 2001). Some types of virus (herpesvirus, cytomegalovirus, poxvirus and members of the retrovirus family) can exploit the chemokine system and subvert the host's defences (Murphy, 2001). Some produce proteins that mimic host chemokines or chemokine receptors, some act as antagonists at chemokine receptors, and some masquerade as growth or angiogenic factors. The AIDS-causing HIV virus is responsible for the most audacious exploitation of the host chemokine system. This virus has a protein (gp120) in its envelope that recognises and binds T-cell receptors for CD4 *and* a chemokine coreceptor that allows it to penetrate the T cell (see Ch. 47).

INTERFERONS

Interferons are considered in more detail below; the colony-stimulating factors are considered in Chapter 22.

There are three classes of interferon, termed *IFN-α, IFN-β* and *IFN-γ*. IFN-α is not a single substance but a family of approximately 20 proteins with similar activities. IFN-α and IFN-β have antiviral activity, and IFN-α also has some antitumour action. Both are released from virus-infected cells and activate antiviral mechanisms in neighbouring cells. IFN-γ has a role in induction of Th1 responses (Fig. 13.3; see also Abbas et al., 1996).

Clinical use of interferons

Interferon-α is used in the treatment of chronic hepatitis B and C, and has some action against *herpes zoster* and in the prevention of the common cold. Antitumour action against some lymphomas and solid tumours has been reported. A variety of dose-related side effects may occur. IFN-β is used in some patients with multiple sclerosis, whereas IFN-γ is used in chronic granulomatous disease in conjunction with antibacterial drugs.

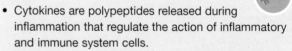

Cytokines

- Cytokines are polypeptides released during inflammation that regulate the action of inflammatory and immune system cells.
- The cytokine superfamily includes the *interferons*, *interleukins*, *tumour necrosis factor* (*TNF*), *growth factors*, *chemokines* and *colony-stimulating factors*.
- Utilising both autocrine or paracrine mechanisms, they exert complex effects on leucocytes, vascular endothelial cells, mast cells, fibroblasts, haemopoietic stem cells and osteoclasts, controlling proliferation, differentiation and/or activation.
- Interleukin (IL)-1 and TNF-α are important primary inflammatory cytokines inducing the formation of other cytokines.
- Interferon (IFN)-α and IFN-β have antiviral activity, and IFN-α is used as an adjunct in the treatment of viral infections. IFN-γ has significant immunoregulatory function and is used in the treatment of multiple sclerosis.

GLOSSARY OF ABBREVIATIONS AND ACRONYMS

APC	antigen-presenting cell
C	complement (as in C3a, C5a, C3b, etc.)
CD4 and CD8	coreceptors in T lymphocytes for MHC molecules classes II and I, respectively
COX-1 and COX-2	isoforms of cyclo-oxygenases
ICAM	intercellular adhesion molecule
IFN	interferon (as in IFN-α, IFN-β, IFN-γ)
IL	interleukin (as in IL-1, IL-2, etc.)
LT	leukotriene (as in LTB$_4$, LTC$_4$, LTD$_4$)
mAb	monoclonal antibody
MCP-1	monocyte chemoattractant protein-1
MHC	major histocompatibility complex

NK	natural killer lymphocyte
NSAID	non-steroidal anti-inflammatory drug
PAF	platelet-activating factor
PAMP	pathogen-associated molecular pattern
PG	prostaglandin (as in PGE$_2$, PGI$_2$, etc.)
RANTES	regulated on activation normal T-cell expressed and secreted
Th	T-helper lymphocyte (occurs as Th1 and Th2)
TLR	Toll receptor
TNF-α	tumour necrosis factor-α
TNF-β	tumour necrosis factor-β

REFERENCES AND FURTHER READING

The innate and adaptive responses

Abbas A K, Murphy K M, Sher A 1996 Functional diversity of helper lymphocytes. Nature 383: 787–793 (*Excellent review, helpful diagrams; commendable coverage of Th1 and Th2 cells and their respective cytokine subsets*)

Adams D H, Lloyd A R 1997 Chemokines: leucocyte recruitment and activation cytokines. Lancet 349: 490–495 (*Commendable review*)

Akira S, Takeda K, Kaisho T 2001 Toll-like receptors: critical proteins linking innate and acquired immunity. Nat Immunol 2: 675–680 (*Article describing the receptors for PAMPs shared by large groups of micro-organisms. Stimulation of these receptors by components of micro-organisms activates innate immunity and is a prerequisite for triggering acquired immunity. Useful diagrams.*)

Brown P 2001 Cinderella goes to the ball. Nature 410: 1018–1020.

Delves P J, Roitt I M 2000 The immune system. N Engl J Med 343: 37–49, 108–117 (*A good overview of the immune system—a minitextbook of major areas in immunology; colourful three-dimensional figures*)

Gabay C, Kushner I 1999 Acute phase proteins and other systemic responses to inflammation. N Engl J Med 340: 448–454 (*Lists the acute-phase proteins and outlines the mechanisms controlling their synthesis and release*)

Kärre K, Welsh R M 1997 Viral decoy vetoes killer cell. Nature 386: 446–447

Kay A B 2001 Allergic diseases and their treatment. N Engl J Med 344: 30–37, 109–113 (*Covers atopy and Th2 cells, the role of Th2 cytokines in allergies, IgE, the main types of allergy, and new therapeutic approaches*)

Mackay C R, Lanzavecchia A, Sallusto F 1999 Chemoattractant receptors and immune responses. Immunologist 7: 112–118 (*Masterly short review covering the role of chemoattractants in orchestrating immune responses—both the innate reaction and the Th1 and Th2 responses*)

Medzhitov R 2001 Toll-like receptors and innate immunity. Nat Rev Immunol 1: 135–145 (*Excellent review of the role of Toll-like receptors in (a) the detection of microbial infection, and (b) the activation of innate non-adaptive responses, which in turn lead to antigen-specific adaptive responses*)

Medzhitov R, Janeway C 2000 Innate immunity. N Engl J Med 343: 338–344 (*Outstanding clear coverage of

the mechanisms involved in innate immunity and its significance for the adaptive immune response*)

Murphy P M 2001 Viral exploitation and subversion of the immune system through chemokine mimicry. Nat Immunol 2: 116–122 (*Excellent description of viral/immune system interaction*)

Panes J, Perry M, Granger D N 1999 Leucocyte–endothelial cell adhesion: avenues for therapeutic intervention. Br J Pharmacol 126: 537–550 (*Brief coverage of the principal cell adhesion molecules and factors affecting leucocyte–endothelial adhesion precedes consideration of potential therapeutic targets*)

Parkin J, Cohen B 2001 An overview of the immune system. Lancet 357: 1777–1789 (*A competent straightforward review covering the role of the immune system in recognising, repelling and eradicating pathogens and in reacting against molecules foreign to the body*)

Romagnani S 1996 Short analytical review: Th1 and Th2 in human diseases. Clin Immunol Immunopathol 80: 225–235 (*Admirable coverage of the pathophysiology of Th1 and Th2 responses*)

Walker C, Zuany-Amorini C 2001 New trends in immunotherapy to prevent atopic disease. Trends Pharmacol Sci 22: 84–91 (*Discusses potential therapies based on recent advances in the understanding of the immune mechanisms of atopy*)

Wills-Karp M, Santeliz J, Karp C L 2001 The germless theory of allergic diseases. Nat Rev Immunol 1: 69–75 (*Discusses the hypothesis that early childhood infections inhibit the tendency to develop allergic disease*)

Mainly mediators

Arrang J M, Garbarg M, Schwartz J C 1983 Autoinhibition of brain histamine release mediated by a novel class (H$_3$) of histamine receptor. Nature 302: 832–834 (*Seminal article on the existence of H$_3$ receptors*)

Casciari J J, Sato H et al. 1996 Tabular lexicon of cytokine structure and function. In: Chabner B A, Longo D N (eds) Cancer chemotherapy and biotherapy, 2nd edn. Lippincott-Raven, Philadelphia, pp. 787–793 (*Useful classification bringing order to a confusing field*)

Coleman R A, Humphrey P A et al. 1993 Prostanoid receptors: their function and classification. In: Vane J, O'Grady J (eds) Therapeutic applications of

prostaglandins. Edward Arnold, London, pp. 15–36 (*Useful coverage; includes structures of prostanoids, their analogues and antagonists—a classification that brought forth order from chaos!*)

Dale M M 1994 Summary of section on mediators. In: Dale M M, Foreman J C, Fan T-P (eds) Textbook of immunopharmacology, 3rd edn. Blackwell Scientific, Oxford, pp. 206–207 (*Considers which mediators meet defined criteria*)

Gerard C, Rollins B 2001 Chemokines and disease. Nat Immunol 2: 108–115 (*Discusses diseases associated with inappropriate activation of the chemokine network, and discusses some therapeutic implications; describes how viruses evade the immune responses by mimicry of the chemokines or their receptors*)

Gutzmer R, Diestel C, Mommert S et al. 2005 Histamine H$_4$ receptor stimulation suppresses IL-12p70 production and mediates chemotaxis in human monocyte-derived dendritic cells. J Immunol 174: 5224–5232

Horuk R 2001 Chemokine receptors. Cytokine Growth Factor Rev 12: 313–335 (*Comprehensive review focusing on recent findings in chemokine receptor research; describes the molecular, physiological and biochemical properties of each chemokine receptor*)

Luster A D 1998 Mechanisms of disease: chemokines—chemotactic cytokines that mediate inflammation. N Engl J Med 338: 436–445 (*Excellent review; outstanding diagrams*)

Mackay C R 2001 Chemokines: immunology's high impact factors. Nat Immunol 2: 95–101 (*Clear, elegant coverage of the role of chemokines in leucocyte–endothelial interaction, control of primary immune responses and T/B cell interaction, T cells in inflammatory diseases, and viral subversion of immune responses*)

Maggi C A 1996 Pharmacology of the efferent function of primary sensory neurones. In: Geppetti P, Holzer P (eds) Neurogenic inflammation. CRC Press, London (*Worthwhile. Covers neurogenic inflammation, the release of neuropeptides from sensory nerves, and inflammatory mediators. Discusses agents that inhibit release and the pharmacological modulation of receptor-mediated release.*)

Mantovani A, Bussolino F, Introna M 1997 Cytokine regulation of endothelial cell function: from molecular level to the bedside. Immunol Today 5: 231–239 (*Pathophysiology of endothelial cell–cytokine interactions; detailed diagrams*)

Rodi D, Couture R et al. 2005 Targeting kinin receptors for the treatment of neurological diseases. Curr Pharm Des 11: 1313–1326 (*An overview of the potential role of kinin receptor antagonists in neurological diseases, dealing particularly with those of immunological origin*)

Samuelsson B 1983 Leukotrienes: mediators of immediate hypersensitivity reactions and inflammation. Science 220: 568–575 (*Seminal article on leukotrienes*)

Szolcsànyi J 1996 Neurogenic inflammation: reevaluation of the axon reflex theory. In: Geppetti P, Holzer P (eds) Neurogenic inflammation. CRC Press, London, pp. 33–42 (*Good coverage of neurogenic inflammation*)

Ulrich H, von Andrian U H, Englehardt B 2003 α_4 Integrins as therapeutic targets in autoimmune disease. N Engl J Med 348: 68–70 (*Editorial commenting on two articles in the journal that describe the use of natalizumab, a recombinant mAb, for the treatment of multiple sclerosis and Crohn's disease; natalizumab binds to α_4 integrins on haemopoietic cells and prevents them from binding to their endothelial receptors*)

Zhu Y, Michalovich D, Wu H et al. 2001 Cloning, expression, and pharmacological characterization of a novel human histamine receptor. Mol Pharmacol 59: 434–441 (*Describes the cloning of the fourth type of histamine receptor, H_4*)

Some anti-inflammatory papers

Bazan N G, Flower R J 2002 Lipid signals in pain control. Nature 420: 135–138 (*Succinct editorial article describing the significance of recent advances in COX pharmacology*)

Black J W, Duncan W A M, Durant G J et al. 1972 Definition and antagonism of histamine H_2-receptors. Nature 236: 385–390 (*Seminal article on H_2 receptors*)

Chung K F 2005 Drugs to suppress cough. Expert Opin Investig Drugs 14: 19–27 (*Useful review of cough treatments, including a section on the role of neurokinin and bradykinin receptor antagonists*)

Gilroy D W, Perretti M 2005 Aspirin and steroids: new mechanistic findings and avenues for drug discovery. Curr Opin Pharmacol 5: 405–411 (*A very interesting review dealing with anti-inflammatory substances that are released during the inflammatory response and that bring about resolution; it also deals with a rather odd effect of aspirin—its ability to boost the production of anti-inflammatory lipoxins. Easy to read and informative.*)

Larsson B M, Kumlin M, Sundblad B M et al. 2006 Effects of 5-lipoxygenase inhibitor zileuton on airway responses to inhaled swine house dust in healthy subjects. Respir Med 100: 226–237 (*A paper dealing with the effects of zileuton, a 5-lipoxygenase inhibitor, on the allergic response in humans; the results are not unequivocally positive, but the study is an interesting one*)

Leveau P, Wang X et al. 2005 Severity of pancreatitis-associated gut barrier dysfunction is reduced following treatment with the PAF inhibitor lexipafant. Biochem Pharmacol 69: 1325–1331 (*A paper dealing with the role of the PAF inhibitor lexipafant in pancreatitis; this is an experimental study using a rat model but provides a useful insight into the potential clinical role of such an antagonist*)

Serhan C N 2005 Lipoxins and aspirin-triggered 15-epi-lipoxins are the first lipid mediators of endogenous anti-inflammation and resolution. Prostaglandins Leukot Essent Fatty Acids 73: 141–162 (*A paper reviewing the lipoxins—anti-inflammatory substances formed by the 5-lipoxygenase enzyme; also discusses the action of aspirin in boosting the synthesis of these compounds and the receptors on which they act. A good review that summarises a lot of work.*)

Vane J R 1971 Inhibition of prostaglandin synthesis as a mechanism of action for aspirin-like drugs. Nat New Biol 231: 232–239 (*Seminal article on the mechanism of action of aspirin as inhibitor of prostanoid synthesis*)

Books

Dale M M, Foreman J C, Fan T-P (eds) 1994 Textbook of immunopharmacology, 3rd edn. Blackwell Scientific, Oxford (*Excellent textbook written with second- and third-year medical and science students in mind; contains many sections relevant to this chapter and the next*)

Janeway C A, Travers P, Nolan A et al. 2004 Immunobiology: the immune system in health and disease, 6th edn. Churchill Livingstone, Edinburgh (*Excellent textbook, good diagrams*)

Roitt I, Brostoff J, Male D 1998 Immunology, 9th edn. Blackwell Science, Oxford (*Excellent textbook; well illustrated*)

Useful web links

http://microvet.arizona.edu/Courses/MIC419/Tutorials/cytokines.html (*This is a useful web site with a series of immunological tutorials. The cytokines module is worth looking at, and it has a good (although not complete) list of the most important members of the family, their targets and function. Also contains other material that is likely to be useful in understanding this chapter.*)

http://www.copewithcytokines.de/ (*A very comprehensive site dealing with practically all known cytokines. Also contains a list of terms, links to reviews, and short pieces on individual cytokines. Worth a look if you are stuck for some information.*)

http://www.biochemweb.org/fenteany/research/cell_migration/movement_movies.html (*If you have never seen a neutrophil in hot pursuit of a bacterium, then you definitely need to look at this online movie. This page also contains links to another segment of the site (http://cellix.imolbio.oeaw.ac.at/Videotour/video_tour.html), a fantastic video tutorial on cell motility in general assembled by the Institute of Molecular Biology at the Austrian Academy of Sciences in Salzburg, Austria. Great fun and highly instructive.*)

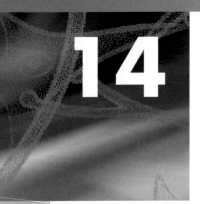

14

Anti-inflammatory and immunosuppressant drugs

OVERVIEW

This chapter deals with the drugs used to treat inflammatory and immune disorders. While generally associated with disorders such as *rheumatoid arthritis,* it has become clear that inappropriate inflammatory or immune reactions form a significant component of many, if not most, of the diseases encountered in the clinic, and consequently anti-inflammatory drugs are extensively employed in virtually all branches of medicine.

The three major groups of drugs are the *non-steroidal anti-inflammatory drugs (NSAIDs);* the *antirheumatoid drugs,* which include the disease-modifying antirheumatic drugs (DMARDs); and the *glucocorticoids.* We describe the therapeutic effects, mechanisms of action, and unwanted effects common to all NSAIDs, and deal in a little more detail with aspirin, paracetamol and drugs that are selective for cyclo-oxygenase (COX)-2. DMARDs comprise a rather heterogeneous group of drugs and include some important new agents. The *glucocorticoids* are covered in Chapter 28, but their immunosuppressive actions are discussed briefly in this chapter. Also considered in this chapter are immunosuppressant drugs used to prevent rejection of organ transplants. Finally, we consider drugs used to treat gout and (although they are not strictly anti-inflammatory agents) the histamine H$_1$ receptor antagonists used to treat certain acute allergic conditions.

NON-STEROIDAL ANTI-INFLAMMATORY DRUGS

The NSAIDs, sometimes called the *aspirin-like drugs,* are among the most widely used of all drugs. There are now more than 50 different NSAIDs on the global market; some of the more important examples are listed in Table 14.1 and some structures in Figure 14.1. They provide symptomatic relief from pain and swelling in chronic joint disease such as occurs in osteo- and rheumatoid arthritis, and in more acute inflammatory conditions such as sports injuries, fractures, sprains and other soft tissue injuries. They also provide relief from postoperative, dental and menstrual pain, and from the pain of headaches and migraine. As several NSAIDs are available over the counter, they are often taken without prescription for other types of minor aches and pains. There are many different formulations available, including tablets, injections and gels. Virtually all NSAIDs, particularly the 'classic' NSAIDs, can have significant unwanted effects, especially in the elderly. Newer agents have fewer adverse actions.

PHARMACOLOGICAL ACTIONS

All the NSAIDs have actions very similar to those of aspirin, the archetypal NSAID, which was introduced into clinical medicine in the 1890s. The three main therapeutic effects are:

- *an anti-inflammatory effect*: modification of the inflammatory reaction
- *an analgesic effect*: reduction of certain types of (especially inflammatory) pain
- *an antipyretic effect*: lowering of body temperature when this is raised in disease (i.e. fever).

In addition, all the NSAIDs share, to a greater or lesser degree, the same types of mechanism-based side effects. These include:

- *gastric irritation,* which may range from simple discomfort to ulcer formation
- an effect on *renal blood flow* in the compromised kidney

Table 14.1   Comparison of some common non-steroidal anti-inflammatory drugs and coxibs

Drug	Type	RD	Gout	MS	PO	Dys	H&M	Comments
Aceclofenac	Phenylacetate	•						–
Acemetacin	Indole ester	•		•	•			Ester of indometacin
Aspirin	Salicylate	•		•	•	•	•	Mainly cardiovascular usage
Celecoxib	Coxib	•						Fewer gastrointestinal effects
Dexketoprofen	Propionate			•	•			–
Diclofenac	Phenylacetate	•	•	•	•			Moderate potency
Diflunisal	Salicylate	•		•	•	•		–
Etodolac	Pyranocarboxylate	•						Possibly fewer gastrointestinal effects
Etoricoxib	Coxib	•	•					–
Fenbufen	Propionate	•		•				–
Fenoprofen	Propionate	•		•				Prodrug activated in liver
Flurbiprofen	Propionate	•		•	•	•	•	–
Ibuprofen	Propionate	•		•	•	•	•	Suitable for children
Indometacin	Indole	•	•	•		•		Suitable for moderate to severe disease
Ketoprofen	Propionate	•	•	•	•	•		Suitable for mild disease
Ketorolac	Pyrrolizine				•			–
Mefenamic acid	Fenamate	•		•	•	•		Moderate activity
Meloxicam	Oxicam	•						Possibly fewer gastrointestinal effects
Nabumetone	Napthylalkenone	•						Prodrug activated in liver
Naproxen	Propionate	•	•	•		•		–
Parecoxib	Coxib				•			Prodrug activated in liver
Piroxicam	Oxicam	•	•	•				–
Sulindac	Indene	•	•	•				Prodrug
Tenoxicam	Oxicam	•		•				–
Tiaprofenic acid	Propionate	•		•				–
Tolfenamic acid	Fenamate						•	–

Dys, dysmenorrhoea; H&M, headache and migraine; MS, musculoskeletal disorders; PO, postoperative pain; RD, rheumatic diseases (e.g. rheumatoid arthritis and osteoarthritis).
(From British Medical Association and Royal Pharmaceutical Society of Great Britain 2005 British National Formulary. BMA and RPSGB, London.)

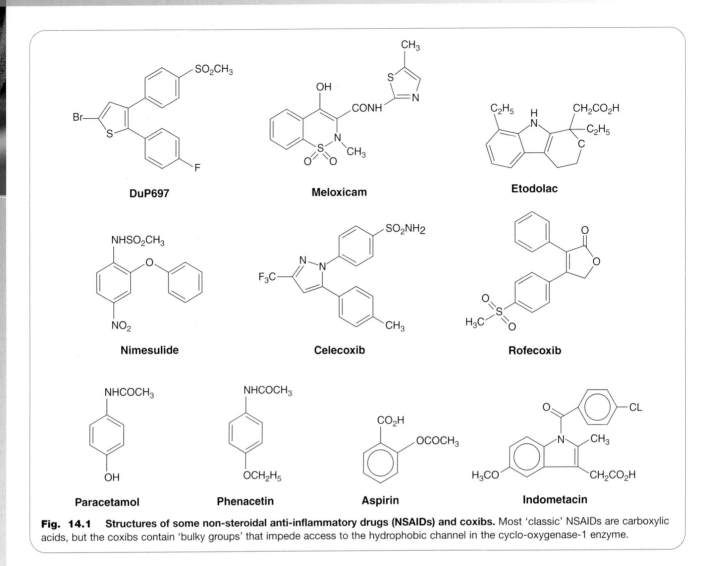

Fig. 14.1   Structures of some non-steroidal anti-inflammatory drugs (NSAIDs) and coxibs. Most 'classic' NSAIDs are carboxylic acids, but the coxibs contain 'bulky groups' that impede access to the hydrophobic channel in the cyclo-oxygenase-1 enzyme.

- a tendency to prolong bleeding through inhibition of *platelet function*
- controversially, it is argued that they may also all—but especially COX-2 selective drugs—increase the likelihood of thrombotic events such as myocardial infarction by inhibiting prostaglandin (PG) I_2 synthesis.

While there are differences between individual drugs, all these effects are generally thought to be related to the primary action of the drugs—inhibition of the *fatty acid COX* enzyme, and thus inhibition of the production of prostaglandins and thromboxanes. There are three known isoforms—COX-1, COX-2 and COX-3—as well as some non-catalytic species (see Table 14.2). As it is not yet certain that COX-3 actually occurs in humans in a functional form, we will confine the discussion mainly to a consideration of COX-1 and COX-2. While they are closely related (> 60% sequence identity) and catalyse the same reaction, it is clear that there are important differences between the expression and role of these two isoforms. COX-1 is a constitutive enzyme expressed in most tissues, including blood platelets. It has a 'housekeeping' role in the body, being involved in tissue homeostasis, and is responsible for the production of prostaglandins involved in, for

example, gastric cytoprotection (see Ch. 25), platelet aggregation (Ch. 21), renal blood flow autoregulation (Ch. 24, p. 374) and the initiation of parturition (Ch. 30).

In contrast, COX-2 is induced in inflammatory cells when they are activated, and the primary inflammatory cytokines—interleukin (IL)-1 and tumour necrosis factor (TNF)-α (see Ch. 13)—are important in this regard. Thus the COX-2 isoform is responsible for the production of the prostanoid mediators of inflammation (Vane & Botting, 2001), although there are some significant exceptions. For example, there is a considerable pool of 'constitutive' COX-2 present in the central nervous system (CNS) and some other tissues, although its function is not yet completely clear.

Most 'traditional' NSAIDs are inhibitors of both isoenzymes, although they vary in the degree to which they inhibit each isoform. It is believed that the anti-inflammatory action (and probably most analgesic actions) of the NSAIDs is related to their inhibition of COX-2, while their unwanted effects—particularly those affecting the gastrointestinal tract—are largely a result of their inhibition of COX-1. Compounds with a selective inhibitory action on COX-2 are now in clinical use, but expectations that these inhibitors would transform the treatment

Table 14.2   The cyclo-oxygenase family: a summary of properties

Gene	Gene product	Tissue expression	Functions	Inhibitors	Comments
COX1	COX-1	Constitutively expressed in most tissues	Platelet aggregation, gastrointestinal protection, some pain, production of vascular prostacyclin	Most 'classic' NSAIDs, some selective inhibitors	First COX to be identified
COX1	COX-3	Brain, heart and aorta; constitutive?	Pain perception	Paracetamol, diclofenac, ibuprofen, dipyrone, phenacetin, antipyrine	Few details presently known
COX1	pCOX-1a[a]	Brain	?	n/a	Not catalytically active
COX1	pCOX-1b	Brain	?	n/a	Not catalytically active
COX2	COX-2	Induced in many tissues by many stimuli, including growth factors, cytokines, oxidative stress, brain hypoxia or seizures, and other forms of injury or stress; constitutively present in brain, kidney and elsewhere	Inflammation, fever, some pain, parturition and renal function. Production of vascular prostacyclin?	Many NSAIDs, COX-2–selective drugs such as the coxibs and others	–
COX2	COX-?	J774 cells during apoptosis	?	Paracetamol	Studied in only one system to date

COX, cyclo-oxygenase; n/a, not applicable; NSAID, non-steroidal anti-inflammatory drug.
[a]p stands for partial; this refers to the fact that the protein is a truncated form.
(Modified from Bazan & Flower 2002.)

of inflammatory conditions have received a setback because of an increase in cardiovascular risk (see below). A broad scheme for classifying the relative selectivity for COX-1/2 of the currently available NSAIDs is given in Table 14.3.

There are few significant differences in pharmacological actions among the currently used NSAIDs, but there are marked differences in toxicity and degree of patient tolerance. Aspirin, however, has other qualitatively different pharmacological actions, and paracetamol is an interesting exception to the general NSAID 'stereotype'. While it is an excellent analgesic and antipyretic, the anti-inflammatory activity of paracetamol is very low and seems to be restricted to a few special cases (e.g. inflammation following dental extraction; see Skjelbred et al., 1984). Paracetamol has been shown to inhibit prostaglandin biosynthesis in some experimental settings (e.g. during fever) but not in others. It was hoped that the discovery of COX-3A (Chandrasekharan et al; 2002), an isoform found in dog brain and that seemed more sensitive to paracetamol, might provide a neat explanation of this anomaly, but it is too soon to tell whether this will be the case.

The main pharmacological actions and the common side effects of the NSAIDs are outlined below, followed by a more detailed coverage of aspirin and paracetamol, an outline of the pharmacology of the selective COX-2 inhibitors, and finally the clinical applications of the group as a whole.

ANTIPYRETIC EFFECT

Normal body temperature is regulated by a centre in the hypothalamus that controls the balance between heat loss and heat production. Fever occurs when there is a disturbance of this hypothalamic 'thermostat', which leads to the set point of body temperature being raised. NSAIDs 'reset' this thermostat. Once there has been a return to the normal set point, the temperature-regulating mechanisms (dilatation of superficial blood vessels, sweating, etc.) then operate to reduce temperature. Normal body temperature in humans is not affected by NSAIDs.

The NSAIDs exert their antipyretic action largely through inhibition of prostaglandin production in the hypothalamus. During an inflammatory reaction, bacterial endotoxins cause the release from macrophages of a pyrogen—IL-1 (Ch. 13)—which stimulates the generation, in the hypothalamus, of E-type prostaglandins that elevate the temperature set point. COX-2 may have a role here, because it is induced by IL-1 in vascular endothelium in the hypothalamus. There is some evidence that

Table 14.3 Cyclo-oxygenase–inhibitory specificity of some common non-steroidal anti-inflammatory drugs and coxibs

Group	Description	Selectivity ratio	Examples
I	Highly COX-1–selective	100–1000	Ketorolac
II	Very COX-1–selective	10–100	Flurbiprofen
III	Weakly COX-1–selective	1–10	Indometacin, aspirin, naproxen, ibuprofen
IVa	Non-selective; full inhibition of both enzymes	1	Fenoprofen
IVb	Non-selective; incomplete inhibition of both enzymes	1	Salicylate
V	Weakly COX-2–selective	1–10	Diflunisal, piroxicam, meclofenamate, sulindac, diclofenac, celecoxib
VI	Very COX-2–selective	10–100	Valdecoxib, etoricoxib
VII	Highly COX-2–selective	100–1000	Rofecoxib[a]

COX, cyclo-oxygenase.
[a]Rofecoxib has been withdrawn from use and is shown here as an illustration only.
(Based on data from Warner T D, Mitchell J A 2004 FASEB J 18: 790–804.)

prostaglandins are not the only mediators of fever, hence NSAIDs may have an additional antipyretic effect by mechanisms as yet unknown.

ANALGESIC EFFECT

The NSAIDs are effective against mild or moderate pain, especially that arising from inflammation or tissue damage. Two sites of action have been identified. First, peripherally, they decrease production of the prostaglandins that sensitise nociceptors to inflammatory mediators such as bradykinin (see Chs 13 and 41) and they are therefore effective in arthritis, bursitis, pain of muscular and vascular origin, toothache, dysmenorrhoea, the pain of postpartum states and the pain of cancer metastases in bone—all conditions that are associated with increased local prostaglandin synthesis. In combination with opioids, they decrease postoperative pain, and in some cases can reduce the requirement for opioids by as much as one-third. Their ability to relieve headache may be related to the abrogation of the vasodilator effect of prostaglandins on the cerebral vasculature.

In addition to these peripheral effects, there is a second, less well-characterised central action, possibly in the spinal cord. Inflammatory lesions increase prostaglandin release within the cord, causing facilitation of transmission from afferent pain fibres to relay neurons in the dorsal horn.

ANTI-INFLAMMATORY EFFECTS

Many mediators coordinate inflammatory and allergic reactions. While some are produced in response to specific stimuli (e.g. histamine in allergic inflammation), there is considerable redundancy, and each facet of the response—vasodilatation,

increased vascular permeability, cell accumulation, etc.—can be produced by several separate mechanisms.

The NSAIDs reduce mainly those components of the inflammatory and immune response in which prostaglandins, mainly derived from COX-2, play a significant part. These include:

- *vasodilatation*
- *oedema* (by an indirect action: the vasodilatation facilitates and potentiates the action of mediators such as histamine that increase the permeability of postcapillary venules—Ch. 13, p. 204)
- *pain* (see above), again potentiating other mediators, such as bradykinin (see Ch. 41, Fig. 41.7).

The NSAIDs suppress the pain, swelling and increased blood flow associated with inflammation but have little or no action on the actual progress of the underlying chronic disease itself. As a class, they are generally without effect on other aspects of inflammation, such as leucocyte migration, lysosomal enzyme release and toxic oxygen radical production, that contribute to tissue damage in chronic inflammatory conditions such as rheumatoid arthritis, vasculitis and nephritis.

MECHANISM OF CYCLO-OXYGENASE INHIBITORY ACTION

Vane and his colleagues established in 1971 that the main actions of NSAIDs were bought about through inhibition of arachidonic acid oxidation by the fatty acid COXs (see Fig. 14.2).

These are bifunctional enzymes, having two distinct catalytic activities. The first, *dioxygenase* step incorporates two molecules of oxygen into the arachidonic (or other fatty acid substrate) chain at C11 and C15, giving rise to the highly unstable endoperoxide

Non-steroidal anti-inflammatory drugs

The NSAIDs have three major pharmacologically desirable actions, stemming from the suppression of prostanoid synthesis in inflammatory cells through inhibition of the cyclo-oxygenase (COX)-2 isoform of the arachidonic acid COX. They are as follow.

- *An anti-inflammatory action*: the decrease in prostaglandin E_2 and prostacyclin reduces vasodilatation and, indirectly, oedema. Accumulation of inflammatory cells is not reduced.
- *An analgesic effect*: decreased prostaglandin generation means less sensitisation of nociceptive nerve endings to inflammatory mediators such as

bradykinin and 5-hydroxytryptamine. Relief of headache is probably a result of decreased prostaglandin-mediated vasodilatation.

- *An antipyretic effect*: interleukin-1 releases prostaglandins in the central nervous system, where they elevate the hypothalamic set point for temperature control, thus causing fever. NSAIDs prevent this. Some important examples are aspirin, ibuprofen, naproxen, indometacin, piroxicam and paracetamol. Newer agents with more selective inhibition of COX-2 (and thus fewer adverse effects on the gastrointestinal tract) include celecoxib and etoricoxib.

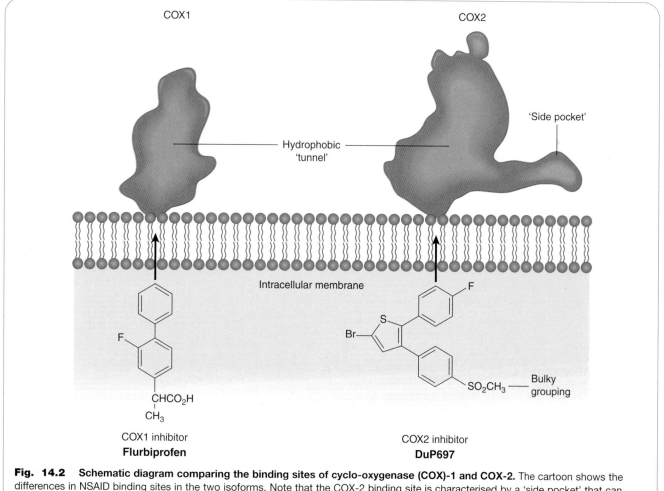

Fig. 14.2 Schematic diagram comparing the binding sites of cyclo-oxygenase (COX)-1 and COX-2. The cartoon shows the differences in NSAID binding sites in the two isoforms. Note that the COX-2 binding site is characterised by a 'side pocket' that can accommodate the bulky groups, such as the methylsulfonyl moiety of the prototype COX-2 inhibitor DuP697, which would impede its access to the COX-1 site. Other NSAIDs, such as flurbiprofen (shown here), can enter the active site of either enzyme. (After Luong et al. 1996 Nat Struct Biol 3: 927–933.)

intermediate *PGG$_2$* with a hydroperoxy group at C15. A second, *peroxidase* function of the enzyme converts this to *PGH$_2$* with a hydroxy group at C15 (see Ch. 13), which can then be transformed in a cell-specific manner by separate *isomerase*, *reductase* or *synthase* enzymes into other prostanoids. Both COX-1 and COX-2 are haem-containing enzymes (see Ch. 8, p. 114) that exist as homodimers in intracellular membranes. Structurally, the isoforms are similar; both have a long hydrophobic channel into which the arachidonic or other substrate fatty acids dock so that the oxygenation reaction can proceed.

Most NSAIDs inhibit only the initial dioxygenation reaction. They are generally 'competitive reversible' inhibitors, but there are differences in their time courses. Generally, these drugs inhibit COX-1 rapidly, but the inhibition of COX-2 is more time-dependent and the inhibition is often irreversible. To block the enzymes, NSAIDs enter the hydrophobic channel, forming hydrogen bonds with an arginine residue at position 120, thus preventing substrate fatty acids from entering into the catalytic domain. However, a single amino acid change (isoleucine to valine at position 523) in the structure of the entrance of this channel in COX-2 results in a bulky side pocket that is not found in COX-1. This is important in understanding why some drugs, especially those with bulky side groups, are more selective for the COX-2 isoform (Fig. 14.2). Aspirin is, however, an anomaly. It enters the active site and acetylates a serine at position 530, irreversibly inactivating COX-1. This is the basis for aspirin's long-lasting effects on platelets (see below).

Other actions besides inhibition of COX may contribute to the anti-inflammatory effects of some NSAIDs. Reactive oxygen radicals produced by neutrophils and macrophages are implicated in tissue damage in some conditions, and some NSAIDs (e.g. **sulindac**) have oxygen radical–scavenging effects as well as COX inhibitory activity, so may decrease tissue damage. Aspirin also inhibits expression of the transcription factor nuclear factor (NF) κB, which has a key role in the transcription of the genes for inflammatory mediators.

COMMON UNWANTED EFFECTS

Because prostaglandins are involved in gastric cytoprotection, platelet aggregation, renal vascular autoregulation and induction of labour, among other effects, it may be reasonably expected that all NSAIDs share, to some extent, a similar profile of mechanism-dependent side effects. While this is true, there may be other additional unwanted effects peculiar to individual members of the group.

Overall, the burden of unwanted side effects is high. Severe gastrointestinal effects alone (perforations, ulcers or bleeding) are said to result in the hospitalisation of over 100 000 people per year in the USA. Some 15% of these patients may die from this iatrogenic disease (Fries, 1998). These figures probably reflect the fact that NSAIDs are used extensively in the elderly, and often for extended periods of time. When the classic NSAIDs are used in joint diseases (which usually necessitates fairly large doses and long-continued use), there is a high incidence of side effects—particularly in the gastrointestinal tract but also in

liver, kidney, spleen, blood and bone marrow. COX-2-selective drugs have less gastrointestinal toxicity (see below).

GASTROINTESTINAL DISTURBANCES

Adverse gastrointestinal events are the commonest unwanted effects of the NSAIDs, and are believed to result mainly from inhibition of gastric COX-1, which is responsible for the synthesis of the prostaglandins that normally inhibit acid secretion and protect the mucosa (see Fig. 25.2).

Common gastrointestinal side effects include gastric discomfort, dyspepsia, diarrhoea (but sometimes constipation), nausea and vomiting, and in some cases gastric bleeding and ulceration. It has been estimated that 34–46% of users of NSAIDs will sustain some gastrointestinal damage that, while it may be asymptomatic, carries a risk of serious haemorrhage and/or perforation (Fries, 1983). The mechanism is dependent on inhibition of COX in the gastric mucosa, and damage is seen whether the drugs are given orally or systemically. However, in some cases (aspirin being a good example) *local* damage to the gastric mucosa caused directly by the drug itself may compound the damage. Figure 14.3 gives the relative risks of gastrointestinal damage with some common NSAIDs. Oral administration of prostaglandin analogues such as **misoprostol** (see Ch. 25) can diminish the gastric damage produced by these agents.

Based on extensive experimental evidence, it had been predicted that COX-2-selective agents would provide good anti-inflammatory and analgesic actions with less gastric damage, and some older drugs (e.g. **meloxicam**) that were believed to be better tolerated in the clinic turned out to have some COX-2 selectivity. Two large prospective studies compared **celecoxib** and **rofecoxib** with standard comparator NSAIDs in patients with arthritis and showed some benefit, although the results were not as clear-cut as had been hoped. Less encouraging, however, was an increase in the incidence of serious cardiovascular incidents seen in these trials (Boers, 2001; FitzGerald & Patrono, 2001). At the time, it was not clear that this was connected with COX-2 inhibition, and two 'coxibs', as they came to be called, were licensed in the USA in 1998 (and in the UK shortly after), with many more in the pipeline. Continuing uncertainty about the cardiovascular risk led to the addition of warning labels on these drugs in 2002, but the results from a long-term trial designed to assess the anticancer activity of rofecoxib showed that the risk of cardio-vascular events increased significantly after 18 months' treatment. As a result of this, the drug was voluntarily withdrawn in 2004. When another coxib, **valdecoxib**, apparently showed similar effects as well as serious skin reactions, this too was withdrawn. At the time of writing, only celecoxib, **parecoxib** and **etoricoxib** remain licensed in the UK (see below).

Some adverse cardiovascular pharmacology may be a feature of coxibs, and indeed, of traditional "non selective" NSAIDs in general. It was originally thought that this might be attributed to a selective reduction of PGI$_2$ synthesis by blood vessels thus indirectly promoting inappropriate platelet deposition, but this idea now seems less likely. Recent studies suggest instead that the cardiovascular risks of COX inhibitors are linked to the development of high blood pressure possibly as a result of the

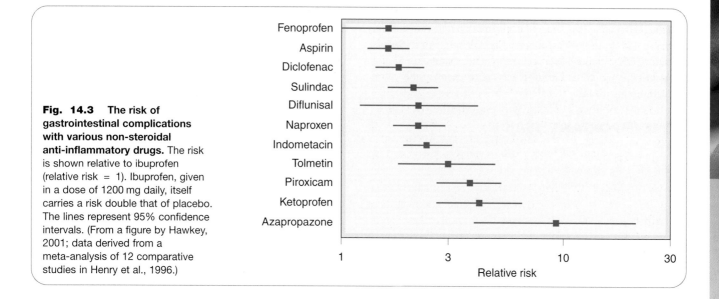

Fig. 14.3 The risk of gastrointestinal complications with various non-steroidal anti-inflammatory drugs. The risk is shown relative to ibuprofen (relative risk = 1). Ibuprofen, given in a dose of 1200 mg daily, itself carries a risk double that of placebo. The lines represent 95% confidence intervals. (From a figure by Hawkey, 2001; data derived from a meta-analysis of 12 comparative studies in Henry et al., 1996.)

inhibition of PGE_2 and PGI_2 production in the kidney. In practice, such high blood pressure is dose and time dependent. Conventional analgesic doses of Celecoxib (for example) produce little or no high blood pressure and pose negligible cardiovascular risk whereas the higher dose regimes that are sometimes used in trials to assess its efficacy in the treatment of cancer, may do so after prolonged treatment. Boers has concluded that 'in patients who do not require platelet inhibition, selective COX-2 inhibitors seem to be a true advance and an attractive alternative to classic NSAIDs combined with gastroprotective strategies', but points out that cardiologists and rheumatologists should routinely consider gastroprotection alongside cardioprotection.

Other ideas have been proposed to explain the gastric side effects of NSAIDs. The administration of COX-1 inhibitors themselves causes COX-2 induction and, on the basis of experimental evidence, Wallace (2000) has argued that *selective* inhibitors of *either* isozyme will cause less gastric damage than non-selective drugs.

SKIN REACTIONS

Rashes are common idiosyncratic unwanted effects of NSAIDs, particularly with mefenamic acid (10–15% frequency) and sulindac (5–10% frequency). They vary from mild erythematous, urticarial and photosensitivity reactions to more serious and potentially fatal diseases including Stevens–Johnson syndrome (which is fortunately rare).

ADVERSE RENAL EFFECTS

Therapeutic doses of NSAIDs in healthy individuals pose little threat to kidney function, but in susceptible patients they cause acute renal insufficiency, which is reversible on stopping the drug (see Ch. 53, p. 755, Table 53.1). This occurs through the inhibition of the biosynthesis of those prostanoids (PGE_2 and PGI_2;

prostacyclin) involved in the maintenance of renal blood flow, specifically in the PGE_2-mediated compensatory vasodilatation that occurs in response to the action of noradrenaline or angiotensin II (see Ch. 24). Neonates and the elderly are especially at risk, as are patients with heart, liver or kidney disease (p. 745), or a reduced circulating blood volume.

Chronic NSAID consumption, especially NSAID 'abuse',[1] can cause *analgesic nephropathy* characterised by chronic nephritis and renal papillary necrosis (Ch. 24, p. 374). **Phenacetin**, now withdrawn, was the main culprit; paracetamol, one of its major metabolites, is much less toxic. Regular use of prescribed doses of NSAIDs is less hazardous for the kidney in this respect than is very heavy and prolonged use of over-the-counter analgesics in a social context (e.g. Swiss workers manufacturing watches would hand round analgesics in the same way as sharing sweets or cigarettes).

OTHER UNWANTED EFFECTS

Other, much less common, unwanted effects of NSAIDs include CNS effects, bone marrow disturbances and liver disorders, the last being more likely if there is already renal impairment.[2] Paracetamol overdose causes liver failure (see below). Approximately 5% of patients exposed to NSAIDs may experience *aspirin-sensitive asthma*. The exact mechanism is unknown, but

---

[1] So called because the availability of NSAIDs in proprietary medicines over the counter, often in combination with other substances, such as caffeine, has tempted some people to consume them, often in prodigious quantities, for every conceivable malady.

[2] An odd side effect of the NSAID diclofenac came to light when a team of scientists investigated the curious decline in the population of several species of vultures in the Indian subcontinent. Dead cattle form an important part of the diet of these birds, and some animals had been treated with diclofenac for veterinary reasons. Apparently, residual amounts of the drug in the carcasses proved uniquely toxic to this species.

233

inhibition of COX is implicated (see Ch. 23). Aspirin is the worst offender, but there is cross-reaction with all other class members, except possibly COX-2 inhibitors (see Ch. 23). All NSAIDs (except COX-2 inhibitors) prevent platelet aggregation and therefore may prolong bleeding. Again, aspirin is the main problem in this regard (see below).

SOME IMPORTANT NSAIDS

Table 14.1 lists commonly used NSAIDs, and the clinical uses of the NSAIDs are summarised in the clinical box. Here we discuss only aspirin and paracetamol.

ASPIRIN

Aspirin (acetylsalicylic acid) was among the earliest drugs synthesised, and is still one of the most commonly consumed drugs worldwide. It is relatively insoluble, but its sodium and calcium salts are readily soluble. A newer related drug is **diflunisal** (Table 14.1).

Aspirin in non-inflammatory conditions

Aspirin—previously thought of as an old anti-inflammatory workhorse—is now approaching the status of a wonder drug that is of benefit not only in inflammation, but in an increasing number of other conditions. These include:

- *cardiovascular disorders*: through the antiplatelet action of low-dose aspirin (Ch. 21)
- *colonic and rectal cancer*: aspirin (and COX-2 inhibitors) may reduce colorectal cancer—clinical trial results are awaited

---

General unwanted effects of NSAIDs

Unwanted effects, many stemming from inhibition of the constitutive housekeeping enzyme cyclo-oxygenase (COX)-1 isoform of COX, are common, particularly in the elderly, and include the following.
- *Dyspepsia, nausea and vomiting.* Gastric damage may occur in chronic users, with risk of haemorrhage. The cause is suppression of gastroprotective prostaglandins in the gastric mucosa.
- *Skin reactions.* Mechanism unknown.
- *Reversible renal insufficiency.* Seen mainly in individuals with compromised renal function when the compensatory prostaglandin E_2-mediated vasodilatation is inhibited.
- *'Analgesic-associated nephropathy'.* This can occur following long-continued high doses of NSAIDs (e.g. paracetamol) and is often irreversible.
- *Liver disorders, bone marrow depression.* Relatively uncommon.
- *Bronchospasm.* Seen in 'aspirin-sensitive' asthmatics.

Clinical uses of NSAIDs

- For *analgesia* (e.g. headache, dysmenorrhoea, backache, bony metastases, postoperative pain):
  - short-term use: **aspirin**, **paracetamol** or **ibuprofen**
  - chronic pain: more potent, longer lasting drugs (e.g. **diflunisal**, **naproxen**, **piroxicam**)
  - to reduce the requirement for narcotic analgesics (e.g. **ketorolac** postoperatively).
- For *anti-inflammatory effects* (e.g. rheumatoid arthritis and related connective tissue disorders, gout and soft tissue disorders).
  - Note that there is substantial individual variation in clinical response to NSAIDs and considerable unpredictable patient preference for one drug rather than another.
- To lower temperature (*antipyretic*): **paracetamol**.

- *Alzheimer's disease*: again, clinical trial results are awaited (Ch. 35)
- *radiation-induced diarrhoea*.

Pharmacokinetic aspects

Aspirin, being a weak acid, is protonated in the acid environment of the stomach, thus facilitating its passage across the mucosa. Most absorption, however, occurs in the ileum, because of the extensive surface area of the microvilli. Aspirin is rapidly (probably within 30 minutes) hydrolysed by esterases in the plasma and the tissues—particularly the liver—yielding **salicylate**. This compound itself has anti-inflammatory actions (indeed, it was the original anti-inflammatory from which aspirin was derived); the mechanism is not clearly understood, although it involves the COX system. Oral salicylate is no longer used for treating inflammation, although it is a component of some topical preparations. Approximately 25% of the salicylate is oxidised; some is conjugated to give the glucuronide or sulfate before excretion, and about 25% is excreted unchanged, the rate of excretion being higher in alkaline urine (see Ch. 8).

The plasma half-life of aspirin will depend on the dose, but the duration of action is not directly related to the plasma half-life because of the irreversible nature of the action of the acetylation reaction by which it inhibits COX activity.

Unwanted effects

Salicylates may produce both local and systemic toxic effects. Aspirin shares many of the general unwanted effects of NSAIDs outlined above. In addition, there are certain specific unwanted effects that occur with aspirin and other salicylates.

- *Salicylism*, characterised by tinnitus, vertigo, decreased hearing, and sometimes also nausea and vomiting, occurs with overdosage of any salicylate.
- *Reye's syndrome*, a rare disorder of children that is characterised by hepatic encephalopathy following an acute

viral illness and a 20–40% mortality. Since the withdrawal of aspirin for paediatric use in the UK, the incidence of Reye's syndrome has fallen dramatically.

Salicylate poisoning is a result of disturbances of the acid–base and the electrolyte balance that may be seen in patients treated with high doses of salicylate-containing drugs and in attempted suicides. These drugs can uncouple oxidative phosphorylation (mainly in skeletal muscle), leading to increased oxygen consumption and thus increased production of carbon dioxide. This stimulates respiration, which is also stimulated by a direct action of the drugs on the respiratory centre. The resulting hyperventilation causes a respiratory alkalosis that is normally compensated by renal mechanisms involving increased bicarbonate excretion. Larger doses can cause a depression of the respiratory centre, which leads eventually to retention of carbon dioxide and thus an increase in plasma carbon dioxide. Because this is superimposed on a reduction in plasma bicarbonate, an uncompensated *respiratory acidosis* will occur. This may be complicated by a *metabolic acidosis*, which results from the accumulation of metabolites of pyruvic, lactic and acetoacetic acids (an indirect consequence of interference with carbohydrate metabolism). The acid load associated with the salicylate itself is quantitatively trivial. Hyperpyrexia secondary to the increased metabolic rate is also likely to be present, and dehydration may follow repeated vomiting.

In the CNS, initial stimulation with excitement is followed eventually by coma and respiratory depression. Disturbances of haemostasis can also occur, mainly as a result of depressed platelet aggregation. Salicylate poisoning is a medical emergency; it is more common, and more serious, in children than in adults. The acid–base disturbance seen in children is usually a metabolic acidosis, whereas that in adults is a respiratory alkalosis.

Some important interactions with other drugs

Aspirin causes a potentially hazardous increase in the effect of **warfarin**, partly by displacing it from plasma proteins (Ch. 52) and partly because its effect on platelets interferes with haemostatic mechanisms (see Ch. 21). Aspirin also interferes with the effect of uricosuric agents such as **probenecid** and **sulfinpyrazone**, and because low doses of aspirin may, on their own, reduce urate excretion, aspirin should not be used in gout.

PARACETAMOL

Paracetamol (called acetaminophen in the USA) is one of the most commonly used non-narcotic analgesic–antipyretic agents, and is a component of many over-the-counter proprietary preparations. In some ways, the drug constitutes an anomaly: while it has excellent analgesic and antipyretic activity, which can be traced to inhibition of CNS prostaglandin synthesis, it has weak anti-inflammatory activity (except in some specific instances) and does not share the gastric or platelet side effects of the other NSAIDs. For this reason, paracetamol is sometimes not classified as an NSAID at all.

A potential solution to this puzzle was supplied by the observation that a further COX isoform, COX-3 (an alternate splice

> ### Aspirin
>
> Aspirin (acetylsalicylic acid) is the oldest non-steroidal anti-inflammatory drug. It acts by irreversibly inactivating both cyclo-oxygenase (COX)-1 and COX-2.
> - In addition to its anti-inflammatory actions, aspirin inhibits platelet aggregation, and its main clinical importance now is in the therapy of myocardial infarction.
> - It is given orally and is rapidly absorbed; 75% is metabolised in the liver.
> - Elimination follows first-order kinetics with low doses (half-life 4 hours), and saturation kinetics with high doses (half-life over 15 hours).
> - Unwanted effects:
>   - with therapeutic doses: some gastric bleeding (usually slight and asymptomatic) is common
>   - with large doses: dizziness, deafness and tinnitus ('salicylism'); compensated respiratory alkalosis may occur
>   - with toxic doses (e.g. from self-poisoning): uncompensated respiratory acidosis with metabolic acidosis may occur, particularly in children
>   - aspirin has been linked with a postviral encephalitis (Reye's syndrome) in children.
> - If given concomitantly with warfarin, aspirin can cause a potentially hazardous increase in the risk of bleeding.

product of COX-1) existed predominantly in the CNS of some species, and that paracetamol, as well as some other drugs with similar properties (e.g. **antipyrine** and **dipyrone**), were selective inhibitors of this enzyme (Chandrasekharan et al. 2002). This elegant idea is still under investigation. Alternative explanations for the ability of paracetamol selectively to inhibit COX in the CNS alone have been provided by Ouellet & Percival (2001) and Boutaud et al. (2002).

Pharmacokinetic aspects

Paracetamol is given orally and is well absorbed, with peak plasma concentrations reached in 30–60 minutes. The plasma half-life of therapeutic doses is 2–4 hours, but with toxic doses it may be extended to 4–8 hours. Paracetamol is inactivated in the liver, being conjugated to give the glucuronide or sulfate.

Unwanted effects

With therapeutic doses, side effects are few and uncommon, although allergic skin reactions sometimes occur. It is possible that regular intake of large doses over a long period may cause kidney damage.

Toxic doses (10–15 grams) cause potentially fatal hepatotoxicity. This occurs when the liver enzymes catalysing the normal conjugation reactions are saturated, causing the drug to be metabolised instead by mixed function oxidases. The resulting toxic metabolite, N-*acetyl*-p-*benzoquinone imine*, is inactivated by conjugation with glutathione, but when glutathione is depleted the toxic intermediate accumulates and reacts with nucleophilic constituents in the cell. This causes necrosis in the liver and also in the kidney tubules.

The initial symptoms of acute paracetamol poisoning are nausea and vomiting, the hepatotoxicity being a delayed manifestation that occurs 24–48 hours later. Further details of the toxic effects of paracetamol are given in Chapter 53. If the patient is seen sufficiently soon after ingestion, the liver damage can be prevented by giving agents that increase glutathione formation in the liver (acetylcysteine intravenously, or methionine orally). If more than 12 hours have passed since the ingestion of a large dose, the antidotes, which themselves can cause adverse effects (nausea, allergic reactions), are less likely to be useful. Regrettably, ingestion of large amounts of paracetamol is a common method of suicide.

AGENTS SELECTIVE FOR CYCLO-OXYGENASE-2

Three coxibs, agents selective for COX-2, are currently available for clinical use in the UK; others may be available elsewhere. Several have been withdrawn, and the overall licensing situation is volatile. Current advice restricts the use of coxibs to patients for whom treatment with conventional NSAIDs would pose a high probability of serious gastrointestinal side effects, and coxibs are prescribed only after an assessment of cardiovascular risk. There is still a possibility that gastrointestinal disturbances will occur with these agents, perhaps because COX-2 has been implicated in the healing of pre-existing ulcers, so inhibition could delay recovery from earlier lesions.

CELECOXIB AND ETORICOXIB

Celecoxib and etoricoxib are licensed in the UK for symptomatic relief in the treatment of osteoarthritis and rheumatoid arthritis. Both are administered orally.

Pharmacokinetic properties

Both drugs have similar pharmacokinetic profiles, being well absorbed with peak plasma concentrations being achieved within 1–3 hours. They are extensively (> 99%) metabolised in the liver, and plasma protein binding is high (> 90%).

Unwanted effects

Common unwanted effects may include headache, dizziness, skin rashes, and peripheral oedema caused by fluid retention. As with all COX-2 inhibitors, consideration should be given to the possibility of serious adverse cardiovascular events. Because of the potential role of COX-2 in the healing of ulcers, the drugs should be avoided, if possible, by patients with pre-existing disease.

PARECOXIB

Parecoxib is a prodrug of valdecoxib. The latter drug has now been withdrawn, but parecoxib is licensed for the short-term treatment of postoperative pain. It is given by intravenous or intramuscular injection.

Pharmacokinetic properties

Following injection, parecoxib is rapidly and virtually completely (> 95%) converted into the active valdecoxib by enzymatic hydrolysis in the liver. Maximum blood levels are achieved within approximately 30–60 minutes, depending on the route of administration. Plasma protein binding is high. Elimination of the active metabolite, valdecoxib, is through hepatic metabolism. Multiple pathways are utilised. About 70% of the total dose is excreted in the urine, with an elimination half-life of approximately 8 hours.

Paracetamol

Paracetamol has potent analgesic and antipyretic actions but rather weaker anti-inflammatory effects than other NSAIDs. It may act through inhibition of a central nervous system–specific cyclo-oxygenase (COX) isoform such as COX-3, although this is not yet conclusive.

- It is given orally and metabolised in the liver (half-life 2–4 hours).
- Toxic doses cause nausea and vomiting, then, after 24–48 hours, potentially fatal liver damage by saturating normal conjugating enzymes, causing the drug to be converted by mixed function oxidases to *N*-acetyl-*p*-benzoquinone imine. If not inactivated by conjugation with glutathione, this compound reacts with cell proteins and kills the cell.
- Agents that increase glutathione (intravenous acetylcysteine or oral methionine) can prevent liver damage if given early.

Clinical uses of histamine H₁ receptor antagonists

- Allergic reactions (see Ch. 13):
  - non-sedating drugs (e.g. **fexofenadine**, **cetirizine**) are used for allergic rhinitis (*hay fever*) and *urticaria*
  - topical preparations may be useful for *insect bites*
  - injectable formulations are useful as an adjunct to adrenaline for severe drug hypersensitivities and emergency treatment of anaphylaxis (see Ch. 23).
- As antiemetics:
  - prevention of motion sickness
  - other causes of nausea, especially labyrinthine disorders.
- For sedation:
  - some H₁ receptor antagonists (e.g. **promethazine**; see Table 14.4) are fairly strong sedatives.

Unwanted effects

The risk of precipitating cardiovascular events should be carefully considered prior to treatment with any COX-2 inhibitor. Skin reactions, some of them serious, have been reported with the active metabolite valdecoxib, and patients should be monitored carefully. The drug should also be given with caution to patients with impaired renal function, and renal failure has been reported in connection with this drug. Postoperative anaemia may also occur.

ANTAGONISTS OF HISTAMINE

There are three groups: H_1, H_2 and H_3 receptor antagonists. The first group was introduced first by Bovet and his colleagues in the 1930s, at a time when histamine receptors had not been classified (indeed, this was possible only *because* these agents were available). For historical reasons then, the generic term *antihistamine* conventionally refers only to the H_1 receptor antagonists that affect various inflammatory and allergic mechanisms, and it is these drugs that are discussed in this section. The main clinical effect of H_2 receptor antagonists is inhibition of gastric secretion, and this is discussed in Chapter 25. Several H_3 receptor agonists and antagonists are now available, and the potential for their clinical use (mainly in CNS conditions) is being explored.

H_1 RECEPTOR ANTAGONISTS (ANTIHISTAMINES)

Details of some characteristic H_1 receptor antagonists are shown in Table 14.4.

Pharmacological actions

Many of the pharmacological actions of the H_1 receptor antagonists follow from the actions of histamine outlined in Chapter 13. In vitro, for example, they decrease histamine-mediated contraction of the smooth muscle of the bronchi, the intestine and the uterus. They inhibit histamine-induced increases in vascular permeability and bronchospasm in the guinea pig in vivo, but are unfortunately of little value in allergic bronchospasm in humans. The clinical uses of H_1 receptor antagonists are summarised in the clinical box.

Some H_1 receptor antagonists have pronounced effects in the CNS. These are usually listed as 'side effects', but they may be more clinically useful than the peripheral H_1 antagonist effects. Some are fairly strong sedatives and may be used for this action (e.g. **diphenhydramine**; see Table 14.4). Several are antiemetic and are used to prevent motion sickness (e.g. **promethazine**; see Ch. 25).

Many H_1 receptor antagonists (e.g. diphenhydramine) also show significant antimuscarinic effects, although their affinity is much lower for muscarinic than for histamine receptors. When selective H_1 receptor antagonism is desired, untrammelled by

Table 14.4 Comparison of some commonly used H1 receptor antagonists

Type	Drug	H	U	R	AE	S	Comments
Non-sedating	Acrivastine	•	•				–
	Cetirizine	•	•				–
	Desloratidine	•	•				Metabolite of loratidine
	Fexofenadine		•	•			Metabolite of terfenadine
	Levocetrizine	•	•				Isomer of cetrizine
	Loratidine	•	•				–
	Mizolastine	•	•				May cause QT interval prolongation
Sedating	Alimemazine		•			•	Used for premedication
	Brompheniramine	•	•			•	–
	Chlorpheniramine	•	•		•	•	–
	Clemastine	•	•			•	–
	Cyproheptadine	•	•			•	Used also for migraine
	Diphenhydramine					•	Mainly used as a mild hypnotic
	Doxylamine					•	Mainly used as an ingredient of proprietary decongestant and other medicines
	Hydroxyzine		•			•	Also used to treat anxiety
	Promethazine	•	•		•	•	Also used for motion sickness
	Triprolidine					•	Mainly used as an ingredient of proprietary decongestant and other medicines

AE, allergic emergency (e.g. anaphylactic shock); H, hay fever; R, rhinitis; S, sedation; U, urticaria and/or pruritis.
(From British Medical Association and Royal Pharmaceutical Society of Great Britain 2005 British National Formulary. BMA and RPSGB, London.)

CNS effects, newer drugs—such as **Cetirizine** (Table 14.4) which do not penetrate the blood–brain barrier—may be used. Some non-sedating antihistamines such as terfenadine, (now withdrawn) can cause serious cardiac dysrhythmias (p. 117). The risk is extremely low but is increased if taken with grapefruit juice or agents that inhibit cytochrome P450 in the liver (see Chs 8 and 52). **Fexofenadine**, the non-toxic, pharmacologically active metabolite of terfenadine, is now available (see p. 117). Other, newer drugs that lack sedative action are **loratadine** and **mizolastine**.

Several H_1 receptor antagonists show weak blockade at α_1 adrenoceptors (an example is the phenothiazine promethazine). **Cyproheptadine** is a 5-hydroxytryptamine antagonist as well as an H_1 receptor antagonist.

Pharmacokinetic aspects

Most H_1 receptor antagonists are given orally, are well absorbed, reach their peak effect in 1–2 hours and are effective for 3–6 hours, although there are exceptions. Most appear to be widely distributed throughout the body, but some do not penetrate the blood–brain barrier, for example the non-sedative drugs mentioned above (see Table 14.4). They are metabolised in the liver and excreted in the urine.

Unwanted effects

What is defined as 'unwanted' will depend to a certain extent on the purpose for which a drug is used. When used to treat allergies, for example, the sedative CNS effects are generally unwanted, but there are other occasions (e.g. in small children approaching bedtime) when such effects are more desirable. Even under these circumstances, other CNS effects, such as dizziness, tinnitus and fatigue, are unwelcome.

The peripheral antimuscarinic actions are always unwanted. The commonest of these is dryness of the mouth, but blurred vision, constipation and retention of urine can also occur. Unwanted effects that are not mechanism-based are also seen; gastrointestinal disturbances are fairly common, while allergic dermatitis can follow topical application.

DRUGS USED IN GOUT

Gout is a metabolic disease in which plasma urate concentration is raised because of overproduction (sometimes linked to indulgence in alcoholic beverages, especially beer, or purine-rich foods such as offal, or increased cell turnover as in haematological malignancies, particularly when treated with cytotoxic drugs; Ch. 51) or impaired excretion of uric acid. It is characterised by very painful intermittent attacks of acute arthritis produced by the deposition of crystals of sodium urate (a product of purine metabolism) in the synovial tissue of joints and elsewhere. An inflammatory response is evoked, involving activation of the kinin, complement and plasmin systems (see Ch. 13 and Fig. 13.1), generation of lipoxygenase products such as leukotriene B_4 (Fig. 13.5), and local accumulation of neutrophil granulocytes. These engulf the crystals by phagocytosis, releasing tissue-damaging toxic oxygen metabolites and subsequently causing lysis of the cells with release of proteolytic enzymes. Urate crystals also induce the production of IL-1 and possibly other cytokines too.

Drugs used to treat gout may act in the following ways:

- by inhibiting uric acid synthesis: **allopurinol** (this is the main prophylactic drug)
- by increasing uric acid excretion (uricosuric agents: probenecid, sulfinpyrazone)
- by inhibiting leucocyte migration into the joint (**colchicine**)
- by a general anti-inflammatory and analgesic effect (NSAIDs).

ALLOPURINOL

Allopurinol is an analogue of hypoxanthine and reduces the synthesis of uric acid by competitive inhibition of *xanthine oxidase* (Fig. 14.4). Some inhibition of *de novo* purine synthesis also occurs. Allopurinol is converted to alloxanthine by xanthine oxidase, and this metabolite, which remains in the tissue for a considerable time, is an effective non-competitive inhibitor of the enzyme. The pharmacological action of allopurinol is largely due to alloxanthine.

Allopurinol reduces the concentration of the relatively insoluble urates and uric acid in tissues, plasma and urine, while increasing the concentration of their more soluble precursors, the xanthines and hypoxanthines. The deposition of urate crystals in tissues (*tophi*) is reversed, and the formation of renal stones is inhibited. Allopurinol is the drug of choice in the long-term treatment of gout, but it is ineffective in the treatment of an acute attack and may even exacerbate the inflammation.

Pharmacokinetic aspects

Allopurinol is given orally and is well absorbed in the gastrointestinal tract. Its half-life is 2–3 hours; it is converted to alloxanthine (Fig. 14.4), which has a half-life of 18–30 hours.

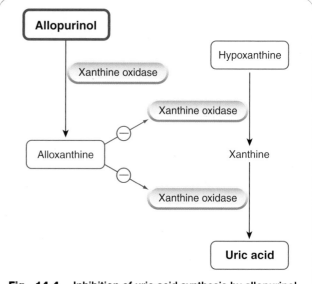

Fig. 14.4 Inhibition of uric acid synthesis by allopurinol. (See text for details.)

Renal excretion is a balance between glomerular filtration and probenecid-sensitive tubular reabsorption.

Unwanted effects

These are few. Gastrointestinal disturbances and allergic reactions (mainly rashes) can occur but usually disappear if the drug is stopped. Potentially fatal skin diseases (Stevens–Johnson syndrome and *toxic epidermal necrolysis*—a horrible disorder where skin peels away in sheets as if scalded) are rare but devastating. Rechallenge is never justified. Acute attacks of gout occur commonly during the early stages of therapy (possibly as a result of physicochemical changes in the surfaces of urate crystals as these start to redissolve), so treatment is never initiated during an acute attack and is usually initiated accompanied by an NSAID.

Drug interactions

Allopurinol increases the effect of **mercaptopurine**, an antimetabolite used in cancer chemotherapy (Ch. 51), and also that of **azathioprine** (an immunosuppressant used to prevent transplant rejection; see below), which is metabolised to mercaptopurine. Allopurinol also enhances the effect of another anticancer drug, **cyclophosphamide** (Ch. 51). The effect of warfarin is increased because its metabolism is inhibited.

URICOSURIC AGENTS

Uricosuric drugs increase uric acid excretion by a direct action on the renal tubule. Examples are probenecid and sulfinpyrazone. They remain useful as prophylaxis for patients with severe recurrent gout who have severe adverse reactions to allopurinol. Sulfinpyrazone has NSAID activity; treatment with uricosuric drugs is initiated with an NSAID, as for allopurinol.

COLCHICINE

Colchicine is an alkaloid extracted from the autumn crocus. It has a specific effect in gouty arthritis and can be used both to prevent and to relieve acute attacks. It prevents migration of neutrophils into the joint, apparently by binding to tubulin, resulting in the depolymerisation of the microtubules and reduced cell motility. Colchicine-treated neutrophils develop a 'drunken walk'. Colchicine may also prevent the production of a putative inflammatory glycoprotein by neutrophils that have phagocytosed urate crystals, and other mechanisms may also be important in bringing about its effects.

Pharmacokinetic aspects

Colchicine is given orally, is well absorbed, and reaches peak concentrations in about 1 hour. It is excreted partly in the gastrointestinal tract and partly in the urine.

Unwanted effects

The acute unwanted effects of colchicine are largely gastrointestinal: nausea, vomiting and abdominal pain. Severe diarrhoea[3] may be a problem, and with large doses may be associated with gastrointestinal haemorrhage and kidney damage. Prolonged treatment can, rarely, cause blood dyscrasias, rashes or peripheral neuropathy.

ANTIRHEUMATOID DRUGS

Arthritic disease is one of the commonest chronic inflammatory conditions in developed countries, and *rheumatoid arthritis* is a common cause of disability. One in three patients with rheumatoid arthritis is likely to become severely disabled. The joint changes, which probably represent an autoimmune reaction, comprise inflammation, proliferation of the synovium, and erosion of cartilage and bone. The primary inflammatory cytokines, IL-1 and TNF-α, have a major role in pathogenesis (Ch. 13).

The drugs most frequently used in therapy are the *DMARDs* and the NSAIDs. Unlike the NSAIDs, which reduce the symptoms, but not the progress, of the disease, the former group may halt or reverse the underlying disease itself. Such claims may be more optimistic than real, but nevertheless these drugs are useful in the treatment of discrete groups of patients. Some immunosuppressants (e.g. azathioprine, **ciclosporin**; see below and Ch. 51) are also used, as are the **glucocorticoids** (covered in Ch. 28). Newer agents, with more specific actions, are the anticytokine drugs.

DISEASE-MODIFYING ANTIRHEUMATIC DRUGS

The term *DMARD* is a latex concept that can be stretched to cover a heterologous group of agents with unrelated chemical structures and different mechanisms of action. Included in this category are **methotrexate**, **sulfasalazine**, **gold** compounds, **penicillamine** and **chloroquine** (see Table 14.5).

The antirheumatoid action of most of these agents was usually discovered through a mixture of serendipity and clinical intuition. When the drugs were introduced, nothing was known about their mechanism of action in these conditions, and decades of in vitro experiments have generally resulted in further bewilderment rather than understanding. DMARDs generally improve symptoms and can reduce disease activity in rheumatoid arthritis, as measured by reduction in number of swollen and tender joints, pain score, disability score, articular index on radiology, and serum concen-

---

[3]Because the therapeutic margin is so small, it used to be said by rheumatologists that 'patients must run before they can walk'.

> ### Drugs used in gout
>
> - To treat an acute attack:
>   - non-steroidal anti-inflammatory drugs have anti-inflammatory action and reduce pain
>   - **colchicine** reduces leucocyte migration into joints.
> - For prophylaxis:
>   - **allopurinol** inhibits uric acid synthesis
>   - probenecid increases uric acid excretion.
> - Drugs used for prophylaxis must not be started until the acute attack has resolved.

Table 14.5 Comparison of some common 'disease-modifying' and immunosuppressive drugs

		Indications				
Drug	Type	RA	JRA	SLE	Severity	Comments
Sodium aurothiomalate	Gold complex	•	•		–	–
Auranofin	Gold complex	•			–	–
Penicillamine	Penicillin metabolite	•			Severe	–
Chloroquine	Antimalarial	•	•	•	Moderate	–
Hydroxychloroquine sulfate	Antimalarial	•	•	•	Moderate	Useful for some skin disorders
Mepacrine	Antimalarial			•	Moderate	–
Methotrexate	Immunomodulator	•			Moderate to severe	Also used in Crohn's disease, psoriasis and cancer treatment
Azathioprine	Immunomodulator	•			–	Also used in transplant rejection
Ciclosporin	Immunomodulator	•			Severe	Used when other therapies fail; some skin diseases; transplant rejection
Cyclophosphamide	Immunomodulator				Severe	–
Leflunamide	Immunomodulator	•			Moderate to severe	Also used in psoriatic arthritis
Adalimumab	Cytokine inhibitor	•			Moderate to severe	Used when other drugs inadequate; often combined with methotrexate
Anakinra	Cytokine inhibitor	•			Moderate to severe	Used when other drugs inadequate; often combined with methotrexate
Etanercept	Cytokine inhibitor	•			–	Used when other drugs inadequate; often combined with methotrexate
Infliximab	Cytokine inhibitor	•			–	Used when other drugs inadequate; often combined with methotrexate; used in psoriasis
Sulfasalazine	NSAID	•			–	Also used in ulcerative colitis

JRA, juvenile rheumatoid arthritis; NSAID, non-steroidal anti-inflammatory drug; RA, rheumatoid arthritis; SLE, systemic lupus erythematosus.
(From British Medical Association and Royal Pharmaceutical Society of Great Britain 2005 British National Formulary. BMA and RPSGB, London.)

tration of acute-phase proteins and of rheumatoid factor (an immunoglobulin [Ig] M antibody against host IgG). However, whether they actually halt the long-term progress of the disease is hotly debated.

The DMARDs were often referred to as *second-line drugs*, with the implication that they are only resorted to when other therapies (e.g. NSAIDs) failed. Today, however, DMARD therapy may be initiated as soon as a definite diagnosis has been reached. Their clinical effects are usually slow (months) in onset, and it is usual to provide NSAID 'cover' during this induction phase. If therapy is successful (and the success rate is not invariably high),

concomitant NSAID (or glucocorticoid) therapy can generally be dramatically reduced. Some DMARDs have a place in the treatment of other chronic inflammatory diseases, whereas others (e.g. penicillamine) are not thought to have a general anti-inflammatory action. Putative mechanisms of action of DMARDs are reviewed by Bondeson (1997).

SULFASALAZINE

Sulfasalazine, a common first-choice DMARD in the UK, produces remission in active rheumatoid arthritis and is also used for chronic inflammatory bowel disease. It may act by scavenging the toxic oxygen metabolites produced by neutrophils. The drug is a combination of **sulfonamide (sulfapyridine)** with a salicylate. It is split into its component parts by bacteria in the colon, the **5-aminosalicylic acid** being the putative radical scavenger. It is poorly absorbed after oral administration. The common side effects are gastrointestinal disturbances, malaise and headache. Skin reactions and leucopenia can occur but are reversible on stopping the drug. The absorption of folic acid is sometimes impaired; this can be countered by giving folic acid supplements. A reversible decrease in sperm count has also been reported. As with other sulfonamides, blood dyscrasias and anaphylactic-type reactions may occur in a few patients.

GOLD COMPOUNDS

Gold is administered in the form of organic complexes; **sodium aurothiomalate** and **auranofin** are the two most common preparations. The effect of gold compounds develops slowly, the maximum action occurring after 3–4 months. Pain and joint swelling subside, and the progression of bone and joint damage diminishes. The mechanism of action is not clear, but auranofin, although not aurothiomalate, inhibits the induction of IL-1 and TNF-α.

Pharmacokinetic aspects
Sodium aurothiomalate is given by deep intramuscular injection; auranofin is given orally. Peak plasma concentrations of the former drug are reached in 2–6 hours. The compounds gradually become concentrated in the tissues, not only in synovial cells in joints but also in liver cells, kidney tubules, the adrenal cortex and macrophages throughout the body. The gold complexes remain in the tissues for some time after treatment is stopped. Excretion is mostly renal, but some is eliminated in the gastrointestinal tract. The half-life is 7 days initially but increases with treatment, so the drug is usually given first at weekly, then at monthly intervals.

Unwanted effects
Unwanted effects with aurothiomalate are seen in about one-third of patients treated, and serious toxic effects in about 1 patient in 10. Unwanted effects with auranofin are less frequent and less severe. Important unwanted effects include skin rashes (which can be severe), mouth ulcers, non-specific flu-like symptoms, proteinuria, thromboctyopenia and blood dyscrasias. Encephalopathy, peripheral neuropathy and hepatitis can occur. If therapy is stopped when the early symptoms appear, the incidence of serious toxic effects is relatively low.

PENICILLAMINE

Penicillamine is dimethylcysteine; it is one of the substances produced by hydrolysis of **penicillin** and appears in the urine after treatment with that drug. The D isomer is used in the therapy of rheumatoid disease. About 75% of patients with rheumatoid arthritis respond to penicillamine. In responders, therapeutic effects are seen within weeks but do not reach a plateau for several months. Penicillamine is thought to modify rheumatoid disease partly by decreasing the immune response, IL-1 generation, and/or partly by an effect on collagen synthesis, preventing the maturation of newly synthesised collagen. However, the precise mechanism of action is still a matter of conjecture. The drug has a highly reactive thiol group and also has metal-chelating properties, which are put to good use in the treatment of *Wilson's disease* (pathological copper deposition causing neurodegeneration) or heavy metal poisoning.

Pharmacokinetic aspects
Penicillamine is given orally, and only half the dose administered is absorbed. It reaches peak plasma concentrations in 1–2 hours and is excreted in the urine. Dosage is started low and increased only gradually to minimise unwanted effects.

Unwanted effects
Unwanted effects occur in about 40% of patients treated and may necessitate cessation of therapy. Anorexia, fever, nausea and vomiting, and disturbances of taste (the last related to the chelation of zinc) are seen but often disappear with continued treatment. Proteinuria occurs in 20% of patients. Rashes and stomatitis are the most common unwanted effects and may resolve if the dosage is lowered, as may dose-related thrombocytopenia. Other bone marrow disorders (leucopenia, aplastic anaemia) are absolute indications for stopping therapy, as are the various autoimmune conditions (e.g. thyroiditis, myasthenia gravis) that sometimes supervene. Because penicillamine is a metal chelator, it should not be given with gold compounds.

HYDROXYCHLOROQUINE

Hydroxychloroquine and chloroquine are 4-aminoquinoline drugs used mainly in the prevention and treatment of malaria (Ch. 49), but they are also used as DMARDs. Chloroquine is usually reserved for cases where other treatments have failed. They are also used in patients with systemic or discoid lupus erythematosus, but are contraindicated in patients with psoriatic arthropathy because they make the skin lesions worse. **Mepacrine** is also sometimes used in discoid lupus. Pharmacological effects do not appear until a month or more after the drug is started, and only about half the patients treated respond. The pharmacokinetic aspects and unwanted effects of chloroquine are dealt with in Chapter 49; screening for ocular toxicity is particularly important.

METHOTREXATE

Methotrexate is a folic acid antagonist with cytotoxic and immunosuppressant activity (see below and Chs 45 and 51) and potent antirheumatoid action. It is commonly a first-choice DMARD. It has a more rapid onset of action than other DMARDs, but treatment has to be closely monitored because of blood dyscrasias (some fatal) and liver cirrhosis. More than 50% of patients continue with it for 5 years or more, whereas about half stop other DMARDs within 2 years because of unwanted effects and lack of efficacy.

- These comprise non-steroidal anti-inflammatory drugs (see key points box on p. 234), disease-modifying antirheumatic drugs (DMARDs) and anticytokine agents.
- DMARDs:
  - include **sulfasalazine**, **methotrexate** (a folate antagonist), **gold** compounds, **chloroquine** (an antimalarial), **penicillamine** and **azathioprine** (an immunosuppressant)
  - are slow-acting drugs and can improve symptoms and reduce the inflammatory process
  - retard progress of the disease but do not halt it entirely.
- Anticytokine agents (e.g. **infliximab**, **etanercept**) are used in *Crohn's disease* (Ch. 25, p. 396) and *psoriatic arthropathy*, as well as in rheumatoid arthritis.

IMMUNOSUPPRESSANT DRUGS

Immunosuppressants are used in the therapy of autoimmune disease and to prevent and/or treat transplant rejection. Because they impair immune responses, they carry the hazard of a decreased response to infections and may facilitate the emergence of malignant cell lines. However, the relationship between these adverse effects and potency in preventing graft rejection varies with different drugs. The clinical use of immunosuppressants is summarised in the clinical box.

Most of these drugs act during the induction phase of the immunological response (see Ch. 13), reducing lymphocyte

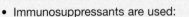

> **Clinical uses of immunosuppressants**

- Immunosuppressants are used:
  - to suppress rejection of transplanted organs and tissues (kidneys, bone marrow, heart, liver, etc.)
  - to suppress graft-versus-host disease in bone marrow transplantation
  - to treat conditions with an autoimmune component in their pathogenesis, including *idiopathic thrombocytopenic purpura*, some forms of *haemolytic anaemia*, some forms of *glomerulonephritis*, *myasthenia gravis*, *systemic lupus erythematosus*, *rheumatoid arthritis*, *psoriasis*, and *ulcerative colitis*.
- Therapy of autoimmune disease often involves a combination of glucocorticoid and cytotoxic agents.
- For transplantation of organs or bone marrow, **ciclosporin** is usually combined with a glucocorticoid, a cytotoxic drug or an antilymphocyte immunoglobulin.

proliferation, although others also inhibit aspects of the effector phase. They can be roughly characterised as:

- drugs that inhibit IL-2 production or action (e.g. ciclosporin, **tacrolimus**)
- drugs that inhibit cytokine gene expression (e.g. the **corticosteroids**)
- drugs that inhibit purine or pyrimidine synthesis (e.g. azathioprine, **mycophenolate mofetil**)
- drugs that block the T-cell surface molecules involved in signalling (e.g. monoclonal antibody–based agents).

CICLOSPORIN

Ciclosporin is a compound first found in fungus. It consists of a cyclic peptide of 11 amino acid residues (including some not found in animals) with potent immunosuppressive activity but no effect on the acute inflammatory reaction per se. Its unusual activity, which, unlike most earlier immunosuppressants, does not involve cytotoxicity, was discovered in 1972 and was crucial for the development of transplant surgery (for a detailed review, see Borel et al., 1996). The drug has numerous actions on several cell types; in general, the actions of relevance to immunosuppression are:

- decreased clonal proliferation of T cells, primarily by inhibiting IL-2 synthesis and possibly also by decreasing expression of IL-2 receptors
- reduced induction, and clonal proliferation, of cytotoxic T cells from CD8[+] precursor T cells
- reduced function of the effector T cells that are responsible for cell-mediated responses (e.g. decreased delayed-type hypersensitivity)
- some reduction of T cell–dependent B-cell responses.

The main action is a relatively selective inhibitory effect on IL-2 gene transcription, although a similar effect on interferon (IFN)-γ and IL-3 has also been reported. Normally, interaction of antigen with a T-helper (Th) cell receptor results in increased intracellular Ca^{2+} (Chs 2 and 13), which in turn stimulates a phosphatase, *calcineurin*; this activates various transcription factors that initiate IL-2 transcription. Ciclosporin binds to *cyclophilin*, a cytosolic protein member of the *immunophilins* (a group of proteins that act as intracellular receptors for such drugs). The drug– immunophilin complex binds to and inhibits calcineurin, thereby preventing activation of Th cells and production of IL-2 (Ch. 13).

Pharmacokinetic aspects

Ciclosporin is poorly absorbed by mouth but can be given orally in a more readily absorbed formulation, or given by intravenous infusion. After oral administration, peak plasma concentrations are usually attained in about 3–4 hours. The plasma half-life is approximately 24 hours. Metabolism occurs in the liver, and most of the metabolites are excreted in the bile. Ciclosporin accumulates in most tissues at concentrations three to four times that seen in the plasma. Some of the drug remains in lymphomyeloid tissue and remains in fat depots for some time after administration has stopped.

Unwanted effects

The commonest and most serious unwanted effect of ciclosporin is nephrotoxicity, which is thought to be unconnected with calcineurin inhibition. It may be a limiting factor in the use of the drug in some patients (see also Ch. 52). Hepatotoxicity and hypertension can also occur. Less important unwanted effects include anorexia, lethargy, hirsutism, tremor, paraesthesia (tingling sensation), gum hypertrophy (especially when coprescribed with calcium antagonists for hypertension; Ch. 18) and gastro-intestinal disturbances. Ciclosporin has no depressant effects on the bone marrow.

TACROLIMUS

Tacrolimus is a macrolide antibiotic of fungal origin with a very similar mechanism of action to ciclosporin, but considerably more potency. The main difference is that the internal receptor for this drug is not cyclophilin but a different immunophilin termed *FKBP* (*FK-binding protein*, so-called because tacrolimus was initially termed *FK506*). The tacrolimus–FKBP complex inhibits calcineurin with the effects described above. **Pimecrolimus** (used topically for atopic eczema) and **sirolimus** (used to prevent organ rejection after transplantation, and also in coating on stents to prevent restenosis; Ch. 7, p. 111) have similar properties.

Pharmacokinetic aspects

Tacrolimus can be given orally, by intravenous injection or as an ointment for topical use in inflammatory disease of the skin. It is 99% metabolised by the liver and has a half-life of approximately 7 hours.

Unwanted effects

The unwanted effects of tacrolimus are similar to those of ciclosporin but are more severe. The incidence of nephrotoxicity and neurotoxicity is higher, but that of hirsutism is lower. Gastrointestinal disturbances and metabolic disturbances (hyperglycaemia) can occur. Thrombocytopenia and hyper-lipidaemia have been reported but respond to reducing the dosage.

GLUCOCORTICOIDS

Immunosuppression by glucocorticoids involves both their effects on the immune response and their anti-inflammatory actions. These are described in Chapter 28, and the sites of action of the agents on cell-mediated immune reactions are indicated in Figure 14.5. Glucocorticoids are immunosuppressant chiefly because, like ciclosporin, they restrain the clonal proliferation of Th cells, through decreasing transcription of the gene for IL-2. However, they also decrease the transcription of many other cytokine genes (including those for TNF-α, IFN-γ, IL-1 and many other interleukins) in both the induction and effector phases of the immune response. These effects on transcription are mediated through inhibition of the action of transcription factors, such as activator protein-1 and NFκB.

AZATHIOPRINE

Azathioprine interferes with purine synthesis and is cytotoxic. It is widely used for immunosuppression, particularly for control of autoimmune diseases such as rheumatoid arthritis and to prevent tissue rejection in transplant surgery. This drug is metabolised to give mercaptopurine, a purine analogue that inhibits DNA synthesis (see Ch. 51). Both cell-mediated and antibody-mediated immune reactions are depressed by this drug, because it inhibits clonal proliferation during the induction phase of the immune response (see Ch. 13) by a cytotoxic action on dividing cells. As is the case with mercaptopurine itself, the main unwanted effect is depression of the bone marrow. Other toxic effects are nausea and vomiting, skin eruptions and a mild hepatotoxicity.

MYCOPHENOLATE MOFETIL

Mycophenolate mofetil is a semisynthetic derivative of a fungal antibiotic. In the body, it is converted to mycophenolic acid, which restrains proliferation of both T and B lymphocytes and reduces the production of cytotoxic T cells by inhibiting *inosine monophosphate dehydrogenase*, an enzyme crucial for *de novo* purine biosynthesis in both T and B cells (other cells can generate purines through another pathway), so the drug has a fairly selective action. It is mainly used to curtail transplant rejection.

Mycophenolate mofetil is given orally and is well absorbed. Magnesium and aluminium hydroxides impair absorption, and **colestyramine** reduces plasma concentrations. The metabolite mycophenolic acid undergoes enterohepatic cycling and is eliminated by the kidney as the inactive glucuronide. Unwanted gastrointestinal effects are common.

LEFLUNOMIDE

Leflunomide has a relatively specific inhibitory effect on activated T cells. It gives rise to a metabolite that inhibits *de novo* synthesis of pyrimidines by inhibiting *dihydroorotate dehydrogenase*. It is orally active and well absorbed from the gastrointestinal tract. It has a long plasma half-life, and the active metabolite undergoes enterohepatic circulation. Unwanted effects include diarrhoea, alopecia, raised liver enzymes and indeed a risk of hepatic failure. The long half-life increases the risk of cumulative toxicity.

ANTICYTOKINE DRUGS

The drugs in this section probably represent the greatest conceptual breakthrough in the treatment of severe chronic inflammation for many years (see Maini, 2005). Using these agents, treatment can, for the first time, be aimed at specific aspects of the disease processes in rheumatoid arthritis. The drugs are 'biopharmaceuticals', that is to say, they are recombinant engineered antibodies and other proteins (see Ch. 55). As such, they are difficult and expensive to produce, and this limits their use. In the UK, their use (on the National Health Service) is restricted to patients who do not respond adequately to other DMARD therapy.

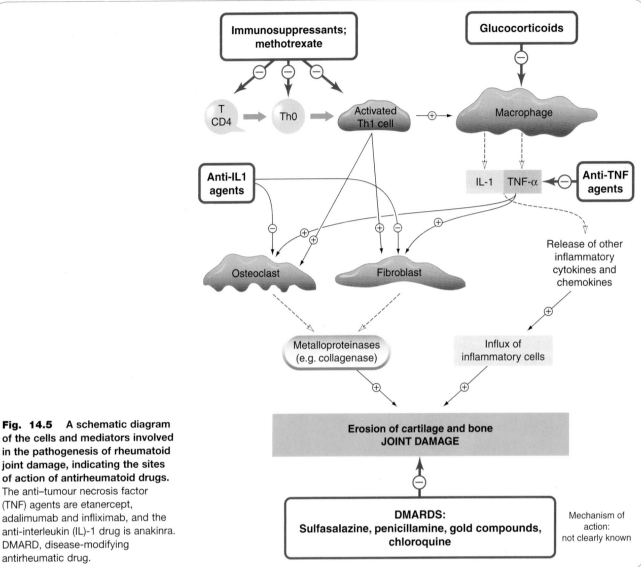

Fig. 14.5 A schematic diagram of the cells and mediators involved in the pathogenesis of rheumatoid joint damage, indicating the sites of action of antirheumatoid drugs. The anti–tumour necrosis factor (TNF) agents are etanercept, adalimumab and infliximab, and the anti-interleukin (IL)-1 drug is anakinra. DMARD, disease-modifying antirheumatic drug.

Immunosuppressants

- Clonal proliferation of T-helper cells can be decreased through inhibition of transcription of interleukin (IL)-2: ciclosporin, tacrolimus and glucocorticoids act in this way.
  - Ciclosporin and tacrolimus are given orally or intravenously; common adverse effect is nephrotoxicity.
  - For glucocorticoids, see pp. 242-243.

- DNA synthesis is inhibited by:
  - azathioprine, through its active metabolite mercaptopurine
  - mycophenolate mofetil, through inhibition of *de novo* purine synthesis.
- T-cell signal transduction events are blocked by basiliximab and daclizumab, which are monoclonal antibodies against the α chain of the IL-2 receptor.

The drugs currently available are **infliximab** and **adalimumab** (chimeric mouse/human monoclonal antibodies against TNF-α), **etanercept** (a TNF receptor fused to the Fc domain of a human IgG molecule) and **anakinra** (an IL-1 antagonist). Infliximab, adalimumab and etenercept bind TNF and inhibit its effects (Fig. 14.5). Etanercept and anakinra function as antagonists, although etanercept can also bind another cytokine, lymphotoxin -α, which may be of relevance for the treatment of juvenile arthritis because this cytokine is found in inflamed tissues in this condition.

Related compounds include **basiliximab** and **daclizumab**, monoclonal antibodies against the α chain of the IL-2 receptor. They exert an immunosuppressant action by blocking this receptor on Th cells (see Ch. 13). They are given by intravenous infusion and can cause serious hypersensitivity reactions.

Pharmacokinetic aspects

Etanercept is given subcutaneously twice a week. Infliximab is used in conjunction with methotrexate therapy and is given intravenously every 6–8 weeks. Adalimumab is given by sub-cutaneous injection in alternate weeks. Anakinra is given daily by subcutaneous injection.

Unwanted effects

Cytokines have an important part to play in the regulation of host defence systems, so one might predict that anticytokine therapy—like any treatment that interferes with immune function—may precipitate latent disease or encourage opportunistic infections. With etanercept, unwanted effects have in general been minimal and consist mainly of reactions at the injection site, although there have been reports of blood dyscrasias and demyelinating CNS disorders. Anakinra is similarly well tolerated. Infliximab and adalimumab have been associated with recurrence of tuberculosis, and there is evidence that long-term use can cause the development of autoantibodies. Despite misgivings, it seems that prolonged inhibition of TNF action does not substantially increase infections or malignancies.

POSSIBLE FUTURE DEVELOPMENTS

At the time of writing, it would seem that the whole area of anti-inflammatory drug development stands at a crossroads. The mainstay treatments for inflammation (e.g. the NSAIDs and the glucocorticoids) are rather 'old' drugs—aspirin, it will be remembered, being synthesised in the final years of the 19th century and the glucocorticoids having been discovered in the late 1940s. Compared with the innovation in some other therapeutic areas, such as the treatment of hypertension, for example, the field seems somewhat impoverished.

A major blow to the NSAID area (and indeed to the pharmaceutical industry in general) has been the recent controversy surrounding the adverse cardiovascular side effects of the COX-2 inhibitors and the withdrawal of several prominent members of this class. The emerging evidence that traditional NSAIDs may also have similar cardiovascular side effects has cast a pall over our existing therapies. At the time of writing, it is too early to say exactly how this awkward situation will be resolved.

One of the few innovations in the beleaguered NSAID area has been the design and synthesis of *nitric oxide (NO)-NSAIDs*—conventional NSAIDs that have NO-donating groups attached to them by ester linkages. The ability of these drugs to release NO following hydrolysis in plasma and tissue fluid is associated with a decreased risk of ulcerogenic events and an improved anti-inflammatory profile, presumably due to the beneficial effects of low concentrations of NO (see Ch. 17). Some of these drugs are currently in clinical trial.

Other techniques for manipulating or inhibiting the production of arachidonic acid metabolites, such as inhibiting phospholipase A_2 or preventing the generation or action of lipoxygenase products, have yet to realise their apparent potential, except in the case of the leukotriene receptor antagonist **montelukast** (see Ch. 23), which has a minor role in the treatment of asthma.

Elsewhere, a lot of attention has been given to inhibitors of leucocyte trafficking, on the premise that this would achieve a comprehensive anti-inflammatory action. The rationale for these developments has arisen from the detailed researches into the integrins, selectins and other adhesion molecules that are involved in the targeting, capture and transmigration of blood-borne leucocytes as they enter an area of inflammation. Several putative compounds have utilised a monoclonal antibody strategy. One of these, **efaluzimab**, which binds the *CD11a* adhesion molecule, has been approved in some countries for the treatment of psoriasis.

Another adhesion molecule that has been targeted is very late antigen (VLA)-4. **Natalizumab** antagonizes this adhesion molecule. It prevents lymphocytes from targeting the plaques in multiple sclerosis, but is used therapeutically only in the rapidly evolving severe relapsing-remitting form of this disease because it can, rarely, precipitate a lethal viral encephalopathy.

The journal *Current Opinion in Pharmacology* has several compendium issues devoted to recent advances in anti-inflammatory therapy for those who wish to research this field in more detail.

REFERENCES AND FURTHER READING

Seminal or original papers

Chandrasekharan N V et al. 2002 COX-3, a cyclooxygenase-1 variant inhibited by acetaminophen and other analgesic/antipyretic drugs: cloning, structure, and expression. Proc Natl Acad Sci USA 99: 13926–13931 (*A new COX isozyme is described: COX-3. In humans, the COX-3 mRNA is expressed most abundantly in cerebral cortex and heart. It is selectively inhibited by analgesic/antipyretic drugs such as paracetamol and is inhibited by some other NSAIDs.*)

Vane J R 1971 Inhibition of prostaglandin synthesis as a mechanism of action for aspirin-like drugs. Nat New Biol 231: 232–239 (*Definitive, seminal article*)

Cyclo-oxygenase pharmacology

Bazan N G 2001 COX-2 as a multifunctional neuronal modulator. Nat Med 7: 414–415 (*Succinct treatment of possible role of COX-2 in the CNS; useful diagrams*)

Bazan N G, Flower R J 2002 Lipid signals in pain control. Nature 420: 135–138. (*Succinct article commenting on the discovery of COX-3*)

Boers M 2001 NSAIDs and selective COX-2 inhibitors: competition between gastroprotection and cardioprotection. Lancet 357: 1222–1223 (*Editorial analysing crisply the results of two major randomised double-blind studies of gastrointestinal toxicity of selective COX-2 inhibitors as compared with non-selective NSAIDs*)

Boutaud O, Aronoff D M, Richardson J H et al. 2002 Determinants of the cellular specificity of acetaminophen as an inhibitor of prostaglandin H_2 synthases. Proc Natl Acad Sci USA 99: 7130–7135

Catella-Lawson F, Reilly M P et al. 2001 Cyclooxygenase inhibitors and the anti-platelet effects of aspirin. N Engl J Med 345: 1809–1817 (*Points out that ibuprofen, but not rofecoxib, paracetamol or diclofenac, given simultaneously with aspirin reduces the antiplatelet effect of aspirin. Excellent diagram. This problem is discussed by Crofford L J, pp. 1844–1845, in the same issue of the journal.*)

de Broe M E, Elseviers M M 1998 Current concepts: analgesic nephropathy. N Engl J Med 338: 446–452 (*Useful review*)

FitzGerald G A, Patrono C 2001 The coxibs, selective inhibitors of cyclooxygenase-2. N Engl J Med 345: 433–442 (*Excellent coverage of the selective COX-2 inhibitors*)

Flower R J 2003 The development of COX-2 inhibitors. Nat Rev Drug Discov 2: 179–191. (*Reviews the work that led up to the development of the COX-2 inhibitors; several useful diagrams*)

Fries J F 1983 Measuring the quality of life in relation to arthritis therapy. Postgrad Med May: 49–56

Fries J F 1998 Quality-of-life considerations with respect to arthritis and nonsteroidal anti-inflammatory drugs. Am J Med 104: 14S–20S; discussion 21S–22S

Harris R E, Beebe-Donk J, Doss H, Burr Doss D 2005 Aspirin, ibuprofen, and other non-steroidal anti-inflammatory drugs in cancer prevention: a critical review of non-selective COX-2 blockade. Oncol Rep 13: 559–583 (*This is an interesting paper that deals with the use of NSAIDs in the treatment of cancer; this is fast emerging as an alternative arena for NSAID therapy*)

Hawkey C J 1999 COX-2 inhibitors. Lancet 353: 307–314 (*Clear, simple description of the structures of COX-1 and COX-2 and the mechanism of action of selective and non-selective inhibitors. Gives details of results with the COX-2-preferential and COX-2-selective inhibitors. Brief coverage of NO-NSAIDs.*)

Hawkey C J 2001 Gastrointestinal toxicity of non-steroid anti-inflammatory drugs. In: Vane J R, Botting R M (eds) Therapeutic roles of selective COX-2 inhibitors. William Harvey Press, London, pp. 355–394 (*Clear, detailed account of the adverse effects of NSAIDs*)

Henry D, Lim L L-Y et al. 1996 Variability in risk of gastrointestinal complications with individual non-steroidal anti-inflammatory drugs: results of a collaborative meta-analysis. Br Med J 312: 1563–1566 (*Substantial analysis of the gastrointestinal effects of non-selective NSAIDs*)

McAdam B F, Catella-Lawson F, Mardini I A et al 1999 Systemic biosynthesis of prostacyclin by cyclooxygenase (COX)-2: the human pharmacology of a selective inhibitor of COX-2. Proc Natl Acad Sci USA 96: 272–277

Melnikova I 2005 Future of COX2 inhibitors. Nat Rev Drug Discov 4: 453–454

Mitchell J A, Warner T D 1999 Cyclo-oxygenase-2: pharmacology, physiology, biochemistry and relevance to NSAID therapy. Br J Pharmacol 128: 1121–1132 (*Lucid review article; covers homeostatic roles of COX-2*)

Ouellet M, Percival M D 2001 Mechanism of acetaminophen inhibition of cyclooxygenase isoforms. Arch Biochem Biophys 387: 273–280

Skjelbred et al. 1984 Post-operative administration of acetaminophen to reduce swelling and other inflammatory events. Curr Ther Res 35: 377–385 (*A study showing that paracetamol can have anti-inflammatory properties under some circumstances*)

Vane J R, Botting R M (eds) 2001 Therapeutic roles of selective COX-2 inhibitors. William Harvey Press, London, p. 584 (*Outstanding multiauthor book covering all aspects of the mechanisms of action, actions, adverse effects and clinical role of COX-2 inhibitors in a range of tissues; excellent coverage*)

Wallace J L 2000 How do NSAIDs cause ulcer disease? Bailliere's Best Pract Res Clin Gastroenterol 14: 147–159

Weir M R, Sperling R S, Reicin A, Gertz B J 2003 Selective COX-2 inhibition and cardiovascular effects: a review of the rofecoxib development program. Am Heart J 146: 591–604 (*Thoughtful review that deals with the problems encountered by the COX-2 inhibitors that culminated in the withdrawal of rofecoxib*)

Whittle B J R 2001 Basis of gastrointestinal toxicity of non-steroid anti-inflammatory drugs. In: Vane J R, Botting R M (eds) Therapeutic roles of selective COX-2 inhibitors. William Harvey Press, London, pp. 329–354 (*Excellent coverage; very good diagrams*)

Wolfe M M 1998 Future trends in the development of safer nonsteroidal anti-inflammatory drugs. Am J Med 105: 44S–52S (*Discusses various trends, emphasising specific COX-2 inhibitors and NO-releasing NSAIDs*)

Wolfe M M, Lichtenstein D R, Singh G 1999 Gastrointestinal toxicity of nonsteroidal antiinflammatory drugs. N Engl J Med 340: 1888–1899 (*Reviews epidemiology of the gastrointestinal complications of NSAIDs, covering the risk factors, the pathogenesis of gastrointestinal tract damage, and treatment; brief discussion of COX-2-selective drugs and NO-NSAIDs*)

Antihistamines

Assanasen P, Naclerio R M 2002 Antiallergic anti-inflammatory effects of H_1-antihistamines in humans. Clin Allergy Immunol 17: 101–139 (*An interesting paper that reviews several alternative mechanisms whereby antihistamines may regulate inflammation*)

Leurs R, Blandina P, Tedford C, Timmerm N H 1998 Therapeutic potential of histamine H_3 receptor agonists and antagonists (*Describes the available H_3 receptor agonists and antagonists, and their effects in a variety of pharmacological models, with discussion of possible therapeutic applications*)

Simons F E R, Simons K J 1994 Drug therapy: the pharmacology and use of H_1-receptor-antagonist drugs. N Engl J Med 23: 1663–1670 (*Effective coverage of the topic*)

Disease-modifying antirheumatic drugs

Alldred A, Emery P 2001 Leflunomide: a novel DMARD for the treatment of rheumatoid arthritis. Expert Opin Pharmacother 2: 125–137 (*Useful review and update of this relatively new DMARD*)

Bondeson J 1997 The mechanisms of action of disease-modifying antirheumatic drugs: a review with emphasis on macrophage signal transduction and the induction of proinflammatory cytokines. Gen Pharmacol 29: 127–150 (*Good detailed review*)

Hochberg M C 1999 Early aggressive DMARD therapy: the key to slowing disease progression in rheumatoid arthritis. Scand J Rheumatol Suppl 112: 3–7 (*Good general review of DMARD therapy and the use of these drugs in treating rheumatoid disease*)

Smolen J S, Kalden J R et al. 1999 Efficacy and safety of leflunomide compared with placebo and sulphasalazine in active rheumatoid arthritis: a double-blind, randomised, multicentre trial. Lancet 353: 259–260 (*Gives details of the results of a clinical trial showing the efficacy of leflunomide*)

Immunosuppressants

Borel J F, Baumann G et al. 1996 In vivo pharmacological effects of ciclosporin and some analogues. Adv Pharmacol 35: 115–246 (*Borel was instrumental in the development of ciclosporin*)

Gummert J F, Ikonen T, Morris R E 1999 Newer immunosuppressive drugs: a review. J Am Soc Nephrol 10: 1366–1380 (*Comprehensive review covering leflunomide, mycophenolate mofetil, sirolimus, tacrolimus and IL-2 receptor antibodies*)

Lipsky J J 1996 Mycophenolate mofetil. Lancet 348: 1357–1359

Mackay I R, Rosen F S 2001 Immunomodulation of autoimmune and inflammatory diseases with intravenous globulin. N Engl J Med 345: 747–755 (*Clear review of mechanisms of action and clinical use of immunoglobulins; simple, clear diagrams*)

Morris R E 1995 Mechanisms of action of new immunosuppressive drugs. Ther Drug Monit 17: 564–569 (*Succinct, edifying review*)

Snyder S H, Sabatini D M 1995 Immunophilins and the nervous system. Nat Med 1: 32–37 (*Good coverage of mechanism of action of ciclosporin and related drugs*)

Monoclonal antibodies and other anticytokine agents

Breedeveld F C 2000 Therapeutic monoclonal antibodies. Lancet 355: 735–740 (*Good review on the clinical potential of monoclonal antibodies*)

Carterton N L 2000 Cytokines in rheumatoid arthritis: trials and tribulations. Mol Med Today 6: 315–323 (*Good review of agents modulating the action of TNF-α and IL-1; simple, clear diagram of cellular action of these cytokines, and summaries of the clinical trials of the agents in tabular form*)

Choy E H S, Panayi G S 2001 Cytokine pathways and joint inflammation in rheumatoid arthritis. N Engl J Med 344: 907–916 (*Clear description of the pathogenesis of rheumatoid arthritis, emphasising the cells and mediators involved in joint damage; excellent diagrams of the interaction of inflammatory cells and of the mechanism of action of anticytokine agents*)

Feldman 2002 Development of anti-TNF therapy for rheumatoid arthritis. Nat Rev Immunol 2: 364–371 (*Excellent review covering the role of cytokines in rheumatoid arthritis, the effects of anti-TNF therapy*)

Kalden J R 2001 How do the biologics fit into the current DMARD armamentarium? J Rheumatol Suppl 62: 27–35 (*Provides a useful perspective on the use of 'biologics' and DMARD therapy*)

Klippel J H K 2000 Biologic therapy for rheumatoid arthritis. N Engl J Med 343: 1640–1641 (*Pithy editorial dealing with the significance of the introduction of the anti-TNF-α agents*)

Maini R N 2005 The 2005 International Symposium on Advances in Targeted Therapies: what have we learned in the 2000s and where are we going? Ann Rheum Dis 64(suppl 4): 106–108 (*An updated review dealing with similar subject matter*)

Maini R N, Taylor P C 2000 Anti-cytokine therapy for rheumatoid arthritis. Annu Rev Med 51: 207–229 (*Detailed review describing the role of cytokines in the pathogenesis of rheumatoid arthritis and the results of clinical trials with anti-TNF and anti-IL-1 therapy*)

O'Dell J R 1999 Anticytokine therapy—a new era in the treatment of rheumatoid arthritis. N Engl J Med 340: 310–312 (*Editorial with excellent coverage of the role of TNF-α in rheumatoid arthritis; summarises the differences between infliximab and etanercept*)

Vincent F, Kirkman R et al. 1998 Interleukin-2-receptor blockade with daclizumab to prevent acute rejection in renal transplantation. N Engl J Med 338: 161–165

New directions

Fiorucci S 2001 NO-releasing NSAIDs are caspase inhibitors. Trends Immunol 22: 232–235 (*Describes* modulation of the immune response by NSAIDs, and the possible mechanism of their action in down-regulating inflammatory cytokines)

Makarov S S 2000 NF-κB as a therapeutic target in chronic inflammation: recent advances. Mol Med Today 6: 441–448 (*This article gives an overview of the NFκB signalling pathway and its role in chronic inflammation, and discusses the feasibility of treatment based on selective suppression of this pathway*)

Ulrich H, von Andrian U H, Englehardt B 2003 α4-Integrins as therapeutic targets in autoimmune disease. N Engl J Med 348: 68–70 (*Editorial commenting on two articles in the journal that describe the use of natalizumab, a recombinant monoclonal antibody, for the treatment of the inflammatory/immune diseases: multiple sclerosis and Crohn's disease. Natalizumab binds to α4-integrins on haemopoietic cells and prevents them from binding to their endothelial receptors.*)

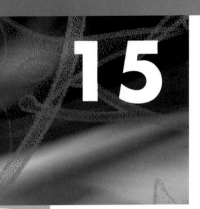

15 Cannabinoids

OVERVIEW

Modern pharmacological interest in cannabinoids dates from the discovery that Δ^9-tetrahydrocannabinol (THC) is the active principle of cannabis, and took off with the discovery of specific cannabinoid receptors—termed CB receptors—and endogenous ligands (*endocannabinoids*), together with mechanisms for their synthesis and elimination. Drugs that act on this endocannabinoid system have considerable therapeutic potential. Here we consider endocannabinoids, cannabinoid receptors, physiological functions, plant-derived cannabinoids, synthetic ligands, pathological mechanisms and potential clinical applications, which are revisited in Ch. 27. More detailed information is given in reviews by DiMarzo et al. (2004), DePetrocellis et al. (2004) and Howlett et al. (2004). The pharmacology of cannabinoids in the central nervous system (CNS) is discussed in Chapters 34, 42 and 43.

ENDOCANNABINOIDS

The discovery of specific cannabinoid receptors led to a search for endogenous mediators. The first success was chalked up by a team that screened fractions of extracted pig brain for ability to displace a radiolabelled cannabinoid receptor ligand (Devane et al., 1992). This led to the purification of N *arachidonylethanolamide*, an *eicosanoid* mediator (see Ch. 13), the structure of which is shown in Figure 15.1. This was christened *anandamide*.[1] Anandamide not only displaced labelled cannabinoid from synaptosomal membranes in the binding assay, but also inhibited electrically evoked twitches of mouse vas deferens, a bioassay for psychotropic cannabinoids (Fig. 15.2). A few years later, a second endocannabinoid, 2-arachidonoyl glycerol (2-AG), was identified, and more recently three further endocannabinoid candidates with distinct CB_1/CB_2 (see below) receptor selectivities have been added to the list (Table 15.1). Endocannabinoids are made 'on demand' like other eicosanoids

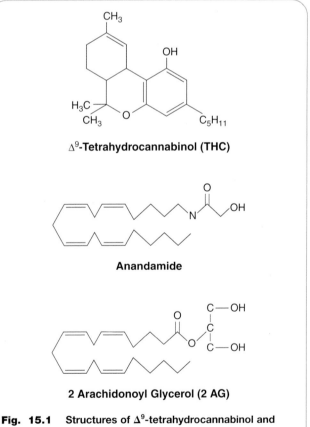

Fig. 15.1   Structures of Δ^9-tetrahydrocannabinol and two endocannabinoids.

---

[1]From a Sanskrit word meaning 'bliss' + amide.

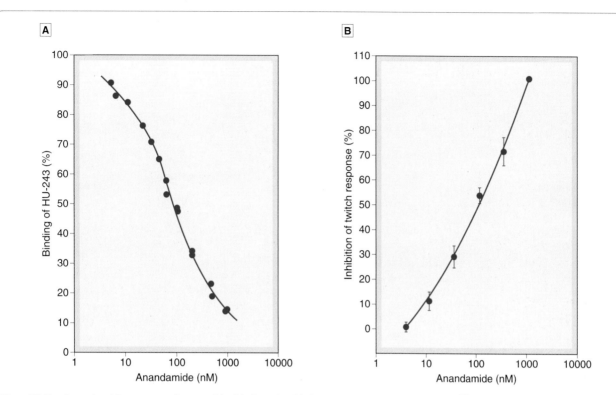

Fig. 15.2 Anandamide as an endocannabinoid. Anandamide is an endogenous cannabinoid. **A** Competitive inhibition of tritiated HU-243 (a cannabinoid receptor ligand) binding to synaptosomal membranes from rat brain by natural anandamide. **B** Inhibition of vas deferens twitch response (a bioassay for cannabinoids) by natural anandamide. Note the similarity between the binding and bioactivity. (Redrawn from Devane et al. 1992.)

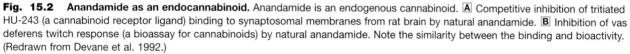

Table 15.1 Definite and possible endocannabinoids

Endocannabinoid	Selectivity
Definite endocannabinoids	
Anandamide	$CB_1 > CB_2$
2-Arachidonoyl glycerol	$CB_1 = CB_2$
Less well-established endocannabinoid candidates	
Virhodamine	$CB_2 > CB_1$
Noladin	$CB_1 \gg CB_2$
N-Arachidonoyl dopamine	$CB_1 \gg CB_2$

(e.g. *prostaglandins* and *leukotrienes*; see Ch. 13), rather than being presynthesised and stored for release when needed.

BIOSYNTHESIS OF ENDOCANNABINOIDS

Biosynthesis of anandamide and of 2-AG is summarised in Figure 15.3.

▼ Anandamide is formed by a distinct phospholipase D (PLD) selective for *N*-acyl-phosphatidylethanolamine (NAPE) but with low affinity for other membrane phospholipids, and known as NAPE-PLD. NAPE-PLD is a zinc metallohydrolase that is stimulated by Ca^{2+} and also by polyamines. Selective inhibitors for NAPE-PLD are being sought. The precursors are produced by an as-yet-uncharacterised but Ca^{2+}-sensitive transacylase that transfers an acyl group from the *sn*-1 position of phospholipids to the nitrogen atom of phosphatidylethanolamine.

2-AG is also produced by hydrolysis of precursors derived from phospholipid metabolism. The key enzymes are two recently cloned *sn*-1-selective diacylglycerol lipases (DAGL-α and DAGL-β), which belong to the family of serine lipases. Both these enzymes, like NAPE-PLD, are Ca^{2+}-sensitive, consistent with intracellular Ca^{2+} acting as the physiological stimulus to endocannabinoid synthesis. The DAGLs are located in axons and presynaptic axon terminals during development, but postsynaptically in dendrites and cell bodies of adult neurons, consistent with a role for 2-AG in neurite growth, and with a role as a retrograde mediator (see below) in adult brain.

Little is known as yet about the biosynthesis of the more recent endocannabinoid candidates noladin, virhodamine and *N*-arachidonoyl dopamine. pH-dependent non-enzymatic interconversion of vihrodamine and anandamide is one possibility, and could result in a switch between CB_2- and CB_1-mediated responses (see Table 15.1).

TERMINATION OF THE ENDOCANNABINOID SIGNAL

Endocannabinoids are rapidly taken up from the extracellular space. Being lipid-soluble, they diffuse through plasma membranes down a concentration gradient. There is also plausible but indirect evidence for a saturable, temperature-dependent, facilitated transport mechanism for anandamide and

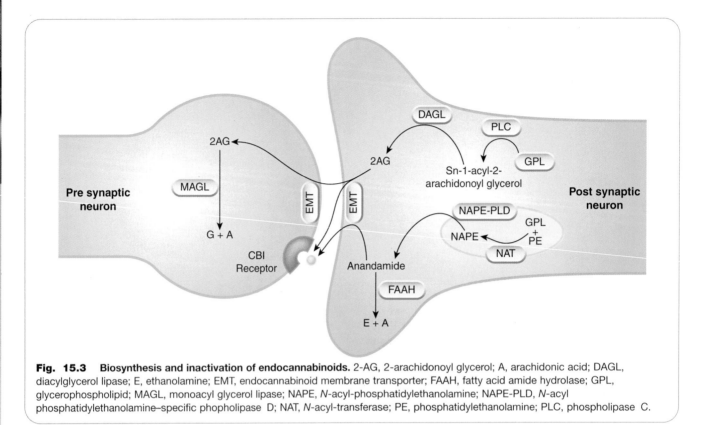

Fig. 15.3 **Biosynthesis and inactivation of endocannabinoids.** 2-AG, 2-arachidonoyl glycerol; A, arachidonic acid; DAGL, diacylglycerol lipase; E, ethanolamine; EMT, endocannabinoid membrane transporter; FAAH, fatty acid amide hydrolase; GPL, glycerophospholipid; MAGL, monoacyl glycerol lipase; NAPE, *N*-acyl-phosphatidylethanolamine; NAPE-PLD, *N*-acyl phosphatidylethanolamine–specific phopholipase D; NAT, *N*-acyl-transferase; PE, phosphatidylethanolamine; PLC, phospholipase C.

2-AG dubbed the 'endocannabinoid membrane transporter'. This has yet to be isolated and cloned, but selective uptake inhibitors (e.g. UCM-707) have been developed. Pathways of endo-cannabinoid metabolism are summarised in Figure 15.3. The key enzyme for anandamide is a microsomal enzyme known as *fatty acid amide hydrolase (FAAH)*. FAAH has been crystallised and is a serine hydrolase. It converts anandamide to arachidonic acid plus ethanolamine and also hydrolyses 2-AG, yielding arachidonic acid and glycerol. Expression of its gene is up-regulated by *leptin* and *progesterone*, and down-regulated by *oestrogen* and *glucocorticoids*.

The phenotype of FAAH 'knockout' mice gives some clues to endocannabinoid physiology; such mice have an increased brain content of anandamide and an increased pain threshold. Selective inhibitors of FAAH have analgesic and anxiolytic properties in mice (see Ch. 37, p. 537, for an explanation of how drugs are tested for anxiolytic properties in rodents). In contrast to anandamide, brain content of 2-AG is not increased in FAAH knockout animals, indicating that another route of metabolism of 2-AG, for example via monoacylglycerol lipase (MAGL), an enzyme that is coexpressed with presynaptic CB$_1$ receptors in the hippocampus, is likely to be important. Other possible routes of metabolism include esterification, acylation and oxidation by cyclo-oxygenase-2 to prostaglandin ethanolamides ('prostamides'), or by 12- or 15-lipoxygenase (see Ch. 13).

CANNABINOID RECEPTORS

Cannabinoids, being highly lipid-soluble, were originally thought to act in a similar way to general anaesthetics. However, in 1988, saturable high-affinity binding of a tritiated cannabinoid was demonstrated in membranes prepared from homogenised rat brain. This led to the identification of specific cannabinoid receptors in brain. These are now termed *CB$_1$ receptors* to distinguish them from the *CB$_2$ receptors* subsequently identified in peripheral tissues. Cannabinoid receptors are typical members of the family of G-protein–coupled receptors (Ch. 3, p. 29). CB$_1$ receptors are linked via G$_{i/o}$ to inhibition of adenylate cyclase and of voltage-operated calcium channels, and to activation of G-protein–sensitive inward-rectifying potassium (GIRK) channels, causing hyperpolarisation (Fig. 15.4). These effects are similar to those mediated by opioid receptors (Ch. 41, p. 598). CB$_1$ receptors are located in the plasma membrane of nerve endings and inhibit transmitter release from presynaptic terminals, which is caused by depolarisation and Ca^{2+} entry (Ch. 4, pp. 67-68). CB receptors also influence gene expression, both directly by activating mitogen-activated protein kinase, and indirectly by reducing the activity of protein kinase A as a result of reduced adenylate cyclase activity (see Ch. 3).

The CB$_1$ receptors are among the most numerous receptors in the brain, their abundance being comparable with receptors for

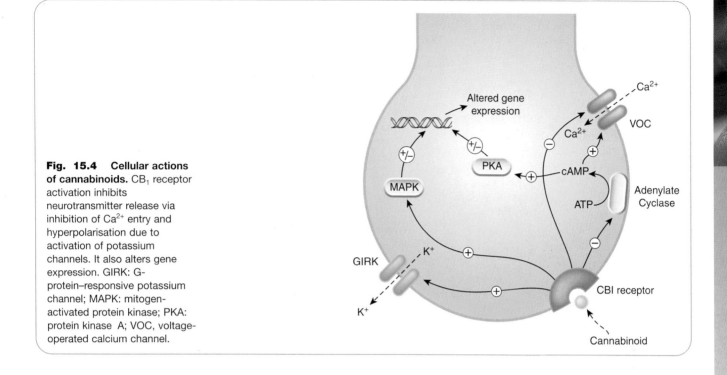

Fig. 15.4 Cellular actions of cannabinoids. CB₁ receptor activation inhibits neurotransmitter release via inhibition of Ca^{2+} entry and hyperpolarisation due to activation of potassium channels. It also alters gene expression. GIRK: G-protein–responsive potassium channel; MAPK: mitogen-activated protein kinase; PKA: protein kinase A; VOC, voltage-operated calcium channel.

glutamate and GABA, the main central excitatory and inhibitory neurotransmitters (Ch. 33). They are not homogeneously distributed, being concentrated in the hippocampus (relevant to effects of cannabinoids on memory), cerebellum (relevant to loss of coordination), hypothalamus (important in control of appetite; see Ch. 27 and below), substantia nigra, mesolimbic dopamine pathways that have been implicated in psychological 'reward' (Ch. 43, p. 621), and in association areas of cerebral cortex. There is a relative paucity of CB₁ receptors in the brain stem, perhaps explaining the lack of serious respiratory or cardiovascular toxicity of the cannabinoids. At a cellular level, CB₁ receptors are localised presynaptically, and inhibit transmitter release as explained above. Like opioids, they can, however, increase the activity of some neuronal pathways by inhibiting inhibitory connections, including GABA-ergic interneurons in the hippocampus and amygdala.

In addition to their well-recognised location in the CNS, CB₁ receptors are also expressed in peripheral tissues, including on endothelial cells and adipocytes. Cannabinoids promote lipogenesis through activation of CB₁ receptors, an action that could contribute to their effect on body weight (Cota et al., 2003).

The peripheral cannabinoid receptor (CB₂ subtype) has only approximately 45% amino acid homology with CB₁ and is located mainly in lymphoid tissue (spleen, tonsils and thymus as well as circulating lymphocytes, monocytes and tissue mast cells). CB₂ receptors are also present on microglia—immune cells in the CNS (Ch. 32, p. 475). The localisation of CB₂ receptors on cells of the immune system was unexpected, but it may account for inhibitory effects of cannabis on immune function. CB₂ receptors differ in their responsiveness to cannabinoid ligands from CB₁ receptors (see Table 15.1). They are linked via $G_{i/o}$ to adenylate cyclase, GIRK channels and mitogen-activated

protein kinase similarly to CB₁, but not to voltage-operated calcium channels (which are not expressed in immune cells). So far, rather little is known about their function. They are present in atherosclerotic lesions (see Ch. 20), and CB₂ agonists have antiatherosclerotic effects (Steffens et al., 2005).

Some endocannabinoids turned out, surprisingly,[2] to activate *vanilloid* receptors, ionotropic receptors that stimulate nociceptive nerve endings (see Ch. 41, p. 593). Other as-yet-unidentified G-protein–coupled receptors are also implicated, because cannabinoids exhibit analgesic actions and activate G-proteins in the brain of CB₁ knockout mice despite the absence of CB₁ receptors.

PHYSIOLOGICAL MECHANISMS

Stimuli that release endocannabinoids, leading to activation of CB₁ receptors and the linkage to downstream events including behavioural or psychological effects, are very incompletely defined. Increased intracellular Ca^{2+} concentration is probably an important cellular trigger because, as mentioned above, Ca^{2+} activates NAPE-PLD and other enzymes involved in endocannabinoid biosynthesis.

Activation of CB receptors is implicated in a phenomenon known as depolarisation-induced suppression of inhibition (DSI). DSI occurs in hippocampal pyramidal cells; when these are depolarised by an excitatory input, this *suppresses* the GABA-

---

[2]Surprising because **capsaicin**, the active principle of chilli peppers, causes intense burning pain, whereas the endocannabinoid anandamide is associated with pleasure, or even bliss ... so perhaps not so surprising after all!

mediated inhibitory input to the pyramidal cells, implying a retrograde flow of information from the depolarised pyramidal cell to inhibitory axons terminating on it. Such a reverse flow of information from post- to presynaptic cell is a feature of other instances of neuronal plasticity, such as 'wind-up' in nociceptive pathways (p. 591, Fig. 41.3) and long-term potentiation in the hippocampus (p. 486, Fig. 33.7), where nitric oxide is implicated as an *excitatory* reverse messenger diffusing from depolarised hippocampal neurons to a glutamate-releasing excitatory axon terminal. DSI is blocked by the CB_1 antagonist **rimonabant**. The presynaptic location of CB_1 receptors and cellular distributions of the DAGL and MAGL enzymes (Fig. 15.3) fit nicely with the idea that the endocannabinoid 2-AG could be a 'retrograde' messenger in DSI (see Fig. 34.9, p. 506).

Neuromodulatory actions of endocannabinoids could influence a wide range of physiological activities, including *nociception*, *cardiovascular*, *respiratory* and *gastrointestinal* function. Hypothalamic hormone interactions could influence *food intake* and *reproductive* function. Effects of endocannabinoids on food intake are of particular interest, because of the importance of obesity (Ch. 27) and the potential of CB receptor antagonists in treating this (see below).

PLANT-DERIVED CANNABINOIDS AND THEIR PHARMACOLOGICAL EFFECTS

Cannabis sativa, the hemp plant, has been used for its psychoactive properties for thousands of years (Ch. 54). Its medicinal use was advocated in antiquity, but serious interest resurfaced only with the identification of THC, see Figure 15.1, as the main psychoactive component in 1964. Cannabis extracts contain numerous related compounds, called cannabinoids, most of which are insoluble in water. The most abundant cannabinoids are THC, its precursor *cannabidiol*, and *cannabinol*, a breakdown product formed spontaneously from THC. Cannabidiol and cannabinol lack the psychoactive properties of THC, but can exhibit anticonvulsant activity and induce hepatic drug metabolism (see Ch. 8, p. 116).

PHARMACOLOGICAL EFFECTS

Δ^9-Tetrahydrocannabinol acts mainly on the CNS, producing a mixture of psychotomimetic and depressant effects, together with various centrally mediated peripheral autonomic effects. The main subjective effects in humans consist of the following:

- Sensations of relaxation and well-being, similar to the effect of ethanol but without the accompanying recklessness and aggression. (Insensitivity to risk is an important feature of alcohol—often a factor in road accidents. Cannabis users are less accident-prone, even though their motor performance is similarly impaired.)
- Feelings of sharpened sensory awareness, with sounds and sights seeming more intense and fantastic.

These effects are similar to, but usually less pronounced than, those produced by psychotomimetic drugs such as **lysergic acid diethylamide** (**LSD**; see Ch. 42). Subjects report that time passes

> ### The endocannabinoid system
>
> - Cannabinoid receptors (CB_1, CB_2) are G-protein–coupled ($G_{i/o}$).
> - Activation of CB_1 inhibits adenylate cyclase and calcium channels, and activates potassium channels, inhibiting synaptic transmission.
> - The peripheral receptor (CB_2) is expressed mainly in cells of the immune system.
> - Selective agonists and antagonists have been developed.
> - Endogenous ligands for CB receptors are known as endocannabinoids. They are eicosanoid mediators (see Ch. 13).
> - The best-established endocannabinoids are *anandamide* and *2-arachidonoyl glycerol* (*2-AG*). They act as 'retrograde' mediators passing information from postsynaptic to presynaptic neurons.
> - The main enzyme that inactivates anandamide is fatty acid amide hydrolase (FAAH).
> - A putative 'endocannabinoid membrane transporter' may transport cannabinoids from postsynaptic neurons, where they are synthesised, to the synaptic cleft, where they access CB_1 receptors, and into presynaptic terminals, where 2-AG is metabolised.
> - FAAH 'knockout' mice have an increased brain content of anandamide and an increased pain threshold; selective inhibitors of FAAH have analgesic and anxiolytic properties, implicating endocannabinoids in nociception and anxiety.
> - **Rimonabant**, an antagonist at CB_1 receptors, causes sustained weight loss and may promote abstinence from tobacco.

extremely slowly. The alarming sensations and paranoid delusions that often occur with LSD are seldom experienced after cannabis. There is, however, evidence that chronic use is associated with an increased incidence of schizophrenia and mood disorder (Henquet et al., 2005).

Central effects that can be directly measured in human and animal studies include:

- impairment of short-term memory and simple learning tasks—subjective feelings of confidence and heightened creativity are not reflected in actual performance
- impairment of motor coordination (e.g. driving performance)
- catalepsy—the retention of fixed unnatural postures
- hypothermia
- analgesia
- antiemetic action
- increased appetite.

The main peripheral effects of cannabis are:

- tachycardia, which can be prevented by drugs that block sympathetic transmission

- vasodilatation, which is particularly marked on the scleral and conjunctival vessels, producing a bloodshot appearance characteristic of cannabis smokers
- reduction of intraocular pressure
- bronchodilatation.

TOLERANCE AND DEPENDENCE

Tolerance to cannabis, and physical dependence, occur only to a minor degree and mainly in heavy users. The abstinence symptoms are similar to those of ethanol or opiate withdrawal, namely nausea, agitation, irritability, confusion, tachycardia and sweating, but are relatively mild and do not result in a compulsive urge to take the drug. Psychological dependence does occur with cannabis, but it is less compelling than with the major drugs of addiction (Ch. 43), and it is arguable whether cannabis should be classified as addictive (see reviews by Abood & Martin, 1992; Maldonado & Rodríguez de Fonseca, 2002).

PHARMACOKINETIC AND ANALYTICAL ASPECTS

The effect of cannabis, taken by smoking, takes about 1 hour to develop fully and lasts for 2–3 hours. A small fraction of THC is converted to *11-hydroxy-THC*, which is more active than THC itself and probably contributes to the pharmacological effect of smoking cannabis, but most is converted to inactive metabolites that are subject to conjugation and enterohepatic recirculation. Being highly lipophilic, THC and its metabolites are sequestered in body fat, and excretion continues for several days after a single dose. Radioimmunoassay of THC is bedevilled by cross-reactivity, and accurate identification and quantification of THC in biological fluids, important for medico-legal reasons, depends on mass spectrometry.

ADVERSE EFFECTS

In overdose, THC is relatively safe, producing drowsiness and confusion but not life-threatening respiratory or cardiovascular depression. In this respect, it is safer than most abused substances, particularly opiates and ethanol. Even in low doses, THC and synthetic derivatives such as **nabilone** (see below) produce euphoria and drowsiness, sometimes accompanied by sensory distortion and hallucinations. These effects, together with legal restrictions on the use of cannabis, have precluded the widespread therapeutic use of cannabinoids.

In rodents, THC produces teratogenic and mutagenic effects, and an increased incidence of chromosome breaks in circulating white cells has been reported in humans. Such breaks are, however, by no means unique to cannabis, and epidemiological studies have not shown an increased risk of fetal malformation or cancer among cannabis users.

SYNTHETIC LIGANDS

Cannabinoid receptor agonists were developed in the 1970s in the hope that they would prove useful non-opioid/non-NSAID

Cannabis

- Main active constituent is Δ^9-tetrahydrocannabinol (THC); a pharmacologically active 11-hydroxy metabolite is also important.
- Actions on the central nervous system include both depressant and psychotomimetic effects.
- Subjective experiences include euphoria and a feeling of relaxation, with sharpened sensory awareness.
- Objective tests show impairment of learning, memory and motor performance, including impaired driving ability.
- THC also shows analgesic and antiemetic activity, as well as causing catalepsy and hypothermia in animal tests.
- Peripheral actions include vasodilatation, reduction of intraocular pressure, and bronchodilatation.
- Cannabinoids are less liable than opiates, nicotine or alcohol to cause dependence but may have long-term psychological effects.

analgesics (cf. Chs 41 and 14, respectively, for limitations of opioids and NSAIDs), but adverse effects, particularly sedation and memory impairment, were problematic. Nevertheless, one such drug, **nabilone**, is sometimes used clinically for nausea and vomiting caused by cytotoxic chemotherapy if this is unresponsive to conventional antiemetics (Ch. 25, pp. 391-392). The cloning of CB_2 receptors, and their absence from healthy brain, led to the synthesis of CB_2-selective agonists in the hope that these would lack the CNS-related adverse effects of plant cannabinoids. Several such drugs are being investigated for possible use in inflammatory and neuropathic pain. See Howlett (2004) for a review of efficacy in CB_1-mediated signal transduction and a discussion of synthetic analogues with a range of agonist selectivities.

The first selective CB_1 receptor antagonist, **rimonabant**, also has *inverse agonist* properties in some systems and shows considerable therapeutic promise (see below). It is in advanced clinical trials for the indications of obesity and tobacco dependence. Synthetic inhibitors of endocannabinoid uptake and/or metabolism (see above) have shown potentially useful effects in animal models of pain, epilepsy, multiple sclerosis, Parkinson's disease, anxiety and diarrhoea.

PATHOLOGICAL INVOLVEMENT

There is evidence, both from experimental animals and from human tissue, that endocannabinoid signalling is abnormal in various neurodegenerative diseases (see Ch. 35). Other diseases where abnormalities of cannabinoid signalling have been reported in human tissue as well as experimental models include *hypotensive shock* (both haemorrhagic and septic; see Ch. 19, pp. 315-316), advanced *cirrhosis* of the liver (where there is evidence that vasodilatation is mediated by endocannabinoids acting on vascular CB_1

receptors—see Batkai et al., 2001), *miscarriage* (see Maccarrone et al., 2000) and *malignant disease* (see Galve-Roperh et al., 2000). It seems likely that in some disorders, endocannabinoid activity is a compensatory mechanism limiting the progression of disease or occurrence of symptoms, whereas in others it may be 'too much of a good thing' and actually contribute to disease progression. Consequently, there may be a place in therapeutics for drugs that potentiate or inhibit the cannabinoid system; see DiMarzo et al. (2004) for a fuller discussion.

CLINICAL APPLICATIONS

Clinical uses of drugs that act on the cannabinoid system remain controversial, but in both the UK and the USA cannabinoids have been used as antiemetics and to encourage weight gain in patients with chronic disease such as HIV-AIDS and malignancy. A substantial randomised controlled trial of THC in patients with multiple sclerosis found no objective evidence of benefit on spasticity but improved mobility (see also Ch. 43, p. 636). Adverse events were generally mild at the doses used—see UK MS Research Group (2003). Other potential clinical uses are given in the clinical box.

The CB_1 receptor antagonist rimonabant, combined with a reduced calorie diet, caused a dose-related weight loss (of approximately one stone at the higher dose) after 12 months' treatment in one placebo-controlled trial (see Fig. 15.5, and see also Ch. 27). Adverse effects at doses used in reported clinical trials have been relatively mild and consist of symptoms such as nausea and diarrhoea, which might be anticipated from

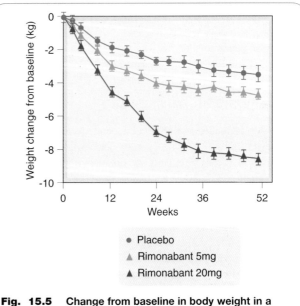

Fig. 15.5 Change from baseline in body weight in a double-blind, placebo-controlled trial of rimonabant versus placebo in 1507 overweight patients. (Redrawn from Van Gaal et al., 2005.)

blocking the actions of a tonically active endocannabinoid system. Long-term psychological effects in clinical trials will be carefully analysed for evidence of anhedonia (i.e. loss of pleasure) and other symptoms of depression or psychological disturbance.

Potential and actual clinical uses of cannabinoid agonists and antagonists

Cannabinoid agonists and antagonists are undergoing evaluation for a wide range of possible indications, including the following.
- Agonists:
  - glaucoma (to reduce pressure in the eye)
  - nausea/vomiting associated with cancer chemotherapy
  - to reduce weight loss in patients with cancer or AIDS
  - neuropathic pain
  - head injury

- Tourette's syndrome (to reduce tics—rapid involuntary movements that are a feature of this disorder)
- Parkinson's disease (to reduce involuntary movements caused as an adverse effect of L-dopa; see Ch. 35, p. 520).
- Antagonists:
  - obesity
  - tobacco dependence
  - drug addiction
  - alcoholism.

REFERENCES AND FURTHER READING

Further reading

DePetrocellis L, Cascio M G, DiMarzo V 2004 The endocannabinoid system: a general view and latest additions. Br J Pharmacol 141: 765–774 (*Reviews the latest 'additions' to the endocannabinoid system, including newer endocannabinoid candidates*)

DiMarzo V, Bifulco M, DePetrocellis L 2004 The endocannabinoid system and its therapeutic exploitation. Nat Rev Drug Discov 3: 771–784 (*Reviews the system, its involvement in pathological conditions and potential for therapeutic drugs*)

Freund T F, Katona I, Piomelli D 2003 Role of endogenous cannabinoids in synaptic signaling. Physiol Rev 83: 1017–1066 (*The fine-grain anatomical distribution of the neuronal cannabinoid receptor CB_1 is described, and possible functions of endocannabinoids as retrograde synaptic signal*) molecules discussed in relation to synaptic plasticity and network activity patterns)

Howlett A C, Breivogel C S, Childers S R et al. 2004 Cannabinoid physiology and pharmacology: 30 years of progress. Neuropharmacology 47(suppl): 345–358 (*Particularly useful account of retrograde signalling and depolarisation-induced suppression of inhibition or excitation*)

Maldonado R, Rodríguez de Fonseca F 2002 Cannabinoid addiction: behavioral models and neural correlates. J Neurosci 22: 3326–3331 (*Deals mainly with animal models and argues that cannabis meets criteria for classification as addictive*)

Wilson R I, Nicoll R A 2002 Endocannabinoid signaling in the brain. Science 296: 678–682

Specific aspects

Abood M E, Martin B R 1992 Neurobiology of marijuana abuse. Trends Pharmacol Sci 13: 201–206 (*There is little evidence that animals will self-administer THC; while marked tolerance develops to marijuana, it has been difficult to demonstrate physical dependence*)

Batkai S et al. 2001 Endocannabinoids acting at vascular CB_1 receptors mediate the vasodilated state in advanced liver cirrhosis. Nat Med 7: 827–832 (*Rats with cirrhosis have low blood pressure, which is elevated by a CB_1 receptor antagonist. Compared with non-cirrhotic controls, in cirrhotic human livers there was a threefold increase in CB_1 receptors on isolated vascular endothelial cells.*)

Cota D et al. 2003 The endogenous cannabinoid system affects energy balance via central orixogenic drive and peripheral lipogenesis. J Clin Invest 112: 423–431 (*Investigation of CB_1 knockout mice, implicating this receptor in regulation of energy homeostasis via both central effect on food intake and on peripheral lipogenesis; see also related commentary by Horvath T L, pp. 323–326 of the same issue, on endocannabinoids and regulation of body fat*)

Devane W A, Hanu L, Breurer A et al. 1992 Isolation and structure of a brain constituent that binds to the cannabinoid receptor. Science 258: 1946–1949 (*Identification of arachidonylethanolamide, extracted from pig brain, both chemically and via a bioassay, as a natural ligand for the cannabinoid receptor; the authors named it* anandamide *after a Sanskrit word meaning 'bliss' + amide*)

Galve-Roperh I, Sánchez C, Cortés M L et al. 2000 Anti-tumoral activity of cannabinoids: involvement of sustained ceramide accumulation and extracellular signal-related kinase activation. Nat Med 6: 313–319 (*Administration of THC into malignant gliomas in rodents induced substantial regression*)

Henquet C, Krabbendam L, Spauwen J et al. 2005 Prospective cohort study of cannabis use, predisposition for psychosis, and psychotic symptoms in young people. Br Med J 330: 11–14 (*Cannabis use moderately increased the risk of psychotic symptoms but had a much stronger effect in young people with evidence of predisposition for psychosis*)

Howlett A C 2004 Efficacy in CB_1 receptor–mediated signal transduction. Br J Pharmacol 142: 1209–1218 (*Review summarising evidence for brain regional differences in CB_1 receptor signal transduction efficacy and agonist selectivity for G-proteins; possible interactions with G_s or G_q—in addition to well-known $G_{i/o}$—are evaluated*)

Karst M, Salim K, Burstein S et al. 2003 Analgesic effect of the synthetic cannabinoid CT-3 on chronic neuropathic pain. A randomized controlled trial. JAMA 290: 1757–1762. (*CT-3, a potent cannabinoid, produces marked antiallodynic and analgesic effects in animals. In a preliminary randomised cross-over study in 21 patients with chronic neuropathic pain, CT-3 was effective in reducing chronic neuropathic pain compared with placebo.*)

Knoller N, Levi L, Shoshan I et al. 2002 Dexanabinol (HU-211) in the treatment of severe closed head injury. Crit Care Med 30: 548–554 (*A randomised, placebo-controlled, phase II clinical trial in 67 patients, injured within 6 hours of treatment. The aim was to investigate safety rather than prove efficacy. Dexanabinol was safe and well tolerated. Actively treated patients had better intracranial pressure/cerebral perfusion pressure control. There was a trend towards improved neurological outcome.*)

Maccarrone M, Valensise H, Bari M et al. 2000 Relation between decreased anandamide hydrolase concentrations in human lymphocytes and miscarriage. Lancet 355: 1326–1329 (*Preliminary study that observed decreased anandamide hydrolase in lymphocytes as an early marker of spontaneous abortion: 'endocannabinoids might be critical in regulating the lymphocyte-dependent cytokine network associated with human fertility and successful pregnancy'*)

Schlicker E, Kathmann M 2001 Modulation of transmitter release via presynaptic cannabinoid receptors. Trends Pharmacol Sci 22: 565–572

(*Reviews effects of cannabinoids in modulating transmitter release in both the central and peripheral nervous systems. Studies using rimonabant or CB_1 receptor-deficient mice suggest that presynaptic cannabinoid receptors are tonically activated by endogenous cannabinoids and/or are constitutively active. 'CB_1-receptor–mediated inhibition of transmitter release might explain ... reinforcing properties and memory impairment caused by cannabinoids.'*)

Steffens S 2005 Low dose oral cannabinoid therapy reduces progression of atherosclerosis in mice. Nature 434: 782–786 (*Oral administration of THC [1 mg/kg per day] resulted in significant inhibition of disease progression in apoE knockout mice. CB_2 receptors were expressed in both human and mouse atherosclerotic plaques. Lymphoid cells isolated from THC-treated mice showed diminished proliferation capacity and decreased interferon secretion. Macrophage chemotaxis, crucial for the development of atherosclerosis, was also inhibited in vitro by THC. All these effects were completely blocked by a specific CB_2 receptor antagonist. Concludes that cannabinoids with activity at the CB_2 receptor may be valuable targets for treating atherosclerosis. See also News and Views, p. 708 of the same issue, for comment by Roth M D.*)

UK MS Research Group 2003 Cannabinoids for treatment of spasticity and other symptoms related to multiple sclerosis (CAMS study): multicentre randomised placebo-controlled trial Lancet 362: 1517–1526 (*Randomised, placebo-controlled trial in 667 patients with stable multiple sclerosis and muscle spasticity. Trial duration was 15 weeks. There was no treatment effect of THC or cannabis extract on the primary outcome of spasticity assessed with a standard rating scale, but there was an improvement in patient-reported spasticity and pain, which might be clinically useful.*)

Van Gaal L F, Rissanen A M, Scheen A J et al. for the RIO-Europe Study Group 2005 Effects of the cannabinoid-1 receptor blocker rimonabant on weight reduction and cardiovascular risk factors in overweight patients: 1-year experience from the RIO-Europe study. Lancet 365: 1389–1397 (*A total of 1507 overweight patients treated with rimonabant 5 or 20 mg or with placebo daily for 1 year in addition to dietary advice: significant dose-related decrease in weight and improvement in cardiovascular risk factors in actively treated patients; adverse effects were mild*)

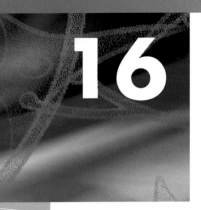

16

Peptides and proteins as mediators

OVERVIEW

Much of today's pharmacology is based on signalling molecules that are of low molecular weight and non-peptide in nature. Since the 1970s, it has emerged that peptides and proteins are at least as important, maybe more so, as signalling molecules. Yet the pharmacological manipulation of peptide signalling is still far less advanced than that of, say, the cholinergic, adrenergic or 5-hydroxytryptamine systems (Chs 10–12). Pharmacology, one could say, has some catching up to do. In this chapter, we give an overview of the main characteristics of peptides and proteins as mediators and as drugs, bringing out the contrasts between these and non-peptides, and we evaluate the present and possible future use of peptides as therapeutic agents. For reviews, with more detail than can be provided here, see Buckel (1996), Cooper et al. (1996), Hökfelt et al. (2000) and Nestler et al. (2001).

HISTORICAL ASPECTS

▼ Despite the fact that some peptide mediators were discovered early in the history of our discipline (e.g. substance P was discovered in the 1930s), pharmacology has historically harboured a strong bias towards non-peptides. One reason for this apparently irrational dislike is that, at one time, most drugs were natural (mainly plant) products. Very few were peptides or acted through what we now recognise as peptide signalling systems. A second reason is that the methodology required to study peptides is of more recent origin. The development of high-performance liquid chromatography and solid-phase peptide synthesis, and the use of antibodies for radioimmunoassay and immunocytochemistry, as well as the the use of molecular biology, have facilitated the development of the area.

In 1953, du Vigneaud made history, and earned a Nobel Prize, by determining the structure and carrying out the synthesis of **oxytocin**, the first peptide mediator to be characterised and the first to be produced commercially for clinical use. The structures of many other mediators, for example substance P, bradykinin and angiotensin, which had been identified as peptides in the 1930s, remained unsolved for many years. While all are small peptides of 11 residues or fewer, determination of their structure, and their total chemical synthesis, was a Herculean effort. The structure of bradykinin was not elucidated until 1960, while that of substance P was published in 1970.

By contrast, the use of contemporary techniques enabled endothelin (a much larger peptide) to be fully characterised, synthesised and cloned within about a year, the complete information being published in a single paper (Yanagisawa et al., 1988). Protein mediators, such as cytokines (Ch. 13) and growth factors (Ch. 22), containing 50 or more residues are still very difficult to synthesise chemically, and major advances must rely largely on molecular biology. The use of recombinant proteins as therapeutic agents—a development driven mainly by the emergent biotechnology industry—is rapidly gaining ground (see Ch. 55). Whereas the discovery of new 'small molecule' mediators has virtually dried up, the discovery of new protein and peptide mediators continues apace. Hökfelt et al. (2000) list 13 neuropeptides that have been discovered since 1990.

GENERAL PRINCIPLES OF PEPTIDE PHARMACOLOGY

STRUCTURE OF PEPTIDES

Peptide and protein mediators vary from 3 to about 200 amino acid residues in size (Fig. 16.1), the arbitrary dividing line between peptides and proteins being about 50 residues. For convenience, in this chapter, we use the term *peptide* to cover both classes. Specific residues in peptides generally undergo post-translational modifications, such as C-terminal *amidation*, *glycosylation*, *acetylation*, *carboxylation*, *sulfation* or *phosphorylation*. They also may contain *intramolecular* disulfide bonds, such that the molecule adopts a partially cyclic conformation, or may comprise two or more separate chains linked by disulfide bonds.

It is difficult to determine the conformation of peptides in solution because they are so flexible, and peptides of less than about 40 residues have proved impossible to crystallise, precluding

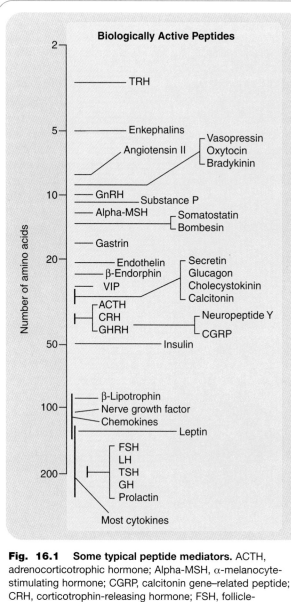

Fig. 16.1 Some typical peptide mediators. ACTH, adrenocorticotrophic hormone; Alpha-MSH, α-melanocyte-stimulating hormone; CGRP, calcitonin gene–related peptide; CRH, corticotrophin-releasing hormone; FSH, follicle-stimulating hormone; GH, growth hormone; GHRH, growth hormone–releasing hormone; GnRH, gonadotrophin-releasing hormone; LH, luteinising hormone; TRH, thyrotrophin-releasing hormone; TSH, thyroid-stimulating hormone; VIP, vasoactive intestinal peptide.

the use of X-ray diffraction methods to study their conformation (although some other techniques, such as nuclear magnetic resonance, have proved helpful). Larger proteins adopt more restricted conformations, but because of their size they generally interact with multiple sites on the receptor. To envisage peptides fitting into a receptor site in a precise 'lock and key' mode is to imagine that you can unlock your front door with a length of cooked spaghetti. Such problems have greatly impeded the rational design of non-peptide analogues (*peptidomimetics*) that mimic the action of peptides at their receptors. The use of random screening methods has (somewhat to the chagrin of the rationalists)

nevertheless led in recent years to the discovery of many non-peptide antagonists—although few agonists—for peptide receptors (see below; Betancur et al., 1997).

TYPES OF PEPTIDE MEDIATOR

Peptide mediators that are secreted by cells and act on surface receptors of the same or other cells can be very broadly divided into four groups:

- *neurotransmitters and neuroendocrine mediators* (discussed further in this chapter)
- *hormones from non-neural sources*: these comprise (a) plasma-derived peptides, notably angiotensin (Ch. 19) and bradykinin (Ch. 13), and (b) substances such as insulin (Ch. 26) endothelin (Ch. 19), atrial natriuretic peptide (Ch. 19) and leptin (Ch. 27)
- *growth factors*: produced by many different cells and tissues that control cell growth and differentiation (see Ch. 22)
- *mediators of the immune system* (cytokines and chemokines; see Ch. 13).

Some important examples of peptide and protein mediators are shown in Figure 16.1.

Role of molecular biology

▼ Because peptide structures are represented directly in the genome, molecular biology has been the key to most of the recent advances in knowledge. It is used in many ways, as in the following examples.

- *Cloning of the genes encoding peptide precursors* has shown how several active peptides can arise from a single precursor protein. Calcitonin gene–related peptide (CGRP) was discovered in this way.
- *Cloning of the genes encoding peptide receptors* has revealed that nearly all belong either to the class of G-protein–coupled receptors or the tyrosine kinase–linked receptors (see Ch. 3). Very few peptides act on ligand-gated channels.
- Several new peptide mediators have been discovered by *screening for ligands of 'orphan receptors'* (see Civelli et al., 2001). Searching in an extract of brain peptides for possible ligands for an opioid receptor–like orphan (called ORL1) led to the identification of the novel neuropeptide *nociceptin* (Meunier et al., 1995). When the gene encoding nociceptin was cloned, it was found also to encode another peptide, *nocistatin*, which had the opposite effects on pain transmission and acted on yet another receptor (see Okuda-Ashitaka & Ito, 2000). The discovery of *orexins* (peptides involved in appetite and obesity; see Ch. 27) arose through similar molecular orienteering.
- The control of precursor synthesis can be studied indirectly by measuring *mRNA*, for which highly sensitive and specific assays have been developed. The technique of *in situ hybridisation* enables the location and abundance of the mRNA to be mapped at microscopic resolution.
- *Transgenic animals* with peptide or receptor genes deleted or overexpressed provide valuable clues to the functions of novel peptides. *Antisense oligonucleotides* (see also Ch. 55, p. 779) can also be used to silence such genes.

PEPTIDES IN THE NERVOUS SYSTEM: COMPARISON WITH CONVENTIONAL TRANSMITTERS

The abundance of neuropeptides in the brain and elsewhere became evident in the 1970–80s, and new examples are still emerging. In most respects, neuropeptide-mediated transmission resembles transmission by 'conventional' non-peptide mediators; the mechanisms for peptide storage and release (summarised in Fig. 16.2), and the receptor mechanisms through which their effects are produced, are essentially the same in both cases. One difference is that the vesicles are loaded with peptide *precursors* in the cell body, the active peptides being generated within the vesicles as they move to the nerve terminals. Following exocytosis, the vesicles cannot be reloaded in situ but must instead be replaced with new preloaded vesicles. Transmitter turnover is therefore less rapid than with conventional mediators, and recapture of the released transmitter does not occur.

As with other chemical mediators, the effects of peptides may be excitatory or inhibitory, pre- or postsynaptic, and exerted over short or long distances from the site of release. There are, however, certain monopolies of function between peptide and non-peptide mediators. For example, peptides do not activate ligand-gated ion channels, and therefore do not function as fast neurotransmitters in the manner of non-peptides such as acetylcholine, glutamate, glycine or GABA (see Chs 10 and 32). Instead, they serve (as do many non-peptides) mainly as neuromodulators, by activating G-protein–coupled receptors. In contrast, the ligands for tyrosine kinase–linked receptors are all peptides or proteins.

In summary, the similarities in function between peptide and non-peptide mediators are more striking than the differences. The main difference stems from the fact that peptides, being gene products, represent variations on a single theme—a linear string of amino acids. Such sequences are much more susceptible to evolutionary change than are the structures of non-peptide mediators, and the number of known peptide mediators now greatly exceeds that of non-peptides. As Iversen pointed out in 1983: 'almost overnight, the number of putative transmitters in the mammalian nervous system has jumped from the ten or so monoamine and amino acid candidates to more than 40'. Since then, no new monoamine transmitters have appeared, but there are at least another 60 peptides.

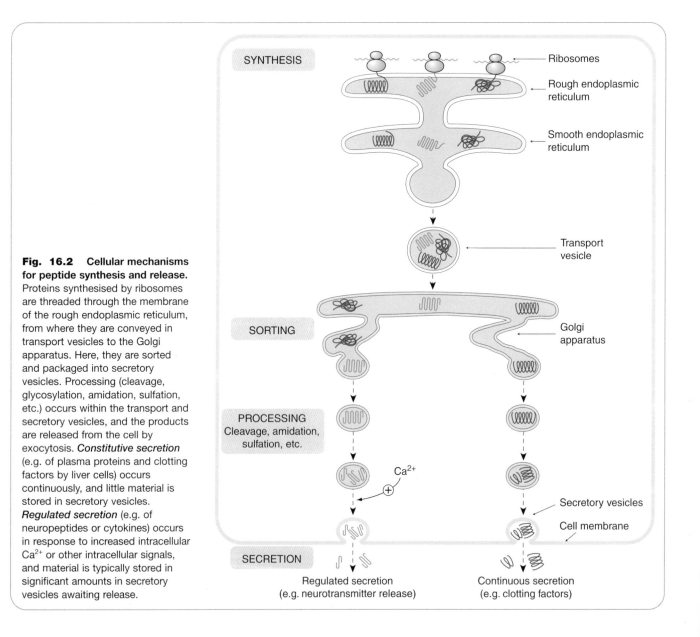

Fig. 16.2 Cellular mechanisms for peptide synthesis and release. Proteins synthesised by ribosomes are threaded through the membrane of the rough endoplasmic reticulum, from where they are conveyed in transport vesicles to the Golgi apparatus. Here, they are sorted and packaged into secretory vesicles. Processing (cleavage, glycosylation, amidation, sulfation, etc.) occurs within the transport and secretory vesicles, and the products are released from the cell by exocytosis. *Constitutive secretion* (e.g. of plasma proteins and clotting factors by liver cells) occurs continuously, and little material is stored in secretory vesicles. *Regulated secretion* (e.g. of neuropeptides or cytokines) occurs in response to increased intracellular Ca^{2+} or other intracellular signals, and material is typically stored in significant amounts in secretory vesicles awaiting release.

The role of peptides as cotransmitters is discussed in Chapter 9. Two well-documented examples (reviewed by Lundberg, 1996) are the parasympathetic nerves innervating the salivary glands (where the secretory response is produced by acetylcholine and the vasodilatation partly by *vasoactive intestinal peptide*) and the sympathetic innervation to many tissues, which releases the vasoconstrictor *neuropeptide Y* in addition to noradrenaline (norepinephrine).

The distinction between neuropeptides and peripherally acting hormones is useful but not absolute. Thus insulin, angiotensin, atrial natriuretic peptide and oxytocin are best known as hormones that are formed, released and act in the periphery. They are, however, also found in the brain, although their role there is uncertain. Similarly, endothelin was first discovered in blood vessels but is now known to occur extensively in the brain as well.

MULTIPLE PHYSIOLOGICAL ROLES OF PEPTIDES

▼ In common with many non-peptide mediators, such as noradrenaline, dopamine, 5-hydroxytryptamine or acetylcholine, the same peptides may function as mediators in several different organs, and intriguingly often appear to subserve some coordinated physiological function. For example, angiotensin acts on the cells of the hypothalamus to release antidiuretic hormone (vasopressin), which in turn causes water retention. Angiotensin also acts elsewhere in the brain to promote drinking behaviour and to increase blood pressure by activation of the sympathetic system; in addition, it releases aldosterone, which causes salt and water retention and acts directly to constrict blood vessels. Each of these effects plays a part in the overall response of the body to water deprivation and reduced circulating volume. There are other examples of what appears to be an orchestrated functional response produced by the various actions of a single mediator, but there are many more examples where the multiple effects seem just to be—multiple effects.

So far, the stream of new information about neuropeptides since the 1970s has led to few useful generalisations about their functional role, and surprisingly few new drugs—with the exception of antihypertensive drugs acting on the renin–angiotensin system (see Ch. 19). For whatever reason, peptide pharmacology has proved to be something of a graveyard for drug discovery projects. For example, substance P antagonists were confidently expected to be effective analgesic drugs based on copious data from animal studies, but proved to have no analgesic activity in humans, although one such drug, **aprepitant**, has been found to have a role in preventing vomiting caused by cisplatin-based cytotoxic chemotherapy (Ch. 51). They also have unexpected anxiolytic properties.

BIOSYNTHESIS AND REGULATION OF PEPTIDES

Peptide structure is, of course, directly coded in the genome, in a manner that the structure of (say) acetylcholine is not, so intracellular manufacture is simpler. Peptide synthesis (Fig. 16.3) begins with the manufacture of a *precursor protein* in which the peptide sequence is embedded, along with specific proteolytic enzymes that excise the active peptide, a process of sculpture rather than synthesis. The precursor protein is packaged into vesicles at the point of synthesis, and the active peptide is formed in situ ready for release (Fig. 16.2). Thus there is no need for specialised biosynthetic pathways, or for uptake or recapturing mechanisms, such as are important for the synthesis and release of non-peptide mediators.

> **Structure and function of peptide mediators**
>
> - Size varies from three to several hundred amino acid residues. Conventionally, molecules of fewer than 50 residues are called peptides, larger molecules being proteins.
> - Neural and endocrine mediators range in size from 3 to over 200 residues. Cytokines, chemokines and growth factors are generally larger than 100 residues.
> - Most known peptide mediators come from the nervous system and endocrine organs. However, some are found in the plasma, and many occur at other sites (e.g. vascular endothelium, heart, cells of the immune system). The same peptide may occur in several places and serve different functions.
> - Small peptides and chemokines act mainly on G-protein–coupled receptors, and act through the same second messenger systems as those used by other mediators. Cytokines and growth factors generally act through tyrosine kinase–linked membrane receptors.
> - Peptides frequently function in the nervous system as cotransmitters with other peptides or with non-peptide transmitters.
> - The number of known peptide mediators now greatly exceeds that of non-peptides.

PEPTIDE PRECURSORS

The precursor protein, or *preprohormone*, usually 100–250 residues in length, consists of an N-terminal *signal sequence* (peptide), followed by a variable stretch of unknown function, and a peptide-containing region in which several copies of active peptide fragments may be contained. Often, several different peptides are found within one precursor, but sometimes there is only one in multiple copies. An extreme example occurs in the invertebrate *Aplysia*, in which the precursor contains 28 copies of the same short peptide. The signal peptide, which is strongly hydrophobic, facilitates insertion of the protein into the endoplasmic reticulum and is then cleaved off at an early stage, yielding the *prohormone*.

The active peptides are usually demarcated within the prohormone sequence by pairs of basic amino acids (Lys-Lys or Lys-Arg), which are cleavage points for the trypsin-like proteases that release the peptides. This *endoproteolytic* cleavage generally occurs in the Golgi apparatus or the secretory vesicles. The enzymes responsible are known as *prohormone convertases*, of which two subtypes (PC1 and PC2) have been studied in detail (see Cullinan et al., 1991). Scrutiny of the prohormone sequence often reveals likely cleavage points that demarcate unknown peptides. In some cases (e.g. CGRP; see below), new peptide mediators have been discovered in this way, but there are many examples where no function has yet been assigned. Whether these peptides are, like strangers at a funeral, waiting to declare their purpose or merely functionless relics, remains a mystery. There are also large

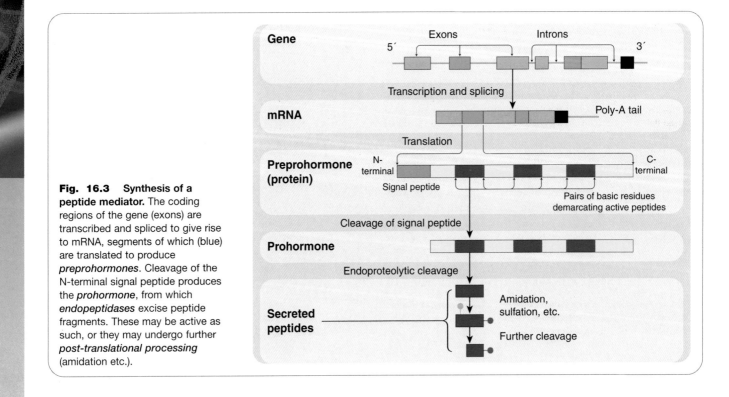

Fig. 16.3 Synthesis of a peptide mediator. The coding regions of the gene (exons) are transcribed and spliced to give rise to mRNA, segments of which (blue) are translated to produce *preprohormones*. Cleavage of the N-terminal signal peptide produces the *prohormone*, from which *endopeptidases* excise peptide fragments. These may be active as such, or they may undergo further *post-translational processing* (amidation etc.).

stretches of the prohormone sequence of unknown function lying between the active peptide fragments.

The abundance of mRNA coding for particular preprohormones, which reflects the level of gene expression, is very sensitive to physiological conditions, and this type of transcriptional control is one of the main mechanisms by which peptide expression and release are regulated over the medium to long term. Inflammation, for example, increases the expression, and hence the release, of various cytokines by immune cells (see Ch. 13). Sensory neurons respond to peripheral inflammation by increased expression of tachykinins, which is important in the genesis of inflammatory pain (see Ch. 41).

DIVERSITY WITHIN PEPTIDE FAMILIES

▼ Peptides commonly occur in families with similar or related sequences and actions. Opioid peptides (see Ch. 41) provide a good example of the representation of such a family at the genomic level. Opioid peptides, defined as peptides with opiate-like pharmacological effects, are coded by

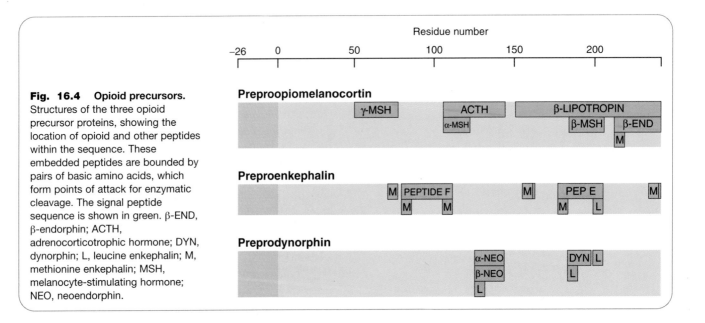

Fig. 16.4 Opioid precursors. Structures of the three opioid precursor proteins, showing the location of opioid and other peptides within the sequence. These embedded peptides are bounded by pairs of basic amino acids, which form points of attack for enzymatic cleavage. The signal peptide sequence is shown in green. β-END, β-endorphin; ACTH, adrenocorticotrophic hormone; DYN, dynorphin; L, leucine enkephalin; M, methionine enkephalin; MSH, melanocyte-stimulating hormone; NEO, neoendorphin.

three distinct genes whose products are, respectively, *prepro-opiomelanocortin* (*POMC*), *preproenkephalin* and *preprodynorphin*. Each of these precursors contains the sequences of a number of opioid peptides (Fig. 16.4). Hughes and Kosterlitz, who discovered the enkephalins in 1975, noticed that the sequence of *met-enkephalin* is contained within that of a pituitary hormone, β-lipotrophin. About this time, three other peptides with morphine-like actions were discovered, α-, β- and γ-endorphin, which also were contained within the β-lipotrophin molecule. It was then found that the enkephalins actually come from the other gene products, *proenkephalin* and *prodynorphin*, POMC itself serving as a source of adrenocorticotrophic hormone (ACTH), melanocyte-stimulating hormones and β-endorphin, but not of enkephalins.

The expression of the precursor proteins varies greatly in different tissues and brain areas. For example, POMC and its peptide products are found mainly in the pituitary and hypothalamus, whereas endorphin, met-enkephalin, leu-enkephalin and dynorphin are more widely distributed. In the spinal cord, dynorphin occurs mainly in interneurons, while the enkephalins are found mainly in long descending pathways from the midbrain to the dorsal horn. Opioid peptides are also produced by many non-neuronal cells, including endocrine and exocrine glands and cells of the immune system, as well as in brain areas distinct from those involved in nociception, and correspondingly they play a regulatory role in many different physiological systems, as reflected in the rather complex pharmacological properties of opiate drugs.

Diversity of members of a peptide family can also arise by *gene splicing* or during *post-translational processing* of the prohormone.

Gene splicing as a source of peptide diversity

▼ Genes contain coding regions (exons) interspersed with non-coding regions (introns), and when the gene is transcribed RNA (hnRNA—*heterologous nuclear RNA*) is spliced to remove the introns and some of the exons, forming the final mRNA that is translated. Control of the splicing process allows a measure of cellular control over the peptides that are produced. Good examples of this are calcitonin/CGRP and substance P/neurokinin A.

The calcitonin gene codes for calcitonin itself (Ch. 31) and also for a completely dissimilar peptide, CGRP. Alternative splicing allows cells to produce either *procalcitonin* (expressed in thyroid cells) or *pro-CGRP* (expressed in many neurons) from the same gene. Substance P and neurokinin A are two closely related tachykinins belonging to the same family, and are encoded on the same gene. Alternative splicing results in the production of two precursor proteins; one of these includes both peptides, the other includes only substance P. The ratio of the two varies widely between tissues, which correspondingly produce either one or both peptides. The control of the splicing process is not well understood.

Post-translational modifications as a source of peptide diversity

▼ Many peptides, such as tachykinins and peptides related to ACTH (see Ch. 28), must undergo enzymatic amidation at the C-terminus to acquire full biological activity. Tissues may also generate peptides of varying length from the same primary sequence by the action of specific peptidases that cut the chain at different points. For example, procholecystokinin (pro-CCK) contains the sequences of at least five CCK-like peptides ranging in length from 4 to 58 amino acid residues, all with the same C-terminal sequence. CCK itself (33 residues) is the main peptide produced by the intestine, whereas the brain produces mainly CCK-8. The opioid precursor, prodynorphin, similarly gives rise to several peptides with a common terminal sequence, the proportions of which vary in different tissues and in different neurons in the brain. In some cases (e.g. the inflammatory mediator bradykinin; Ch. 13), peptide cleavage occurring after release generates a new active peptide (des-Arg⁹-bradykinin), which acts on a different receptor, both peptides contributing differently to the inflammatory response.

PEPTIDE TRAFFICKING AND SECRETION

The basic mechanisms by which peptides are synthesised, packaged into vesicles, processed and secreted are summarised in Figure 16.2 (see review by Perone et al., 1997). Two secretory pathways exist, for *constitutive* and *regulated* secretion, respectively. Constitutively secreted proteins (e.g. plasma proteins, some clotting factors) are not stored in appreciable amounts, and secretion is coupled to synthesis. Regulated secretion is, as with many hormones and transmitters, controlled mainly by intracellular Ca^{2+} (see Ch. 4), and peptides awaiting release are stored in cytoplasmic vesicles. Specific protein–protein interactions appear to be responsible for the sorting of different proteins into different vesicles, and for their selective release. Identification of the specific 'trafficking' proteins involved in particular secretory pathways may yield novel drug targets for the selective control of secretion, but the prospect is still some way off, and conventional receptor–based pharmacology will be the basis for shorter term therapeutic developments.

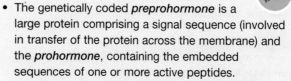

Biosynthesis and release of peptides

- The genetically coded *preprohormone* is a large protein comprising a signal sequence (involved in transfer of the protein across the membrane) and the *prohormone*, containing the embedded sequences of one or more active peptides.
- The active peptides are produced intracellularly by selective enzymic cleavage, centred on pairs of adjacent Arg or Lys residues. In most cases, the active peptides are stored (often in vesicles) in a releasable form.
- A single precursor gene may give rise to several peptides by selective mRNA splicing before translation, by selective cleavage of the prohormone, or by post-translational modification.
- Peptides and proteins are located in intracellular vesicles, which are budded off from the endoplasmic reticulum and Golgi apparatus.
- After sorting and post-translational processing of the peptide products, the vesicles differentiate into secretory vesicles, which discharge their contents by exocytosis.
- With *constitutive release* (e.g. plasma proteins, clotting factors), secretory vesicles are discharged as soon as they are formed, and secretion is continuous. With *regulated release* (neuropeptides and endocrine peptides), exocytosis is controlled by intracellular Ca^{2+}, as with release of conventional transmitters.
- There are many examples of closely related peptides, presumably produced by divergent evolution from a single gene, with different locations and physiological functions.

PEPTIDE ANTAGONISTS

Although selective antagonists are available for the great majority of non-peptide receptors, only a few peptide antagonists are so far in clinical use, although their therapeutic potential is considerable (see Betancur et al., 1997). Substitution into endogenous peptides of unnatural amino acids, such as D-amino acids, sometimes produces excellent antagonists. This strategy was successful in the case of substance P, angiotensin and bradykinin. However, for reasons discussed below, such peptide antagonists are of little use therapeutically, so effort has been channelled instead into discovering non-peptides that bind to peptide receptors. In a few cases, 'peptoids' have been produced by modifying the peptide backbone, while retaining as far as possible the disposition of the side-chain groups that are responsible for binding to the receptor. Such compounds have been developed as antagonists for several peptide receptors (e.g. CCK and neuropeptide Y). In other cases, random screening of large compound libraries has succeeded where rational approaches failed, resulting in highly potent and selective antagonists, some of which are in use, or under development, as therapeutic agents. The most important peptide receptor antagonists in clinical use, all of them non-peptides, are:

- **naloxone**, **naltrexone** (μ-opioid receptors): used to antagonise opiate effects (see Ch. 41)
- **losartan**, **valsartan**, **ibresartan**, etc. (angiotensin AT_1 receptors): used as antihypertensive drugs (see Ch. 19)
- **bosentan** (endothelin ET_1/ET_2 receptors).

Antagonists for many other peptides, including bradykinin, substance P, CGRP, corticotrophin-releasing factor, neuropeptide Y, neurotensin, oxytocin, antidiuretic hormone and somatostatin, have been discovered but, with some notable exceptions (e.g. the oxytocin antagonist **atosiban**; see Ch. 30), have not yet been developed for clinical use. Details can be found in Alexander et al. (2006) and in the review by Betancur et al. (1997).

Few, if any, *agonists* at peptide receptors have been discovered by random screening, and morphine-like compounds are probably the most important clinical examples of non-peptide agonists at peptide receptors. It is becoming increasingly clear, however, that some peptide receptors are 'promiscuous', in that they can bind both peptide and non-peptide ligands. A recent example is that of the FPR family of G-protein–coupled receptors, some of which recognise both the bacterial tripeptide *fMLP* and also the anti-inflammatory lipid *lipoxin A_4*. Binding of the two ligands probably occurs at different receptor domains. Understanding of what makes non-peptides chemically recognisable by peptide receptors remains elusive, much to the frustration of medicinal chemists who would dearly like to be able to design such compounds de novo. There remain many peptide mediators for which no antagonists are known, but strenuous efforts are being made to fill this gap in the hope of developing new therapeutic agents.

Not surprisingly, it has proved easier to find synthetic compounds that block receptors for small peptides (e.g. most neuropeptides), which have only a few points of attachment, than for large peptides and proteins (e.g. cytokines and growth factors), which interact with the receptor at many points. These receptors are not easily fooled by small molecules, and efforts to target them therapeutically rely on protein-based approaches (see below).

PROTEINS AND PEPTIDES AS DRUGS

Many proteins, including antibodies, decoy receptors, cytokines, enzymes and clotting factors, are registered for use as therapeutic agents in specific conditions; they are mainly given by injection but occasionally by other routes (see Table 16.1). Many of the proteins currently in therapeutic use are functional human proteins prepared by recombinant technology, which are used to supplement the action of endogenous mediators. Although their preparation requires advanced technology, such proteins are relatively straightforward to develop as drugs, because they rarely cause toxicity and have a more predictable therapeutic effect than synthetic drugs. 'Designer proteins'—genetically engineered variants of natural proteins—for specific purposes are already a reality. Examples include 'humanised antibodies' and fusion proteins consisting of an antibody (targeted, for example, at a tumour antigen) or a peptide (e.g. bombesin or somatostatin, which bind to receptors on tumour cells) linked to a toxin (such as ricin or diphtheria toxin) to kill the target cells (see Ch. 51). Many ingenious ideas are being explored, and some prophets anticipate the dawn of a new era of therapeutics, as the hegemony of small-molecule therapeutics begins to fade. Pharmacologists, needless to say, are somewhat sceptical, but nobody can afford to ignore the potential of biotechnology-based therapeutics in the future. A full discussion of this exciting area is provided in Chapter 55.

Smaller peptides are used therapeutically mainly when there is simply no viable alternative (e.g. insulin and its designer variants, Ch. 26) but, in general, peptides make bad drugs. There are several reasons for this.

- Most must be administered by injection or nasal spray, because they are poorly absorbed or metabolised in the gut. (An important exception is ciclosporin, discussed in Ch. 14, which contains so many unnatural amino acids that no peptidase will touch it.)
- They are expensive to manufacture.
- They usually have a short biological half-life because of hydrolysis by plasma and tissue peptidases, although there are exceptions to this.
- They do not penetrate the blood–brain barrier.

A list of some important therapeutic proteins and peptides is given in Table 16.1.

CONCLUDING REMARKS

The physiology and pharmacology of peptides—particularly neuropeptides—has stimulated a large amount of research since the early 1980s, and the flow of data continues unabated. With more than a dozen major families of peptides, and a host of minor players, it is beyond the scope of this book to cover them individually or in detail. Instead, we will introduce information on peptide pharmacology wherever it has relevance to the physiology and pharmacology under discussion. Examples are bradykinin (Ch. 13) and monoclonal antibodies (Chs 14 and 55) in inflammation; endothelins and angiotensin in cardiovascular regulation (Ch. 19); tachykinins in asthma (Ch. 23); tachykinins and opioid peptides in nociception (Ch. 41); and leptin, neuropeptide Y and orexins in obesity (Ch. 27). Useful general accounts of peptide pharmacology include Sherman et al. (1989), Hökfelt et al. (1991, 2000), Cooper et al. (1996) and Nestler et al. (2001).

Peptides and proteins as drugs

- Despite the large number of known peptide mediators, only a few peptides, mostly close analogues of endogenous mediators, are currently useful as drugs.
- In most cases, peptides make poor drugs, because:
  - they are poorly absorbed when given orally
  - they have a short duration of action because of rapid degradation in vivo
  - they do not cross the blood–brain barrier
  - they are expensive and difficult to manufacture.
- Peptide antagonists were slow to be discovered, but many are now available for experimental purposes and in development as therapeutic agents.

- Important peptide antagonists used clinically include *naloxone*, *losartan* and *bosentan*.
- Protein-based therapeutic agents are limited in number and include hormones (e.g. *insulin*, *growth hormone*), clotting factors, cytokines, antibodies and enzymes. In many cases, these are produced using recombinant technology.
- 'Designer proteins' prepared by recombinant techniques are expected to play an increasing therapeutic role in the future.

Table 16.1 Some peptide and protein drugs

Drug	Use	Route
Peptides		
Captopril/enalapril (peptide-related)	Hypertension, heart failure (Ch. 19)	Oral
Antidiuretic hormone, desmopressin and lypressin	Diabetes insipidus (Ch. 24)	Intranasal, injection
Oxytocin	Induction of labour (Ch. 30)	Injection
Gonadotrophin-releasing hormone analogues (e.g. buserelin)	Infertility, suppression of ovulation (Ch. 30), prostate and breast tumours	Intranasal, injection
Adrenocorticotrophic hormone	Diagnosis of adrenal insufficiency (Ch. 28)	Injection
Thyroid-stimulating hormone/thyrotrophin-releasing hormone	Diagnosis of thyroid disease (Ch. 29)	Injection
Calcitonin	Paget's disease of bone (Ch. 31)	Intranasal, injection
Insulin	Diabetes (Ch. 26)	Injection
Somatostatin, octreotide	Acromegaly, gastrointestinal tract tumours (Ch. 25)	Intranasal, injection
Growth hormone	Dwarfism (Ch. 28)	Injection
Ciclosporin	Immunosuppression (Ch. 13)	Oral
F(ab) fragment	Digoxin overdose	Injection
Proteins		
Streptokinase, tissue plasminogen activator	Thromboembolism (Ch. 21)	Injection
Asparaginase	Tumour chemotherapy (Ch. 51)	Injection

Table 16.1 (cont'd)   Some peptide and protein drugs

Drug	Use	Route
DNAase	Cystic fibrosis (Ch. 23)	Inhalation
Glucocerebrosidase	Gaucher's disease	Injection
Proteins Interferons	Tumour chemotherapy (Chs 13 and 51), multiple sclerosis (Ch. 35)	Injection
Erythropoietin, granulocyte colony-stimulating factor, etc.	Anaemia (Ch. 22)	Injection
Clotting factors	Clotting disorders (Ch. 21)	Injection
Monoclonal antibodies (e.g. anti–tumour necrosis factor-α)	Inflammatory diseases (Ch. 13)	Injection
Antibodies, vaccines, etc.	Infectious diseases	Injection or oral
Enfurvitide	HIV infection (Ch. 47)	Injection

REFERENCES AND FURTHER READING

Alexander S P, Mathie A, Peters J A (eds) 2006 Guide to receptors and channels, 2nd edn. Br J Pharmacol 147(suppl 3): S1–S168 (*Comprehensive summary of receptors, including peptide receptors, and compounds that act on them*)

Betancur C, Azzi M, Rostene W 1997 Nonpeptide antagonists of neuropeptide receptors. Trends Pharmacol Sci 18: 372–386 (*Describes success in finding non-peptide antagonists—for a long time elusive—and their possible therapeutic uses*)

Bristow A F 1991 The current status of therapeutic peptides and proteins. In: Hider R C, Barlow D (eds) Polypeptide and protein drugs. Ellis Horwood, Chichester (*Review article*)

Bruckdorfer T, Marder O, Albericio F 2004 From production of peptides in milligram amounts for research to multi-tons quantities for drugs of the future. Curr Pharm Biotechnol 5: 29–43 (*Deals with the considerable technical problems in scaling up the synthesis of peptide drugs, and gives the example of enfurvitide, the anti-AIDs drug that was the first peptide to be produced in multiton amounts; it is a remarkable story, even if you are not a chemical engineering geek*)

Buckel P 1996 Recombinant proteins for therapy. Trends Pharmacol Sci 17: 450–456 (*Good account of therapeutic proteins*)

Civelli O, Nothacker H-P, Saito Y et al. 2001 Novel neurotransmitters as natural ligands of orphan

G-protein–coupled receptors. Trends Neurosci 24: 230–237 (*Describes how new peptide mediators have been discovered by screening orphan receptors*)

Cooper J R, Bloom F E, Roth R H 1996 Biochemical basis of neuropharmacology. Oxford University Press, New York (*Excellent standard textbook*)

Cullinan W E, Day N C, Schafer M K et al. 1991 Neuroanatomical and functional studies of peptide precursor–processing enzymes. Enzyme 45: 285–300 (*Review of enzyme mechanisms involved in neuropeptide processing*)

Hökfelt T 1991 Neuropeptides in perspective: the last ten years. Neuron 7: 867–879 (*Excellent overview by a neuropeptide pioneer*)

Hökfelt T, Broberger C, Xu Z-Q D et al. 2000 Neuropeptides—an overview. Neuropharmacology 39: 1337–1356 (*Excellent summary of developments at the millennium*)

Lundberg J M 1996 Pharmacology of co-transmission in the autonomic nervous system: integrative aspects on amines, neuropeptides, adenosine triphosphate, amino acids and nitric oxide. Pharmacol Rev 48: 114–192

Meunier J-C, Mollereau C, Toll L et al. 1995 Isolation and structure of the endogenous agonist of opioid receptor–like ORL1 receptor. Nature 377: 532–535 (*Describes the discovery of an opioid-like peptide ligand for a hitherto 'orphan' receptor*)

Mizejewski G J 2001 Peptides as receptor ligand drugs and their relationship to G-coupled signal transduction. Expert Opin Investig Drugs 10: 1063–1073 (*Useful general review of peptide therapeutics, dealing with many issues including the advantages and disadvantages of peptides as drugs and their potential use in anticancer therapy*)

Nestler E J, Hyman S E, Malenka R C 2001 Molecular neuropharmacology. McGraw-Hill, New York (*Good modern textbook*)

Okuda-Ashitaka E, Ito S 2000 Nocistatin: a novel neuropeptide encoded by the gene for the nociceptin/orphanin FQ precursors. Peptides 21: 1101–1109

Perone M J, Windeatt S, Castro M G 1997 Intracellular trafficking of prohormones and proneuropeptides: cell type–specific sorting and targeting. Exp Physiol 82: 609–628 (*Excellent review of mechanisms by which cells manage to avoid getting their many neuropeptides confused*)

Sherman T G, Akil H, Watson S J 1989 The molecular biology of neuropeptides. Disc Neurosci 6: 1–58 (*General review*)

Yanagisawa M, Kurihara H, Kimura S et al. 1988 A novel potent vasoconstrictor peptide produced by vascular endothelial cells. Nature 332: 411–415 (*The discovery of endothelin—a remarkable tour de force*)

Nitric oxide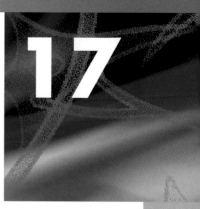

OVERVIEW

Nitric oxide (NO) is a ubiquitous mediator with diverse functions. It is generated from L-arginine by nitric oxide synthase (NOS), an enzyme that occurs in endothelial, neuronal and inducible isoforms. In this chapter, we concentrate on general aspects of NO, especially its biosynthesis, degradation and effects. We touch on recent evidence that it can act as a circulating as well as a local mediator, and conclude with a brief consideration of the therapeutic potential of drugs that act on the L-arginine/NO pathway.

INTRODUCTION

Nitric oxide, a free radical gas, is formed in the atmosphere during lightning storms. Less dramatically, but with far-reaching biological consequences, it is also formed in an enzyme-catalysed reaction between molecular oxygen and L-arginine. The convergence of several lines of research led to the realisation that NO is a key signalling molecule in the cardiovascular and nervous systems, and that it has a role in host defence.

A physiological function of NO was discovered in the vasculature when it was shown that the endothelium-derived relaxing factor described by Furchgott & Zawadzki (1980)

(Fig. 17.1) is NO (Fig. 17.2). NO is the endogenous activator of soluble guanylate cyclase, leading to the formation of cyclic GMP (cGMP), an important 'second messenger' (Ch. 3) in many cells, including nerves, smooth muscle, monocytes and platelets. Nitrogen and oxygen are neighbours in the periodic table, and NO shares several properties with O_2, in particular a high affinity for haem and other iron–sulfur groups. This is important for activation of guanylate cyclase, which contains a haem group, and for the inactivation of NO by haemoglobin (see below).

The role of NO in specific settings is described in other chapters: the endothelium in Chapter 19, the autonomic nervous system in Chapter 9, as a chemical transmitter and mediator of excitotoxicity in the central nervous system (CNS) in Chapters 32–35, and in the innate mediator-derived reactions of acute inflammation and the immune response in Chapter 13. Therapeutic uses of organic nitrates and of nitroprusside (NO donors) are described in Chapters 18 and 19.

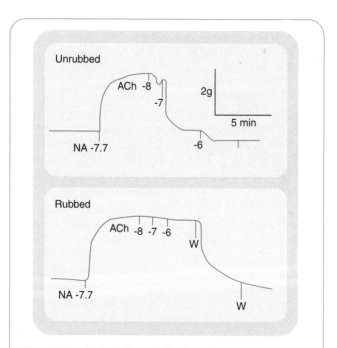

Fig. 17.1 Endothelium-derived relaxing factor.
Acetylcholine (ACh) relaxes a strip of rabbit aorta precontracted with noradrenaline (NA) if the endothelium is intact ('unrubbed': upper panel), but not if it has been removed by gentle rubbing ('rubbed': lower panel). The numbers are logarithms of molar concentrations of drugs. (From Furchgott & Zawadzki, 1980.)

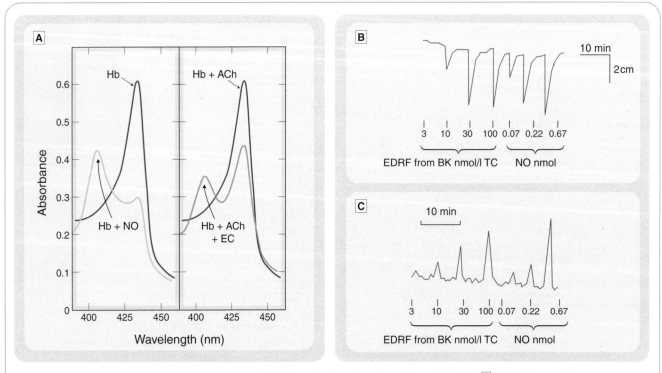

Fig. 17.2 Endothelium-derived relaxing factor (EDRF) is closely related to nitric oxide (NO). A EDRF released from aortic endothelial cells (EC) by acetylcholine (ACh) (right-hand panel) has the same effect on the absorption spectrum of deoxyhaemoglobin (Hb) as does authentic NO (left panel). B EDRF is released from a column of cultured endothelial cells by bradykinin (BK 3–100 nmol) applied through the column of cells (TC) and relaxes a de-endothelialised precontracted bioassay strip, as does authentic NO (upper trace). C A chemical assay of NO based on chemiluminescence shows that similar concentrations of NO are present in the EDRF released from the column of cells as in equiactive authentic NO solutions. (From: A Ignarro et al. 1987 Circ Res 61: 866–879; (B and C) Palmer et al. 1987 Nature 327: 524–526.)

BIOSYNTHESIS OF NITRIC OXIDE AND ITS CONTROL

Nitric oxide synthase enzymes are central to the control of NO biosynthesis. There are three known isoforms: an *inducible* form (iNOS or NOS-II; expressed in macrophages and Kupffer cells, neutrophils, fibroblasts, vascular smooth muscle and endothelial cells in response to pathological stimuli such as invading microorganisms) and two so-called *constitutive* forms, which are present under physiological conditions in endothelium (eNOS or NOS-III) and in neurons (nNOS or NOS-I). eNOS is not restricted to endothelium. It is also present in cardiac myocytes, renal mesangial cells, osteoblasts and osteoclasts, airway epithelium and, in small amounts, platelets. The constitutive enzymes generate small amounts of NO, whereas iNOS produces much greater amounts both because of its high activity and because of the large amounts in which it is present, at least in pathological states associated with cytokine release.[1]

▼ All three NOS isoenzymes are dimers. They are structurally and functionally complex, bearing similarities to the cytochrome P450 enzymes (described in Ch. 8, p. 114) that are so important in drug metabolism. Each isoform contains iron protoporphyrin IX (haem), flavin adenine dinucleotide (FAD), flavin mononucleotide (FMN) and tetrahydrobiopterin (H₄B) as bound prosthetic groups. They also bind l-arginine, reduced nicotinamide adenine dinucleotide phosphate (NADPH) and calcium–calmodulin. These prosthetic groups and ligands control the assembly of the enzyme into the active dimer. Calcium–calmodulin regulates electron transfer within the molecule.

Both nNOS and iNOS are soluble cytosolic enzymes, and eNOS is dually acylated by *N*-myristoylation and cysteine palmitoylation; these post-translational modifications lead to its association with membranes in the Golgi apparatus and in *caveolae*, specialised cholesterol-rich microdomains in the plasma membrane derived from the Golgi apparatus. In the caveolae, eNOS is associated with *caveolin*, a transmembrane protein involved in signal transduction. Association of eNOS with caveolin is reversible, dissociation from caveolin activating the enzyme. Oxidised low-density lipoprotein (oxLDL) displaces eNOS from caveolae by binding to endothelial cell CD36 receptors. This depletes the caveolae of cholesterol, disturbing eNOS function.

▼ The nitrogen atom in NO is derived from the terminal guanidino group of L-arginine. NOS enzymes are functionally 'bimodal', in that they combine oxygenase and reductase activities associated with distinct structural domains. The oxygenase domain contains haem, while the

---

[1]It is possible that some of the NO made in healthy animals under basal conditions is derived from the action of iNOS, just as the inducible form of cyclo-oxygenase is active under basal conditions (Ch. 13)—whether this is because there is some iNOS expressed even when there is no pathology, or because there is always enough 'pathology', for example gut microflora, to induce it, is a moot point.

reductase domain binds calcium–calmodulin, FMN, FAD and NADPH. NOS enzymes are the only flavohaem enzymes that use H_4B as a redox cofactor. The crystal structure of the NOS heme (oxygenase) domain in iNOS and eNOS has revealed how l-arginine, heme and H4B bind in the active site. By analogy with cytochrome P450, it is believed that the flavins accept electrons from NADPH and transfer them to the haem iron, which binds oxygen and catalyses the stepwise oxidation of L-arginine, via a hydroxyl-arginine intermediate, to NO and citrulline. In pathological states, the enzyme can undergo structural change leading to electron transfer between substrates, enzyme cofactors and products becoming 'uncoupled', so that electrons are transferred to molecular oxygen, leading to the synthesis of superoxide anion rather than NO. This is important, as superoxide anion is a reactive oxygen species and reacts with NO to form a toxic product (peroxynitrite anion, see p. 268 below).

L-Arginine is usually present in excess in endothelial cell cytoplasm, so the rate of production of NO is determined by the activity of the enzyme rather than by substrate availability. Nevertheless, very high doses of L-arginine can restore endothelial NO biosynthesis in some pathological states (e.g. hypercholesterolaemia; see below) in which endothelial function is impaired. Possible explanations for this paradox include:

- compartmentation: i.e. existence of a distinct pool of substrate in a cell compartment with access to the synthase enzyme, which can become depleted despite apparently plentiful total cytoplasmic arginine concentrations
- competition with endogenous inhibitors of NOS such as asymmetric dimethylarginine (ADMA; see below), which is elevated in plasma from patients with hypercholesterolaemia
- reassembly/reactivation of enzyme in which transfer of electrons has become uncoupled from L-arginine
- relative depletion of arginine, which can inhibit NOS activity by inhibiting translation of iNOS mRNA.

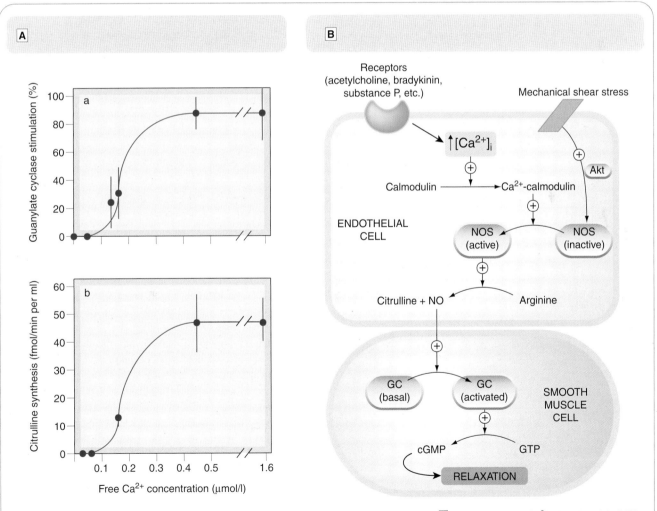

Fig. 17.3 Control of constitutive nitric oxide synthase (NOS) by calcium–calmodulin. Ⓐ Dependence on Ca^{2+} of nitric oxide (NO) and citrulline synthesis from L-arginine by rat brain synaptosomal cytosol. Rates of synthesis of NO from L-arginine were determined by stimulation of guanylate cyclase (GC) (a) or by synthesis of [3H]-citrulline from L-[3H]-arginine (b). Ⓑ Regulation of GC in smooth muscle by NO formed in adjacent endothelium. Akt is a protein kinase that phosphorylates NOS, making it more sensitive to calcium–calmodulin. (From: (A) Knowles R G et al. 1989 Proc Natl Acad Sci USA 86: 5159–5162.)

The activity of constitutive isoforms of NOS is controlled by intracellular calcium–calmodulin (Fig. 17.3). Control is exerted in two ways:

- many endothelium-dependent agonists (e.g. acetylcholine, bradykinin, substance P) increase the cytoplasmic concentration of calcium ions, $[Ca^{2+}]_i$; the consequent increase in calcium–calmodulin activates eNOS or nNOS
- phosphorylation of specific residues on eNOS renders it more or less active at a given concentration of calcium–calmodulin; this can alter NO synthesis in the absence of any change in $[Ca^{2+}]_i$.

The main physiological stimulus controlling endothelial NO synthesis in resistance vessels is probably *shear stress*. This is sensed by endothelial mechanoreceptors and transduced via a serine–threonine protein kinase called *Akt* or *protein kinase B*. Agonists that increase cAMP in endothelial cells (e.g. β_2 agonists) also increase eNOS activity, but via protein kinase A–mediated phosphorylation,[2] whereas protein kinase C *reduces* eNOS activity by phosphorylating residues in the calmodulin-binding domain, thereby reducing the binding of calmodulin. Insulin increases eNOS activity via tyrosine kinase activation (and also increases the expression of nNOS in diabetic mice).

In contrast to constitutive NOS isoforms, the activity of iNOS is independent of $[Ca^{2+}]_i$. Although iNOS contains a binding site for calcium–calmodulin, the very high affinity of this site for its ligand means that iNOS is activated even at the low values of $[Ca^{2+}]_i$ present under resting conditions. The enzyme is induced by bacterial lipopolysaccharide and/or cytokines synthesised in response to lipopolysaccharide, notably interferon-γ, the antiviral effect of which can be explained by this action. Tumour necrosis factor-α and interleukin-1 do not alone induce iNOS, but they each synergise with interferon-γ in this regard (see Ch. 13). Induction of iNOS is inhibited by glucocorticoids and by several cytokines, including transforming growth factor-β. There are important species differences in the inducibility of iNOS, which is less readily induced in human than in mouse cells.

DEGRADATION AND CARRIAGE OF NITRIC OXIDE

Nitric oxide reacts with oxygen to form N_2O_4, which combines with water to produce a mixture of nitric and nitrous acids. Nitrite ions are oxidised to nitrate by oxyhaemoglobin. These reactions are summarised as follow.

$$2NO + O_2 \rightarrow N_2O_4 \qquad (17.1)$$

$$N_2O_4 + H_2O \rightarrow NO_3^- + NO_2^- + 2H^+ \qquad (17.2)$$

$$NO_2^- + HbO \rightarrow NO_3^- + Hb \qquad (17.3)$$

Low concentrations of NO are relatively stable in air because the reaction shown in equation 17.1 is second order. Consequently,

---

[2]The β_2 agonists, which have endothelium-dependent as well as endothelium-independent relaxing effects, work partly in this way.

Nitric oxide: synthesis, inactivation and carriage

- Nitric oxide (NO) is synthesised from L-arginine and molecular O_2 by nitric oxide synthase (NOS).
- NOS exists in three isoforms: inducible, and constitutive endothelial and neuronal forms (respectively iNOS, eNOS and nNOS). NOSs are dimeric flavoproteins, contain tetrahydrobiopterin and have homology with cytochrome P450. The constitutive enzymes are activated by calcium–calmodulin. Sensitivity to calcium–calmodulin is controlled by phosphorylation of specific residues on the enzymes.
- iNOS is induced in macrophages and other cells by interferon-γ.
- nNOS is present in the central nervous system (see Chs 32–35) and in non-noradrenergic non-cholinergic nerves (see Ch. 9).
- eNOS is present in platelets and other cells in addition to endothelium.
- NO is inactivated by combination with the haem of haemoglobin or by oxidation to nitrite and nitrate, which are excreted in urine.
- NO is unstable but can react reversibly with cysteine residues (e.g. in globin or albumin) to form stable nitrosothiols; as a result, red cells can act as an O_2-regulated source of NO. NO released in this way escapes inactivation by haem by being exported via cysteine residues in the anion exchange protein in red cell membranes.

small amounts of NO produced in the lung escape degradation and can be detected in exhaled air. In contrast, NO reacts very rapidly with even low concentrations of superoxide anion (O_2^-) to produce peroxynitrite anion ($ONOO^-$), which is responsible for some of its toxic effects.

Endothelium-derived NO acts locally on underlying vascular smooth muscle or on adherent monocytes or platelets. The potential for action at a distance is neatly demonstrated by *Rhodnius prolixus*, a blood-sucking insect that produces a salivary vasodilator/platelet inhibitor with the properties of a nitro-vasodilator. This consists of a mixture of nitrosylated haemoproteins, which bind NO in the salivary glands of the insect but release it in the tissues of its prey. The consequent vasodilatation and inhibition of platelet activation presumably facilitates extraction of the bug's meal in liquid form. A strong, but still controversial, case has been made that NO can also act at a distance in the mammalian circulation via reversible interactions with haemoglobin. Here we describe this proposal only in broad outline; readers who require a more detailed account are directed to reviews by Singel & Stamler (2005) and, for a sceptical view, Schechter & Gladwyn (2003).

Haem has an affinity for NO > 10 000 times greater than for oxygen. In the absence of oxygen, NO bound to haem is relatively stable, but in the presence of oxygen NO is converted to nitrate and the haem iron oxidised to methaemoglobin. Distinct from this inactivation reaction, a specific cysteine residue in globin combines *reversibly* with NO under physiological conditions. The resulting *S*-nitrosylated haemoglobin is believed to be involved in various NO-related activities, including the control of vascular resistance, blood pressure and respiration. Key features of the proposed mechanism include the following.

- Nitrosylation of haemoglobin is reversible.
- It depends on the state of oxygenation of the haemoglobin, which consequently takes up NO in the lungs and releases it in tissues, in concert with release of oxygen. Haemoglobin acts as an O_2 sensor and could regulate vascular tone (and hence tissue perfusion) in response to the local partial pressure of O_2 by releasing NO in this way. This mechanism is impaired in *sickle cell* disease (a common inherited disorder caused by a molecular variant of haemoglobin).
- NO is not released into the cytoplasm of erythrocytes (where it would promptly be inactivated by haem), but is transported out of the red cells via cysteine residues in the haemoglobin-binding cytoplasmic domain of an anion exchanger called AE1.[3]
- *S*-nitrosylated albumin also constitutes a source of circulating NO bioactivity. An alternative view is that nitrite anion, rather than nitrosylated protein, is the main intravascular NO storage molecule (see Kim-Shapiro et al., 2006).

---

[3]AE1 is responsible for the exchange of chloride and bicarbonate ions across the cell membrane, the 'Hamburger shift' beloved of red cell physiologists. It is the most abundant protein in red cell membranes.

EFFECTS OF NITRIC OXIDE

Nitric oxide reacts with various metals, thiols and oxygen species, thereby modifying proteins, DNA and lipids. One of its most important biochemical effects (see Ch. 3) is activation of *soluble guanylate cyclase*, a heterodimer present as distinct isoenzymes in vascular and nervous tissue. Guanylate cyclase synthesises the second messenger cGMP. NO activates the enzyme by combining with its haem group, and many physiological effects of low concentrations of NO are mediated by cGMP. These effects are prevented by inhibitors of guanylate cyclase (e.g. 1H-[1,2,4]-oxadiazole-[4,3-α]-quinoxalin-1-one, ODQ), which are useful investigational tools. NO activates soluble guanylate cyclase in intact cells (neurons and platelets) extremely rapidly, and activation is followed by desensitisation to a steady-state level. This contrasts with its effect on the isolated enzyme, which is slower but more sustained. Guanylate cyclase contains another regulatory site, which is NO-independent. This is activated by several investigational drugs (e.g. BAY 41-2272 and YC-1) that potentiate NO and have therapeutic promise.

Effects of cGMP are terminated by phosphodiesterase enzymes. **Sildenafil** and **tadalafil** are inhibitors of phosphodiesterase type V that are used to treat erectile dysfunction, because they potentiate NO actions in the corpora cavernosa of the penis by this mechanism (see Ch. 30, p. 458). NO also combines with haem groups in other biologically important proteins (e.g. cytochrome *c* oxidase, where it competes with oxygen, contributing to the control of cellular respiration). Cytotoxic and/or cytoprotective effects of higher concentrations of NO relate to its chemistry as a free radical (see Ch. 35). Some physiological and pathological effects of NO are shown in Table 17.1.

Table 17.1 Postulated roles of endogenous nitric oxide

System	Physiological role	Pathological role	
		Excess production	*Inadequate production or action*
Cardiovascular Endothelium/vascular smooth muscle	Control of blood pressure and regional blood flow	Hypotension (septic shock)	Atherogenesis, thrombosis (e.g. in hypercholesterolaemia, diabetes mellitus)
Platelets	Limitation of adhesion/aggregation	–	–
Host defence Macrophages, neutrophils, leucocytes	Defence against viruses, bacteria, fungi, protozoa, parasites	–	–
Nervous system Central	Neurotransmission, long-term potentiation, plasticity (memory, appetite, nociception)	Excitotoxicity (Ch. 35) (e.g. ischaemic stroke, Huntington's disease, AIDS dementia)	–
Peripheral	Neurotransmission (e.g. gastric emptying, penile erection)	–	Hypertrophic pyloric stenosis, erectile dysfunction

BIOCHEMICAL AND CELLULAR ASPECTS

Pharmacological effects of NO can be studied with NO gas dissolved in deoxygenated salt solution. More conveniently, but less directly, various donors of NO, such as **nitroprusside**, S-*nitrosoacetylpenicillamine* (*SNAP*) or S-*nitrosoglutathione* (*SNOG*) have been used as surrogates. This has pitfalls; for example, ascorbic acid potentiates SNAP but inhibits responses to authentic NO.[4]

Nitric oxide can activate guanylate cyclase in the same cells that produce it, giving rise to *autocrine* effects, for example on the barrier function of the endothelium. NO also diffuses from its site of synthesis and activates guanylate cyclase in neighbouring cells. The resulting increase in cGMP affects protein kinase G, cyclic nucleotide phosphodiesterases, ion channels and possibly other proteins. This inhibits the $[Ca^{2+}]_i$-induced smooth muscle contraction and platelet aggregation that occur in response to agonists. NO also hyperpolarises vascular smooth muscle, as a consequence of potassium channel activation. NO inhibits monocyte adhesion and migration, adhesion and aggregation of platelets, and smooth muscle and fibroblast proliferation. These cellular effects probably underlie the antiatherosclerotic action of NO (see Ch. 20, p. 321).

Large amounts of NO (released following induction of NOS or excessive stimulation of NMDA receptors in the brain; see pp. 510–512) cause cytotoxic effects (either directly or via peroxynitrite anions). These contribute to host defence, but also to the neuronal destruction that occurs when there is overstimulation of NMDA receptors by glutamate (see Chs 33 and 35). Paradoxically, NO is also cytoprotective under some circumstances (see Ch. 35).

VASCULAR EFFECTS (SEE ALSO CH. 19, P. 306)

The endothelial L-arginine/NO pathway is tonically active in resistance vessels, reducing peripheral vascular resistance and hence systemic blood pressure. Mutant mice that lack the gene coding for eNOS are hypertensive, consistent with a role for NO biosynthesis in the physiological control of blood pressure. Increased endothelial NO generation may contribute to the generalised vasodilatation that occurs during pregnancy.

NEURONAL EFFECTS (SEE CH. 9, P. 139, TABLE 9.2 AND FIG. 9.7, AND CH. 34, P. 504)

Nitric oxide is a non-noradrenergic non-cholinergic (NANC) neurotransmitter in many tissues (Ch. 9), and is important in the upper airways, gastrointestinal tract and control of penile erection (Chs 23, 25 and 30). It is implicated in the control of neuronal development and of synaptic plasticity in the CNS (Chs 32 and 34). Mice carrying a mutation disrupting the gene coding nNOS have grossly distended stomachs similar to those seen human hypertrophic pyloric stenosis (a disorder characterised by pyloric hypertrophy causing gastric outflow obstruction, which occurs in approximately 1 in 150 male infants and is corrected surgically). nNOS knockout mice resist stroke damage caused by middle cerebral artery ligation but are aggressive and oversexed (characteristics that may not be unambiguously disadvantageous, at least in the context of natural selection!).

HOST DEFENCE (SEE CH. 13, P. 221)

Cytotoxic and/or cytostatic effects of NO are implicated in primitive non-specific host defence mechanisms against numerous pathogens, including viruses, bacteria, fungi, protozoa and parasites, and against tumour cells. The importance of this is evidenced by the susceptibility to *Leishmania major* (to which wild-type mice are highly resistant) of mice lacking iNOS. Mechanisms whereby NO damages invading pathogens include nitrosylation of nucleic acids and combination with haem-containing enzymes, such as the mitochondrial enzymes involved in cell respiration.

THERAPEUTIC APPROACHES
NITRIC OXIDE

Inhalation of high concentrations of NO (as occurred when cylinders of nitrous oxide, N_2O, for anaesthesia were accidentally contaminated) causes acute pulmonary oedema and methaemoglobinaemia, but concentrations below 50 ppm (parts per million) are not toxic. NO (5–300 ppm) inhibits bronchoconstriction (at least in guinea pigs), but the main action of inhaled NO is pulmonary vasodilatation. Inspired NO acts preferentially on ventilated alveoli, and could therefore be therapeutically useful in *respiratory distress syndrome*. This condition has a high mortality and is caused by diverse insults (e.g. infection). It is

---

Actions of nitric oxide

- Nitric oxide (NO) acts by:
  - combining with haem in guanylate cyclase, activating the enzyme, increasing cGMP and thereby lowering $[Ca^{2+}]_i$
  - combining with haem groups in other proteins (e.g. cytochrome *c* oxidase)
  - combining with superoxide anion to yield the cytotoxic peroxynitrite anion
  - nitrosation of proteins, lipids and nucleic acids.
- Effects of NO include:
  - vasodilatation, inhibition of platelet and monocyte adhesion and aggregation, inhibition of smooth muscle proliferation, protection against atheroma
  - synaptic effects in the peripheral and central nervous system (see Chs 9 and 32–35)
  - host defence and cytotoxic effects on pathogens (see Ch. 13)
  - cytoprotection.

---

[4]Ascorbic acid releases NO from SNAP but accelerates NO degradation in solution, which could explain this divergence.

characterised by intrapulmonary 'shunting' (i.e. pulmonary arterial blood entering the pulmonary vein without passing through capillaries in contact with ventilated alveoli), resulting in arterial hypoxaemia, and by acute pulmonary arterial hypertension. Inhaled NO dilates blood vessels in ventilated alveoli (which are exposed to the inspired gas) and thus reduces shunting. NO is used in intensive care units to reduce pulmonary hypertension and to improve oxygen delivery in patients with respiratory distress syndrome, but it is not known whether this improves long-term survival in these severely ill patients. **Ethyl nitrite** gas has been investigated in newborns (who are at much increased risk of respiratory distress syndrome because of their immature lungs) as a potentially less toxic alternative.

NITRIC OXIDE DONORS

Nitrovasodilators have been used therapeutically for over a century. The common mode of action of these drugs is as a source of NO (Chs 18 and 19). There is interest in the potential for selectivity of nitrovasodilators; for instance, **glyceryl trinitrate** is more potent on vascular smooth muscle than on platelets, whereas *SNOG* selectively inhibits platelet function.

INHIBITION OF NITRIC OXIDE SYNTHESIS

Drugs can inhibit NO synthesis or action by several mechanisms. Arginine analogues compete with arginine for NOS. Several such compounds, for example N^G-monomethyl-L-arginine (L-NMMA) and N^G-nitro-L-arginine methyl ester (L-NAME), have proved of great value as experimental tools. One such compound, *ADMA*, is approximately equipotent with L-NMMA. It is present in human plasma and is excreted in urine. Its plasma concentration correlates with vascular mortality in patients receiving haemodialysis for chronic renal failure, and is increased in people with hypercholesterolaemia (see p. 266, above). In addition to urinary excretion, ADMA is also eliminated by metabolism to citrulline and methylamine by *dimethylarginine dimethylamino hydrolase (DDAH)*, an enzyme that exists in two isoforms, each with a functionally essential reactive cysteine residue in the active site that is subject to control by nitrosylation. Inhibition of DDAH by NO causes feedback inhibition of the L-arginine/NO pathway by allowing cytoplasmic accumulation of ADMA. Conversely, activation of DDAH could potentiate the L-arginine/NO pathway—see Figure 17.4.

Infusion of a low dose of L-NMMA into the brachial artery causes local vasoconstriction (Fig. 17.5), owing to inhibition of the basal production of NO in resistance vessels of the infused arm, without influencing blood pressure or causing other systemic effects, whereas intravenous L-NMMA causes vasoconstriction in renal, mesenteric, cerebral and striated muscle resistance vessels, increases blood pressure and causes reflex bradycardia.

There is therapeutic interest in selective inhibitors of different isoforms of NOS. Drugs for long-term treatment should not inhibit eNOS, to avoid adverse cardiovascular effects. Selective inhibitors of iNOS versus the two constitutive forms have been described (e.g. *N*-iminoethyl-L-lysine), and have potential for the treatment of inflammatory and other conditions in which iNOS

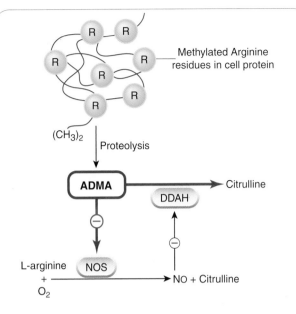

Fig. 17.4 **Effect of asymmetric dimethylarginine (ADMA).** DDAH, dimethylarginine dimethylamino hydrolase; NO, nitric oxide; NOS, nitric oxide synthase.

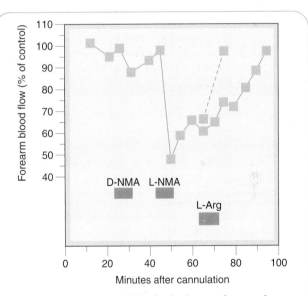

Fig. 17.5 **Basal blood flow in the human forearm is influenced by nitric oxide (NO) biosynthesis.** Forearm blood flow is expressed as a percentage of the flow in the non-cannulated control arm (which does not change). Brachial artery infusion of the D-isomer of the arginine analogue N^G-monomethyl-L-arginine (D-NMA) has no effect, while the L-isomer (L-NMA) causes vasoconstriction. L-Arginine (L-Arg) accelerates recovery from such vasoconstriction (dashed line). (From Vallance et al. 1989 Lancet ii: 997–1000.)

has been implicated (e.g. asthma). 7-Nitroindazole inhibits nNOS and, following intraperitoneal administration to mice, inhibits nociception without altering arterial blood pressure; this selectivity apparently results from an incompletely understood pharmacokinetic effect relating to access of the drug to NOS in brain.

An endogenous protein inhibitor of nNOS (termed *PIN*) works by an entirely different mechanism, namely destabilising the NOS dimer.

POTENTIATION OF NITRIC OXIDE

Several means whereby the L-arginine/NO pathway could be enhanced are under investigation. Some of these rely on existing drugs of proven value in other contexts. The hope (as yet unproven) is that, by potentiating NO, they will prevent atherosclerosis or its thrombotic complications or have other beneficial effects attributed to NO. Possibilities include:

- selective NO donors as 'replacement' therapy (see above)
- dietary supplementation with L-arginine (see above)
- antioxidants (to reduce concentrations of reactive oxygen species and hence stabilise NO; Ch. 20)
- drugs that restore endothelial function in patients with metabolic risk factors for vascular disease (e.g. angiotensin-converting enzyme inhibitors, statins, insulin, oestrogens; Chs 19, 20, 26 and 30)
- β_2-adrenoceptor agonists and related drugs (e.g. **nebivolol**, a β_1-adrenoceptor antagonist that is metabolised to an active metabolite that activates the L-arginine/NO pathway)
- phosphodiesterase type V inhibitors (e.g. **sildenafil**; see above and Ch. 30).

CLINICAL CONDITIONS IN WHICH NITRIC OXIDE MAY PLAY A PART

The wide distribution of NOS enzymes and diverse actions of NO suggest that abnormalities in the L-arginine/NO pathway could be important in disease. Either increased or reduced production could play a part, and hypotheses abound. Evidence is harder to come by but has been sought using various indirect approaches, including:

- analysing nitrate and/or cGMP in urine: these are bedevilled, respectively, by dietary nitrate and by membrane-bound guanylate cyclase (which is stimulated by natriuretic peptides; see Ch. 18)

- a considerable refinement is to administer [^{15}N]-arginine and use mass spectrometry to measure the enrichment of ^{15}N over naturally abundant [^{14}N]-nitrate in urine
- measuring NO in exhaled air
- measuring effects of NOS inhibitors (e.g. L-NMMA)
- comparing responses to endothelium-dependent agonists (e.g. acetylcholine) and endothelium-independent agonists (e.g. nitroprusside)
- measuring responses to increased blood flow ('flow-mediated dilatation'), which are largely mediated by NO
- studying histochemical appearances and pharmacological responses in vitro of tissue obtained at operation (e.g. coronary artery surgery).

All these methods have limitations, and the dust is far from settled. Nevertheless, it seems clear that the L-arginine/NO pathway is indeed a player in the pathogenesis of several important diseases, opening the way to new therapeutic approaches. Some pathological roles of excessive or reduced NO production are summarised in Table 17.1. We touch only briefly on these clinical conditions, and would caution the reader that not all of these exciting possibilities are likely to withstand the test of time!

Sepsis can cause multiple organ failure. Whereas NO benefits host defence by killing invading organisms, excessive NO causes harmful hypotension. Disappointingly, however, L-NMMA worsened survival in one controlled clinical trial. Chronic low-grade endotoxaemia occurs in patients with hepatic cirrhosis. Systemic vasodilatation is typical in such patients. Urinary excretion of cGMP is increased, and vasodilatation may be a consequence of induction of NOS leading to increased NO synthesis. Nitrosative stress and nitration of proteins in airway epithelium may contribute to steroid resistance in asthma, and the ineffectiveness of glucocorticoids in chronic obstructive pulmonary disease (see Ch. 23, pp. 365–366).

Nitric oxide biosynthesis is reduced in patients with *hypercholesterolaemia* and some other disorders that predispose to atheromatous vascular disease, including cigarette smoking and *diabetes mellitus*. In hypercholesterolaemia, evidence of

---

Inhibition of the L-arginine/nitric oxide pathway

- Glucocorticoids inhibit biosynthesis of inducible (but not constitutive) nitric oxide synthase (NOS).
- Synthetic arginine analogues (e.g. L-NMMA, L-NAME; see text) compete with arginine and are useful experimental tools.
- Endogenous NOS inhibitors include ADMA (see text) and PIN (a protein that inhibits NOS dimerisation).
- Isoform-selective inhibitors have therapeutic potential.

Nitric oxide in pathophysiology

- Nitric oxide (NO) is synthesised under physiological and pathological circumstances.
- Either reduced or increased NO production can contribute to disease.
- Underproduction of neuronal NO is reported in babies with hypertrophic pyloric stenosis. Endothelial NO production is reduced in patients with hypercholesterolaemia and some other risk factors for atherosclerosis, and this may contribute to atherogenesis.
- Overproduction of NO may be important in neurodegenerative diseases (see Ch. 35) and in septic shock.

blunted NO release in forearm and coronary vascular beds is supported by evidence that this can be corrected by lowering plasma cholesterol (with a statin; see Ch. 20) or by supplementation with L-arginine.

Endothelial dysfunction in diabetic patients with *erectile dysfunction* occurs in tissue from the corpora cavernosum of the penis, as evidenced by blunted relaxation to acetylcholine despite preserved responses to nitroprusside (Fig. 17.6). Vasoconstrictor responses to intra-arterial L-NMMA are reduced in forearm vasculature of *insulin-dependent diabetics*, especially in patients

with traces of albumin in their urine ('microalbuminuria': early evidence of glomerular endothelial dysfunction), suggesting that basal NO synthesis may be reduced throughout their circulation.

It is thought that failure to increase endogenous NO biosynthesis normally during pregnancy contributes to *eclampsia*. This is a hypertensive disorder that accounts for many maternal deaths and in which the normal vasodilatation seen in healthy pregnancy is lost.

Excessive NMDA receptor activation increases NO synthesis, which contributes to several forms of neurological damage (see Ch. 35). nNOS is absent in pyloric tissue from babies with idiopathic hypertrophic pyloric stenosis.[5]

Established clinical uses of drugs that influence the L-arginine/NO system are summarised in the clinical box.

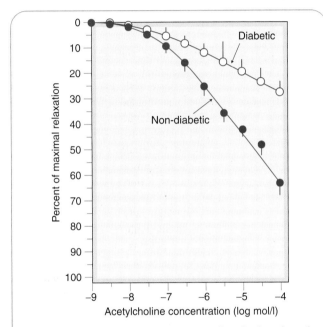

Fig. 17.6 **Impaired endothelium-mediated relaxation of penile smooth muscle from diabetic men with erectile dysfunction.** Mean (± SE) relaxation responses to acetylcholine in corpora cavernosa tissue (obtained at the time of performing surgical implants to treat impotence) from 16 diabetic men and 22 non-diabetic subjects. (Data from Saenz de Tejada et al. 1989 N Engl J Med 320: 1025–1030.)

Nitric oxide in therapeutics

- Nitric oxide (NO) donors (e.g. **nitroprusside** and **organic nitrovasodilators**) are well established (see Ch. 19, clinical box, p. 310).
- Type V phosphodiesterase inhibitors (e.g. **sildenafil**, **tadalafil**) potentiate the action of NO. They are used:
  — to treat *erectile dysfunction* (Ch. 30)
  — other possible uses (e.g. *pulmonary hypertension*, *gastric stasis*) are being investigated.
- Inhaled NO is used in adult and neonatal respiratory distress syndrome.
- Inhibition of NO biosynthesis (e.g. by L-NMMA; see text) is being investigated in disorders where there is overproduction of NO (e.g. inflammation and neurodegenerative disease). Disappointingly, L-NMMA increases mortality in one such condition (sepsis).

---

[5]Are such individuals 'nNOS gene knockout humans'? What of their subsequent development?

REFERENCES AND FURTHER READING

Biochemical aspects

Alderton W K, Cooper C E, Knowles R G 2001 Nitric oxide synthases: structure, function and inhibition. Biochem J 357: 593–615

Bellamy T C, Wood J, Goodwin D A, Garthwaite J 2000 Rapid desensitization of the nitric oxide receptor, soluble guanylyl cyclase, underlies diversity of cellular cGMP responses. Proc Natl Acad Sci USA 97: 2928–2933 (*In its natural environment, soluble guanylate cyclase behaves much more like a neurotransmitter receptor than had been expected from previous enzymological studies; rapid desensitisation is likely to be important under physiological conditions*)

Davis K L, Martin E, Turko I V, Murad F 2001 Novel effects of nitric oxide. Annu Rev Pharmacol Toxicol 41: 203–236 (*Reviews non–cGMP-mediated effects of NO, including modifications of proteins, lipids and nucleic acids*)

Fleming I, Busse R 2003 Molecular mechanisms involved in the regulation of the endothelial nitric oxide synthase. Am J Physiol 284: R1–R12

Fulton D, Fontana J, Sowa G et al. 2002 Localization of endothelial nitric-oxide synthase phosphorylated on serine 1179 and nitric oxide in Golgi and plasma membrane defines the existence of two pools of active enzyme. J Biol Chem 277: 4277–4284 (*Activated, phosphorylated eNOS resides in caveolin-enriched plasmalemma and Golgi membranes; both pools are VEGF-regulated to produce NO*)

Hess D T, Matsumoto A, Kim S O et al. 2005 Protein S-nitrosylation: purview and parameters. Nature Rev Mol Cell Biol 6: 150–166

Jaffrey S R, Snyder S 1996 PIN: an associated protein inhibitor of neuronal nitric oxide synthase. Science 274: 774–777 (*Works by destabilising the nNOS dimer*)

Kim-Shapiro D B, Schechter A N, Gladwin M T 2006 Unraveling the reactions of nitric oxide, nitrite, and

hemoglobin in physiology and therapeutics. Arterioscler Thromb Vasc Biol 26: 697–705 (*Reviews recent evidence that nitrite anion may be the main intravascular NO storage molecule; cf. Singel & Stamler, 2005, below*)

Krumenacker J, Hanafy K A, Murad F 2004 Regulation of nitric oxide and soluble guanylyl cyclase. Brain Res Bull 62: 505–515

Lee J, Ryu H, Ferrante R J et al. 2003 Translational control of inducible nitric oxide synthase expression by arginine can explain the arginine paradox. Proc Natl Acad Sci USA 100: 4843–4848 (*Inhibition of NOS activity by arginine depletion in stimulated astrocyte cultures occurs via inhibition of translation of iNOS mRNA, and provides one explanation for the 'arginine paradox' while indicating a distinct mechanism by which substrate can regulate the activity of its associated enzyme*)

Liu J, Garcia-Cardena G, Sessa W C 1996 Palmitoylation of endothelial nitric oxide synthase is necessary for optimal stimulated release of nitric oxide: implications for caveolae localization. Biochemistry 35: 13277–13281 (*N-Myristoylation of eNOS is necessary for its association and targeting into the Golgi complex, whereas palmitoylation influences its targeting to caveolae*)

Matsubara M, Hayashi N, Jing T, Titani K 2003 Regulation of endothelial nitric oxide synthase by protein kinase C. J Biochem 133: 773–781 (*Protein kinase C inhibits eNOS activity by changing the binding of calmodulin to the enzyme*)

Moore P K, Handy R C L 1997 Selective inhibitors of nitric oxide synthase—is no NOS really good NOS for the nervous system? Trends Pharmacol Sci 18: 204–211 (*Emphasis on compounds with selectivity for the neuronal isoform*)

Pawloski J R, Hess D T, Stamler J S 2001 Export by red cells of nitric oxide bioactivity. Nature 409: 622–626 (*Movement of NO from red blood cells via anion exchange protein AE1; see also editorial by Gross S S, pp. 577–578*)

Ribiero J M C, Hazzard J M H, Nussenzveig R H et al. 1993 Reversible binding of nitric oxide by a salivary haem protein from a blood sucking insect. Science 260: 539–541 (*Action at a distance*)

Russwurm M, Koesling D 2004 Guanylyl cyclase: NO hits its target. Free Radic Enzymol Signal Dis 71: 51–63

Schechter A N, Gladwin M T 2003 Hemoglobin and the paracrine and endocrine functions of nitric oxide. N Engl J Med 348: 1483–1485 (*see also dissenting correspondence in New Engl J Med 394: 402–406*)

Shaul P W 2002 Regulation of endothelial nitric oxide synthase: location, location, location. Annu Rev Physiol 64: 749–774

Singel D J, Stamler J S 2005 Chemical physiology of blood flow regulation by red blood cells: the role of nitric oxide and S-nitrosohemoglobin. Annu Rev Physiol 67: 99–145

Stasch J P, Becker E M, Alonso-Alija C et al. 2001 NO-independent regulatory site on soluble guanylate cyclase. Nature 410: 212–215 (*Reports the discovery of a regulatory site on soluble guanylate cyclase; a pyrazolopyridine, BAY 41-2272, potently stimulates the cyclase through this site by a mechanism that is independent of NO, resulting in antiplatelet activity, hypotension and increased survival in a low-NO rat model of hypertension*)

Stuehr D J, Santolini J, Wang Z Q et al. 2004 Update on mechanism and catalytic regulation in the NO synthases. J Biol Chem 279: 36167–36170

Vallance P, Leiper J 2002 Blocking NO synthesis: how, where and why? Nat Rev Drug Discov 1: 939–950

Xu W M, Charles I G, Moncada S 2005 Nitric oxide: orchestrating hypoxia regulation through mitochondrial respiration and the endoplasmic reticulum stress response. Cell Res 15: 63–65

Physiological aspects

Chiavegatto S, Nelson R J 2003 Interaction of nitric oxide and serotonin in aggressive behavior. Horm Behav 44: 233–241 (*'NO appears to play an important role in normal brain 5-HT function and may have significant implications for the treatment of psychiatric disorders characterised by aggressive and impulsive behaviors.'*)

Esplugues J V 2002 NO as a signalling molecule in the nervous system. Br J Pharmacol 135: 1079–1095

Furchgott R F, Zawadzki J V 1980 The obligatory role of endothelial cells in the relaxation of arterial smooth muscle by acetylcholine. Nature 288: 373–376 (*Classic*)

Huang P L, Huang Z, Mashimo H et al. 1995 Hypertension in mice lacking the gene for endothelial nitric oxide synthase. Nature 377: 239–242 (*Absent EDRF activity in aorta, and hypertension in the mutant mice*)

Nelson R J, Demas G E, Huang P L et al. 1995 Behavioural abnormalities in male mice lacking neuronal nitric oxide synthase. Nature 378: 383–386 (*'A large increase in aggressive behaviour and excess, inappropriate sexual behaviour in nNOS knockout mice'*)

Toda N, Okamura T 2003 The pharmacology of nitric oxide in the peripheral nervous system of blood vessels. Pharmacol Rev 55: 271–324

Vallance P, Leiper J 2004 Cardiovascular biology of the asymmetric dimethylarginine:dimethylarginine dimethylaminohydrolase pathway. Arterioscler Thromb Vasc Biol 24: 1023–1030

Walford G, Loscalzo J 2003 Nitric oxide in vascular biology. J Thromb Haemost 1: 2112–2118 (*Review*)

Pathological aspects

Boger R H, Tsikas D, Bode-Boger S M et al. 2004 Hypercholesterolemia impairs basal nitric oxide synthase turnover rate: a study investigating the conversion of L-[guanidino-^{15}N$_2$]-arginine to N-15-labeled nitrate by gas chromatography-mass spectrometry. Nitric Oxide Biol Chem 11: 1–8 (*The mechanism of impaired NOS activity in hypercholesterolaemia most likely involves inhibition of NOS by ADMA*)

Karupiah G, Xie Q, Buller M L et al. 1993 Inhibition of viral replication by interferon-induced nitric oxide synthase. Science 261: 1445–1448

Ricciardolo F L M, Sterk P J, Gaston B et al. 2004 Nitric oxide in health and disease of the respiratory system. Physiol Rev 84: 731–765

Shaul P W 2003 Endothelial nitric oxide synthase, caveolae and the development of atherosclerosis. J Physiol (Lond) 547: 21–33 (*oxLDL displaces eNOS from caveolae by binding to endothelial cell CD36 receptors and by depleting caveolae cholesterol content, resulting in the disruption of eNOS activation; the adverse effects of oxLDL are prevented by high-density lipoprotein and could be involved in early phases of atherogenesis*)

Vanderwinden J-M, Mailleux P, Schiffmann S N et al. 1992 Nitric oxide synthase activity in infantile hypertrophic pyloric stenosis. N Engl J Med 327: 511–515

Watkins C C, Sawa A, Jaffrey S et al. 2000 Insulin restores neuronal nitric oxide synthase expression and function that is lost in diabetic gastropathy. J Clin Invest 106: 373–384 (*Diabetic mice manifest pronounced reduction in pyloric nNOS. The decline of nNOS does not result from loss of myenteric neurons.*

nNOS expression and pyloric function are restored to normal levels by insulin treatment. Delayed gastric emptying can be reversed with a phosphodiesterase inhibitor, sildenafil, in diabetic mice.*)

Wei X-Q, Charles I G, Smith A et al. 1995 Altered immune responses in mice lacking inducible nitric oxide synthase. Nature 375: 408–411 (*Homozygotes lacking iNOS were uniformly susceptible to infection by Leishmania major*)

Zoccali C et al. 2001 Plasma concentration of asymmetrical dimethylarginine and mortality in patients with end-stage renal disease: a prospective study. Lancet 358: 2113–2117 (*Accumulation of ADMA appears to be an important risk factor for cardiovascular disease in chronic renal failure*)

Clinical aspects

Broeders M A W, Doevendans P A, Bekkers B C A M et al. 2000 Nebivolol: a third generation β-blocker that augments vascular nitric oxide release by endothelial β$_2$-adrenergic receptor–mediated nitric oxide production. Circulation 102: 677–684 (*This highly β$_1$-selective antagonist causes vasodilation through β$_2$-adrenergic receptor–mediated stimulation of the L-arginine/NO pathway*)

Griffiths M J D, Evans T W 2005 Drug therapy: inhaled nitric oxide therapy in adults. N Engl J Med 353: 2683–2695 (*Concludes that, on the available evidence, inhaled NO is not effective in patients with acute lung injury, but that it may be useful as a short-term measure in acute hypoxia ± pulmonary hypertension*)

Kharitonov S A, Barnes P J 2003 Nitric oxide, nitrotyrosine, and nitric oxide modulators in asthma and chronic obstructive pulmonary disease. Curr Allergy Asthma Rep 3: 121–129

Malmstrom R E, Tornberg D C, Settergren G et al. 2003 Endogenous nitric oxide release by vasoactive drugs monitored in exhaled air. Am J Respir Crit Care Med 168: 114–120 (*In humans, acetylcholine evokes a dose-dependent increase of NO in exhaled air; NO release by vasoactive agonists can be measured online in the exhaled air of pigs and humans*)

Moya M P, Gow A J, Califf R M et al. 2002 Inhaled ethyl nitrite gas for persistent pulmonary hypertension of the newborn. Lancet 360: 141–143 (*'Ethyl nitrite can improve oxygenation and systemic haemodynamics in neonates, and seems to reduce rebound hypoxaemia and production of toxic byproducts.'*)

Pawloski J R, Hess D T, Stamler J S 2005 Impaired vasodilation by red blood cells in sickle cell disease. Proc Natl Acad Sci USA 102: 2531–2536 (*Sickle red cells are deficient in membrane S-nitrosothiol and impaired in their ability to mediate hypoxic vasodilation; the magnitudes of these impairments correlate with the clinical severity of disease*)

Steudel W, Kirmse M, Weimann J et al. 2000 Exhaled nitric oxide production by nitric oxide synthase-deficient mice. Am J Respir Crit Care Med 162: 1262–1267 (*iNOS-deficient mice exhale NO at a similar rate to wild-type animals, but eNOS- and nNOS-deficient animals both exhale more rather than less NO than the wild types; iNOS apparently contributes importantly to exhaled NO exhalation in healthy mice*)

DRUGS AFFECTING MAJOR ORGAN SYSTEMS

The heart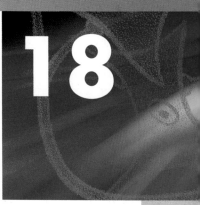

OVERVIEW

In this chapter, we review briefly the physiology of cardiac function in terms of electrophysiology, of contraction, of oxygen consumption and coronary blood flow, and of autonomic control. This provides a basis for understanding effects of drugs on the heart and their place in treating cardiac disease. The main drugs considered are antidysrhythmic drugs, drugs that increase the force of contraction of the heart (especially digoxin), and antianginal drugs. The commonest forms of heart disease are caused by atheroma in the coronary arteries, and thrombosis on ruptured atheromatous plaques; drugs to treat and prevent these are considered in Chapters 20 and 21. Heart failure is mainly treated indirectly by drugs that work on vascular smooth muscle, discussed in Chapter 19, by diuretics (Ch. 24) and β-adrenoceptor antagonists (Ch. 11).

INTRODUCTION

In this chapter, we consider effects of drugs on the heart under three main headings:

- rate and rhythm
- myocardial contraction
- metabolism and blood flow.

The effects of drugs on these aspects of cardiac function are not, of course, independent of each other. For example, if a drug affects the electrical properties of the myocardial cell membrane, it is likely to influence both cardiac rhythm and myocardial contraction. Similarly, a drug that affects contraction will inevitably alter metabolism and blood flow as well. Nevertheless, from a therapeutic point of view, these three classes of effect represent distinct clinical objectives in relation to the treatment, respectively, of cardiac dysrhythmias, cardiac failure and coronary insufficiency (as occurs during angina pectoris or myocardial infarction).

PHYSIOLOGY OF CARDIAC FUNCTION
CARDIAC RATE AND RHYTHM

The chambers of the heart normally contract in a coordinated manner, pumping blood efficiently by a route determined by the valves. Coordination of contraction is achieved by a specialised conducting system. Physiological sinus rhythm is characterised by impulses arising in the sinoatrial (SA) node and conducted in sequence through the atria, the atrioventricular (AV) node, bundle of His, Purkinje fibres and ventricles. Cardiac cells owe their electrical excitability to voltage-sensitive plasma membrane channels selective for various ions, including Na^+, K^+ and Ca^{2+}, the structure and function of which are described in Chapter 4. Electrophysiological features of cardiac muscle that distinguish it from other excitable tissues include:

- pacemaker activity
- absence of fast Na^+ current in SA and AV nodes, where slow inward Ca^{2+} current initiates action potentials
- long action potential ('plateau') and refractory period
- influx of Ca^{2+} during the plateau.

Thus several of the special features of cardiac rhythm relate to Ca^{2+} currents. The heart contains *intracellular* calcium channels (i.e. the large ryanodine receptors and smaller inositol trisphosphate–activated calcium channels described in Chapter 4 and important in myocardial contraction) and *voltage-dependent* calcium channels in the plasma membrane, which are important in controlling cardiac rate and rhythm. The main type of voltage-dependent calcium channel in adult working myocardium is the

L-type channel, which is also important in vascular smooth muscle; L-type channels are important in specialised conducting regions as well as in working myocardium.

The action potential of an idealised cardiac muscle cell is shown in Figure 18.1A and is divided into five phases: 0 (fast depolarisation), 1 (partial repolarisation), 2 (plateau), 3 (repolarisation) and 4 (pacemaker).

▼ Ionic mechanisms underlying these phases can be summarised as follows.

Phase 0, rapid depolarisation, occurs when the membrane potential reaches a critical firing threshold (about -60 mV), at which the inward current of Na^+ flowing through the voltage-dependent sodium channels becomes large enough to produce a regenerative ('all or nothing') depolarisation. This mechanism is the same as that responsible for action potential generation in neurons (see Ch. 4). Activation of sodium channels by membrane depolarisation is transient, and if the membrane remains depolarised for more than a few milliseconds, they close again (inactivation). They are therefore closed during the plateau of the action potential and remain unavailable for the initiation of another action potential until the membrane repolarises.

Phase 1, partial repolarisation, occurs as the Na^+ current is inactivated. There may also be a transient voltage-sensitive outward current.

Phase 2, the *plateau*, results from an inward Ca^{2+} current. Calcium channels show a pattern of voltage-sensitive activation and inactivation qualitatively similar to sodium channels, but with a much slower time course. The plateau is assisted by a special property of the cardiac muscle membrane known as inward-going rectification, which means that the K^+ conductance falls to a low level when the membrane is depolarised. Because of this, there is little tendency for outward K^+ current to restore the resting membrane potential during the plateau, so a relatively small inward Ca^{2+} current suffices to maintain the plateau.

Phase 3, repolarisation, occurs as the Ca^{2+} current inactivates and a delayed outwardly rectifying K^+ current (analogous to but much slower than the K^+ current that causes repolarisation in nerve fibres; Ch. 4) activates, causing outward K^+ current. This is augmented by another K^+ current, which is activated by high intracellular Ca^{2+} concentrations, $[Ca^{2+}]_i$, during the plateau, and sometimes also by other K^+ currents, including one through channels activated by acetylcholine (see below) and another that is activated by arachidonic acid, which is liberated under pathological conditions such as myocardial infarction.

Phase 4, the *pacemaker potential*, is a gradual depolarisation during diastole. Pacemaker activity is normally found only in nodal and conducting tissue. The pacemaker potential is caused by a combination of increasing inward currents and declining outward currents during diastole. It is usually most rapid in cells of the SA node, which therefore acts as pacemaker for the whole heart. Cells in the SA node have a greater background conductance to Na^+ than do atrial or ventricular myocytes, leading to a greater background inward current. In addition, inactivation of voltage-dependent calcium channels wears off during diastole, resulting in increasing inward Ca^{2+} current during late diastole. Activation of T-type calcium channels during late diastole contributes to pacemaker activity in the SA node. The negative membrane potential early in diastole activates a cation channel that is permeable to Na^+ and K^+, giving rise to another inward current, called I_f.[1] An inhibitor of this current, **ivabradine**, slows the heart and is used therapeutically (see below, p. 292).

Several voltage- and time-dependent outward currents play a part as well: delayed rectifier K^+ current (I_K), which is activated during the action potential, is turned off by the negative membrane potential early in diastole. Current from the electrogenic Na^+/K^+ pump also contributes to the outward current during the pacemaker potential.

Figure 18.1B shows the action potential configuration in different parts of the heart. Phase 0 is absent in the nodal regions, where the conduction velocity is correspondingly slow (~ 5 cm/s) compared with other regions such as the Purkinje fibres (conduction velocity ~ 200 cm/s), which propagate the action potential rapidly to the ventricles. Regions that lack a fast inward current have a much longer refractory period than fast-conducting regions. This is because recovery of the slow inward current following its inactivation during the action potential takes a considerable time (a few hundred milliseconds), and the refractory period outlasts the action potential. With fast-conducting fibres, recovery from inactivation of the Na^+ current is quick, and the cell becomes excitable again as soon as it is repolarised.

The orderly pattern of sinus rhythm can become disrupted either by heart disease or by the action of drugs or circulating hormones, and an important therapeutic use of drugs is to restore a normal cardiac rhythm where it has become disturbed. The commonest cause of cardiac dysrhythmia is ischaemic heart disease, and many deaths following myocardial infarction result from ventricular fibrillation rather than directly from contractile failure. For a more detailed coverage, 'from cell to bedside', readers are referred to an authoritative textbook such as that of Zipes & Jalife (2004).

DISTURBANCES OF CARDIAC RHYTHM

Clinically, dysrhythmias are classified according to:

- the site of origin of the abnormality—atrial, junctional or ventricular
- whether the rate is increased (tachycardia) or decreased (bradycardia).

They may cause palpitations (awareness of the heartbeat) or symptoms from cerebral hypoperfusion (feeling faint or losing consciousness). Their diagnosis depends on the surface electrocardiogram (ECG), and details are beyond the scope of this book—see Braunwald & Opie (2001). The commonest types of tachyarrhythmia are atrial fibrillation, where the heartbeat is completely irregular, and supraventricular tachycardia (SVT), where the heartbeat is rapid but regular. Occasional ectopic beats (ventricular as well as supraventricular) are common. Sustained ventricular tachyarrhythmias are much less common but much more serious; they include ventricular tachycardia and ventricular fibrillation, where the electrical activity in the ventricles is completely chaotic and cardiac output ceases. Bradyarrhythmias include various kinds of heart block (e.g. at the AV or SA node) and complete cessation of electrical activity ('asystolic arrest'). It is often unclear which of the various mechanisms discussed below are responsible. These cellular mechanisms nevertheless provide a useful starting point for understanding how antidysrhythmic drugs work. Four basic phenomena underlie disturbances of cardiac rhythm:

---

[1] 'f' for 'funny', because it is unusual for cation channels to be activated by hyperpolarisation; electrophysiologists are renowned for a peculiar sense of humour!

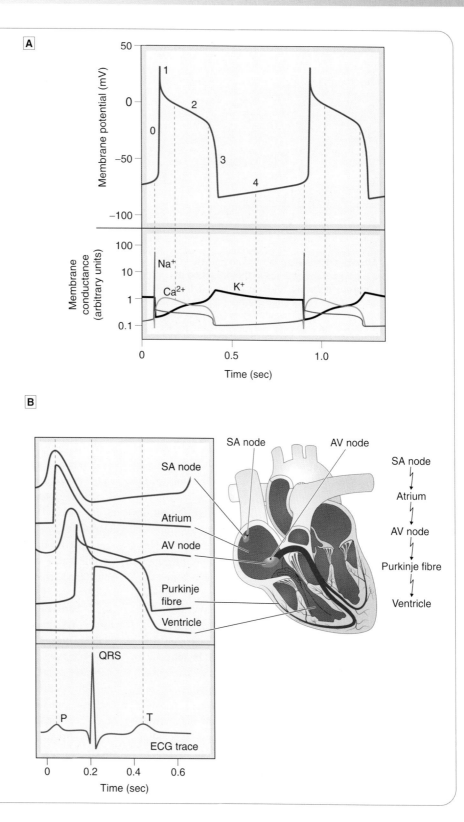

Fig. 18.1 The cardiac action potential. A Phases of the action potential: 0, rapid depolarisation; 1, partial repolarisation; 2, plateau; 3, repolarisation; 4, pacemaker depolarisation. The lower panel shows the accompanying changes in membrane conductance for Na⁺, K⁺ and Ca²⁺. B Conduction of the impulse through the heart, with the corresponding electrocardiogram (ECG) trace. Note that the longest delay occurs at the atrioventricular (AV) node, where the action potential has a characteristically slow waveform. SA, sinoatrial. (Adapted from: (A) Noble D 1975 The initiation of the heartbeat. Oxford University Press, Oxford.)

- delayed after-depolarisation
- re-entry
- ectopic pacemaker activity
- heart block.

The main cause of *delayed after-depolarisation* is abnormally raised $[Ca^{2+}]_i$, which triggers inward current and hence a train of abnormal action potentials (Fig. 18.2). After-depolarisation is the result of a net inward current, known as the transient inward current. A rise in $[Ca^{2+}]_i$ activates Na^+/Ca^{2+} exchange. This transfers one Ca^{2+} out of the cell in exchange for entry of three Na^+, resulting in a net influx of one positive charge and hence membrane depolarisation. Additionally, Ca^{2+} opens non-selective cation

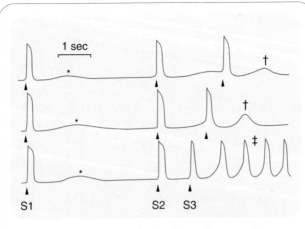

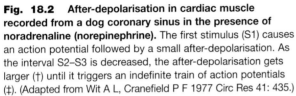

Fig. 18.2   After-depolarisation in cardiac muscle recorded from a dog coronary sinus in the presence of noradrenaline (norepinephrine). The first stimulus (S1) causes an action potential followed by a small after-depolarisation. As the interval S2–S3 is decreased, the after-depolarisation gets larger (†) until it triggers an indefinite train of action potentials (‡). (Adapted from Wit A L, Cranefield P F 1977 Circ Res 41: 435.)

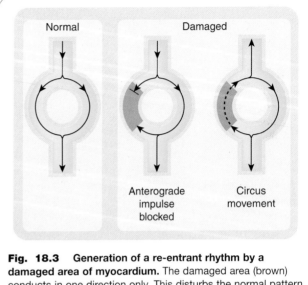

Fig. 18.3   Generation of a re-entrant rhythm by a damaged area of myocardium. The damaged area (brown) conducts in one direction only. This disturbs the normal pattern of conduction and permits continuous circulation of the impulse to occur.

channels in the plasma membrane, causing depolarisation analogous to the endplate potential at the neuromuscular junction (Ch. 10). Consequently, hypercalcaemia can delay repolarisation. This is recognised clinically from prolongation of the QT interval in the ECG. Hypokalaemia also prolongs the QT interval (via an effect on the gating of cardiac delayed rectifier potassium channels). Many drugs, including ones whose principal effects are on other systems, delay cardiac repolarisation as a result of effects on electrolyte concentrations or from binding to potassium or other cardiac channels (see Roden, 2004). This increases Ca^{2+} entry during the prolonged action potential, leading to after-depolarisation. Prolongation of the QT interval, which carries a risk of causing dangerous ventricular dysrhythmias, is a concern in drug development (see section below, *Class III drugs*, and see Ch. 53).

In normal cardiac rhythm, the conducted impulse dies out after it has activated the ventricles because it is surrounded by refractory tissue, which it has just traversed. *Re-entry* (Fig. 18.3) describes the situation in which the impulse re-excites regions of the myocardium after the refractory period has subsided, causing continuous circulation of action potentials. It can result from anatomical anomalies or, more commonly, from myocardial damage. Re-entry underlies many types of dysrhythmia, the pattern depending on the site of the re-entrant circuit, which may be in the atria, ventricles or nodal tissue. A simple ring of tissue can give rise to a re-entrant rhythm if a transient or unidirectional conduction block is present. Normally, an impulse originating at any point in the ring will propagate in both directions and die out when the two impulses meet, but if a damaged area causes either a transient block (so that one impulse is blocked but the second can get through; Fig. 18.3) or a unidirectional block, continuous circulation of the impulse can occur. This is known as circus movement and was first demonstrated experimentally on rings of jellyfish tissue many years ago.

Although the physiological pacemaker resides in the SA node, other cardiac tissues can take on pacemaker activity. This provides a safety mechanism in the event of failure of the SA node but can also trigger tachyarrhythmias. *Ectopic pacemaker activity* is encouraged by sympathetic activity and by partial depolarisation, which may occur during ischaemia. Catecholamines, acting on β_1 adrenoceptors (see below), increase the rate of depolarisation during phase IV and can cause normally quiescent parts of the heart to take on a spontaneous rhythm. Several tachyarrhythmias (e.g. paroxysmal atrial fibrillation) can be triggered by circumstances associated with increased sympathetic activity. Pain (e.g. during myocardial infarction) increases sympathetic discharge and releases adrenaline (epinephrine) from the adrenal gland. Partial depolarisation resulting from ischaemic damage also causes abnormal pacemaker activity.

Heart block results from fibrosis of, or ischaemic damage to, the conducting system (often in the AV node). In complete heart block, the atria and ventricles beat independently of one another, the ventricles beating at a slow rate determined by whatever pacemaker picks up distal to the block. Sporadic complete failure of AV conduction causes sudden periods of unconsciousness (Stokes–Adams attacks) and is treated by implanting an artificial pacemaker.

CARDIAC CONTRACTION

Cardiac output is the product of heart rate and mean left ventricular stroke volume (i.e. the volume of blood ejected from the ventricle with each heartbeat). Heart rate is controlled by the autonomic nervous system (Chs 10 and 11, and see below, pp. 283–285). Stroke volume is determined by a combination of factors, including some intrinsic to the heart itself and other haemodynamic factors extrinsic to the heart. Intrinsic factors regulate myocardial contractility via $[Ca^{2+}]_i$ and ATP, and are

- Dysrhythmias arise because of:
  - delayed after-depolarisation, which triggers ectopic beats
  - re-entry, resulting from partial conduction block
  - ectopic pacemaker activity
  - heart block.
- Delayed after-depolarisation is caused by an inward current associated with abnormally raised intracellular Ca^{2+}.
- Re-entry is facilitated when parts of the myocardium are depolarised as a result of disease.
- Ectopic pacemaker activity is encouraged by sympathetic activity.
- Heart block results from disease in the conducting system, especially the atrioventricular node.
- Clinically, dysrhythmias are divided:
  - according to their site of origin (supraventricular and ventricular)
  - according to whether the heart rate is increased or decreased (tachycardia or bradycardia).

sensitive to various drugs and pathological processes. Extrinsic circulatory factors include the elasticity and contractile state of arteries and veins, and the volume and viscosity of the blood, which together determine cardiac load (preload and afterload). Drugs that influence these circulatory factors are of paramount importance in treating patients with heart failure. They are covered in Chapter 19.

MYOCARDIAL CONTRACTILITY AND VIABILITY

The contractile machinery of myocardial striated muscle is basically the same as that of voluntary striated muscle (Ch. 4). It involves binding of Ca^{2+} to troponin C; this changes the conformation of the troponin complex, permitting cross-bridging of myosin to actin and initiating contraction.

Many effects of drugs on cardiac contractility can be explained in terms of actions on $[Ca^{2+}]_i$, via effects on calcium channels in plasma membrane or sarcoplasmic reticulum, or on the Na^+/K^+ pump, which indirectly influences the Na^+/Ca^{2+} pump (see below, pp. 291–292). Other factors that affect the force of contraction are the availability of oxygen and a source of metabolic energy such as free fatty acids. Myocardial *stunning*—contractile dysfunction that persists after ischaemia and reperfusion despite restoration of blood flow and absence of cardiac necrosis—is incompletely understood but can be clinically important. Its converse is known as *ischaemic preconditioning*; this means an improved ability to withstand ischaemia following previous ischaemic episodes. This potentially beneficial state could also be clinically important. There is some evidence that it is mediated by *adenosine* (see Ch. 2), which accumulates as ATP is depleted. Exogenous adenosine affords protection similar to that

caused by ischaemic preconditioning, and blockade of adenosine receptors prevents the protective effect of preconditioning (see Saurin et al., 2000; Linden, 2001). There is considerable interest in developing strategies to minimise harmful effects of ischaemia while maximising preconditioning.

VENTRICULAR FUNCTION CURVES AND HEART FAILURE

The force of contraction of the heart is determined partly by its intrinsic contractility (which, as described above, depends on $[Ca^{2+}]_i$ and availability of ATP), and partly by extrinsic haemodynamic factors that affect end-diastolic volume and hence the resting length of the muscle fibres. The end-diastolic volume is determined by the end-diastolic pressure, and its effect on stroke work is expressed in the Frank–Starling law of the heart, which reflects an inherent property of the contractile system. The Frank–Starling law can be represented as a ventricular function curve (Fig. 18.4). The area enclosed by the pressure–volume curve during the cardiac cycle provides a measure of ventricular stroke work. It is approximated by the product of stroke volume and mean arterial pressure. As Starling showed, factors extrinsic to the heart affect its performance in various ways, two patterns of response to increased load being particularly important.

- Increased cardiac filling pressure (*preload*), whether caused by increased blood volume or by venoconstriction, increases

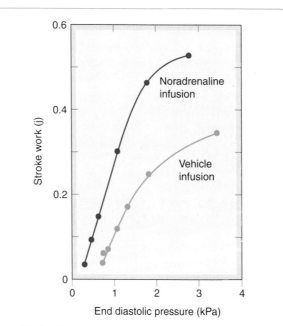

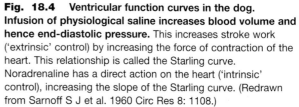

Fig. 18.4   Ventricular function curves in the dog. Infusion of physiological saline increases blood volume and hence end-diastolic pressure. This increases stroke work ('extrinsic' control) by increasing the force of contraction of the heart. This relationship is called the Starling curve. Noradrenaline has a direct action on the heart ('intrinsic' control), increasing the slope of the Starling curve. (Redrawn from Sarnoff S J et al. 1960 Circ Res 8: 1108.)

ventricular end-diastolic volume. This increases stroke volume and hence cardiac output and mean arterial pressure. Cardiac work and cardiac oxygen consumption both increase.

- Arterial and arteriolar vasoconstriction increases *afterload*. End-diastolic volume and hence stroke work are initially unchanged, but constant stroke work in the face of increased vascular resistance causes reduced stroke volume and hence increased end-diastolic volume. This in turn increases stroke work, until a steady state is re-established with increased end-diastolic volume and the same cardiac output as before. As with increased preload, cardiac work and cardiac oxygen consumption both increase.

Normal ventricular filling pressure is only a few centimetres of water, on the steep part of the ventricular function curve, so a large increase in stroke work can be achieved with only a small increase in filling pressure. The Starling mechanism plays little part in controlling cardiac output in healthy subjects (e.g. during exercise), because changes in contractility, mainly as a result of changes in sympathetic activity, achieve the necessary regulation without any increase in ventricular filling pressure (Fig. 18.4). In contrast, the denervated heart in patients who have received a heart transplant relies on the Starling mechanism to increase cardiac output during exercise.

In *heart failure*, the cardiac output is insufficient to meet the circulatory needs of the body, initially only when these are increased during exercise but ultimately, as disease progresses, also at rest. It has many causes, most commonly ischaemic heart disease. In patients with heart failure (see Ch. 19), the heart may be unable to deliver as much blood as the tissues require, even when its contractility is increased by sympathetic activity. Under these conditions, the basal (i.e. at rest) ventricular function curve is greatly depressed, and there is insufficient reserve, in the sense of extra contractility that can be achieved by sympathetic activity, to enable cardiac output to be maintained during exercise without a large increase in central venous pressure (Fig. 18.4). Oedema of peripheral tissues (causing swelling of the legs) and the lungs (causing breathlessness) is an important consequence of cardiac failure. It is caused by the increased venous pressure, and retention of Na^+ (see Ch. 19).

MYOCARDIAL OXYGEN CONSUMPTION AND CORONARY BLOOD FLOW

Relative to its large metabolic needs, the heart is one of the most poorly perfused tissues in the body. Coronary flow is, under normal circumstances, closely related to myocardial oxygen consumption, and both change over a nearly 10-fold range between conditions of rest and maximal exercise.

PHYSIOLOGICAL FACTORS

The main physiological factors that regulate coronary flow are:

- physical factors
- vascular control by metabolites
- neural and humoral control.

Myocardial contraction

- Controlling factors are:
  — intrinsic myocardial contractility
  — extrinsic circulatory factors.
- Myocardial contractility depends critically on intracellular Ca^{2+}, and hence on:
  —Ca^{2+} entry across the cell membrane
  —Ca^{2+} storage in the sarcoplasmic reticulum.
- The main factors controlling Ca^{2+} entry are:
  — activity of voltage-gated calcium channels
  — intracellular Na^+, which affects Ca^{2+}/Na^+ exchange.
- Catecholamines, cardiac glycosides, and other mediators and drugs influence these factors.
- Extrinsic control of cardiac contraction is through the dependence of stroke work on the end-diastolic volume, expressed in the Frank–Starling law.
- Cardiac work is affected independently by afterload (i.e. peripheral resistance and arterial compliance) and preload (i.e. central venous pressure).

Physical factors

During systole, the pressure exerted by the myocardium on vessels that pass through it equals or exceeds the perfusion pressure, so coronary flow occurs only during diastole. Diastole is shortened more than systole during tachycardia, reducing the period available for myocardial perfusion. During diastole, the effective perfusion pressure is equal to the difference between the aortic and ventricular pressures (Fig. 18.5). If diastolic aortic pressure falls or diastolic ventricular pressure increases, perfusion pressure falls and so (unless other control mechanisms can compensate) does coronary blood flow. Stenosis of the aortic

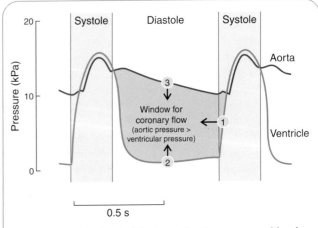

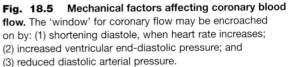

Fig. 18.5 Mechanical factors affecting coronary blood flow. The 'window' for coronary flow may be encroached on by: (1) shortening diastole, when heart rate increases; (2) increased ventricular end-diastolic pressure; and (3) reduced diastolic arterial pressure.

valve reduces aortic pressure but increases left ventricular pressure upstream of the narrowed valve, and often causes ischaemic chest pain (*angina*) even in the absence of coronary artery disease.

Vascular control by metabolites/mediators

Vascular control by metabolites is the most important mechanism by which coronary flow is regulated. A reduction in arterial partial pressure of oxygen (Po_2) causes marked vasodilatation of coronary vessels in situ but has little effect on isolated strips of coronary artery. This suggests that it is a change in the pattern of metabolites produced by the myocardial cells, rather than the change in Po_2 per se, that controls the state of the coronary vessels, a popular candidate for the dilator metabolite being adenosine (see Ch. 12).

Neural and humoral control

Coronary vessels have a dense sympathetic innervation, but sympathetic nerves (like circulating catecholamines) exert only a small direct effect on the coronary circulation. Large coronary vessels possess α-adrenoceptors that mediate vasoconstriction, whereas smaller vessels have β$_2$-adrenoceptors that have a dilator effect. Coronary vessels are also innervated by purinergic, peptidergic and nitrergic nerves. Normally, neural and endocrine effects on coronary vasculature are overshadowed by the vascular response to altered mechanical and metabolic activity.

AUTONOMIC TRANSMITTERS

Many aspects of autonomic pharmacology have been discussed in Chapters 9–11; here, we mention only aspects that particularly concern the heart.

AUTONOMIC CONTROL OF THE HEART

The sympathetic and parasympathetic systems each exert a tonic effect on the heart at rest. They influence each of the aspects of cardiac function that have been discussed above, namely rate and rhythm, myocardial contraction, and myocardial metabolism and blood flow.

Sympathetic system

The main effects of sympathetic activity on the heart are:

- increased force of contraction (positive *inotropic* effect; Fig. 18.6)
- increased heart rate (positive *chronotropic* effect; Fig. 18.7)
- increased automaticity
- repolarisation and restoration of function following generalised cardiac depolarisation
- reduced cardiac efficiency (i.e. oxygen consumption is increased more than cardiac work).

These effects all result from activation of β$_1$-adrenoceptors. The β$_1$ effects of catecholamines on the heart, although complex, probably all occur through increased intracellular cAMP (see Ch. 3). cAMP activates protein kinase A, which phosphorylates sites on the α$_1$ subunits of calcium channels. This increases the probability that the channels will open, increasing inward Ca^{2+} current and hence force of cardiac contraction (Fig. 18.6). Activation of β$_1$-adrenoceptors also increases the Ca^{2+} sensitivity of the contractile machinery, possibly by phosphorylating troponin C; furthermore, it facilitates Ca^{2+} capture by the sarcoplasmic reticulum, thereby increasing the amount of Ca^{2+} available for release by the action potential. The net result of catecholamine action is to elevate and steepen the ventricular function curve (Fig. 18.4). The increase in heart rate results from an increased slope of the pacemaker potential (Figs 18.1 and 18.7). Increased Ca^{2+} entry also increases automaticity because of the effect of $[Ca^{2+}]_i$ on the transient inward current, which can result in a train of action potentials following a single stimulus (Fig. 18.2).

Activation of β$_1$-adrenoceptors repolarises damaged or hypoxic myocardium by stimulating the Na^+/K^+ pump. This can

---

Coronary flow, ischaemia and infarction

- The heart has a smaller blood supply in relation to its oxygen consumption than most organs.
- Coronary flow is controlled mainly by:
  - physical factors, including transmural pressure during systole
  - vasodilator metabolites.
- Autonomic innervation is less important.
- Coronary ischaemia is usually the result of atherosclerosis and causes angina. Sudden ischaemia is usually caused by thrombosis and may result in cardiac infarction.
- Coronary spasm sometimes causes angina (variant angina).
- Cellular Ca^{2+} overload results from ischaemia and may be responsible for:
  - cell death
  - dysrhythmias.

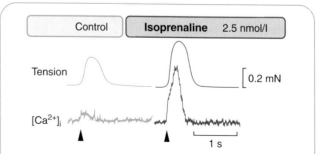

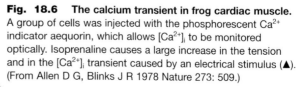

Fig. 18.6 The calcium transient in frog cardiac muscle. A group of cells was injected with the phosphorescent Ca^{2+} indicator aequorin, which allows $[Ca^{2+}]_i$ to be monitored optically. Isoprenaline causes a large increase in the tension and in the $[Ca^{2+}]_i$ transient caused by an electrical stimulus (▲). (From Allen D G, Blinks J R 1978 Nature 273: 509.)

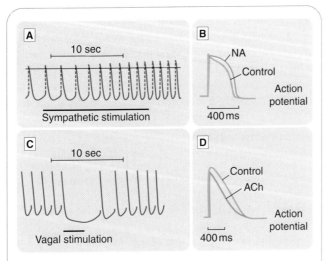

Fig. 18.7 Autonomic regulation of the heartbeat. A and B. Effects of sympathetic stimulation and noradrenaline (NA). C and D. Effects of parasympathetic stimulation and acetylcholine (ACh). Sympathetic stimulation (A) increases the slope of the pacemaker potential and increases heart rate, whereas parasympathetic stimulation (C) abolishes the pacemaker potential, hyperpolarises the membrane and temporarily stops the heart (frog sinus venosus). NA (B) prolongs the action potential, while ACh (D) shortens it (frog atrium). (From: (A and C) Hutter O F, Trautwein W 1956 J Gen Physiol 39: 715; (B) Reuter H 1974 J Physiol 242: 429; (D) Giles W R, Noble S J 1976 J Physiol 261: 103.)

restore function if asystole has occurred following myocardial infarction, and **adrenaline** is one of the most important drugs used during cardiac arrest.

The reduction of cardiac efficiency by catecholamines is important because it means that the oxygen requirement of the myocardium increases. This limits the use of β agonists such as adrenaline and **dobutamine** for circulatory shock (Ch. 19). Myocardial infarction activates the sympathetic nervous system (Fig. 18.8), which has the undesirable effect of increasing the oxygen needs of the damaged myocardium.

Parasympathetic system

Parasympathetic activity produces effects that are, in general, opposite to those of sympathetic activation. However, in contrast to sympathetic activity, the parasympathetic nervous system has little effect on contractility, its main effects being on rate and rhythm, namely:

- cardiac slowing and reduced automaticity
- inhibition of AV conduction.

These effects result from occupation of muscarinic (M_2) acetylcholine receptors, which are abundant in nodal and atrial tissue but sparse in the ventricles. These receptors are negatively coupled to adenylate cyclase and thus reduce cAMP formation, acting to inhibit the slow Ca^{2+} current, in opposition to β_1 adrenoceptors. M_2 receptors also open a potassium channel (called K_{ACh}). The resulting increase in K^+ permeability produces

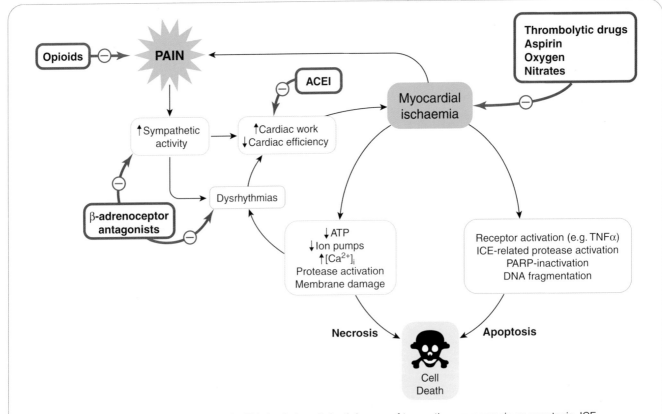

Fig. 18.8 Effects of myocardial ischaemia. This leads to cell death by one of two pathways: necrosis or apoptosis. ICE, interleukin-1–converting enzyme; PARP, poly-[ADP-ribose]-polymerase; TNF-α, tumour necrosis factor-α.

a hyperpolarising current that opposes the inward pacemaker current, slowing the heart and reducing automaticity (see Fig. 18.7). Vagal activity is often increased during myocardial infarction, both in association with vagal afferent stimulation and as a side effect of opioids used to control the pain, and parasympathetic effects are important in predisposing to acute dysrhythmias.

Vagal stimulation decreases the force of contraction of the atria associated with marked shortening of the action potential (Fig. 18.7). Increased K^+ permeability and reduced Ca^{2+} current both contribute to conduction block at the AV node, where propagation depends on the Ca^{2+} current. Shortening the atrial action potential reduces the refractory period, which can lead to re-entrant arrhythmias. Coronary vessels lack cholinergic innervation; consequently, the parasympathetic nervous system has little effect on coronary artery tone (see Ch. 10).[2]

CARDIAC NATRIURETIC PEPTIDES

Atrial cells have a specialised endocrine function in relation to the cardiovascular system. They contain secretory granules, and store and release atrial natriuretic peptide (ANP). This has powerful effects on the kidney and vascular system. Release of ANP occurs during volume overload in response to stretching of the atria. Saline infusion is sufficient to evoke ANP release. Two related natriuretic peptides (B and C) are found, respectively, in ventricular muscle and vascular endothelium. The plasma concentration of B-type natriuretic hormone (BNP) is predictably increased in patients with heart failure and is increasingly used as an aid to diagnosis.

The main effects of natriuretic peptides are to increase Na^+ and water excretion by the kidney; relax vascular smooth muscle (except efferent arterioles of renal glomeruli; see below); increase vascular permeability; and inhibit the release and/or actions of several hormones and mediators, including aldosterone, angiotensin II, endothelin and antidiuretic hormone. They exert their effects by combining with membrane receptors (natriuretic peptide receptors, NPRs, which exist in at least two subtypes, designated A and B).[3]

Both NPR-A and NPR-B incorporate a catalytic guanylate cyclase moiety (see Ch. 3). Binding of one of the natriuretic peptides to either receptor leads to intracellular generation of cGMP. This is the same response as that produced by organic nitrates (see later) and endothelium-derived nitric oxide (Ch. 17), which, however, achieve this by interacting with soluble rather than membrane-bound guanylate cyclase. Renal glomerular

> ### Autonomic control of the heart
>
> - Sympathetic activity, acting through β_1 adrenoceptors, increases heart rate, contractility and automaticity, but reduces cardiac efficiency (in relation to oxygen consumption).
> - The β_1 adrenoceptors act by increasing cAMP formation, which increases Ca^{2+} currents.
> - Parasympathetic activity, acting through muscarinic M_2 receptors, causes cardiac slowing, decreased force of contraction (atria only), and inhibition of atrioventricular conduction.
> - M_2 receptors inhibit cAMP formation and also open potassium channels, causing hyperpolarisation.

afferent arterioles are dilated by ANP but efferent arterioles are constricted, so filtration pressure is increased, leading to increased glomerular filtration and enhanced Na^+ excretion. Elsewhere, natriuretic peptides cause vasorelaxation and reduce blood pressure. Their therapeutic potential is considered in Chapter 19.

ISCHAEMIC HEART DISEASE

Atheromatous deposits are ubiquitous in the coronary arteries of adults living in developed countries. They are asymptomatic for most of the natural history of the disease (see Ch. 20), but can progress insidiously, culminating in acute myocardial infarction and its complications, including dysrhythmia and heart failure. Details of ischemic heart disease are beyond the scope of this book, and up-to-date accounts (e.g. Braunwald, 2005) are available for those seeking pathological and clinical information. Here, we merely set the scene for understanding the place of drugs that affect cardiac function in treating this most common form of heart disease.

Important consequences of coronary atherosclerosis include:

- angina (ischaemic chest pain)
- myocardial infarction.

ANGINA

Angina occurs when the oxygen supply to the myocardium is insufficient for its needs. The pain has a characteristic distribution in the chest, arm and neck, and is brought on by exertion, cold or excitement. A similar type of pain occurs in skeletal muscle when it is made to contract while its blood supply is interrupted, and Lewis showed many years ago that chemical factors released by ischaemic muscle are responsible. Possible candidates include K^+, H^+ and *adenosine* (Ch. 12), all of which stimulate nociceptors (see Ch. 41). It is possible that the same mediator that causes coronary vasodilatation is responsible, at higher concentration, for initiating pain.

Three kinds of angina are recognised clinically: stable, unstable and variant.

---

[2]The Creator has, however, thoughtfully provided coronary *endothelium* with muscarinic receptors linked to nitric oxide synthesis (see Chs 17 and 19), presumably for the delectation of vascular pharmacologists.

[3]The nomenclature of natriuretic peptides and their receptors is peculiarly obtuse. The peptides are named 'A' for atrial, 'B' for brain—despite being present mainly in cardiac ventricle—and 'C' for A, B, C...; NPRs are named NPR-A, which preferentially binds ANP; NPR-B, which binds C natriuretic peptide preferentially; and NPR-C for 'clearance' receptor, because until recently clearance via cellular uptake and degradation by lysosomal enzymes was the only definite known function of this binding site.

Stable angina. This is predictable chest pain on exertion. It is produced by an increased demand on the heart and is caused by a fixed narrowing of the coronary vessels, almost always by atheroma. Symptomatic therapy is directed at altering cardiac work with organic nitrates, β-adrenoceptor antagonists and/or calcium antagonists (as described below), together with treatment of the underlying atheromatous disease, usually including a statin (Ch. 20), and prophylaxis against thrombosis with an antiplatelet drug, usually **aspirin** (Ch. 21).

Unstable angina. This is characterised by pain that occurs with less and less exertion, culminating in pain at rest. The pathology is similar to that involved in myocardial infarction, namely platelet–fibrin thrombus associated with a ruptured atheromatous plaque, but without complete occlusion of the vessel. The risk of infarction is substantial, and the main aim of therapy is to reduce this. Aspirin approximately halves the risk of myocardial infarction in this setting, and **heparin** and **platelet glycoprotein receptor antagonists** add to this benefit (Ch. 21).

Variant angina. This is uncommon. It occurs at rest and is caused by coronary artery spasm, again usually in association with atheromatous disease. Therapy is with coronary artery vasodilators (e.g. organic nitrates, calcium antagonists).

MYOCARDIAL INFARCTION

Myocardial infarction occurs when a coronary artery has been blocked by thrombus. This may be fatal and is a common cause of death, usually as a result of mechanical failure of the ventricle or from dysrhythmia. Cardiac myocytes rely on aerobic metabolism. If the supply of oxygen remains below a critical value, a sequence of events leading to cell death (by *necrosis* or *apoptosis*) ensues (see Ch. 5 for a fuller account of apoptosis). The sequences leading from vascular occlusion to cell death via the two pathways are illustrated in Figure 18.8. The relative importance of necrosis and apoptosis in myocardial cell death in clinically distinct settings is unknown, but it has been suggested that apoptosis may be an adaptive process in hypoperfused regions, sacrificing some jeopardised myocytes but thereby avoiding the disturbance of membrane function and risk of dysrhythmia inherent in necrosis. Consequently, it is currently unknown if pharmacological approaches to promote or inhibit this pathway could be clinically beneficial.

Prevention of irreversible ischaemic damage following an episode of coronary thrombosis is an important therapeutic aim. The main possibilities among existing therapeutic drugs, shown in Figure 18.8, are:

- thrombolytic and antiplatelet drugs (aspirin and clopidogrel) to open the blocked artery and prevent their reocclusion (see Ch. 21)
- oxygen
- opioids to prevent pain and reduce excessive sympathetic activity
- β-adrenoceptor antagonists
- angiotensin-converting enzyme (ACE) inhibitors (see Ch. 19).

The latter two classes of drug reduce cardiac work and thereby the metabolic needs of the heart. The β-adrenoceptor antagonists

have an important benefit during chronic treatment in reducing dysrhythmic deaths, and are widely used in patients with unstable angina; they increase the risk of cardiogenic shock if given during acute infarction to patients with signs of heart failure, but are started as soon as is haemodynamically prudent (COMMIT Collaborative Group, 2005). Several clinical trials have demonstrated that ACE inhibitors improve survival if given to patients shortly after myocardial infarction, especially if there is even a modest degree of myocardial dysfunction. It is possible (see Ch. 19 for a discussion of the differences between angiotensin receptor antagonists—*sartans*—and ACE inhibitors) that sartans could prove similarly beneficial.

Despite several encouraging small trials of *organic nitrates*, a large randomised controlled trial (the Fourth International Study of Infarct Survival, ISIS-4, 1994) showed that these drugs do not improve outcome in patients with myocardial infarction, although they are useful in preventing or treating anginal pain (see below). *Calcium antagonists*, which reduce cardiac work (via arteriolar vasodilatation and afterload reduction) and block Ca^{2+} entry into cardiac myocytes, have been disappointing, and several clinical trials of short-acting dihydropyridines (e.g. **nifedipine**) were halted when adverse trends were evident. **Trimetazidine**, a 3-ketoacyl-CoA thiolase inhibitor, is believed to protect the heart from ischaemia by switching cardiac metabolism from fatty acid to glucose oxidation, but its place (if any) in therapeutics is yet to be established (see Marzilli, 2003; and Lee et al., 2004).

DRUGS THAT AFFECT CARDIAC FUNCTION

Drugs that have a major action on the heart can be divided into three groups.

- *Drugs that affect myocardial cells directly.* These include:
  —autonomic neurotransmitters and related drugs
  —antidysrhythmic drugs
  —cardiac glycosides and other inotropic drugs
  —miscellaneous drugs and hormones; these are dealt with elsewhere (e.g. **doxorubicin**, Ch. 51; thyroxine, Ch. 29; glucagon, Ch. 26).
- *Drugs that affect cardiac function indirectly.* These have actions elsewhere in the vascular system. Some antianginal drugs (e.g. nitrates) fall into this category, as do most drugs that are used to treat heart failure (e.g. diuretics and ACE inhibitors).
- *Calcium antagonists.* These affect cardiac function by a direct action on myocardial cells and also indirectly by relaxing arterioles.

ANTIDYSRHYTHMIC DRUGS

A classification of antidysrhythmic drugs based on their electrophysiological effects was proposed by Vaughan Williams in 1970. It provides a good starting point for discussing mechanisms, although many useful drugs do not fit neatly into this classification (Table 18.1). Furthermore, emergency treatment of serious dysrhythmias is usually by physical means (e.g. pacing or electrical cardioversion by applying a direct current shock to the chest or via an implanted device) rather than drugs.

There are four classes (see Table 18.2).

- *Class I*: drugs that block voltage-sensitive sodium channels. They are subdivided: Ia, Ib and Ic (see below).
- *Class II*: β-adrenoceptor antagonists.
- *Class III*: drugs that substantially prolong the cardiac action potential.
- *Class IV*: calcium antagonists.

The phase of the action potential on which each of these classes of drug have their main effect is shown in Figure 18.9.

Table 18.1 Antidysrhythmic drugs unclassified in the Vaughan Williams system

Drug	Use
Atropine	Sinus bradycardia
Adrenaline (epinephrine)	Cardiac arrest
Isoprenaline	Heart block
Digoxin	Rapid atrial fibrillation
Adenosine	Supraventricular tachycardia
Calcium chloride	Ventricular tachycardia due to hyperkalaemia
Magnesium chloride	Ventricular fibrillation, digoxin toxicity

Table 18.2 Summary of antidysrhythmic drugs (Vaughan Williams classification)

Class	Example(s)	Mechanism
Ia	Disopyramide	Sodium channel block (intermediate dissociation)
Ib	Lidocaine	Sodium channel block (fast dissociation)
Ic	Flecainide	Sodium channel block (slow dissociation)
II	Propranolol	β-Adrenoceptor antagonism
III	Amiodarone, sotalol	Potassium channel block
IV	Verapamil	Calcium channel block

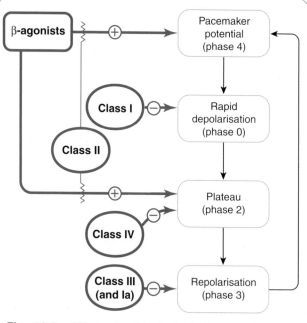

Fig. 18.9 Effects of antidysrhythmic drugs on the different phases (as defined in Fig. 18.1) of the cardiac action potential.

MECHANISMS OF ACTION

Class I drugs

Class I drugs block sodium channels, just as local anaesthetics do, by binding to sites in the α subunit (see Chs 4 and 44). Because this inhibits action potential propagation in many excitable cells, it has been referred to as 'membrane-stabilising' activity, a phrase best avoided now that the ionic mechanism is understood. Their characteristic effect on the action potential is to reduce the maximum rate of depolarisation during phase 0.

The reason for further subdivision of these drugs into classes Ia, Ib and Ic is that the earliest examples, **quinidine** and **procainamide** (class Ia), have different effects from many of the more recently developed drugs, even though all share the same basic mechanism of action. A partial explanation for these functional differences comes from electrophysiological studies of the characteristics of the sodium channel block produced by different class I drugs.

The central concept is of *use-dependent channel block*. It is this characteristic that enables all class I drugs to block the high-frequency excitation of the myocardium that occurs in tachyarrhythmias, without preventing the heart from beating at normal frequencies. Sodium channels exist in three distinct functional states: resting, open and refractory (see Ch. 4). Channels switch rapidly from resting to open in response to depolarisation; this is known as activation. Maintained depolarisation, as in ischaemic muscle, causes channels to change more slowly from open to refractory (inactivation), and the membrane must then be repolarised for a time to restore the channel to the resting state before it can be activated again. Class I drugs bind to channels most strongly when they are in either the open or the refractory state, less strongly to channels in the resting state. Their action therefore shows the property of 'use dependence' (i.e. the more frequently the channels are activated, the greater the degree of block produced).

Class Ib drugs, for example **lidocaine**, associate and dissociate rapidly within the timeframe of the normal heartbeat. The drug binds to open channels during phase 0 of the action potential (affecting the rate of rise very little, but leaving many of the channels blocked by the time the action potential reaches its peak). Dissociation occurs in time for the next action potential, provided the cardiac rhythm is normal. A premature beat, however, will be aborted because the channels are still blocked. Furthermore, class Ib drugs bind selectively to refractory channels and thus block preferentially when the cells are depolarised, for example in ischaemia.

Class Ic drugs, such as **flecainide** and **encainide**, associate and dissociate much more slowly, thus reaching a steady-state level of block that does not vary appreciably during the cardiac cycle; they also show only a marginal preference for refractory channels, so are not specific for damaged myocardium. Therefore they cause a rather general reduction in excitability and do not discriminate particularly against occasional premature beats, as class Ib drugs do, but will suppress re-entrant rhythms that depend on unidirectional or intermittent conduction pathways operating at a low margin of safety (e.g. some forms of paroxysmal atrial fibrillation). They markedly inhibit conduction through the His–Purkinje system.

Class Ia, the oldest group (e.g. **quinidine**, **procainamide**, **disopyramide**), lies midway in its properties between Ib and Ic but, in addition, prolongs repolarisation, albeit less markedly than class III drugs (see below).

Class II drugs

Class II drugs comprise the β-adrenoceptor antagonists (e.g. **propranolol**).

Adrenaline can cause dysrhythmias by its effects on the pacemaker potential and on the slow inward Ca^{2+} current (see above). Ventricular dysrhythmias following myocardial infarction are partly the result of increased sympathetic activity (see Fig. 18.8), providing a rationale for using β-adrenoceptor antagonists in this setting. AV conduction depends critically on sympathetic activity; β-adrenoceptor antagonists increase the refractory period of the AV node and can therefore prevent recurrent attacks of SVT. The β-adrenoceptor antagonists are also used to prevent paroxysmal attacks of atrial fibrillation when these occur in the setting of sympathetic activation.

Class III drugs

The class III category was originally based on the unusual behaviour of a single drug, **amiodarone** (see below), although others with similar properties (e.g. **sotalol**) have since been described. Both amiodarone and sotalol have more than one mechanism of antidysrhythmic action. The special feature that defines them as class III drugs is that they substantially prolong the cardiac action potential. The mechanism of this effect is not fully understood, but it involves blocking some of the potassium channels involved in cardiac repolarisation, including the outward

(delayed) rectifier. Action potential prolongation increases the refractory period, accounting for powerful and varied anti-dysrhythmic activity, for example by interrupting re-entrant tachycardias and suppressing ectopic activity. However, all drugs that prolong the cardiac action potential (detected clinically as prolonged QT interval on the ECG; see above) can paradoxically also have proarrhythmic effects, notably a polymorphic form of ventricular tachycardia called (somewhat whimsically) *torsade de pointes* (because the appearance of the ECG trace is said to be reminiscent of this ballet sequence). This occurs particularly in patients taking other drugs that can prolong QT, including several antipsychotic drugs; those with disturbances of electrolytes involved in repolarisation (e.g. hypokalaemia, hypercalcaemia); or individuals with hereditary prolonged QT (Ward–Romano syndrome).[4] The mechanism of the dysrhythmia is not fully understood; possibilities include increased dispersion of repolarisation (i.e. lack of spatial homogeneity) and increased Ca^{2+} entry during the prolonged action potential, leading to increased after-depolarisation.

Class IV drugs

Class IV agents act by blocking voltage-sensitive calcium channels. Class IV drugs in therapeutic use as antidysrhythmic drugs (e.g. **verapamil**) act on L-type channels. Class IV drugs slow conduction in the SA and AV nodes where action potential propagation depends on slow inward Ca^{2+} current, slowing the heart and terminating SVT by causing partial AV block. They shorten the plateau of the action potential and reduce the force of contraction. Reduced Ca^{2+} entry reduces after-depolarisation and thus suppresses premature ectopic beats.

DETAILS OF INDIVIDUAL DRUGS

Quinidine, procainamide and disopyramide (class Ia)

Quinidine and **procainamide** are pharmacologically similar. They are now mainly of historical interest. **Disopyramide** resembles quinidine, including in its marked atropine-like effects, which result in blurred vision, dry mouth, constipation and urinary retention. It has more negative inotropic action than quinidine but is less likely to cause hypersensitivity reactions.

Lidocaine (class Ib)

Lidocaine, also well-known as a local anaesthetic (see Ch. 44) is given by intravenous infusion to treat and prevent ventricular dysrhythmias in the immediate aftermath of myocardial infarction. It is almost completely extracted from the portal circulation by

---

[4]A 3-year-old girl began to have blackouts, which decreased in frequency with age. Her ECG showed a prolonged QT interval. When 18 years of age, she lost consciousness running for a bus. When she was 19, she became quite emotional as a participant in a live television audience and died suddenly. The molecular basis of this rare inherited disorder is now known. It is caused by a mutation in either the gene coding for a particular potassium channel—called *HERG*—or another gene, *SCN5A*, which codes for the sodium channel and disruption of which results in a loss of inactivation of the Na^+ current (see Welsh & Hoshi, 1995, for a commentary).

hepatic first-pass metabolism (Ch. 8), and so cannot usefully be administered orally. Its plasma half-life is normally about 2 hours, but its elimination is slowed if hepatic blood flow is reduced, for example by reduced cardiac output following myocardial infarction or by drugs that reduce cardiac contractility (e.g. β-adrenoceptor antagonists). Dosage must be reduced accordingly to prevent accumulation and toxicity. Indeed, its clearance has been used to estimate hepatic blood flow, analogous to the use of *para*-aminohippurate clearance to measure renal blood flow.

The adverse effects of lidocaine are mainly due to its actions on the central nervous system and include drowsiness, disorientation and convulsions. Because of its relatively short half-life, the plasma concentration can be adjusted fairly rapidly by varying the infusion rate.

Phenytoin (class Ib)

Phenytoin is an antiepileptic drug (Ch. 40); it has antidysrhythmic actions on the heart, but its clinical use for this indication is obsolete.

Flecainide and encainide (class Ic)

Flecainide and **encainide** suppress ventricular ectopic beats. They are long acting and reduce the frequency of ventricular ectopic beats when administered orally. However, in clinical trials, they *increase* the incidence of sudden death associated with ventricular fibrillation after myocardial infarction, so they are no longer used in this setting. This counter-intuitive result had a profound impact on the way clinicians and drug regulators view the use of seemingly reasonable intermediate end points (in this case, reduction of frequency of ventricular ectopic beats) as evidence of efficacy in clinical trials. Currently, the main use of flecainide is in prophylaxis against paroxysmal atrial fibrillation.

β-Adrenoceptor antagonists (class II)

The most important β-adrenoceptor antagonists are described in Chapter 11. Their clinical use for rhythm disorders is shown in

---

> **Clinical uses of class I antidysrhythmic drugs**
>
>
> - **Class Ia** (e.g. **disopyramide**)
>   - ventricular dysrhythmias
>   - prevention of recurrent paroxysmal atrial fibrillation triggered by vagal overactivity.
> - **Class Ib** (e.g. intravenous **lidocaine**)
>   - treatment and prevention of ventricular tachycardia and fibrillation during and immediately after myocardial infarction.
> - **Class Ic**
>   - to prevent paroxysmal atrial fibrillation (**flecainide**)
>   - recurrent tachyarrhythmias associated with abnormal conducting pathways (e.g. Wolff–Parkinson–White syndrome).

> **Clinical uses of class II antidysrhythmic drugs (e.g. propranolol, timolol)**
>
>
> - To reduce mortality following *myocardial infarction*.
> - To prevent recurrence of tachyarrhythmias (e.g. paroxysmal atrial fibrillation) provoked by increased sympathetic activity.

---

the clinical box. **Propranolol**, like several other drugs of this type, has some class I action in addition to blocking β adrenoceptors. This may contribute to its antidysrhythmic effects, although probably not very much, because an isomer with little β antagonist activity has little antidysrhythmic activity, despite similar activity as a class I agent.

Adverse effects are described in Chapter 11, the most important being worsening bronchospasm in patients with asthma, a negative inotropic effect, bradycardia and fatigue. It was hoped that the use of β₁-selective drugs (e.g. **metoprolol**, **atenolol**) would reduce the risk of bronchospasm, but their selectivity is insufficient to achieve this goal in clinical practice, although the once-a-day convenience of several such drugs has led to their widespread use in patients without lung disease.

Amiodarone and sotalol (class III)

Amiodarone is highly effective at suppressing dysrhythmias (see the clinical box). Like other drugs that interfere with cardiac repolarisation, it is important to monitor plasma electrolyte concentrations during its use to avoid precipitating torsades de pointes. Unfortunately, it has several peculiarities in addition to its main pharmacological action on potassium channels, that complicate its use. It is extensively bound in tissues, has a long elimination half-life (10–100 days) and accumulates in the body during repeated dosing (see p. 104). For this reason, a loading dose is used, and for life-threatening dysrhythmias this is given intravenously via a central vein (it causes phlebitis if given into a peripheral vessel). Adverse effects are numerous and important; they include photosensitive skin rashes and a slate-grey/bluish discoloration of the skin; thyroid abnormalities (hypo- and hyper-, connected with its high iodine content); pulmonary fibrosis, which is slow in onset but may be irreversible; corneal deposits; and neurological and gastrointestinal disturbances, including hepatitis.

Sotalol is a non-selective β-adrenoceptor antagonist, this activity residing in the L isomer. Unlike other β antagonists, it prolongs the cardiac action potential and the QT interval by delaying the slow outward K⁺ current. This class III activity is present in both L and D isomers. Racemic sotalol (the form prescribed) appears to be somewhat less effective than amiodarone in preventing chronic malignant ventricular tachyarrhythmias. It shares the ability of amiodarone to cause torsades de pointes but lacks its other adverse effects; it is valuable in patients in whom β-adrenoceptor antagonists are not contraindicated. As with amiodarone, close monitoring of plasma electrolytes is important during its use.

> ### Clinical uses of class III antidysrhythmic drugs
>
> - **Amiodarone**: tachycardia associated with the Wolff–Parkinson–White syndrome. It is also effective in many other supraventricular and ventricular tachyarrhythmias but has serious adverse effects.
> - (Racemic) **sotalol** combines class III with class II actions. It is used in paroxysmal supraventricular dysrhythmias and suppresses ventricular ectopic beats and short runs of ventricular tachycardia.

> ### Clinical uses of class IV antidysrhythmic drugs
>
> - **Verapamil** is the main drug. It is used:
>   - to prevent recurrence of paroxysmal *supraventricular tachycardia* (*SVT*)
>   - to reduce the ventricular rate in patients with *atrial fibrillation,* provided they do not have Wolff–Parkinson–White or a related disorder.
> - Verapamil was previously given intravenously to terminate SVT; it is now seldom used for this because **adenosine** is safer.

Verapamil and diltiazem (class IV)

Verapamil is given by mouth. (Intravenous preparations are available but are dangerous and almost never needed.) It has a plasma half-life of 6–8 hours and is subject to quite extensive first-pass metabolism, which is more marked for the isomer that is responsible for its cardiac effects. A slow-release preparation is available for once-daily use, but it is less effective when used for prevention of dysrhythmia than the regular preparation because the bioavailability of the cardioactive isomer is reduced through the presentation of a steady low concentration to the drug-metabolising enzymes in the liver. If verapamil is added to **digoxin** in patients with poorly controlled atrial fibrillation, the dose of digoxin should be reduced and plasma digoxin concentration checked after a few days, because verapamil both displaces digoxin from tissue-binding sites and reduces its renal elimination, hence predisposing to digoxin accumulation and toxicity (see Ch. 52).

Verapamil is contraindicated in patients with Wolff–Parkinson–White syndrome, and is ineffective and dangerous in ventricular dysrhythmias. Adverse effects of verapamil and **diltiazem** are described below in the section on calcium channel antagonists.

Diltiazem is similar to verapamil but has relatively more smooth muscle–relaxing effect and produces less bradycardia.

Adenosine (unclassified in the Vaughan Williams classification)

Adenosine is produced endogenously and is an important chemical mediator (Ch. 12) with effects on breathing, on cardiac muscle and afferent nerves, and on platelets, in addition to the effects on cardiac conducting tissue that underlie its therapeutic use. The A_1 receptor is responsible for its effect on the AV node. These receptors are linked to the same cardiac potassium channel (K_{ACh}) that is activated by acetylcholine, and adenosine hyperpolarises cardiac conducting tissue and slows the rate of rise of the pacemaker potential accordingly. It is used intravenously to terminate SVT if this rhythm persists despite manoeuvres such as carotid artery massage designed to increase vagal tone. It has largely replaced verapamil for this purpose, because it is safer owing to its effect being short-lived. This is a consequence of its pharmacokinetics: it is taken up via a specific nucleoside transporter by red blood cells and is metabolised by enzymes on the lumenal surface of vascular endothelium. Consequently, the effects of a bolus dose of adenosine last only 20–30 seconds. Once SVT has terminated, the patient usually remains in sinus rhythm, even though adenosine is no longer present in plasma, but the unwanted effects resolve very rapidly. These include chest pain, shortness of breath, dizziness and nausea. **Theophylline** and other xanthine alkaloids block adenosine receptors and inhibit the actions of intravenous adenosine, whereas **dipyridamole** (a vasodilator and antiplatelet drug; see below and Ch. 21) blocks the nucleoside uptake mechanism, potentiating adenosine and prolonging its adverse effects. Both these interactions are clinically important.

DRUGS THAT INCREASE MYOCARDIAL CONTRACTION

CARDIAC GLYCOSIDES

Cardiac glycosides come from foxgloves (*Digitalis* spp.) and related plants. Withering (1775) wrote on the use of the foxglove: 'it has a power over the motion of the heart to a degree yet unobserved in any other medicine...' There is evidence in mammals of an endogenous digitalis-like factor closely similar to another cardiac glycoside, **ouabain**, and this is of potential physiological and pathological significance (see Schoner, 2002).

Chemistry

▼ Foxgloves contain several cardiac glycosides with similar actions. **Digoxin** is the most important therapeutically. Ouabain is similar but shorter acting. The basic chemical structure of glycosides consists of three components: a sugar moiety, a steroid and a lactone. The sugar moiety consists of unusual 1–4 linked monosaccharides. The lactone ring is essential for activity, and substituted lactones can retain biological activity even when the steroid moiety is removed.

Actions and adverse effects

The main actions of glycosides are on the heart, but some of their adverse effects are extracardiac, including nausea, vomiting, diarrhoea and confusion. The cardiac effects are:

- cardiac slowing and reduced rate of conduction through the AV node
- increased force of contraction

- disturbances of rhythm, especially:
  —block of AV conduction
  —increased ectopic pacemaker activity.

Adverse effects are common and can be severe. One of the main drawbacks of glycosides in clinical use is the narrow margin between effectiveness and toxicity.

Mechanism

The main mechanisms of action of cardiac glycosides are increased vagal activity and inhibition of the Na⁺/K⁺ pump. Cardiac glycosides bind to a site on the extracellular aspect of the α subunit of the Na⁺/K⁺ ATPase (which is an αβ heterodimer), and are useful experimental tools for studying this important transport system.

Rate and rhythm

Cardiac glycosides slow AV conduction by increasing vagal outflow via central nervous system activity. Their beneficial effect in established rapid atrial fibrillation results partly from this. If ventricular rate is excessively rapid, the time available for diastolic filling is inadequate. Increasing the refractory period of the AV node reduces ventricular rate. The atrial dysrhythmia is unaffected, but the pumping efficiency of the heart improves owing to improved ventricular filling. SVT can be terminated by cardiac glycosides, which slow AV conduction, although other drugs are usually employed for this indication (see below).

Larger doses of glycosides disturb sinus rhythm. This can occur at plasma concentrations of digoxin within, or only slightly above, the therapeutic range. Slowing of AV conduction can progress to AV block. Glycosides can also cause ectopic beats. Because Na⁺/K⁺ exchange is electrogenic, inhibition of the pump by glycosides causes depolarisation, predisposing to disturbances of cardiac rhythm. Furthermore, the increased $[Ca^{2+}]_i$ causes increased after-depolarisation, leading first to coupled beats (*bigeminy*), in which a normal ventricular beat is followed by an ectopic beat; this is followed by ventricular tachycardia and eventually by ventricular fibrillation.

Force of contraction

Glycosides cause a large increase in twitch tension in isolated preparations of cardiac muscle. Unlike catecholamines, they do not accelerate relaxation (compare Fig. 18.6 with Fig. 18.10). Increased tension is caused by an increased $[Ca^{2+}]_i$ transient (Fig. 18.10). The action potential is only slightly affected and the slow inward current little changed, so the increased $[Ca^{2+}]_i$ transient probably reflects a greater release of Ca^{2+} from intracellular stores. The most likely mechanism is as follows (see also Ch. 4).

1. Glycosides inhibit the Na⁺/K⁺ pump.
2. Increased $[Na^+]_i$ slows extrusion of Ca^{2+} via the Na⁺/Ca²⁺ exchange transporter. Increasing $[Na^+]_i$ reduces the inwardly directed gradient for Na⁺; the smaller this gradient, the slower is extrusion of Ca^{2+} by Na⁺/Ca²⁺ exchange.
3. Increased $[Ca^{2+}]_i$ is stored in the sarcoplasmic reticulum, and thus increases the amount of Ca^{2+} released by each action potential.

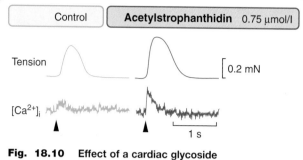
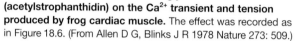

Fig. 18.10 Effect of a cardiac glycoside (acetylstrophanthidin) on the Ca^{2+} transient and tension produced by frog cardiac muscle. The effect was recorded as in Figure 18.6. (From Allen D G, Blinks J R 1978 Nature 273: 509.)

The effect of extracellular potassium

Effects of cardiac glycosides are increased if plasma [K⁺] decreases, because of reduced competition at the K⁺-binding site on the Na⁺/K⁺ ATPase. This is clinically important, because diuretics (Ch. 24) are often used to treat heart failure, and most of them decrease plasma [K⁺], thereby increasing the risk of glycoside-induced dysrhythmia.

Pharmacokinetic aspects

Digoxin is administered by mouth or, in urgent situations, intravenously. It is a very polar molecule; elimination is mainly by renal excretion and involves P-glycoprotein (p. 102), leading to clinically significant interactions with other drugs used to treat heart failure, such as **spironolactone**, and with antidysrhythmic drugs such as **verapamil** and **amiodarone**. Elimination half-time is approximately 36 hours in patients with normal renal function, but considerably longer in elderly patients and those with overt renal failure, in whom reduced doses are needed. A loading dose is used in urgent situations. The therapeutic range of plasma concentrations, below which digoxin is unlikely to be effective and above which the risk of toxicity increases substantially, is fairly well defined (1–2.6 nmol/l). Determination of plasma digoxin concentration is useful when lack of efficacy or toxicity is suspected.

Clinical use

Clinical uses of digoxin are summarised in the clinical box.

OTHER DRUGS THAT INCREASE MYOCARDIAL CONTRACTILITY

Certain β₁-adrenoceptor agonists, for example **dobutamine**, are used to treat acute but potentially reversible heart failure (e.g. following cardiac surgery or in some cases of cardiogenic or septic shock) on the basis of their positive inotropic action. Dobutamine, for reasons that are not well understood, produces less tachycardia than other β₁ agonists. It is administered intravenously. **Glucagon** also increases myocardial contractility by increasing synthesis of cAMP, and has been used in patients with acute cardiac dysfunction owing to overdosage of β-adrenoceptor antagonists (see the glucagon clinical box on p. 402).

Inhibitors of the heart-specific subtype (type III) of phosphodiesterase, the enzyme responsible for the intracellular

> **Clinical uses of cardiac glycosides (e.g. digoxin)**
>
> - To slow ventricular rate in rapid persistent *atrial fibrillation*.
> - Treatment of heart failure in patients who remain symptomatic despite optimal use of diuretics and angiotensin-converting enzyme inhibitors (Ch. 19).

degradation of cAMP, increase myocardial contractility. Consequently, like β-adrenoceptor agonists, they increase intracellular cAMP but cause dysrhythmias for the same reason. Compounds in this group include **amrinone** and **milrinone**, which are chemically and pharmacologically very similar. They improve haemodynamic indices in patients with heart failure but paradoxically worsen survival, presumably because of dysrhythmias. This dichotomy has had a sobering effect on clinicians and drug regulatory authorities.

ANTIANGINAL DRUGS

The mechanism of anginal pain is discussed above (p. 285). Angina is managed by using drugs that improve perfusion of the myocardium or reduce its metabolic demand, or both. Two of the main groups of drugs, *organic nitrates* and *calcium antagonists*, are vasodilators and produce both these effects. The third group, β-adrenoceptor antagonists, slow heart rate and hence reduce metabolic demand. Organic nitrates and calcium antagonists are described below. The β-adrenoceptor antagonists are covered in Chapter 11, except for their antidysrhythmic actions, which are described above. Very recently, **ivabradine**, which slows the heart by inhibiting the sinus node I_f current (see above, p. 278) has been introduced as an alternative to β-adrenoceptor antagonists in patients in whom these are not tolerated or are contraindicated.

ORGANIC NITRATES

The ability of organic nitrates (see also Chs 17 and 19) to relieve angina was discovered by Lauder Brunton, a distinguished British physician, in 1867. He had found that angina could be partly relieved by bleeding, and also knew that **amyl nitrite**, which had been synthesised 10 years earlier, caused flushing and tachycardia, with a fall in blood pressure, when its vapour was inhaled. He thought that the effect of bleeding resulted from hypotension, and found that amyl nitrite inhalation worked much better. Amyl nitrite has now been replaced by **glyceryl trinitrate** (nitroglycerin).[5] Efforts to increase the duration of action of glyceryl trinitrate

have led to the synthesis of several related organic nitrates, of which the most important is **isosorbide mononitrate**.

Actions

Organic nitrates relax vascular and some other (e.g. oesophageal and biliary) smooth muscles. They cause marked venorelaxation, with a consequent reduction in central venous pressure (reduced preload). In healthy subjects, this reduces stroke volume. Venous pooling occurs on standing and can cause postural hypotension and dizziness. Therapeutic doses have less effect on small resistance arteries than on veins, but there is a marked effect on larger muscular arteries. This reduces pulse wave reflection from arterial branches (as appreciated in the 19th century by Murrell but neglected for many years thereafter), and consequently reduces central (aortic) pressure and cardiac afterload (see Ch. 19 for more detail on the role of these factors in determining cardiac work). The direct effect on coronary artery tone opposes coronary artery spasm in variant angina. With larger doses, resistance arteries and arterioles dilate, and arterial pressure falls. Nevertheless, coronary flow is increased as a result of coronary vasodilatation. Myocardial oxygen consumption is reduced because of the reductions in both cardiac preload and afterload. This, together with the increased coronary blood flow, causes a large increase in the oxygen content of coronary sinus blood. Studies in experimental animals have shown that glyceryl trinitrate diverts blood from normal to ischaemic areas of myocardium. The mechanism involves dilatation of collateral vessels that bypass narrowed coronary artery segments (Fig. 18.11).

▼ It is interesting to compare this effect with that of other vasodilators, notably **dipyridamole**, which dilate arterioles but not collaterals. Dipyridamole is at least as effective as nitrates in increasing coronary flow in normal subjects but actually *worsens* angina. This is probably because arterioles in an ischaemic region are fully dilated by the ischaemia, and drug-induced dilatation of the arterioles in normal areas has the effect of diverting blood away from the ischaemic areas (Fig. 18.11), producing what is termed a vascular *steal*. This effect is exploited in a pharmacological 'stress' test for coronary arterial disease, in which dipyridamole is administered intravenously to patients in whom this diagnosis is suspected but who cannot exercise, while monitoring myocardial perfusion and the ECG.

In summary, the antianginal action of nitrates involves:

- reduced cardiac oxygen consumption, secondary to reduced cardiac preload and afterload
- redistribution of coronary flow towards ischaemic areas via collaterals
- relief of coronary spasm.

In addition to its effects on smooth muscle, nitric oxide increases the rate of relaxation of *cardiac* muscle (dubbed a 'lusiotropic' action). It is probable that organic nitrates mimic this action, which could be important in patients with impaired diastolic function, a common accompaniment of hypertension and of heart failure.

Mechanism of action

Organic nitrates are metabolised with release of nitric oxide. At concentrations achieved during therapeutic use, this involves an enzymic step and possibly a reaction with tissue sulfhydryl (−SH) groups. Nitric oxide activates soluble guanylate cyclase

---

[5]Nobel discovered how to stabilise nitroglycerin with kieselguhr, enabling him to exploit its explosive properties in dynamite, the manufacture of which earned him the fortune with which he endowed the eponymous prizes.

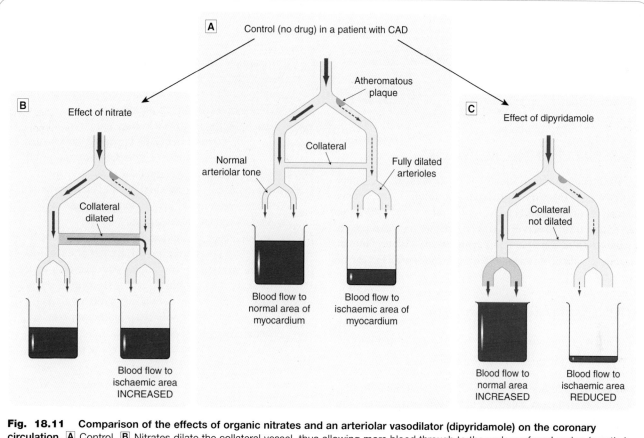

Fig. 18.11 **Comparison of the effects of organic nitrates and an arteriolar vasodilator (dipyridamole) on the coronary circulation.** A Control. B Nitrates dilate the collateral vessel, thus allowing more blood through to the underperfused region (mostly by diversion from the adequately perfused area). Dipyridamole dilates arterioles, increasing flow through the normal area at the expense of the ischaemic area (in which the arterioles are anyway fully dilated). CAD, coronary artery disease.

(see Ch. 17), increasing formation of cGMP, which activates protein kinase G and leads to a cascade of effects in smooth muscle culminating in dephosphorylation of myosin light chains and sequestration of intracellular Ca^{2+}, with consequent relaxation.

Tolerance and unwanted effects

Repeated administration of nitrates to smooth muscle preparations in vitro results in diminished relaxation, possibly partly because of depletion of free –SH groups, although attempts to prevent tolerance by agents that restore tissue –SH groups have not been clinically useful. Tolerance to the antianginal effect of nitrates does not occur to a clinically important extent with ordinary formulations of short-acting drugs (e.g. glyceryl trinitrate), but does occur with longer-acting drugs (e.g. isosorbide mononitrate) or when glyceryl trinitrate is administered by prolonged intravenous infusion or by frequent application of slow-release transdermal patches (see below).

The main adverse effects of nitrates are a direct consequence of their main pharmacological actions, and include postural hypotension and headache. This was the cause of 'Monday morning sickness' among workers in explosives factories. Tolerance to these effects develops quite quickly but wears off after a brief nitrate-free interval (which is why the symptoms appeared on Mondays and not later in the week). Formation of methaemoglobin, an oxidation product of haemoglobin that is ineffective as an oxygen carrier, seldom occurs when nitrates are used clinically but is induced deliberately with **amyl nitrite** in the treatment of cyanide poisoning, because methaemoglobin binds cyanide ions.

Pharmacokinetic and pharmaceutical aspects

Glyceryl trinitrate is rapidly inactivated by hepatic metabolism. It is well absorbed from the mouth and is taken as a tablet under the tongue or as a sublingual spray, producing its effects within a few minutes. If swallowed, it is ineffective because of first-pass metabolism. Given sublingually, the trinitrate is converted to di- and mononitrates. Its effective duration of action is approximately 30 minutes. It is quite well absorbed through the skin, and a more sustained effect can be achieved by applying it as a transdermal patch. Once a bottle of the tablets has been opened, its shelf life is quite short because the volatile active substance evaporates; spray preparations avoid this problem.

Isosorbide mononitrate is longer acting than glyceryl trinitrate (half-life approximately 4 hours) but has similar pharmacological actions. It is swallowed rather than taken sublingually, and is taken twice a day for prophylaxis (usually in the morning and at lunch, to allow a nitrate-free period during the night, when patients are not exerting themselves, to avoid tolerance). It is also available in slow-release form for once-daily use in the morning.

Clinical use

The clinical use of organic nitrates is summarised in the clinical box.

POTASSIUM CHANNEL ACTIVATORS

Nicorandil combines activation of the potassium K_{ATP} channel (see Chs 4 and 26) with nitrovasodilator (nitric oxide donor) actions. It is both an arterial and a venous dilator, and causes the expected unwanted effects of headache, flushing and dizziness. It is used for patients who remain symptomatic despite optimal management with other drugs, often while they await surgery or angioplasty.

β-ADRENOCEPTOR ANTAGONISTS

β-Adrenoceptor antagonists (see Ch. 11) are important in prophylaxis of angina, and in treating patients with unstable angina. They work for these indications by reducing cardiac oxygen consumption. In addition, they reduce the risk of death following myocardial infarction, probably via their antidysrhythmic action. Their effects on coronary vessels are of minor importance, although these drugs are avoided in variant angina because of the theoretical risk that they will increase coronary spasm. Their very diverse clinical uses are summarised in the clinical box on p. 182.

CALCIUM ANTAGONISTS

The term *calcium antagonists* is often used for drugs that block cellular entry of Ca^{2+} through calcium channels rather than its intracellular actions (Ch. 4). Some authors use the term Ca^{2+} *entry blockers* to make this distinction clearer. Therapeutically important calcium antagonists act on L-type channels. L-type calcium antagonists comprise three chemically distinct classes: *phenylalkylamines* (e.g. **verapamil**), *dihydropyridines* (e.g. **nifedipine**, **amlodipine**) and *benzothiazepines* (e.g. **diltiazem**).

Mechanism of action: types of calcium channel

The properties of voltage-gated calcium channels have been studied in great detail by voltage-clamp and patch clamp techniques (see Ch. 2). Drugs of each of the three chemical classes mentioned above all bind the α_1 subunit of the cardiac L-type calcium channel but at distinct sites, which interact allosterically with each other and with the gating machinery of the channel to prevent its opening (see below), thus reducing Ca^{2+} entry. Many calcium antagonists show properties of use dependence (i.e. they block more effectively in those cells in which the calcium channels are most active; see the discussion of class I antidysrhythmic drugs above). For the same reason, they also show voltage-dependent blocking actions, blocking more strongly when the membrane is depolarised, causing calcium channel opening and inactivation.

Organic nitrates

- Important compounds include **glyceryl trinitrate** and longer-acting **isosorbide mononitrate**.
- These drugs are powerful vasodilators, acting on veins to reduce cardiac preload and reducing arterial wave reflection to reduce afterload.
- Act via nitric oxide, to which they are metabolised. Nitric oxide stimulates cGMP formation and hence activates protein kinase G, affecting both contractile proteins (myosin light chains) and Ca^{2+} regulation.
- Tolerance occurs experimentally and is important clinically with frequent use of long-acting drugs or sustained-release preparations.
- Effectiveness in angina results partly from reduced cardiac load and partly from dilatation of collateral coronary vessels, causing more effective distribution of coronary flow. Dilatation of constricted coronary vessels is particularly beneficial in variant angina.
- Serious unwanted effects are uncommon; headache and postural hypotension may occur initially. Overdose can, rarely, cause methaemoglobinaemia.

Clinical uses of organic nitrates

- *Stable angina*:
  - prevention (e.g. daily **isosorbide mononitrate**, or **glyceryl trinitrate** sublingually immediately before exertion)
  - treatment (sublingual glyceryl trinitrate).
- *Unstable angina*: intravenous glyceryl trinitrate
- *Acute heart failure*: intravenous glyceryl trinitrate
- *Chronic heart failure*: isosorbide mononitrate, with hydralazine in patients of African origin (Ch. 19).
- Uses related to relaxation of other smooth muscles (e.g. uterine, biliary) are being investigated.

▼ Dihydropyridines affect calcium channel function in a complex way, not simply by physical plugging of the pore. This became clear when some dihydropyridines, exemplified by BAY K 8644, were found to bind to the same site but to act in the converse way; that is, to promote the opening of voltage-gated calcium channels. Thus BAY K 8644 produces effects opposite to those of the clinically used dihydropyridines, namely an increase in the force of cardiac contraction, and constriction of blood vessels; it is competitively antagonised by nifedipine. Studies on the response of single calcium channels to a step depolarisation of the membrane suggest that channels can exist in one of three distinct states, termed 'modes' (Fig. 18.12). When a channel is in mode 0, it does not open in response to depolarisation; in mode 1, depolarisation produces a low opening probability, and each opening is brief. In mode 2, depolarisation produces a very high opening probability, and single openings are prolonged. Under normal conditions, about 70% of the channels at any one moment exist in mode 1, with only 1% or less in mode 2; each channel switches randomly and quite slowly between the

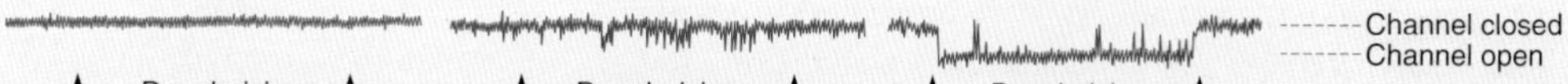

Mode	Mode 0	Mode 1	Mode 2	
	▲—Depolarising—▲ step	▲—Depolarising—▲ step	▲—Depolarising—▲ step	---- Channel closed ---- Channel open
Opening probability	Zero	Low	High	
Favoured by	DHP antagonists		DHP agonists	
% of time normally spent in this mode	<1%	~70%	~30%	

Fig. 18.12 **Mode behaviour of calcium channels.** The traces are patch clamp recordings (see Ch. 2) of the opening of single calcium channels (downward deflections) in a patch of membrane from a cardiac muscle cell. A depolarising step is imposed close to the start of each trace, causing an increase in the opening probability of the channel. When the channel is in mode 1 (centre), this causes a few brief openings to occur; in mode 2 (right), the channel stays open for most of the time during the depolarising step; in mode 0 (left), it fails to open at all. Under normal conditions, the channel spends most of its time in modes 1 and 2, and only rarely enters mode 0. (Redrawn from Hess et al. 1984 Nature 311: 538–544.)

three modes. Dihydropyridines of the antagonist type bind selectively to channels in mode 0, thus favouring this non-opening state, whereas agonists bind selectively to channels in mode 2 (Fig. 18.12). This type of two-directional modulation resembles the phenomenon seen with the GABA/benzodiazepine interaction (Ch. 37), and invites speculation about possible endogenous dihydropyridine-like mediator(s) with a regulatory effect on Ca^{2+} entry.

Mibefradil is distinctive in that it blocks T- as well as L-type channels at therapeutic concentrations, but it was withdrawn from therapeutic use because it caused adverse drug interactions by interfering with drug metabolism.

Pharmacological effects

The main effects of calcium antagonists, as used therapeutically, are on cardiac and smooth muscle. **Verapamil** preferentially affects the heart, whereas most of the dihydropyridines (e.g. **nifedipine**) exert a greater effect on smooth muscle than on the heart. **Diltiazem** is intermediate in its actions.

Cardiac actions

The antidysrhythmic effects of **verapamil** and **diltiazem** have been discussed above. Calcium antagonists can cause AV block and cardiac slowing by their actions on conducting tissues, but this is offset by a reflex increase in sympathetic activity secondary to their vasodilator action. For example, **nifedipine** typically causes reflex tachycardia; **diltiazem** causes little or no change in heart rate and **verapamil** slows the heart rate. Calcium antagonists also have a negative inotropic effect, which results from the inhibition of the slow inward current during the action potential plateau. Despite this, the cardiac output usually stays constant or increases because of the reduction in peripheral resistance. Again, there are clinically important differences between the different classes of drug, with verapamil having the most marked negative inotropic action, and therefore being contraindicated in heart failure, as are most other calcium antagonists, although amlodipine does not worsen cardiovascular mortality in patients with severe chronic heart failure.

Vascular smooth muscle

Calcium antagonists cause generalised arterial/arteriolar dilatation, thereby reducing blood pressure, but do not much affect the veins. They affect all vascular beds, although regional effects vary considerably between different drugs. They cause coronary vasodilatation and are used in patients with coronary artery spasm (variant angina). Other types of smooth muscle (e.g. biliary tract, urinary tract and uterus) are also relaxed by calcium antagonists, but these effects are less important therapeutically than their actions on vascular smooth muscle, although they do cause adverse effects (see below).

Protection of ischaemic tissues

There are theoretical reasons (see Fig. 18.8) why calcium antagonists might exert a cytoprotective effect in ischaemic tissues and thus be of use in treating heart attack and stroke (see Ch. 35). However, randomised clinical trials have been disappointing, with little or no evidence of beneficial (or harmful) effects of calcium antagonists on cardiovascular morbidity or mortality in patient groups other than patients with hypertension, in whom calcium antagonists have beneficial effects comparable with those of other drugs that lower blood pressure to similar extents. **Nimodipine** has some selectivity for cerebral vasculature and is sometimes used in the hope of reducing cerebral vasospasm following subarachnoid haemorrhage.

Pharmacokinetics

Calcium antagonists in clinical use are all well absorbed from the gastrointestinal tract, and are given by mouth except for some special indications, such as following subarachnoid haemorrhage, for which intravenous preparations are available. They are extensively metabolised. Pharmacokinetic differences between different drugs and different pharmaceutical preparations are clinically important, because they determine the dose interval and also the intensity of some of the unwanted effects, such as headache and flushing (see below). Amlodipine has a long elimination half-life and is given once daily, whereas nifedipine, diltiazem and verapamil have shorter elimination half-lives and are either given more frequently or are formulated in various slow-release preparations to permit once-daily dosing.

Unwanted effects

Most of the unwanted effects of calcium antagonists are extensions of their main pharmacological actions. Short-acting dihydropyridines cause flushing and headache because of their vasodilator action, and in chronic use dihydropyridines often cause ankle swelling related to arteriolar dilatation and increased permeability of postcapillary venules. Verapamil can cause constipation, probably because of effects on calcium channels in gastrointestinal nerves or smooth muscle. Effects on cardiac rhythm (e.g. heart block) and force of contraction (e.g. worsening heart failure) are discussed above.

Apart from these predictable effects, calcium channel antagonists, as a class, appear rather free from idiosyncratic adverse effects.

Clinical uses

The main clinical uses of calcium antagonists are summarised in the clinical box below.

Calcium antagonists

- Block Ca^{2+} entry by preventing opening of voltage-gated L-type calcium channels.
- There are three main L-type antagonists, typified by verapamil, diltiazem and dihydropyridines (e.g. nifedipine).
- Mainly affect heart and smooth muscle, inhibiting the Ca^{2+} entry caused by depolarisation in these tissues.
- Selectivity between heart and smooth muscle varies: verapamil is relatively cardioselective, nifedipine is relatively smooth muscle–selective, and diltiazem is intermediate.
- Vasodilator effect (mainly dihydropyridines) is mainly on resistance vessels, reducing afterload. Calcium antagonists dilate coronary vessels, which is important in variant angina.
- Effects on heart (verapamil, diltiazem): antidysrhythmic action (mainly atrial tachycardias), because of impaired atrioventricular conduction; reduced contractility.
- Clinical uses:
  — antidysrhythmic (mainly verapamil)
  — angina (e.g. diltiazem)
  — hypertension (mainly dihydropyridines).
- Unwanted effects include headache, constipation (verapamil) and ankle oedema (dihydropyridines). There is a risk of causing cardiac failure or heart block, especially with verapamil.

Clinical uses of calcium antagonists

- Dysrhythmias (**verapamil**):
  — to slow ventricular rate in rapid *atrial fibrillation*
  — to prevent recurrence of *supraventricular tachycardia* (*SVT*) (intravenous administration of verapamil to terminate SVT attacks has been replaced by use of adenosine).
- *Hypertension*: usually a dihydropyridine drug (e.g. **amlodipine** or slow-release **nifedipine**; Ch. 19).
- To prevent *angina* (e.g. dihydropyridine or **diltiazem**).

REFERENCES AND FURTHER READING

Further reading

Braunwald E 2005 Cardiology: how did we get here, where are we today and where are we going? Can J Cardiol 21: 1015–1017

Braunwald E, Opie L H 2001 Drugs for the heart. Saunders, Philadelphia

Vaughan Williams E M 1989 Classification of antiarrhythmic actions. In: Vaughan Williams E M (ed) Antiarrhythmic drugs. Handbook of experimental pharmacology, vol. 89. Springer-Verlag, Berlin (*For a different approach see Circulation 1994, 84: 1848*)

Zipes D, Jalife J 2004 Cardiac electrophysiology: from cell to bedside, 4th edn. Saunders, Philadelphia (*Comprehensive textbook*)

Specific aspects

Physiological and pathophysiological aspects

Ingwall J S 2004 Transgenesis and cardiac energetics: new insights into cardiac metabolism. J Mol Cell Cardiol 37: 613–623

Linden J 2001 Molecular approach to adenosine receptors: receptor-mediated mechanisms of tissue protection. Annu Rev Pharmacol Toxicol 41: 775–787 (*Adenosine in cardiac ischaemicpreconditioning*)

Opie L H 1999 Cardiac metabolism in ischemic heart disease. Arch Mal Coeur Vaiss 92: 1755–1760

Rockman H A, Koch W J, Lefkowitz R J 2002 Seven-transmembrane–spanning receptors and heart function. Nature 415: 206–212

Saurin A T, Rakhit R D, Marber M S 2000 Therapeutic potential of ischaemic preconditioning. Br J Clin Pharmacol 50: 87–97 (*Adenosine etc.*)

Schoner W 2002 Endogenous cardiac glycosides, a new class of steroid hormones. Eur J Biochem 269: 2440–2448

Trochu J N, Bouhour J B, Kaley G, Hintze T H 2000 Role of endothelium-derived nitric oxide in the regulation of cardiac oxygen metabolism—implications in health and disease. Circ Res 87: 1108–1117 (*Evaluates the role of nitric oxide in the control of mitochondrial respiration, with special emphasis on its effect on cardiac metabolism*)

Welsh M J, Hoshi T 1995 Molecular cardiology—ion channels lose the rhythm. Nature 376: 640–641 (*Commentary on Ward–Romano syndrome*)

Winslow R L, Cortassa S, Greenstein J L 2005 Using models of the myocyte for functional interpretation of cardiac proteomic data. J Physiol (Lond) 563: 73–81 (*Shows how altered expression of sarcoplasmic reticulum Ca^{2+} ATPase influences cardiac action potential duration, and how phosphorylation of L-type calcium channels affects the properties of excitation–contraction coupling and risk for arrhythmia, using a computational model*)

Pathological aspects

Falk R H 2001 Atrial fibrillation. N Engl J Med 344: 1067–1078

Therapeutic aspects

Camm A J, Garratt C J 1991 Adenosine and supraventricular tachycardia. N Engl J Med 325: 1621–1628 (*Discusses its role as an endogenous mediator and its pharmacology and clinical use*)

COMMIT Collaborative Group 2005 Early intravenous then oral metoprolol in 45,852 patients with acute myocardial infarction: randomised placebo-controlled trial. Lancet 366: 1622–1632 (*Early β blockade reduced ventricular fibrillation and reinfarction, benefits that were offset by increased cardiogenic shock in patients with signs of heart failure; see*

accompanying comment by Sabatine M S, pp. 1587–1589 in the same issue)

Digitalis Investigation Group 1997 The effect of digoxin on mortality and morbidity in patients with heart failure. N Engl J Med 336: 525–533 (*Digoxin did not affect overall mortality, but reduced hospitalisations over an average follow-up of approximately 3 years—the inference is that it improves symptoms*)

ISIS-4 Collaborative Group 1995 ISIS-4: a randomised factorial trial assessing early oral captopril, oral mononitrate, and intravenous magnesium sulphate in 58 050 patients with suspected acute myocardial infarction. Lancet 345: 669–685 (*Impressive trial: disappointing results! Magnesium was ineffective; oral nitrate did not reduce 1-month mortality*)

Kochegarov A A 2003 Pharmacological modulators of voltage-gated calcium channels and their therapeutical application. Cell Calcium 33: 145–162

Lee L, Horowitz J, Frenneaux M 2004 Metabolic manipulation in ischaemic heart disease, a novel approach to treatment. Eur Heart J 25: 634–641 (*Reviews four metabolic antianginal drugs: perhexiline, trimetazidine, ranolazine and etomoxir*)

Marzilli M 2003 Cardioprotective effects of trimetazidine: a review. Curr Med Res Opin 19: 661–672 (*Reviews metabolic effects of this 3-ketoacyl-CoA thiolase inhibitor and its lack of haemodynamic effects in stable angina pectoris*)

Podrid P J 1999 Redefining the role of antiarrhythmic drugs. N Engl J Med 340: 1910–1911 (*Discusses studies with ibutilide and sotalol, which 'highlight what may become the primary indication for anti-arrhythmic drug therapy; as an adjunct to non-pharmacologic therapy for relief of symptoms and improvement in the quality of life.'*)

Prospective Randomised Amlodipine Survival Evaluation Study Group 1996 Effect of amlodipine on morbidity and mortality in severe chronic heart failure. N Engl J Med 335: 1107–1114 (*No adverse or beneficial effect on survival in the group as a whole*)

Rahimtoola S H 2004 Digitalis therapy for patients in clinical heart failure. Circulation 109: 2942–2946 (*Review*)

Roden D M 2004 Drug therapy: drug-induced prolongation of the QT interval. N Engl J Med 350: 1013–1022 (*Adverse effect of great concern in drug development; see also Ch 53*)

Roy D, Talajic M, Dorian P et al. 2000 Amiodarone to prevent recurrence of atrial fibrillation. N Engl J Med 342: 913–920 (*Low-dose amiodarone was more effective than sotalol or propafenone*)

Ruskin J N 1989 The cardiac arrhythmia suppression trial (CAST). N Engl J Med 321: 386–388 (*Enormously influential trial showing increased mortality with active treatment despite suppression of dysrhythmia*)

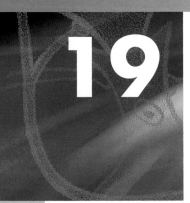

19

The vascular system

OVERVIEW

This chapter is concerned with the pharmacology of blood vessels. The walls of arteries, arterioles, venules and veins contain smooth muscle whose contractile state is controlled by circulating hormones and by mediators released locally from sympathetic nerve terminals (Ch. 9) and endothelial cells. These work mainly by regulating Ca^{2+} in vascular smooth muscle cells, as described in Chapter 4. In the present chapter, we first consider the control of vascular smooth muscle by the endothelium and by the renin–angiotensin system, followed by the actions of vasoconstrictor and vasodilator drugs. Finally, we briefly consider clinical uses of vasoactive drugs in some important diseases, namely hypertension (pulmonary as well as systemic), heart failure, shock, peripheral vascular disease and Raynaud's disease. The use of vasoactive drugs to treat angina is covered in Chapter 18.

VASCULAR STRUCTURE AND FUNCTION

Blood is ejected with each heartbeat from the left ventricle into the aorta, whence it flows rapidly to the organs via large conduit arteries. Successive branching leads via muscular arteries to arterioles (endothelium surrounded by a layer of smooth muscle only one cell thick) and capillaries, where gas and nutrient exchanges occur. Capillaries coalesce to form postcapillary venules, venules and progressively larger veins leading, via the vena cava, to the right heart. Deoxygenated blood ejected from the right ventricle travels through the pulmonary artery, pulmonary capillaries and pulmonary veins back to the left atrium.[1] Small muscular arteries and arterioles are the main resistance vessels, while veins are capacity vessels that contain a large fraction of the total blood volume. In terms of cardiac function, therefore, arteries and arterioles regulate the *afterload*, while veins and pulmonary vessels regulate the *preload* of the ventricles.

Viscoelastic properties of large arteries determine arterial compliance (i.e. the degree to which the volume of the arterial system increases as the pressure increases). This is an important factor in a circulatory system that is driven by an intermittent pump such as the heart. Blood ejected from the left ventricle is accommodated, in the first instance, by distension of the aorta, which absorbs the pulsations and delivers a relatively steady flow to the tissues. The greater the compliance of the aorta, the more effectively are fluctuations damped out,[2] and the smaller the oscillations of arterial pressure with each heartbeat (i.e. the difference between the systolic and diastolic pressure, known as the 'pulse pressure'). Reflection of the pressure wave from branch points in the vascular tree also sustains arterial pressure during diastole. In young people, this helps to preserve a steady perfusion of vital organs, such as the kidney, during diastole. However, excessive reflection can pathologically augment aortic systolic pressure.

---

[1]William Harvey (physician to King Charles I) inferred the circulation of the blood on the basis of superbly elegant quantitative experiments long before the invention of the microscope enabled visual confirmation of the tiny vessels he had predicted. This intellectual triumph did his medical standing no good at all, and Aubrey wrote that 'he fell mightily in his practice, and was regarded by the vulgar as crack-brained'. Plus ça change...

[2]This cushioning action is called the 'windkessel' effect. The same principle was used to deliver a steady rather than intermittent flow from old-fashioned fire pumps.

This results from stiffening of the aorta due to loss of elastin during ageing, especially in people with hypertension. Elastin is replaced by inelastic collagen. Cardiac work (see Ch. 18) can be reduced by increasing arterial compliance or by reducing arterial wave reflection, even if the cardiac output and mean arterial pressure are unchanged. Over around 55 years of age, pulse pressure and aortic stiffness are important risk factors for cardiac disease.

Actions of drugs on the vascular system can be broken down into effects on:

- total systemic ('peripheral') vascular resistance, which is one of the main determinants of arterial pressure and is relevant to the treatment of hypertension
- the resistance of individual vascular beds, which determines the local distribution of blood flow to and within different organs; such effects are relevant to the drug treatment of angina (Ch. 18), Raynaud's phenomenon, pulmonary hypertension and circulatory shock
- aortic compliance and pulse wave reflection, which are relevant to the treatment of cardiac failure and angina
- venous tone and blood volume (the 'fullness' of the circulation), which together determine the central venous pressure and are relevant to the treatment of cardiac failure and angina; diuretics (which reduce blood volume) are discussed in Chapter 24
- atheroma (Ch. 20) and thrombosis (Ch. 21).

CONTROL OF VASCULAR SMOOTH MUSCLE TONE

Like other muscle cells, vascular smooth muscle contracts when $[Ca^{2+}]_i$ rises, but the coupling between $[Ca^{2+}]_i$ and contraction is less tight than in striated or cardiac muscle (Ch. 4). Vasoconstrictors and vasodilators act by increasing or reducing $[Ca^{2+}]_i$, and/or by altering the sensitivity of the contractile machinery to $[Ca^{2+}]_i$. Figure 4.10 (p. 67) summarises cellular mechanisms that are involved in the control of smooth muscle contraction and relaxation.

THE VASCULAR ENDOTHELIUM

A new chapter in our understanding of vascular control opened with the discovery that vascular endothelium acts not only as a passive barrier between plasma and extracellular fluid, but also as a source of numerous potent mediators. These actively control the contraction of the underlying smooth muscle as well as influencing platelet and mononuclear cell function: the roles of the endothelium in haemostasis and thrombosis are discussed in Chapter 21. Several distinct classes of mediator are involved (Fig. 19.1).

- *Prostanoids* (see Ch. 13). The discovery by Bunting, Gryglewski, Moncada & Vane (1976) of *prostaglandin (PG) I_2* (also known as prostacyclin) ushered in this era. This mediator, acting on I prostanoid receptors (Ch. 13), relaxes smooth muscle and inhibits platelet aggregation by activating adenylate cyclase. Endothelial cells from microvessels synthesise PGE_2, which is a direct vasodilator and also

> **Vascular smooth muscle**
>
> - Vascular smooth muscle is controlled by mediators secreted by sympathetic nerves (Chs 9 and 11) and vascular endothelium, and by circulating hormones.
> - Smooth muscle cell contraction is initiated by a rise in $[Ca^{2+}]_i$, which activates myosin light-chain kinase, causing phosphorylation of myosin, or by sensitisation of the myofilaments to Ca^{2+} by inhibition of myosin phosphatase (see Ch. 4).
> - Agents cause contraction via one or more mechanism:
>   - release of intracellular Ca^{2+} via inositol trisphosphate
>   - depolarising the membrane, opening voltage-gated calcium channels and causing Ca^{2+} entry
>   - increasing sensitivity to Ca^{2+} via actions on myosin light-chain kinase and/or myosin phosphatase (Ch. 4, Fig. 4.9)
> - Agents cause relaxation by:
>   - inhibiting Ca^{2+} entry through voltage-gated calcium channels either directly (e.g. **nifedipine**) or indirectly by hyperpolarising the membrane (e.g. potassium channel activators such as **cromakalim**)
>   - increasing intracellular cAMP or cGMP; cAMP inactivates myosin light-chain kinase and facilitates Ca^{2+} efflux, cGMP opposes agonist-induced increases in $[Ca^{2+}]_i$.

inhibits noradrenaline (norepinephrine) release from sympathetic nerve terminals, while lacking the effect of PGI_2 on platelets. Prostaglandin endoperoxide intermediates (PGG_2, PGH_2) are endothelium-derived contracting factors acting via thromboxane (T prostanoid) receptors.

- *Nitric oxide (NO)* (see Ch. 17). Endothelium-derived relaxing factor (EDRF) was discovered by Furchgott and Zawadzki in 1980, and identified as NO by the groups of Moncada and of Ignarro (see Fig. 17.2, p. 266). These discoveries enormously expanded our understanding of the role of the endothelium. NO activates guanylate cyclase. It is released continuously in resistance vessels, giving rise to vasodilator tone and contributing to the physiological control of blood pressure. As well as causing vascular relaxation, it inhibits vascular smooth muscle cell proliferation, inhibits platelet adhesion and aggregation, and inhibits monocyte adhesion and migration; consequently, it may protect blood vessels from atherosclerosis and thrombosis (see Chs 20 and 21).

- *Peptides.* The endothelium secretes several vasoactive peptides. *C-natriuretic peptide* (Ch. 18, p. 285) and *adrenomedulin* (a vasodilator peptide originally discovered in an adrenal tumour—phaeochromocytoma—but expressed in many tissues, including vascular endothelium) are vasodilators

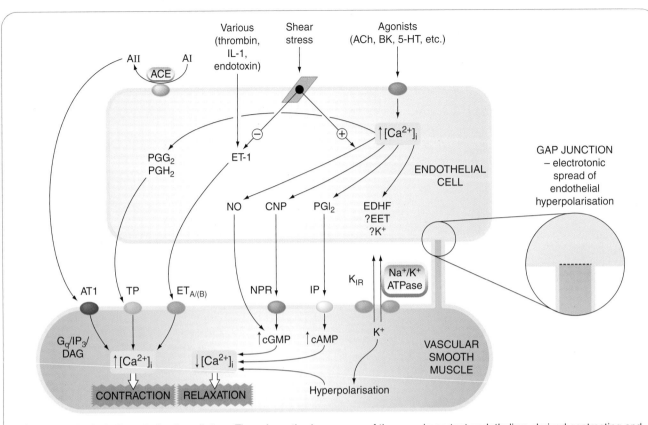

Fig. 19.1 Endothelium-derived mediators. The schematic shows some of the more important endothelium-derived contracting and relaxing mediators; many (if not all) of the vasoconstrictors also cause smooth muscle mitogenesis, while vasodilators commonly inhibit mitogenesis. 5-HT, 5-hydroxytryptamine; A, angiotensin; ACE, angiotensin-converting enzyme; ACh, acetylcholine; AT_1, angiotensin AT_1 receptor; BK, bradykinin; CNP, C-natriuretic peptide; DAG, diacylglycerol; EDHF, endothelium-derived hyperpolarising factor; EET, epoxyeicosatetraenoic acid; ET-1, endothelin-1; $ET_{A/(B)}$, endothelium A (and B) receptors; G_q, G-protein; IL-1, interleukin-1; IP, I prostanoid receptor; IP_3, inosinol 1,4,5-trisphosphate; K_{IR}, inward rectifying potassium channel; Na^+/K^+ ATPase, electrogenic pump; NPR, natriuretic peptide receptor; PG, prostaglandin; TP, T prostanoid receptor.

working, respectively, through cGMP and cAMP. *Angiotensin II*, formed by *angiotensin-converting enzyme (ACE)* on the surface of endothelial cells (see below), and *endothelin* are potent endothelium-derived vasoconstrictor peptides.

- *Endothelium-derived hyperpolarising factor(s) (EDHFs).* Endothelium-dependent dilatation in response to several mediators (including acetylcholine and bradykinin) persists in some vessels despite complete inhibition of prostaglandin and NO synthesis. Such relaxation is accompanied by endothelium-dependent hyperpolarisation of vascular smooth muscle, and is abolished by an unusual combination of Ca^{2+}-dependent potassium channel–blocking toxins (*apamin* plus *charybdotoxin*), but not by these toxins individually. Such hyperpolarising/relaxant responses are caused by EDHFs distinct from prostanoids and NO.[3] EDHF becomes progressively important, compared with NO, in progressively smaller arteries. Its chemical identity (or identities) remains elusive, but there are currently three main contenders, which

are not necessarily mutually exclusive. These are (i) epoxyeicosanoids synthesised from arachidonic acid by an isoform of cytochrome P450; (ii) electrotonic spread of hyperpolarisation from endothelium to vascular smooth muscle by gap junctions; and (iii) K^+ released from endothelium, which paradoxically hyperpolarises vascular smooth muscle by activating inwardly rectifying potassium channels (which can be blocked by barium ions) and an electrogenic Na^+/K^+ pump (which can be blocked by **ouabain** or other cardiac glycosides; p. 291).

In addition to secreting this array of vasoactive mediators, endothelial cells express several enzymes and transport mechanisms on their plasma membranes that act on circulating hormones and are important targets of drug action. ACE is a particularly important example (see below).

Many endothelium-derived mediators are mutually antagonistic, conjuring an image of opposing rugby football players swaying back and forth in a scrum; in moments of exasperation, one sometimes wonders whether all this makes sense or whether the designer simply could not make up his mind! An important distinction is made between mechanisms that are tonically active

---

[3]Confusingly, PGI_2 and NO do each hyperpolarise vascular smooth muscle, and this can contribute to their relaxant effects.

in resistance vessels under basal conditions, as is the case with the *noradrenergic nervous system* (Ch. 11), NO (Ch. 17), and possibly *endothelin*, and those that operate mainly in response to injury, inflammation, etc., as with PGI$_2$. Some of the latter group may be functionally redundant, perhaps representing vestiges of mechanisms that were important to our evolutionary forebears, or they may simply be taking a breather on the touchline and are ready to rejoin the fray if called on by the occurrence of some vascular insult. Evidence for such a 'back-up' role comes, for example, from mice that lack the I prostanoid receptor for PGI$_2$, and that have a normal blood pressure and do not develop spontaneous thrombosis, but are more susceptible to vasoconstrictor and thrombotic stimuli than their wild-type litter mates (Murata et al., 1997). Such redundancy complicates interpretation of experiments using mutant gene 'knockout' animals. For example, whereas acetylcholine relaxes arterioles (from muscle) of wild-type mice mainly by releasing NO, it also relaxes vessels from 'eNOS knockout' mice (which lack the gene for the endothelial NO synthase, eNOS) by releasing EDHF in place of NO.

The endothelium in angiogenesis

As touched on in Chapter 7 (pp. 98-99), the barrier function of vascular endothelium differs markedly in different organs, and its development during angiogenesis is controlled by several growth factors, including non-specific ones such as vascular endothelial growth factor (VEGF) and tissue-specific factors such as endocrine gland VEGF. These are involved in repair processes but also in pathological situations, including tumour growth and neovascularisation in the eye (an important cause of blindness in patients with diabetes mellitus). These factors and their receptors are potentially fruitful targets for drug development and new therapies (including gene therapies; Ch. 55, p. 773).

ENDOTHELIN

Discovery, biosynthesis and secretion

Hickey et al. described a vasoconstrictor factor produced by cultured endothelial cells in 1985. This was identified as endothelin, a 21-residue peptide, by Yanagisawa et al. (1988), who achieved the isolation, analysis and cloning of the gene for this peptide in an impressively short space of time.

▼ Three genes encode different sequences (ET-1, ET-2 and ET-3), each with a distinctive 'shepherd's crook' structure produced by two internal disulfide bonds. These isoforms are differently expressed in organs such as brain and adrenal glands (Table 19.1), suggesting that endothelins have functions beyond the cardiovascular system, and this is supported by observations of mice in which the gene coding for ET-1 is disrupted (see below). ET-1 is the only endothelin present in endothelial cells, and is also expressed in many other tissues. Its synthesis and actions are summarised schematically in Figure 19.2. ET-2 is much less widely distributed: it is present in kidney and intestine. ET-3 is present in brain, lung, intestine and adrenal gland. ET-1 is synthesised from a 212-residue precursor molecule (prepro-ET), which is processed to 'big ET-1' and finally cleaved by an endothelin-converting enzyme to yield ET-1. Cleavage occurs not at the usual Lys–Arg or Arg–Arg position, but at a Trp–Val pair, implying a very atypical endopeptidase. The converting enzyme is a metalloprotease and is inhibited by **phosphoramidon**. Big ET-1 is converted to ET-1 intracellularly and also on the surface of endothelial and smooth muscle cells.

Table 19.1 Distribution of endothelins and endothelin receptors in various tissues[a]

Tissues	Endothelin			Endothelin receptor	
	1	**2**	**3**	**ET$_A$**	**ET$_B$**
Vascular tissue					
Endothelium	++++				+
Smooth muscle	+			++	
Brain	+++		+	+	+++
Kidney	++	++	+	+	++
Intestines	+	+	+++	+	+++
Adrenal gland	+		+++	+	++

[a]Levels of expression of endothelins or the receptor mRNA and/or immunoreactive endothelins: ++++, highest; +++, high; ++, moderate; +, low.
(Adapted from: Masaki T 1993 Endocr Rev 14: 256–268.)

Stimuli to endothelin synthesis include many noxious vasoconstrictor mediators released by trauma or inflammation, including activated platelets, endotoxin, thrombin, various cytokines and growth factors, angiotensin II, antidiuretic hormone (ADH) (arginine–vasopressin), adrenaline (epinephrine), insulin, hypoxia and low shear stress. Inhibitors of ET synthesis include NO, natriuretic peptides, PGE$_2$, PGI$_2$, heparin and high shear stress. It was originally believed that ET-1 is generated entirely *de novo* and not stored intracellularly, but secretion of ET-1 can occur more rapidly (e.g. in response to stretch) than would be expected if it were always freshly synthesised, and there is evidence that preformed ET-1 can be stored in endothelial cells, although probably not in granules. Release mechanisms of such stored ET-1 are poorly understood. ET-1 concentration in plasma is low (< 5 pmol/l) compared with concentrations that activate endothelin receptors, but concentrations in the extracellular space between endothelium and vascular smooth muscle are presumably much higher, and endothelin receptor antagonists (see below) cause vasodilatation when infused directly into the brachial artery, consistent with tonic ET-1-mediated vasoconstrictor activity in resistance vasculature. ET-1 has an elimination half life of < 5 minutes, despite a much longer duration of action, and clearance occurs mainly in the lung and kidneys.

Endothelin receptors and responses

There are two types of endothelin receptor, designated ET$_A$ and ET$_B$ (Table 19.2), both of which are G-protein–coupled (Ch. 3). The predominant overall response is vasoconstriction.

▼ Endothelin-1 preferentially activates ET$_A$ receptors. Messenger RNA for the ET$_A$ receptor is expressed in many human tissues, including vascular smooth muscle, heart, lung and kidney. It is not expressed in endothelium. ET$_A$-mediated responses include *vasoconstriction, bronchoconstriction* and *aldosterone secretion*. ET$_A$ receptors are coupled to phospholipase C, which stimulates Na$^+$/H$^+$ exchange, protein kinase C and mitogenesis, as well as causing vasoconstriction through inositol trisphosphate–mediated

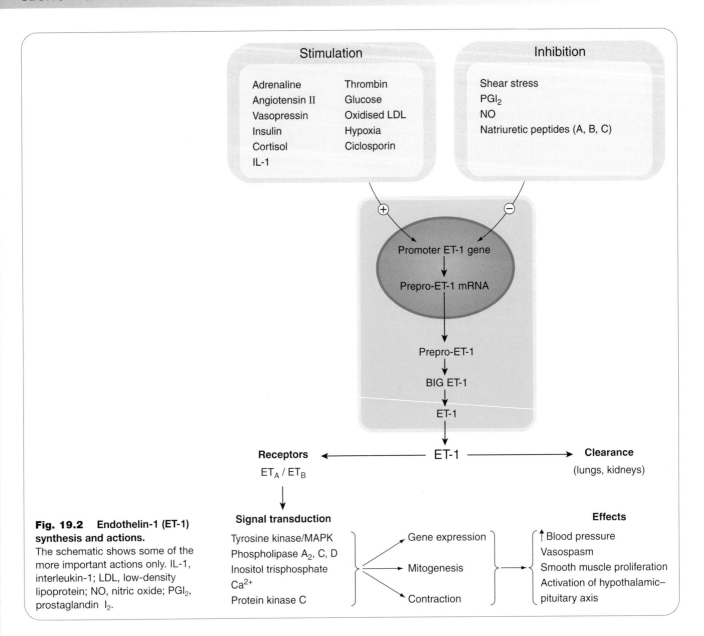

Fig. 19.2 **Endothelin-1 (ET-1) synthesis and actions.** The schematic shows some of the more important actions only. IL-1, interleukin-1; LDL, low-density lipoprotein; NO, nitric oxide; PGI$_2$, prostaglandin I$_2$.

Table 19.2 **Endothelin receptors**

Receptor	Affinity	Pharmacological response
ET$_A$	ET-1 = ET-2 > ET-3	Vasoconstriction, bronchoconstriction, stimulation of aldosterone secretion
ET$_B$	ET-1 = ET-2 = ET-3	Vasodilatation, inhibition of ex vivo platelet aggregation

(From: Masaki T 1993 Endocr Rev 14: 256–268.)

Ca^{2+} release (Ch. 3). There are several selective ET$_A$-receptor antagonists, including **BQ-123** (a cyclic pentapeptide) and several orally active non-peptide drugs (e.g. **bosentan**, a mixed ET$_A$/ET$_B$ antagonist used in treating pulmonary arterial hypertension—see below). ET$_B$ receptors are activated to a similar extent by each of the three endothelin isoforms, but **sarafotoxin S6c** (a 21-residue peptide that shares the shepherd's crook structure of the endothelins and was isolated from the venom of the burrowing asp) is a selective agonist and has proved useful as a pharmacological tool for studying the ET$_B$ receptor. Messenger RNA for the ET$_B$ receptor is mainly expressed in brain (especially cerebral cortex and cerebellum), with moderate expression in aorta, heart, lung, kidney and adrenals. In contrast to the ET$_A$ receptor, it is highly expressed in endothelium, where it may initiate *vasodilatation* by stimulating NO and PGI$_2$ production, but it is also present in vascular smooth muscle, where it initiates vasoconstriction like the ET$_A$ receptor.

Functions of endothelin

Endothelin-1 is a paracrine mediator rather than a circulating hormone, although it stimulates secretion of several hormones (see below). Administration of an ET$_A$-receptor antagonist or of

phosphoramidon into the brachial artery increases forearm blood flow, suggesting that ET-1 may contribute to vasoconstrictor tone and the control of peripheral vascular resistance (Haynes & Webb, 1994). Endothelins have several other possible functions, including roles in:

- release of various hormones, including atrial natriuretic peptide, aldosterone, adrenaline, and hypothalamic and pituitary hormones
- thyroglobulin synthesis (the concentration of ET-1 in thyroid follicles is extremely high)
- control of uteroplacental blood flow (ET-1 is present in very high concentrations in amniotic fluid)
- renal and cerebral vasospasm (Fig. 19.3)
- development of the cardiorespiratory systems (the *ET-1* gene has been disrupted experimentally; pharyngeal arch tissues develop abnormally in such mice and homozygotes die of respiratory failure at birth).

THE RENIN–ANGIOTENSIN SYSTEM

The renin–angiotensin system synergises with the sympathetic nervous system, for example by increasing the release of noradrenaline from sympathetic nerve terminals. It stimulates aldosterone secretion and plays a central role in the control of Na^+ excretion and fluid volume, as well as of vascular tone.

Renin is a proteolytic enzyme that is secreted by the *juxtaglomerular apparatus* (see p. 370, Fig. 24.2). The control of renin secretion (Fig. 19.4) is only partly understood. It is secreted in response to various physiological stimuli, including a fall in Na^+ concentration in the distal tubule and a fall in renal perfusion pressure. The Na^+ concentration in the distal tubule is sensed by the macula densa (a specialised part of the distal tubule apposed to the juxtaglomerular apparatus). Renal sympathetic nerve activity, β-adrenoceptor agonists and PGI_2 all stimulate renin secretion directly, whereas angiotensin II causes feedback inhibition. Atrial natriuretic peptide (Ch. 18, p. 285) also inhibits renin secretion.

The role of the endothelium in controlling vascular smooth muscle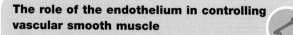

- Endothelial cells release vasoactive mediators including prostaglandin I_2 and nitric oxide (NO) (vasodilators), and endothelin (vasoconstrictor).
- Many vasodilators (e.g. acetylcholine and bradykinin) act via endothelial NO production. The NO derives from arginine and is produced when $[Ca^{2+}]_i$ increases in the endothelial cell, or the sensitivity of endothelial NO synthase to Ca^{2+} is increased (see Fig. 17.3, p. 267).
- NO relaxes smooth muscle by increasing cGMP formation.
- Endothelin is a potent and long-acting vasoconstrictor peptide released from endothelial cells by many chemical and physical factors. It is not confined to blood vessels, and it has several functional roles.

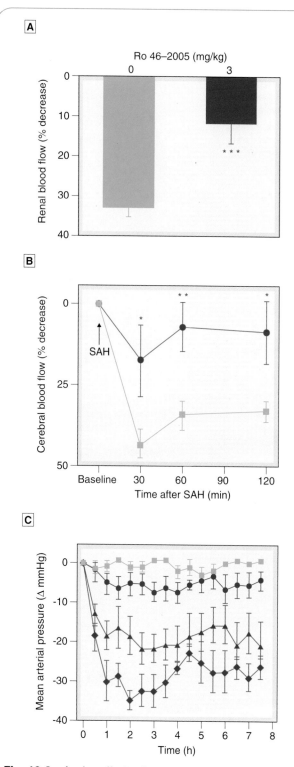

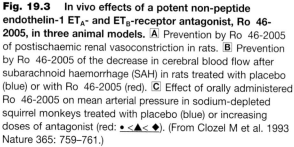

Fig. 19.3 In vivo effects of a potent non-peptide endothelin-1 ET_A- and ET_B-receptor antagonist, Ro 46-2005, in three animal models. **A** Prevention by Ro 46-2005 of postischaemic renal vasoconstriction in rats. **B** Prevention by Ro 46-2005 of the decrease in cerebral blood flow after subarachnoid haemorrhage (SAH) in rats treated with placebo (blue) or with Ro 46-2005 (red). **C** Effect of orally administered Ro 46-2005 on mean arterial pressure in sodium-depleted squirrel monkeys treated with placebo (blue) or increasing doses of antagonist (red: ● < ▲ < ◆). (From Clozel M et al. 1993 Nature 365: 759–761.)

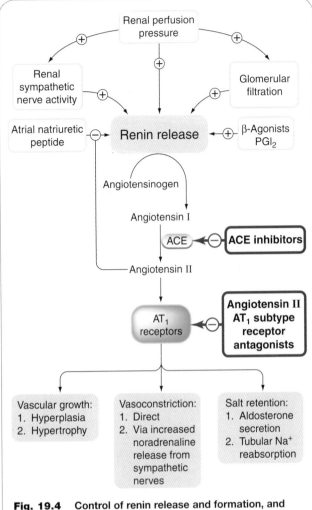

Fig. 19.4 Control of renin release and formation, and action of angiotensin II. Sites of action of drugs that inhibit the cascade are shown. ACE, angiotensin-converting enzyme; AT$_1$, angiotensin II receptor subtype 1.

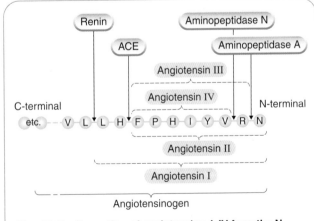

Fig. 19.5 Formation of angiotensins I–IV from the N-terminal of the precursor protein angiotensinogen.

Renin is cleared rapidly from plasma. It acts on angiotensinogen (a plasma globulin made in the liver), splitting off a decapeptide, *angiotensin I*, from the N-terminal end of the protein.

Angiotensin I has no appreciable activity per se, but is converted by ACE to an octapeptide, *angiotensin II*, which is a potent vasoconstrictor. Angiotensin II is a substrate for enzymes (aminopeptidase A and N) that remove single amino acid residues, giving rise, respectively, to angiotensin III and angiotensin IV (Fig. 19.5). These had been regarded as of little importance, but it is now known that angiotensin III stimulates aldosterone secretion and is involved in thirst. Angiotensin IV also has distinct actions, probably via its own receptor, including release of plasminogen activator inhibitor-1 from the endothelium (Ch. 21). Receptors for angiotensin IV have a distinctive distribution, including the hypothalamus.

Angiotensin-converting enzyme is a membrane-bound enzyme on the surface of endothelial cells, and is particularly abundant in the lung, which has a vast surface area of vascular endothelium.[4] The common isoform of ACE is also present in other vascular tissues, including heart, brain, striated muscle and kidney, and is not restricted to endothelial cells.[5] Consequently, local formation of angiotensin II can occur in different vascular beds, and it provides local control independent of blood-borne angiotensin II. ACE inactivates bradykinin (see Ch. 13—Fig. 13.13 and p. 221) and several other peptides. This may contribute to the pharmacological actions of ACE inhibitors, as discussed below. The main actions of angiotensin II are mediated via AT$_1$ and/ or AT$_2$ receptors, which belong to the family of G-protein–coupled receptors. Effects mediated by AT$_1$ receptors include:

- generalised vasoconstriction, especially marked in efferent arterioles of the kidney
- increased release of noradrenaline from sympathetic nerve terminals, reinforcing vasoconstriction and increasing the rate and force of contraction of the heart
- stimulation of proximal tubular reabsorption of Na$^+$
- secretion of aldosterone from the adrenal cortex (see Ch. 28)
- cell growth in the heart and in arteries.[6]

The AT$_2$ receptors have also been cloned. They are expressed during fetal life and in distinct brain regions in adults. Studies of mice in which the gene for the AT$_2$ receptor has been disrupted suggest that it may be involved in growth, development and exploratory behaviour. Cardiovascular effects of AT$_2$ receptors (inhibition of cell growth and lowering of blood pressure) appear to be relatively subtle and oppose those of AT$_1$ receptors.

The renin–angiotensin–aldosterone pathway is important in the pathogenesis of heart failure, and several very important classes of therapeutic drug act by inhibiting it at various points (see below).

---

[4]Approximately that of a football field.

[5]A different isoform of ACE is also present in testis, and male mice lacking this ACE have markedly reduced fertility.

[6]These effects are initiated by the G-protein–coupled AT$_1$ receptor acting via the same intracellular tyrosine phosphorylation pathways as are used by cytokines, for example the Jak/Stat pathway (Ch. 3; Marrero et al. 1995 Nature 375: 247–250).

VASOACTIVE DRUGS

Drugs can affect vascular smooth muscle by acting either directly on smooth muscle cells, or indirectly, for example on endothelial cells, on sympathetic nerve terminals or on the central nervous system (CNS) (Table 19.3). Another type of indirect action is exemplified by ACE inhibitors. Mechanisms of directly acting vasoconstrictors and vasodilators are summarised in Figure 4.10 (p. 67). Many indirectly acting drugs are discussed in other chapters (see Table 19.3). We concentrate here on agents that are not covered elsewhere.

VASOCONSTRICTOR DRUGS

The α_1-adrenoceptor agonists and drugs that release noradrenaline from sympathetic nerve terminals or inhibit its reuptake (*sympathomimetic amines*) cause vasoconstriction and are discussed in Chapter 11. Some eicosanoids (e.g. *thromboxane A_2*; see Chs 13 and 21) and several peptides, notably *endothelin, angiotensin* and *ADH*, are also predominantly vasoconstrictor. **Sumatriptan** and ergot alkaloids acting on certain 5-hydroxytryptamine receptors (5-HT$_2$ and 5-HT$_{1D}$) also cause vasoconstriction (Ch. 12).

ANGIOTENSIN II

The physiological role of the renin–angiotensin system is described above. Angiotensin II is roughly 40 times as potent as noradrenaline in raising blood pressure. Like α_1-adrenoceptor agonists, it constricts mainly cutaneous, splanchnic and renal vasculature, with less effect on blood flow to brain and skeletal muscle. It has no routine clinical uses, its therapeutic importance lying in the fact that other drugs (e.g. **captopril** and **losartan**; see below) affect the cardiovascular system by reducing its production or action.

ANTIDIURETIC HORMONE

Antidiuretic hormone (also known as vasopressin) is a posterior pituitary peptide hormone (Ch. 28, pp. 425-426). It is important for its antidiuretic action on the kidney (Ch. 24, p. 372) but is also a powerful vasoconstrictor in skin and some other vascular beds. Its effects are initiated by two distinct receptors (V_1 and V_2). Water retention is mediated through V_2 receptors, occurs at low plasma concentrations of ADH, and involves activation of adenylate cyclase in renal collecting ducts. Vasoconstriction is mediated through V_1 receptors, requires higher concentrations of ADH, and involves activation of phospholipase C (see Ch. 3). ADH causes generalised vasoconstriction, including the coeliac, mesenteric and coronary vessels. It also affects other (e.g. gastro-intestinal and uterine) smooth muscle and causes abdominal cramps for this reason. It is sometimes used to treat patients with bleeding oesophageal varices and portal hypertension before more definitive treatment, although many gastroenterologists prefer to use **octreotide** (unlicensed indication; see Ch. 28—also Ch. 26 and Ch. 51) for this. It may also have a place in treating hypotensive shock (see below, p. 316).

ENDOTHELIN

Endothelins are discussed above in the context of their physiological roles; as explained, they have vasodilator and vaso-constrictor actions, but vasoconstriction predominates. Intravenous administration causes transient vasodilatation followed by pro-found and very long-lived vasoconstriction. The endothelins are even more potent vasoconstrictors than angiotensin II. As yet, they have no clinical uses and their pharmacological importance, like that of angiotensin II, will probably lie in drugs that affect the cardiovascular system by reducing their production or actions.

VASODILATOR DRUGS

Many vasodilators are clinically important, being used to treat common conditions including hypertension, cardiac failure and angina pectoris.

DIRECTLY ACTING VASODILATORS

Targets on which drugs act to relax vascular smooth muscle include plasma membrane voltage-dependent calcium channels, sarcoplasmic reticulum channels (Ca^{2+} release or reuptake), and enzymes that determine Ca^{2+} sensitivity of the contractile proteins (see Fig. 4.10, p. 67). A pyridine drug, **Y27632**, causes vaso-relaxation by inhibiting a Rho-associated protein kinase, thereby selectively inhibiting smooth muscle contraction by inhibiting Ca^{2+} sensitisation.

Calcium antagonists

L-type calcium antagonists are discussed in Chapter 18 (pp. 294-296). They cause generalised arterial vasodilatation, although individual agents exhibit distinct patterns of regional potency. Dihydropyridines (e.g. **nifedipine**) act preferentially on vascular smooth muscle, whereas **verapamil** acts also on the heart; **diltiazem** is intermediate in specificity. Consequently, rapid acting dihydropyridines usually produce reflex tachycardia as a result of

Vasoconstrictor substances

- The main groups are sympathomimetic amines (direct and indirect; Ch. 11), certain eicosanoids (especially thromboxane A_2; Ch. 13), peptides (angiotensin II, antidiuretic hormone [ADH] and endothelin; Ch. 16) and a group of miscellaneous drugs (e.g. ergot alkaloids; Ch. 12).
- Clinical uses include local applications (e.g. nasal decongestion, coadministration with local anaesthetics). Sympathomimetic amines and ADH are used in circulatory shock. Adrenaline is life-saving in anaphylactic shock and in cardiac arrest. ADH may be used to stop bleeding from oesophageal varices in patients with portal hypertension caused by liver disease.

Table 19.3   Classification of vasoactive drugs that act indirectly

Site	Mechanism	Examples	Chapter(s) for further details
Vasoconstrictors			
Sympathetic nerves	Noradrenaline (norepinephrine) release	Tyramine	11
	Blocks noradrenaline reuptake	Cocaine	11
Endothelium	Endothelin release	Angiotensin II (in part)	This chapter
Vasodilators			
Sympathetic nerves	Inhibits noradrenaline release	Prostaglandin E_2, guanethidine	9, 11 and 13
Endothelium	Nitric oxide release	Acetylcholine, substance P	17
Central nervous system	Vasomotor inhibition	Anaesthetics	36
Enzymes	Angiotensin-converting enzyme inhibition	Captopril	This chapter

lowering the blood pressure, whereas verapamil and diltiazem do not because, although they also lower blood pressure, they slow the cardiac pacemaker by their direct action on the heart.

Drugs that activate potassium channels (see also Ch. 18, pp. 294-295)

Some drugs (e.g. **cromakalim** and **minoxidil**) relax smooth muscle by selectively increasing the membrane permeability to K^+ by K_{ATP} channel activation. This hyperpolarises the cells and switches off voltage-dependent calcium channels. Patch clamp recording (see Fig. 19.6 and p. 32) demonstrated that these drugs open a high-conductance potassium channel. This discovery coincided with studies demonstrating the existence of ATP-sensitive potassium channels in various cells. In cardiac muscle and pancreatic islet insulin-secreting B cells, for example, intracellular ATP closes these potassium channels, thus causing depolarisation.[7] Potassium channel activators work by antagonising the action of intracellular ATP on these channels (Fig. 19.6), thus opening them and causing hyperpolarisation and relaxation.

Minoxidil is a very potent and long-acting vasodilator, used as a drug of last resort in treating severe hypertension unresponsive to other drugs. It causes hirsutism (its active metabolite is actually used as a rub-on cream to treat baldness). This is unacceptable to most women. It also causes marked salt and water retention, and is usually prescribed with a loop diuretic. It causes reflex tachycardia, and a β-adrenoceptor antagonist is used to prevent this. **Cromakalim** and its active isomer **lemakalim** are also K_{ATP} channel activators. **Nicorandil** (Ch. 18, p. 294) combines K_{ATP} channel activation with NO donor activity, and is used in refractory angina. **Levosimendan** combines K_{ATP} channel activation with sensitisation of the cardiac contractile mechanism to Ca^{2+} by

binding troponin (Ch. 18, p. 281), and is used in decompensated heart failure (see below, p. 314).

Drugs that act via cyclic nucleotides

Cyclase activation

Many drugs relax vascular smooth muscle by increasing the cellular concentration of either cGMP or cAMP. For example, NO, nitrates and the natriuretic peptides act through cGMP (see Chs 17 and 18); BAY41-2272, a pyrazolopyridine, activates soluble guanylate cyclase via an NO-independent site (see Ch. 17, p. 269). The *β₂ agonists, adenosine* and *PGI₂* increase cytoplasmic cAMP (see Chs 11–13). *Dopamine* has mixed vasodilator and vasoconstrictor actions. It selectively dilates renal vessels, where it increases cAMP by activating adenylate cyclase. It is the precursor of noradrenaline (Ch. 11), and is also a transmitter in its own right in the brain (Ch. 34) and probably also in the periphery (Ch. 9). The proposal that dopamine might serve a role as a peripheral transmitter came from observations that stimulation of sympathetic nerves to the kidney causes vasodilatation that is not affected by adrenoceptor antagonists, but is blocked by dopamine receptor antagonists such as **haloperidol**. Dopamine, when administered as an intravenous infusion, produces a mixture of cardiovascular effects resulting from agonist actions on α and β adrenoceptors, as well as on dopamine receptors. Blood pressure increases slightly, but the main effects are vasodilatation in the renal circulation and increased cardiac output. Dopamine was widely used in intensive care units in patients in whom renal failure associated with decreased renal perfusion appeared imminent; despite its beneficial effect on renal haemodynamics, it does not, however, improve survival in these circumstances and this use is obsolete. **Nesiritide**, a recombinant form of human B-type natriuretic peptide (BNP) (see Ch. 18, p. 285), has been approved in the USA for the treatment of acutely decompensated heart failure, but a pooled analysis of randomised controlled trials has suggested that it too may increase mortality (Sackner-Bernstein et al., 2005).

---

[7]This mechanism forms an important link between the metabolic state of the cell and membrane function, and sulfonylurea drugs cause insulin secretion by mimicking the action of ATP on these channels (see Ch. 26). Conversely, some potassium channel activators increase blood glucose by inhibiting insulin secretion from the pancreas.

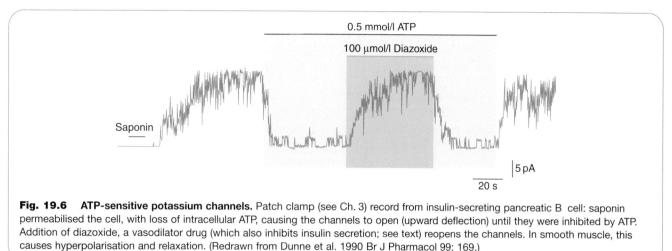

Fig. 19.6   ATP-sensitive potassium channels. Patch clamp (see Ch. 3) record from insulin-secreting pancreatic B cell: saponin permeabilised the cell, with loss of intracellular ATP, causing the channels to open (upward deflection) until they were inhibited by ATP. Addition of diazoxide, a vasodilator drug (which also inhibits insulin secretion; see text) reopens the channels. In smooth muscle, this causes hyperpolarisation and relaxation. (Redrawn from Dunne et al. 1990 Br J Pharmacol 99: 169.)

Nitroprusside (nitroferricyanide) is a powerful vasodilator with little effect outside the vascular system. It reacts with tissue sulfhydryl groups under physiological conditions to yield NO. Unlike the organic nitrates, which preferentially dilate capacitance vessels and muscular arteries, it acts equally on arterial and venous smooth muscle. Its clinical usefulness is limited because it must be given intravenously. In solution, particularly when exposed to light, nitroprusside hydrolyses with formation of cyanide. The intravenous solution must therefore be made up freshly from dry powder and protected from light (usually by covering the container with foil). Nitroprusside is rapidly converted to thiocyanate in the body, its plasma half-life being only a few minutes, so it must be given as a continuous infusion with careful monitoring to avoid hypotension. Prolonged use causes thiocyanate accumulation and toxicity (weakness, nausea and inhibition of thyroid function); consequently, nitroprusside is useful only for short-term treatment (usually up to 72 hours maximum). It is used in intensive care units for hypertensive emergencies, to produce controlled hypotension during surgery, and to reduce cardiac work during the reversible cardiac dysfunction that occurs after cardiopulmonary bypass surgery.

Phosphodiesterase inhibition
Phosphodiesterases (PDEs; see Ch. 3) include at least 14 distinct isoenzymes. Methylxanthines (e.g. **theophylline**) and **papaverine** are non-selective PDE inhibitors (and have other actions too). Methylxanthines exert their main effects on bronchial smooth muscle and on the CNS, and are discussed in Chapters 23 and 42. In addition to inhibiting PDE, some methylxanthines are also purine receptor antagonists. They are not used clinically as vasodilators. Papaverine is chemically related to **morphine**, and indeed is produced by opium poppies (see Ch. 41, p. 596). Pharmacologically, it is quite unlike morphine, however, its main action being to relax smooth muscle in blood vessels and elsewhere. Its mechanism is poorly understood but seems to involve a combination of PDE inhibition and block of calcium channels. Selective PDE type III inhibitors (e.g. **milrinone, amrinone**) increase cytoplasmic cAMP in cardiac muscle. They have a positive inotropic effect but, despite short-term haemodynamic improvement,

> **Vasodilator drugs**
>
> - Vasodilators act:
>   — to increase local tissue blood flow
>   — to reduce arterial pressure
>   — to reduce central venous pressure.
> - Net effect is a reduction of cardiac preload (reduced filling pressure) and afterload (reduced vascular resistance), hence reduction of cardiac work.
> - Main uses are:
>   — antihypertensive therapy (e.g. AT^1 antagonists, calcium antagonists and α_1 antagonists)
>   — treatment/prophylaxis of angina (e.g. calcium antagonists, nitrates)
>   — treatment of cardiac failure (e.g. angiotensin-converting enzyme inhibitors, AT_1 antagonists).

increase mortality in heart failure, possibly by causing dysrhythmias (p. 292). **Cilostazol**, a related drug, improves symptoms in patients with peripheral vascular disease (see below). **Dipyridamole** can provoke angina (p. 293) and is used to prevent stroke (p. 342). Selective PDE type V inhibitors (e.g. **sildenafil**) inhibit the breakdown of cGMP. Penile erection is caused by increased activity in nitrergic nerves in the pelvis. These release NO, which activates guanylate cyclase in smooth muscle in the corpora cavernosa. Taken by mouth about an hour before sexual stimulation, sildenafil increases penile erection by potentiating this pathway. It has revolutionised treatment of erectile dysfunction (see Ch. 30) and has therapeutic potential via potentiation of other NO-mediated activities (Ch. 17), including pulmonary hypertension (see below).

VASODILATORS WITH UNKNOWN MECHANISM OF ACTION

Hydralazine
Hydralazine acts mainly on arteries and arterioles, causing a fall in blood pressure accompanied by reflex tachycardia and an

increased cardiac output. It interferes with the action of inositol trisphosphate on Ca^{2+} release from the sarcoplasmic reticulum. Its original clinical use was in hypertension. It is still used for short-term treatment of severe hypertension in pregnancy but can cause an immune disorder resembling *systemic lupus erythematosus*,[8] so alternative agents are now usually preferred for long-term treatment of hypertension. Recent evidence has, however, suggested that it has a place in treating heart failure in patients of African origin (see below).

Ethanol

Ethanol (see Ch. 43) dilates cutaneous vessels, causing the familiar drunkard's flush. Several general anaesthetics (e.g. **propofol**) cause vasodilatation as an unwanted effect (Ch. 36).

INDIRECTLY ACTING VASODILATOR DRUGS

The two main groups of indirectly acting vasodilator drugs are inhibitors of:

- sympathetic vasoconstriction
- the renin–angiotensin system.

The central control of sympathetically mediated vasoconstriction is believed to involve not only α_2 adrenoceptors but also another class of receptor, termed the *imidazoline I_1 receptor*, present in the brain stem in the rostral ventrolateral medulla. Drugs can inhibit the sympathetic pathway at any point from the CNS to the peripheral sympathetic nerve terminal (see Ch. 11). In addition, many vasodilators (e.g. acetylcholine, bradykinin, substance P) exert some or all of their effects by stimulating biosynthesis of vasodilator prostaglandins or of NO (or of both) by vascular endothelium (see above and Ch. 17), thereby causing functional antagonism of the constrictor tone caused by sympathetic nerves and angiotensin II. Endothelin receptor antagonists including **bosentan** lower systemic and pulmonary arterial pressure.

We concentrate here on the renin–angiotensin–aldosterone system. This can be inhibited at several points:

- renin release: β-adrenoceptor antagonists inhibit renin release (although their other actions can result in a small *increase* in peripheral vascular resistance)
- renin activity: renin inhibitors
- ACE: ACE inhibitors
- angiotensin II type 1 (AT_1) receptors: AT_1-receptor antagonists
- aldosterone receptors: aldosterone receptor antagonists.

All such drugs can increase plasma K^+ concentration by reducing aldosterone secretion or action.

Renin inhibitors

Orally active renin inhibitors (e.g. **enalkiren**) reduce plasma renin activity, but their effects on blood pressure in patients with hypertension have been disappointing.

Angiotensin-converting enzyme inhibitors

Several specific ACE inhibitors have been developed, the first of which was **captopril** (Fig. 19.7). ACE cleaves the C-terminal pair of amino acids from peptide substrates. Its active site contains a zinc atom. The development of captopril was one of the first examples of successful drug design based on a chemical knowledge of the target molecule. Various small peptides had been found to be weak inhibitors of the enzyme,[9] but these were unsuitable as drugs because of their low potency and poor oral absorption. Captopril was designed to combine the steric properties of such peptide antagonists in a non-peptide molecule. It contains a sulfhydryl group appropriately placed to bind the zinc atom, coupled to a proline residue that binds the site on the enzyme that normally accommodates the terminal leucine of angiotensin I (Fig. 19.7). Several ACE inhibitors, differing in duration of action and tissue distribution, are used clinically, including **enalapril**, **lisinopril**, **ramipril**, **perindopril** and **trandolapril**.

Pharmacological effects

Captopril is a powerful inhibitor of the effects of angiotensin I in the whole animal. It causes only a small fall in arterial pressure in normal animals or human subjects who are consuming the amount of salt contained in a usual western diet, but a much larger fall in hypertensive patients, particularly those in whom renin secretion is enhanced (e.g. in patients receiving diuretics). ACE inhibitors affect capacitance and resistance vessels, and reduce cardiac load as well as arterial pressure. They do not affect cardiac contractility, so cardiac output normally increases. They act preferentially on angiotensin-sensitive vascular beds, which include those of the kidney, heart and brain. This selectivity may be important in sustaining adequate perfusion of these vital organs in the face of reduced perfusion pressure. Critical *renal artery stenosis*[10] represents an exception to this, where ACE inhibition results in a fall of glomerular filtration rate (see below).

Clinical uses

Clinical uses of ACE inhibitors are summarised in the clinical box.

Clinical uses of angiotensin-converting enzyme inhibitors

- Hypertension.
- Cardiac failure.
- Following myocardial infarction (especially when there is ventricular dysfunction).
- In people at high risk of ischaemic heart disease.
- Diabetic nephropathy.
- Progressive renal insufficiency.

---

[8]An autoimmune disease affecting one or more tissues, including joints, skin and pleural membranes. It is characterised by antibodies directed against DNA.

[9]The lead compound was a nonapeptide derived from the venom of *Bothrops jacaraca*—a South American snake. It was originally characterised as a bradykinin-potentiating peptide, an indirect effect of inhibiting ACE, which inactivates bradykinin (see Ch. 13).

[10]Severe narrowing of the renal artery, for example that caused by atheroma (Ch. 20).

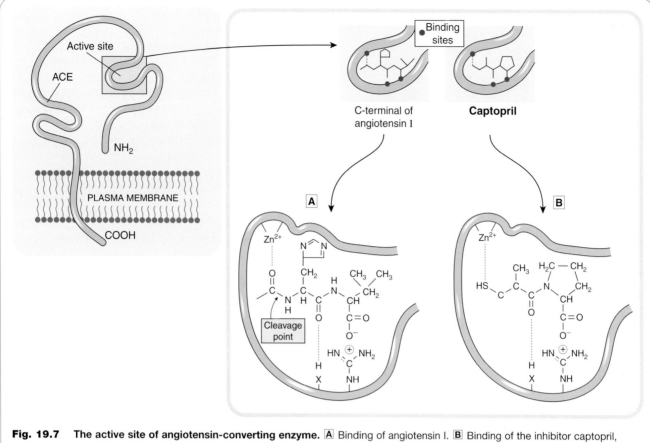

Fig. 19.7 **The active site of angiotensin-converting enzyme.** [A] Binding of angiotensin I. [B] Binding of the inhibitor captopril, which is an analogue of the terminal dipeptide of angiotensin I.

Unwanted effects

Captopril was initially used in doses that, in retrospect, were excessive. In these large doses, it caused rashes, taste disturbance, neutropenia and heavy proteinuria. This pattern of adverse effects also occurs during treatment with **penicillamine** (Ch. 14), which also contains a sulfhydryl group, and it has been argued that these effects are attributable to this chemical feature of the molecule rather than to ACE inhibition as such. Other ACE inhibitors that do not possess a sulfhydryl group do not cause these effects. In contrast, adverse effects that are directly related to ACE inhibition are common to all drugs of this class. These include hypotension, especially after the first dose and especially in patients with heart failure who have been treated with loop diuretics, in whom the renin–angiotensin system is highly activated. A dry cough, possibly the result of accumulation of bradykinin (Ch. 16), is the commonest persistent adverse effect. Patients with severe bilateral renal artery stenosis predictably develop renal failure if treated with ACE inhibitors, because glomerular filtration in the face of low afferent arteriolar pressure is maintained by angiotensin II, which constricts the efferent arteriole; hyperkalaemia may be severe owing to reduced aldosterone secretion. Such renal failure is reversible provided that it is recognised promptly and the ACE inhibitor stopped.

Angiotensin II receptor subtype 1 antagonists (sartans)

Losartan, **candesartan**, **valsartan** and **irbesartan** (*sartans*) are non-peptide, orally active AT_1 receptor antagonists. These differ predictably from ACE inhibitors in their pharmacological properties (Fig. 19.8) but behave rather similarly to ACE inhibitors in clinical practice, apart from not causing cough—consistent with the 'bradykinin accumulation' explanation of this side effect, mentioned above. ACE is not the only enzyme capable of forming angiotensin II, *chymase* (which is not inhibited by ACE inhibitors) providing one alternative route. It is not known if alternative pathways of angiotensin II formation are important in vivo, but if so, then AT_1 receptor antagonists could be more effective than ACE inhibitors in such situations. It is not known whether any of the beneficial effects of ACE inhibitors are bradykinin/NO-mediated, so it is unwise to assume that AT_1 receptor antagonists will necessarily share all the therapeutic properties of ACE inhibitors. Experience with **valsartan** and **candesartan** (a longer-acting drug) in patients with heart failure has, however, been positive, as has experience with **irbesartan**, in limiting the progression of diabetic nephropathy.

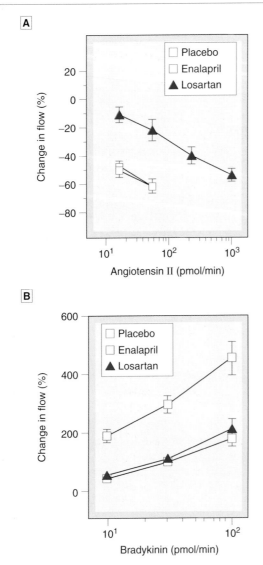

Fig. 19.8 **Comparison of effects of angiotensin-converting enzyme inhibition and angiotensin receptor blockade in the human forearm vasculature.** A Effect of brachial artery infusion of angiotensin II on forearm blood flow after oral administration of placebo, enalapril (10 mg) or losartan (100 mg). B Effect of brachial artery infusion of bradykinin, as in A. (From Cockcroft J R et al. 1993 J Cardiovasc Pharmacol 22: 579–584.)

CLINICAL USES OF VASOACTIVE DRUGS

It is beyond the scope of this book to provide a detailed account of the clinical uses of vasoactive drugs, but it is nonetheless useful to consider briefly the treatment of certain important disorders. The conditions that will be discussed are:

- systemic hypertension
- cardiac failure
- shock
- peripheral vascular disease
- Raynaud's disease
- pulmonary hypertension.

Types of vasodilator drug

Directly acting vasodilators

- Calcium antagonists (e.g. **nifedipine**, **diltiazem**, **verapamil**): block Ca^{2+} entry in response to depolarisation. Common adverse effects include ankle swelling and (especially with verapamil) constipation.
- K_{ATP} channel activators (e.g. **minoxidil**): open membrane potassium channels, causing hyperpolarisation. Ankle swelling and increased hair growth are common.
- Drugs that *increase cytoplasmic cyclic nucleotide* concentrations by:
  — increasing adenylyl cyclase activity, for example prostacyclin (**epoprostenol**), β_2-adrenoceptor agonists, adenosine
  — increasing guanylyl cyclase activity: nitrates (e.g. **glyceryl trinitrate**, **nitroprusside**)
  — inhibiting phosphodiesterase activity (e.g. **sildenafil**).

Indirectly acting vasodilators

- Drugs that interfere with the sympathetic nervous system (e.g. α_1-adrenoceptor antagonists). Postural hypotension is a common adverse effect.
- Drugs that block the renin–angiotensin system:
  — renin inhibitors (e.g. **enalkiren**)
  — angiotensin-converting enzyme inhibitors (e.g. **enalapril**); dry cough may be troublesome
  — AT_1 receptor antagonists (e.g. **losartan**).
- Drugs or mediators that stimulate endothelial NO release (e.g. acetylcholine, bradykinin).
- Drugs that block the endothelin system:
  — endothelin synthesis (e.g. **phosphoramidon**)
  — endothelin action (e.g. **bosentan**).

Vasodilators whose mechanism is uncertain

- Miscellaneous drugs including alcohol, **propofol** (Ch. 36) and **hydralazine**.

Clinical uses of angiotensin II subtype 1 receptor antagonists (sartans)

The AT_1 antagonists are extremely well tolerated. Their uses include the following.

- Hypertension, especially in:
  — young patients (who have higher renin than older ones)
  — hypertensive diabetic patients
  — hypertension complicated by left ventricular hypertrophy.
- Heart failure
- Diabetic nephropathy.

SYSTEMIC HYPERTENSION

Systemic hypertension is a common disorder that, if not effectively treated, results in a greatly increased probability of coronary thrombosis, strokes and renal failure. Until about 1950, there was no effective treatment, and the development of antihypertensive drugs, which restore healthy life expectancy, has been a major therapeutic success story.

There are a few recognisable and surgically treatable causes of hypertension, such as *phaeochromocytoma*,[11] steroid-secreting tumours of the adrenal cortex, renal artery stenosis and so on, but most cases involve no obvious cause and are grouped as *essential hypertension* (so-called because it was originally, albeit incorrectly, thought that the raised blood pressure was 'essential' to maintain adequate tissue perfusion). Increased cardiac output may be an early feature, but by the time it is diagnosed (commonly in middle life) there is usually increased peripheral resistance and the cardiac output is normal. Blood pressure control is intimately related to the kidneys, as demonstrated by transplantation experiments in which kidneys are transplanted from or to animals with genetic hypertension, or to humans requiring renal transplantation: hypertension 'goes with' the kidney from a hypertensive donor, and donating a kidney from a normotensive to a hypertensive corrects hypertension in the recipient (see also Ch. 24). Persistently raised arterial pressure leads to hypertrophy of the left ventricle and remodelling of resistance arteries, with narrowing of the lumen. The raised peripheral vascular resistance calls into play various physiological responses involving the cardiovascular system, nervous system and kidney. Such vicious circles provide targets for pharmacological attack.

Figure 19.9 summarises physiological mechanisms that control arterial blood pressure and shows sites at which antihypertensive drugs act. The main systems include the *sympathetic nervous system*, the *renin–angiotensin–aldosterone* system and *tonically active endothelium–derived autacoids* (NO and probably ET-1; see above). Remodelling of resistance arteries in response to the raised pressure reduces the ratio of lumen diameter to wall thickness and increases the peripheral vascular resistance. The role of cellular growth factors (including angiotensin II) and inhibitors of growth (e.g. NO) in the evolution of these structural changes is of great interest to vascular biologists, and is potentially of importance to the therapeutic use of drugs such as ACE inhibitors.

Contrary to the earlier view that hypertension was 'essential' to sustain life, reducing arterial blood pressure greatly improves the prognosis of patients with hypertension. Controlling hypertension (which is asymptomatic) without producing unacceptable side effects is therefore an important clinical need, which is, in general, well catered for by modern drugs. Treatment involves non-pharmacological measures (e.g. increased exercise, reduced dietary salt and saturated fat with increased fruit and fibre, weight and alcohol reduction) followed by the staged introduction of drugs, starting with those of proven benefit and least likely to produce side effects. Some of the drugs that were used to lower blood pressure in the early days of antihypertensive therapy, including *ganglion blockers*, *adrenergic neuron blockers* and **reserpine** (see Ch. 11), produced a fearsome array of adverse effects and are now obsolete. The preferred regimens have changed progressively as better-tolerated drugs have become available. One rational strategy with some evidence to support it, and recommended by the current British Hypertension Society guidelines, is to start treatment with either an ACE inhibitor or an AT_1 antagonist in patients who are likely to have normal or raised plasma renin (i.e. younger white people), and with either a thiazide diuretic or a calcium antagonist in older people and people of African origin (who are more likely to have low plasma renin). If the target blood pressure is not achieved but the drug is well tolerated, then a drug of the other group is added. It is best not to increase the dose of any one drug excessively, as this often causes adverse effects and engages homeostatic control mechanisms (e.g. renin release by a diuretic) that limit efficacy.

β-Adrenoceptor antagonists are less well tolerated than ACE inhibitors or AT_1 antagonists, and the evidence supporting their routine use is less strong than for other classes of antihypertensive drugs. They are useful for hypertensive patients with some additional indication for β blockade, such as angina or heart failure.

Addition of a third or fourth drug (e.g. to sartan/diuretic or sartan/calcium antagonist combination) is often needed, and a long-acting α_1 antagonist (Ch. 11, p. 180) such as **doxazosin** is one option in this setting. The α_1 antagonists additionally improve symptoms of prostatism,[12] enabling one to kill two birds with one stone in older men with the common disorder of benign prostatic hypertrophy, albeit at the expense of some postural hypotension, which is the main unwanted effect of these agents. Doxazosin is used once daily and has a mild but theoretically desirable effect on plasma lipids (reducing the ratio of low- to high-density lipoproteins; see Ch. 20). **Spironolactone** (a competitive antagonist of aldosterone; Ch. 24, p. 379) has staged something of a comeback in treating severe hypertension, with the realisation that this is often associated with an excess of circulating aldosterone relative to renin. Careful monitoring of plasma K^+ concentration is required, because spironolactone inhibits urinary K^+ excretion as well as causing oestrogen-related adverse effects (see p. 379), but it is usually well tolerated in low doses. **Methyldopa** (p. 184) is now used mainly for hypertension during pregnancy because of the lack of documented adverse effects on the baby (in contrast to ACE inhibitors, sartans and standard β-adrenoceptor antagonists, which are contraindicated during pregnancy). **Clonidine** (a centrally acting α_2 agonist; clinical box, p. 179) is now seldom used. **Moxonidine**, a centrally acting agonist at imidazoline I_1 receptors that causes less drowsiness than α_2 agonists, is licensed for mild or moderate hypertension, but there is little evidence from clinical end-point trials to support its use. **Minoxidil**, combined with a diuretic and β-adrenoceptor antagonist, is sometimes effective where other

---

[11]Catecholamine-secreting tumours of chromaffin tissue, usually the adrenal medulla (Ch. 11).

[12]Difficulty starting the stream, poor stream, terminal dribbling, and needing to get up often in the night to pass urine—all depressingly common in ageing men.

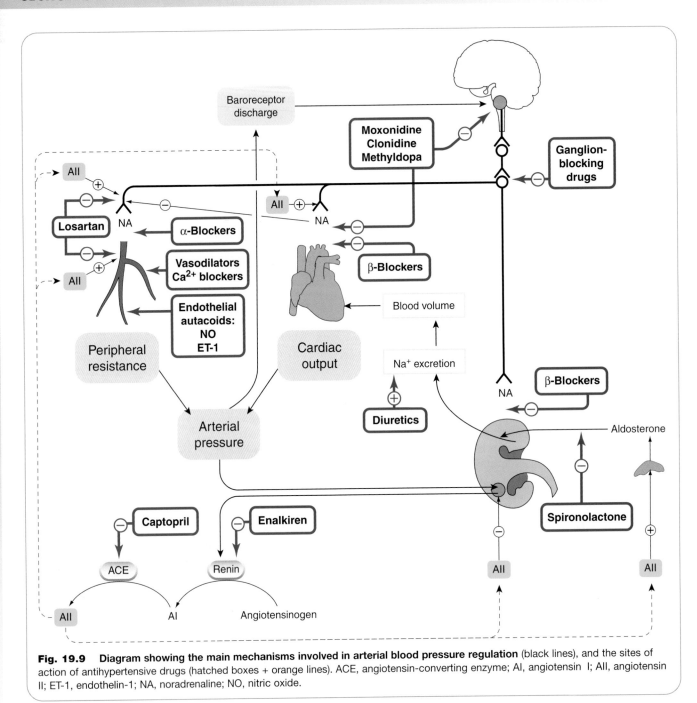

Fig. 19.9 **Diagram showing the main mechanisms involved in arterial blood pressure regulation** (black lines), and the sites of action of antihypertensive drugs (hatched boxes + orange lines). ACE, angiotensin-converting enzyme; AI, angiotensin I; AII, angiotensin II; ET-1, endothelin-1; NA, noradrenaline; NO, nitric oxide.

drugs have failed in severe hypertension resistant to other drugs. **Fenoldopam**, a selective dopamine D_1 receptor agonist, is approved in the USA for the short-term management in hospital of severe hypertension. Its effect is similar in magnitude to that of intravenous **nitroprusside**, but it lacks thiocyanate-associated toxicity and is slower in onset and offset.

Commonly used antihypertensive drugs and their common adverse effects are summarised in Table 19.4.

CARDIAC FAILURE

The underlying abnormality in *cardiac failure* (see also Ch. 18) is a cardiac output that is inadequate to meet the metabolic

demands of the body during exercise (and ultimately also at rest). It may be caused by disease of the myocardium itself (most commonly ischaemic heart disease), or by circulatory factors such as volume overload (e.g. leaky valves, or arteriovenous shunts caused by congenital defects)[13] or pressure overload (e.g. stenosed-narrowed valves, arterial or pulmonary hypertension). Some of these underlying causes are surgically correctable, and in some either the underlying disease (e.g. hyperthyroidism; Ch. 29), or

[13]So-called 'hole in the heart' babies have a defect in the atrial or ventricular septum, leading to shunting of blood from high- to low-pressure parts of the circulation.

Table 19.4 Common antihypertensive drugs and their adverse effects

Drug	Adverse effects[a]		
	Postural hypotension	*Impotence*	*Other*
Thiazide diuretics[b] (e.g. bendroflumethiazide)	±	++	Urinary frequency, gout, glucose intolerance, $K^+ \downarrow$, $Na^+ \downarrow$
Angiotensin-converting enzyme inhibitors (e.g. ramipril, lisinopril)	±	–	First-dose hypotension, dry cough, reversible renal dysfunction in patients with bilateral renal artery stenosis, fetal toxicity
AT_1 antagonists (e.g. losartan, candesartan)	–	–	Reversible renal dysfunction in patients with bilateral renal artery stenosis, fetal toxicity
Ca^{2+} antagonists (e.g. nifedipine, amlodipine)	–	±	Ankle oedema
β-Adrenoceptor antagonists[c] (e.g. metoprolol)	–	+	Bronchospasm, fatigue, cold hands/feet, bradycardia
$α_1$-Adrenoceptor antagonists[c] (e.g. doxazosin)	++	–	First-dose hypotension

[a]± indicates that the adverse effect occurs in special circumstances only (e.g. postural hypotension occurs with a thiazide diuretic only if the patient is dehydrated for some other reason or is taking some additional drug.)
[b]See Chapter 24.
[c]See Chapter 11.

an aggravating factor such as anaemia (Ch. 22) or atrial fibrillation (Ch. 18), is treatable with drugs. Here, we focus on drugs used to treat heart failure irrespective of the underlying cause. When cardiac output is insufficient to meet metabolic demand, an increase in fluid volume occurs, partly because increased venous pressure causes increased formation of tissue fluid, and partly because reduced renal blood flow activates the renin–angiotensin–aldosterone system, causing Na^+ and water retention. Irrespective of the cause, the outlook for adults with cardiac failure is grim: 50% of those with the most severe grade are dead in 6 months, and of those with 'mild/moderate' disease 50% are dead in 5 years. Non-drug measures, including dietary salt restriction, are important, but drugs are needed to improve symptoms of oedema, fatigue and breathlessness, and to improve prognosis.

A highly simplified diagram of the sequence of events is shown in Figure 19.10. A common theme is that several of the feedbacks that are activated are 'counter-regulatory'—i.e. they make the situation worse not better. This occurs because the body fails to distinguish the haemodynamic state of heart failure from haemorrhage, in which release of vasoconstrictors such as angiotensin II and ADH would be appropriate.[14] ACE inhibitors and AT_1, β-adrenoceptor and aldosterone antagonists interrupt these counter-regulatory neurohormonal mechanisms and have each been shown to prolong life in heart failure, although prognosis remains poor despite optimal management.

Drugs used to treat heart failure act in various complementary ways to do the following.

Increase natriuresis. Diuretics, especially loop diuretics (Ch. 24), are important in increasing salt and water excretion, especially if there is pulmonary oedema. In chronic heart failure, drugs that have been shown to improve prognosis were all studied in patients treated with diuretics.

Inhibit the renin–angiotensin–aldosterone system. The renin–angiotensin–aldosterone system is inappropriately activated in patients with cardiac failure, especially when they are treated with diuretics. The β-adrenoceptor antagonists inhibit renin secretion and are used in clinically stable patients with chronic heart failure (see below). ACE inhibitors and AT_1 antagonists block the formation of angiotensin II and inhibit its action, respectively, thereby reducing vascular resistance, improving tissue perfusion and reducing cardiac afterload. They also cause natriuresis by inhibiting secretion of aldosterone and by reducing the direct stimulatory effect of angiotensin II on reabsorption of Na^+ and HCO_3^- in the early part of the proximal convoluted tubule. Most important of all, they prolong life. The question of whether ACE inhibitors and AT_1 antagonists can usefully be combined is being evaluated. Angiotensin II is not the only stimulus to aldosterone secretion, and during chronic treatment with ACE inhibitors, circulating aldosterone concentrations return towards pretreatment values (a phenomenon known as 'aldosterone escape'). This provided a rationale for studying the effect of combining **spironolactone** (an aldosterone antagonist; see Ch. 24) with ACE inhibitor treatment, and this further reduces mortality. **Eplerenone** is a recently licensed aldosterone antagonist with less oestrogen-like adverse effects than spironolactone; it

[14]Natural selection presumably favoured mechanisms that would benefit young hunter gatherers at risk of haemorrhage; middle-aged or elderly people at high risk of heart failure are past their reproductive prime.

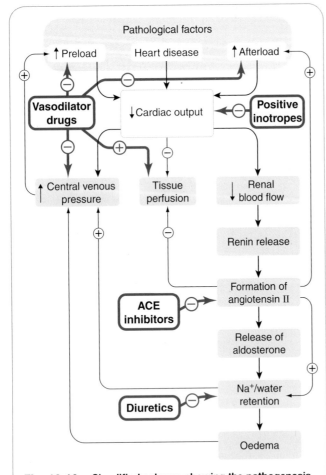

Fig. 19.10 **Simplified scheme showing the pathogenesis of heart failure, and the sites of action of some of the drugs used to treat it.** The symptoms of heart failure are produced by reduced tissue perfusion, oedema and increased central venous pressure. ACE, angiotensin-converting enzyme.

common in severe heart failure.[15] **Tolvaptan** is an orally active non-peptide selective V_2 receptor antagonist that has shown promise in patients with heart failure and hyponatraemia. Its effect (if any) on mortality is unknown, and it is not yet licensed for general use.

Relax vascular smooth muscle. **Glyceryl trinitrate** (Ch. 18, pp. 292-294) is infused intravenously to treat acute cardiac failure. Its venodilator effect reduces venous pressure, and its effects on arterial compliance and wave reflection reduce cardiac work. The combination of **hydralazine** (to reduce afterload) with a long-acting organic nitrate (to reduce preload) in patients with chronic heart failure improved survival in a randomised controlled trial known as VHeFT (Vasodilator Heart Failure Trial). Retrospective analysis of this trial suggested that the benefit was restricted to black patients, and a prospective study in African-American patients with severe heart failure receiving standard treatment indicated that addition of hydralazine and isosorbide dinitrate caused a substantial (and significant) reduction in mortality. This evidence has been accepted by the US Food and Drug Administration, but people of African origin are genetically very heterogeneous, and it is unknown what other groups will benefit from such treatment.

Increase the force of cardiac contraction. Cardiac glycosides (Ch. 18, pp. 291-292) are used either in patients with heart failure who also have chronic rapid atrial fibrillation, or in patients who remain symptomatic despite treatment with diuretic and ACE inhibitor. **Digoxin** does not reduce mortality in heart failure patients in sinus rhythm who are otherwise optimally treated, but does improve symptoms and reduce the need for hospital admission. In contrast, PDE inhibitors (e.g. **amrinone**, **milrinone**; see Ch. 18, p. 292) increase cardiac output acutely but increase mortality in heart failure, probably through cardiac dysrhythmias. **Dobutamine** (a β_1-selective adrenoceptor agonist; see Ch. 18, p. 291) is used intravenously when a rapid response is needed in the short term, for example following heart surgery. **Levosimendan**, a positive inotrope with additional vasodilator properties attributed, respectively, to sensitisation of cardiac muscle to $[Ca^{2+}]_i$ and activation of K_{ATP} in vascular smooth muscle (p. 306), is showing promise in the treatment of severe heart failure and circulatory shock (below).

SHOCK AND HYPOTENSIVE STATES

Shock is a medical emergency characterised by inadequate perfusion of vital organs, usually because of a very low arterial blood pressure. This leads to anaerobic metabolism and hence to increased lactate production. Mortality is extremely high, even with optimal treatment in an intensive care unit. Shock can be caused by various insults, including haemorrhage, burns, bacterial infections, anaphylaxis (Ch. 13) and myocardial infarction (Fig. 19.11). Reduced effective circulating blood volume (hypovolaemia) may be caused either directly by bleeding or by

too has been shown to improve survival in patients with heart failure when added to conventional therapy. Patients with impaired renal function were excluded from these trials, and careful monitoring of plasma K^+ concentration is important when they are treated with an ACE inhibitor or an AT_1 antagonist in combination with an aldosterone antagonist.

Antagonise β adrenoceptors. Heart failure is accompanied by potentially harmful activation of the sympathetic nervous system as well as of the renin–angiotensin system, providing a rationale for using β-adrenoceptor antagonists for this disorder. Most clinicians have been very wary of this approach because of the negative inotropic action of these drugs, but when started in low doses that are increased slowly, **metoprolol**, **carvedilol** and **bisoprolol** have each been shown convincingly to improve survival when added to other treatment in clinically stable patients with chronic heart failure.

Inhibit ADH. ADH, also known as vasopressin (above, p. 305; Ch. 24, p. 372; and Ch. 28 pp. 425-426), is released inappropriately in heart failure and may contribute to the hyponatraemia that is

---

[15]Inappropriate secretion of ADH causes hyponatraemia because the kidney fails to excrete water while continuing to excrete sodium ions, while drinking, which is largely determined by habit in addition to thirst, continues. This leads to reduction of the plasma sodium concentration as a result of dilution.

Drugs used in chronic heart failure

- Loop diuretics, for example **furosemide** (Ch. 24, pp. 375-377).
- Angiotensin-converting enzyme inhibitors (e.g. **captopril**, **enalapril**).
- Angiotensin II subtype 1 receptor antagonists (e.g. **valsartan**, **candesartan**).
- β-adrenoceptor antagonists (e.g. **metoprolol**, **bisoprolol**, **carvedilol**), introduced in low dose in stable patients.
- Aldosterone receptor antagonists (e.g. **spironolactone**, Ch. 24, p. 379; and **eplerenone**).
- **Digoxin** (see Ch. 18, pp. 291-292), especially for heart failure associated with established rapid atrial fibrillation. It is also indicated in patients who remain symptomatic despite optimal treatment.
- Organic nitrates (e.g. **isosorbide mononitrate**) reduce preload, and **hydralazine** reduces afterload. Used in combination, these prolong life in African-Americans.

movement of fluid from the plasma to the gut lumen or tissues. The physiological (homeostatic) response to this is complex: vasodilatation in a vital organ (e.g. brain, heart or kidney) favours perfusion of that organ, but at the expense of a further reduction in blood pressure, which leads to reduced perfusion of other organs. Ideally, there is a balance between vasoconstriction in non-essential vascular beds and vasodilatation in vital ones. The dividing line between the normal physiological response to blood loss and clinical shock is that in shock tissue hypoxia produces secondary effects that magnify rather than correct the primary disturbance. Therefore patients with established shock have profound and inappropriate vasodilatation in non-essential organs, and this is difficult to correct with vasoconstrictor drugs. The release of mediators (e.g. histamine, 5-hydroxytryptamine, bradykinin, prostaglandins, cytokines including interleukins and tumour necrosis factor, NO, and undoubtedly many more as-yet-unidentified substances) that cause capillary dilatation and leakiness is the opposite of what is required to improve function in this setting. Mediators promoting vasodilatation in shock converge on two main mechanisms:

- activation of ATP-sensitive potassium channels in vascular smooth muscle by reduced cytoplasmic ATP and increased lactate and protons

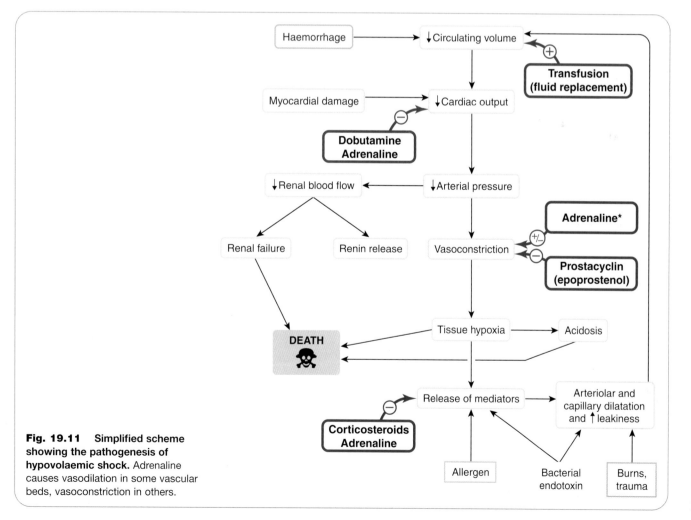

Fig. 19.11 Simplified scheme showing the pathogenesis of hypovolaemic shock. Adrenaline causes vasodilation in some vascular beds, vasoconstriction in others.

- increased synthesis of NO, which activates myosin light-chain phosphatase and activates K_{Ca} channels.

A third key mechanism seems to be a relative deficiency of ADH, which is secreted acutely in response to haemorrhage but subsequently declines, probably because of depletion from the neurohypophysis (see Ch. 28, pp. 425-426).

Patients with shock are not a homogeneous population, making it hard to perform valid clinical trials, and in contrast to hypertension and heart failure there is very little evidence to support treatment strategies based on hard clinical end points (such as improved survival). Hypoperfusion leads to multiple organ failure, and intensive therapy specialists spend much effort supporting the circulations of such patients with cocktails of vasoactive drugs designed to optimise flow to vital organs. Trials of antagonists designed to block or neutralise endotoxin, interleukins, tumour necrosis factor and the inducible form of NO synthase have so far been disappointing. *Volume replacement* is of benefit if there is hypovolaemia; *antibiotics* are essential if there is persistent infection; **adrenaline** can be life-saving in anaphylaxis; a preparation of recombinant *activated protein C*, **drotrecogin alpha (activated)** (see Ch 21, p. 334) improves mortality in severe septic shock with multiple organ failure and is licensed for this indication; *ADH* may be effective in increasing blood pressure even when there is resistance to adrenaline; *corticosteroids* suppress the formation of NO and of prostaglandins but are not of proven benefit once shock is established; **epoprostenol** (PGI_2) may be useful in patients with inappropriate platelet activation (e.g. meningococcal sepsis); positive inotropes, including **adrenaline** and **dobutamine**, may help in individual patients.

PERIPHERAL VASCULAR DISEASE

When atheroma involves peripheral arteries, the commonest symptom is pain in the legs on walking (*claudication*), followed by pain at rest, and in severe cases gangrene of the feet or legs. Treatment is often surgical (surgical reconstruction or amputation) or by *angioplasty* (disruption of atheroma by inflation of a balloon surrounding the tip of a catheter). Other vascular beds (e.g. coronary, cerebral and renal) are often also affected by atheromatous disease in patients with peripheral vascular disease. Drug treatment includes antiplatelet drugs (e.g. **aspirin**, **clopidogrel**; see Ch. 21), a statin (e.g. **simvastatin**; see Ch. 20) and an ACE inhibitor (e.g. **ramipril**; see above). These reduce the excess risk of ischaemic coronary and cerebral events. Additionally, several placebo-controlled studies have demonstrated that **cilostazol**, a type III PDE inhibitor (see above, p. 307), improves pain-free and maximum walking distance in such patients, but its effect on mortality is unknown.

RAYNAUD'S DISEASE

Inappropriate vasoconstriction of small arteries and arterioles gives rise to Raynaud's phenomenon (blanching of the fingers during vasoconstriction, followed by blueness owing to deoxygenation of the static blood and redness from reactive hyperaemia following return of blood flow). This can be mild, but if severe causes ulceration and gangrene of the fingers. It can occur in isolation (Raynaud's disease) or in association with a number of other diseases, including several so-called connective tissue diseases (e.g. systemic sclerosis, systemic lupus erythematosus). Treatment of Raynaud's phenomenon involves stopping smoking and avoiding the cold; β-adrenoceptor antagonists are contraindicated. Vasodilators (e.g. **nifedipine**; see Ch. 18, pp. 295-296) are of some benefit in severe cases, but treatment is difficult.

PULMONARY HYPERTENSION

After birth, pulmonary vascular resistance is much lower than systemic vascular resistance, and systolic pulmonary artery pressure in adults is normally approximately 20 mmHg.[16]

Pulmonary artery pressure is much less easy to measure than is systemic pressure, requiring cardiac catheterisation. If pulmonary artery pressure is raised, this usually causes some leak of the tricuspid valve, allowing regurgitation of blood from the right ventricle to the right atrium. This phenomenon, detectable by ultrasonography, can be used to estimate the pulmonary artery pressure indirectly. Because of the difficulty in measuring pulmonary artery pressure, only severe and symptomatic pulmonary hypertension usually gets diagnosed. Such pulmonary hypertension may be *idiopathic* (i.e. of unknown cause, analogous to essential hypertension in the systemic circulation), or *associated* with some other disease. Increased pulmonary pressure can result from an increased cardiac output (such as occurs for example in patients with hepatic cirrhosis—where vasodilatation may accompany intermittent subclinical exposure to bacterial endotoxin—or in patients with congenital connections between the systemic and pulmonary circulations that lead to increased flow of blood in the low-pressure pulmonary circuit as a consequence of 'shunting' of blood from high to low pressure). Alternatively, vasoconstriction and/or structural narrowing of the pulmonary resistance arteries increase pulmonary arterial pressure, even if flow (cardiac output) is maintained constant. In some situations, both increased cardiac output and increased pulmonary vascular resistance are present. A clinical classification has been proposed by the World Health Organization (see http://www.who.int/cardiovascular_diseases/en/).

In contrast to systemic hypertension, pulmonary hypertension associated with other diseases is much more common than idiopathic pulmonary hypertension, which is a rare, severe and progressive disease. Onset of idiopathic pulmonary hypertension is usually in the thirties, with progressive shortness of breath and fatigue. Women are affected more commonly than men. Approximately 10% of patients have Raynaud's phenomenon

---

[16]In fetal life, pulmonary vascular resistance is high; failure to adapt appropriately at birth is associated with prematurity, lack of pulmonary surfactant, and hypoxaemia. The resulting pulmonary hypertension is treated by paediatric intensivists with measures including replacement of surfactant and ventilatory support, sometimes including inhaled NO—see Ch. 17, pp. 270-271.

(see above). Endothelial dysfunction (see above) p. 299, Ch. 20 p. 321, and Ch. 21 pp. 333-334 is implicated in its aetiology. *Familial* primary pulmonary hypertension is caused by mutations in the gene coding for a receptor related to transforming growth factor-β called bone morphogenetic protein receptor type 2 (*BMPR-2*).

Drugs (e.g. anorexic drugs including **dexfenfluramine**) and toxins (e.g. *monocrotaline*) can cause pulmonary hypertension. Occlusion of the pulmonary arteries, for example with recurrent pulmonary emboli (Ch. 21, p. 335), causes pulmonary hypertension. Pulmonary emboli or thrombi formed in situ as a result of endothelial dysfunction (Ch. 21, pp. 333-334) commonly accompany pulmonary hypertension—both the idiopathic form and when associated with other pathologies. Consequently, anticoagulation (see Ch. 21) is an important part of treatment. Aggregates of sickled red cells in patients with *sickle cell anaemia* (Ch. 22) can occlude small pulmonary arteries during sickling crises and increase pulmonary artery pressure, exacerbated by the increased cardiac output associated with chronic anaemia.

Increased pulmonary vascular resistance may, alternatively, result from vasoconstriction and/or structural changes in the walls of pulmonary resistance arteries. Many of the diseases (e.g. systemic sclerosis) associated with Raynaud's phenomenon mentioned in the section above are also associated with pulmonary hypertension, and there are case reports where pulmonary hypertension was observed in discrete episodes, presumably as a result of vasoconstriction occurring in the pulmonary circulation rather than (or as well as) in the skin of the fingers. Vasoconstriction may precede cellular proliferation and medial hypertrophy in the pulmonary vasculature. Treatment with vasodilators such as the calcium antagonist **nifedipine** is of some use, but vasodilators that also have an antiproliferative action (e.g. **epoprostenol**, drugs that potentiate NO, or drugs that antagonise endothelin) are more promising—see below.

Several diseases affect the pulmonary vasculature directly (e.g. *sarcoidosis*, *histiocytosis X* and *schistosomiasis*[17]) and can cause pulmonary hypertension. In addition, pulmonary vessels are unique in *constricting* in response to hypoxia; physiologically, this enables the lung to match poorly ventilated areas with reduced perfusion, but when hypoxia is generalised it causes pulmonary hypertension.[18] Consequently, *any* lung disease that causes hypoxaemia of sufficient severity will be complicated by pulmonary hypertension, even if the pulmonary vasculature is not directly involved, and oxygen treatment is indicated to correct this. The mechanism of pulmonary hypoxic vasoconstriction remains elusive, but both an increase in $[Ca^{2+}]_i$ and increased sensitivity to Ca^{2+}, possibly mediated by Rho kinase (see above, p. 305) have been implicated.

---

[17]Respectively, a granulomatous disease with histological features related to those of tuberculosis, infiltration of various tissues with abnormal histiocytes, and an infection with a parasite that is endemic in the Nile delta and has a life cycle shared between humans and snails—see Ch. 50, p. 713.

[18]Glover and Newson were commissioned by cattle ranchers to study high mountain disease in cattle in Colorado in 1913, leading to the recognition that chronic hypoxia causes pulmonary hypertension, medial hypertrophy of the small pulmonary arteries, and right ventricular hypertrophy.

Drug treatment

Drugs used in treating pulmonary arterial hypertension are shown in the clinical box. It follows from the above discussion that treatment is often that of the underlying disease. In addition to *anticoagulation* and inhaled *oxygen*, **digoxin** (Ch. 18) and *diuretics* (Ch. 24) can provide symptomatic improvement. Recently, several direct and indirect vasodilators have been shown to have useful clinical effects, including improved exercise tolerance and slowing of disease progression. Continuous intravenous **epoprostenol** (see Ch. 13), inhaled **iloprost** (a stable analogue of prostacyclin, sometimes administered by inhalation of a mist of nebulised solution, in the same way as for several of the drugs used to treat asthma, Ch. 23), subcutaneous **treprostinil** and oral **bosentan** (see above, pp. 301-303) are all used clinically. The choice of drug is influenced by the stage of the disease (usually classified using a system modified from that used in heart failure—the New York Heart Association–World Health Organization classification—where I is very mild and IV severe). Oral treatment (e.g. bosentan) is used for the less severe and parenteral (subcutaneous treprostinil, intravenous epoprostenol) for the more severe. Survival may be improved by epoprostenol (see Fig. 19.12). Inhaled NO is

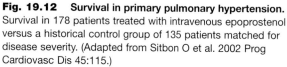

Drugs used in pulmonary hypertension

- Oral anticoagulants (Ch. 21).
- Diuretics (Ch. 24).
- Oxygen.
- Digoxin (Ch. 18).
- Calcium channel blockers (Ch. 18).
- Epoprostenol (Ch. 13).
- Prostanoid analogues (iloprost, treprostinil, beraprost).
- Bosentan.
- Phosphodiesterase V inhibitor (sildenafil).

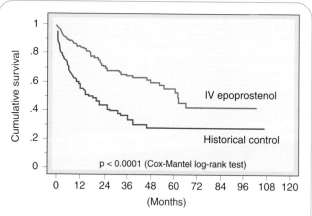

Fig. 19.12 Survival in primary pulmonary hypertension. Survival in 178 patients treated with intravenous epoprostenol versus a historical control group of 135 patients matched for disease severity. (Adapted from Sitbon O et al. 2002 Prog Cardiovasc Dis 45:115.)

mentioned above in the context of pulmonary hypertensive crises, for example in the newborn. PDE V inhibitors (e.g. **sildenafil**) potentiate the action of NO by blocking the metabolism of cGMP (Ch. 17, p. 269) and show promise in idiopathic pulmonary hypertension.

Unwanted effects

Adverse effects of the prostaglandin analogues relate mainly to systemic vasodilatation (e.g. flushing, hypotension, syncope); **bosentan** causes dose-related increases in liver transaminases; unwanted effects of **sildenafil** are on page 459.

Clinical disorders for which vasoactive drugs are important

- *Systemic hypertension:*
  - secondary to underlying disease (e.g. renal or endocrine)
  - primary 'essential' hypertension, an important risk factor for atheromatous disease (Ch. 20). Treatment reduces the excess risk of stroke or myocardial infarction, the main classes of drugs being *A*, angiotensin-converting enzyme (ACE) inhibitors or AT_1 receptor antagonists; *B*, β-adrenoceptor antagonists; *C*, calcium antagonists; and *D*, diuretics.
- *Cardiac failure.* Several diseases (most commonly ischaemic heart disease) impair the ability of the heart to deliver an output adequate to metabolic needs. Symptoms of oedema can be improved with diuretics. Life expectancy is reduced but can be improved by treatment of haemodynamically stable patients with:
  - ACE inhibitors and/or AT_1 receptor antagonists
  - β-adrenoceptor antagonists (e.g. **carvedilol, bisoprolol**)

- aldosterone antagonists (e.g. **spironolactone**).
- *Shock.* Several diseases (e.g. overwhelming bacterial infections, Ch. 46; anaphylactic reactions, Ch. 23) lead to inappropriate vasodilatation, hypotension and reduced tissue perfusion with raised circulating concentrations of lactic acid. Pressors (e.g. **adrenaline**) are used.
- *Peripheral vascular disease.* Atheromatous plaques in the arteries of the legs are often associated with atheroma in other vascular territories. Statins (Ch. 20) and antiplatelet drugs (Ch. 21) are important.
- *Raynaud's disease.* Inappropriate vasoconstriction in small arteries in the hands causes blanching of the fingers followed by blueness and pain. **Nifedipine** or other vasodilators are used.
- *Pulmonary hypertension,* which can be:
  - *idiopathic* (a rare disorder): **epoprostenol, iloprost, bosentan** and **sildenafil** are of benefit in selected patients
  - *associated* with hypoxic lung disease.

REFERENCES AND FURTHER READING

Vascular structure and function, control of vascular smooth muscle tone

Guimarães S, Moura D 2001 Vascular adrenoceptors: an update. Pharmacol Rev 53: 319–356 (*Functional perspective*)

Quayle J M, Nelson M T, Standen N B 1997 ATP-sensitive and inwardly rectifying potassium channels in smooth muscle. Physiol Rev 77: 1165–1232 (*Reviews these potassium channels, both of which are important in controlling the contractile state of vascular smooth muscle*)

Stasch J-P et al. 2001 NO-independent regulatory site on soluble guanylate cyclase. Nature 410: 212–415 (*An activator of this site, BAY 41-2242, relaxes vascular smooth muscle, inhibits platelet aggregation and lowers blood pressure in the spontaneously hypertensive rat*)

Uehata M, Ishizaki T, Satoh H et al. 1997 Calcium sensitization of smooth muscle mediated by a Rho-associated protein kinase in hypertension. Nature 389: 990–994 (*A pyridine derivative, Y-27632, selectively inhibits smooth muscle contraction by inhibiting Ca^{2+} sensitisation via the Rho-associated protein kinase pathway, and lowers blood pressure in several experimental models of hypertension*)

Ward J P T, Knock G A, Snetkov V A, Aaronson P I 2004 Protein kinases in vascular smooth muscle tone—role in the pulmonary vasculature and hypoxic pulmonary vasoconstriction. Pharmacol Ther 104:

207–231 (*Concludes that the strongest evidence for direct involvement of protein kinases in the mechanisms of hypoxic pulmonary vasoconstriction concerns a central role for Rho kinase in Ca^{2+} sensitisation*)

Vascular endothelium (see Ch. 17 for further reading on nitric oxide)

Prostacyclin

Bunting S, Gryglewski R, Moncada S, Vane JR 1976 Arterial walls generate from prostaglandin endoperoxides a substance (prostaglandin X) which relaxes strips of mesenteric and celiac arteries and inhibits platelet aggregation. Prostaglandins 12: 897–913 (*Classic*)

Murata T, Ushikubi F, Matsuoka T et al. 1997 Altered pain perception and inflammatory response in mice lacking prostacyclin receptor. Nature 388: 678–682 (*I prostanoid receptor–deficient mice are viable, reproductive and normotensive; however, their susceptibility to thrombosis is increased ... the results establish that prostacyclin is an endogenous antithrombotic agent*)

Endothelium-derived hyperpolarising factor

Busse R, Edwards G, Feletou M et al. 2002 EDHF: bringing the concepts together. Trends Pharmacol Sci 23: 374–380 (*Consensus on EDHF? Potassium ions are important*)

Huang A, Sun D, Smith C J et al. 2000 In eNOS knockout mice skeletal muscle arteriolar dilation to acetylcholine is mediated by EDHF. Am J Physiol 278: H762–H768 (*Where NO is absent, EDHF compensates*)

Angiogenesis

Carmeliet P, Jain R K 2000 Angiogenesis in cancer and other diseases. Nature 407: 249–257 (*New approaches to treatment of cancer and other diseases, via a growing number of pro- and antiangiogenic molecules; see also (in same issue) Yancopoulos G D et al. 2000 Vascular specific growth factors and blood vessel formation, pp. 242–248*)

Endothelin

Bagnall A J, Webb D J 2000 The endothelin system: physiology. In: Vallance P J T, Webb D J (eds) Vascular endothelium in human physiology and pathophysiology. Harwood Academic, Singapore, pp. 31–60

Haynes W G, Webb D J 1994 Contribution of endogenous generation of endothelin-1 to basal vascular tone. Lancet 344: 852–854 (*Demonstrated a contribution in humans of endogenous endothelin-1 to peripheral vascular tone by local intra-arterial administration of phosphoramidon and an ET_A antagonist*)

Hickey K A, Rubanyi G, Paul R J, Highsmith R F 1985 Characterization of a coronary vasoconstrictor produced by cultured endothelial cells. Am J Physiol 248(part 1): C550–C556 (*Key discovery*)

Kedzierski R M, Yanagisawa M 2001 Endothelin system: the double-edged sword in health and disease. Annu Rev Pharmacol Toxicol 41: 851–876 (*Review by one of the discoverers of endothelin*)

Kirchengast M, Luz M 2005 Endothelin receptor antagonists—clinical realities and future directions. J Cardiovasc Pharmacol 5: 182–191 (*Critically reviews clinical data on endothelin receptor antagonism in cardiovascular indications against the background of preclinical research*)

Yanagisawa M, Kurihara H, Kimura S et al. 1988 A novel potent vasoconstrictor peptide produced by vascular endothelial cells. Nature 332: 411–415 (*Tour de force*)

Renin–angiotensin system

Burnier M, Brunner H R 2000 Angiotensin II receptor antagonists. Lancet 355: 637–645 (*Reviews this class of drugs*)

Cai H, Griendling K K, Harrison D G 2003 The vascular NAD(P)H oxidases as therapeutic targets in cardiovascular diseases. Trends Pharmacol Sci 24: 471–478 (*Reactive oxygen species produced following angiotensin II-mediated stimulation of NAD(P)H oxidases signal through pathways such as mitogen-activated protein kinases, tyrosine kinases and transcription factors, and lead to inflammation, hypertrophy, remodelling and angiogenesis. Studies in mice deficient in NAD(P)H oxidase subunits show that reactive oxygen species produced by these oxidases contribute to cardiovascular diseases including atherosclerosis and hypertension.*)

Heart Outcomes Prevention Evaluation Study Investigators 2000 Effects of an angiotensin-converting enzyme inhibitor, ramipril, on cardiovascular events in high-risk patients. N Engl J Med 342: 145–153 (*Ramipril significantly lowers rates of death, myocardial infarction and stroke in a wide range of high-risk patients*)

Hein L, Barsh G S, Pratt R E et al. 1995 Behavioural and cardiovascular effects of disrupting the angiotensin II type-2 receptor gene in mice. Nature 377: 744–747 ('*The AT_2 receptor plays a role in the CNS and in cardiovascular functions that are mediated by the renin–angiotensin system.*' Pause for thought for clinicians inclined to prescribe ACE inhibitors and AT_1 receptor antagonists interchangeably.)

Ichiki T, Labosky P A, Shiota C et al. 1995 Effects on blood pressure and exploratory behaviour of mice lacking angiotensin II type-2 receptor. Nature 377: 748–750 (*Angiotensin II activates AT_1 and AT_2, which have mutually counteracting haemodynamic effects; AT_2 regulates CNS functions, including behaviour*)

Watanabe T, Barker T A, Berk B C 2005 Angiotensin II and the endothelium—diverse signals and effects. Hypertension 45: 163–169 (*Reviews the renin–angiotensin system in the endothelium based on the diverse signals and effects mediated by multiple angiotensin I- and angiotensin II-derived peptides, multiple angiotensin-metabolising enzymes, multiple receptors, and vascular bed-specific intracellular signals*)

Vasoactive drugs

Vasoconstrictor drugs

Antidiuretic hormone

Holmes C L, Russell J A 2004 Vasopressin. Semin Respir Crit Care Med 25: 705–711 ('*A deficiency of vasopressin exists in some shock states and replacement of physiological levels of vasopressin can restore vascular tone. Vasopressin is therefore emerging as a rational therapy for vasodilatory shock.*' Reviews rationale, evidence and uncertainties for using vasopressin in shock.)

Vasodilator drugs (see Ch. 18 for further reading on calcium antagonists)

Indirect

Chan C K S, Burke S L, Zhu H et al. 2005 Imidazoline receptors associated with noradrenergic terminals in the rostral ventrolateral medulla mediate the hypotensive responses of moxonidine but not clonidine. Neuroscience 132: 991–1007 (*The hypotensive and bradycardic actions of moxonidine but not clonidine are mediated through imidazoline receptors and depend on noradrenergic CNS pathways; noradrenergic innervation may be associated with imidazoline receptor protein*)

Weber M A 2001 Vasopeptidase inhibitors. Lancet 358: 1525–1532 (*Reviews this new class of drug, for example omapatrilat, that inhibits both neutral endopeptidase and ACE; omapatrilat is more effective than other antihypertensive drugs and encouraging in heart failure. The frequency of angiooedema 'remains to be established', as do effects on clinical end points.*)

Clinical uses

Hypertension

Murphy M B, Murray C, Shorten G D 2001 Fenoldopam—a selective peripheral dopamine receptor agonist for treatment of severe hypertension. N Engl J Med 345: 1548–1557 (*Similar effectiveness as that of nitroprusside but without thiocyanate toxicity or instability in light; however, it is slower in onset and offset than nitroprusside*)

Chronic heart failure

Background reading

Jessup M, Brozena S. 2003 Heart failure. N Engl J Med 348: 2007–2018

References

Azizi M, Menard J 2004 Combined blockade of the renin–angiotensin system with angiotensin-converting enzyme inhibitors and angiotensin II type 1 receptor antagonists. Circulation 109: 2492–2499 (*Discusses rationale*)

de Lemos J A, McGuire D K, Drazner M H 2003 B-type natriuretic peptide in cardiovascular disease. Lancet 362: 316–322 (*BNP is an important diagnostic tool and possible therapeutic agent in heart failure. Reviews the physiology of the natriuretic peptide system, measurement of circulating concentrations of BNP ... to diagnose heart failure and assess prognosis in patients with cardiac abnormalities, and use of recombinant human BNP—nesiritide—and vasopeptidase inhibitors to treat heart failure.*)

Gheorghiade M, Gattis W A, O'Connor C M et al. 2004 Effects of tolvaptan, a vasopressin antagonist, in patients hospitalized with worsening heart failure—a randomized controlled trial. JAMA 291: 1963–1971 (*tolvaptan + standard therapy has promise for heart failure*)

McMurray J J V 2005 Val-HeFT: do angiotensin-receptor blockers benefit heart failure patients already receiving ACE inhibitor therapy? Nat Clin Pract Cardiovasc Med 2: 128–129

MERIT-HF Study Group 1999 Effect of metoprolol CR/XL in chronic heart failure: Metoprolol CR/XL Randomized Intervention Trial in Congestive Heart Failure (MERIT-HF). Lancet 353: 2001–2007 (*Randomised trial in 3991 patients: addition of metoprolol to standard optimum treatment substantially improved survival; see also accompanying editorial entitled* Benefit of β blockers for heart failure: proven in 1999 *by N Sharpe for references to other β blocker/heart failure trials*)

Sackner-Bernstein J D, Kowalski M, Fox M, Aaronson K 2005 Short-term risk of death after treatment with nesiritide for decompensated heart failure—a pooled

analysis of randomized controlled trials. JAMA 293: 1900–1905 ('*Nesiritide—i.e. BNP—may be associated with an increased risk of death after treatment for acutely decompensated heart failure. The possibility of an increased risk of death should be investigated in a large-scale, adequately powered, controlled trial before routine use of nesiritide for acutely decompensated heart failure.*')

Taylor A L, Ziesche S, Yancy C et al. 2004 Combination of isosorbide dinitrate and hydralazine in blacks with heart failure. N Engl J Med 351: 2049–2057 (*Addition of a fixed dose of isosorbide dinitrate plus hydralazine to standard therapy for heart failure including neurohormonal blockers increased survival among black patients with advanced heart failure*)

Topol E J 2005 Nesiritide—not verified. N Engl J Med 353: 113–116 (*Critical perspective*)

Shock

Further reading

Landry D W, Oliver J A 2001 Mechanisms of disease: the pathogenesis of vasodilatory shock. N Engl J Med 345: 588–595 (*Reviews mechanisms promoting inappropriate vasodilation in shock, including activation of ATP-sensitive potassium channels, increased synthesis of NO and depletion of ADH*)

References

Australian and New Zealand Intensive Care Society Clinical Trials Group 2000 Low-dose dopamine in patients with early renal dysfunction: a placebo-controlled randomized trial. Lancet 356: 2139–2143 (*No clinically significant protection; see also accompanying editorial,* Renal-dose dopamine: will the message now get through?)

Bernard G R et al. 2001 Efficacy and safety of recombinant human activated protein C for severe sepsis. N Engl J Med 344: 699–709 (*Continuous intravenous infusion of activated protein C, a vitamin K–dependent anticoagulant that promotes fibrinolysis, inhibits thrombosis and is anti-inflammatory, significantly reduced risk of death at 28 days, from 30.8 to 24.7%*)

Peripheral vascular disease

Hiatt W R 2001 Medical treatment of peripheral arterial disease and claudication. N Engl J Med 344: 1608–1621 (*Discusses risk factor modification, summarises evidence for efficacy of cilostazol, and describes rationale for several investigational drugs, for example propionyl levocarnitine*)

Raynaud's disease and pulmonary hypertension

Further reading

Rich S, McLaughlin V V 2005 Chapter 67. In: Zipes D P, Libby P, Bonow R O, Braunwald E (eds) Braunwald's heart disease, 7th edn. Elsevier, Philadelphia, pp. 1807–1842

Task-force on Diagnosis and Treatment of Pulmonary Arterial Hypertension of the European Society of Cardiology 2004 Guidelines on diagnosis and treatment of pulmonary arterial hypertension. Eur Heart J 25: 2243–2278

References

Abe K, Shimokawa H, Morikawa K et al. 2004 Long-term treatment with a Rho-kinase inhibitor improves monocrotaline-induced fatal pulmonary hypertension in rats. Circ Res 94: 385–393 (*The Rho-kinase–mediated pathway is involved in the pathogenesis of pulmonary hypertension, suggesting that this molecule could be a novel therapeutic target for this fatal disorder.*)

Badesch D B, Abman S H, Ahearn G S et al. 2004 Medical therapy for pulmonary arterial hypertension—

ACCP evidence-based clinical practice guidelines. Chest 126(suppl): 35S–62S (*Evidence-based treatment recommendations for physicians involved in the care of these complex patients*)

Beppu H, Ichinose F, Kawai N et al. 2004 BMPR-II heterozygous mice have mild pulmonary hypertension and an impaired pulmonary vascular remodeling response to prolonged hypoxia. Am J Physiol Lung Cell Mol Physiol 287: L1241–L1247 ('*Heterozygous mutations of the bone morphogenetic protein type II receptor, BMPR-II, gene have been identified in patients with primary pulmonary hypertension ... in mice, mutation of one copy of the BMPR-II gene causes pulmonary hypertension but impairs the ability of the pulmonary vasculature to remodel in response to prolonged hypoxic breathing.*')

Channick R N et al. 2001 Effects of the dual endothelin-receptor antagonist bosentan in patients with pulmonary hypertension. Lancet 358: 1119–1123 (*Bosentan increased exercise capacity and reduced pulmonary vascular resistance in a 12-week double-blind placebo-controlled study of 32 patients with this serious disorder for which previous therapies have been unsatisfactory*)

Higenbottam T, Laude L, Emery C, Essener M 2004 Pulmonary hypertension as a result of drug therapy. Clin Chest Med 25: 123–131 (*Reviews anorectic drug-induced pulmonary arterial hypertension and considers mechanisms*)

Humbert M, Sitbon O, Simonneau G 2004 Drug therapy: treatment of pulmonary arterial hypertension. N Engl J Med 351: 1425–1436

Lee A J, Chiao T B, Tsang M P 2005 Sildenafil for pulmonary hypertension. Ann Pharmacother 39: 869–884 (*Sildenafil is a promising and well-tolerated treatment for pulmonary hypertension; well-designed trials are needed*)

McLaughlin V V, Sitbon O, Badesch D B et al. 2005 Survival with first-line bosentan in patients with primary pulmonary hypertension. Eur Respir J 25: 244–249 (*Bosentan improved survival in patients with advanced primary pulmonary hypertension*)

Napoli C, Loscalzo J 2004 Nitric oxide and other novel therapies for pulmonary hypertension. J Cardiovasc Pharmacol Ther 9: 1–8 (*Focus on endothelial NO, NO replacement and related therapies*)

Papp Z, Csapo K, Pollesello P et al. 2005 Pharmacological mechanisms contributing to the clinical efficacy of levosimendan. Cardiovasc Drug Rev 23: 71–98 (*Levosimendan is a Ca^{2+} sensitiser, binding to troponin C in the myocardium and, additionally, opening ATP-sensitive potassium channels in vascular smooth muscle. Clinical studies have suggested long-term benefits on mortality following short-term administration in patients with decompensated heart failure.*)

Runo J R, Loyd J E 2003 Primary pulmonary hypertension. Lancet 361: 1533–1544 ('*Without treatment, the disorder progresses in most cases to right heart failure and death. With current therapies such as epoprostenol, progression of disease is slowed, but not halted. Many promising new therapeutic options, including prostacyclin analogues, endothelin-l receptor antagonists, and phosphodiesterase inhibitors, improve clinical function and haemodynamic measures and may prolong survival.*')

West J, Fagan K, Steudel W et al. 2004 Pulmonary hypertension in transgenic mice expressing a dominant-negative BMPRII gene in smooth muscle. Circ Res 94: 1109–1114 (*Bone morphogenetic peptides, BMPs, a family of cytokines critical to normal development, are implicated in the pathogenesis of familial pulmonary arterial hypertension; deletion of BMPRII results in early fetal death. To study BMP signalling in postnatal vascular disease, these authors constructed a smooth muscle–specific transgenic mouse expressing a dominant-negative BMPRII under control of a tetracycline gene switch. When the mutation was activated after birth, mice developed increased pulmonary artery pressure, indicating that loss of BMPRII signalling is sufficient to produce the pulmonary hypertensive phenotype.*)

Zhao L, Mason N A, Morrell N W et al. 2001 Sildenafil inhibits hypoxia-induced pulmonary hypertension. Circulation 104: 424–428

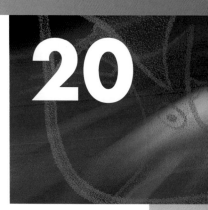

Atherosclerosis and lipoprotein metabolism

20

OVERVIEW

Atheromatous disease is ubiquitous and underlies the commonest causes of death (myocardial infarction caused by thrombosis—Chapter 21—which occurs on ruptured atheromatous plaque) and disability (stroke, heart failure) in industrial societies. Hypertension is one of the most important risk factors for atheroma, and is discussed in Chapter 19. Here, we consider other risk factors, especially dyslipidaemia,[1] which, like hypertension, is amenable to drug therapy. We describe briefly the processes of atherogenesis and of lipid transport as a basis for understanding the actions of lipid-lowering drugs. Important agents (*statins, fibrates, cholesterol absorption inhibitors, nicotinic acid derivatives, fish oil derivatives*) are described, with emphasis on the statins, which reduce the incidence of arterial disease and prolong life.

ATHEROGENESIS

Atheroma is a *focal* disease of the intima of large and medium-sized arteries. Lesions evolve over decades, during most of which time they are clinically silent, the occurrence of symptoms signalling advanced disease. Presymptomatic lesions are often difficult to detect non-invasively, although ultrasound is useful in relatively static and superficial arteries (e.g. the carotids), and associated changes such as reduced aortic compliance and arterial calcium deposition can be detected by measuring, respectively, aortic pulse wave velocity and coronary artery calcification. Until recently, there have been no good subprimate models, but transgenic mice (see Ch. 6) deficient in apolipoproteins or receptors that play key roles in lipoprotein metabolism have transformed this scene. Nevertheless, most of our current understanding of atherogenesis comes from human epidemiology and pathology, and from clinical investigations.

Epidemiological studies have identified numerous risk factors for atheromatous disease. Some of these cannot be altered (e.g. a family history of ischaemic heart disease), but others are modifiable (see Table 20.1) and are potential targets for therapeutic drugs. Clinical trials have shown that improving risk factors can reduce the consequences of atheromatous disease. For example, drugs that reduce the concentration of low-density lipoprotein cholesterol (LDL-C) in plasma reduce the incidence of myocardial infarction. Many risk factors cause endothelial dysfunction (see Ch. 19, pp. 299-301), evidenced by reduced vasodilator responses to acetylcholine or to increased blood flow (so-called 'flow-mediated dilatation', a response that is inhibited by drugs that block nitric oxide, NO, synthesis; Ch. 17, pp. 271-272). Healthy endothelium produces NO and other mediators that protect against atheroma, so it is likely that the adverse effects on endothelium of many metabolic risk factors are a common pathway to atherogenesis.

Atherogenesis involves the following.

1. Endothelial dysfunction, with altered prostaglandin (PG) I_2 (prostacyclin; Ch. 13) and NO (Ch. 17) biosynthesis.
2. Injury of dysfunctional endothelium leads to expression of adhesion molecules. This encourages monocyte attachment and migration of monocytes from the lumen into the intima. Lesions have a predilection for regions of disturbed flow such as the origins of aortic branches.
3. Low-density lipoprotein (LDL) particles are transported into the vessel wall. Endothelial cells and monocytes/macrophages

---

[1]The term *dyslipidaemia* is preferred to *hyperlipidaemia* because a *low* plasma concentration of high-density lipoprotein cholesterol is believed to be harmful and is a novel therapeutic target.

Table 20.1 Modifiable risk factors for atheromatous disease

Raised low-density lipoprotein cholesterol

Reduced high-density lipoprotein cholesterol

Hypertension (Ch. 19)

Diabetes mellitus (Ch. 26)

Cigarette smoking (Ch. 54)

Obesity (Ch. 27)

Physical inactivity

Raised C-reactive protein[a]

Raised coagulation factors (e.g. factor VII, fibrinogen)

Raised homocysteine

Raised lipoprotein(a)[b]

[a]Strongly associated with atheromatous disease but unknown if this is causal.
[b]Potentially modifiable but strongly genetically determined: nicotinic acid does lower lipoprotein(a).

Atheromatous disease

- Atheroma is a focal disease of large and medium-sized arteries. Atheromatous plaques are almost universally present in members of economically developed countries, progress insidiously over many decades, and underlie the commonest causes of death (myocardial infarction) and disability (e.g. stroke) in these countries.
- Fatty streaks are the earliest structurally apparent lesion and progress to fibrous and/or fatty plaques. Symptoms depend on the vascular bed and occur only when blood flow through the vessel is reduced below that needed to meet the metabolic demands of tissues downstream from the obstruction.
- Important modifiable risk factors include hypertension (Ch. 19), dyslipidaemia (this chapter) and smoking (Ch. 43).
- The pathophysiology is of chronic inflammation in response to injury. Endothelial dysfunction leads to loss of protective mechanisms, monocyte/macrophage and T-cell migration, uptake of low-density lipoprotein (LDL) cholesterol and its oxidation, uptake of oxidised LDL by macrophages, smooth muscle cell migration and proliferation, and deposition of collagen.
- Plaque rupture leads to platelet activation and thrombosis (Ch. 21).

generate free radicals that oxidise LDL (oxLDL), resulting in lipid peroxidation.

4. The oxLDL is taken up by macrophages via 'scavenger' receptors. Such macrophages are called foam cells because of their 'foamy' histological appearance, resulting from accumulation of cytoplasmic lipid. Uptake of oxLDL activates macrophages and releases proinflammatory cytokines. Foam cells are pathognomonic of atheroma. Macrophage chemotaxis is inhibited by *tetrahydrocannabinol*, and CB_2 receptor agonists have potential as antiatherosclerotic drugs (see Ch. 15).

5. Subendothelial collections of foam cells and T lymphocytes form fatty streaks.

6. Cholesterol can be mobilised from the artery wall and transported in plasma in the form of high-density lipoprotein cholesterol (HDL-C).

7. Activated platelets, macrophages and endothelial cells release cytokines and growth factors, causing proliferation of smooth muscle and deposition of connective tissue components. This inflammatory fibroproliferative response leads to a dense fibrous cap overlying a lipid-rich core, the whole structure comprising the atheromatous plaque.

8. A plaque can rupture, forming a substrate for *thrombosis* (see Ch. 21, Figs 21.1 and 21.10). The presence of large numbers of macrophages predisposes to plaque rupture, whereas vascular smooth muscle and matrix proteins stabilise the plaque.

PREVENTION OF ATHEROMATOUS DISEASE

Drug treatment is often justified, to supplement healthy habits. Treatment of hypertension (Ch. 19) and, to a lesser extent, diabetes mellitus (Ch. 26) reduces the incidence of symptomatic atheromatous disease, and antithrombotic drugs (Ch. 21) reduce arterial thrombosis. Reducing LDL-C is highly effective and is the main subject of this present chapter, but several other steps in atherogenesis are also potential targets for pharmacological attack. *Angiotensin-converting enzyme inhibitors* (Ch. 19) improve endothelial function and prolong life in patients with atheromatous disease. Other drugs that also increase NO biosynthesis or availability are under investigation. Moderate *alcohol* consumption increases HDL-C, and epidemiological evidence favours moderate alcohol consumption in older people.[2]

▼ Regular exercise also increases circulating HDL-C; drug treatment to increase HDL-C is less established than drugs that lower LDL-C, because until recently such drugs (e.g. *fibrates and nicotinic acid derivatives*—see below) have had only modest effects on HDL-C, accompanied by effects on LDL-C and triglycerides that complicate interpretation of clinical trials. However, in subjects with low HDL-C, inhibition of cholesteryl ester transfer protein (CETP; see below) with **torcetrapib** markedly

---

[2]'Sinful, ginful, rum-soaked men, survive for three score years and ten'—or longer, we rather hope...

increases HDL-C (Brousseau et al., 2004). Torcetrapib is being developed in combination with a statin. ApoA-I Milano is a variant of apolipoprotein A-I identified in individuals in rural Italy with very low levels of HDL but *low* arterial disease prevalence. Infusion of recombinant ApoA-I Milano–phospholipid complexes produces rapid regression of atherosclerosis in animal models, and administered intravenously caused regression of atherosclerosis in patients with acute coronary syndrome (Nissen et al., 2003).

Antioxidants (e.g. vitamin C and vitamin E) are of interest, both because of evidence that they improve endothelial function in patients with increased oxidant stress, and because of epidemiological evidence that a diet rich in antioxidants is associated with reduced risk of coronary artery disease. Results from clinical trials have been negative, however, and several antioxidants reduce HDL-C. *Oestrogen*, used to prevent symptoms of the menopause (Ch. 30) and to prevent postmenopausal osteoporosis, has antioxidant properties and exerts other vascular effects that could be beneficial. Epidemiological evidence suggested that women who use such hormone replacement are at reduced risk of atheromatous disease, but controlled trials show significant *adverse* effects on cardiovascular mortality (Ch. 30 and see commentary by Dubey et al., 2004). Drug treatment to lower C-reactive protein has been mooted, but it is possible that elevated C-reactive protein is a marker of vascular inflammation rather than playing an active part in disease progression. Other anti-inflammatory measures are being investigated; for example, an acyl coenzyme A: cholesterol acyltransferase (ACAT) inhibitor, **avasimibe**, reduces circulating tumour necrosis factor-α levels in hypercholesterolaemic subjects without much effect on plasma lipids, and improves resistance vessel endothelial function (Kharbanda et al., 2005), but it may not improve coronary atherosclerosis (Tardif et al., 2004). Other novel therapies in development were reviewed recently (Wierzbicki, 2004).

Plasma homocysteine can be lowered by supplementing the diet with *folic acid*, and it will be interesting to see whether countries such as the USA, which have introduced folate supplements to prevent congenital neural tube defects (see Ch. 53, p. 759), experience a reduced incidence of atheromatous disease.

In contrast to this somewhat unclear (albeit exciting) picture, drugs that lower plasma LDL-C are of proven benefit in preventing coronary artery disease. To understand how such drugs work, it is necessary to address how lipids are handled in the body.

LIPOPROTEIN TRANSPORT IN THE BLOOD

Lipids and cholesterol are transported through the bloodstream as macromolecular complexes of lipid and protein known as lipoproteins. These consist of a central core of hydrophobic lipid (including triglycerides and cholesteryl esters) encased in a hydrophilic coat of polar phospholipid, free cholesterol and apolipoprotein. There are four main classes of lipoprotein, differing in the relative proportion of the core lipids and in the type of apoprotein. They also differ in size and density, and this latter property, as measured by ultracentrifugation, is the basis for their classification into:

- HDL-C particles
- LDL-C particles
- very low-density lipoprotein (VLDL) particles
- chylomicrons.

Each class of lipoprotein has a specific role in lipid transport, and there are different pathways for exogenous and for endogenous

lipids, as well as a pathway for reverse cholesterol transport (Fig. 20.1). The pathways are distinguished by the main *apoproteins* (apoB-48, apoB-100 and apoA1, respectively) that are ligands for the key receptors. In the exogenous pathway, cholesterol and triglycerides absorbed from the ileum are transported as chylomicrons (diameter 100–1000 nm), in lymph and then blood, to capillaries in muscle and adipose tissue. Here, triglycerides are hydrolysed by lipoprotein lipase, and the tissues take up the resulting free fatty acids and glycerol. The chylomicron remnants (diameter 30–50 nm), still containing their full complement of cholesteryl esters, pass to the liver, bind to receptors on hepatocytes and undergo endocytosis. Cholesterol liberated in hepatocytes is stored, oxidised to bile acids, secreted unaltered in bile, or can enter the endogenous pathway.

In the endogenous pathway, cholesterol and newly synthesised triglycerides are transported from the liver as VLDL (diameter 30–80 nm) to muscle and adipose tissue, where triglyceride is hydrolysed to fatty acids and glycerol; these enter the tissues as described above. During this process, the lipoprotein particles become smaller (diameter 20–30 nm) but retain a full complement of cholesteryl esters. Consequently, they increase in density to intermediate-density cholesterol and ultimately LDL-C particles. LDL-C provides the source of cholesterol for incorporation into cell membranes and for synthesis of steroids (see Chs 28 and 30) but is also key in atherogenesis, as described above. Cells take up LDL-C by endocytosis via LDL receptors that recognise LDL apolipoproteins. Some drugs (notably statins; see below) reduce circulating LDL-C by inhibiting endogenous cholesterol synthesis and stimulating the synthesis of hepatic LDL receptors. Cholesterol can return to plasma from the tissues in HDL particles (diameter 7–20 nm). Cholesterol is esterified with long-chain fatty acids in HDL particles, and the resulting cholesteryl esters are transferred to VLDL or LDL particles by a transfer protein present in the plasma and known as cholesteryl ester transfer protein (CETP). Lipoprotein(a), or Lp(a), is a species of LDL that is strongly associated with atherosclerosis and is localised in atherosclerotic lesions. Lp(a) contains a unique apoprotein, apo(a), with structural similarities to *plasminogen* (Ch. 21, p. 344). Lp(a) competes with and inhibits the binding of plasminogen to its receptors on the endothelial cell. Plasminogen is normally the substrate for *plasminogen activator*, which is secreted by and bound to endothelial cells, generating the fibrinolytic enzyme *plasmin* (see Fig. 21.10). The effect of the binding of Lp(a) is that less plasmin is generated, fibrinolysis is inhibited and thrombosis promoted.

There is currently much interest in four lipid transfer proteins that have been implicated in atherogenesis. *ACAT* (acyl coenzyme A: cholesterol acyltransferase), which is expressed in two forms, catalyses the intracellular synthesis of cholesteryl ester in macrophages, adrenal cortex, gut and liver. *LCAT* (*lecithin cholesterol acyltransferase*) catalyses cholesteryl ester synthesis in HDL particles. *CETP* and *PLTP* (*phospholipid transfer protein*) are involved in transfer of cholesterol between different classes of lipoprotein particle in plasma. **Tamoxifen**, used in the treatment and prevention of breast cancer (Ch. 51, p. 729; also discussed in Ch. 30 on p. 449), was recently discovered to be a potent ACAT inhibitor (De Medina et al., 2004). So far, the most promising therapeutic approach has been inhibition of CETP: **torcetrapib**

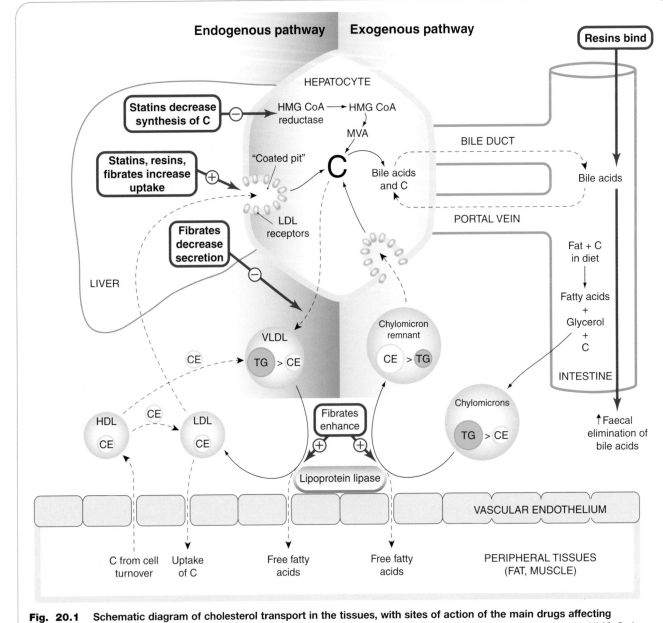

Fig. 20.1 **Schematic diagram of cholesterol transport in the tissues, with sites of action of the main drugs affecting lipoprotein metabolism.** ACoA, acetyl-coenzyme A; C, cholesterol; CE, cholesteryl ester; HDL, high-density lipoprotein; HMG-CoA reductase, 3-hydroxy-3-methylglutaryl-coenzyme A reductase; LDL, low-density lipoprotein; MVA, mevalonate; TG, triglyceride; VLDL, very low-density lipoprotein.

(mentioned above) increases HDL-C and is in a late stage of development.

DYSLIPIDAEMIA

The normal range of plasma total cholesterol concentration varies in different populations (e.g. in the UK 25–30% of middle-aged people have serum cholesterol concentrations > 6.5 mmol/l, in contrast to a much lower prevalence in China). There are smooth gradations of increased cardiovascular risk with increased LDL-C and with reduced HDL-C. Dyslipidaemia may be *primary* or *secondary*. The primary forms are due to a combination of

diet and genetics (often but not always polygenic). They are classified, according to which lipoprotein particle is raised, into six phenotypes (the Frederickson classification; Table 20.2). An especially great risk of ischaemic heart disease occurs in a subset of primary type IIa hyperlipoproteinaemia caused by single-gene defects of LDL receptors; this is known as *familial hyper-cholesterolaemia*, and the serum cholesterol concentration in affected adults is typically > 8 mmol/l in heterozygotes and 12–25 mmol/l in homozygotes. Study of familial hyper-cholesterolaemia enabled Brown & Goldstein (1986) to define the LDL receptor pathway of cholesterol homeostasis (for which they shared a Nobel Prize).

Table 20.2 Frederickson/World Health Organization classification of hyperlipoproteinaemia

Type	Lipoprotein elevated	Cholesterol	Triglycerides	Atherosclerosis risk	Drug treatment
I	Chylomicrons	+	+++	NE	None
IIa	LDL	++	NE	High	Statin ± ezetimibe
IIb	LDL + VLDL	++	++	High	Fibrates, statin, nicotinic acid
III	βVLDL	++	++	Moderate	Fibrates
IV	VLDL	+	++	Moderate	Fibrates
V	Chylomicrons + VLDL	+	++	NE	Fibrate, niacin, fish oil and statin combinations

+, increased concentration; LDL, low-density lipoprotein; NE, not elevated; VLDL, very low-density lipoprotein; βVLDL, a qualitatively abnormal form of VLDL identified by its pattern on electrophoresis.

Secondary forms of dyslipidaemia are a consequence of other conditions, such as diabetes mellitus, alcoholism, nephrotic syndrome, chronic renal failure, hypothyroidism, liver disease and administration of drugs, for example **isotretinoin** (an isomer of vitamin A given by mouth as well as topically in the treatment of severe acne), **tamoxifen** (Mikhailidis et al., 1997, and see above), **ciclosporin** (Ch. 14) and *protease inhibitors* used to treat infection with human immunodeficiency virus (Ch. 47).

LIPID-LOWERING DRUGS

Several drugs decrease plasma LDL-C. Drug therapy is used in addition to dietary measures and correction of other modifiable cardiovascular risk factors. The selection of patients to be treated with drugs remains controversial, not least for reasons of cost: the benefit is greatest for those who are at greatest risk, including those with symptomatic atherosclerotic disease (referred to as *secondary prevention*) and those with several cardiovascular risk factors, as well as those with the highest plasma concentrations of cholesterol.

The main agents used clinically are:

- statins: 3-hydroxy-3-methylglutaryl-coenzyme A (HMG-CoA) reductase inhibitors
- fibrates
- inhibitors of cholesterol absorption
- nicotinic acid or its derivatives
- fish oil derivatives.

Fish oil lowers plasma triglyceride concentration but can increase plasma cholesterol.

STATINS: HMG-CoA REDUCTASE INHIBITORS

The rate-limiting enzyme in cholesterol synthesis is HMG-CoA reductase, which catalyses the conversion of HMG-CoA to mevalonic acid (see Fig. 20.1). **Simvastatin**, **lovastatin** and **pravastatin** are specific, reversible, competitive HMG-CoA reductase

Lipoprotein metabolism and dyslipidaemia

- Lipids, including cholesterol and triglycerides, are transported in the plasma as lipoproteins, of which there are four classes.
  - Chylomicrons transport triglycerides and cholesterol from the gastrointestinal tract to the tissues, where triglyceride is split by lipoprotein lipase, releasing free fatty acids and glycerol. These are taken up in muscle and adipose tissue. Chylomicron remnants are taken up in the liver, where cholesterol is stored, secreted in bile, oxidised to bile acids or converted into
  - very low density lipoproteins (VLDL), which transport cholesterol and newly synthesised triglycerides to the tissues, where triglycerides are removed as before, leaving
  - low-density lipoprotein (LDL) particles with a large component of cholesterol; some LDL cholesterol is taken up by the tissues and some by the liver, by endocytosis via specific LDL receptors.
  - High-density lipoprotein (HDL) particles adsorb cholesterol derived from cell breakdown in tissues (including arteries) and transfer it to VLDL and LDL particles.
- Hyperlipidaemias can be *primary,* or *secondary* to a disease (e.g. hypothyroidism). They are classified according to which lipoprotein particle is raised into six phenotypes (the Frederickson classification). The higher the LDL cholesterol, and the lower the HDL cholesterol, the higher the risk of ischaemic heart disease.

inhibitors with K_i values of approximately 1 nmol/l. **Atorvastatin** and **rosuvastatin** are long-lasting inhibitors. Decreased hepatic cholesterol synthesis *up-regulates* LDL receptor synthesis, increasing LDL-C clearance from plasma into liver cells. The main biochemical effect of statins is therefore to reduce plasma LDL-C. There is also some reduction in plasma triglyceride and increase in HDL-C. Several large randomised placebo-controlled trials of the effects of HMG-CoA reductase inhibitors on morbidity and mortality have been positive.

▼ The *Scandinavian Simvastatin Survival Study (4S)* recruited patients with ischaemic heart disease and plasma cholesterol of 5.5–8.0 mmol/l; simvastatin lowered serum LDL-C by 35% and death by 30% (Fig. 20.2). This was accounted for by a 42% reduction in death from coronary disease over the median follow-up period of 5.4 years. Other large trials have confirmed reduced mortality both in patients with established ischaemic heart disease (e.g. the *Cholesterol and Recurrent Events, CARE, Trial*) and in healthy people at risk of coronary disease, with a wide range of plasma cholesterol values and other risk factors, and treated with different statins (e.g. the *West of Scotland Coronary Prevention Study* [*WOSCOPS*], the *Heart Protection Study* and the *Anglo-Scandinavian Cardiac Outcomes Trial* [*ASCOT*]). Intensive lowering of LDL-C with atorvastatin 80 mg had a greater effect on event rate than did a 10-mg dose in a recent randomised comparison, but with a greater incidence of abnormally raised plasma transaminase activity (LaRosa et al., 2005). In secondary prevention trials of statins, cardiovascular event rate is approximately linearly related to the achieved plasma LDL-C over a concentration range from approximately 1.8 to 4.9 mmol/l, and the event rate falls on the same line in placebo and statin-treated patients.

Other actions of statins

Products of the mevalonate pathway prenylate or farnesylate several important membrane-bound enzymes (e.g. endothelial NO synthase; see Ch. 17). These fatty groups serve as anchors, localising the enzyme in organelles such as caveoli and Golgi apparatus. Consequently, there is currently great interest in actions of statins that are unrelated, or indirectly related, to their effect on plasma LDL-C (sometimes referred to as *pleiotropic*

effects). Some of these actions are undesirable (e.g. HMG-CoA reductase guides migrating primordial germ cells, and statin use is contraindicated during pregnancy), but some offer therapeutic promise, for example in Alzheimer's disease (Sparks et al., 2005) and prevention of prostate cancer (Shannon et al., 2005). Such actions include:

- improved endothelial function
- reduced vascular inflammation
- reduced platelet aggregability
- increased neovascularisation of ischaemic tissue
- increased circulating endothelial progenitor cells
- stabilisation of atherosclerotic plaque
- antithrombotic actions
- enhanced fibrinolysis
- inhibition of germ cell migration during development
- immune suppression
- protection against sepsis.

The extent to which these effects contribute to the antiatheromatous actions of statins is unknown.

Pharmacokinetics

Short-acting statins are given by mouth at night to reduce peak cholesterol synthesis in the early morning. They are well absorbed and extracted by the liver, their site of action, and are subject to extensive presystemic metabolism via cytochrome P450 and glucuronidation pathways. Simvastatin is an inactive lactone prodrug; it is metabolised in the liver to its active form, the corresponding β-hydroxy fatty acid.

Adverse effects

Statins are well tolerated; mild unwanted effects include myalgia, gastrointestinal disturbance, raised concentrations of liver enzymes in plasma, insomnia and rash. More serious adverse effects are rare but include severe myositis (*rhabdomyolysis*) and *angio-oedema*. Myositis is a class effect of statins, occurs also with other lipid-lowering drugs (especially fibrates) and is dose-related.[3] It is commoner in patients with small lean body mass or uncorrected hypothyroidism.

Clinical uses

See the clinical box.

FIBRATES

Several fibric acid derivatives (*fibrates*) are available, including **bezafibrate**, **ciprofibrate**, **gemfibrozil**, **fenofibrate** and **clofibrate**. These cause a marked reduction in circulating VLDL, and hence triglyceride, with a modest (approximately 10%) reduction in LDL-C and an approximately 10% increase in HDL-C. In one study, gemfibrozil reduced coronary heart disease by approximately one-third compared with placebo in middle-aged men with primary

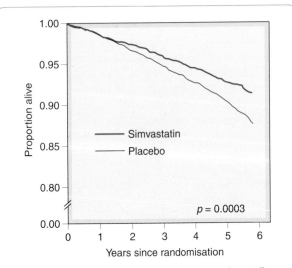

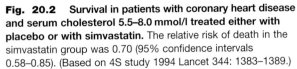

Fig. 20.2 **Survival in patients with coronary heart disease and serum cholesterol 5.5–8.0 mmol/l treated either with placebo or with simvastatin.** The relative risk of death in the simvastatin group was 0.70 (95% confidence intervals 0.58–0.85). (Based on 4S study 1994 Lancet 344: 1383–1389.)

---

[3]**Cerivastatin**, a potent statin introduced at relatively high dose, was withdrawn because of severe myositis occurring particularly in patients treated with **gemfibrozil**—discussed later in the chapter.

> ### Clinical uses of HMG-CoA reductase inhibitors (statins, e.g. simvastatin. atorvastatin)
>
> - *Secondary prevention* of myocardial infarction and stroke in patients who have symptomatic atherosclerotic disease (e.g. *angina, transient ischaemic attacks,* or following *myocardial infarction* or *stroke*).
> - *Primary prevention* of arterial disease in patients who are at high risk because of elevated serum cholesterol concentration, especially if there are other risk factors for atherosclerosis. Tables (available for example in the British National Formulary) are used to target treatment to those at greatest risk.
> - **Atorvastatin** lowers serum cholesterol in patients with homozygous familial hypercholesterolaemia.
> - In severe drug-resistant dyslipidaemia (e.g. heterozygous familial hypercholesterolaemia), **ezetimibe** is combined with statin treatment.

hyperlipoproteinaemia. An HDL-C intervention trial performed by the US Veterans Affairs Department in some 2500 men with coronary heart disease and low HDL-C together with *low* LDL-C showed that gemfibrozil increased HDL-C and reduced coronary disease and stroke. Event rates were linked to changes in HDL-C but not to triglycerides or to LDL-C, suggesting that increasing HDL-C with a fibrate reduces vascular risk.

The mechanism of action of fibrates is complex (see Fig. 20.1). They are agonists for a subset of lipid-controlled gene regulatory elements (*PPARs*[4]), PPARα, which are members of the super-family of nuclear receptors (Ch. 3); in humans, the main effects are to increase transcription of the genes for *lipoprotein lipase*, apoA1 and apoA5. They increase hepatic LDL-C uptake. In addition to effects on lipoproteins, fibrates reduce plasma C-reactive protein and fibrinogen, improve glucose tolerance, and inhibit vascular smooth muscle inflammation by inhibiting the expression of the transcription factor nuclear factor κB (see Ch. 28, p. 428). As with the pleiotropic effects of statins (see above), there is great interest in these actions, although again it is unknown if they are clinically important.

Adverse effects

Myositis is unusual but can be severe (*rhabdomyolysis*), with myoglobinuria and acute renal failure. It occurs particularly in patients with renal impairment, because of reduced protein binding and impaired drug elimination. Fibrates should be avoided in such patients and also in alcoholic individuals, who are predisposed to hypertriglyceridaemia but are at risk of rhabdomyolysis.[5] Myositis can also be caused (rarely) by statins (see above), and the combined use of fibrates with this class of drugs is therefore generally inadvisable (although it is sometimes undertaken by specialists). Gastrointestinal symptoms, pruritus and rash are more common than with statins. **Clofibrate** predisposes to gallstones, and its use is therefore limited to patients who have had a cholecystectomy (i.e. removal of the gall bladder).

Clinical use

See the clinical box.

DRUGS THAT INHIBIT CHOLESTEROL ABSORPTION

Historically, *bile acid–binding resins* were the only agents available to reduce cholesterol absorption and were among the few means to lower plasma cholesterol. Decreased absorption of exogenous cholesterol and increased metabolism of endogenous cholesterol into bile acids in the liver lead to increased expression of LDL receptors on hepatocytes, and hence to increased clearance of LDL-C from the blood and a reduced concentration of LDL-C in plasma. Such resins (see below) reduce the incidence of myocardial infarction, but their effect is modest and they are bulky, unpalatable and cause diarrhoea. With the introduction of statins, their role in treating dyslipidaemia was relegated largely to additional treatment in patients with severe disease (e.g. familial hypercholesterolaemia).

▼ Subsequently, plant *sterols* and *stanols* have been marketed; these are isolated from wood pulp and used to make margarines or yoghurts. They modestly reduce plasma cholesterol and are tastier than resins.[6] Their

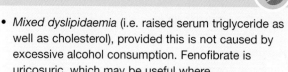

> ### Clinical uses of fibrates (e.g. gemfibrozil, fenofibrate)
>
> - *Mixed dyslipidaemia* (i.e. raised serum triglyceride as well as cholesterol), provided this is not caused by excessive alcohol consumption. Fenofibrate is uricosuric, which may be useful where hyperuricaemia coexists with mixed dyslipidaemia.
> - In patients with *low high-density lipoprotein* and *high risk of atheromatous disease* (often type 2 diabetic patients; see Ch. 26).
> - Combined with other lipid-lowering drugs in patients with severe treatment-resistant dyslipidaemia. This may, however, increase the risk of rhabdomyolysis.

---

[4]Standing for peroxisome proliferator-activated receptors—don't ask! (Peroxisomes are organelles that are not present in human cells, so something of a misnomer!) Thiazolidinedione drugs used in treating diabetes act on related PPARγ receptors; see Chapter 26.

[5]For several reasons, including a tendency to lie immobile for prolonged periods followed by generalised convulsions—'rum fits'—and delirium tremens.

[6]This is not, however, saying much.

mechanism is unclear; sitostanol in the gut lumen competes with cholesterol for an enterocyte cholesterol uptake receptor called NPC1L1,[7] and sitosterol interferes with cholesterol transfer within the enterocyte. Stanol supplements worsen homozygous *sitosterolaemia*, a rare autosomal recessive disease characterised by increased intestinal absorption of plant sterols, decreased hepatic excretion into bile and raised plasma phytosterols, tuberous xanthomas (potato-like accumulations of lipid-rich material in tendons) and atherosclerosis.

EZETIMIBE

Ezetimibe is one of a group of azetidinone cholesterol absorption inhibitors, and is indicated as an adjunct to diet and statins in hypercholesterolaemia. It specifically inhibits absorption of cholesterol (and of plant stanols) from the duodenum by blocking NPC1L1 in the brush border of enterocytes, without affecting the absorption of fat-soluble vitamins, triglycerides or bile acids. It is truly a drug in the sense defined in Chapter 2 (p. 8), in contrast to resins, which act by combining with bile acids rather than by binding to receptors; ezetimibe is consequently very much more convenient to take because of its high potency (a daily dose of 10 mg compared with a dose of resin of up to 36 g of **colestyramine**—a difference of 3600-fold), and represents a very real advance as a substitute for resins as supplementary treatment to statins in patients with severe dyslipidaemia. Its mechanism is distinct from that of phytosterol and phytostanol esters, which interfere with the micellar presentation of sterols to the cell surface.

Pharmacokinetic aspects

Ezetimibe is administered by mouth and is absorbed into intestinal epithelial cells, where it localises to the brush border, which is its presumed site of action. It is also extensively (> 80%) metabolised to ezetimibe–glucuronide, which is pharmacologically active. Total ('parent' plus glucuronide) ezetimibe concentrations reach a maximum 1–2 hours after administration, followed by enterohepatic recycling and slow elimination. The terminal half-life is approximately 22 hours. It enters milk (at least in animal studies) and, in contrast to resins, is therefore contraindicated for women who are breast feeding.

Adverse effects

Ezetimibe is generally well tolerated but can cause diarrhoea, abdominal pain or headache; rash and angio-oedema have been reported.

Clinical use

See clinical box.

BILE ACID–BINDING RESINS

Colestyramine and **colestipol** are anion exchange resins. Taken by mouth, they sequester bile acids in the intestine and prevent their reabsorption and enterohepatic recirculation (Fig. 20.1). The concentration of HDL-C is unchanged, and they cause an unwanted increase in triglycerides. The American Lipid Research Clinics' trial of middle-aged men with primary hypercholesterolaemia showed that addition of a resin to dietary treatment caused a mean 13% fall in plasma cholesterol and a 20–25% fall in coronary heart disease over 7 years.

Unwanted effects

Because resins are not absorbed, systemic toxicity is low but gastrointestinal symptoms—especially diarrhoea—are common and dose-related. Resins are bulky and unappetising. They interfere with the absorption of fat-soluble vitamins, and of drugs such as **chlorothiazide** (Chs 19 and 24), **digoxin** (Ch. 18) and **warfarin** (Ch. 21), which should therefore be taken at least 1 hour before or 4–6 hours after the resin.

Clinical use

They have been superseded by ezetimibe in treating dyslipidaemia in adults; for other uses, see the clinical box.

NICOTINIC ACID DERIVATIVES

Nicotinic acid is a vitamin, and as such is essential for many important metabolic processes. Quite separately from this, it has been used in gram quantities as a lipid-lowering agent. Nicotinamide inhibits hepatic triglyceride production and VLDL secretion (see Fig. 20.1), with reductions in triglyceride and LDL-C including Lp(a), and increase in HDL-C. The mechanism is poorly understood but is believed to be initiated by an effect on lipolysis via a G-protein–coupled orphan receptor called HM74A and present in adipocyte membranes (see review by Karpe & Frayn, 2004). It also influences hepatic diacylglycerol transferase. Long-term administration to survivors of myocardial infarction reduced mortality in the Coronary Drug Project trial, but unwanted effects limit its clinical use. A *modified-release preparation* is better tolerated, with preserved lipid effects, marginal adverse effects on glycaemia and liver function, and efficacy on intermediate (angiographic and ultrasound) end points; it is a real, if modest, advance.

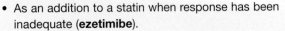

Clinical use of drugs that reduce cholesterol absorption: ezetimibe or bile acid–binding resins (e.g. colestyramine)

- As an addition to a statin when response has been inadequate (**ezetimibe**).
- For hypercholesterolaemia when a statin is contraindicated.
- Uses unrelated to atherosclerosis, including:
  - pruritus in patients with partial biliary obstruction (bile acid–binding resin)
  - bile acid diarrhoea, for example caused by diabetic neuropathy (bile acid–binding resin).

[7]For Niemann-Pick C1-like protein-1

Adverse effects

Adverse effects include flushing, palpitations and gastrointestinal disturbances. Flushing is associated with production of PGD_2 (Ch. 13) and is reduced by taking the dose 30 minutes after **aspirin**. High doses can disturb liver function, impair glucose tolerance, and precipitate gout by increasing circulating urate concentration.

FISH OIL DERIVATIVES

Omega-3 marine triglycerides reduce plasma triglyceride concentrations but increase cholesterol. Plasma triglyceride concentrations are less strongly associated with coronary artery disease than is cholesterol, but there is epidemiological evidence that eating fish regularly does reduce ischaemic heart disease, and dietary supplementation with n-3 polyunsaturated fatty acids (PUFA) improves survival in patients who have recently had a myocardial infarction (GISSI-Prevenzione Investigators, 1999). The mechanism may be the potent antiarrhythmic effects of PUFA (reviewed by Leaf et al., 2003). The mechanism of action of fish oil on plasma triglyceride concentrations is unknown. Fish oil is rich in PUFA, including eicosapentaenoic and docosahexaenoic acid, and it has other potentially important effects including inhibition of platelet function, prolongation of bleeding time, anti-inflammatory effects and reduction of plasma fibrinogen. Eicosapentaenoic acid substitutes for arachidonic acid in cell membranes and gives rise to 3-series prostaglandins and thromboxanes (that is, prostanoids with three double bonds in their side-chains rather than the usual two), and 5-series leukotrienes. This probably accounts for their effects on haemostasis, because thromboxane A_3 is much less active as a platelet-aggregating agent than is thromboxane A_2, whereas PGI_3 is similar in potency to PGI_2 as an inhibitor of platelet function. The alteration in leukotriene biosynthesis probably underlies the anti-inflammatory effects of fish oil. Fish oil is contraindicated in patients with type IIa hyperlipoproteinaemia because of the increase in LDL-C that it causes. A preparation of **omega 3-acid ethyl esters** is licensed in the UK for prevention of recurrent events after myocardial infarction in addition to treatment of hypertriglyceridaemia; it causes less increase in LDL-C and fewer problems with fishy odour, weight gain and dyspepsia than the older fish oil preparations.

REFERENCES AND FURTHER READING

Atherosclerosis

Brown M S, Goldstein J L 1986 A receptor-mediated pathway for cholesterol homeostasis. Science 232: 34–47 (*Classic from these Nobel Prize winners; see also Goldstein J L, Brown M S 1990 Regulation of the mevalonate pathway. Nature 343: 425–430*)

Davies M J, Woolf N 1993 Atherosclerosis: what is it and why does it occur? Br Heart J 69: S3–S11 (*Review of pathology/pathogenesis*)

Glass C K, Witztum J L 2001 Atherosclerosis. The Road Ahead. Cell 104: 503–516

McCully K S 1996 Homocysteine and vascular disease. Nat Med 2: 386–389 (*Discusses therapeutic promise of increased dietary folate and vitamin B_6*)

Miles L A, Fless G M, Levin E G et al. 1989 A potential basis for the thrombotic risks associated with

lipoprotein(a). Nature 339: 301–303 (*See also comment: Scott J 1989 Thrombogenesis linked to atherogenesis at last? Nature 341: 22–33*)

Ross R 1999 Atherosclerosis—an inflammatory disease. N Engl J Med 340: 115–126

Stein O, Stein Y 2005 Lipid transfer proteins (LTP) and atherosclerosis. Atherosclerosis 178: 217–230 (*Reviews four lipid transfer proteins—ACAT, CETP, LCAT and PLTP—and the therapeutic potential of modulating them*)

Lipoprotein metabolism and dyslipidaemias

Gervois P, Torra I P, Fruchart J C, Staels B 2000 Regulation of lipid and lipoprotein metabolism by PPAR activators. Clin Chem Lab Med 38: 3–11 (*Review*)

Statins

Almog Y, Shefer A, Novack V et al. 2004 Prior statin therapy is associated with a decreased rate of severe sepsis. Circulation 110: 880–885 (*Statin therapy was associated with a reduced rate of severe sepsis and intensive care unit admission—a role for statins in the prevention of sepsis?*)

LaRosa J C et al. for the Treating to New Targets (TNT) Investigators 2005 Intensive lipid lowering with atorvastatin in patients with stable coronary disease. N Engl J Med 352: 1425–1435 (*Intensive lipid-lowering therapy atorvastatin 80 mg daily in coronary heart disease patients provided significant clinical benefit beyond that afforded by 10 mg; this occurred with a greater incidence of elevated aminotransferase levels*)

Liao J K, Laufs U 2005 Pleiotropic effects of statins. Annu Rev Pharmacol Toxicol 45: 89–118 ('*Many pleiotropic effects are mediated by inhibition of isoprenoids, which serve as lipid attachments for intracellular signalling molecules. In particular, inhibition of small GTP-binding proteins, Rho, Ras, and Rac, whose proper membrane localisation and function are dependent on isoprenylation, may play an important role in mediating the pleiotropic effects of statins.*')

Merx M W, Liehn E A, Graf J et al. 2005 Statin treatment after onset of sepsis in a murine model improves survival. Circulation 112: 117–124 (*Statins offer the potential of effective sepsis treatment*)

Reid I R et al. 2001 Effect of pravastatin on the frequency of fracture in the LIPID study. Lancet 357: 509–512 (*No support for the hypothesis that statins reduce fracture risk; clinical trials aimed primarily at osteoporosis in at-risk subjects and using more sensitive measures of bone density are awaited*)

Ridker P M for the Air Force/Texas Coronary Atherosclerosis Prevention Study Investigators 2001 Measurement of C-reactive protein for the targeting of statin therapy in the primary prevention of acute events. N Engl J Med 344: 1959–1965 (*Statins may be effective in preventing coronary events in people with unremarkable serum lipid concentrations but with elevated C-reactive protein, a marker of inflammation and risk factor for coronary disease; see also accompanying editorial, Munford R S, Statins and the acute phase response, pp. 2016–2018*)

Shannon J et al. 2005 Statins and prostate cancer risk: a case-control study. Am J Epidemiol 162: 318–325 (*Statin use was associated with a reduction in prostate cancer risk—odds ratio, 0.38; 95% confidence interval, 0.21, 0.69—especially of more aggressive prostate cancer*)

Sparks D L et al. 2005 Atorvastatin for the treatment of mild to moderate Alzheimer disease. Preliminary results. Arch Neurol 62: 753–757 (*Laboratory evidence of cholesterol-induced production of amyloid, along with epidemiological evidence, provided a rationale; individuals with mild to moderate Alzheimer's disease were studied, with encouraging pilot data*)

Undas A, Brummel K E, Musial J et al. 2001 Simvastatin depresses blood clotting by activation of prothrombin, factor V, and factor XIII and by enhancing factor Va inactivation. Circulation 103: 2248–2253 (*Simvastatin effects on blood clotting independent of cholesterol reduction*)

Van Doren M, Broihier H T, Moore L A, Lehman R 1998 HMG-CoA reductase guides migrating primordial germ cells. Nature 396: 466–469 (*Regulated expression of HMG-CoA reductase provides spatial guide to migrating primordial germ cells*)

Vasa M et al. 2001 Increase in circulating endothelial progenitor cells by statin therapy in patients with stable coronary artery disease. Circulation 103: 2885–2890 (*May participate in repair after ischaemic injury*)

Other therapies

Nicotinic acid

Canner P L, Furberg C D, Terrin M L, McGovern M E 2005 Benefits of niacin by glycemic status in patients with healed myocardial infarction (from the Coronary Drug Project). Am J Cardiol 95: 254–257 (*The Coronary Drug Project, conducted during 1966 to 1974, was a randomised, double-blind, placebo-controlled trial in 8341 men with previous myocardial infarction; nicotinic acid significantly reduced total mortality during 6.2 years' treatment plus an additional 9 years of post-trial follow-up*)

Karpe F, Frayn K N 2004 The nicotinic acid receptor—a new mechanism for an old drug. Lancet 363: 1892–1894 (*Brief review of recent evidence that nicotinic acid acts via a G-protein–coupled orphan receptor*)

Taylor A J, Sullenberger L E, Lee H J et al. 2004 Arterial biology for the investigation of the treatment effects of reducing cholesterol (ARBITER) 2—A double-blind, placebo-controlled study of extended-release niacin on atherosclerosis progression in secondary prevention patients treated with statins. Circulation 110: 3512–3517 (*A double-blind randomised placebo-controlled study of once-daily extended-release nicotinic acid 1 g added to background statin therapy in 167 patients with coronary heart disease and low HDL-C. The primary end point was the change in common carotid intima media thickness after 1 year. Nicotinic acid slowed the progression of atherosclerosis.*)

Fibrates

Rubins H B et al. 2001 Reduction in stroke with gemfibrozil in men with coronary heart disease and low HDL cholesterol. The Veterans Affairs HDL Intervention Trial (VA-HIT). Circulation 103: 2828–2833 (*Evidence that increasing HDL-C reduces stroke*)

Fish oil

GISSI-Prevenzione Investigators (Gruppo Italiano per lo Studio della Sopravvivenza nell'Infarto Miocardico) 1999 Dietary supplementation with n-3 polyunsaturated fatty acids and vitamin E after myocardial infarction: results of the GISSI-Prevenzione trial (*11 324 patients surviving myocardial infarction were randomly assigned supplements of n-3 PUFA, 1 g daily, vitamin E, both or neither for 3.5 years. The primary end point was death, non-fatal myocardial infarction and stroke combined. Dietary supplementation with n-3 PUFA led to a clinically important and statistically significant benefit. Vitamin E had no benefit.*)

Leaf A, Kang J X, Xiao Y F, Billman G E 2003 Clinical prevention of sudden cardiac death by n-3 polyunsaturated fatty acids and mechanism of prevention of arrhythmias by n-3 fish oils. Circulation 107: 2646–2652 (*Reviews antiarrhythmic action of PUFA, including electrophysiological effects on voltage-dependent sodium and L-type calcium channels*)

Ezetimibe

Clader J W 2005 Ezetimibe and other azetidinone cholesterol absorption inhibitors. Curr Top Med Chem 5: 243–256 (*Summarises the medicinal chemistry of the azetidinone cholesterol absorption inhibitors as a class, with emphasis on the discovery of ezetimibe and structure action relations*)

Kosoglou T, Statkevich P, Johnson-Levonas A O et al. 2005 Ezetimibe—a review of its metabolism, pharmacokinetics and drug interactions. Clin Pharmacokinetics 44: 467–494

Potential therapies

Brousseau M E et al. 2004 Effects of an inhibitor of cholesteryl ester transfer protein on HDL cholesterol. N Engl J Med 350: 1505–1515 (*In subjects with low HDL-C, CETP inhibition with torcetrapib markedly increased HDL-C and also decreased LDL-C. See also editorial comment: Brewer H B 2004 Increasing HDL cholesterol levels. N Engl J Med 350: 1491–1494*)

De Medina P et al. 2004 Tamoxifen is a potent inhibitor of cholesterol esterification and prevents the formation of foam cells. J Pharmacol Exp Ther 308: 1542–1548 (*Molecular modelling revealed similarity between tamoxifen and ACAT inhibitor, pointing to atheroprotective possibilities—but see Mikhailidis et al., 1997, in the Clinical aspects section below*)

Kharbanda R K, Wallace S, Walton B et al. 2005 Systemic acyl-CoA: cholesterol acyltransferase inhibition reduces inflammation and improves vascular function in hypercholesterolemia. Circulation 111: 804–807 (*Systemic ACAT inhibition reduced tumour necrosis factor-α levels in hypercholesterolaemic subjects and improved resistance vessel endothelial function, with small effects on circulating cholesterol*)

Nissen S E et al. 2003 Effect of recombinant ApoA-I Milano on coronary atherosclerosis in patients with acute coronary syndromes. A randomized controlled trial. JAMA 290: 2292–2300 (*Assessed the effect of intravenous recombinant ApoA-I Milano–phospholipid complexes, ETC-216, on atheroma burden measured by intravascular ultrasound in patients with acute coronary syndromes. Five doses at weekly intervals produced significant regression. These encouraging results require confirmation.*)

Tardif J C et al. 2004 Effects of the acyl coenzyme A: cholesterol acyltransferase inhibitor avasimibe on human atherosclerotic lesions. Circulation 110: 3372–3377 (*Avasimibe did not favourably alter coronary atherosclerosis as assessed by intravascular ultrasound and mildly increased LDL-C*)

Wierzbicki A S 2004 Lipid lowering therapies in development. Expert Opin Investig Drugs 13: 1405–1408

Clinical aspects

Dubey R K, Imthurn B, Zacharia L C, Jackson E K 2004 Hormone replacement therapy and cardiovascular disease—what went wrong and where do we go from here? Hypertension 44: 789–795 ('*Observational studies in humans and experimental studies in animals and isolated cells supported the widely held belief that hormone replacement therapy protects the cardiovascular system from disease. To nearly everyone's astonishment, the Women's Health Initiative Study and the Heart and Estrogen/Progestin Replacement Study overturned the conclusion that hormone replacement therapy protects the cardiovascular system and, in fact, supported the opposite view that such therapy may actually increase the risk of cardiovascular disease.*')

Durrington P N 2005 Hyperlipidaemia: diagnosis and management, 3rd edn. Hodder Arnold, London (*Extremely readable, authoritative book*)

Mikhailidis D P, Ganotakis E S, Georgoulias V A et al. 1997 Tamoxifen-induced hypertriglyceridaemia: seven case reports and suggestions for remedial action. Oncology Rep 4: 625–628 (*In general, tamoxifen improves the lipid profile; however, in some individuals it can cause severe hypertriglyceridaemia*)

Haemostasis and thrombosis

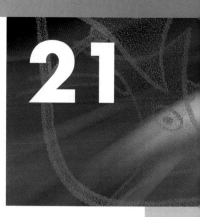

21

OVERVIEW

This chapter summarises the main features of blood coagulation, platelet function and fibrinolysis. These processes underlie haemostasis and thrombosis, and provide a basis for understanding haemorrhagic disorders (e.g. haemophilia) and thrombotic diseases both of arteries (e.g. thrombotic stroke, myocardial infarction) and of veins (e.g. deep vein thrombosis). Drugs that act on the coagulation cascade, on platelets and on fibrinolysis are considered. Anticoagulants, antiplatelet drugs and fibrinolytic drugs are especially important clinically because of the prevalence of thrombotic disease, and are emphasised for this reason.

INTRODUCTION

Haemostasis is the arrest of blood loss from damaged blood vessels and is essential to life. A wound causes vasoconstriction, accompanied by:

• adhesion and activation of platelets
• fibrin formation.

Platelet activation leads to the formation of a haemostatic plug, which stops the bleeding and is subsequently reinforced by fibrin. The relative importance of each process depends on the type of vessel (arterial, venous or capillary) that has been injured.

Thrombosis is the pathological formation of a 'haemostatic' plug within the vasculature in the absence of bleeding. Over a century ago, Rudolph Virchow defined three predisposing factors, still known as Virchow's triad. This comprises *injury to the vessel wall*—for example when an atheromatous plaque ruptures or becomes eroded; *altered blood flow*—for example in the left atrial appendage of the heart during atrial fibrillation, or in the veins of the legs while sitting cramped up on a long journey; and *abnormal coagulability of the blood*—as occurs, for example, in the later stages of pregnancy or during treatment with certain oral contraceptives (see Ch. 30). Increased coagulability of the blood can be inherited and is referred to as thrombophilia. A *thrombus*, which forms in vivo, should be distinguished from a *clot*, which forms in static blood in vitro. Clots are amorphous, consisting of a diffuse fibrin meshwork in which red and white blood cells are trapped indiscriminately. By contrast, arterial and venous thrombi each have a distinct structure.

An *arterial thrombus* (see Fig. 21.1) is composed of so-called white thrombus consisting mainly of platelets and leucocytes in a fibrin mesh. It is usually associated with *atherosclerosis*. It interrupts blood flow, causing ischaemia or death (infarction) of the tissue beyond. *Venous thrombus* is composed of 'red thrombus' and consists of a small white head and a large jelly-like red tail, similar in composition to a blood clot, which streams away in the flow. Thrombus can break away, forming an *embolus*; this may lodge in the lungs or, if it comes from the left heart or a carotid artery, in the brain or other organs, causing death or other disaster.

Drug therapy to promote haemostasis is rarely necessary, being required only when this essential process is defective (e.g. coagulation factors in haemophilia or following excessive anticoagulant therapy), or when it proves difficult to staunch haemorrhage following surgery or for menorrhagia (e.g. antifibrinolytic and haemostatic drugs; see below). Drug therapy to treat or prevent thrombosis or thromboembolism, by comparison, is extensively used because such diseases are common as well as serious. Drugs affect haemostasis and thrombosis in three distinct ways, by affecting:

• blood coagulation (fibrin formation)
• platelet function
• fibrin removal (fibrinolysis).

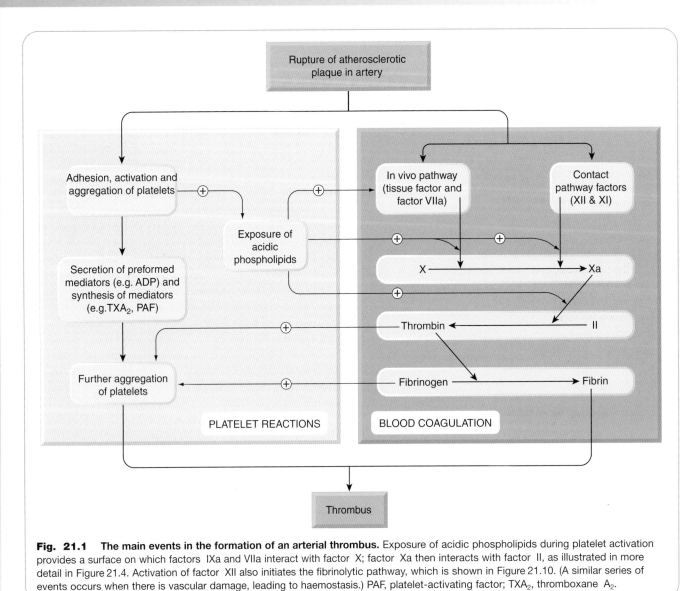

Fig. 21.1   The main events in the formation of an arterial thrombus. Exposure of acidic phospholipids during platelet activation provides a surface on which factors IXa and VIIa interact with factor X; factor Xa then interacts with factor II, as illustrated in more detail in Figure 21.4. Activation of factor XII also initiates the fibrinolytic pathway, which is shown in Figure 21.10. (A similar series of events occurs when there is vascular damage, leading to haemostasis.) PAF, platelet-activating factor; TXA_2, thromboxane A_2.

BLOOD COAGULATION

COAGULATION CASCADE

Blood coagulation means the conversion of fluid blood to a solid gel or clot. The main event is the conversion by thrombin of soluble fibrinogen to insoluble strands of fibrin, the last step in a complex enzyme cascade. The components (called factors) are present in blood as inactive precursors (zymogens) of proteolytic enzymes and cofactors. They are activated by proteolysis, the active forms being designated by the suffix 'a'. Factors XIIa, XIa, Xa, IXa and thrombin (IIa) are all serine proteases. Activation of a small amount of one factor catalyses the formation of larger amounts of the next factor, which catalyses the formation of still larger amounts of the next, and so on; consequently, the cascade provides a mechanism of amplification.[1] As might be expected,

this accelerating enzyme cascade has to be controlled by inhibitors, because otherwise all the blood in the body would solidify within minutes of the initiation of haemostasis. One of the most important inhibitors is *antithrombin III*, which neutralises all the serine proteases in the cascade. Vascular endothelium also actively limits thrombus extension (see below).

There are two main pathways of fibrin formation (Fig. 21.2), one traditionally termed 'intrinsic' (because all the components are present in the blood) and the other 'extrinsic' (because some components come from outside the blood). The extrinsic pathway is especially important in controlling blood coagulation and can accurately be called the in vivo pathway. The intrinsic pathway (better called the contact pathway) is activated when shed blood comes into contact with an artificial surface such as glass.

▼ The in vivo (extrinsic) pathway is initiated by 'tissue factor'. This is the cellular receptor for factor VII, which, in the presence of Ca^{2+}, undergoes an active site transition. This results in rapid autocatalytic activation of factor VII to VIIa. The tissue factor–VIIa complex activates factors IX and X. Acidic phospholipids function as *surface catalysts*.

---

[1]Coagulation of 100 ml of blood requires 0.2 mg of factor VIII, 2 mg of factor X, 15 mg of prothrombin and 250 mg of fibrinogen.

- Haemostasis is the arrest of blood loss from damaged vessels and is essential to survival. The main phenomena are:
  — platelet adhesion and activation
  — blood coagulation (fibrin formation).
- Thrombosis is a pathological condition resulting from inappropriate activation of haemostatic mechanisms:
  — venous thrombosis is usually associated with stasis of blood; a venous thrombus has a small platelet component and a large component of fibrin
  — arterial thrombosis is usually associated with atherosclerosis, and the thrombus has a large platelet component.
- A portion of a thrombus may break away, travel as an embolus and lodge downstream, causing ischaemia and infarction.

They are provided during platelet activation, which exposes acidic phospholipids (especially phosphatidylserine), and these activate various clotting factors, closely juxtaposing them in functional complexes. Platelets also contribute by secreting coagulation factors, including factor Va and fibrinogen. Coagulation is sustained by further generation of factor Xa by IXa–VIIIa–Ca^{2+}–phospholipid complex. This is needed because the tissue factor–VIIa complex is rapidly inactivated in plasma by tissue factor pathway inhibitor and by antithrombin III. Factor Xa, in the presence of Ca^{2+}, phospholipid and factor Va, activates prothrombin to *thrombin*, the main enzyme of the cascade. The *contact* (intrinsic) pathway commences when factor XII (Hageman factor) adheres to a negatively charged surface and converges with the in vivo pathway at the stage of factor X activation (see Fig. 21.2). The proximal part of this pathway is not crucial for blood coagulation in vivo. The two pathways are not entirely separate even before they converge, and various positive feedbacks promote coagulation.

The role of thrombin

Thrombin (factor IIa) cleaves fibrinogen, producing fragments that polymerise to form fibrin. It also activates factor XIII, a fibrinoligase, which strengthens fibrin-to-fibrin links, thereby stabilising the coagulum. In addition to coagulation, thrombin also causes platelet aggregation, stimulates cell proliferation and modulates smooth muscle contraction. Paradoxically, it can inhibit as well as promote coagulation (see below). Effects of thrombin on platelets and smooth muscle are initiated by interaction with specific protease-activated receptors (PARs), which belong to the superfamily of G-protein–coupled receptors. PARs initiate cellular responses that contribute not only to haemostasis and thrombosis, but also to inflammation and perhaps angiogenesis. The signal transduction mechanism is unusual: receptor activation requires proteolysis by thrombin of the extracellular N-terminal domain of the receptor, revealing a new N-terminal sequence that acts as a 'tethered agonist' (see Fig. 3.7, p. 35).

VASCULAR ENDOTHELIUM IN HAEMOSTASIS AND THROMBOSIS

Vascular endothelium, the container of the circulating blood, can change from a non-thrombogenic to a thrombogenic structure in response to different demands. Normally, it provides a non-thrombogenic surface by virtue of surface *heparan sulfate*, a glycosaminoglycan related to **heparin**, which is, like heparin, a cofactor for antithrombin III. Endothelium thus plays an essential role in preventing intravascular platelet activation and coagulation. However, it also plays an active part in haemostasis, synthesising and storing several key haemostatic components; von Willebrand factor,[2] tissue factor and plasminogen activator inhibitor (PAI)-1 are particularly important. PAI-1 is secreted in response to *angiotensin IV*, receptors for which are present on endothelial cells, providing a link between the renin–angiotensin system (see Ch. 19) and thrombosis. These *prothrombotic factors* are involved,

The clotting system consists of a cascade of proteolytic enzymes and cofactors.
- Inactive precursors are activated in series, each giving rise to more of the next.
- The last enzyme, thrombin, derived from prothrombin (II), converts soluble fibrinogen (I) to an insoluble meshwork of fibrin in which blood cells are trapped, forming the clot.
- There are two pathways in the cascade:
  — the extrinsic pathway, which operates in vivo
  — the intrinsic or contact pathway, which operates in vitro.
- Both pathways result in activation of factor X, which then converts prothrombin to thrombin.
- Calcium ions and a negatively charged phospholipid (PL) are essential for three steps, namely the actions of:
  — factor IXa on X
  — factor VIIa on X
  — factor Xa on II.
- PL is provided by activated platelets adhering to the damaged vessel.
- Some factors promote coagulation by binding to PL and a serine protease factor; for example, factor Va in the activation of II by Xa, or VIIIa in the activation of X by IXa.
- Blood coagulation is controlled by:
  — enzyme inhibitors (e.g. antithrombin III)
  — fibrinolysis.

---

[2]Von Willebrand factor is a glycoprotein that is missing in a hereditary haemorrhagic disorder called von Willebrand's disease. It is synthesised by vascular endothelial cells (the presence of immunoreactive von Willebrand factor is an identifying feature of these cells in culture) and is also present in platelets.

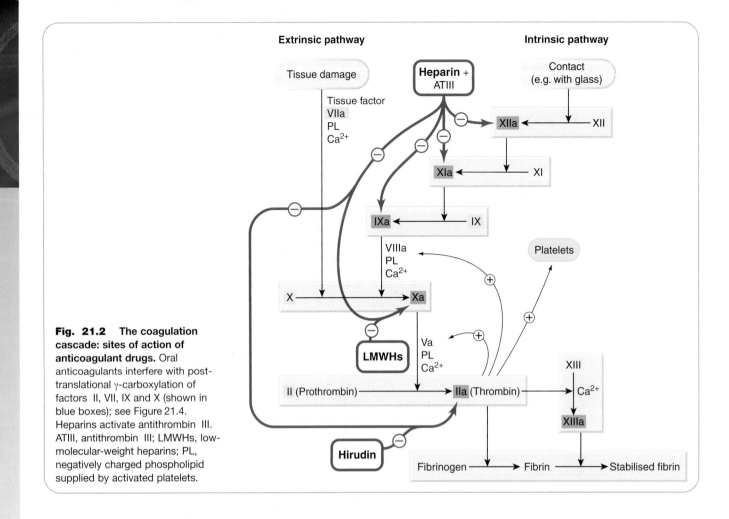

Fig. 21.2 **The coagulation cascade: sites of action of anticoagulant drugs.** Oral anticoagulants interfere with post-translational γ-carboxylation of factors II, VII, IX and X (shown in blue boxes); see Figure 21.4. Heparins activate antithrombin III. ATIII, antithrombin III; LMWHs, low-molecular-weight heparins; PL, negatively charged phospholipid supplied by activated platelets.

respectively, in platelet adhesion and in coagulation and clot stabilisation. However, the endothelium is also implicated in *thrombus limitation*. Thus it generates *prostaglandin (PG) I_2 (prostacyclin;* Ch. 13) and *nitric oxide (NO;* Ch. 17); converts the platelet agonist ADP to *adenosine,* which inhibits platelet function (Ch. 12); synthesises *tissue plasminogen activator (tPA;* see below); and expresses *thrombomodulin,* a receptor for thrombin. After combination with thrombomodulin, thrombin activates *protein C,* a vitamin K–dependent anticoagulant. Activated protein C, helped by its cofactor protein S, inactivates factors Va and VIIa. This is known to be physiologically important, because a naturally occurring mutation of the gene coding for factor V (factor V Leiden), which confers resistance to activated protein C, results in the commonest recognised form of inherited thrombophilia. A synthetic form of activated protein C, **drotrecogin alpha (activated),** is licensed for the treatment of severe septic shock with multiple organ failure (Ch. 19).

Endotoxin and cytokines, including tumour necrosis factor, tilt the balance of prothrombotic and antithrombotic endothelial functions towards thrombosis by causing loss of heparan and expression of tissue factor, and impair endothelial NO function. If other mechanisms limiting coagulation are also faulty or become exhausted, *disseminated intravascular coagulation* can result. This is a serious complication of sepsis and of certain malignancies, and the main treatment is to correct the underlying disease.

DRUGS THAT ACT ON THE COAGULATION CASCADE

Drugs are used to modify the cascade either when there is a *defect in coagulation* or when there is *unwanted coagulation*.

COAGULATION DEFECTS

Genetically determined deficiencies of clotting factors are rare. Examples are *classic haemophilia,* caused by lack of factor VIII, and an even rarer form of haemophilia (haemophilia B or Christmas disease) caused by lack of factor IX (also called Christmas factor). Missing factors can be supplied by giving fresh plasma or concentrated preparations of factor VIII or factor IX. In the past, these have transmitted viral infections including HIV and hepatitis B and C (Ch. 47). Pure forms of several human factors are now available, synthesised by recombinant technology, but are difficult to manufacture because of the need for post-translational modification in mammalian cells, and they are expensive.

Acquired clotting defects are more common than hereditary ones. These include liver disease, vitamin K deficiency (universal in neonates) and excessive oral anticoagulant therapy, each of which may require treatment with vitamin K.

VITAMIN K

Vitamin K (for *Koagulation* in German) is a fat-soluble vitamin occurring naturally in plants (Fig. 21.3). It is essential for the formation of clotting factors II, VII, IX and X. These are all glycoproteins with several *γ-carboxyglutamic acid* (*Gla*) residues. γ-Carboxylation occurs *after* the synthesis of the chain, and the carboxylase enzyme requires vitamin K as a cofactor. The role of the vitamin is clarified by considering the interaction of factors Xa and prothrombin (factor II) with Ca^{2+} and phospholipid, as shown in Figure 21.4. Binding does not occur in the absence of γ-carboxylation. The reduced form of vitamin K is an essential cofactor in the carboxylation of glutamate residues (Fig. 21.5). Similar considerations apply to the proteolytic activation of factor X by IXa and by VIIa (see Fig. 21.2).

There are several other vitamin K–dependent Gla proteins, including proteins C and S (see above) and osteocalcin in bone. The effect of the vitamin on osteoporosis is under investigation.

Administration and pharmacokinetic aspects

Natural vitamin K (*phytomenadione*) may be given orally or by injection. If given by mouth, it requires bile salts for absorption, and this occurs by a saturable energy-requiring process in the proximal small intestine. A synthetic preparation, menadiol sodium phosphate, is also available. It is water-soluble and does not require bile salts for its absorption. This synthetic compound takes longer to act than phytomenadione. There is very little storage of vitamin K in the body. It is metabolised to more polar substances that are excreted in the urine and the bile.

Clinical uses

Clinical uses of vitamin K are summarised in the clinical box.

THROMBOSIS

Thrombotic and thromboembolic disease is common and has severe consequences, including myocardial infarction, stroke, deep vein thrombosis and pulmonary embolus. The main drugs used for platelet-rich 'white' thrombi are the antiplatelet drugs (notably **aspirin**) and fibrinolytic drugs, which are considered below. The main drugs used to prevent or treat 'red' thrombus are:

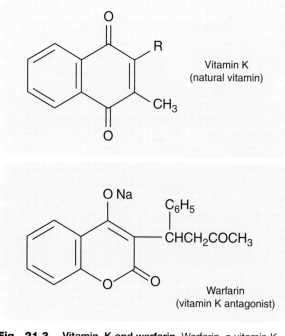

Fig. 21.3 Vitamin K and warfarin. Warfarin, a vitamin K antagonist, is an oral anticoagulant. It competes with vitamin K (note the similarity in their structures) for the reductase enzyme that activates vitamin K (see Fig. 21.5).

- injectable anticoagulants (**heparin** and newer thrombin inhibitors)
- oral anticoagulants (**warfarin** and related compounds).

Heparins act immediately, whereas oral anticoagulants take several days to exert their effect. Consequently, patients with venous thrombosis are treated immediately with an injectable anticoagulant, which is continued until the effect of warfarin has become established.

Clinical use of vitamin K

- Treatment and/or prevention of bleeding:
  - from excessive oral anticoagulation (e.g. by **warfarin**)
  - in babies: to prevent *haemorrhagic disease of the newborn*.
- For vitamin K deficiencies in adults:
  - *sprue, coeliac disease, steatorrhoea*
  - lack of bile (e.g. with *obstructive jaundice*).

Clinical use of anticoagulants

- **Heparin** (often as **low-molecular-weight heparin**) is used acutely. **Warfarin** is used for prolonged therapy. Anticoagulants are used to prevent:
  - *deep vein thrombosis* (e.g. perioperatively)
  - extension of established deep vein thrombosis
  - *pulmonary embolus*
  - thrombosis and embolisation in patients with atrial fibrillation (Ch.18)
  - thrombosis on *prosthetic heart valves*
  - clotting in *extracorporeal circulations* (e.g. during haemodialysis)
  - myocardial infarction in patients with *unstable angina*.

INJECTABLE ANTICOAGULANTS

Heparin (including low-molecular-weight heparins)

Heparin was discovered in 1916 by a second-year medical student at Johns Hopkins Hospital. He was attempting to extract thromboplastic (i.e. coagulant) substances from various tissues during a vacation project, but found instead a powerful anticoagulant activity.[3] This was named *heparin*, because it was first extracted from liver.

Heparin is not a single substance but a family of sulfated glycosaminoglycans (mucopolysaccharides). It is present together with histamine in the granules of mast cells. Commercial preparations are extracted from beef lung or hog intestine and, because preparations differ in potency, assayed biologically against an agreed

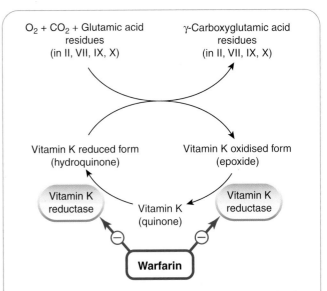

Fig. 21.5 Mechanism of vitamin K and of warfarin. After the peptide chains in clotting factors II, VII, IX and X have been synthesised, reduced vitamin K (the hydroquinone) acts as a cofactor in the conversion of glutamic acid (Glu) to γ-carboxyglutamic acid (Gla). During this reaction, the reduced form of vitamin K is converted to the epoxide, which in turn is reduced to the quinone and then the hydroquinone.

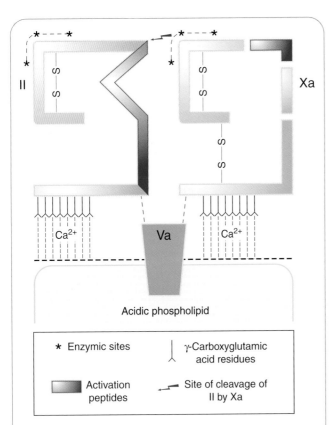

Fig. 21.4 Activation of prothrombin (factor II) by factor Xa. The complex of factor Va with a negatively charged phospholipid surface (supplied by aggregating platelets) forms a binding site for factor Xa and prothrombin (II), which have peptide chains (shown schematically) that are similar to one another. Platelets thus serve as a localising focus. Calcium ions are essential for binding. Xa activates prothrombin, liberating thrombin (shown in grey). (Modified from Jackson C M 1978 Br J Haematol 39: 1.)

international standard: doses are specified in units of activity rather than of mass.

Heparin fragments (e.g. **enoxaparin**, **dalteparin**) or a synthetic pentasaccharide (**fondaparinux**), referred to as low-molecular-weight heparins (LMWHs), are used increasingly in place of unfractionated heparin.

Mechanism

Heparin inhibits coagulation, both in vivo and in vitro, by activating antithrombin III (see above). Antithrombin III inhibits thrombin and other serine proteases by binding to the active serine site. Heparin modifies this interaction by binding, via a unique pentasaccharide sequence, to antithrombin III, changing its conformation and accelerating its rate of action.

Thrombin is considerably more sensitive to the inhibitory effect of the heparin–antithrombin III complex than is factor X. To inhibit thrombin, it is necessary for heparin to bind to the enzyme as well as to antithrombin III; to inhibit factor X, it is necessary only for heparin to bind to antithrombin III (Fig. 21.6). Antithrombin III deficiency is very rare but can cause thrombophilia and resistance to heparin therapy.

The LMWHs increase the action of antithrombin III on factor Xa but not its action on thrombin, because the molecules are too small to bind to both enzyme and inhibitor, essential for inhibition of thrombin but not for that of factor Xa (Fig. 21.6).

Administration and pharmacokinetic aspects

Heparin is not absorbed from the gut because of its charge and large size, and it is therefore given intravenously or subcutaneously (intramuscular injections would cause haematomas).

---

[3]This kind of good fortune also favoured Vane and his colleagues in their discovery of PGI₂ (Chs 13 and 19), where they were looking for one kind of biological activity and found another. More specific chemical assays (Ch. 6), for all their strengths, cannot throw up this kind of unexpected discovery.

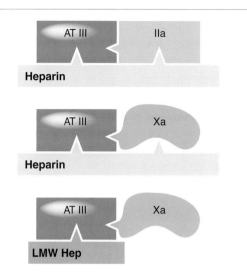

Fig. 21.6 Action of heparins. The schematic shows interactions of heparins, antithrombin III (AT III) and clotting factors. To increase the inactivation of thrombin (IIa) by AT III, heparin needs to interact with both substances (top), but to speed up its effect on factor Xa it need only interact with AT III (middle). Low-molecular-weight heparins (LMW Hep) increase the action of AT III on factor Xa (bottom), but cannot increase the action of AT III on thrombin because they cannot bind both simultaneously. (Modified from Hirsh J, Levine M 1992 Blood 79: 1–17.)

▼ After intravenous injection of a bolus dose, there is a phase of rapid elimination followed by a more gradual disappearance owing both to saturable processes (involving binding to sites on endothelial cells and macrophages) and slower first-order processes including renal excretion. As a result, once the dose exceeds the saturating concentration, a greater proportion is dealt with by these slower processes, and the apparent half-life increases with increasing dose (saturation kinetics; see Ch. 8).

Heparin acts immediately following intravenous administration, but the onset is delayed by up to 60 minutes when it is given subcutaneously. The elimination half-life is approximately 40–90 minutes. In urgent situations, it is therefore usual to start treatment with a bolus intravenous dose, followed by a constant-rate infusion. The activated partial thromboplastin time (APTT), or some other in vitro clotting test, is measured and the dose of unfractionated heparin adjusted to achieve a value within a target range (e.g. 1.5–2.5 times control).

Low-molecular-weight heparins are given subcutaneously. They have a longer elimination half-life than unfractionated heparin, and this is independent of dose (first-order kinetics), so the effects are more predictable and dosing less frequent (once or twice a day). LMWHs do not prolong the APTT; unlike unfractionated heparin, the effect of a standard dose is sufficiently predictable that monitoring is not required routinely. They are eliminated mainly by renal excretion, and unfractionated heparin is preferred in renal failure. In general, they are at least as safe and effective as unfractionated heparin and are more convenient to use, because patients can be taught to inject themselves at home and there is generally no need for blood tests and dose adjustment.

Unwanted effects

Haemorrhage. The main hazard is haemorrhage, which is treated by stopping therapy and, if necessary, giving **protamine** sulfate. This heparin antagonist is a strongly basic protein that forms an inactive complex with heparin; it is given intravenously. The dose is estimated from the dose of heparin that has been administered recently, and it is important not to give too much, as this can itself cause bleeding. If necessary, an in vitro neutralisation test is performed on a sample of blood from the patient to provide a more precise indication of the required dose.

Thrombosis. This is an uncommon but serious adverse effect of heparin and, as with *warfarin necrosis* (see below), may be misattributed to the natural history of the disease for which heparin is being administered. Paradoxically, it is associated with *heparin-induced thrombocytopenia* (*HIT*). A transitory early decrease in platelet numbers is not uncommon, and is not clinically important. More serious thrombocytopenia occurring 2–14 days after the start of therapy is uncommon and is caused by IgM or IgG antibodies against complexes of heparin and platelet factor 4. Circulating immune complexes bind to Fc receptors (see Ch. 13) on circulating platelets, thereby activating them and releasing more platelet factor 4 and causing thrombocytopenia. Antibody also binds to platelet factor 4 complexed with glycosaminoglycans on the surface of endothelial cells, leading to immune injury of the vessel wall, thrombosis and disseminated intravascular coagulation. LMWHs are less liable than standard heparin to activate platelets to release platelet factor 4, and they bind less avidly to platelet factor 4. Consequently, LMWHs are less likely than unfractionated heparin to cause thrombocytopenia and thrombosis. If antibodies to heparin–platelet factor 4 complexes have formed, however, it is to be expected that LMWHs could trigger these immunologically mediated adverse effects. Management of patients with thromboembolic disease who develop HIT is therefore usually with either **danaparoid** or with a direct thrombin inhibitor (see below). **Danaparoid** is a low-molecular-weight heparinoid consisting of a mixture of heparan, dermatan and chondroitin sulfates, with well-established antithrombotic activity.

Osteoporosis with spontaneous fractures has been reported with long-term (6 months or more) treatment with heparin (usually during pregnancy, when warfarin is contraindicated or problematic—see below). Its explanation is unknown.

Hypoaldosteronism (with consequent hyperkalaemia) has been described.

Hypersensitivity reactions are rare with heparin but more common with **protamine**. (Protamine sensitivity also occurs in patients treated with protamine zinc insulin; see p. 404. Protamine is extracted from fish roe, and sensitivity to protamine occurs in some people with fish allergy.)

ANTITHROMBIN III–INDEPENDENT ANTICOAGULANTS

Hirudins are direct thrombin inhibitors derived from the anticoagulant present in saliva from the medicinal leech. **Hirudin** itself has been synthesised by recombinant DNA techniques, but clinical trials, including Global Use of Strategies to Open Occluded Coronary Arteries (GUSTO)-2 and Thrombolysis in Myocardial

Infarction (TIMI)-9, have been somewhat disappointing. **Lepirudin** is a related polypeptide that binds irreversibly both to the fibrin-binding and catalytic sites on thrombin. **Argatroban** is a synthetic low-molecular-weight inhibitor that binds irreversibly to the catalytic site alone. Each of these agents is effective for preventing and treating thrombosis in HIT. Lepirudin can itself provoke antibody synthesis. **Melagatran** is a related inhibitor that can be administered subcutaneously. A prodrug form of melagatran, **ximelagatran**, is an orally active direct thrombin inhibitor. It can be administered in a standard dose twice daily. In large clinical trials, it has proved to be similarly effective as **warfarin** in preventing stroke in patients with atrial fibrillation, and it may well be safer than warfarin. Disappointingly, it caused abnormal liver function in around 6% of patients, and its licensing has been delayed in consequence. **Bivalirudin**, another hirudin analogue, is used by cardiologists in selected patients undergoing percutaneous coronary interventions.

▼ Various other approaches are being explored. These include several naturally occurring anticoagulants (tissue factor pathway inhibitor, thrombomodulin and protein C) synthesised by recombinant technology. A particularly ingenious approach is the development of thrombin agonists that are selective for the anticoagulant properties of thrombin. One such modified thrombin, differing by a single amino acid substitution, has substrate specificity for protein C. It produces anticoagulation in monkeys without prolonging bleeding times, suggesting that it may be less likely than standard anticoagulants to cause bleeding (Gibbs, 1995; Pineda et al 2004).

VITAMIN K ANTAGONISTS: WARFARIN

▼ Oral anticoagulants were discovered as an indirect result of a change in agricultural policy in North America in the 1920s. Sweet clover was substituted for corn in cattle feed, and an epidemic of deaths of cattle from haemorrhage ensued. This turned out to be caused by *bishydroxycoumarin* in spoiled sweet clover, and it led to the discovery of **warfarin** (named for the <u>W</u>isconsin <u>A</u>lumni <u>R</u>esearch <u>F</u>oundation). One of the first uses to which this was put was as a rat poison, but for the past 50 years it has been the standard anticoagulant for the treatment and prevention of thromboembolic disease.

Warfarin (Fig. 21.3) is the most important oral anticoagulant; alternatives with a similar mechanism of action, for example **phenindione**, are now used only in rare patients who experience idiosyncratic adverse reactions to warfarin. Warfarin and other vitamin K antagonists require frequent blood tests to individualise dose, and are consequently inconvenient as well as having a low margin of safety; hopes that the oral direct thrombin inhibitor ximelagatran (see above) would replace warfarin for some at least of its many indications have been put on hold as a result of hepatotoxicity.

Mechanism of action

Vitamin K antagonists act only in vivo and have no effect on clotting if added to blood in vitro. They interfere with the post-translational γ-carboxylation of glutamic acid residues in clotting factors II, VII, IX and X. They do this by inhibiting enzymic reduction of vitamin K to its active hydroquinone form (Fig. 21.5). Inhibition is competitive (reflecting the structural similarity between warfarin and vitamin K, Fig. 21.3). Their effect takes several days to develop because of the time taken for

degradation of preformed carboxylated clotting factors. Their onset of action thus depends on the elimination half-lives of the relevant factors. Factor VII, with a half-life of 6 hours, is affected first, then IX, X and II, with half-lives of 24, 40 and 60 hours, respectively.

Administration and pharmacokinetic aspects

Warfarin is absorbed rapidly and completely from the gut after oral administration. It has a small distribution volume, being strongly bound to plasma albumin (see Ch. 7). The peak concentration in the blood occurs within an hour of ingestion, but because of the mechanism of action this does not coincide with the peak pharmacological effect, which occurs about 48 hours later. The effect on *prothrombin time* (*PT*, see below) of a single dose starts after approximately 12–16 hours and lasts 4–5 days. Warfarin is metabolised by the hepatic mixed function oxidase P450 system, and its half-life is very variable, being of the order of 40 hours in many individuals.

Warfarin crosses the placenta and is not given in the first months of pregnancy because it is teratogenic, nor in the later stages because it can cause intracranial haemorrhage in the baby during delivery. It appears in milk during lactation. This could theoretically be important because newborn infants are naturally deficient in vitamin K. However, infants are routinely prescribed vitamin K to prevent haemorrhagic disease (see above), so warfarin treatment of the mother does not generally pose a risk to the breast-fed infant.

The therapeutic use of warfarin requires a careful balance between giving too little, leaving unwanted coagulation unchecked, and giving too much, thereby causing haemorrhage. Therapy is complicated not only because the effect of each dose is maximal some 2 days after its administration, but also because numerous medical and environmental conditions modify sensitivity to warfarin, including interactions with other drugs (see Ch. 52). The effect of warfarin is monitored by measuring PT, which is expressed as an *international normalised ratio* (*INR*).

▼ The PT is the time taken for clotting of citrated plasma after the addition of Ca^{2+} and standardised reference thromboplastin; it is expressed as the ratio (PT ratio) of the PT of the patient to the PT of a pool of plasma from healthy subjects on no medication. Because of the variability of thromboplastins, different results are obtained in different laboratories. To standardise PT measurements internationally, each thromboplastin is assigned an international sensitivity index (ISI), and the patient's PT is expressed as an INR, where INR = (PT ratio)^{ISI}. This kind of normalisation procedure shocks purists but provides similar results when a patient moves from, say, Birmingham to Baltimore, permitting warfarin dose adjustment independent of laboratory. Pragmatic haematologists argue that the proof of the pudding is in the eating!

The dose of warfarin is usually adjusted to give an INR of 2–4, the precise target depending on the clinical situation. The duration of treatment also varies, but for several indications (e.g. to prevent thromboembolism in chronic atrial fibrillation) treatment is long term.

Factors that potentiate oral anticoagulants

Various diseases and drugs potentiate warfarin, increasing the risk of haemorrhage.

Disease

Liver disease interferes with the synthesis of clotting factors; conditions in which there is a high metabolic rate, such as fever and thyrotoxicosis, increase the effect of anticoagulants by increasing degradation of clotting factors.

Drugs (see also Chs 8 and 52)

Many drugs potentiate warfarin.

Agents that inhibit hepatic drug metabolism. Examples include **cimetidine**, **imipramine**, **co-trimoxazole**, **chloramphenicol**, **ciprofloxacin**, **metronidazole**, **amiodarone** and many antifungal azoles. Stereoselective effects (warfarin is a racemate, and its isomers are metabolised differently from one another) are described in Chapter 52.

Drugs that inhibit platelet function. **Aspirin** increases the risk of bleeding if given during warfarin therapy, although this combination can be used safely with careful monitoring (e.g. Turpie, 1993). Other non-steroidal anti-inflammatory drugs (NSAIDs) also increase the risk of bleeding, partly by their effect on platelet thromboxane synthesis (Ch. 14) and, in the case of some NSAIDs, also by inhibiting warfarin metabolism as above. Some antibiotics, including **moxalactam** and **carbenicillin**, inhibit platelet function.

Drugs that displace warfarin from binding sites on plasma albumin. Some of the NSAIDs and **chloral hydrate**, for example, result in a transient increase in the concentration of free warfarin in plasma. This mechanism seldom causes clinically important effects, unless accompanied in addition by inhibition of warfarin metabolism, as with **phenylbutazone** (Ch. 52).

Drugs that inhibit reduction of vitamin K. Such drugs include the *cephalosporins*.

Drugs that decrease the availability of vitamin K. Broad-spectrum antibiotics and some *sulfonamides* (see Ch. 46) depress the intestinal flora that normally synthesise vitamin K_2 (a form of vitamin K made by gut bacteria); this has little effect unless there is concurrent dietary deficiency.

Factors that lessen the effect of oral anticoagulants

Physiological state/disease

There is a decreased response to warfarin in conditions (e.g. *pregnancy*) where there is increased coagulation factor synthesis. Similarly, the effect of oral anticoagulants is lessened in *hypothyroidism*, which is associated with reduced degradation of coagulation factors.

Drugs (see also Chs 8 and 52)

Several drugs reduce the effectiveness of warfarin; this leads to increased doses being used to achieve the target INR. If the dose of warfarin is not reduced when the interacting drug is discontinued, this can result in over-anticoagulation and haemorrhage.

Vitamin K. This vitamin is a component of some parenteral feeds and vitamin preparations.

Drugs that induce hepatic P450 enzymes. Enzyme induction (e.g. by **rifampicin**, **carbamazepine**, **barbiturates**, **griseofulvin**) increases the rate of degradation of warfarin. Induction may wane only slowly after the inducing drug is discontinued, making it difficult to adjust the dose appropriately.

Drugs that reduce absorption. Drugs that bind warfarin in the gut, for example **colestyramine**, reduce its absorption.

Unwanted effects

Haemorrhage (especially into the bowel or the brain) is the main hazard. Depending on the urgency of the situation, treatment may consist of withholding warfarin (for minor problems), administration of vitamin K, or fresh plasma or coagulation factor concentrates (for life-threatening bleeding). Oral anticoagulants are teratogenic. Hepatotoxicity occurs but is uncommon. Necrosis of soft tissues (e.g. breast or buttock) owing to thrombosis in venules occurs shortly after starting treatment and is attributed to inhibition of biosynthesis of protein C, which has a shorter elimination half-life than do the vitamin K–dependent coagulation factors; this results in a procoagulant state soon after starting treatment. This is a rare but serious adverse effect. Treatment with heparin is usually started before warfarin, avoiding this problem except in individuals experiencing HIT as an adverse effect of heparin (see above).

Clinical use

The clinical use of anticoagulants is summarised in the box on page 335.

PLATELET ADHESION AND ACTIVATION

Platelets maintain the integrity of the circulation: a low platelet count results in *thrombocytopenic purpura*.[4]

When platelets are activated, they undergo a sequence of reactions that are essential for haemostasis, important for the healing of damaged blood vessels, and play a part in inflammation (see Ch. 13). These reactions, several of which are redundant (in the sense that if one pathway of activation is blocked another is available) and several autocatalytic, include:

- *adhesion* following vascular damage (via von Willebrand factor bridging between subendothelial macromolecules and glycoprotein (GP) Ib receptors on the platelet surface)[5]
- *shape change* (from smooth discs to spiny spheres with protruding pseudopodia)
- *secretion* of the granule contents (including platelet agonists, such as ADP and 5-hydroxytryptamine, and coagulation factors and growth factors, such as platelet-derived growth factor)
- *biosynthesis of labile mediators* such as platelet-activating factor and thromboxane (TX) A_2 (see Fig. 21.7)
- *aggregation*, which is promoted by various agonists, including collagen, thrombin, ADP, 5-hydroxytryptamine and TXA_2, acting on specific receptors on the platelet surface; activation by agonists leads to expression of GPIIb/IIIa

---

[4]*Purpura* means a purple rash caused by multiple spontaneous bleeding points in the skin. When this is caused by reduced circulating platelets, bleeding can occur into other organs, including the gut and brain.

[5]Various platelet membrane glycoproteins are receptors or binding sites for adhesive proteins such as von Willebrand factor or fibrinogen.

Drugs affecting blood coagulation

Procoagulant drugs: vitamin K
- Reduced vitamin K is a cofactor in the post-translational γ-carboxylation of glutamic acid (Glu) residues in each of factors II, VII, IX and X. The γ-carboxylated glutamic acid (Gla) residues are essential for the interaction of these factors with Ca^{2+} and negatively charged phospholipid.

Injectable anticoagulants (e.g. heparin, low-molecular-weight heparins)
- Potentiate antithrombin III, a natural inhibitor that inactivates Xa and thrombin.
- Act both in vivo and in vitro.
- Anticoagulant activity results from a unique pentasaccharide sequence with high affinity for antithrombin III.
- Heparin therapy is monitored via activated partial thromboplastin time, and dose individualised.
- Low-molecular-weight heparins have the same effect on factor X as heparin but less effect on thrombin; therapeutic efficacy is similar to heparin but monitoring and dose individualisation are not needed. Patients can administer them subcutaneously at home.

Oral anticoagulants (e.g. warfarin)
- Inhibit the reduction of vitamin K, thus inhibiting the γ-carboxylation of Glu in II, VII, IX and X.
- Act only in vivo, and their effect is delayed until preformed clotting factors are depleted.
- Many factors modify their action; drug interactions are especially important.
- There is wide variation in response; their effect is monitored by measuring the international normalised ratio (INR) and the dose individualised accordingly.

Platelet function

- Healthy vascular endothelium prevents platelet adhesion.
- Platelets adhere to diseased or damaged areas and become activated, i.e. they change shape, exposing negatively charged phospholipids and glycoprotein (GP) IIb/IIIa receptors, and synthesise and/or release various mediators, for example thromboxane A2 and ADP, which activate other platelets, causing aggregation.
- Aggregation entails fibrinogen binding to GPIIb/IIIa receptors on adjacent platelets.
- Activated platelets constitute a focus for fibrin formation.
- Chemotactic factors and growth factors necessary for repair, but also implicated in atherogenesis, are released during platelet activation.

Antiplatelet drugs

- **Aspirin** inhibits cyclo-oxygenase irreversibly. The balance between prostaglandin (PG) I_2 (an inhibitor of aggregation generated by vascular endothelium) and thromboxane (a stimulant of aggregation generated by platelets) is thus altered, because the endothelium can synthesise more enzyme but platelets cannot. Aspirin is very important clinically.
- **Clopidogrel** is a prodrug. Given by mouth, it inhibits platelet responses to ADP. Its actions are additive with aspirin.
- Antagonists of GPIIb/IIIa receptors include a monoclonal antibody (**abciximab**) and several oligopeptides (e.g. **tirofiban**). They inhibit diverse agonists, for example ADP and thromboxane (TX) A_2, because different pathways of activation converge on GPIIb/IIIa receptors. They are used intravenously for short-term treatment.
- **Dipyridamole** is a phosphodiesterase inhibitor. It is used in addition to aspirin.
- **Epoprostenol** (synthetic PGI_2) is chemically unstable. Given as an intravenous infusion, it acts on I Prostanoid (IP) phosphate receptors on vascular smooth muscle and platelets (Ch. 15), stimulating adenylate cyclase and thereby causing vasodilatation and inhibiting aggregation caused by any pathway (e.g. ADP and TXA_2).
- Agents that inhibit TXA_2 synthesis or block TXA_2 receptors, or have both actions, are available but are not used clinically.

receptors that bind fibrinogen, and this links adjacent platelets, sticking them together (aggregation)

- *exposure of acidic phospholipid* on the platelet surface, promoting thrombin formation (and hence further platelet activation via thrombin receptors and fibrin formation via cleavage of fibrinogen; see above).

These processes are essential for haemostasis but may be inappropriately triggered if the artery wall is diseased, most commonly with atherosclerosis, resulting in thrombosis (Fig. 21.7).

ANTIPLATELET DRUGS

Platelets play such a critical role in thromboembolic disease that it is no surprise that antiplatelet drugs are of great therapeutic value. Clinical trials of **aspirin** radically altered clinical practice, and more recently drugs that inhibit ADP and GPIIb/IIIa have also been found to be therapeutically useful. Sites of action of antiplatelet drugs are shown in Figure 21.7.

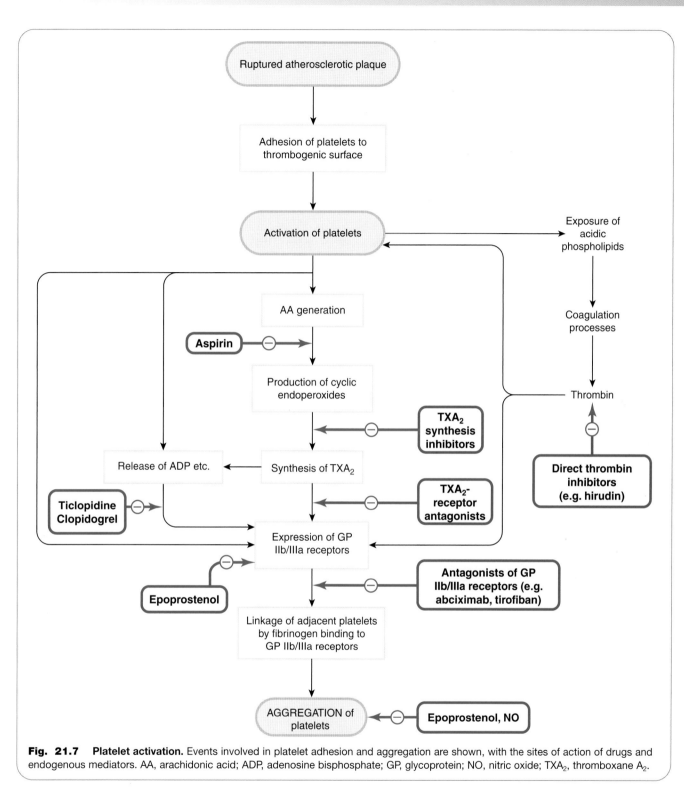

Fig. 21.7 Platelet activation. Events involved in platelet adhesion and aggregation are shown, with the sites of action of drugs and endogenous mediators. AA, arachidonic acid; ADP, adenosine bisphosphate; GP, glycoprotein; NO, nitric oxide; TXA$_2$, thromboxane A$_2$.

ASPIRIN

Aspirin (see Ch. 14, pp. 234-235) alters the balance between TXA$_2$, which promotes aggregation, and PGI$_2$, which inhibits it. Aspirin inactivates cyclo-oxygenase (COX)—acting mainly on the constitutive form COX-1—by irreversibly acetylating a serine residue in its active site. This reduces both TXA$_2$ synthesis in platelets and PGI$_2$ synthesis in endothelium. Oral administration is relatively selective for platelets because of presystemic elimination (see p. 117). Furthermore, vascular endothelial cells can synthesise new enzyme via regeneration of COX-1 and via COX-2, whereas platelets (which contain only COX-1 and have no nuclei) cannot. After administration of aspirin, TXA$_2$ synthesis does not recover until the affected cohort of platelets is replaced in 7–10 days. Consequently, low doses of aspirin given once every 24 or 48 hours decrease the synthesis of TXA_2 without drastically reducing PGI_2 synthesis. Clinical trials have demonstrated the efficacy of aspirin in several clinical settings (e.g. Fig. 21.8), with similar efficacy over a dose range of 50–1500 mg per day, all of which doses nearly completely abolish platelet thromboxane biosynthesis (see the clinical box on p. 343). Adverse effects of aspirin, mainly on the gastrointestinal tract (pp. 232-234), are, however, clearly dose-related, so a low dose (often 75 mg once daily) is usually recommended for thromboprophylaxis. Treatment failure can occur despite taking aspirin, and there is currently interest in the possibility that some patients exhibit a syndrome of 'aspirin resistance', although the mechanism and possible importance of this remains controversial (see Sanderson et al., 2005, for a review). Other non-steroidal drugs (e.g. **sulfinpyrazone**, for which there is supportive trial evidence) may have similar antithrombotic effects to aspirin, but they differ from aspirin in several potentially important ways (notably in being reversible rather than irreversible inhibitors of COX), so it is unwise to assume this in the absence of clinical trials.

DIPYRIDAMOLE

The value of **dipyridamole**—a phosphodiesterase inhibitor (see Ch. 19, p. 307)—has been clarified by the European Stroke Prevention Study 2 in patients with a history of ischaemic stroke or transient cerebral ischaemic attack. This showed that a modified-release form of dipyridamole reduced the risk of stroke and

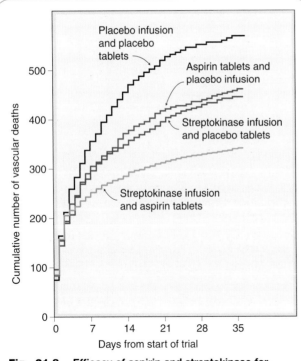

Fig. 21.8 Efficacy of aspirin and streptokinase for myocardial infarction. The curves show cumulative vascular mortality in patients treated with placebo, aspirin alone, streptokinase alone or a combined aspirin–streptokinase regimen. (ISIS-2 trial 1988 Lancet ii: 350–360.)

death in such patients by around 15%—a similar effect to that of aspirin (25 mg twice daily).[6] The beneficial effects of aspirin and dipyridamole were additive. Headache was the commonest adverse effect of dipyridamole; unlike aspirin, it caused no excess risk of bleeding.

THIENOPYRIDINE DERIVATIVES

Ticlopidine inhibits ADP-dependent aggregation. Its action is slow in onset, taking 3–7 days to reach maximal effect, and it works through an active metabolite that blocks platelet P_{2Y12} receptors (see Ch. 12, p. 199). Its efficacy in reducing stroke is similar to that of aspirin, but idiosyncratic unwanted effects, including severe blood dyscrasias (especially neutropenia), have limited its long-term use.

Clopidogrel is structurally related to ticlopidine and also inhibits ADP-induced aggregation through an active metabolite. Like ticlopidine, it can cause rash or diarrhoea, but neutropenia is no more common than with aspirin. Clopidogrel was slightly more effective than aspirin in reducing a composite outcome of ischaemic stroke, myocardial infarction or vascular death in one large trial. Because ADP antagonists inhibit a separate pathway of platelet activation than that which is inhibited by aspirin, their effects add to those of aspirin. Clinical trials of adding clopidogrel to aspirin in patients with acute coronary syndromes[7] (see Fig. 21.9) and (in a megatrial of over 45 000 patients) in patients with acute myocardial infarction (COMMIT Collaborative Group, 2005) have confirmed that combined treatment reduces mortality. Pretreatment with clopidogrel and aspirin followed by long-term therapy is also effective in patients with ischaemic heart disease undergoing percutaneous coronary interventions.

GLYCOPROTEIN IIB/IIIA RECEPTOR ANTAGONISTS

Antagonists of the GPIIb/IIIa receptor have the theoretical attraction that they inhibit all pathways of platelet activation (because these all converge on activation of GPIIb/IIIa receptors). A hybrid murine–human monoclonal antibody Fab fragment directed against the GPIIb/IIIa receptor, which rejoices in the catchy little name of **abciximab**, is licensed for use in high-risk patients undergoing coronary angioplasty, as an adjunct to heparin and aspirin. It reduces the risk of restenosis at the expense of an increased risk of bleeding. Immunogenicity limits its use to a single administration.

Tirofiban and **eptifibatide** are cyclic peptides based on the Arg-Gly-Asp ('RGD') sequence that is common to ligands for

---

[6]This dose regimen of aspirin is unconventional, being somewhat lower than the 75 mg once daily commonly used in thromboprophylaxis.

[7]Acute coronary syndromes include unstable angina (p. 286) and myocardial infarction that has not extended through the wall of the heart. The clinical picture is similar to transmural infarction, but there is no ST segment elevation on the electrocardiogram.

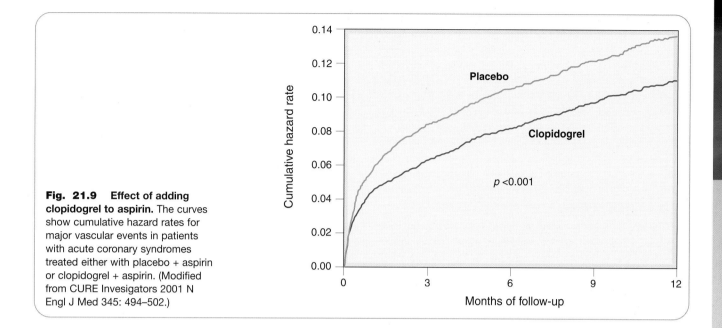

Fig. 21.9 Effect of adding clopidogrel to aspirin. The curves show cumulative hazard rates for major vascular events in patients with acute coronary syndromes treated either with placebo + aspirin or clopidogrel + aspirin. (Modified from CURE Invesigators 2001 N Engl J Med 345: 494–502.)

GPIIb/IIIa receptors. Given intravenously, these agents reduce early events in acute coronary syndrome[8] when given as an adjunct to aspirin and a heparin preparation, but long-term oral therapy with GPIIb/IIIa receptor antagonists is not effective and may be harmful. Unsurprisingly, they increase the risk of bleeding.

OTHER ANTIPLATELET DRUGS

Epoprostenol (PGI_2) may be administered into blood entering the dialysis circuit to prevent thrombosis during haemodialysis, especially in patients in whom heparin is contraindicated. It is also used in severe pulmonary hypertension (Ch. 19, pp. 316-318) and circulatory shock. It is unstable under physiological conditions and has a half-life of around 3 minutes, so it is administered by an intravenous infusion pump. Adverse effects related to its vasodilator action include flushing, headache and hypotension.

▼ *Thromboxane A_2-receptor ('TP') antagonists* (e.g. GR32191) are unlikely to be more effective than low-dose aspirin but could have fewer adverse effects. *TXA$_2$ synthesis inhibitors* ('TXSI', e.g. dazoxiben, an analogue of imidazole) increase PGI_2 synthesis, as a consequence of diversion of endoperoxide intermediates from TXA_2 synthesis to PGI_2 synthesis, as well as reducing TXA_2 production. However, they only weakly inhibit platelet function in vitro, probably because prostaglandin endoperoxides (e.g. PGH_2) are agonists at thromboxane receptors. Compounds that have both TXA_2 synthetase inhibition as well as TXA_2 receptor–blocking activity offer a better possibility of selectively inhibiting thromboxane synthesis while increasing PGI_2 synthesis, and drugs with this combination of activities (e.g. **ridogrel**) are in development.

---

[8]The UK National Institute for Clinical Excellence belied suspicions that it was actually an institute for rationing the use of expensive drugs by endorsing GPIIb/IIIa antagonist in acute coronary syndromes when a percutaneous invention is desirable but has to be delayed.

Clinical use of antiplatelet drugs

The clinical use of antiplatelet drugs is summarised in the clinical box below.

Clinical uses of antiplatelet drugs

- The main drug is **aspirin**. Other drugs with distinct actions (e.g. **dipyridamole**, **clopidogrel**) can have additive effects, or be used in patients who are intolerant of aspirin. Uses of antiplatelet drugs relate mainly to arterial thrombosis and include:
  - *acute myocardial infarction*
  - high risk of myocardial infarction, including a history of *myocardial infarction, angina* or *intermittent claudication* (see Ch. 19)
  - following *coronary artery bypass grafting*
  - *unstable coronary syndromes* (**clopidogrel** is added to **aspirin**)
  - following coronary artery *angioplasty* and/or *stenting* (intravenous glycoprotein IIb/IIIa antagonists, e.g. **abciximab**, are used in some patients in addition to aspirin)
  - *transient cerebral ischaemic attack* ('ministrokes') or *thrombotic stroke,* to prevent recurrence (**dipyridamole** can be added to **aspirin**)
  - *atrial fibrillation,* if oral anticoagulation is contraindicated.
- Other antiplatelet drugs (e.g. **epoprostenol** [PGI_2]; see Ch. 13) have specialised clinical applications (e.g. in *haemodialysis* or *haemofiltration*, Ch. 24, or in *pulmonary hypertension*, Ch. 19).

FIBRINOLYSIS (THROMBOLYSIS)

When the coagulation system is activated, the fibrinolytic system is also set in motion via several endogenous *plasminogen activators*, including tPA, urokinase-type plasminogen activator, kallikrein and neutrophil elastase. tPA is inhibited by a structurally related lipoprotein, lipoprotein(a), increased concentrations of which constitute an independent risk factor for myocardial infarction (Ch. 20, p. 323). Plasminogen is deposited on the fibrin strands within a thrombus. Plasminogen activators are serine proteases and are unstable in circulating blood. They diffuse into thrombus and cleave plasminogen to release plasmin (see Fig. 21.10).

▼ Plasmin is trypsin-like, acting on Arg-Lys bonds, and thus digests not only fibrin but fibrinogen; factors II, V and VIII; and many other proteins. It is formed locally and acts on the fibrin meshwork, generating fibrin degradation products and lysing the clot. Its action is localised to the clot, because plasminogen activators are effective mainly on plasminogen adsorbed to fibrin; any plasmin that escapes into the circulation is inactivated by plasmin inhibitors, including PAI-1 (see above and Ch. 19, p. 304), which protect us from digesting ourselves from within.

Drugs affect this system by increasing or inhibiting fibrinolysis (*fibrinolytic* and *antifibrinolytic* drugs, respectively).

FIBRINOLYTIC DRUGS

Figure 21.10 summarises the interaction of the fibrinolytic system with the coagulation cascade and platelet activation, and the action of drugs that modify this. Several fibrinolytic (thrombolytic) drugs are used clinically, principally to reopen the occluded coronary artery in patients with acute myocardial infarction, less commonly in patients with life-threatening venous thrombosis or pulmonary embolism.

Streptokinase is a protein extracted from cultures of streptococci. It activates plasminogen. Infused intravenously, it reduces mortality in acute myocardial infarction, and this beneficial effect is additive with aspirin (Fig. 21.8). Its action is blocked by anti-

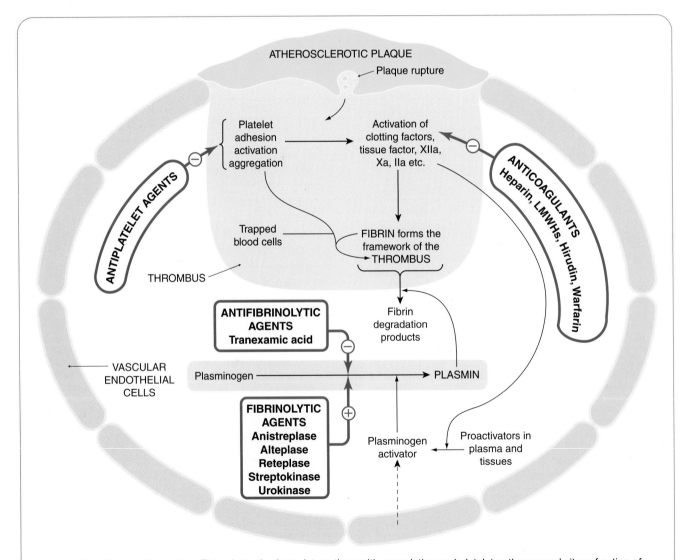

Fig. 21.10 **Fibrinolytic system.** The schematic shows interactions with coagulation and platelet pathways and sites of action of drugs that modify these systems. LMHs, low-molecular-weight heparins. For more details of platelet activation and the coagulation cascade, refer to Figures 21.1, 21.2 and 21.7.

bodies, which appear about 4 days or more after the initial dose. At least 1 year must elapse before it is used again.

Alteplase and duteplase are, respectively, single- and double-chain recombinant tPA. They are more active on fibrin-bound plasminogen than on plasma plasminogen, and are therefore said to be 'clot-selective'. Recombinant tPA is not antigenic, and can be used in patients likely to have antibodies to streptokinase. Because of their short half-lives, they must be given as intravenous infusions. Reteplase is similar but has a longer elimination half-life, allowing for bolus administration and making for simplicity of administration. It is available for clinical use in myocardial infarction.

Unwanted effects and contraindications

The main hazard of all fibrinolytic agents is bleeding, including gastrointestinal haemorrhage and stroke. If serious, this can be treated with **tranexamic acid** (see below), fresh plasma or coagulation factors. Streptokinase can cause allergic reactions and low-grade fever. Streptokinase causes a burst of plasmin formation, generating kinins (see Ch. 13), and can cause hypotension by this mechanism.

Contraindications to the use of these agents are active internal bleeding, haemorrhagic cerebrovascular disease, bleeding diatheses, pregnancy, uncontrolled hypertension, invasive procedures in which haemostasis is important, and recent trauma—including vigorous cardiopulmonary resuscitation.

Which fibrinolytic agent is best?

Several large placebo-controlled studies in patients with myocardial infarction have shown convincingly that fibrinolytic drugs reduce mortality if given within 12 hours of the onset of symptoms, and that the sooner they are administered the better is the result. Much has been written as to which drug is best, but an authoritative review (Collins et al., 1997) concluded that:

...the choice of fibrinolytic drug makes little difference to the overall probability of stroke-free survival, because the regimens that dissolve coronary thrombi more rapidly produce greater risks of cerebral haemorrhage... It is ... important that any uncertainties about which fibrinolytic regimen or dose of aspirin to use do not engender uncertainty about whether to use fibrinolytic and antiplatelet therapies routinely.

The important thing is to open up the thrombosed coronary artery as swiftly as possible. If facilities are available to do this mechanically (percutaneous coronary intervention), this is at least as good as using a lytic drug.

Clinical use

The clinical use of fibrinolytic agents is summarised in the clinical box.

ANTIFIBRINOLYTIC AND HAEMOSTATIC DRUGS

Tranexamic acid inhibits plasminogen activation and thus prevents fibrinolysis. It can be given orally or by intravenous injection. It is used to treat various conditions in which there is bleeding or risk of bleeding, such as haemorrhage following prostatectomy or dental extraction, in menorrhagia (excessive menstrual blood loss) and for life-threatening bleeding following thrombolytic drug administration. It is also used in patients with the rare disorder of hereditary angio-oedema.

Aprotinin inhibits proteolytic enzymes and is used for hyperplasminaemia caused by fibrinolytic drug overdose and in patients at risk of major blood loss during cardiac surgery.

Fibrinolysis and drugs modifying fibrinolysis

- A fibrinolytic cascade is initiated concomitantly with the coagulation cascade, resulting in the formation within the coagulum of plasmin, which digests fibrin.
- Various agents promote the formation of plasmin from its precursor plasminogen, for example **streptokinase**, and tissue plasminogen activators (tPAs) such as **alteplase**, **duteplase** and **reteplase**. Most are infused; reteplase can be given as a bolus injection.
- Some drugs (e.g. **tranexamic acid**, **aprotinin**) inhibit fibrinolysis.

Clinical uses of fibrinolytic drugs

The main drugs are **streptokinase** and **tissue plasminogen activators (tPAs)**, for example **tenecteplase**.
- The main use is in *acute myocardial infarction*, with ST segment elevation on the ECG within 12 hours of onset (the earlier the better!)
- Other uses include:
  — *acute thrombotic stroke* within 3 hours of onset (tPA), in selected patients
  — clearing *thrombosed shunts* and cannulae
  — acute *arterial thromboembolism*
  — *life-threatening deep vein thrombosis* and *pulmonary embolism* (streptokinase, given promptly).

REFERENCES AND FURTHER READING

Blood coagulation and anticoagulants
Bates S M, Weitz J I 2003 Emerging anticoagulant drugs. Arterioscler Thromb Vasc Biol 23: 1491–1500

Clouse L H, Comp P C 1987 The regulation of hemostasis: the protein C system. N Engl J Med 314: 1298–1304

Coughlin S R 2000 Thrombin signalling and protease-activated receptors. Nature 407: 258–264 (*Reviews cellular actions of thrombin via PARs; see also Brass*

S 2001 Platelets and proteases Nature 413: 26–27)

Dager W E 2004 Ximelagatran: a new antithrombotic option in atrial fibrillation. J Cardiovasc Pharmacol Ther 9: 151–162 (*Many patients with atrial fibrillation do not receive warfarin because of the difficulties in dosing and maintaining desirable target goals. Ximelagatran, 36 mg p.o. twice daily, is non-inferior to warfarin for thromboprophylaxis against stroke or systemic embolism in atrial fibrillation.*)

Furie B, Furie B C 1992 Molecular and cellular biology of blood coagulation. N Engl J Med 326: 800–806

Gibbs C S 1995 Conversion of thrombin into an anticoagulant by protein engineering. Nature 387: 413–416 (*A single amino acid substitution shifts thrombin's specificity in favour of the anticoagulant protein C; see also accompanying editorial: Griffin J H 1992 The thrombin paradox. Nature 387: 337–338*)

Gurm H S, Bhatt D L 2005 Thrombin, an ideal target for pharmacological inhibition: a review of direct thrombin inhibitors. Am Heart J 149: S43–S53

Hirsh J 1991 Heparin. N Engl J Med 324: 1565–1574

Hirsh J 1991 Oral anticoagulant drugs. N Engl J Med 324: 1865–1873

Hirsh J, O'Donnell M, Weitz J I 2005 New anticoagulants. Blood 105: 453–463 (*'Limitations of existing anticoagulants, vitamin K antagonist and heparins, have led to the development of newer anticoagulant therapies... New anticoagulants under evaluation include: inhibitors of the factor VIIa/tissue factor pathway; factor Xa inhibitors, both indirect and direct; activated protein C and soluble thrombomodulin; and direct thrombin inhibitors. Several of the direct inhibitors of factor Xa and thrombin are orally active. The greatest clinical need is for an oral anticoagulant to replace warfarin for long-term prevention and treatment of patients with venous and arterial thrombosis.'*)

Ibbotson T, Perry C M 2002 Danaparoid—a review of its use in thromboembolic and coagulation disorders. Drugs 62: 2283–2314 (*Danaparoid is an effective anticoagulant that has undergone clinical evaluation in a wide range of disease indications; discusses use in HIT*)

Pineda A O et al. 2004 The anticoagulant thrombin mutant W215A/E217A has a collapsed primary specificity pocket. J Biol Chem 279: 39824–39828 (*The thrombin mutant W215A/E217A features a drastically impaired catalytic activity, but activates the anticoagulant protein C in the presence of thrombomodulin. Describes the X-ray crystal structures of its free form and its complex with the active site inhibitor H-D-Phe-Pro-Arg- CH2Cl (PPACK), which explain the altered catalytic activity of the mutant.*)

Endothelium, platelets and antiplatelet agents

CAPRIE Steering Committee 1996 A randomised, blinded trial of clopidogrel versus aspirin in patients at risk of ischaemic events (CAPRIE). Lancet 348: 1329–1339 (*19 185 patients randomised; clopidogrel was marginally more effective than aspirin, with an overall safety profile at least as good as that of aspirin*)

Chew D P, Bhatt D, Sapp S, Topol E J 2001 Increased mortality with oral platelet glycoprotein IIb/IIIa antagonists: a meta-analysis of phase III multicenter trials. Circulation 103: 201–206

COMMIT Collaborative Group 2005 Addition of clopidogrel to aspirin in 45 852 patients with acute myocardial infarction: randomised placebo-controlled trial. Lancet 366: 1607–1621 (*Clopidogrel reduced the risk of death, myocardial infarction or stroke combined, and of mortality alone; see accompanying comment by Sabatine M S, pp. 1587–1589 in the same issue*)

CURE Investigators 2001 Effects of clopidogrel in addition to aspirin in patients with acute coronary syndromes without ST-segment elevation. N Engl J Med 345: 494–502 (*A total of 12 562 patients randomised; primary outcome occurred in 9.4% of patients in the clopidogrel + aspirin group and in 11.3% of those in the placebo + aspirin group, a relative risk of 0.72–0.90, P < 0.001*)

EPIC Investigators 1994 Use of a monoclonal antibody directed against the platelet glycoprotein IIb/IIIa receptor in high-risk coronary angioplasty. N Engl J Med 330: 956–961 (*Ischaemic complications were reduced by 35% at the cost of increased bleeding*)

Mehta S R for the CURE Investigators 2001 Effects of pretreatment with clopidogrel and aspirin followed by long-term therapy in patients undergoing percutaneous coronary intervention: the PCI-CURE study. Lancet 358: 527–533 (*Positive study showing additive effect of clopidogrel + aspirin*)

Patrono C, Coller B, FitzGerald G A et al. 2004 Platelet-active drugs: the relationships among dose, effectiveness, and side effects. Chest 126: 234S–264S

Sanderson S, Emery J, Baglin T, Kinmonth A L 2005 Narrative review: aspirin resistance and its clinical implications. Ann Intern Med 142: 370–380

Ware J A, Heisted D D 1993 Platelet-endothelium interactions. N Engl J Med 328: 628–635

Thrombolysis and antifibrinolytic agents

Fears R 1990 Biochemical pharmacology and therapeutic aspects of thrombolytic agents. Pharmacol Rev 42: 201–224

Mannuccio M 1998 Hemostatic drugs. N Engl J Med 333: 245–253

Special Writing Group of the Stroke Council of the American Health Association 1996 Guidelines for thrombolytic therapy for acute stroke: a supplement to the guidelines for the management of patients with acute ischemic stroke. Stroke 27: 1711–1718

(*Recommends using tPA in selected patients within the first 3 hours of ischaemic stroke*)

Clinical and general aspects

Aster R H 1995 Heparin-induced thrombocytopenia and thrombosis. N Engl J Med 332: 1374–1376 (*Succinct and lucid editorial; see also accompanying paper, pp. 1330–1335*)

Collins R, Peto R, Baigent C, Sleight P 1997 Aspirin, heparin and thrombolytic therapy in suspected acute myocardial infarction. N Engl J Med 336: 847–860 (*Unbiased and authoritative overview; includes a section on 'general problems of unduly selective emphasis'—fighting stuff!*)

Diener H, Cunha L, Forbes C et al. 1996 European Stroke Prevention Study 2. Dipyridamole and acetylsalicylic acid in the secondary prevention of stroke. J Neurol Sci 143: 1–14 (*Slow-release dipyridamole 200 mg twice daily was as effective as aspirin 25 mg twice daily, and the effects of aspirin and dipyridamole were additive*)

Donnan G A, Dewey H M, Chambers B R 2004 Warfarin for atrial fibrillation: the end of an era? Lancet Neurol 3: 305–308 (*Direct thrombin inhibitors such as ximelagatran are not inferior to warfarin and, based on results from the Stroke Prevention Using an Oral Thrombin Inhibitor in Atrial Fibrillation [SPORTIF] III and V trials, are perhaps safer, with no need for long-term monitoring and dose adjustment; however, the side effect of raised liver enzymes in 6% of patients needs to be resolved*)

Goldhaber S Z 2004 Pulmonary embolism. Lancet 363: 1295–1305

Kyrle P A, Eichinger S 2005 Deep vein thrombosis. Lancet 365: 1163–1174

Levine M 1995 A comparison of low-molecular-weight heparin administered primarily at home with unfractionated heparin administered in the hospital for proximal deep vein thrombosis. N Engl J Med 334: 677–681 (*Concludes that LMWH can be used safely and effectively at home; this has potentially very important implications for patient care*)

Markus H S 2005 Current treatments in neurology: stroke. J Neurol 252: 260–267

Turpie A G G 1993 A comparison of aspirin with placebo in patients treated with warfarin after heart-valve replacement. N Engl J Med 329: 524–529 (*Considerable benefit of combined treatment with aspirin and warfarin—meticulous monitoring mandatory!*)

Warkentin T E 2003 Management of heparin-induced thrombocytopenia: a critical comparison of lepirudin and argatroban. Thromb Res 110: 73–82 (*A direct thrombin inhibitor should be given alone during acute HIT, with oral anticoagulants deferred until substantial resolution of the thrombocytopenia has occurred*)

The haemopoietic system

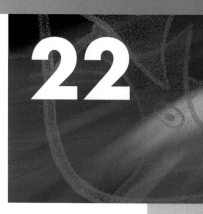

22

OVERVIEW

In this chapter, we summarise the different kinds of anaemia and cover the main haematinic agents used to treat them, namely iron, folic acid and vitamin B$_{12}$. We also cover erythropoietin, a growth factor specific for red blood cells used to treat anaemia of chronic disease, and several other haemopoietic factors, known as colony-stimulating factors (CSFs), which are used to increase numbers of circulating white blood cells.

THE HAEMOPOIETIC SYSTEM

The main components of the haemopoietic system are the blood, bone marrow, lymph nodes and thymus, with the spleen, liver and kidneys as important accessory organs. Blood consists of formed elements (red and white blood cells and platelets) and plasma. It has diverse functions, including key roles in host defence (Ch. 13) and haemostasis (Ch. 21). This present chapter deals mainly with red cells, which have the principal function of carrying oxygen. Their oxygen-carrying power depends on their haemoglobin content. The most important site of formation of red blood cells in adults is the bone marrow, whereas the spleen acts as their grave-yard. Red cell loss in healthy adults is precisely balanced by production of new cells. The liver stores vitamin B$_{12}$ and is involved in the process of breakdown of the haemoglobin liberated when red blood cells are destroyed. The kidney manufactures erythropoietin. Cells from various organs synthesise and release CSFs, which regulate the production of leucocytes and platelets. The

function of platelets is discussed in Chapter 21, and that of leucocytes in Chapter 13. Drugs used in the chemotherapy of leukemias, a very important part of oncology, are described in Chapter 51.

TYPES OF ANAEMIA

Anaemia is defined as a reduced concentration of haemoglobin in the blood. It may give rise to fatigue but, especially if it is chronic, is often surprisingly asymptomatic. The commonest cause is blood loss related to menstruation and child bearing, but there are several different types of anaemia and several different diagnostic levels. Determining indices of red cell size and haemoglobin content and microscopical examination of a stained blood smear of blood allow characterisation into:

- hypochromic, microcytic anaemia (small red cells with low haemoglobin; caused by iron deficiency)
- macrocytic anaemia (large red cells, few in number)
- normochromic normocytic anaemia (fewer normal-sized red cells, each with a normal haemoglobin content)
- mixed pictures.

Further evaluation may include determination of concentrations of ferritin, iron, vitamin B$_{12}$ and folic acid in serum (*haematinics*), and microscopic examination of smears of bone marrow. This leads to more precise diagnostic groupings of anaemias into:

- deficiency of nutrients necessary for haemopoiesis, most importantly:
  —iron
  —folic acid and vitamin B$_{12}$
  —pyridoxine, vitamin C.
- depression of the bone marrow, caused by:
  —toxins (e.g. drugs used in chemotherapy)
  —radiation therapy
  —diseases of the bone marrow of unknown origin (e.g. idiopathic aplastic anaemia, leukaemias)
  —reduced production of, or responsiveness to, erythropoietin (e.g. chronic renal failure, rheumatoid arthritis, AIDS).
- excessive destruction of red blood cells (i.e. haemolytic anaemia); this has many causes, including haemoglobinopathies (such as sickle cell anaemia), adverse reactions to drugs, and inappropriate immune reactions.

It is important to note that the use of haematinic agents is often only an adjunct to treatment of the underlying cause of the

347

anaemia—for example surgery for colon cancer (a common cause of iron deficiency) or anthelminthic drugs for patients with hookworm (a frequent cause of anaemia in parts of Africa and Asia; Ch. 50). Sometimes treatment consists of stopping an offending drug, for example a non-steroidal anti-inflammatory drug that causes blood loss from the stomach (Ch. 14).

HAEMATINIC AGENTS

IRON

Iron is a transition metal with two important properties relevant to its biological role:

- ability to exist in several oxidation states
- ability to form stable coordination complexes.

The body of a 70-kg man contains about 4 g of iron, 65% of which circulates in the blood as haemoglobin. About one-half of the remainder is stored in the liver, spleen and bone marrow, chiefly as *ferritin* and *haemosiderin*. The iron in these molecules is available for haemoglobin synthesis. The rest, which is not available for haemoglobin synthesis, is present in myoglobin, cytochromes and various enzymes.

The distribution of iron in an average adult man is shown in Table 22.1. The corresponding values for a woman would be about 55% of these. Because most of the iron in the body is either part of—or destined to be part of—haemoglobin, the most obvious clinical result of iron deficiency is anaemia, and the only indication for therapy with iron is for treatment or prophylaxis of iron deficiency anaemia.

Haemoglobin is made up of four protein chain subunits (globins), each of which contains one haem moiety. Haem consists of a tetrapyrrole porphyrin ring containing ferrous (Fe^{2+}) iron. Each haem group can carry one oxygen molecule, which is bound reversibly to Fe^{2+} and to a histidine residue in the globin chain. This reversible binding is the basis of oxygen transport.

Iron turnover and balance

Both the normal physiological turnover of iron and *pharmacokinetic factors* affecting iron when it is given therapeutically will be dealt with here. The normal daily requirement for iron is approximately 5 mg for men, and 15 mg for growing children and for menstruating women. A pregnant woman needs between 2 and 10 times this amount because of the demands of the fetus and increased requirements of the mother.[1] The average diet in Western Europe provides 15–20 mg of iron daily, mostly in meat. Iron in meat is generally present as haem, and about 20–40% of haem iron is available for absorption.

▼ Humans are adapted to absorb iron in the form of haem. It is thought that one reason why modern humans have problems in maintaining iron balance (there are an estimated 500 million people with iron deficiency in the world) is that the change from hunting to grain cultivation 10 000 years ago led to cereals, which have a relatively small amount of utilisable iron, being substituted for meat in the diet.

Non-haem iron in food is mainly in the ferric state, and this needs to be converted to ferrous iron for absorption. Ferric iron, and to a lesser extent ferrous iron, has low solubility at the neutral pH of the intestine; however, in the stomach iron dissolves and binds to mucoprotein. In the presence of ascorbic acid, fructose and various amino acids, iron is detached from the carrier, forming soluble low-molecular-weight complexes that enable it to remain in soluble form in the intestine. Ascorbic acid stimulates iron absorption partly by forming soluble iron–ascorbate chelates and partly by reducing ferric iron to the more soluble ferrous form.

Tetracycline forms an insoluble iron chelate, resulting in impaired uptake of both substances.

The amount of iron in the diet and the various factors affecting its availability are thus important determinants in absorption, but the regulation of iron absorption is a function of the intestinal mucosa, influenced by the body's iron stores. Because there is no mechanism whereby iron excretion is regulated, the absorptive mechanism has a central role in iron balance as it is the sole mechanism by which body iron is controlled.

The site of iron absorption is the duodenum and upper jejunum, and absorption is a two-stage process involving first a rapid uptake across the brush border and then transfer into the plasma from the interior of the epithelial cells. The second stage, which is rate limiting, is energy-dependent. Haem iron in the diet is absorbed as intact haem, and the iron is released in the mucosal cell by the action of haem oxidase. Non-haem iron is absorbed in the ferrous state. Within the cell, ferrous iron is oxidised to ferric iron, which is bound to an intracellular carrier, a transferrin-like protein; the iron is then either held in storage in the mucosal cell as ferritin (if body stores of iron are high) or passed on to the plasma (if iron stores are low).

Table 22.1 The distribution of iron in the body of a healthy 70-kg man

Protein	Tissue	Iron content (mg)
Haemoglobin	Erythrocytes	2600
Myoglobin	Muscle	400
Enzymes (cytochromes, catalase, guanylate cyclase, etc.)	Liver and other tissues	25
Transferrin	Plasma and extracellular fluid	8
Ferritin and haemosiderin	Liver Spleen Bone marrow	410 48 300

(Data from Jacobs A, Worwood M 1982 Chapter 5. In: Hardisty R M, Weatherall D J [eds] Blood and its disorders. Blackwell Scientific, Oxford.)

---

[1]Each pregnancy 'costs' the mother 680 mg of iron, equivalent to 1300 ml of blood, owing to the demands of the fetus, plus requirements of the expanded blood volume and blood loss at delivery.

Iron is carried in the plasma bound to *transferrin*, a β-globulin with two binding sites for ferric iron, which is normally only 30% saturated. Plasma contains 4 mg of iron at any one time, but the daily turnover is about 30 mg (Fig. 22.1). Most of the iron that enters the plasma is derived from mononuclear phagocytes, following the degradation of time-expired erythrocytes. Intestinal absorption and mobilisation of iron from storage depots contribute only small amounts. Most of the iron that leaves the plasma each day is used for haemoglobin synthesis by red cell precursors. These cells have receptors that bind transferrin molecules, releasing them after the iron has been taken up.

Iron is stored in two forms: soluble *ferritin* and insoluble *haemosiderin*. Ferritin is found in all cells, the mononuclear phagocytes of liver, spleen and bone marrow containing especially high concentrations. It is also present in plasma. The precursor of ferritin, *apoferritin*, is a large protein of molecular weight 450 000, composed of 24 identical polypeptide subunits that enclose a cavity in which up to 4500 iron molecules can be stored. Apoferritin takes up ferrous iron, oxidises it and deposits the ferric iron in its core. In this form, it constitutes ferritin, the primary storage form of iron, from which the iron is most readily available. The lifespan of this iron-laden protein is only a few days. Haemosiderin is a degraded form of ferritin in which the iron cores of several ferritin molecules have aggregated, following partial disintegration of the outer protein shells.

The ferritin in plasma has virtually no iron associated with it. It is in equilibrium with the storage ferritin in cells, and its concentration in plasma provides an estimate of total body iron stores.

The body has no means of actively excreting iron. Small amounts leave the body through *desquamation* (peeling off) of mucosal cells containing ferritin, and even smaller amounts leave in the bile, sweat and urine. A total of about 1 mg is lost daily. Iron balance is therefore critically dependent on the active absorption mechanism in the intestinal mucosa. This absorption is influenced by the iron stores in the body, but the precise mechanism of this control is still a matter of debate; the amount of ferritin in the intestinal mucosa may be important, as may the balance between ferritin and the transferrin-like carrier molecule in these cells. The daily movement of iron in the body is illustrated in Figure 22.1.

The clinical use of iron is given in the clinical box.

Administration

Iron is usually given orally but may be given parenterally in special circumstances.

Several different preparations of ferrous iron salts are available for oral administration. The main one is **ferrous sulfate**, which has an elemental iron content of 200 µg/mg. Others are ferrous succinate, ferrous gluconate and ferrous fumarate. These are all absorbed to a comparable extent.

Parenteral iron may be necessary in individuals who are not able to absorb oral iron because of malabsorption syndromes, or as a result of surgical procedures or inflammatory conditions involving the gastrointestinal tract. It is also used for patients who do not tolerate oral preparations, and patients with chronic renal failure receiving treatment with erythropoietin (see below). The preparations used are **iron-dextran** or **iron-sucrose**. Iron-dextran can be given by deep intramuscular injection or slow intravenous infusion; iron-sucrose is given by slow intravenous infusion. A small initial dose is given because of the risk of anaphylactoid reaction.

Unwanted effects

The unwanted effects of oral iron administration are dose-related and include nausea, abdominal cramps and diarrhoea. Parenteral iron can cause anaphylactoid reactions (cf. p. 212).

Acute iron toxicity, usually seen in young children who have swallowed attractively coloured iron tablets in mistake for sweets, occurs after ingestion of large quantities of iron salts. This can result in severe necrotising gastritis with vomiting, haemorrhage and diarrhoea, followed by circulatory collapse.

Chronic iron toxicity or iron overload is virtually always caused by conditions other than ingestion of iron salts, for example chronic haemolytic anaemias such as the thalassaemias (a large group of genetic disorders of globin chain synthesis) or repeated blood transfusions.

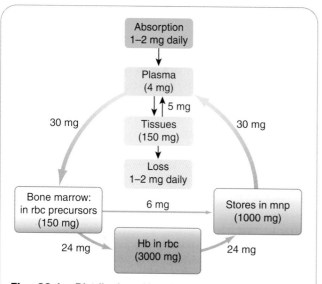

Fig. 22.1   Distribution of iron in the body. The quantities by the arrows indicate the usual amounts transferred each day. Hb, haemoglobin; mnp, mononuclear phagocytes; rbc, red blood cells.

Clinical uses of iron salts

• To treat *iron deficiency anaemia*, which can be caused by:
  – *chronic blood loss* (e.g. with menorrhagia, hookworm, colon cancer)
  – *increased demand* (e.g. in pregnancy and early infancy)
  – *inadequate dietary intake* (uncommon in developed countries)
  – *inadequate absorption* (e.g. following gastrectomy).

The treatment of acute and chronic iron toxicity involves the use of iron chelators such as **desferrioxamine**. This is not absorbed from the gut but is nonetheless given intragastrically following acute overdose (to bind iron in the bowel lumen and prevent its absorption) as well as intramuscularly and, if necessary, intravenously. In severe poisoning, it is given by slow intravenous infusion. Desferrioxamine forms a complex with ferric iron and, unlike unbound iron, this is excreted in the urine. **Deferiprone**, an orally absorbed iron chelator, is an alternative treatment for iron overload in patients with thalassaemia major who are unable to take desferrioxamine. Agranulocytosis and other blood dyscrasias are serious potential adverse effects.

FOLIC ACID AND VITAMIN B₁₂

Vitamin B₁₂ and **folic acid** are essential constituents of the human diet, being necessary for DNA synthesis and consequently for cell proliferation. Their biochemical actions are interdependent (see below), and treatment of vitamin B₁₂ deficiency with folic acid corrects some, but not all, of the features of vitamin B₁₂ deficiency. Deficiency of either vitamin B₁₂ or folic acid affects tissues with a rapid cell turnover, particularly bone marrow, but vitamin B₁₂ deficiency also causes important disorders of nerves, which are not corrected (or may even be made worse) by treatment with folic acid. Deficiency of either vitamin causes *megaloblastic haemopoiesis*, in which there is disordered erythroblast differentiation and defective erythropoiesis in the bone marrow. Large abnormal erythrocyte precursors appear in the marrow,

each with a high RNA:DNA ratio as a result of decreased DNA synthesis. The circulating erythrocytes (*macrocytes*) are large fragile cells, often distorted in shape. Mild leucopenia and thrombocytopenia usually accompany the anaemia, and the nuclei of polymorphonuclear leucocytes are abnormal (hypersegmented). Neurological disorders caused by deficiency of vitamin B₁₂ include *peripheral neuropathy* and *dementia*, as well as *subacute combined² degeneration* of the spinal cord.

Folic acid deficiency is caused by dietary insufficiency, especially in settings of increased demand (e.g. during pregnancy, or because of chronic haemolysis in patients with haemoglobinopathies). Vitamin B₁₂ deficiency, however, is usually caused by decreased absorption, caused either by a lack of intrinsic factor (see below) or by conditions that interfere with its absorption in the terminal ileum, for example resection of diseased ileum in patients with Crohn's disease (a chronic inflammatory bowel disease that can affect this part of the gut). Intrinsic factor is a glycoprotein secreted by the stomach and is essential for vitamin B₁₂ absorption. It is lacking in patients with *pernicious anaemia* and in individuals who have had total gastrectomies. In pernicious anaemia, there is atrophic gastritis caused by autoimmune injury of the stomach, and antibodies to gastric parietal cells are often present in the plasma of such patients.

FOLIC ACID

Folic acid (pteroylglutamic acid) consists of a pteridine ring, *para*-aminobenzoic acid and glutamic acid. Some aspects of folate structure and metabolism are dealt with in Chapters 45 and 51, because several important antibacterial and anticancer drugs are antimetabolites that interfere with folate synthesis in microorganisms. Liver and green vegetables are rich sources of folate. In healthy non-pregnant adults, the daily requirement is about 200 μg daily, but this is increased during pregnancy.

Actions

Dihydrofolate (FH₂) and tetrahydrofolate (FH₄) act as carriers and donors of methyl groups (1-carbon transfers) in a number of important metabolic pathways. For example, FH₄ is essential for DNA synthesis because of its role as cofactor in the synthesis of purines and pyrimidines. It is also necessary for reactions involved in amino acid metabolism. The active FH₄ form is maintained by *dihydrofolate reductase*. This important enzyme reduces dietary folic acid to FH₄ and regenerates FH₄ from FH₂ (see Figs 22.2 and 22.3). Folate antagonists (e.g. **trimethoprim**, **methotrexate**) are important antibacterial and anticancer drugs, and work by inhibiting dihydrofolate reductase (see also Chs 46, 49 and 51). Methotrexate is also used as a disease modifying drug for *rheumatoid arthritis* (p. 241) and for treating severe forms of *psoriasis*—a common skin disorder characterised by scaly lesions.

Tetrahydrofolate is especially important for the conversion of deoxyuridylate monophosphate to deoxythymidylate monophosphate. This is rate-limiting in mammalian DNA synthesis and is

> **Iron**
>
> - Iron is important for the synthesis of haemoglobin, myoglobin, cytochromes and other enzymes.
> - Ferric iron (Fe³⁺) must be converted to ferrous iron (Fe²⁺) for absorption in the gastrointestinal tract.
> - Absorption involves active transport into mucosal cells in jejunum and upper ileum, from where it can be transported into the plasma and/or stored intracellularly as ferritin.
> - Total body iron is controlled exclusively by absorption; in iron deficiency, more is transported into plasma than is stored as ferritin in jejunal mucosa.
> - Iron loss occurs mainly by sloughing of ferritin-containing mucosal cells.
> - Iron in plasma is bound to transferrin, and most is used for erythropoiesis. Some is stored as ferritin in other tissues. Iron from time-expired erythrocytes enters the plasma for reuse.
> - The main therapeutic preparation is ferrous sulfate; iron-sucrose can be given as an intravenous infusion.
> - Unwanted effects include gastrointestinal disturbances. Severe toxic effects occur if large doses are ingested; these can be countered by desferrioxamine, an iron chelator.

---

²'Combined' because the lateral as well as the dorsal columns are involved, giving rise to motor as well as sensory symptoms.

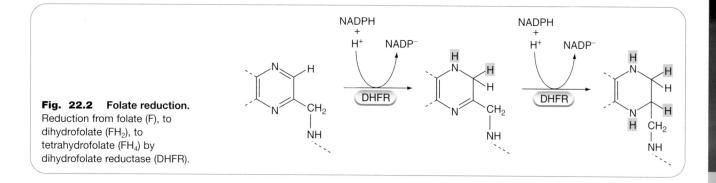

Fig. 22.2 Folate reduction. Reduction from folate (F), to dihydrofolate (FH$_2$), to tetrahydrofolate (FH$_4$) by dihydrofolate reductase (DHFR).

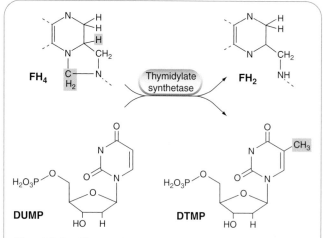

Fig. 22.3 The synthesis of 2-deoxythymidylate (DTMP). DTMP is synthesised by the transfer of a methyl group from tetrahydrofolate (FH$_4$) to 2-deoxyuridylate (DUMP), the FH$_4$ being oxidised to dihydrofolate (FH$_2$) in the process.

Unwanted effects

Unwanted effects do not occur even with large doses of folic acid—except possibly in the presence of vitamin B$_{12}$ deficiency, because if the vitamin deficiency is treated with folic acid, the blood picture may improve and give the appearance of cure while the neurological lesions get worse. It is therefore important to determine whether a megaloblastic anaemia is caused by a folate or a vitamin B$_{12}$ deficiency. This could have been important in the setting of supplementation of bread with folate, which is used in the USA as a public health measure to reduce the number of neural tube defects. There is a theoretical risk of precipitating neuropathy in the small group of people with undiagnosed pernicious anaemia by such measures, but such problems have not been noted.

catalysed by thymidylate synthetase, with FH$_4$ acting as methyl donor (Fig. 22.3).

Pharmacokinetic aspects

Folates in food are in the form of polyglutamates. These are converted to monoglutamates before absorption, and are transported in blood as such. They are converted back into polyglutamates, which are considerably more active than monoglutamates, in the tissues. Therapeutically, folic acid is given orally (or, in exceptional circumstances, parenterally) and is absorbed in the ileum. Methyl-FH$_4$ is the form in which folate is usually carried in blood and which enters cells. It is functionally inactive until it is demethylated in a vitamin B$_{12}$–dependent reaction (see below). This is because (unlike FH$_2$, FH$_4$ and formyl-FH$_4$) methyl-FH$_4$ is a poor substrate for polyglutamate formation. This has relevance for the effect of vitamin B$_{12}$ deficiency on folate metabolism, as is explained below. Folate is taken up into hepatocytes and bone marrow cells by active transport. Within the cells, folic acid is reduced and formylated before being converted to the active polyglutamate form. **Folinic acid**, a synthetic FH$_4$, is converted much more rapidly to the polyglutamate form.

> **Clinical uses of folic acid and hydroxocobalamin**
>
> **Folic acid**
> - Treatment of *megaloblastic anaemia* resulting from folate deficiency, which can be caused by:
>   - *poor diet* (common in alcoholic individuals)
>   - *malabsorption* syndromes
>   - drugs (e.g. **phenytoin**).
> - Treatment or prevention of toxicity from **methotrexate**, a folate antagonist (see Ch. 51).
> - Prophylactically in individuals at hazard from developing folate deficiency, for example:
>   - *pregnant women* and *before conception* (especially if there is a risk of birth defects)
>   - *premature infants*
>   - patients with severe chronic *haemolytic anaemias*, including haemoglobinopathies (e.g. sickle cell anaemia).
>
> **Hydroxocobalamin (vitamin B$_{12}$)**
> - Treatment of *pernicious anaemia* and other causes of vitamin B12 deficiency.
> - Prophylactically after surgical operations that remove the site of production of intrinsic factor (the stomach) or of vitamin B$_{12}$ absorption (the terminal ileum).

Clinical use

The clinical use of folic acid is given in the box opposite (p. 351).

VITAMIN B$_{12}$

Vitamin B$_{12}$ is a complex cobalamin compound. The vitamin B$_{12}$ used medically is **hydroxocobalamin**. The principal dietary sources of vitamin B$_{12}$ are meat (particularly liver), eggs and dairy products. All cobalamins, dietary and therapeutic, must be converted to *methylcobalamin* (methyl-B$_{12}$) or 5′-*deoxyadenosylcobalamin* (ado-B$_{12}$) for activity in the body. The average daily diet in Western Europe contains 5–25 μg of vitamin B$_{12}$, and the daily requirement is 2–3 μg. Absorption requires intrinsic factor (p. 350), which forms a one-to-one complex with vitamin B$_{12}$. A healthy stomach secretes a large excess of intrinsic factor, but this is not true in patients with addisonian *pernicious anaemia* (an autoimmune disorder where the lining of the stomach atrophies), or following total gastrectomy. Vitamin B$_{12}$, complexed with intrinsic factor, is absorbed by active transport.

Vitamin B$_{12}$ is carried in the plasma by binding proteins called *transcobalamins*. The vitamin is stored mainly in the liver, the total amount in the body being about 4 mg. This store is so large compared with the daily requirement, that if vitamin B$_{12}$ absorption is stopped suddenly—as after a total gastrectomy—it takes 2–4 years for evidence of deficiency to become manifest.

Actions

Vitamin B$_{12}$ is required for two main biochemical reactions in humans:

- the conversion of methyl-FH$_4$ to FH$_4$
- isomerisation of methylmalonyl-CoA to succinyl-CoA.

The conversion of methyl-FH$_4$ to FH$_4$

The role of vitamin B$_{12}$ in folate coenzyme synthesis is illustrated in Figure 22.4. It is through these mechanisms that the metabolic activities of vitamin B$_{12}$ and folic acid are linked and implicated in the synthesis of DNA. It is also through this pathway that folate/vitamin B$_{12}$ treatment can lower plasma homocysteine concentration. Because increased homocysteine concentrations may have undesirable vascular effects (Ch. 20, Table 20.1, p. 322), this has potential therapeutic and public health implications.

▼ The reaction involves conversion of both methyl-FH$_4$ to FH$_4$ and homocysteine to methionine. The enzyme that accomplishes this is homocysteine–methionine methyltransferase; the reaction requires vitamin B$_{12}$ as cofactor and methyl-FH$_4$ as methyl donor. Methyl-FH$_4$ donates the methyl group to B$_{12}$, the cofactor. The methyl group is then transferred to homocysteine to form methionine (Fig. 22.4). This vitamin B$_{12}$–dependent reaction generates active FH$_4$ from inactive methyl-FH$_4$ and converts homocysteine to methionine.

Vitamin B$_{12}$ deficiency thus traps folate in the inactive methyl-FH$_4$ form, thereby depleting the folate polyglutamate coenzymes needed for DNA synthesis (see above).

Vitamin B$_{12}$–dependent methionine synthesis also affects the synthesis of folate polyglutamate coenzymes by an additional mechanism. The preferred substrate for polyglutamate synthesis is formyl-FH$_4$, and the conversion of FH$_4$ to formyl-FH$_4$ requires a formate donor such as methionine.

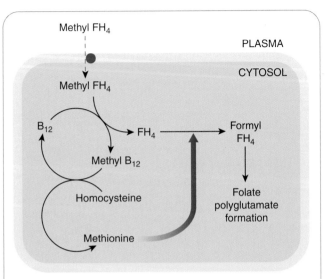

Fig. 22.4   The role of vitamin B$_{12}$ in the synthesis of folate polyglutamate. Methyltetrahydrofolate (Methyl FH$_4$) enters cells by active transport. The methyl group is transferred to homocysteine to form methionine via vitamin B$_{12}$, which is bound to the apoenzyme homocysteine–methionine methyltransferase. (Vitamin B$_{12}$ is shown as 'B$_{12}$' and as 'methyl B$_{12}$', but the enzyme is not shown.) Methionine is important in the donation of formate (shown by the curved red arrow) for the conversion of tetrahydrofolate (FH$_4$) to formyl tetrahydrofolate (formyl FH$_4$), which is the preferred substrate for the formation of folate polyglutamates.

Isomerisation of methylmalonyl-CoA to succinyl-CoA

This isomerisation reaction is part of a route by which propionate is converted to succinate. Through this pathway, cholesterol, odd-chain fatty acids, some amino acids and thymine can be used for gluconeogenesis or for energy production via the tricarboxylic acid cycle. Coenzyme B$_{12}$ (ado-B$_{12}$) is an essential cofactor, so methylmalonyl-CoA accumulates in vitamin B$_{12}$ deficiency. This distorts the pattern of fatty acid synthesis in neural tissue and may be the basis of neuropathy in vitamin B$_{12}$ deficiency.

Administration and pharmacokinetic aspects

When vitamin B$_{12}$ is used therapeutically (as hydroxocobalamin), it is almost always given by injection because, as explained above, vitamin B$_{12}$ deficiency is a result of malabsorption. Plasma transport and distribution of therapeutically administered vitamin B$_{12}$ are described above.

Patients with pernicious anaemia require lifelong therapy. Unwanted effects do not occur. Clinical use of vitamin B$_{12}$ is summarised in the box.

HAEMOPOIETIC GROWTH FACTORS

Every 60 seconds, a human being must generate about 120 million granulocytes and 150 million erythrocytes, as well as numerous mononuclear cells and platelets. The cells responsible for this remarkable productivity are derived from a relatively

Vitamin B₁₂ and folic acid

Both vitamin B_{12} and folic acid are needed for DNA synthesis. Deficiencies particularly affect erythropoiesis, causing macrocytic megaloblastic anaemia.

Folic acid
- Folic acid consists of a pteridine ring, *p*-aminobenzoic acid and a glutamate residue.
- There is active uptake into cells and reduction to tetrahydrofolate (FH_4) by dihydrofolate reductase; extra glutamates are then added.
- Folate polyglutamate is a cofactor (a carrier of 1-carbon units) in the synthesis of purines and pyrimidines (especially thymidylate).

Vitamin B₁₂ (hydroxocobalamin)
- Vitamin B_{12} needs an *intrinsic factor* (a glycoprotein) secreted by gastric parietal cells for absorption in terminal ileum. It is stored in the liver.
- It is required for:
  — conversion of methyl-FH_4 (inactive form of FH_4) to active formyl-FH_4, which, after polyglutamation, is a cofactor in the synthesis of purines and pyrimidines (see above)
  — isomerisation of methylmalonyl-CoA to succinyl-CoA.
- Deficiency occurs most often in pernicious anaemia, which results from malabsorption caused by lack of intrinsic factor from the stomach. It causes neurological disease as well as anaemia.
- Vitamin B_{12} is given by injection to treat pernicious anaemia.

Haemopoietic growth factors

Erythropoietin
- Regulates red cell production.
- Is given intravenously, subcutaneously, intraperitoneally.
- Can cause transient flu-like symptoms, hypertension, iron deficiency and increased blood viscosity.
- Is available as epoetin.

Granulocyte colony-stimulating factor
- Stimulates neutrophil progenitors.
- Is available as **filgrastim**, **pegfilgrastim** or **lenograstim**; it is given parenterally.

CSF (**molgrasmostim**) are used clinically; **thrombopoietin** is in development. Some of the other haemopoietic growth factors (e.g. interleukin-1, interleukin-2 and various other cytokines) are covered in Chapter 13.

ERYTHROPOIETIN

Erythropoietin is produced in juxtatubular cells in the kidney and also in macrophages; its action is to stimulate committed erythroid progenitor cells to proliferate and generate erythrocytes (Fig. 22.5). Two forms of recombinant human erythropoietin, **epoetin alfa** and **epoetin beta**, are available. These are clinically indistinguishable and are referred to here simply as epoetin. **Darbopoietin**, a hyperglycosylated form of epoetin, has a longer half-life and can be administered less frequently.

The clinical use of epoetin is given in the box below.

Pharmacokinetic aspects

Epoetin and darbopoietin can be given intravenously or subcutaneously, the response being greatest after subcutaneous injection and fastest after intravenous injection.

small number of self-renewing, pluripotent stem cells laid down during embryogenesis. Maintenance of haemopoiesis necessitates a balance between self-renewal on the one hand, and differentiation into the various types of blood cell on the other. The factors involved in controlling this balance are the *haemopoietic growth factors*, which direct the division and maturation of the progeny of these cells down eight possible lines of development (Fig. 22.5). These cytokine growth factors are highly potent glycoproteins, acting at concentrations of 10^{-12}–10^{-10} mol/l. They are present in plasma at very low concentrations under basal conditions, but on stimulation their concentrations can increase within hours by 1000-fold or more. *Erythropoietin* regulates the red cell line, and the signal for its production is blood loss and/or low tissue oxygen tension. CSFs regulate the myeloid divisions of the white cell line, and the main stimulus for their production is infection (see also Ch. 13).

The genes for several haemopoietic factors have been cloned, and recombinant erythropoietin (**epoetin**), recombinant granulocyte CSF (**filgrastim, lenograstim**) and granulocyte–macrophage

Clinical uses of epoetin

- Anaemia of chronic *renal failure.*
- Anaemia during *chemotherapy* for cancer.
- Prevention of the anaemia that occurs in *premature infants.*
- To increase the yield of autologous blood before *blood donation.*
- Anaemia of *AIDS* (exacerbated by **zidovudine**).
- Anaemia of *chronic inflammatory conditions* such as rheumatoid arthritis (investigational).

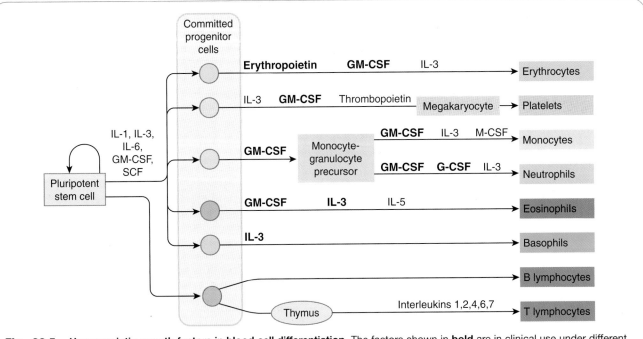

Fig. 22.5 **Haemopoietic growth factors in blood cell differentiation.** The factors shown in **bold** are in clinical use under different names (see text). Most T cells generated in the thymus die by apoptosis; those that emerge are either CD4 or CD8 T cells. The colours used for the mature blood cells reflect how they appear in common staining preparations (and after which some are named). CSF, colony-stimulating factor; G-CSF, granulocyte CSF; GM-CSF, granulocyte–macrophage CSF; IL-1, interleukin-1; IL-3, interleukin-3 or multi-CSF; M-CSF, macrophage CSF; SCF, stem cell factor. (See also Ch. 13.)

Unwanted effects

Transient influenza-like symptoms are common. Hypertension is also common and can cause encephalopathy with headache, disorientation and sometimes convulsions. Iron deficiency can be induced because more iron is required for the enhanced erythro-poiesis. Blood viscosity increases as the haematocrit (i.e. the fraction of the blood that is occupied by red blood cells) rises, increasing the risk of thrombosis, especially during dialysis. There have been rare reports of pure red cell aplasia, possibly connected with development of antibodies directed against erythropoietin.

COLONY-STIMULATING FACTORS

The CSFs are so-called because they stimulate the formation of maturing colonies of leucocytes in semisolid medium in vitro. CSFs are classified as cytokines (see Ch. 13). They not only stimulate particular committed progenitor cells to proliferate (Fig. 22.5) but also cause irreversible differentiation. The responding precursor cells have membrane receptors for specific CSFs and may express receptors for more than one factor, thus permitting collaborative interactions between factors.

Granulocyte CSF is produced mainly by monocytes, fibroblasts and endothelial cells, and controls primarily the development of neutrophils. Recombinant forms (**filgrastim**, which is not glycosylated, and glycosylated **lenograstim**) are used therapeutically. **Pegfilgrastim** is a derivative of filgrastim conjugated with polyethylene glycol (*pegylated*) with a prolonged duration of action.

Actions

Granulocyte CSF acts only on the neutrophil line (Fig. 22.5)—increasing the proliferation and maturation of neutrophils, stimulating their release from bone marrow storage pools and enhancing their function.

The clinical use of granulocyte CSFs is given in the box.

> **Clinical uses of the colony-stimulating factors**
>
> Colony-stimulating factors are used in specialist centres:
> - to reduce the severity/duration of neutropenia induced by cytotoxic drugs during:
>   - anticancer *chemotherapy*
>   - intensive chemotherapy necessitating autologous *bone marrow rescue*
>   - following *bone marrow transplant*.
> - to harvest *progenitor cells*.
> - to expand the number of harvested progenitor cells ex vivo before reinfusing them.
> - for persistent neutropenia in *advanced HIV infection*.
> - in *aplastic anaemia*.

Pharmacokinetic aspects and unwanted effects

Filgrastim and **lenograstim** are given either subcutaneously or by intravenous infusion. **Pegfilgrastim** is administered subcutaneously. Gastrointestinal effects, fever, bone pain, myalgia and rash are recognised adverse effects; less common effects include pulmonary infiltrates and enlargement of liver or spleen.

THROMBOPOIETIN

Thrombopoietin stimulates proliferation of the progenitor cells of the platelet lineage and strikingly increases platelet production. Recombinant thrombopoietin is being tested clinically.

REFERENCES AND FURTHER READING

General

Clarke R, Armitage J 2000 Vitamin supplements and cardiovascular risk: review of the randomized trials of homocysteine-lowering vitamin supplements. Semin Thromb Hemost 26: 341–348

Fishman S M, Christian P, West K P 2000 The role of vitamins in the prevention and control of anaemia. Public Health Nutr 3: 125–150

Goodenough L T, Monk T G, Andriole G L 1997 Erythropoietin therapy. N Engl J Med 336: 933–938

Hoelzer D 1997 Haemopoietic growth factors—not whether, but when and where. N Engl J Med 336: 1822–1824 (*Edifying editorial comment*)

Kurzrock R 2005 Thrombopoietic factors in chronic bone marrow failure states: the platelet problem revisited. Clin Cancer Res 11: 1361–1367 (*Slow progress*)

Levin J 1997 Thrombopoietin—clinically realised? N Engl J Med 336: 434–436 (*A useful editorial*)

Nimer S D 1997 Platelet stimulating agents—off the launch pad. Nat Med 3: 154–155 (*Thrombopoietic growth factors prove useful in clinical trials*)

Spivak J L 1993 Recombinant erythropoietin. Annu Rev Med 44: 243–253

Iron and iron deficiency

Andrews N C 1999 Disorders of iron metabolism N Engl J Med 341: 1986–1995

Finch C A, Hueber S H 1982 Perspectives in iron metabolism. N Engl J Med 306: 1520–1528 (*Good background article on iron*)

Frewin R, Henson A, Provan D 1997 ABC of clinical haematology: iron deficiency anaemia. Br Med J 314: 360–363

Hoffbrand A V, Herbert V 1999 Nutritional anemias. Semin Hematol 36(suppl 7): 13–23

Lieu P T, Heiskala M, Peterson P A, Yang Y 2001 The roles of iron in health and disease. Mol Aspects Med 22: 1–87

Provan D, Weatherall D 2000 Red cells II: acquired anaemias and polycythaemia. Lancet 355: 1260–1268

Toh B-H, van Driel I R, Gleeson P A 1997 Pernicious anaemia. N Engl J Med 337: 1441–1448 (*Immunopathogenesis of pernicious anaemia; excellent figures*)

Folic acid and vitamin B12 and their deficiencies

Botto L D et al. 2005 International retrospective cohort study of neural tube defects in relation to folic acid recommendations: are the recommendations working? Br Med J 330: 571–573 (*Not as well as might be hoped*)

Refsum H 2001 Folate, vitamin B_{12} and homocysteine in relation to birth defects and pregnancy outcome. Br J Nutr 85(suppl 2): S109–S113

Steinberg S E 1984 Mechanisms of folate homeostasis. Am J Physiol 246: G319–G324 (*Good background article on folate*)

Wald N J, Bower C 1994 Folic acid, pernicious anaemia, and prevention of neural tube defects. Lancet 343: 307

Colony-stimulating factors

Dale D C 1995 Where now for colony-stimulating factors? Lancet 346: 135–136

Lieschke G J, Burges A W 1992 Granulocyte colony-stimulating factor and granulocyte-macrophage colony-stimulating factor. N Engl J Med 327: 1–35, 99–106 (*Worthwhile, comprehensive reviews*)

Petros W P 1996 Colony-stimulating factors. In: Chabner B A, Longo D L (eds) Cancer chemotherapy and biotherapy, 2nd edn. Lippincott-Raven, Philadelphia, pp. 639–654 (*Covers mechanism of action, biological effects and clinical pharmacology*)

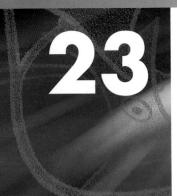

23

The respiratory system

OVERVIEW

In this chapter, we cover some basic aspects of the physiology of the respiratory system as a prelude to pulmonary diseases and drugs used in their treatment. We devote most of the chapter to asthma, dealing first with factors involved in its pathogenesis and then the main drugs used in its treatment—the bronchodilators and anti-inflammatory agents. We address chronic obstructive pulmonary disease (COPD). There are short sections on allergic emergencies, surfactants and the treatment of cough. Other important pulmonary diseases, such as bacterial infections (e.g. tuberculosis and acute pneumonias) and malignancies, are addressed in Chapters 46 and 51, respectively, or are not yet amenable to drug treatment (e.g. occupational and interstitial lung diseases). Antihistamines, important in treatment of hay fever, are covered in Chapter 13. Pulmonary hypertension is covered in Chapter 19.

THE REGULATION OF RESPIRATION

Respiration is controlled by spontaneous rhythmic discharges from the respiratory centre in the medulla, modulated by input from pontine and higher central nervous system (CNS) centres

and vagal afferents from the lungs. Various chemical factors affect the respiratory centre, including the partial pressure of carbon dioxide in arterial blood ($P_A\text{co}_2$) by an action on medullary chemoreceptors, and of oxygen ($P_A\text{o}_2$) by an action on the chemoreceptors in the carotid bodies.

Some voluntary control can be superimposed on the automatic regulation of breathing, implying connections between the cortex and the motor neurons innervating the muscles of respiration. Bulbar poliomyelitis and certain lesions in the brain stem result in loss of the automatic regulation of respiration without loss of voluntary regulation.[1]

REGULATION OF MUSCULATURE, BLOOD VESSELS AND GLANDS OF THE AIRWAYS

Efferent pathways controlling the airways include cholinergic parasympathetic nerves and non-noradrenergic non-cholinergic (NANC) inhibitory nerves. Inflammatory mediators (see Ch. 13) and NANC bronchoconstrictor mediators also have a role in diseased airways. The afferent pathways include three different types of sensory receptor, described below.

The tone of bronchial muscle influences the airways resistance, which is also affected by the state of the mucosa and activity of the glands in patients with asthma and bronchitis. Airway resistance can be measured indirectly by instruments that record the volume or flow of forced expiration. FEV_1 is the forced expiratory volume in 1 second. The peak expiratory flow rate (PEFR) is the maximal flow (expressed as l/min) after a full inhalation; this is simpler to measure at the bedside than FEV_1, which it follows closely.

EFFERENT PATHWAYS

Autonomic innervation
The autonomic innervation of human airways is reviewed by van der Velden & Hulsmann (1999).

Parasympathetic innervation. Parasympathetic innervation of bronchial smooth muscle predominates. Parasympathetic ganglia are embedded in the walls of the bronchi and bronchioles, and the

---

[1]Referred to as Ondine's curse. Ondine was a water nymph who fell in love with a mortal. When he was unfaithful to her, the king of the water nymphs put a curse on him—that he must stay awake in order to breathe. When exhaustion finally supervened and he fell asleep, he died.

postganglionic fibres innervate airway smooth muscle, vascular smooth muscle and glands. Three types of muscarinic (M) receptors are present (see Ch. 10, Table 10.2). M_3 receptors are pharmacologically the most important. They are found on bronchial smooth muscle and glands, and mediate bronchoconstriction and mucus secretion. M_1 receptors are localised in ganglia and on postsynaptic cells, and facilitate nicotinic neurotransmission, whereas M_2 receptors are inhibitory *autoreceptors* mediating negative feedback on acetylcholine release by postganglionic cholinergic nerves. Stimulation of the vagus causes bronchoconstriction—mainly in the larger airways. The possible clinical relevance of the heterogeneity of muscarinic receptors in the airways is discussed below (on p. 363).

Sympathetic innervation. Sympathetic nerves innervate tracheobronchial blood vessels and glands, but not human airway smooth muscle. β-Adrenoceptors are, however, abundantly expressed on human airway smooth muscle (as well as mast cells, epithelium, glands and alveoli) and β agonists relax bronchial smooth muscle, inhibit mediator release from mast cells, and increase mucociliary clearance (see below). In humans, virtually all the β-adrenoceptors in the airways are of the $β_2$ variety.

Non-noradrenergic non-cholinergic nerves. Inhibitory NANC nerves, releasing *vasoactive intestinal peptide* (Ch. 9, Table 9.2) and *nitric oxide* (*NO*; Ch. 17, p. 270), are important neural bronchodilator pathways in human airways. *Excitatory* NANC nerves are also present in human airways. In animal models, they cause an inflammatory response consisting of bronchoconstriction, mucus secretion, increased vascular permeability, cough and vasodilatation. Neuropeptides released from excitatory NANC nerves initiate this *neurogenic inflammation* (see p. 222) and influence the recruitment, proliferation and activation of inflammatory cells that can, in turn, modulate neuronal function. The main excitatory neuropeptides in the lung are the tachykinins *substance P* and *neurokinin A*—see Chapter 41, p. 596.

SENSORY RECEPTORS AND AFFERENT PATHWAYS

Slowly adapting stretch receptors control respiration via the respiratory centre. Unmyelinated sensory C fibres and rapidly adapting irritant receptors associated with myelinated vagal fibres are also important.

Physical or chemical stimuli, acting on irritant receptors on myelinated fibres in the upper airways and/or C-fibre receptors in the lower airways, cause coughing, bronchoconstriction and mucus secretion. Such stimuli include cold air and irritants such as ammonia, sulfur dioxide, cigarette smoke and the experimental tool *capsaicin* (Ch. 41, p. 593), as well as endogenous inflammatory mediators.

PULMONARY DISEASE AND ITS TREATMENT

Common symptoms of pulmonary disease include shortness of breath, wheeze, chest pain, and cough with or without sputum production or haemoptysis—blood in the sputum. Ideally, treatment

> ### Regulation of airway muscle, blood vessels and glands
>
> **Afferent pathways**
> - Irritant receptors and C fibres respond to exogenous chemicals, inflammatory mediators and physical stimuli (e.g. cold air).
>
> **Efferent pathways**
> - Parasympathetic nerves cause bronchoconstriction and mucus secretion through M_3 receptors.
> - Sympathetic nerves innervate blood vessels and glands, but not airway smooth muscle.
> - $β_2$-adrenoceptor agonists relax airway smooth muscle. This is pharmacologically important.
> - Inhibitory non-noradrenergic non-cholinergic (NANC) nerves relax airway smooth muscle by releasing nitric oxide and vasoactive intestinal peptide.
> - Excitatory NANC nerves cause neuroinflammation by releasing tachykinins: substance P and neurokinin A.

is of the underlying disease, but sometimes symptomatic treatment, for example of cough, is all that is possible. The lung is an important target organ of many diseases addressed elsewhere in this book, including infections (Chs 46–50), malignancy (Ch. 51), and occupational and rheumatological diseases; drugs (e.g. **amiodarone**, p. 290; **methotrexate**, p. 241) can adversely affect the pulmonary interstitium. Heart failure leads to pulmonary oedema (Ch. 19). Thromboembolic disease (Ch. 21) and pulmonary hypertension (Ch. 19) affect the pulmonary circulation. In this present chapter, we concentrate on two important diseases of the airways: asthma and COPD.

BRONCHIAL ASTHMA

Asthma is the commonest chronic disease in children in economically developed countries, and is also common in adults. It is increasing in prevalence and severity. It is an inflammatory condition in which there is recurrent reversible airways obstruction in response to irritant stimuli that are too weak to affect non-asthmatic subjects. The obstruction usually causes wheeze and merits drug treatment, although the natural history of asthma includes spontaneous remissions.[2] Reversibility of airways obstruction in asthma contrasts with COPD, where the obstruction is either not reversible or at best incompletely reversible, by bronchodilators.

---

[2]William Osler, 19th century doyen of American and British clinicians, wrote that 'the asthmatic pants into old age'—this at a time when the most effective drug that he could offer was to smoke stramonium cigarettes, a herbal remedy the antimuscarinic effects of which were offset by direct irritation from the smoke.

CHARACTERISTICS OF ASTHMA

Asthmatic patients experience intermittent attacks of wheezing, shortness of breath—with difficulty especially in breathing *out*, and sometimes cough. As explained above, acute attacks are reversible, but the underlying pathological disorder can progress in older patients to a chronic state superficially resembling COPD.

Acute severe asthma (also known as *status asthmaticus*) is not easily reversed and causes hypoxaemia. Hospitalisation is necessary, as the condition, which can be fatal, requires prompt and energetic treatment.

Asthma is characterised by:

- inflammation of the airways
- bronchial hyper-reactivity
- reversible airways obstruction.

The term *bronchial hyper-reactivity* (or *hyper-responsiveness*) refers to abnormal sensitivity to a wide range of stimuli, such as irritant chemicals, cold air, and stimulant drugs, all of which can result in bronchoconstriction. In allergic asthma, these features may be initiated by sensitisation to allergen(s), but once established asthma attacks can be triggered by various stimuli such as viral infection, exercise (in which the stimulus may be cold air and/or drying of the airways), and atmospheric pollutants such as sulfur dioxide. Immunological desensitisation to allergens such as pollen or dust mites is popular in some countries but is not superior to conventional inhaled drug treatment.

The pathogenesis of asthma involves both genetic and environmental factors, and the asthmatic attack itself consists, in many subjects, of two main phases: an immediate and a late (or delayed) phase (see Fig. 23.1).

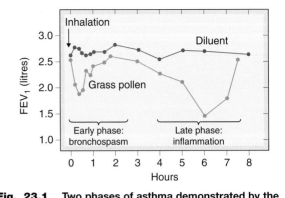

Fig. 23.1 **Two phases of asthma demonstrated by the changes in forced expiratory volume in 1 second (FEV₁) after inhalation of grass pollen in an allergic subject.** (From Cockcroft D W 1983 Lancet ii: 253.)

Numerous cells and mediators play a part in the pathogenesis of asthma, and the full details of the complex events involved are still a matter of debate (Walter & Holtzman, 2005). The following simplified account is intended to provide a basis for understanding the rational use of drugs in the treatment of asthma.

PATHOGENESIS OF ASTHMA

Asthmatics have activated T cells, with a Th2 profile of cytokine production (see Ch. 13 and Fig. 13.3), in their bronchial mucosa. How these cells are activated is not fully understood, but allergens (Fig. 23.2) are one mechanism. The Th2 cytokines that are released do the following.

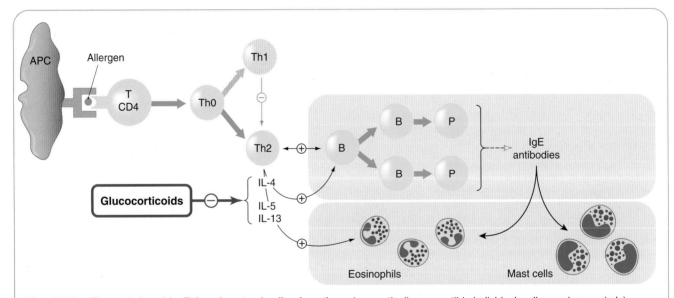

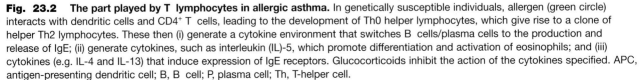

Fig. 23.2 **The part played by T lymphocytes in allergic asthma.** In genetically susceptible individuals, allergen (green circle) interacts with dendritic cells and CD4⁺ T cells, leading to the development of Th0 helper lymphocytes, which give rise to a clone of helper Th2 lymphocytes. These then (i) generate a cytokine environment that switches B cells/plasma cells to the production and release of IgE; (ii) generate cytokines, such as interleukin (IL)-5, which promote differentiation and activation of eosinophils; and (iii) cytokines (e.g. IL-4 and IL-13) that induce expression of IgE receptors. Glucocorticoids inhibit the action of the cytokines specified. APC, antigen-presenting dendritic cell; B, B cell; P, plasma cell; Th, T-helper cell.

Asthma

- Asthma is defined as recurrent reversible airway obstruction, with attacks of wheeze, shortness of breath and often nocturnal cough. Severe attacks cause hypoxaemia and are life-threatening.
- Essential features include:
  — airways inflammation, which causes
  — bronchial hyper-responsiveness, which in turn results in
  — recurrent reversible airway obstruction.
- Pathogenesis involves exposure of genetically disposed individuals to allergens; activation of Th2 lymphocytes and cytokine generation promote:
  — differentiation and activation of eosinophils
  — IgE production and release
  — expression of IgE receptors on mast cells and eosinophils.
- Important mediators include leukotriene B_4 and cysteinyl leukotrienes (C_4 and D_4); interleukins IL-4, IL-5, IL-13; and tissue-damaging eosinophil proteins.
- Antiasthmatic drugs include:
  — bronchodilators
  — anti-inflammatory agents.
- Treatment is monitored by measuring forced expiratory volume in 1 second (**FEV₁**) or peak expiratory flow rate and, in acute severe disease, oxygen saturation and arterial blood gases.

- Attract other inflammatory granulocytes, especially eosinophils, to the mucosal surface. Interleukin (IL)-5 and granulocyte–macrophage colony-stimulating factor prime eosinophils to produce cysteinyl leukotrienes, and to release granule proteins that damage the epithelium. This damage is one cause of bronchial hyper-responsiveness.
- Promote IgE synthesis and responsiveness in some asthmatics (IL-4 and IL-13 'switch' B cells to IgE synthesis and cause expression of IgE receptors on mast cells and eosinophils; they also enhance adhesion of eosinophils to endothelium).

Some asthmatics, in addition to these mechanisms, are also *atopic*—i.e. they make allergen-specific IgE that binds to mast cells in the airways. Inhaled allergen cross-links IgE molecules on mast cells, triggering degranulation with release of histamine and leukotriene B₄, both of which are powerful bronchoconstrictors to which asthmatics are especially sensitive because of their airways hyper-responsiveness. This provides a mechanism for acute exacerbation of asthma in atopic individuals exposed to allergen. The effectiveness of **omalizumab** (an anti-IgE antibody; see below, p. 364) serves to emphasise the importance of IgE in the pathogenesis of asthma as well as in other allergic diseases. Noxious gases (e.g. sulfur dioxide, ozone) and airway dehydration can also cause mast cell degranulation.

Clinicians often refer to atopic or 'extrinsic' asthma and non-atopic or 'intrinsic' asthma; we prefer the terms *allergic* and *non-allergic*.

The immediate phase of the asthmatic attack

In allergic asthma, the immediate phase (i.e. the initial response to allergen provocation) occurs abruptly and is mainly caused by spasm of the bronchial smooth muscle. Allergen interaction with mast cell–fixed IgE causes release of several spasmogens: histamine, leukotriene B₄ (Ch. 13) and prostaglandin (PG) D₂.

Other mediators released include IL-4, IL-5, IL-13, macrophage inflammatory protein-1α and tumour necrosis factor (TNF)-α.

Various chemotaxins and chemokines (see Ch. 13) attract leucocytes—particularly eosinophils and mononuclear cells—into the area, setting the stage for the delayed phase (Fig. 23.3).

The late phase

The late phase or delayed response (see Figs 23.1 and 23.3) may be nocturnal. It is, in essence, a progressing inflammatory reaction, initiation of which occurred during the first phase, the influx of Th2 lymphocytes being of particular importance. The inflammatory cells include activated eosinophils. These release cysteinyl leukotrienes; interleukins IL-3, IL-5 and IL-8; and the toxic proteins, eosinophil cationic protein, major basic protein and eosinophil-derived neurotoxin. These play an important part in the events of the late phase, the toxic proteins causing damage and loss of epithelium (see for example Larche et al., 2003; Kay, 2005). Other putative mediators of the inflammatory process in the delayed phase are adenosine (acting on the A_1 receptor; see Ch. 12), induced NO (see Ch. 17) and the neuropeptides (see Chs 13 and 16).

Growth factors released from inflammatory cells act on smooth muscle cells, causing hypertrophy and hyperplasia, and the smooth muscle can itself release proinflammatory mediators and autocrine growth factors (Chs 5 and 13). Figure 23.4 shows schematically the changes that take place in the bronchioles. Epithelial cell loss means that irritant receptors and C fibres are more accessible to irritant stimuli—an important mechanism of bronchial hyper-reactivity.

'Aspirin-sensitive' asthma

Non-steroidal anti-inflammatory drugs (NSAIDs), especially **aspirin**, can precipitate asthma in sensitive individuals. Such *aspirin-sensitive asthma* is relatively uncommon (< 10% of asthmatic subjects), and is often associated with nasal polyps. Individuals sensitive to one NSAID are usually also sensitive to other chemically unrelated cyclo-oxygenase (COX) inhibitors, including sometimes **paracetamol**, but not highly selective COX-2 inhibitors (Ch. 14, pp. 236-237). Abnormal *leukotriene* (Ch. 13) production and sensitivity are implicated. Patients with aspirin-sensitive asthma produce more *cysteinyl leukotriene* and have greater airway hyper-responsiveness to inhaled cysteinyl leukotrienes than aspirin-tolerant asthmatics. Such airway hyper-responsiveness reflects elevated expression of cysteinyl leukotriene receptors on inflammatory cells, and this is down-regulated by aspirin desensitisation (Sousa et al., 2002). In addition, aspirin and similar drugs directly activate eosinophils

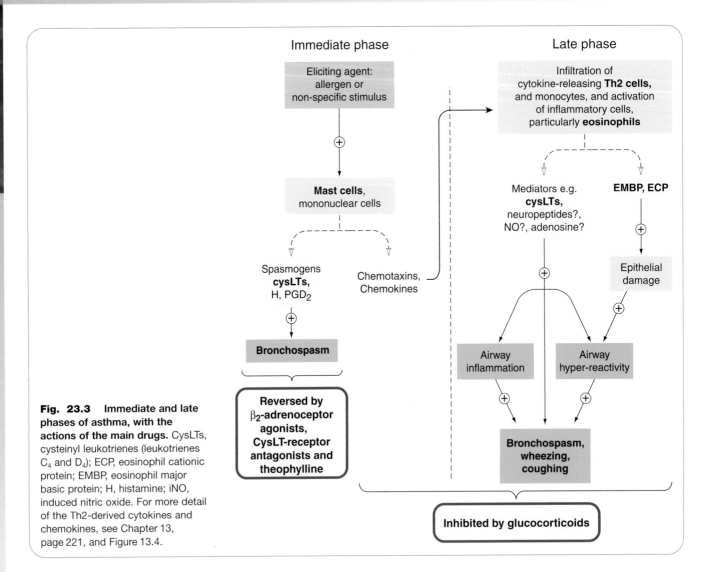

Fig. 23.3 **Immediate and late phases of asthma, with the actions of the main drugs.** CysLTs, cysteinyl leukotrienes (leukotrienes C_4 and D_4); ECP, eosinophil cationic protein; EMBP, eosinophil major basic protein; H, histamine; iNO, induced nitric oxide. For more detail of the Th2-derived cytokines and chemokines, see Chapter 13, page 221, and Figure 13.4.

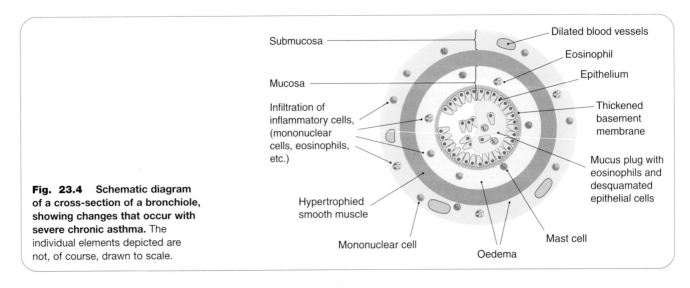

Fig. 23.4 **Schematic diagram of a cross-section of a bronchiole, showing changes that occur with severe chronic asthma.** The individual elements depicted are not, of course, drawn to scale.

and mast cells in these patients through IgE-independent mechanisms.

DRUGS USED TO TREAT ASTHMA

There are two categories of antiasthma drugs: *bronchodilators* and *anti-inflammatory agents*. Bronchodilators reverse the bronchospasm of the immediate phase; anti-inflammatory agents inhibit or prevent the inflammatory components of both phases (Fig. 23.3). These two categories are not mutually exclusive: some drugs classified as bronchodilators also have some anti-inflammatory effect.

How best to use these drugs to treat asthma is complex. A guideline (see British Thoracic Society, updated in 2004) specifies five therapeutic steps for adults and children with chronic asthma. Very mild disease may be controlled with short-acting bronchodilator alone (step 1), but if patients need this more than once a day a regular inhaled corticosteroid should be added (step 2). If the asthma remains uncontrolled, the next step is to add a long-acting bronchodilator (**salmeterol** or **formoterol**); this minimises the need for increased doses of inhaled corticosteroid (step 3). **Theophylline** and *leukotriene antagonists*, such as **montelukast**, also exert a corticosteroid-sparing effect, but this is less reliable. One or other is added in for patients with more severe asthma who remain symptomatic and/or the dose of inhaled corticosteroid increased to the maximum recommended (step 4). If the patient's condition is still poorly controlled, it may be necessary to add a regular oral corticosteroid (e.g. **prednisolone**)—step 5. *Corticosteroids* are the mainstay of therapy because they are the only asthma drugs that potently inhibit T-cell activation, and thus the inflammatory response, in the asthmatic airways. **Cromoglicate** (see below) has only a weak effect and is now seldom used.

BRONCHODILATORS

The main drugs used as bronchodilators are β_2-*adrenoceptor agonists*; others include xanthines, cysteinyl leukotriene receptor antagonists and muscarinic receptor antagonists.

β-Adrenoceptor agonists

The β_2-adrenoceptor agonists are dealt with in detail in Chapter 11. Their primary effect in asthma is to dilate the bronchi by a direct action on the β_2 adrenoceptors on the smooth muscle. Being physiological antagonists of bronchoconstrictors (see Ch. 2, p. 17), they relax bronchial muscle whatever the spasmogens involved. They also inhibit mediator release from mast cells and TNF-α release from monocytes, and increase mucus clearance by an action on cilia.

The β_2-adrenoceptor agonists are usually given by inhalation of aerosol, powder or nebulised solution, but some may be given orally or by injection. A metered-dose inhaler is used for aerosol preparations.

Two categories of β_2-adrenoceptor agonists are used in asthma.

- Short-acting agents: **salbutamol** and **terbutaline**. These are given by inhalation; the maximum effect occurs within 30 minutes and the duration of action is 3–5 hours; they are usually used on an 'as needed' basis to control symptoms.

> **Antiasthma drugs: bronchodilators**
>
> - β_2-Adrenoceptor agonists (e.g. **salbutamol**) are first-line drugs (for details, see Ch. 11).
>   - They act as physiological antagonists of the spasmogenic mediators but have little or no effect on the bronchial hyper-reactivity.
>   - Salbutamol is given by inhalation; its effects start immediately and last 3–5 hours, and it can also be given by intravenous infusion in status asthmaticus.
>   - **Salmeterol** or **formoterol** are given regularly by inhalation; their duration of action is 8–12 hours.
> - **Theophylline** (often formulated as **aminophylline**) is a third-line drug for asthma. Theophylline:
>   - is a methylxanthine
>   - inhibits phosphodiesterase and blocks adenosine receptors
>   - has a narrow therapeutic window: unwanted effects include cardiac dysrhythmia, seizures and gastrointestinal disturbances
>   - is given intravenously (by *slow* infusion) for status asthmaticus, or orally (as a sustained-release preparation) as add-on therapy to inhaled corticosteroids and long-acting β_2 agonists (step 4)
>   - is metabolised in the liver by P450; liver dysfunction and viral infections increase its plasma concentration and half-life (normally approximately 12 hours)
>   - interacts importantly with other drugs; some (e.g. some antibiotics) increase the half-life of theophylline, others (e.g. anticonvulsants) decrease it.
> - Cysteinyl leukotriene receptor antagonists (e.g. **montelukast**) are third-line drugs for asthma. They:
>   - competitively antagonise cysteinyl leukotrienes at CysLT$_1$ receptors
>   - are used mainly as add-on therapy to inhaled corticosteroids and long-acting β_2 agonists (step 4).

- Longer-acting agents: e.g. **salmeterol** and **formoterol**. These are given by inhalation, and the duration of action is 8–12 hours. They are not used 'as needed' but are given regularly, twice daily, as adjunctive therapy in patients whose asthma is inadequately controlled by glucocorticoids.

Unwanted effects

The unwanted effects of β_2-adrenoceptor agonists result from systemic absorption and are given in Chapter 11. In the context of their use in asthma, the commonest adverse effect is *tremor*, other unwanted effects including tachycardia and cardiac dysrhythmia.

Clinical uses

Clinical uses are summarised in the clinical box.

Clinical use of β₂-adrenoceptor agonists as bronchodilators

- Short-acting drugs (**salbutamol** or **terbutaline**, usually by inhalation) to prevent or treat wheeze in patients with reversible obstructive airways disease.
- Long-acting drugs (**salmeterol, formoterol**) to prevent bronchospasm (e.g. at night or with exercise) in patients requiring long-term bronchodilator therapy.

Xanthine drugs

There are three pharmacologically active, naturally occurring methylxanthines: *theophylline*, *theobromine* and *caffeine* (see also Ch. 19, p. 307, and Ch. 42). **Theophylline** (1,3-dimethylxanthine), which is also used as theophylline ethylenediamine (known as **aminophylline**), is the main therapeutic drug of this class. Theophylline has a bronchodilator action, although it is more likely to cause side effects (tachycardia, agitation, seizures) than the β₂-adrenoceptor agonists and has a less favourable risk:benefit ratio.

Actions

Antiasthmatic. Methylxanthines have long been used as bronchodilators.[3]

Central nervous system. Methylxanthines stimulate the CNS, increasing alertness (see Ch. 42). They can cause tremor and nervousness, and can interfere with sleep and have a stimulant action on respiration. This may be useful in patients with COPD and reduced respiration evidenced by a tendency to retain CO_2 (see below).

Cardiovascular. Methylxanthines stimulate the heart (see Ch. 18), having positive chronotropic and inotropic actions, while relaxing vascular smooth muscle (Ch. 19). They cause generalised vasodilatation but constrict cerebral blood vessels.

Kidney. Methylxanthines are weak diuretics, although this effect is not therapeutically useful.

Mechanisms of action

The ways in which the xanthine drugs produce effects in asthma are still unclear.

The relaxant effect on smooth muscle has been attributed to inhibition of the phosphodiesterase (PDE) isoenzymes, with resultant increase in cAMP and/or cGMP (see Fig. 4.10, p. 67). However, the concentrations necessary to inhibit the isolated enzymes exceed the therapeutic range of plasma concentrations.

Competitive antagonism of *adenosine* at adenosine A₁ and A₂ receptors (Ch. 12) may contribute, but the PDE inhibitor **enprofylline**, which is a potent bronchodilator, is not an adenosine antagonist.

Type IV PDE is implicated in inflammatory cells (see below), and non-specific methylxanthines may have some anti-inflammatory effect. (**Roflumilast**, a type IV PDE inhibitor, is mentioned below in the context of COPD.)

Unwanted effects

When theophylline is used in asthma, its other effects (CNS, cardiovascular, gastrointestinal and diuretic) are unwanted side effects. Furthermore, the therapeutic plasma concentration range is 30–100 µmol/l, and adverse effects are common with concentrations greater than 110 µmol/l; thus, there is a relatively narrow therapeutic window. Measurements of its concentration in plasma are useful for optimising dosage of aminophylline. Serious cardiovascular and CNS effects can occur when the plasma concentration exceeds 200 µmol/l. The most serious cardiovascular effect is dysrhythmia, which can be fatal. Seizures can occur with theophylline concentrations at or slightly above the upper limit of the therapeutic range, and can be fatal in patients with impaired respiration due to severe asthma.

Pharmacokinetic aspects

Methylxanthines are given orally in sustained-release preparations. Aminophylline can also be given by *slow* intravenous injection of a loading dose followed by intravenous infusion.

Theophylline is well absorbed from the gastrointestinal tract. It is metabolised by the P450 system in the liver, and the elimination half-life is about 8 hours in adults but varies widely in different subjects.

The half-life of theophylline is increased in liver disease, cardiac failure and viral infections, and is decreased in heavy cigarette smokers and drinkers (as a result of enzyme induction). Theophylline is influenced by many unwanted drug interactions: its plasma concentration is decreased by drugs that induce P450 enzymes (including **rifampicin**, **phenobarbital**, **phenytoin** and **carbamazepine**—see Chs 46 and 40, also Ch. 8, p. 116, and Ch. 52, p. 747, for more on induction of microsomal enzymes). The concentration is increased by drugs that inhibit P450 enzymes, such as **erythromycin**, **clarithromycin**, **ciprofloxacin**, **diltiazem** and **fluconazole** (see Chs 46, 19 and 48, also Ch. 52, p. 747, for more on enzyme inhibition). This is important in view of the narrow therapeutic window; antibiotics such as clarithromycin are often started when asthmatics are hospitalised because of a severe attack precipitated by a chest infection, and if the dose of theophylline is unaltered severe toxicity can result.

The clinical use of theophylline is summarised in the box.

Muscarinic receptor antagonists

Muscarinic receptor antagonists are dealt with in detail in Chapter 10. The main compound used as a bronchodilator is **ipratropium**. **Tiotropium** is also available; it is a longer-acting

Clinical use of theophylline

- As a second-line drug, in addition to steroids, in patients whose *asthma* does not respond adequately to β₂-adrenoceptor agonists.
- Intravenously (as **aminophylline,** a combination of theophylline with ethylenediamine to increase its solubility in water) in *acute severe asthma.*

---

[3]Over 200 years ago, William Withering recommended 'coffee made very strong' as a remedy for asthma.

drug used in maintenance treatment of COPD (see below). Ipratropium is seldom used on a regular basis in asthma but can be useful for cough caused by irritant stimuli in such patients.

Ipratropium is a quaternary derivative of *N*-isopropylatropine. It does not discriminate between muscarinic receptor subtypes (see Ch. 10), and it is possible that its blockade of M_2 autoreceptors on the cholinergic nerves increases acetylcholine release and reduces the effectiveness of its antagonism at the M_3 receptors on the smooth muscle. It is not particularly effective against allergen challenge, but it inhibits the augmentation of mucus secretion that occurs in asthma and may increase the mucociliary clearance of bronchial secretions. It has no effect on the late inflammatory phase of asthma.

It is given by aerosol inhalation. As a quaternary nitrogen compound, it is highly polar and is not well absorbed into the circulation (Ch. 7, p. 99), and thus does not have much action at muscarinic receptors other than those in the bronchi. The maximum effect occurs after approximately 30 minutes and persists for 3–5 hours. It has few unwanted effects and is, in general, safe and well tolerated. It can be used with β_2-adrenoceptor agonists. See the clinical box for clinical uses.

Cysteinyl leukotriene receptor antagonists

All the cysteinyl leukotrienes (LTC_4, LTD_4 and LTE_4) act on the same high-affinity cysteinyl leukotriene receptor termed *CysLT₁* (see Chs 13 and 14). Two receptors have been cloned, $CysLT_1$ and $CysLT_2$, and both are expressed in respiratory mucosa and infiltrating inflammatory cells, but the functional significance of each is unclear. The 'lukast' drugs (**montelukast** and **zafirlukast**) antagonise only $CysLT_1$.

Pharmacological actions

Lukasts reduce acute reactions to aspirin in sensitive patients, but have not been shown to be particularly effective for aspirin-sensitive asthma (see above, p. 359) in the clinic. They inhibit exercise-induced asthma and decrease both early and late responses to inhaled allergen. They relax the airways in mild asthma but are less effective than salbutamol. Their action is additive with β_2-adrenoceptor agonists. They also reduce sputum eosinophilia, but so far there is no clear evidence that they modify the underlying inflammatory process in chronic asthma.

Clinical use of inhaled muscarinic receptor antagonists (e.g. ipratropium)

- For *asthma,* as an adjunct to β_2-adrenoceptor agonists and steroids.
- For some patients with *chronic obstructive pulmonary disease,* especially long-acting drugs (e.g. **tiotropium**).
- For bronchospasm precipitated by β_2-adrenoceptor antagonists.
- For clinical uses of muscarinic receptor antagonists in other organ systems see clinical box in Chapter 10 (p. 156).

Unwanted effects

These are few, consisting mainly of headache and gastrointestinal disturbances. They have, rarely, been associated with the emergence of Churg–Strauss syndrome,[4] but the consensus is that this is because of withdrawal of concomitant corticosteroid therapy that had masked this disease.

Pharmacokinetic aspects

Both drugs are given orally, **montelukast** once daily, **zafirlukast** twice.

Clinical use

They are used in combination with an inhaled corticosteroid, usually at step 3, when regular long-acting β_2 agonists are inadequately effective.

Histamine H₁-receptor antagonists

Although mast cell mediators play a part in the immediate phase of allergic asthma (Fig. 23.3) and in some types of exercise-induced asthma, histamine H_1-receptor antagonists have no routine place in therapy, although they may be modestly effective in mild atopic asthma, especially when this is precipitated by acute histamine release in patients with concomitant allergy such as severe hay fever.

ANTI-INFLAMMATORY AGENTS

The main drugs used for their anti-inflammatory action in asthma are the **glucocorticoids**.

Glucocorticoids

Glucocorticoids are dealt with in detail in Chapter 28. They are not bronchodilators, but prevent the progression of chronic asthma and are effective in acute severe asthma (see below).[5]

Actions and mechanism

The basis of the anti-inflammatory action of glucocorticoids is discussed on page 428. An important action, of relevance for asthma, is that they decrease formation of cytokines (Fig. 13.3), in particular the Th2 cytokines that recruit and activate eosinophils and are responsible for promoting the production of IgE and the expression of IgE receptors (p. 358 and Ch. 13). Glucocorticoids also inhibit the generation of the vasodilators PGE_2 and PGI_2, by inhibiting induction of COX-2 (Fig. 13.5). By inducing *annexin 1*[6] (p. 428), they could inhibit production of leukotrienes and platelet-activating factor, although there is currently no direct evidence that the release of this protein is involved in the antiasthma effects of glucocorticoids.

---

[4]This uncommon but severe syndrome is characterised by systemic vasculitis, eosinophilia, and a history of asthma, sinusitis and rhinitis.

[5]In 1900, Solis-Cohen reported that dried bovine adrenals had antiasthma activity. He noted that the extract did not serve acutely 'to cut short the paroxysm' but was 'useful in averting recurrence of paroxysms'. Mistaken for the first report on the effect of adrenaline, his astute observation was probably the first on the efficacy of steroids in asthma.

[6]Previously known as *lipocortin-1*—the nomenclature was changed in order to comply with the latest genomics data, which indicate there are approximately 30 members of this family!

Corticosteroids inhibit the allergen-induced influx of eosinophils into the lung. Glucocorticoids up-regulate β_2 adrenoceptors, decrease microvascular permeability, and indirectly reduce mediator release from eosinophils by inhibiting the production of cytokines (e.g. IL-5 and granulocyte–macrophage colony-stimulating factor) that activate eosinophils. Reduced synthesis of IL-3 (the cytokine that regulates mast cell production) may explain why long-term steroid treatment eventually reduces the number of mast cells in the respiratory mucosa, and hence suppresses the early-phase response to allergens and exercise.

Glucocorticoid resistance. Glucocorticoids are sometimes ineffective, even in high doses, for reasons that are incompletely understood (see for example review by Adcock & Ito, 2004). Many individual mechanisms could contribute to this. The phenomenon has been linked to the number of glucocorticoid receptors, but in some situations other mechanisms are clearly in play—for example reduced activity of histone deacetylase (HDAC) may be important in cigarette smokers (see below, p. 365).

The main compounds used are **beclometasone**, **budesonide**, **fluticasone**, **mometasone** and **ciclesonide**. These are given by inhalation with a metered-dose or dry powder inhaler, the full effect on bronchial hyper-responsiveness being attained only after weeks or months of therapy.

Unwanted effects

Serious unwanted effects are uncommon with *inhaled* steroids. Oropharyngeal candidiasis (thrush; Ch. 48) can occur (T lymphocytes are important in protection against fungal infection), as can sore throat and croaky voice, but use of 'spacing' devices, which decrease oropharyngeal deposition of the drug and increase airway deposition, reduces these problems. Regular high doses can produce some adrenal suppression, particularly in children, and necessitate carrying a 'steroid card' (Ch. 28). This is less likely with **fluticasone**, **mometasone** and **ciclesonide**, as these drugs are poorly absorbed from the gastrointestinal tract and undergo almost complete presystemic metabolism. The unwanted effects of oral glucocorticoids are given in Chapter 28, page 433 and Figure 28.7.

Cromoglicate and nedocromil

These drugs are now hardly used for the treatment of asthma. Although very safe, they have only weak anti-inflammatory effects and short duration of action. They can be used topically for allergic conjunctivitis or rhinitis. They are not bronchodilators, having no direct effects on smooth muscle, nor do they inhibit the actions of any of the known smooth muscle stimulants. Given prophylactically, they reduce both the immediate and late-phase asthmatic responses and reduce bronchial hyper-reactivity.

Mechanism

Their mechanism of action is not fully understood. Cromoglicate is a 'mast cell stabiliser', preventing histamine release from mast cells. However, this is not the basis of its action in asthma, because compounds have been produced that are more potent than cromoglicate at inhibiting mast cell histamine release but are ineffective against asthma.

Cromoglicate depresses the exaggerated neuronal reflexes that are triggered by stimulation of the 'irritant receptors'; it suppresses

---

> **Clinical use of glucocorticoids in asthma**
>
> - Patients who require regular bronchodilators should be considered for glucocorticoid treatment (e.g. with inhaled **beclometasone**).
> - More severely affected patients are treated with high-potency inhaled drugs (e.g. **budesonide**).
> - Patients with acute exacerbations of asthma may require intravenous **hydocortisone** and oral **prednisolone**.
> - A 'rescue course' of oral **prednisolone** may be needed at any stage of severity if the clinical condition is deteriorating rapidly.
> - Prolonged treatment with oral prednisolone, in addition to inhaled bronchodilators and steroids, is needed by a few severely asthmatic patients.

---

the response of sensory C fibres to capsaicin and may inhibit the release of T-cell cytokines. Various other effects on the inflammatory cells and mediators involved in asthma have been described.

Anti-IgE treatment

Omalizumab is a humanised monoclonal anti-IgE antibody. It is effective in patients with allergic asthma as well as in allergic rhinitis. It is of considerable theoretical interest (see above, p. 359, and review by Holgate et al., 2005), but it is very expensive and its place in therapeutics is still unclear.

SEVERE ACUTE ASTHMA (STATUS ASTHMATICUS)

Severe acute asthma is a medical emergency requiring hospitalisation. Treatment includes **oxygen** (in high concentration, usually $\geq 60\%$), inhalation of **salbutamol** given by nebuliser, and intravenous **hydrocortisone** followed by a course of oral **prednisolone**. Additional measures occasionally used include nebulised **ipratropium**, intravenous **salbutamol** or **aminophylline**, and antibiotics (if bacterial infection is present). Monitoring is by PEFR or FEV_1, and by measurement of arterial blood gases and oxygen saturation. Oxygen saturation can be measured continuously and non-invasively by means of an oximeter clipped over a finger.

ALLERGIC EMERGENCIES

Anaphylaxis (Ch. 19) and *angio-oedema* are emergencies involving acute airways obstruction; **adrenaline** (**epinephrine**) is potentially life-saving. It is administered intramuscularly (or occasionally intravenously, as in anaphylaxis occurring in association with general anaesthesia). Patients at risk of acute anaphylaxis, for example from food or insect sting allergy, may self-administer intramuscular adrenaline using a spring-loaded syringe. Oxygen, an antihistamine such as **chlorphenamine**, and **hydrocortisone** are also indicated.

Angio-oedema is the intermittent occurrence of focal swelling of the skin or intra-abdominal organs caused by plasma leakage

Antiasthma drugs: anti-inflammatory agents

Glucocorticoids (for details see Ch. 28)
- These reduce the inflammatory component in chronic asthma and are life-saving in status asthmaticus (acute severe asthma).
- They do not prevent the immediate response to allergen or other challenges.
- The mechanism of action involves decreased formation of cytokines, particularly those generated by Th2 lymphocytes (see key points box on p. 359), decreased activation of eosinophils and other inflammatory cells.
- They are given by inhalation (e.g. **beclometasone**); systemic unwanted effects are uncommon at moderate doses, but oral thrush and voice problems can occur. Systemic effects can occur with high doses but are less likely with **mometasone** because of its presystemic metabolism. In deteriorating asthma, an oral glucocorticoid (e.g. **prednisolone**) or intravenous **hydrocortisone** is also given.

from capillaries. Most often, it is mild and 'idiopathic', but it can occur as part of acute allergic reactions, when it is generally accompanied by urticaria—'hives'—caused by histamine release from mast cells. If the larynx is involved, it is life-threatening; swelling in the peritoneal cavity can be very painful and mimic a surgical emergency. It can be caused by drugs, especially *angiotensin-converting enzyme inhibitors*—perhaps because they block the inactivation of peptides such as bradykinin (Ch. 19)—and by **aspirin** and related drugs in patients who are aspirin-sensitive (see above, p. 359, and Ch. 14, p. 233). The hereditary form is associated with lack of C1 esterase inhibitor—C1 esterase is an enzyme that degrades the complement component C1 (see Ch. 13, Fig. 13.1). **Tranexamic acid** (Ch. 21, p. 345) or **danazol** (Ch. 30, p. 453) may be used to prevent attacks in patients with *hereditary angioneurotic oedema*, and administration of C1 esterase inhibitor or fresh plasma can terminate acute attacks.

CHRONIC OBSTRUCTIVE PULMONARY DISEASE

Chronic obstructive pulmonary disease is a major global health problem. Cigarette smoking is the main cause, and is increasing in the developing world as a result of targeting by the tobacco industry. Air pollution, also aetiologically important, is also increasing, and there is a huge unmet need for effective drugs. Despite this, COPD has received relatively little attention compared with asthma.

Clinical features. The clinical picture starts with attacks of morning cough during the winter, and progresses to chronic cough with intermittent exacerbations, often initiated by a cold, when the sputum becomes purulent ('chronic bronchitis'). There is progressive breathlessness. Some patients have a reversible component of airflow obstruction identifiable by an improved FEV_1 following a dose of bronchodilator. Pulmonary hypertension

(Ch. 19) is a late complication, causing symptoms of heart failure (*cor pulmonale*). Exacerbations may be complicated by type 1 or type 2 respiratory failure (i.e. reduced $P_{A_{O_2}}$ alone or with increased $P_{A_{CO_2}}$, respectively) requiring hospitalisation and intensive care. Tracheostomy and artificial ventilation, while prolonging survival, may serve only to return the patient to a miserable life.

Pathogenesis. There is small airways fibrosis, resulting in obstruction, and/or destruction of alveoli and of elastin fibres in the lung parenchyma. The latter features are hallmarks of emphysema,[7] thought to be caused by proteases, including elastase, released during the inflammatory response. Small airways obstruction and emphysema vary independently of one another. The explanation for this variation is unknown. It is emphysema that causes respiratory failure, because it destroys the alveoli, impairing gas transfer. There is chronic inflammation, predominantly in small airways and lung parenchyma, characterised by increased numbers of macrophages, neutrophils, and T lymphocytes. The inflammatory mediators have not been as clearly defined as in asthma. Lipid mediators, inflammatory peptides, reactive oxygen and nitrogen species, chemokines, cytokines and growth factors are all implicated (Barnes, 2004).

Principles of treatment. Stopping smoking (Ch. 43) slows the progress of COPD. Patients should be immunised against influenza and *Pneumococcus*, because superimposed infections with these organisms are potentially lethal. Glucocorticoids are generally ineffective, in contrast to asthma, but a trial of glucocorticoid treatment is worthwhile because asthma may coexist with COPD and have been overlooked. This contrast with asthma is puzzling, because in both diseases multiple inflammatory genes are activated, which might be expected to be turned off by glucocorticoids. Inflammatory gene activation results from acetylation of nuclear histones around which DNA is wound. Acetylation opens up the chromatin structure, allowing gene transcription and synthesis of inflammatory proteins to proceed. HDAC is a key molecule in suppressing production of proinflammatory cytokines. Corticosteroids recruit HDAC to activated genes, reversing acetylation and switching off inflammatory gene transcription (Barnes et al., 2004). There is a link between the severity of COPD (but not of asthma) and reduced HDAC activity in lung tissue (Ito et al., 2005); furthermore, HDAC activity is inhibited by smoking-related oxidative stress, which may explain the lack of effectiveness of glucocorticoids in COPD.

Long-acting bronchodilators have been a worthwhile if modest advance in the treatment of COPD, but do not deal with the underlying inflammation. No currently licensed treatments reduce the progression of COPD or suppress the inflammation in small airways and lung parenchyma. Several new treatments that target the inflammatory process are in clinical development (Barnes & Stockley, 2005). Some, such as chemokine antagonists, are directed against the influx of inflammatory cells into the airways and lung parenchyma, whereas others target inflammatory cytokines such as TNF-α. PDE IV inhibitors (e.g. **roflumilast**; Rabe et al., 2005)

---

[7]Emphysema is a pathological condition sometimes associated with COPD, in which lung parenchyma is destroyed and replaced by air spaces that coalesce to form *bullae*—blister-like air-filled spaces in the lung tissue.

show some promise. Other drugs that inhibit cell signalling (see Chs 3 and 5) include inhibitors of p38 mitogen-activated protein kinase, nuclear factor κB and phosphoinositide-3 kinase-γ. More specific approaches are to give antioxidants, inhibitors of inducible NO synthase and leukotriene B_4 antagonists. Other treatments have the potential to combat mucus hypersecretion, and there is a search for serine proteinase and matrix metalloproteinase inhibitors to prevent lung destruction and the development of emphysema.

Specific aspects of treatment. Short- and long-acting inhaled bronchodilators can provide useful palliation in patients with a reversible component. The main short-acting drugs are **ipratropium** (see p. 363) and **salbutamol** (p. 361); long-acting drugs include **tiotropium** (p. 362) and **salmeterol** or **formoterol** (p. 361). **Theophylline** (p. 362) can be given by mouth but is of uncertain benefit. Its respiratory stimulant effect may be useful for patients who tend to retain CO_2. Other respiratory stimulants (e.g. **doxapram;** see Ch. 42) are sometimes used briefly in acute respiratory failure (e.g. postoperatively) but have largely been replaced by ventilatory support (intermittent positive-pressure ventilation).

Long-term **oxygen** therapy administered at home prolongs life in patients with severe disease and hypoxaemia (at least if they refrain from smoking—an oxygen fire is not a pleasant way to go, especially for one's neighbours!).

Acute exacerbations. Acute exacerbations of COPD are treated with *inhaled O_2* in a concentration (initially, at least) of only 24% O_2, i.e. only just above atmospheric O_2 concentration (approximately 20%). The need for caution is because of the risk of precipitating CO_2 retention as a consequence of terminating the hypoxic drive to respiration. Blood gases and tissue oxygen saturation are monitored, and inspired O_2 subsequently adjusted accordingly. Broad-spectrum *antibiotics* (e.g. **cefuroxime**; Ch. 46) including activity against *Haemophilus influenzae* are used if there is evidence of infection. Inhaled bronchodilators may provide some symptomatic improvement.

A systemically active glucocorticoid (intravenous **hydrocortisone** or oral **prednisolone**) is also administered routinely, although efficacy is modest. Inhaled steroids do not influence the progressive decline in lung function in patients with COPD, but do improve the quality of life, probably as a result of a modest reduction in hospital admissions.

SURFACTANTS

Pulmonary surfactants are not true drugs in Ehrlich's sense (Ch. 2, p. 8), acting as a result of their physicochemical properties within the airways rather than by binding to specific receptors. They are effective in the prophylaxis and management of respiratory distress syndrome in newborn babies, especially if premature. Examples include **beractant** and **poractant alpha**, which are derivatives of the physiologically produced pulmonary surfactant protein that is important in preventing collapse of the alveoli. They are administered directly into the tracheobronchial tree via the endotracheal tube. (The mothers of premature infants are sometimes treated with *glucocorticoids* before birth in an attempt to accelerate maturation of the fetal lung and minimise incidence of this disorder.)

COUGH

Cough is a protective reflex that removes foreign material and secretions from the bronchi and bronchioles. It is a very common adverse effect of *angiotensin-converting enzyme inhibitors*, in which case the treatment is usually to substitute an alternative drug, notably an angiotensin receptor antagonist, less likely to cause this adverse effect (Ch. 19, p. 309). It can be triggered by inflammation in the respiratory tract, for example by undiagnosed asthma or chronic reflux with aspiration, or by neoplasia. In these cases, cough suppressant (*antitussant*) drugs are sometimes useful, for example for the dry painful cough associated with bronchial carcinoma, where opioids are invaluable. Antitussive drugs are to be avoided in cases of chronic pulmonary infection, as they can cause undesirable thickening and retention of sputum, and in asthma because of the risk of respiratory depression.

DRUGS USED FOR COUGH

Antitussive drugs act by an ill-defined effect in the brain stem, depressing an even more poorly defined 'cough centre'. All opioid *narcotic analgesics* (see Ch. 41) have antitussive actions in doses below those required for pain relief. Those used as cough suppressants are members of the group with minimal analgesic actions and addictive properties. New opioid analogues that suppress cough by inhibiting release of excitatory neuropeptides through an action on μ receptors (see Table 41.1) on sensory nerves in the bronchi are being assessed.

Codeine (methylmorphine) is a weak opioid (see Ch. 41) with considerably less addiction liability than the main opioids, and is a mild cough suppressant. It decreases secretions in the bronchioles, which thickens sputum, and inhibits ciliary activity. Constipation is common (see Chs 25 and 41). **Dextromethorphan** and **pholcodine** are believed to have fewer adverse effects.

REFERENCES AND FURTHER READING

Background material

Erb K J 1999 Atopic disorders: a default pathway in the absence of infection. Immunol Today 20: 317–322 (*Discusses the hypothesis that the decline of infectious diseases in the developed world could account for an increase in atopic disorders, stressing the role of the Th1-type immune response to infection in*

inhibiting the development of atopy; useful diagrams)

Kirstein S L, Insel P A 2004 Autonomic nervous system pharmacogenomics: a progress report. Pharmacol Rev 56: 31–52 (*Reviews recent ideas regarding pharmacogenomics of components of the autonomic nervous system*)

Small K M, McGraw D W, Liggett S B 2003 Pharmacology and physiology of human adrenergic receptor polymorphisms. Annu Rev Pharmacol Toxicol 43: 381–411 (*Reviews the consequences of adrenergic receptor polymorphisms in terms of signalling, human physiology and disease, and response to therapy*)

Stephens N L 2001 Airway smooth muscle. Lung 179: 333–373

Van der Velden V H J, Hulsmann A R 1999 Autonomic innervation of human airways: structure, function, and pathophysiology in asthma. Neuroimmunomodulation 6: 145–159 (*Review*)

Asthma

Adcock I M, Ito K 2004 Steroid resistance in asthma: a major problem requiring novel solutions or a non-issue? Curr Opin Pharmacol 4: 257–262 (*'Once issues of diagnosis, compliance and psychological disorder have been resolved, true steroid resistance is unlikely to be an issue for most clinicians, who will rarely, if ever, see these patients. However, management of those few patients with true steroid resistance will require novel therapies.'*)

Berry M et al. 2005 Alveolar nitric oxide in adults with asthma: evidence of distal lung inflammation in refractory asthma. Eur Respir J 25: 986–991 (*Alveolar NO as a measure of distal airway inflammation*)

British Thoracic Society 2004 British guideline on management of asthma 2004 update. http://www.brit-thoracic.org.uk

Chatila T A 2004 Interleukin-4 receptor signaling pathways in asthma pathogenesis. Trends Mol Med 10: 493–499

Cormican L J, Farooque S, Altmann D R et al. 2005 Improvements in an oral aspirin challenge protocol for the diagnosis of aspirin hypersensitivity. Clin Exp Allergy 35: 717–722

Corry D B 2002 Emerging immune targets for the therapy of asthma. Nat Rev Drug Discov 1: 55–64 (*Reviews the pathophysiology of asthma and discusses potential immune targets. Excellent diagrams. Annotated references.*)

Gale E A M 2002 The role of mast cells in the pathophysiology of asthma. N Engl J Med 346: 1742–1743 (*Stresses the role of smooth muscle in the pathophysiology of asthma and discusses the inter-relationship of mast cells and smooth muscle*)

Kay A B 2005 The role of eosinophils in the pathogenesis of asthma. Trends Mol Med 11: 148–152 (*The eosinophil is firmly back on the asthma stage, strengthening the case for developing effective eosinophil-depleting agents*)

Kleeberger S R, Peden D 2005 Gene–environment interactions in asthma and other respiratory diseases. Annu Rev Med 56: 383–400

Larche M, Robinson D S, Kay A B 2003 The role of T lymphocytes in the pathogenesis of asthma. J Allergy Clin Immunol 111: 450–463 (*Several Th2 cytokines have the potential to modulate airway inflammation, particularly IL-13, which induces airway hyper-responsiveness independently of IgE and eosinophilia in animal models*)

Lucaks N W 2001 Role of chemokines in the pathogenesis of asthma. Nat Rev Immunol 1: 108–116 (*Excellent coverage of the chemokines involved in asthma, with detailed table of chemokines and good diagrams*)

Luster A D, Tager A M 2004 T-cell trafficking in asthma: lipid mediators grease the way. Nat Rev Immunol 4: 711–724

Pelaia G et al. 2005 Mitogen-activated protein kinases and asthma. J Cell Physiol 202: 642–653 (*Reviews involvement of mitogen-activated protein kinases in asthma pathogenesis, and discusses their possible role as molecular targets for antiasthma drugs*)

Persson C G A 1997 Centennial notions of asthma as an eosinophilic, desquamative, exudative, and steroid-sensitive disease. Lancet 349: 1021–1024 (*A review of astute early observations of the pathogenesis of asthma that foreshadowed modern understanding of the disease*)

Spina D, Page CP 2002 Asthma: time for a rethink. Trends Pharmacol Sci 23: 311–315 (*Discusses the role of alterations in the function of the afferent nerves to the airways in bronchial hyper-responsiveness*)

Walter M J, Holtzman M J 2005 A centennial history of research on asthma pathogenesis. Am J Respir Cell Mol Biol 32: 483–489

Wills-Karp M 2004 Interleukin-13 in asthma pathogenesis. Immunol Rev 202: 175–190

Chronic obstructive pulmonary disease

Barnes P J 2004 Mediators of chronic obstructive pulmonary disease. Pharmacol Rev 56: 515–548 (*'The identification of inflammatory mediators and understanding their interactions is important for the development of anti-inflammatory treatments for this important disease.'*)

Barnes P J, Ito K, Adcock I M 2004 Corticosteroid resistance in chronic obstructive pulmonary disease: inactivation of histone deacetylase. Lancet 363: 731–733 (*Hypothesis that in patients with COPD, HDAC is impaired by cigarette smoking and oxidative stress, leading to reduced responsiveness to corticosteroids; see also Ito et al., 2005, below*)

Barnes P J, Stockley R A 2005 COPD: current therapeutic interventions and future approaches. Eur Respir J 25: 1084–1106 (*Long-acting bronchodilators have been an important advance for COPD but do not deal with the underlying inflammatory process. No currently available treatments reduce the progression of COPD. New approaches, for example chemokine antagonists, PDE IV inhibitors, inhibitors of p38 mitogen-activated protein kinase, nuclear factor-κB and phosphoinositide-3 kinase-γ, are reviewed.*)

Ito K et al. 2005 Decreased histone deacetylase activity in chronic obstructive pulmonary disease. N Engl J Med 352: 1967–1976 (*There is a link between the severity of COPD and the reduction in HDAC activity in the peripheral lung tissue; HDAC is a key molecule in the repression of production of proinflammatory cytokines in alveolar macrophages*)

Puchelle E, Vargaftig B B 2001 Chronic obstructive pulmonary disease: an old disease with novel concepts and drug strategies. Trends Pharmacol Sci 22: 495–498 (*Report of meeting on chronic lung disease*)

Cough

Morice A H, Kastelik J A, Thompson R 2001 Cough challenge in the assessment of cough reflex. Br J Clin Pharmacol 52: 365–375

Reynolds S M, Mackenzie A J, Spina D, Page C P 2004 The pharmacology of cough. Trends Pharmacol Sci 25: 569–576 (*Discusses the pathophysiological mechanisms of cough and implications for developing new antitussive drugs*)

Drugs and therapeutic aspects

Barnes P J 2004 New drugs for asthma. Nat Rev Drug Discov 3: 831–844

Barnes P J, Hansel T T 2004 Prospects for new drugs for chronic obstructive pulmonary disease. Lancet 364: 985–996

Beavo J A 2006 Phosphodiesterases: isoforms and selective inhibition. Annu Rev Pharmacol Toxicol 46 (in press)

Ben-Noun L 2000 Drug-induced respiratory disorders: incidence, prevention and management. Drug Saf 23: 143–164 (*Diverse pulmonary adverse drug effects*)

Chrystyn H 2001 Methods to identify drug deposition in the lungs following inhalation. Br J Clin Pharmacol 51: 289–299

Giri S N 2003 Novel pharmacological approaches to manage interstitial lung fibrosis in the twenty first century. Annu Rev Pharmacol Toxicol 43: 73–95 (*Reviews approaches including maintaining intracellular nicotinamide adenine dinucleotide [NAD$^+$] and ATP, blocking transforming growth factor-β and integrins, platelet-activating factor receptor antagonists and NO synthase inhibitors*)

Green R H, Pavord I D 2001 Leukotriene antagonists and symptom control in chronic persistent asthma. Lancet 357: 1991–1992 (*Editorial discussing briefly the significance of studies of leukotriene receptor antagonists for drug treatment of asthma*)

Holgate S T, Djukanovic R, Casale T, Bousquet J 2005 Anti-immunoglobulin E treatment with omalizumab in allergic diseases: an update on anti-inflammatory activity and clinical efficacy. Clin Exp Allergy 35: 408–416 (*Reviews mechanism and clinical studies*)

Leff A R 2001 Regulation of leukotrienes in the management of asthma: biology and clinical therapy. Annu Rev Med 52: 1–14 (*Discusses the role of leukotrienes in the pathogenesis of bronchoconstriction and the pharmacology of antagonists at the cysteinyl leukotriene receptor*)

Lewis J F, Veldhuizen R 2003 The role of exogenous surfactant in the treatment of acute lung injury. Annu Rev Physiol 65: 613–642

Rabe K F et al. 2005 Roflumilast—an oral anti-inflammatory treatment for chronic obstructive pulmonary disease: a randomized controlled trial. Lancet 366: 563–571 (*This type IV PDE inhibitor improved lung function and reduced exacerbations compared to placebo; the improvement was modest, and it remains to be proved that it relates to an anti-inflammatory rather than a bronchodilator action*)

Sears M R, Lotvall J 2005 Past, present and future—β$_2$-adrenoceptor agonists in asthma management. Respir Med 99: 152–170 (*'Tolerance to the bronchoprotective effects of long-acting β$_2$ agonists and cross-tolerance to the bronchodilator effects of short-acting β$_2$ agonists is apparent despite use of inhaled corticosteroids. The role of β$_2$ receptor polymorphisms in the development of tolerance has yet to be fully determined. Formoterol is unique in having both a long-lasting bronchodilator effect and a fast onset of action.'*)

Sousa A R, Parikh A, Scadding G et al. 2002 Leukotriene-receptor expression on nasal mucosal inflammatory cells in aspirin-sensitive rhinosinusitis. N Engl J Med 347: 1493–1499. (*Demonstrated elevated numbers of nasal inflammatory leucocytes expressing the CysLT$_1$ receptor in biopsy specimens from aspirin-sensitive patients with chronic rhinosinusitis as compared with non-aspirin-sensitive control subjects, and down-regulation of receptor expression after desensitisation to aspirin*)

Tattersfield A E, Harrison T W 2001 Exacerbations of asthma—still room for improvement. Lancet 358: 599–601 (*Editorial discussing optimal treatment of acute asthma*)

Walker C, Zuany-Amorim C 2001 New trends in immunotherapy to prevent atopic diseases. Trends Pharmacol Sci 22: 84–90 (*Possible development of new treatments for atopic diseases based on recent understanding of the role of Th2 cells and Th2 cytokines in allergy; very clear diagram*)

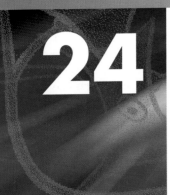

24 The kidney

OVERVIEW

The main drugs that work by altering renal function—the diuretics—are crucial for the management of cardiovascular disease (Chs 18 and 19). The kidneys are the main organ by which drugs and their metabolites are eliminated from the body (Ch. 8), and so when they fail dosing regimens of many drugs must be adapted. Furthermore, they are a target for various kinds of drug toxicity (Ch. 53). In the present chapter, we set the scene for describing drugs that affect renal function with a brief outline of renal physiology based on the functional unit of the kidney—the nephron. Subsequent emphasis is on diuretics—drugs that increase the excretion of Na⁺ ions and water. We also consider briefly other drugs that are used in treating renal failure and urinary tract disorders. Antihypertensive drugs (commonly indicated in kidney disease) are covered in Chapter 19, immunosuppressant drugs (effective in several of the diseases that can cause renal failure, and crucial for maintaining the health of patients who have received a kidney transplant) in Chapter 14, and antibacterial drugs (used to treat renal and urinary tract infections) in Chapter 46.

OUTLINE OF RENAL FUNCTION

The main function of the kidney is to maintain the constancy of the 'interior environment' by eliminating waste products and by regulating the volume, electrolyte content and pH of the extracellular fluid in the face of varying dietary intake and varying environmental (e.g. climatic) demands.

The kidneys receive about a quarter of the cardiac output. From the several hundred litres of plasma that flow through them each day, they filter (in a 70-kg human) approximately 120 litres per day, 11 times the total extracellular fluid volume. This filtrate is similar to plasma apart from the absence of protein. As it passes through the renal tubule, about 99% of the filtered water, and much of the filtered sodium ions, are reabsorbed, and some substances are secreted into it from the blood. Eventually, approximately 1.5 litres is voided as urine per 24 hours under usual conditions (Table 24.1).

Each kidney consists of an outer cortex, an inner medulla and a hollow pelvis, which empties into the ureter. The functional unit is the nephron, of which there are approximately 1.4×10^6 in each kidney (approximately half this number in people with hypertension: Keller et al., 2003), with considerable variation between individuals and an age-related decline.

THE STRUCTURE AND FUNCTION OF THE NEPHRON

Each nephron consists of a *glomerulus, proximal tubule*—comprising convoluted and straight segments, *loop of Henle, distal convoluted tubule* and *collecting duct*—Figure 24.1. The glomerulus comprises a tuft of capillaries projecting into a dilated end of the renal tubule. Most nephrons lie largely or entirely in the cortex. The remaining 12%, called the juxtamedullary nephrons, have their glomeruli and convoluted tubules next to the junction of the medulla and cortex, and their loops of Henle pass deep into the medulla. In juxtamedullary nephrons, part of the

Table 24.1 Reabsorption of fluid and solute in the kidney[a]

	Filtered/ day	Excreted/ day[b]	Percentage reabsorbed
Na⁺ (mmol)	25 000	150	99+
K⁺ (mmol)	600	90	93+
Cl⁻ (mmol)	18 000	150	99+
HCO₃⁻ (mmol)	4900	0	100
Total solute (mosmol)	54 000	700	87
H₂O (litres)	180	~1.5	99+

[a]Typical values for a healthy young adult: renal blood flow, 1200 ml/min (20–25% of cardiac output); renal plasma flow, 660 ml/min; glomerular filtration rate, 125 ml/min.
[b]These are typical figures for an individual eating a western diet. The kidney excretes more or less of each of these substances to maintain the constancy of the internal milieu, so on a low-sodium diet (for instance in the Yanomami Indians of the upper Amazon basin), NaCl excretion may be reduced to below 10 mmol/day! At the other extreme, individuals living in some fishing communities in Japan eat (and therefore excrete) several hundred mmol/day.

thick ascending limb of the loop of Henle (as well as the thin part of the loop) lies in the medulla; the part of the medulla containing the thick ascending limb is known as the outer stripe of the medulla, as opposed to the inner stripe, which contains thin segments only (the difference is visible to the naked eye).

THE BLOOD SUPPLY TO THE NEPHRON

Nephrons possess the special characteristic of having two capillary beds in series with each other (see Fig. 24.1). The afferent arteriole of each *cortical nephron* branches to form the glomerulus; glomerular capillaries coalesce into the efferent arteriole, which, in turn, branches to form a second capillary network in the cortex, around the convoluted tubules and loops of Henle, before converging on venules and thence on renal veins. By contrast, efferent arterioles of *juxtamedullary nephrons* lead to vessel loops that pass deep into the medulla with the thin loops of Henle. These loops are called *vasa recta* and play a key role in counter-current exchange (see p. 373).

THE JUXTAGLOMERULAR APPARATUS

A conjunction of afferent arteriole, efferent arteriole and distal convoluted tubule near the glomerulus forms the juxtaglomerular apparatus (Fig. 24.2). At this site, there are specialised cells in both the afferent arteriole and in the tubule. The latter, termed

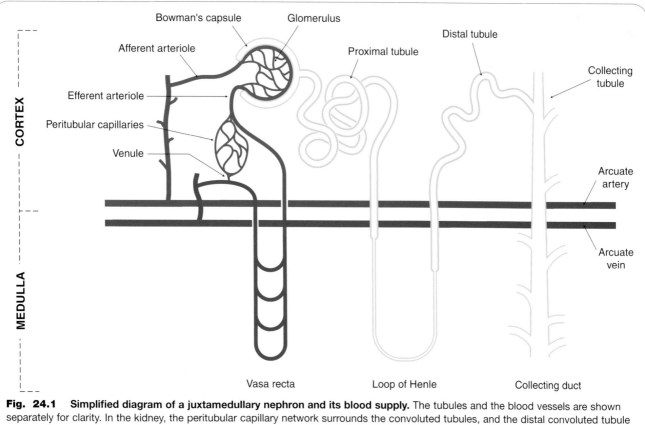

Fig. 24.1 **Simplified diagram of a juxtamedullary nephron and its blood supply.** The tubules and the blood vessels are shown separately for clarity. In the kidney, the peritubular capillary network surrounds the convoluted tubules, and the distal convoluted tubule passes close to the glomerulus, between the afferent and efferent arterioles. (This last is shown in more detail in Fig. 24.2.)

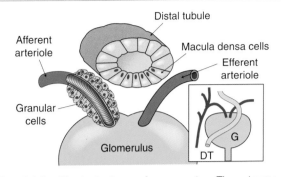
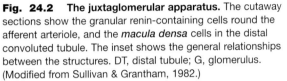

Fig. 24.2   The juxtaglomerular apparatus. The cutaway sections show the granular renin-containing cells round the afferent arteriole, and the *macula densa* cells in the distal convoluted tubule. The inset shows the general relationships between the structures. DT, distal tubule; G, glomerulus. (Modified from Sullivan & Grantham, 1982.)

macula densa cells, respond to changes in the rate of flow and the composition of tubule fluid, and they control renin release from the specialised granular renin-containing cells in the afferent arteriole (Ch. 19). Other mediators also influence renin secretion, including β_2 agonists, vasodilator *prostaglandins* and feedback inhibition from *angiotensin II* acting on AT_1 receptors (see Fig. 19.4). The role of the juxtaglomerular apparatus in the control of Na^+ balance is dealt with below, and its cardiovascular role is considered in Chapter 19.

GLOMERULAR FILTRATION

Fluid is driven from the capillaries into the tubular capsule (Bowman's capsule) by hydrodynamic force opposed by the oncotic pressure of the plasma proteins to which the glomerular capillaries are impermeable. All the low-molecular-weight constituents of plasma appear in the filtrate, while albumin and larger proteins are retained in the blood.

TUBULAR FUNCTION

The apex (lumenal surface) of each tubular cell is surrounded by a tight junction, as in all epithelia. This is a specialised region of membrane that separates the intercellular space from the lumen (see Figs 24.7–24.10, below). The movement of ions and water across the epithelium can occur *through* cells (the transcellular pathway) and *between* cells through the tight junctions (the paracellular pathway).

THE PROXIMAL CONVOLUTED TUBULE

The epithelium of the proximal convoluted tubule is 'leaky', i.e. the tight junctions in the proximal tubule are not so 'tight' after all, being permeable to ions and water, and permitting passive flow in either direction. This prevents the build-up of large concentration gradients; thus, although approximately 60–70% of Na^+ reabsorption occurs in the proximal tubule, this transfer is

accompanied by passive absorption of water so that fluid leaving the proximal tubule remains approximately isotonic to the filtrate entering Bowman's capsule.

Some of the transport processes in the proximal tubule are shown in Figures 24.3–24.5. The most important mechanism for Na^+ entry into proximal tubular cells from the filtrate occurs by Na^+/H^+ exchange (Fig. 24.5). Intracellular carbonic anhydrase is essential for production of H^+ for secretion into the lumen. Na^+ is reabsorbed in exchange for H^+, and transported out of the cells into the interstitium and thence into the blood by a Na^+/K^+ ATPase (sodium pump) in the basolateral membrane. This is the main active transport mechanism of the nephron in terms of energy consumption. Both Na^+/H^+ and Na^+/K^+ exchange are instances of *antiport* systems—that is, ones in which substances are exchanged with each other in opposite directions across a membrane, in distinction from *symporters*, where coupled transport takes place in the same direction (see below).

Bicarbonate is normally completely reabsorbed in the proximal tubule. This is achieved by combination with protons, yielding carbonic acid, which dissociates to form carbon dioxide and water—a reaction catalysed by carbonic anhydrase present in the lumenal brush border of the proximal tubule cells (Fig. 24.5)—followed by passive reabsorption of the dissolved carbon dioxide. The selective removal of sodium bicarbonate, with accompanying water, in the early proximal tubule causes a secondary rise in the concentration of chloride ions. Diffusion of chloride down its concentration gradient via the paracellular shunt leads, in turn, to a lumen positive potential difference that favours reabsorption of sodium. The other mechanism involved in movement via the paracellular route is that sodium ions are secreted by Na^+/K^+

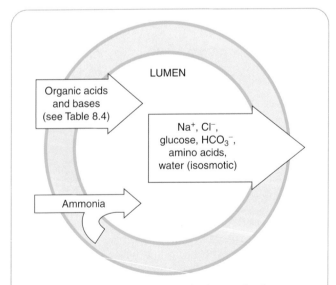

Fig. 24.3   Transport processes in the proximal convoluted tubule. The main driving force for the absorption of solutes and water from the lumen is the Na^+/K^+ ATPase in the basolateral membrane of the tubule cells. Many drugs are secreted into the proximal tubule (see Ch. 8). (Redrawn from Burg, 1985.)

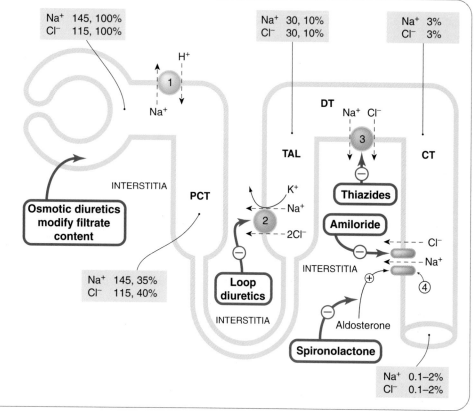

Fig. 24.4 **Schematic showing the absorption of sodium and chloride in the nephron and the main sites of action of drugs.** Cells are depicted as an orange border round the yellow tubular lumen. Mechanisms of ion absorption at the apical margin of the tubule cell: (1) Na^+/H^+ exchange; (2) $Na^+/K^+/2Cl^-$ cotransport; (3) Na^+/Cl^- cotransport, (4) Na^+ entry through sodium channels. Sodium is pumped out of the cells into the interstitium by the Na^+/K^+ ATPase in the basolateral margin of the tubular cells (not shown). The numbers in the boxes give the concentration of ions as millimoles per litre of filtrate, and the percentage of filtered ions still remaining in the tubular fluid at the sites specified. CT, collecting tubule; DT, distal tubule; PCT, proximal convoluted tubule; TAL, thick ascending loop. (Data from Greger, 2000.)

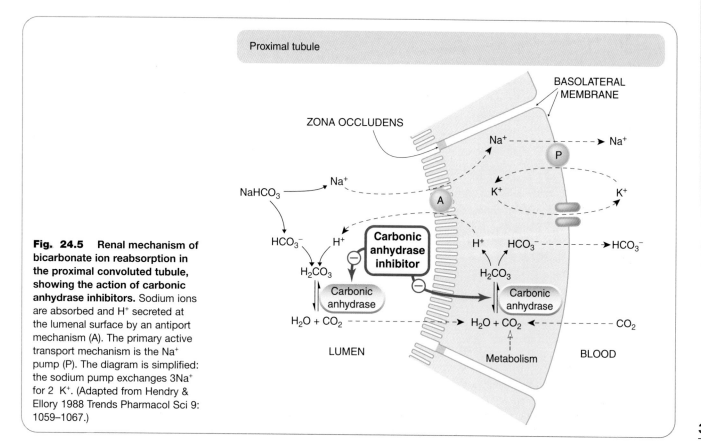

Fig. 24.5 **Renal mechanism of bicarbonate ion reabsorption in the proximal convoluted tubule, showing the action of carbonic anhydrase inhibitors.** Sodium ions are absorbed and H^+ secreted at the lumenal surface by an antiport mechanism (A). The primary active transport mechanism is the Na^+ pump (P). The diagram is simplified: the sodium pump exchanges $3Na^+$ for $2 K^+$. (Adapted from Hendry & Ellory 1988 Trends Pharmacol Sci 9: 1059–1067.)

ATPase into the lateral intercellular space, slightly raising its osmolality because of its 3:2 stoichiometry. This leads to osmotic movement of water across the tight junction, in turn causing sodium reabsorption by convection (solvent drag).

Many organic acids and bases are actively secreted into the tubule from the blood by specific transporters (see below, Fig. 24.3 and Ch. 8).

After passage through the proximal tubule, tubular fluid (now 30–40% of the original volume of the filtrate) passes on to the loop of Henle.

THE LOOP OF HENLE

The loop of Henle consists of a descending and an ascending portion (Figs 24.1 and 24.4), the ascending portion having both thick and thin segments. Up to 30% of filtered Na^+ is reabsorbed by this part of the nephron, which enables the kidney to excrete urine that is either more or less concentrated than plasma, and hence to regulate the osmotic balance of the body as a whole.

The *descending* limb is permeable to water, which exits passively because the interstitial fluid of the medulla is kept hypertonic by the counter-current concentrating system (p. 373). In juxtamedullary nephrons with long loops, there is extensive movement of water out of the tubule so that the fluid eventually reaching the tip of the loop has a high osmolality—normally approximately 1200 mosmol/kg, but up to 1500 mosmol/kg under conditions of dehydration—compared with plasma and extracellular fluid, which is approximately 300 mosmol/kg.[1] The hypertonic milieu of medulla, through which the collecting ducts of all nephrons pass on the way to the renal pelvis, is important in providing a mechanism by which the osmolarity of the urine is controlled (see below).

The *ascending* limb has very low permeability to water, i.e. the tight junctions really are 'tight', enabling the build-up of a substantial concentration gradient across the wall of the tubule. It is here, in the thick ascending limb of the loop of Henle, that 20–30% of filtered Na^+ is reabsorbed. There is active reabsorption of NaCl, unaccompanied by water, reducing the osmolarity of the tubular fluid and making the interstitial fluid of the medulla hypertonic. Ions move into the cell across the apical membrane by a $Na^+/K^+/2\ Cl^-$ symporter (see p. 370 above for the distinction between symport and antiport systems). The energy for this is derived from the electrochemical gradient for Na^+ produced by the Na^+/K^+ ATPase in the basolateral membrane. Chloride exits the cell into the circulation, partly by diffusion through chloride channels and partly by a symport mechanism with K^+. Most of the K^+ taken into the cell by the $Na^+/K^+/2Cl^-$ cotransporter returns to the lumen through apical potassium channels, but some K^+ is reabsorbed, along with Mg^{2+} and Ca^{2+}.

Reabsorption of salt from the thick ascending limb is not balanced by reabsorption of water, so tubular fluid is *hypotonic* with respect to plasma as it leaves the thick ascending limb and

enters the distal convoluted tubule (Fig. 24.4). The thick ascending limb is therefore sometimes referred to as the 'diluting segment'.

THE DISTAL TUBULE

In the early distal tubule, NaCl reabsorption, coupled with impermeability of the *zonula occludens* to water, further dilutes the tubular fluid. Transport is driven by Na^+/K^+ ATPase in the basolateral membrane. This lowers cytoplasmic Na^+ concentration, and consequently Na^+ enters the cell from the lumen down its concentration gradient, accompanied by Cl^-, by means of an electroneutral Na^+/Cl^- carrier (Fig. 24.8).

The excretion of Ca^{2+} is regulated in this part of the nephron, *parathormone* and *calcitriol* both increasing Ca^{2+} reabsorption (see Ch. 31).

THE COLLECTING TUBULE AND COLLECTING DUCT

Distal convoluted tubules empty into collecting tubules, which coalesce to form collecting ducts (Fig. 24.1). Collecting tubules include principal cells, which reabsorb Na^+ and secrete K^+, and two populations of intercalated cells, α and β, which secrete acid and base, respectively.

The tight junctions in this portion of the nephron are impermeable to water and ions. The movement of ions and water in this segment is under independent hormonal control: absorption of NaCl by *aldosterone* (Ch. 19), and absorption of water by *antidiuretic hormone (ADH)*, also termed *vasopressin* (Ch. 28).

Aldosterone enhances Na^+ reabsorption and promotes K^+ excretion. It promotes Na^+ reabsorption by:

- a rapid effect, stimulating Na^+/H^+ exchange by an action on *membrane* aldosterone receptors[2]
- a delayed effect, via nuclear receptors (see Chs 3 and 28), directing the synthesis of a specific protein mediator that activates sodium channels in the apical membrane
- long-term effects, by increasing the number of basolateral Na^+ pumps.

Antidiuretic hormone is secreted by the posterior pituitary (Ch. 28) and binds V_2 receptors in the *basolateral* membranes, increasing expression of *aquaporin* (water channels; see Ch. 7) in the *apical* membranes. This renders this part of the nephron permeable to water, allowing passive reabsorption of water as the collecting duct traverses the hyperosmotic region of the medulla, and hence the excretion of *concentrated urine*. Conversely, in the absence of ADH collecting duct epithelium is impermeable to water, so hypotonic fluid that leaves the distal tubule remains hypotonic as it passes down the collecting ducts, leading to the excretion of *dilute urine*.

Ethanol (see p. 629) inhibits the secretion of ADH, causing a water diuresis (possibly familiar to some of our readers) as a kind

---

[1]These figures are for humans; some other species, notably the desert rat, can do much better, with urine osmolalities up to 5000 mosmol/kg.

[2]A mechanism distinct from regulation of gene transcription, which is the normal transduction mechanism for steroid hormones (Chs 3 and 28).

of transient *diabetes insipidus*—a disorder in which patients excrete large volumes of dilute urine because of failure to secrete ADH (pp. 425–426). Several drugs inhibit the *action* of ADH: **lithium** (used in psychiatric disorders; see Ch. 38), **demeclocycline** (a tetracycline used not as an antibiotic—Chapter 46—but rather to treat conditions, such as some lung cancers, associated with inappropriate secretion of ADH), **colchicine** (Ch. 14) and *vinca alkaloids* (Ch. 51). All these drugs can cause acquired forms of *nephrogenic diabetes insipidus*—i.e. diabetes insipidus caused not by a failure to secrete ADH but by a failure of the renal collecting ducts to respond to its action. Nephrogenic diabetes insipidus can also be caused by two genetic disorders (mutations of the V_2 receptor in the rare X-linked variety, and mutations of aquaporin-2 in the even rarer autosomal recessive variety).

THE MEDULLARY COUNTER-CURRENT MULTIPLIER AND EXCHANGER

The loops of Henle of the juxtamedullary nephrons function as counter-current multipliers, and the vasa recta as counter-current exchangers. NaCl is actively reabsorbed in the thick ascending limb, causing hypertonicity of the interstitium. In the descending limb, water moves out and the tubular fluid becomes progressively more concentrated as it approaches the bend. The resulting osmotic gradient ranges from isotonicity (300 mosmol/l) at the cortical boundary to ≥ 1500 mosmol/l in the deepest part of the renal papilla. This gradient is the key consequence of the counter-current multiplier system, the main principle being that small horizontal osmotic gradients 'stack up' to produce a large vertical gradient. Urea contributes to the gradient because it is more slowly reabsorbed than water and may be added to fluid in the descending limb, so its concentration rises along the nephron until it reaches the collecting tubules, where it diffuses out into the interstitium. It is thus 'trapped' in the inner medulla.

The vertical osmotic gradient would be rapidly dissipated if solute in the medullary interstitium were carried away by brisk blood flow. This does not happen because the vasa recta function as passive *counter-current exchangers*: water effectively 'short-circuits' the deepest parts of the vasa recta by leaving these vessels as they descend into the medulla, re-entering them as they ascend and exit the medulla, and thus preserving the concentration gradient built up in the medullary interstitium by the active counter-current multiplier.

ACID–BASE BALANCE

The kidneys (together with the lungs; Ch. 23, p. 356) regulate the H^+ concentration of body fluids. Acid or alkaline urine can be excreted according to need, the usual requirement being to form acid urine to eliminate phosphoric and sulfuric acids generated during the metabolism of nucleic acids, and sulfur-containing amino acids consumed in the diet. Consequently, metabolic acidosis is a common accompaniment of renal failure. Carbonic anhydrase is essential for acid–base control both because of its lumenal and cellular roles in the proximal tubule (see above), and because intracellular carbonic anhydrase is essential for distal tubular urine acidification.

Renal tubular function

- Protein-free filtrate enters via Bowman's capsule.
- Na^+/K^+ ATPase in the basolateral membrane is the main *active* transporter. It provides the gradients for passive transporters in the apical membranes.
- 60–70% of the filtered Na^+ and > 90% of HCO_3 is absorbed in the proximal tubule.
- Carbonic anhydrase is key for $NaHCO_3$ reabsorption and distal tubular urine acidification.
- The thick ascending limb of Henle's loop is impermeable to water; 20–30% of the filtered NaCl is actively reabsorbed in this segment.
- Ions are reabsorbed from tubular fluid by a $Na^+/K^+/2\ Cl^-$ cotransporter in the apical membranes of the thick ascending limb.
- $Na^+/K^+/2\ Cl^-$ cotransport is inhibited by *loop diuretics*.
- Filtrate is diluted as it traverses the thick ascending limb as ions are reabsorbed, so that it is hypotonic when it leaves.
- The tubular counter-current multiplier actively generates a concentration gradient—small horizontal differences in solute concentration between tubular fluid and interstitium are multiplied vertically. The deeper in the medulla, the more concentrated is the interstitial fluid.
- Medullary hypertonicity is preserved passively by counter-current exchange in the vasa recta.
- Na^+/Cl^- cotransport (inhibited by thiazide diuretics) reabsorbs 5–10% of filtered Na^+ in the distal tubule.
- K^+ is secreted into tubular fluid in the distal tubule and the collecting tubules and collecting ducts.
- In the absence of antidiuretic hormone (ADH), collecting tubule and collecting duct have low permeability to salt and water. ADH increases water permeability.
- Na^+ is reabsorbed from collecting duct through epithelial sodium channels.
- These are stimulated by *aldosterone* and inhibited by **amiloride**. K^+ or H^+ is secreted into the tubule in exchange for Na^+ in this distal region.

POTASSIUM BALANCE

Extracellular K^+—critically important for excitable tissue function; see Chapter 4, page 63-64—is tightly controlled through regulation of K^+ excretion by the kidney. Urinary K^+ excretion matches dietary intake, usually approximately 50–100 mmol in 24 hours in western countries. Most diuretics cause K^+ loss (see below). This causes potentially important drug interactions (see Ch. 52, p. 746) if they are coadministered with *cardiac glycosides* or *class III antidysrhythmic drugs* (whose toxicity is increased by low plasma K^+; see Ch. 19).

Potassium ions are transported into collecting duct—and collecting tubule—cells from blood and interstitial fluid by Na^+/K^+ ATPase in the basolateral membrane, and leak into the lumen through a K^+-selective ion channel. Na^+ passes from tubular fluid through sodium channels in the apical membrane down the electrochemical gradient created by the Na^+/K^+ ATPase; a lumen-negative potential difference across the cell results, increasing the driving force for K^+ secretion into the lumen. Thus K^+ secretion is coupled to Na^+ reabsorption.

Consequently, K^+ is lost when:

- more Na^+ reaches the collecting duct, as occurs with any diuretic acting proximal to the collecting duct
- Na^+ reabsorption in the collecting duct is increased directly (e.g. in hyperaldosteronism).

K^+ is retained when:

- Na^+ reabsorption in the collecting duct is decreased, for example by **amiloride** or **triamterene**, which block the sodium channel in this part of the nephron, or **spironolactone** or **eplerenone**, which antagonise aldosterone (see p. 379).

EXCRETION OF ORGANIC MOLECULES

There are distinct mechanisms (see Ch. 8, Table 8.4) for secreting organic anions and cations into the proximal tubular lumen. Secreted anions include several important drugs, for example *thiazides*, **furosemide**, **salicylate** (Ch. 14), and most *penicillins* and *cephalosporins* (Ch. 46). Similarly, several secreted organic cations are important drugs, for example **triamterene**, **amiloride**, **atropine** (Ch. 10), **morphine** (Ch. 41) and **quinine** (Ch. 49). Both anion and cation transport mechanisms are, like other renal ion transport processes, indirectly powered by active transport of Na^+ and K^+, the energy being derived from Na^+/K^+ ATPase in the basolateral membrane.

Organic anions are exchanged with α-ketoglutarate by an antiport (see p. 370 above for an explanation of antiport/symport) in the basolateral membrane, and diffuse passively into the tubular lumen (Fig. 24.3).

Organic cations diffuse into the cell from the interstitium and are then actively transported into the tubular lumen in exchange for H^+.

NATRIURETIC PEPTIDES

Endogenous A, B and C natriuretic peptides (ANP, BNP and CNP; see Ch. 18, p. 285, and Ch. 19, p. 306) are involved in the regulation of Na^+ excretion. They are released from the heart in response to stretch (A and B), from endothelium (C) and from brain (B). They activate the particulate form of guanylate cyclase (Ch. 3, p. 29), and cause natriuresis both by renal haemodynamic effects (increasing glomerular capillary pressure by dilating afferent and constricting efferent arterioles) and by direct tubular actions. The tubular actions include the inhibition of angiotensin II–stimulated Na^+ and water reabsorption in the proximal convoluted tubule, and of the action of ADH in promoting water reabsorption in the collecting tubule.

Within the kidney, the post-translational processing of ANP prohormone differs from that in other tissues, resulting in an additional four amino acids being added to the amino terminus of ANP to yield a related peptide, *urodilatin*, that promotes Na^+ excretion by acting on receptors on the lumenal side of the collecting duct cells (Vesely, 2003).

PROSTAGLANDINS AND RENAL FUNCTION

Prostaglandins (see Ch. 13) generated in the kidney modulate its haemodynamic and excretory functions. The main renal prostaglandins in humans are vasodilator and natriuretic, namely prostaglandin (PG) E_2 in the medulla and PGI_2 (prostacyclin) in glomeruli. Factors that stimulate their synthesis include ischaemia, angiotensin II, ADH and bradykinin.

Influence on haemodynamics

Prostaglandin biosynthesis is low under basal conditions. However, when vasoconstrictors (e.g. angiotensin II, noradrenaline [norepinephrine]) are released, PGE_2 and PGI_2 modulate their effects on the kidney by causing compensatory vasodilatation.

Influence on the renal control of NaCl and water

The influence of renal prostaglandins on salt balance and haemodynamics can be inferred from the effects of drugs that inhibit prostaglandin synthesis. Non-steroidal anti-inflammatory drugs (NSAIDs, which inhibit prostaglandin production; see Ch. 14) have little or no effect on renal function in healthy people, but predictably cause acute renal failure in clinical conditions in which renal blood flow depends on vasodilator prostaglandin biosynthesis. These include *cirrhosis of the liver*, *heart failure*, *nephrotic syndrome*, *glomerulonephritis* and *extracellular volume contraction* (see Ch. 53, Table 53.1 and pp. 754–755). Volume contraction stimulates the renin–angiotensin–aldosterone system, and the rise in angiotensin II causes glomerular prostaglandin synthesis (see above) without which glomerular blood flow and glomerular filtration rate would be compromised due to the unopposed vasoconstrictor action of angiotensin II on the afferent and efferent arterioles. NSAIDs consequently cause renal failure in states of extracellular volume contraction (Cuzzolin et al., 2001). NSAIDs increase blood pressure in patients treated for *hypertension* by impairing vasodilatation and salt excretion. They exacerbate salt and water retention in patients with *heart failure* (see Ch. 19, pp. 313–314), partly by this same direct mechanism.[3]

---

[3]Additionally, NSAIDs make many of the diuretics used to treat heart failure less effective by competing with them for the weak acid secretory mechanism mentioned above; loop diuretics and thiazides act from within the lumen by inhibiting exchange mechanisms—see later in this chapter—so blocking their secretion into the lumen reduces their effectiveness by reducing their concentration at their site of action.

DRUGS ACTING ON THE KIDNEY

DIURETICS

Diuretics increase the excretion of Na$^+$ and water. They decrease the reabsorption of Na$^+$ and (usually) Cl$^-$ from the filtrate, increased water loss being secondary to the increased excretion of NaCl (*natriuresis*). This can be achieved by:

- a direct action on the cells of the nephron
- indirectly, by modifying the content of the filtrate.

Because a very large proportion of salt (NaCl) and water that passes into the tubule in the glomerulus is reabsorbed (Table 24.1), a small *decrease* in reabsorption can cause a marked *increase* in Na$^+$ excretion. A summary diagram of the mechanisms and sites of action of various diuretics is given in Figure 24.4.

Note that the diuretics that have a direct action on the cells of the nephron (with the exception of **spironolactone**) act from within the tubular lumen and reach their sites of action by being secreted into the proximal tubule.

DIURETICS ACTING DIRECTLY ON CELLS OF THE NEPHRON

Drugs that cause NaCl loss by an action on cells must obviously affect those parts of the nephron where solute reabsorption occurs. Most Na$^+$ absorption occurs in the proximal tubule (see above, p. 370), so it may seem surprising that *carbonic anhydrase inhibitors*—the only class of diuretic drugs that acts on the proximal tubule—are not particularly potent. This is because they inhibit NaHCO$_3$ rather than NaCl absorption, and HCO$_3^-$ normally has only approximately one-quarter the abundance of Cl$^-$ in the glomerular filtrate, and because of the important sodium-reabsorbing sites further down the nephron, which increase in activity in the face of mild volume contraction, attenuating the effect of diuretics acting proximal to them. Plasma HCO$_3^-$ concentration declines during chronic use of these drugs because of the increased urinary excretion of HCO$_3^-$ (see below), further limiting the diuretic potency of carbonic anhydrase inhibitors. Instead, the main therapeutically useful diuretics act on the:

- thick ascending loop of Henle
- early distal tubule
- collecting tubules and ducts.

For a more detailed review of the actions and clinical uses of the diuretics, see Greger et al. (2005).

Diuretics acting on the proximal tubule

Carbonic anhydrase inhibitors—for example **acetazolamide** (Fig. 24.5)—increase excretion of bicarbonate with accompanying Na$^+$, K$^+$ and water, resulting in an increased flow of an alkaline urine and metabolic acidosis. These agents, although not now used as diuretics, are still used in the treatment of glaucoma to reduce the formation of aqueous humour, and also in some unusual types of infantile epilepsy.

Urinary loss of bicarbonate depletes extracellular bicarbonate, and the diuretic effect of carbonic anhydrase inhibitors is consequently self-limiting.

Their mechanism of action is shown in Figure 24.5.

Loop diuretics

Loop diuretics are the most powerful diuretics, capable of causing the excretion of 15–25% of filtered Na$^+$ (see Fig. 24.6 for comparison with a thiazide). Their action is often described—in a phrase that conjures up a rather uncomfortable picture—as causing 'torrential urine flow'. The main example is **furosemide**; **bumetanide** is an alternative agent. These drugs act on the thick ascending limb, inhibiting the Na$^+$/K$^+$/2Cl$^-$ carrier in the lumenal membrane (see above and Figs 24.4 and 24.7) by combining with its Cl$^-$ binding site.

Loop diuretics also have incompletely understood vascular actions. Intravenous administration of furosemide to patients with pulmonary oedema caused by acute heart failure (see Ch. 19, p. 313) causes a therapeutically useful vasodilator effect before the onset of the diuretic effect. Possible mechanisms that have been invoked include decreased vascular responsiveness to vasoconstrictors such as angiotensin II and noradrenaline; increased formation of vasodilating prostaglandins (see above, p. 374); decreased production of the endogenous ouabain-like natriuretic hormone (Na$^+$/K$^+$ ATPase inhibitor; see Ch. 18, p. 291), which has vasoconstrictor properties; and potassium channel–opening effects in resistance arteries (see Greger et al., 2005).

Loop diuretics increase the delivery of Na$^+$ to the distal nephron, causing loss of H$^+$ and K$^+$. Because Cl$^-$ but not HCO$_3^-$ is

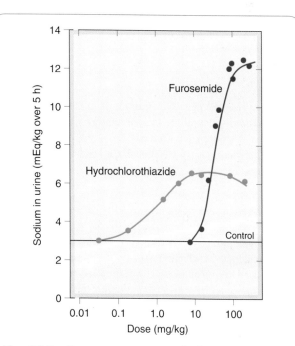

Fig. 24.6 Dose–response curves for furosemide (frusemide) and hydrochlorothiazide, showing differences in potency and maximum effect 'ceiling'. Note that these doses are not used clinically. (Adapted from Timmerman R J et al. 1964 Curr Ther Res 6: 88.)

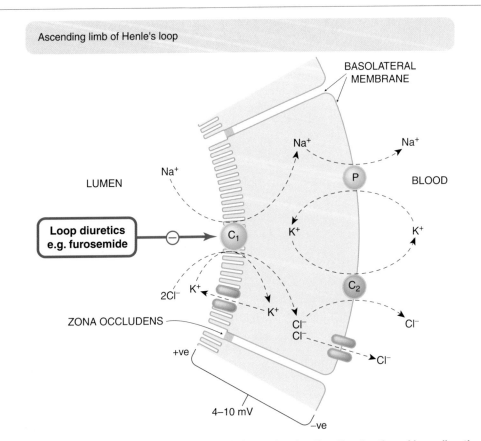

Fig. 24.7 **Ion transport in the thick ascending limb of Henle's loop, showing the site of action of loop diuretics.** The sodium pump (P) is the main primary active transport mechanism, and Na^+, K^+ and Cl^- enter by a cotransport system (C_1). Chloride leaves the cell both through basolateral chloride channels and by an electroneutral K^+/Cl^- cotransport system (C_2). Some K^+ returns to the lumen via potassium channels in the apical membrane, and some Na^+ is absorbed paracellularly through the *zonula occludens*. The diagram is simplified: the sodium pump exchanges 3 Na^+ for 2 K^+. (Based on Greger, 2000.)

lost in the urine, the plasma concentration of HCO_3^- increases as plasma volume is reduced—a form of metabolic alkalosis therefore referred to as 'contraction alkalosis'.

Loop diuretics *increase* excretion of Ca^{2+} and Mg^{2+} and *decrease* excretion of uric acid.

Pharmacokinetic aspects
Loop diuretics are normally readily absorbed from the gastrointestinal tract, and are usually given by mouth. They may also be given intravenously in urgent situations (e.g. acute pulmonary oedema) or when intestinal absorption is impaired, for example as a result of reduced intestinal perfusion in patients with chronic *congestive heart failure*, who can become resistant to the action of orally administered diuretics. Given orally, they act within 1 hour; given intravenously, they produce a peak effect within 30 minutes. Loop diuretics are strongly bound to plasma protein, and so do not pass directly into the glomerular filtrate. They reach their site of action—the lumenal membrane of the cells of the thick ascending limb—by being secreted in the proximal convoluted tubule by the organic acid transport mechanism; the fraction thus secreted is excreted in the urine.

In *nephrotic syndrome*,[4] loop diuretics become bound to albumin in the tubular fluid, and consequently are not available to act on the $Na^+/K^+/2Cl^-$ carrier—another cause of diuretic resistance. Molecular variation in the $Na^+/K^+/2Cl^-$ carrier may also be important in some cases of diuretic resistance (Shankar & Brater, 2003).

The fraction not excreted in the urine is metabolised, mainly in liver—**bumetanide** by cytochrome P450 pathways and **furosemide** being glucuronidated. The plasma half-lives are about 90 minutes (longer in renal failure), and the duration of action 3–6 hours. The clinical use of loop diuretics is given in the box.

---

[4]Several diseases that damage renal glomeruli impair their ability to retain plasma albumin, causing massive loss of albumin in the urine and a reduced concentration of albumin in the plasma, which can in turn cause peripheral oedema. This constellation is referred to as *nephrotic syndrome*.

Clinical uses of loop diuretics (e.g. furosemide)

- Loop diuretics are used (cautiously!), in conjunction with dietary salt restriction and often with other classes of diuretic, in the treatment of *salt and water overload* associated with:
  — acute *pulmonary oedema*
  — *chronic heart failure*
  — cirrhosis of the liver complicated by *ascites*
  — *nephrotic syndrome*
  — *renal failure.*
- Treatment of *hypertension* complicated by renal impairment (thiazides are preferred if renal function is preserved).
- Treatment of *hypercalcaemia* after replacement of plasma volume with intravenous NaCl solution.

Unwanted effects

Unwanted effects directly related to the renal action of loop diuretics are common.[5] Excessive Na^+ loss and diuresis are common, especially in elderly patients, and can cause *hypovolaemia* and *hypotension*. Potassium loss, resulting in low plasma K^+ (*hypokalaemia*), and metabolic alkalosis are common. Hypokalaemia increases the effects and toxicity of several drugs (e.g. **digoxin**, p. 292, and type III antidysrhythmic drugs, pp. 288-289), so this is potentially a clinically important source of drug interaction (Ch. 52, p. 746). If necessary, hypokalaemia can be averted or treated by concomitant use of K^+-sparing diuretics (see below), sometimes with supplementary potassium replacement. *Hypomagnesaemia* is less often recognised but can also be clinically important. *Hyperuricaemia* is common and can precipitate acute gout (see Ch. 14, pp. 238-239).

Unwanted effects *unrelated* to the *renal* actions of the drugs are infrequent. They include predictable reactions related to the main action of these drugs, and unpredictable idiosyncratic reactions (see Ch. 52, pp. 754-755). Dose-related hearing loss (compounded by concomitant use of other ototoxic drugs such as aminoglycoside antibiotics) is explained by the main action of loop diuretics: $Na^+/K^+/2\,Cl^-$ cotransport is important in the basolateral membrane of the stria vascularis in the inner ear, and babies with some forms of Bartter's syndrome (mentioned earlier) have associated deafness. It occurs only at much higher doses than usually needed to produce diuresis, because renal secretion of loop diuretics concentrates them at their site of action in the nephron, as explained above.

---

[5]Such unwanted effects are re-enacted in extreme form in Bartter's syndrome type 1, a rare autosomal recessive single gene disorder of the $Na^+/K^+/2\,Cl^-$ transporter, whose features include polyhydramnios—caused by fetal polyuria—and, postnatally, renal salt loss, low blood pressure, hypokalaemic metabolic alkalosis and hypercalciuria.

Idiosyncratic allergic reactions (e.g. rashes, bone marrow depression) are uncommon.

Diuretics acting on the distal tubule

Diuretics acting on the distal tubule include *thiazides* and related drugs. Widely used thiazides include **bendroflumethiazide** (bendrofluazide) and **hydrochlorothiazide**. Chemically distinct drugs with similar actions include **chlortalidone**, **indapamide** and **metolazone**.

Thiazides are less powerful than loop diuretics (Fig. 24.6) but are preferred in treating uncomplicated hypertension (Ch. 19). They are better tolerated than loop diuretics, and in clinical trials have been shown to reduce risks of stroke and heart attack associated with hypertension. In the largest trial (ALLHAT 2002), chlortalidone performed as well as newer antihypertensive drugs (an angiotensin-converting enzyme [ACE] inhibitor and a calcium antagonist). They bind to the Cl^- site of the distal tubular Na^+/Cl^- cotransport system, inhibiting its action (Figs 24.4 and 24.8) and causing natriuresis with loss of sodium and chloride ions. The resulting contraction in blood volume stimulates renin secretion, leading to angiotensin formation and aldosterone secretion (Ch. 19, see Figs 19.4 and 19.9). This homeostatic mechanism limits the effect of the diuretic on the blood pressure, resulting in an in vivo dose–hypotensive response relationship with only a very gentle gradient during chronic dosing. Potassium loss (by mechanisms explained on p. 374) can be important, as can loss of Mg^{2+}. Excretion of uric acid is decreased, and hypochloraemic alkalosis can occur. Effects of thiazides on Na^+, K^+, H^+ and Mg^{2+} balance are thus qualitatively similar to those of loop diuretics, but smaller in magnitude. In contrast to loop diuretics, however, thiazides *reduce* Ca^{2+} excretion. This could favour thiazides over loop diuretics in terms of bone metabolism during long-term use in older patients (Reid et al., 2000; Rejnmark et al., 2003; Schoofs et al., 2003). The mechanism underlying hypocalciuria caused by thiazide diuretics may be enhanced passive Ca^{2+} transport in the proximal tubule rather than active Ca^{2+} transport in the distal tubule (Nijenhuis et al., 2005).

Although milder than loop diuretics when used alone, coadministration of thiazide with loop diuretics has a synergistic effect, because the loop diuretic delivers a greater fraction of the filtered load of Na^+ to the site of action of the thiazide in the distal tubule.

Thiazide diuretics have an incompletely understood vasodilator action and can cause hyperglycaemia. When used in the treatment of hypertension (Ch. 19), the initial fall in blood pressure results from the decreased blood volume caused by diuresis, but the later phase is also related to an action on vascular smooth muscle. Note that **diazoxide**, a non-diuretic thiazide, has powerful vasodilator effects caused by activation of K_{ATP} channels implicated in the control of membrane potential in vascular smooth muscle and in insulin secretion (Ch. 4, p. 64). It markedly increases blood sugar, an effect opposite to that of chemically related sulfonylureas such as **glibenclamide** that inhibit K_{ATP} channels and are used to treat diabetes (see Ch. 26). **Indapamide** is said to lower blood pressure with less metabolic disturbance than related drugs, possibly because it is marketed at a lower equivalent dose.

Thiazide diuretics have a paradoxical effect in diabetes insipidus, where they reduce the volume of urine by interfering

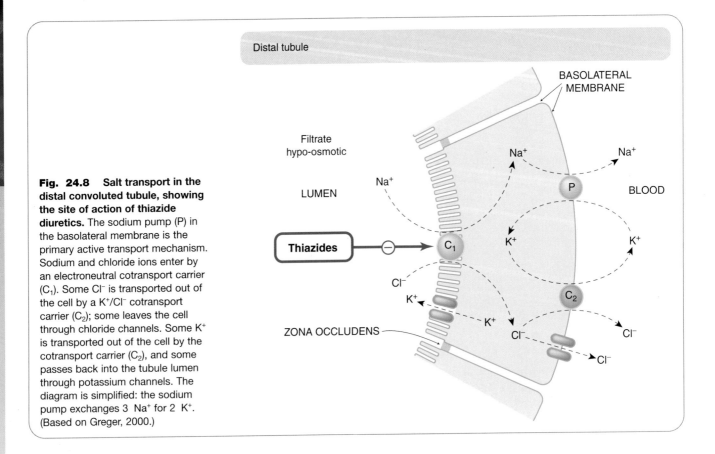

Distal tubule

Fig. 24.8 Salt transport in the distal convoluted tubule, showing the site of action of thiazide diuretics. The sodium pump (P) in the basolateral membrane is the primary active transport mechanism. Sodium and chloride ions enter by an electroneutral cotransport carrier (C_1). Some Cl^- is transported out of the cell by a K^+/Cl^- cotransport carrier (C_2); some leaves the cell through chloride channels. Some K^+ is transported out of the cell by the cotransport carrier (C_2), and some passes back into the tubule lumen through potassium channels. The diagram is simplified: the sodium pump exchanges 3 Na^+ for 2 K^+. (Based on Greger, 2000.)

with the production of hypotonic fluid in the distal tubule, and hence reduce the ability of the kidney to secrete hypotonic urine (i.e. they reduce free water clearance).

Pharmacokinetic aspects

Thiazides and related drugs are effective orally, being well absorbed from the gastrointestinal tract. All are excreted in the urine, mainly by tubular secretion (see p. 374), for which they compete with uric acid. With the shorter-acting drugs such as **bendroflumethiazide**, the maximum effect is at about 4–6 hours and duration is 8–12 hours. **Chlortalidone** has a longer duration of action.

The clinical use of thiazide diuretics is given in the clinical box.

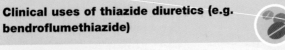

Clinical uses of thiazide diuretics (e.g. bendroflumethiazide)

- *Hypertension.*
- Mild *heart failure* (loop diuretics are usually preferred).
- Severe resistant *oedema* (**metolazone**, especially, is used, together with loop diuretics).
- To prevent recurrent stone formation in *idiopathic hypercalciuria.*
- *Nephrogenic diabetes insipidus.*

Unwanted effects

Mild unwanted effects are common. These re-enact the features of *Gitelman's syndrome*, a rare monogenetic disorder due to an inactivating mutation in the thiazide-sensitive Na^+/Cl^- cotransporter in the distal tubule. The clinical features are milder than Bartter's syndrome (which affects the $Na^+/K^+/2\ Cl^-$ cotransporter—see above), but as in Bartter's syndrome include renal salt loss, low blood pressure and hypokalaemic metabolic alkalosis; hypocalciuria is a feature, in contrast to Bartter's syndrome, and hypomagnesaemia is characteristic. In patients treated with thiazides, symptoms are usually limited to the inconvenience of a mildly increased frequency of micturition. Hypocalciuria may be beneficial as regards bone metabolism (see above) and stone formation. *Hyponatraemia* is potentially serious, especially in the elderly. *Hypokalaemia* can be a cause of adverse drug interaction (see above under loop diuretics) and can precipitate encephalopathy in patients with severe liver disease.

The commonest unwanted effect not obviously related to the main renal actions of the thiazides is *erectile dysfunction*. This emerged in an analysis of reasons given by patients for withdrawing from blinded treatment in the Medical Research Council mild hypertension trial, where (to the surprise of the investigators) it was significantly worse than placebo and β-adrenoceptor antagonists. Thiazide-associated erectile dysfunction is reversible; it is less common with the low doses used in current practice but remains a problem. Other dose-related problems include *hyperuricaemia* precipitating gout and *hyperglycaemia* (which does not, however, contraindicate their use in low dose in patients with diabetes mellitus; Ch. 26, pp. 402-403). Idiosyncratic reactions (e.g. rashes, blood dyscrasias, pancreatitis and acute pulmonary oedema) are rare but can be serious.

Aldosterone antagonists

Spironolactone and its recently marketed analogue **eplerenone** (see Weinberger, 2004, for a review) have very limited diuretic action when used singly, because distal Na^+/K^+ exchange—the site on which they act—accounts for reabsorption of only 2% of filtered Na^+. They do, however, have marked antihypertensive effects (Ch. 19), prolong survival in selected patients with heart failure (Ch. 19), and can prevent hypokalaemia when combined with loop diuretics or with thiazides. They compete with *aldosterone* (p. 372) for its intracellular receptors (see Ch. 28), thereby inhibiting distal Na^+ retention and K^+ secretion (see Figs 24.4 and 24.9). Eplerenone differs from spironolactone by replacement of a 17-α-thioacetyl group with a carbomethoxy group.

Pharmacokinetic aspects

Spironolactone is well absorbed from the gut. Its plasma half-life is only 10 minutes, but its active metabolite, **canrenone**, has a plasma half-life of 16 hours. The action of spironolactone is largely attributable to canrenone. Consistent with this, its onset of action is slow, taking several days to develop. **Eplerenone** has a shorter elimination half-life than canrenone and has no active metabolites. It is administered by mouth once daily.

Unwanted effects

Aldosterone antagonists predispose to *hyperkalaemia*, which is potentially fatal. Potassium supplements must not be coprescribed, and close monitoring of plasma creatinine and electrolytes is needed if these drugs are used for patients with impaired renal function, especially if other drugs that can increase plasma potassium, such as *ACE inhibitors, angiotensin receptor antagonists (sartans)* (Ch. 19) or *β-adrenoceptor antagonists* (Ch. 18) are also prescribed—as they often are for patients with heart failure (Ch. 19). Gastrointestinal upset is quite common. Actions of spironolactone/canrenone on progesterone and androgen receptors in tissues other than the kidney can result in gynaecomastia, menstrual disorders and testicular atrophy. Eplerenone has lower affinity for these receptors, and such oestrogen-like side effects are less common with licensed doses of this drug.

The clinical use of potassium-sparing diuretics is given in the clinical box.

Triamterene and amiloride

Like aldosterone antagonists, **triamterene** and **amiloride** have only limited diuretic efficacy, because they also act in the distal nephron, where only a small fraction of Na^+ reabsorption occurs. They act on the collecting tubules and collecting ducts, inhibiting Na^+ reabsorption by blocking lumenal sodium channels (see Ch. 4) and decreasing K^+ excretion (see Figs 24.4 and 24.9).

They can be given with K^+-losing diuretics (e.g. loop diuretics, thiazides) in order to maintain potassium balance.

Pharmacokinetic aspects

Triamterene is well absorbed in the gastrointestinal tract. Its onset of action is within 2 hours, and its duration of action

> **Clinical uses of potassium-sparing diuretics (e.g. amiloride, spironolactone)**
>
> - With K^+-losing (i.e. loop or thiazide) diuretics to prevent K^+ loss, where hypokalaemia is especially hazardous (e.g. patients requiring **digoxin** or **amiodarone**; see Ch. 18).
> - **Spironolactone** or **eplerenone** is used:
>   - in *heart failure,* where either of these improves survival (see Ch.19)
>   - in primary *hyperaldosteronism* (Conn's syndrome)
>   - in *resistant essential hypertension* (especially low-renin hypertension)
>   - in *secondary hyperaldosteronism* caused by hepatic cirrhosis complicated by ascites.

12–16 hours. It is partly metabolised in the liver and partly excreted unchanged in the urine. **Amiloride** is less well absorbed and has a slower onset, with a peak action at 6 hours and duration of about 24 hours. Most of the drug is excreted unchanged in the urine.

Unwanted effects

The main unwanted effect, *hyperkalaemia*, is related to the pharmacological action of these drugs and can be dangerous, especially in patients with renal impairment or receiving other drugs that can increase plasma K^+ (see above). Gastrointestinal disturbances have been reported but are infrequent. Triamterene has been identified in kidney stones, but its aetiological role is uncertain. Idiosyncratic reactions, for example rashes, are uncommon.

The clinical use of triamterene and amiloride is given in the box on potassium-sparing diuretics.

DIURETICS THAT ACT INDIRECTLY BY MODIFYING THE CONTENT OF THE FILTRATE

Osmotic diuretics

Osmotic diuretics are pharmacologically inert substances (e.g. **mannitol**) that are filtered in the glomerulus but not reabsorbed by the nephron (see Fig. 24.4).[6] To cause a diuresis, they must constitute an appreciable fraction of the osmolarity of tubular fluid. Within the nephron, their main effect is exerted on those parts of the nephron that are freely permeable to water: the proximal tubule, descending limb of the loop, and (in the presence of ADH;

---

[6]In hyperglycaemia, glucose acts as an osmotic diuretic once plasma glucose exceeds the renal reabsorptive threshold (usually approximately 12 mmol/l), accounting for the cardinal symptom of polyuria in diabetes mellitus; see Chapter 26.

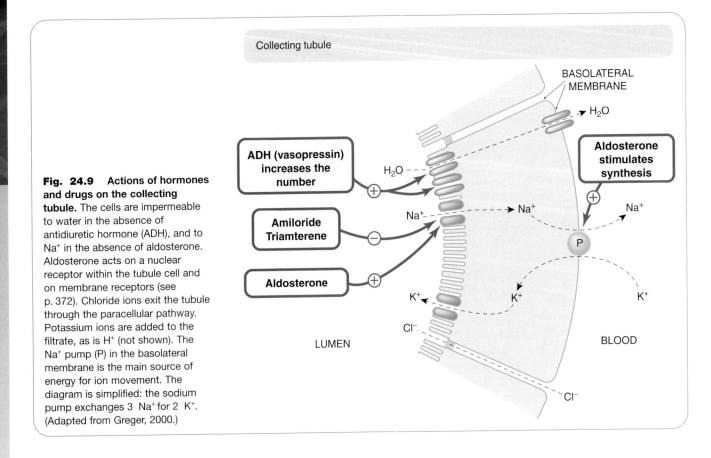

Fig. 24.9 Actions of hormones and drugs on the collecting tubule. The cells are impermeable to water in the absence of antidiuretic hormone (ADH), and to Na⁺ in the absence of aldosterone. Aldosterone acts on a nuclear receptor within the tubule cell and on membrane receptors (see p. 372). Chloride ions exit the tubule through the paracellular pathway. Potassium ions are added to the filtrate, as is H⁺ (not shown). The Na⁺ pump (P) in the basolateral membrane is the main source of energy for ion movement. The diagram is simplified: the sodium pump exchanges 3 Na⁺ for 2 K⁺. (Adapted from Greger, 2000.)

see above) the collecting tubules. Passive water reabsorption is reduced by the presence of non-reabsorbable solute within the tubule; consequently a larger volume of fluid remains within the proximal tubule. This has the secondary effect of reducing Na⁺ reabsorption.

Therefore the main effect of osmotic diuretics is to increase the amount of water excreted, with a smaller increase in Na⁺ excretion. They are *not* useful in treating conditions such as heart failure associated with Na⁺ retention but have much more limited therapeutic indications, including emergency treatment of acutely raised intracranial or intraocular pressure. Such treatment has nothing to do with the kidney, but relies on the increase in plasma osmolarity by solutes that do not enter the brain or eye; this results in extraction of water from these compartments.

In acute renal failure, which can occur as a result of haemorrhage, injury or systemic infections, the glomerular filtration rate is reduced, and absorption of NaCl and water in the proximal tubule becomes almost complete, so that more distal parts of the nephron virtually 'dry up', and urine flow ceases. Protein is deposited in the tubules and may impede the flow of fluid. Osmotic diuretics (e.g. **mannitol** in a dose of 12–15 g) can limit these effects, at least if given in the earliest stages, albeit while increasing intravascular volume and risking left ventricular failure.

Osmotic diuretics are given intravenously.

Unwanted effects include transient expansion of the extra-cellular fluid volume (with a risk of causing left ventricular failure) and hyponatraemia. Headache, nausea and vomiting can occur.

DRUGS THAT ALTER THE PH OF THE URINE

It is possible, by the use of pharmacological agents, to produce urinary pH values ranging from approximately 5 to 8.5.

AGENTS THAT INCREASE URINARY PH

Carbonic anhydrase inhibitors alkalinise urine by blocking bicarbonate reabsorption (see above). *Citrate* (given by mouth as a mixture of sodium and potassium salts) is metabolised via the Krebs cycle with generation of bicarbonate, which is excreted to give an alkaline urine. This may have some antibacterial effects, as well as improving dysuria (a common symptom of bladder infection, consisting of a burning sensation while passing urine). Additionally, some citrate is excreted in the urine as such and inhibits urinary stone formation. Alkalinisation is important in preventing certain weak acid drugs with limited aqueous solubility, for example *sulfonamides* (now seldom used as antibacterial drugs but important in treating *Pneumocystis* infection with high-dose **co-trimoxazole**—Ch. 49, p. 710—and in using **sulfasalazine** in the management of inflammatory bowel disease—p. 395, and as a disease-modifying anti-rheumatoid drug—p. 239-240), from crystallising in the urine; it also decreases the formation of uric acid and cystine stones by favouring the charged anionic form that is more water-soluble (Ch. 7, p. 100).

Diuretics

- Normally, < 1% of filtered Na^+ is excreted.
- Diuretics increase the excretion of salt (NaCl or $NaHCO_3$) and water.
- Loop diuretics, thiazides and K^+-sparing diuretics are the main therapeutic drugs.
- Loop diuretics (e.g. **furosemide**) cause copious urine production. They inhibit the $Na^+/K^+/2\ Cl^-$ cotransporter in the thick ascending loop of Henle. They are used to treat heart failure and other diseases complicated by salt and water retention. Hypovolaemia and hypokalaemia are important unwanted effects.
- Thiazides (e.g. **bendroflumethiazide**) are less potent than loop diuretics. They inhibit the Na^+/Cl^- cotransporter in the distal convoluted tubule. They are used to treat hypertension. Erectile dysfunction is an important adverse effect. Hypokalaemia and other metabolic effects can occur.
- Potassium-sparing diuretics:
  - act in the distal nephron and collecting tubules; they are very weak diuretics but effective in some forms of hypertension and heart failure, and they can prevent hypokalaemia caused by loop diuretics or thiazides
  - **spironolactone** and **eplerenone** compete with aldosterone for its receptor
  - **amiloride** and **triamterene** act by blocking the sodium channels controlled by aldosterone's protein mediator.

Alkalinising the urine increases the excretion of drugs that are weak acids (e.g. salicylates and some barbiturates). Sodium bicarbonate is sometimes used to treat salicylate overdose (Ch. 8).

Note that Na^+ overload is dangerous in cardiac failure, and that overload with either Na^+ or K^+ is harmful in renal insufficiency.

AGENTS THAT DECREASE URINARY PH

Urinary pH can be decreased with ammonium chloride, but this is now rarely, if ever, used clinically except in a specialised test for renal tubular acidosis.

DRUGS THAT ALTER THE EXCRETION OF ORGANIC MOLECULES

Uric acid metabolism and excretion is relevant in the treatment of gout, and a few points about its excretion are made here.

Uric acid is derived from the catabolism of purines, and is present in plasma mainly as ionised urate. In humans, it passes freely into the glomerular filtrate, and most is then reabsorbed in the proximal tubule while a small amount is secreted into the tubule by the anion-secreting mechanism (see p. 374). The net result is excretion of approximately 8–12% of filtered urate. The secretory mechanism is generally inhibited by low doses of drugs that affect uric acid excretion (see below), whereas higher doses are needed to block reabsorption. Such drugs therefore tend to cause retention of uric acid at low doses, while promoting its excretion at higher doses. Normal plasma urate concentration is approximately 0.24 mmol/l. In some individuals, the plasma concentration is high, predisposing to gout. In this disorder, urate crystals are deposited in joints and soft tissues,[7] resulting in acute arthritis and chalky tophi characteristic of this condition. Drugs that increase the elimination of urate (uricosuric agents, e.g. **probenecid** and **sulfinpyrazone**) may be useful in such patients, although these have largely been supplanted by **allopurinol**, which inhibits urate synthesis (Ch. 14, pp. 238-239).

Probenecid inhibits the reabsorption of urate in the proximal tubule, increasing its excretion. It has the opposite effect on penicillin, inhibiting its secretion into the tubules and raising its plasma concentration. Given orally, probenecid is well absorbed in the gastrointestinal tract, maximal concentrations in the plasma occurring in about 3 hours. Approximately 90% is bound to plasma albumin. Free drug passes into the glomerular filtrate but more is actively secreted into the proximal tubule, whence it may diffuse back because of its high lipid solubility (see also Ch. 8).

Sulfinpyrazone is a congener of **phenylbutazone** (see Ch. 14) with a powerful inhibitory effect on uric acid reabsorption in the proximal tubule. It is absorbed from the gastrointestinal tract, is highly protein-bound in the plasma and is secreted into the proximal tubule.

The main effect of uricosuric drugs is to block urate reabsorption and lower plasma urate concentration. Both probenecid and sulfinpyrazone inhibit the secretion as well as the reabsorption of urate and, if given in subtherapeutic doses, can actually increase plasma urate concentrations.

Usual therapeutic doses of *salicylates*, in contrast, selectively *inhibit* urate secretion, *increasing* blood urate concentration. They exacerbate gouty arthritis and antagonise the effects of more powerful uricosuric agents. (But note that salicylates become uricosuric themselves at the very high doses used in the past to treat rheumatoid arthritis.)

Some inorganic agents inhibit secretion of other drugs by the acid carrier system. Thus probenecid, as specified above, inhibits penicillin excretion, and at one time was used to enhance the action of penicillin antibiotics (e.g. in single-dose treatment of gonorrhoea). It is currently licensed in the UK to prevent nephrotoxicity caused by **cidofovir** (Ch. 47), an antiviral drug used to treat cytomegallovirus retinitis in AIDS patients for whom other antiviral drugs are inappropriate. It is given with probenecid to prevent its concentration within the tubular lumen, and intravenous hydration, without which it causes tubular toxicity.

---

[7]The distribution is determined by body temperature: crystals come out of solution in cool extremities such as the joints of the big toe—the classic site for acute gout—and the pinna of the ear, a common site for gouty tophi.

DRUGS USED IN RENAL FAILURE

A huge spectrum of congenital and acquired diseases damage the kidneys. Despite their diversity, these lead ultimately to common end points of acute or chronic renal failure. The management of these states depends crucially on various forms of artificial dialysis or filtration, and on renal transplantation. Dialysis depends on anticoagulation with **heparin** (Ch. 21) and/or **epoprostenol** (Ch. 13), and transplantation on immunosuppression (Ch. 14). These are outside the scope of this book—interested readers should consult a nephrology textbook such as the *Oxford Textbook of Nephrology* (3rd edition, 2005). Hypertension is both a cause and a consequence of renal impairment, so its treatment with *anti-hypertensive* drugs (Ch. 19) is extremely important in the context of renal disease. ACE inhibitors and angiotensin II antagonists are used as renoprotective agents to prevent progression of chronic renal impairment in proteinuric patients, where their benefit is over and above their effects on blood pressure (see Brunner, 1992, and clinical boxes on ACE inhibitors and sartans in Ch. 19). The excess mortality in patients with chronic renal disease is attributable largely to cardiovascular disease, and aggressive management of dyslipidaemia (Ch. 20) is of great importance. *Immunosuppressant* drugs are effective in halting the progression of some systemic diseases (e.g. Wegener's granulomatosis) that can cause renal failure. They are covered in Chapter 14. *Erythropoietin* (Ch. 22, pp. 353-354) is used to treat the anaemia of chronic renal failure. Vitamin D preparations (**calcitriol** or **alphacalcidol**) used to treat the osteodystrophy of chronic renal failure are covered in Chapter 31 (p. 468). *Antibacterial* drugs are crucial in treating renal and urinary tract infections, and are dealt with in Chapter 46.

Dosing regimens of many drugs must be adapted to prevent accumulation and toxicity in patients with renal failure, as described in detail in clinical texts (see Carmichael, 2005). Here we cover briefly preparations used to treat or prevent two other common and important aspects of chronic renal failure, namely *hyperphosphataemia* and *hyperkalaemia*.

HYPERPHOSPHATAEMIA

Phosphate metabolism is closely linked with that of calcium and is discussed in Chapter 31 (pp. 463-464). Phosphate, at concentrations commonly occurring in chronic renal insufficiency, causes vascular smooth muscle cell differentiation into osteoblast-like cells able to sustain mineralisation. Molecular identification of phosphate transporters, transporter regulators, and genes associated with familial and acquired hypo- and hyperphosphataemias has transformed current understanding of phosphate homeostasis.

Hyperphosphataemia (plasma phosphate concentration > 1.45 mmol/l) is common in renal failure. It may be asymptomatic, but an acute increase in plasma phosphate causes symptoms by causing acute hypocalcaemia. In chronic hyperphosphataemia, hypocalcaemia is corrected by compensatory mechanisms, but calcium phosphate precipitates in tissues if the calcium phosphate concentration product (Ca × P) exceeds a threshold of approximately 5.6 (when the concentration of each ion is expressed in mmol/l). Large calcium phosphate deposits around joints limit mobility but otherwise cause surprisingly few symptoms. Conjunctival calcification can cause conjunctivitis ('uraemic red eye'). Calcification of the aortic valve can cause stenosis. *Acute calciphylaxis* is a syndrome characterised by abrupt metastatic calcification in subcutaneous tissues and small vessels, leading to extensive soft tissue necrosis. Hyperphosphataemia is the major trigger for the onset of hyperparathyroidism in early chronic renal failure, and leads to renal osteodystrophy.

Phosphate binders

These effects of hyperphosphataemia have led to the widespread use of phosphate-binding preparations in renal failure; approximately half of patients on chronic haemodialysis are treated with such drugs. The antacid **aluminium hydroxide** (Ch. 25, p. 388) binds phosphate in the gastrointestinal tract, reducing its absorption, but may increase plasma aluminium in dialysis patients. There is huge sensitivity to this in the nephrology community, because before Kerr identified the cause in Newcastle, the use of alum as a water purifier in municipal water supplies led to a horrible and untreatable neurodegenerative condition known as 'dialysis dementia', and also to a particularly painful and refractory form of bone disease. Calcium-containing phosphate-binding agents (e.g. **calcium carbonate**) are widely used. They are contraindicated in hypercalcaemia or hypercalciuria but until recently have been believed to be otherwise safe. However, calcium salts may predispose to tissue calcification (including of artery walls), and calcium-containing phosphate binders may actually contribute to the very high death rates from cardiovascular disease in dialysis patients (Goldsmith et al., 2004).

An *anion exchange resin*, **sevelamer**, lowers plasma phosphate. This is not absorbed and has an additional effect in lowering low-density lipoprotein cholesterol. It is given in gram doses by mouth three times a day with meals. Its adverse effects are gastrointestinal disturbance, and it is contraindicated in bowel obstruction.

In a 2-year randomised study of haemodialysis patients, calcium carbonate was associated with greater progression of arterial calcification than sevelamer (Asmus et al., 2005), and if early reports of positive results on cardiovascular mortality in a randomised controlled trial of sevelamer (Dialysis Clinical Outcomes Revisited) are borne out, this may prove to be of considerable importance.

HYPERKALAEMIA

Severe hyperkalaemia is life-threatening. It is commonly associated with potassium ion retention because of renal failure, especially if there is concomitant hypoaldosteronism (e.g. in Addison's disease; Ch. 28, p. 427) or more commonly because of drugs that interfere with renin secretion (e.g. β-adrenoceptor antagonists; Ch. 11, p. 180), or with angiotensin II formation or action (i.e. ACE inhibitors and angiotensin receptor antagonists; Ch. 19, pp. 308-310), or blockade of distal tubular potassium ion excretion (above, p. 379).

Prompt treatment is indicated if the plasma K⁺ concentration is > 6.5 mmol/l. Cardiac toxicity is counteracted directly by administering *calcium gluconate* intravenously (Table 18.1, p. 287), and by measures that shift K⁺ into the intracellular compartment, for example glucose plus **insulin** (Ch. 26, clinical box on p. 405).

Salbutamol (**albuterol**), administered intravenously or by inhalation, also causes cellular K^+ uptake and is used for this indication (e.g. Murdoch et al., 1991); it acts synergistically with insulin. Intravenous sodium bicarbonate is also often recommended, and moves potassium into cells. Removal of excessive potassium from the body can be achieved by *cation exchange resins* such as **sodium** or **calcium polystyrene sulfonate** administered by mouth (in combination with **sorbitol** to prevent severe constipation) or as an enema. Dialysis is often needed.

DRUGS USED IN URINARY TRACT DISORDERS

Bed wetting (enuresis) is normal in very young children and persists in around 5% of children aged 10. Disordered micturition is also extremely common in adults of either sex, and becomes more so with advancing age. Associated structural problems (e.g. prostatic hypertrophy, uterine prolapse) may warrant surgical intervention, and urinary infection—curable with antibiotics—may have been overlooked. However, many cases of incontinence (socially devastating) are functional, and should in principle be amenable to drugs acting on urinary tract smooth muscle or on the nerves controlling this. Currently available treatment is, however, disappointing, perhaps because it is not easy to prevent incontinence without causing urinary retention.

Nocturnal enuresis in children aged 10 or more may warrant **desmopressin** (oral or nasal; Ch. 28, p. 426) combined with restricting fluid intake, in addition to practical measures such as an enuresis alarm. Tricyclic antidepressants such as **amitryptyline** (Ch. 39) are sometimes used for up to 3 months, but adverse effects including behaviour disturbance can occur, and relapse is common after stopping treatment.

Symptoms from benign prostatic hypertrophy may be improved by α_1-adrenoceptor antagonists, for example **doxazosin** and **tamsulosin** (Ch. 11, p. 179), or by a 5-α-reductase inhibitor such as **finasteride** (Ch. 30, p. 453).

Incontinence in adults and caused by neurogenic detrusor muscle instability is managed by conservative measures such as pelvic floor exercises combined with muscarinic receptor antagonists (Ch. 10, p. 153) such as **oxybutinin**, **tolterodine**, **propiverine** or **trospium**, but the dose is limited by their adverse effects.

REFERENCES AND FURTHER READING

Physiological aspects (molecular/cellular)

Agre P 2004 Aquaporin water channels (Nobel lecture). Angewandte Chemie—International Edition 43: 4278–4290

Berkhin E B, Humphreys M H 2001 Regulation of renal tubular secretion of organic compounds. Kidney Int 59: 17–30 (*Reviews the literature on physiological and pharmacological aspects of anion and cation transport, and discusses factors believed to regulate this*)

Burg M G 1985 Renal handling of sodium, chloride, water, amino acids and glucose. In: Brenner B M, Rector F C (eds) The kidney, 3rd edn. Saunders, Philadelphia, pp. 145–175

Gamba G 2005 Molecular physiology and pathophysiology of electroneutral cation–chloride cotransporters. Physiol Rev 85: 423–493 (*Comprehensive review of the molecular biology, structure–function relationships, and physiological and pathophysiological roles of each cotransporter*)

Greger R 2000 Physiology of sodium transport. Am J Med Sci 319: 51–62 (*Outstanding article. Covers not only Na^+ transport but also, briefly, that of K^+, H^+, Cl^-, HCO_3^-, Ca^{2+}, Mg^{2+} and some organic substances in each of the main parts of the nephron. Discusses regulatory factors, pathophysiological aspects and pharmacological principles.*)

Reilly R F, Ellison D H 2000 Mammalian distal tubule: physiology, pathophysiology, and molecular anatomy. Physiol Rev 80: 277–313 (*Comprehensive review*)

Sullivan L P, Grantham J J 1982 The physiology of the kidney, 2nd edn. Lea & Febiger, Philadelphia

Pathological aspects

Keller G, Zimmer G, Mall G et al. 2003 Nephron numbers in patients with primary hypertension. N Engl J Med 348: 101–108 (*Aged 35–59 + matched normotensive controls, all of whom died in road accidents; elegant morphometry*)

Vesely D L 2003 Natriuretic peptides and acute renal failure. Am J Physiol Renal Physiol 285: F167–F177 (*Review*)

Drugs and therapeutic aspects

Diuretics

Brater D C 2000 Pharmacology of diuretics. Am J Med Sci 319: 38–50 (*Pharmacodynamics, clinical pharmacology and adverse effects of diuretics*)

Greger R, Lang F, Sebekova K, Heidland A 2005 Action and clinical use of diuretics. In: Davison A M et al. (eds) Oxford textbook of clinical nephrology, 3rd edn. Oxford University Press, Oxford, pp. 2619–2648 (*Succinct authoritative account of cellular mechanisms; strong on clinical uses*)

Reid I R, Ames R W et al. 2000 Hydrochlorothiazide reduces loss of cortical bone in normal postmenopausal women: a randomized controlled trial. Am J Med 109: 362–370 (*Thiazides may be useful in prevention but not treatment of postmenopausal osteoporosis; see also, in the same issue, Sebastien A, pp. 429–430*)

Rejnmark L et al. 2003 Dose–effect relations of loop- and thiazide-diuretics on calcium homeostasis: a randomized, double-blinded Latin-square multiple cross-over study in postmenopausal osteopenic women. Eur J Clin Invest 33: 41–50 (*The effects of a loop diuretic, but not a thiazide, on calcium homeostasis are potentially harmful to bone*)

Schoofs M W C J et al. 2003 Thiazide diuretics and the risk for hip fracture. Ann Intern Med 139: 476–482 (*Rotterdam study: thiazide diuretics protected against hip fracture, but protection disappears after use is discontinued*)

Shankar S S, Brater D C 2003 Loop diuretics: from the Na–K–2 Cl transporter to clinical use. Am J Physiol Renal Physiol 284: F11–F21 (*Reviews pharmacokinetics and pharmacodynamics of loop diuretics in health and in edematous disorders; the authors hypothesise that altered expression or activity of the $Na^+/K^+/2Cl^-$ transporter possibly accounts for reduced diuretic responsiveness*)

Weinberger M H 2004 Eplerenone—a new selective aldosterone receptor antagonist. Drugs Today 40: 481–485 (*Review*)

Ca^{2+}/PO_4^- (see also Diuretics section, above)

Asmus H G et al. 2005 Two year comparison of sevelamer and calcium carbonate effects on cardiovascular calcification and bone density. Nephrol Dial Transplant 20: 1653–1661 (*Less progression of vascular calcification with sevelamer*)

Cozzolino M, Brancaccio D, Gallieni M, Slatopolsky E 2005 Pathogenesis of vascular calcification in chronic kidney disease. Kidney Int 68: 429–436 (*Reviews hyperphosphatemia and hypercalcemia as independent risk factors for higher incidence of cardiovascular events in patients with chronic kidney disease: '...hyperphosphatemia accelerates the progression of secondary hyperparathyroidism with the concomitant bone loss, possibly linked to vascular calcium-phosphate precipitation'*)

Goldsmith D, Ritz E, Covic A 2004 Vascular calcification: a stiff challenge for the nephrologist—does preventing bone disease cause arterial disease? Kidney Int 66: 1315–1333 (*Potential danger of using calcium salts as phosphate binders in patients with chronic renal failure*)

Antihypertensives and renal protection

ALLHAT Officers and Coordinators for the ALLHAT Collaborative Research Group. The Antihypertensive and Lipid-Lowering Treatment to Prevent Heart Attack Trial 2002 Major outcomes in high-risk hypertensive patients randomized to angiotensin-converting enzyme inhibitor or calcium channel blocker vs diuretic: the Antihypertensive and Lipid-Lowering Treatment to Prevent Heart Attack Trial (ALLHAT). JAMA 288: 2981–2997 (*Massive trial; see also Appel L J for editorial comment: 'The verdict from ALLHAT—thiazide diuretics are the preferred initial therapy for hypertension' JAMA 288: 3039–3042*)

Brunner H R 1992 ACE inhibitors in renal disease. Kidney Int 42: 463–479 (*Effects beyond those attributable to lowering blood pressure*)

Nijenhuis T et al. 2005 Enhanced passive Ca^{2+} reabsorption and reduced Mg^{2+} channel abundance explains thiazide-induced hypocalciuria and hypomagnesemia. J Clin Invest 115: 1651–1658 (*Micropuncture studies in mouse knockouts showing that enhanced passive Ca^{2+} transport in the proximal tubule rather than active Ca^{2+} transport in distal convolution explains thiazide-induced hypocalciuria*)

Sodium and potassium ion disorders

Coca S G, Perazella M A, Buller G K 2005 The cardiovascular implications of hypokalemia. Am J Kidney Dis 45: 233–247 (*The recent discovery that aldosterone antagonists decrease pathological injury of myocardium and endothelium has focused interest on their mechanism; this review addresses the relative benefits of modulating potassium balance versus non-renal effects of aldosterone blockade*)

Kumar S, Berl T 1998 Sodium. Lancet 352: 220–228 (*Sodium homeostasis, its disorders and treatment*)

Lee W, Kim R B 2003 Transporters and renal drug elimination. Annu Rev Pharmacol Toxicol 44: 137–166 (*Review*)

Murdoch I A, Dos Anjos R, Haycock G B 1991 Treatment of hyperkalaemia with intravenous salbutamol. Arch Dis Child 66: 527–528 (*First description of this approach in children*)

Drug utilisation in kidney disease

Carmichael D J S 2005 Handling of drugs in kidney disease. In: Davison A M et al. (eds) Oxford textbook of clinical nephrology, 3rd edn. Oxford University Press, Oxford, pp. 2599–2618 (*Principles and practice of dose adjustment in patients with renal failure*)

Nephrotoxicity

Cuzzolin L, Dal Cere M, Fanos V 2001 NSAID-induced nephrotoxicity from the fetus to the child. Drug Saf 24: 9–18 (*NSAID nephrotoxicity in extracellular volume contraction*)

The gastrointestinal tract

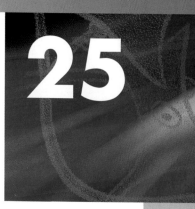

25

OVERVIEW

In addition to its main function of digestion and absorption of food, the gastrointestinal tract is one of the major endocrine systems in the body and has its own integrative neuronal network, the enteric nervous system (see Ch. 9), which contains almost the same number of neurons as the spinal cord. It is also the site of many common pathologies, ranging from simple dyspepsia to complex autoimmune conditions such as Crohn's disease. Medicines for treating these gastrointestinal disorders comprise some 8% of all prescriptions. In this chapter, we briefly review the physiological control of gastrointestinal function and then discuss the pharmacological characteristics of drugs affecting gastric secretion and motility.

THE INNERVATION AND HORMONES OF THE GASTROINTESTINAL TRACT

The blood vessels and the glands (exocrine, endocrine and paracrine) that comprise the gastrointestinal tract are under both neuronal and hormonal control.

NEURONAL CONTROL

There are two principal intramural plexuses in the tract: the *myenteric* plexus (Auerbach's plexus) between the outer, longitudinal and the middle, circular muscle layers, and the *submucous* plexus (Meissner's plexus) on the lumenal side of the circular muscle layer. These plexuses are interconnected, and their ganglion cells receive preganglionic parasympathetic fibres from the vagus, which are mostly cholinergic and excitatory, although a few are inhibitory. Incoming sympathetic fibres are largely postganglionic, and these, in addition to innervating blood vessels, smooth muscle and some glandular cells directly, may terminate in these plexuses, where they inhibit acetylcholine secretion (see Ch. 9).

The neurons within the plexuses constitute the *enteric nervous system* and secrete not only acetylcholine and noradrenaline (norepinephrine), but also 5-hydroxytryptamine, purines, nitric oxide and a variety of pharmacologically active peptides (see Chs 10–12, 16 and 17). The enteric plexus also contains sensory neurons, which respond to mechanical and chemical stimuli.

HORMONAL CONTROL

The hormones of the gastrointestinal tract include both endocrine and paracrine secretions. The endocrine secretions (i.e. substances released into the bloodstream) are mainly peptidic in nature and are synthesised by endocrine cells in the mucosa. Important examples include gastrin and cholecystokinin. The paracrine secretions include many regulatory peptides released from special cells found throughout the wall of the tract. These hormones act on nearby cells, and in the stomach the most important of these is histamine. Some of these paracrine factors also function as neurotransmitters.

Orally administered drugs are absorbed in the gastrointestinal tract (Ch. 7). The main functions of the gastrointestinal tract that are important from the viewpoint of pharmacological intervention are:

- gastric secretion
- vomiting (emesis)

- the motility of the bowel and the expulsion of the faeces
- the formation and excretion of bile.

GASTRIC SECRETION

The stomach secretes about 2.5 litres of gastric juice daily. The principal exocrine secretions are proenzymes such as *prorennin* and *pepsinogen* elaborated by the *chief* or *peptic* cells, and hydrochloric acid (HCl) and intrinsic factor (see Ch. 22) secreted by the *parietal* or *oxyntic* cells. Mucus-secreting cells abound among the surface cells of the gastric mucosa. Bicarbonate ions are also secreted and are trapped in the mucus, creating a gel-like protective barrier that maintains the mucosal surface at a pH of 6–7 in the face of a much more acidic environment (pH 1–2) in the lumen. Alcohol and bile can disrupt this layer. Locally produced 'cytoprotective' prostaglandins stimulate the secretion of both mucus and bicarbonate.

Disturbances in these secretory and protective mechanisms are thought to be involved in the pathogenesis of peptic ulcer, and the therapy of this condition includes drugs that modify each of these factors.

THE REGULATION OF ACID SECRETION BY PARIETAL CELLS

The regulation of acid secretion by parietal cells is especially important in the pathogenesis of peptic ulcer, and constitutes a particular target for drug action. The secretion of the parietal cells is an isotonic solution of HCl (150 mmol/l) with a pH less than 1, the concentration of hydrogen ions being more than a million times higher than that of the plasma. The Cl^- is actively transported into *canaliculi* in the cells that communicate with the lumen of the gastric glands and thus with the stomach itself. This Cl^- secretion is accompanied by K^+, which is then exchanged for H^+ from within the cell by a K^+/H^+ ATPase (Fig. 25.1). Carbonic anhydrase catalyses the combination of carbon dioxide and water to give carbonic acid, which dissociates into H^+ and bicarbonate ions. The latter exchanges across the basal membrane of the parietal cell for Cl^-. The principal stimuli acting on the parietal cells are:

- gastrin (a stimulatory hormone)
- acetylcholine (a stimulatory neurotransmitter)
- histamine (a stimulatory local hormone)
- prostaglandins E_2 and I_2 (local hormones that inhibit acid secretion).

Figure 25.2 summarises the actions of these chemical mediators.

Gastrin

Gastrin is a peptide hormone synthesised in endocrine cells of the mucosa of the gastric antrum and duodenum, and secreted into the portal blood. Its main action is stimulation of the secretion of acid by the parietal cells, but there is controversy about the precise mechanism of stimulatory action (discussed below). Gastrin receptors on the parietal cells have been demonstrated using the radioactively labelled hormone. These receptors are blocked by the experimental drug *proglumide* (Fig. 25.2), which inhibits gastrin action.

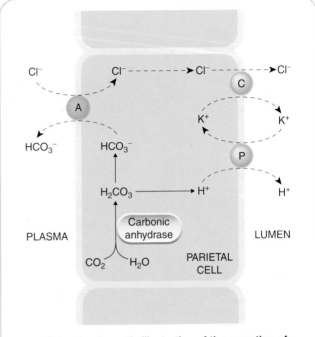

Fig. 25.1 A schematic illustration of the secretion of hydrochloric acid by the gastric parietal cell. Secretion involves a proton pump (P), which is an H^+/K^+ ATPase, a symport carrier (C) for K^+ and Cl^-, and an antiport (A), which exchanges Cl^- and HCO_3^-. An additional Na^+/H^+ antiport situated at the interface with the plasma may also have a role (not shown).

Gastrin also indirectly increases pepsinogen secretion, stimulates blood flow and increases gastric motility. Release of this hormone is controlled both by neuronal transmitters and blood-borne mediators, as well as the chemistry of the stomach contents. Amino acids and small peptides directly stimulate the gastrin-secreting cells, as do milk and solutions of calcium salts, explaining why it is inappropriate to use calcium-containing salts as antacids.

Acetylcholine

Acetylcholine is released from (e.g. vagal) neurons and stimulates specific muscarinic receptors on the surface of the parietal cells and on the surface of histamine-containing cells (see Ch. 10).

Histamine

Histamine is discussed in Chapter 13, and only those aspects of its pharmacology relevant to gastric secretion will be dealt with here. Within the stomach, mast cells (or histamine-containing cells similar to mast cells) lying close to the parietal cell release a steady basal release of histamine, which is further increased by gastrin and acetylcholine. The hormone acts on parietal cell H_2 receptors, which are responsive to histamine concentrations that are below the threshold required for vascular H_2 receptor activation.

The coordinated role of acetylcholine, histamine and gastrin in regulating acid secretion

The exact mechanism of action of the three secretagogues on the parietal cell is not entirely clear. A general scheme is given in

Secretion of gastric acid, mucus and bicarbonate

- The control of the gastrointestinal tract is through nervous and humoral mechanisms.
  - Acid is secreted from gastric parietal cells by a proton pump (K⁺/H⁺ ATPase).
  - The three endogenous secretagogues for acid are histamine, acetylcholine and gastrin.
  - Prostaglandins E_2 and I_2 inhibit acid, stimulate mucus and bicarbonate secretion, and dilate mucosal blood vessels.
- The genesis of peptic ulcers involves:
  - infection of the gastric mucosa with *Helicobacter pylori*.
  - an imbalance between the mucosal-damaging (acid, pepsin) and the mucosal-protecting agents (mucus, bicarbonate, prostaglandins E_2 and I_2, and nitric oxide).

Figure 25.2, which summarises the two main theories: the 'single-cell' or 'permission' hypothesis, and the 'two-cell' or 'transmission' hypothesis. According to the former concept, the parietal cell itself has H_2 receptors for histamine and muscarinic M_2 receptors for acetylcholine, as well as receptors for gastrin itself. Acid secretion follows after the synergistic stimulation of H_2 receptors (which increases cAMP), and M_2 and gastrin receptors (which increase cytosolic Ca^{2+}). Arguing against this is the observation that **cimetidine** (an H_2 receptor antagonist) can block the action of all stimuli under some circumstances. This was accounted for in terms of potentiating interactions at the postreceptor level. According to the alternative, two-cell hypothesis, which has more explanatory power, gastrin and acetylcholine act on parietal cells but also on a second cell type that then releases histamine that further stimulates the parietal cells.

This problem has been thoroughly investigated in several species and discussed in depth by Shankley et al. (1992). Some inter- and even intraspecies specificity was observed in the histamine dependence of the gastrin response. Their overall conclusion is that both models can operate side by side; that histamine released by muscarinic stimulation or gastrin may integrate the local secretory and circulatory responses to these hormones; and that interactions between histamine, acetycholine and gastrin regulate H^+ secretion by the parietal cell itself.

DRUGS USED TO INHIBIT OR NEUTRALISE GASTRIC ACID SECRETION

The principal clinical indications for reducing acid secretion are *peptic ulceration* (both duodenal and gastric), *reflux oesophagitis* (in which gastric juice causes damage to the oesophagus) and the

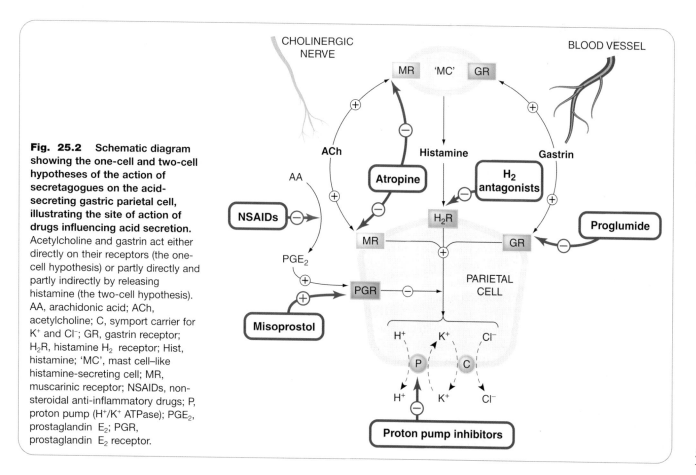

Fig. 25.2 Schematic diagram showing the one-cell and two-cell hypotheses of the action of secretagogues on the acid-secreting gastric parietal cell, illustrating the site of action of drugs influencing acid secretion. Acetylcholine and gastrin act either directly on their receptors (the one-cell hypothesis) or partly directly and partly indirectly by releasing histamine (the two-cell hypothesis). AA, arachidonic acid; ACh, acetylcholine; C, symport carrier for K⁺ and Cl⁻; GR, gastrin receptor; H₂R, histamine H₂ receptor; Hist, histamine; 'MC', mast cell–like histamine-secreting cell; MR, muscarinic receptor; NSAIDs, non-steroidal anti-inflammatory drugs; P, proton pump (H⁺/K⁺ ATPase); PGE₂, prostaglandin E₂; PGR, prostaglandin E₂ receptor.

Zollinger–Ellison syndrome (a rare condition that is caused by a gastrin-producing tumour).

The reason why peptic ulcers develop is not fully understood, although infection of the stomach mucosa with *Helicobacter pylori*[1]—a Gram-negative bacillus that causes chronic gastritis—is now generally considered to be a major cause, especially of duodenal ulcer. Treatment of *H. pylori* infection is discussed below.

Prostaglandins (mainly E_2 and I_2), synthesised in the gastric mucosa mainly by cyclo-oxygenase-1, stimulate mucus and bicarbonate secretion, decrease acid secretion and cause vasodilatation, all of which serve to protect the stomach against damage. This probably explains the ability of many non-specific non-steroidal anti-inflammatory drugs (NSAIDs: inhibitors of prostaglandin formation; see Ch. 14) to cause gastric bleeding and erosions. More selective cyclo-oxygenase-2 inhibitors such as celecoxib and rofecoxib appear to cause less stomach damage (but see Ch. 14 for a discussion of this issue).

Therapy of peptic ulcer and reflux oesophagitis aims to decrease the secretion of gastric acid with H_2 receptor antagonists or proton pump inhibitors, and/or to neutralise secreted acid with antacids (see Huang & Hunt, 2001). These treatments are often coupled with measures to eradicate *H. pylori* (see Horn, 2000).

ANTACIDS

Antacids are the simplest of all the therapies for treating the symptoms of excessive gastric acid secretion. They directly neutralise acid, thus raising the gastric pH; this also has the effect of inhibiting the activity of peptic enzymes, which practically ceases at pH 5. Given in sufficient quantity for long enough, they can produce healing of duodenal ulcers but are less effective for gastric ulcers.

Most antacids in common use are salts of magnesium and aluminium. Magnesium salts cause diarrhoea and aluminium salts constipation, so mixtures of these two can, happily, be used to preserve normal bowel function. Some preparations of these substances (e.g. magnesium trisilicate mixture and some proprietary aluminium preparations) contain high concentrations of sodium and should not be given to patients on a sodium-restricted diet. Numerous antacid preparations are available; a few of the more significant are given below.

Magnesium hydroxide is an insoluble powder that forms magnesium chloride in the stomach. It does not produce systemic alkalosis, because Mg^{2+} is poorly absorbed from the gut. Another salt, **magnesium trisilicate**, is an insoluble powder that reacts slowly with the gastric juice, forming magnesium chloride and colloidal silica. This agent has a prolonged antacid effect, and it also adsorbs pepsin.

Aluminium hydroxide gel forms aluminium chloride in the stomach; when this reaches the intestine, the chloride is released and is reabsorbed. Aluminium hydroxide raises the pH of the gastric juice to about 4, and also adsorbs pepsin. Its action is

gradual, and its effect continues for several hours.[2] Colloidal aluminium hydroxide combines with phosphates in the gastrointestinal tract, and the increased excretion of phosphate in the faeces that occurs results in decreased excretion of phosphate via the kidney. This effect has been used in treating patients with chronic renal failure (see Ch. 24, p. 382).

▼ **Sodium bicarbonate** acts rapidly and is said to raise the pH of gastric juice to about 7.4. Carbon dioxide is liberated, and this causes eructation (belching). The carbon dioxide stimulates gastrin secretion and can result in a secondary rise in acid secretion. Because some sodium bicarbonate is absorbed in the intestine, large doses or frequent administration of this antacid can cause alkalosis, the onset of which can be insidious. To avoid this possibility, sodium bicarbonate should not be prescribed for long-term treatment, nor should it be given to patients who are on a sodium-restricted diet.

Alginates or **simeticone** are sometimes combined with antacids. The former are believed to increase the viscosity and adherence of mucus to the oesophageal mucosa, forming a protective barrier (see also below), whereas the latter is a surface active compound that, by preventing 'foaming', can relieve bloating and flatulence.

The clinical use of antacids is given in the box below.

HISTAMINE H₂ RECEPTOR ANTAGONISTS

The histamine H_2 receptor antagonists competitively inhibit histamine actions at all H_2 receptors, but their main clinical use is

---

> **Clinical use of agents affecting gastric acidity**
>
> - Histamine H_2 receptor antagonists (e.g. **ranitidine**):
>   - *peptic ulcer*
>   - *reflux oesophagitis.*
> - Proton pump inhibitors (e.g. **omeprazole, lansoprasole**):
>   - *peptic ulcer*
>   - *reflux oesophagitis*
>   - as one component of therapy for *Helicobacter pylori* infection
>   - *Zollinger–Ellison* syndrome (a rare condition caused by gastrin-secreting tumours)
> - Antacids (e.g. **magnesium trisilicate, aluminium hydroxide, alginates**):
>   - *dyspepsia*
>   - symptomatic relief in *peptic ulcer* or (alginate) *oesophageal reflux.*
> - **Bismuth chelate**:
>   - as one component of therapy for *H. pylori* infection.

---

[1]Helicobacter pylori infection in the stomach has been classified as a class 1 (definite) carcinogen for gastric cancer.

[2]There was a suggestion–no longer widely believed–that if aluminium was absorbed, it could trigger Alzheimer's disease. In fact, aluminium is not absorbed to any significant extent during administration of aluminium hydroxide, but some perhaps overly cautious practitioners may prefer to use other antacids.

as inhibitors of gastric acid secretion. They can inhibit histamine-, gastrin- and acetylcholine-stimulated acid secretion; pepsin secretion also falls with the reduction in volume of gastric juice. These agents not only decrease both basal and food-stimulated acid secretion by 90% or more, but numerous clinical trials indicate that they also promote healing of duodenal ulcers. However, relapses are likely to follow after cessation of treatment.

The drugs used are cimetidine, **ranitidine** (sometimes in combination with bismuth; see below), **nizatidine** and **famotidine**. The effect of cimetidine on gastric secretion in human subjects is shown in Figure 25.3. The clinical use of H$_2$ receptor antagonists is given in the clinical box on page 388.

Pharmacokinetic aspects and unwanted effects

The drugs are generally given orally and are well absorbed, although preparations for intramuscular and intravenous use are also available (except famotidine). Dosage regimens vary depending on the condition under treatment. Low-dosage over-the-counter formulations of cimetidine, ranitidine and famotidine are available to the general public for short-term uses, without prescription, from pharmacies.

Unwanted effects are rare. Diarrhoea, dizziness, muscle pains, alopecia, transient rashes and *hypergastrinaemia* have been reported. Cimetidine sometimes causes *gynaecomastia* in men and, rarely, a decrease in sexual function. This is probably caused by a modest affinity for androgen receptors. Cimetidine also inhibits cytochrome P450, and can retard the metabolism (and thus potentiate the action) of a range of drugs including oral anticoagulants and tricyclic antidepressants. It can cause confusion in the elderly.

PROTON PUMP INHIBITORS

The first proton pump inhibitor was the substituted benzimidazole **omeprazole**, which irreversibly inhibits the H$^+$/K$^+$ ATPase (the proton pump), the terminal step in the acid secretory pathway (see Figs 25.1 and 25.2). Both basal and stimulated gastric acid secretion (Fig. 25.4) is reduced. The drug is a weak base, and accumulates in the acid environment of the canaliculi of the stimulated parietal cell where it is activated. This preferential accumulation means that it has a specific effect on these cells. Other proton pump inhibitors include **esomeprazole** (the (*S*) isomer of omeprazole), **lansoprazole**, **pantoprazole** and **rabeprazole**. The clinical use of these inhibitors is given in the clinical box on page 388.

Pharmacokinetic aspects and unwanted effects

Oral administration is the most common route of administration, although some injectable preparations are available. Omeprazole is given orally, but as it degrades rapidly at low pH it is administered as capsules containing enteric-coated granules. It is absorbed and, from the blood, passes into the parietal cells and then into the canaliculi. Increased doses give disproportionately higher increases in plasma concentration (possibly because its inhibitory effect on acid secretion improves its own bioavailability). Although its

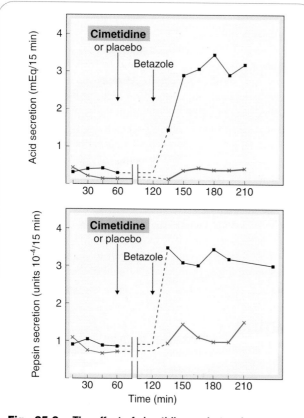

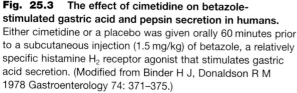

Fig. 25.3 **The effect of cimetidine on betazole-stimulated gastric acid and pepsin secretion in humans.** Either cimetidine or a placebo was given orally 60 minutes prior to a subcutaneous injection (1.5 mg/kg) of betazole, a relatively specific histamine H$_2$ receptor agonist that stimulates gastric acid secretion. (Modified from Binder H J, Donaldson R M 1978 Gastroenterology 74: 371–375.)

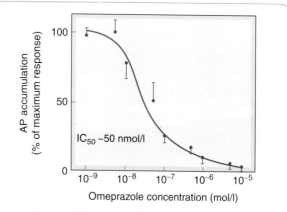

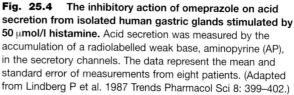

Fig. 25.4 **The inhibitory action of omeprazole on acid secretion from isolated human gastric glands stimulated by 50 μmol/l histamine.** Acid secretion was measured by the accumulation of a radiolabelled weak base, aminopyrine (AP), in the secretory channels. The data represent the mean and standard error of measurements from eight patients. (Adapted from Lindberg P et al. 1987 Trends Pharmacol Sci 8: 399–402.)

half-life is about 1 hour, a single daily dose affects acid secretion for 2–3 days, because it accumulates in the canaliculi and inhibits H^+/K^+ ATPase irreversibly. With daily dosage, there is an increasing antisecretory effect for up to 5 days, after which a plateau is reached.

Unwanted effects of this class of drugs are uncommon. They may include headache, diarrhoea (both sometimes severe) and rashes. Dizziness, somnolence, mental confusion, impotence, gynaecomastia, and pain in muscles and joints have been reported. Proton pump inhibitors should be used with caution in patients with liver disease, or in women who are pregnant or breast feeding. The use of these drugs may 'mask' the symptoms of gastric cancer.

TREATMENT OF *HELICOBACTER PYLORI* INFECTION

Helicobacter pylori infection has been implicated as a causative factor in the production of gastric and, more particularly, duodenal ulcers, as well as a risk factor for gastric cancer. Indeed, some would argue that infectious gastroduodenitis is actually the chief clinical entity with ulcers, and gastric cancer its prominent sequela. Certainly, eradication of *H. pylori* infection promotes rapid and long-term healing of ulcers, and it is routine practice to test for the organism in patients presenting with suggestive symptoms. If the test is positive, then the organism can generally be eradicated with a 1- or 2-week regimen of 'triple therapy'. A further test can be used to confirm eradication.

Triple therapy usually comprises a proton pump inhibitor in combination with the antibacterials **amoxicillin** and **metronidazole** or **clarithromycin**, although other combinations are also used. Sometimes, particularly in the case of the 2-week regimen, bismuth-containing preparations are added. The antibiotics are covered in Chapter 46, and bismuth chelates are considered below. While elimination of the bacillus can produce long-term remission of ulcers, reinfection with the organism can occur.

DRUGS THAT PROTECT THE MUCOSA

Some agents, termed *cytoprotective*, are said to enhance endogenous mucosal protection mechanisms (see above) and/or to provide a physical barrier over the surface of the ulcer.

Bismuth chelate

Bismuth chelate (colloidal bismuth subcitrate, tripotassium dicitratobismuthate) is used in combination regimens to treat *H. pylori*. It has toxic effects on the bacillus, and may also prevent its adherence to the mucosa or inhibit its bacterial proteolytic enzymes. It is also believed to have other mucosa-protecting actions, including coating of the ulcer base, adsorbing pepsin, enhancing local prostaglandin synthesis and stimulating bicarbonate secretion. The small amount of bismuth that is actually absorbed is excreted in the urine. If renal excretion is impaired, the raised plasma concentrations of bismuth can result in encephalopathy.

Unwanted effects include nausea and vomiting, and blackening of the tongue and faeces.

Sucralfate

Sucralfate is a complex of aluminium hydroxide and sulfated sucrose, which releases aluminium in the presence of acid. The residual complex carries a strong negative charge and binds to cationic groups in proteins, glycoproteins, etc. It can form complex gels with mucus, an action that is thought to decrease the degradation of mucus by pepsin and to limit the diffusion of H^+. Sucralfate can also inhibit the action of pepsin and stimulate secretion of mucus, bicarbonate and prostaglandins from the gastric mucosa. All these actions contribute to its mucosa-protecting action.

Sucralfate is given orally, and in the acid environment of the stomach the polymerised product forms a viscous paste; about 30% is still present in the stomach 3 hours after administration. It reduces the absorption of a number of other drugs, including fluoroquinolone antibiotics, **theophylline**, **tetracycline**, **digoxin** and **amitriptyline**. Because it requires an acid environment for activation, antacids given concurrently or prior to its administration will reduce its efficacy.

Unwanted effects are few, the most common being constipation, which occurs in up to 15% of patients treated. Less common effects include dry mouth, nausea, vomiting, headache and rashes. It should be used with caution in pregnancy, when breast feeding, or in patients for whom enteral feeding is in progress.

Misoprostol

Prostaglandins of the E and I series have a generally protective action in the gastrointestinal tract, and a deficiency in endogenous prostaglandin production (after ingestion of a NSAID, for example) may contribute to ulcer formation. **Misoprostol** is a stable analogue of prostaglandin E_1. It is given orally and is used to promote the healing of ulcers or to prevent the gastric damage that can occur with chronic use of NSAIDs. It exerts a direct action on the parietal cell (Fig. 25.2), inhibiting the basal secretion of gastric acid as well as the stimulation of production seen in response to food, histamine, pentagastrin and caffeine. It also increases mucosal blood flow and augments the secretion of mucus and bicarbonate.

Unwanted effects include diarrhoea and abdominal cramps; uterine contractions can also occur, so the drug should not be given during pregnancy (unless deliberately to induce a therapeutic abortion; see Ch. 30). Prostaglandins and NSAIDs are discussed fully in Chapters 13 and 14.

VOMITING

The act of vomiting is a physical event that results in the forceful evacuation of gastric contents through the mouth. It is often preceded by nausea (a feeling of 'queaziness' or of impending vomiting), and may be accompanied by retching (repetitive contraction of the abdominal muscles with or without actual discharge of vomit). Vomiting can be a valuable (indeed life-saving) physiological response to the ingestion of a toxic substance (e.g. alcohol), but it is also an unwanted side effect of many clinically used drugs, notably those used for cancer chemotherapy as well as opioids, general anaesthetics and digoxin. Vomiting also occurs in motion sickness and during early pregnancy, and also accompanies numerous disease states (e.g. migraine) as well as bacterial and viral infections.

THE REFLEX MECHANISM OF VOMITING

Vomiting is regulated centrally by the *vomiting centre* and the *chemoreceptor trigger zone (CTZ)*, both of which lie in the medulla. The CTZ is sensitive to chemical stimuli and is the main site of action of many emetic and antiemetic drugs. The blood–brain barrier in the neighbourhood of the CTZ is relatively permeable, allowing circulating mediators to act directly on this centre. The CTZ also regulates motion sickness, a condition caused by conflicting spatial signals arising from the vestibular apparatus and the eye. Impulses from the CTZ pass to those areas of the brain stem—known collectively as the vomiting centre—that control and integrate the visceral and somatic functions involved in vomiting.

An outline of the pathways involved in the control of vomiting is given in Figure 25.5 and reviewed in detail by Hornby (2001). The main neurotransmitters are acetylcholine, histamine, 5-hydroxytryptamine and dopamine, and receptors for these transmitters have been demonstrated in the relevant areas (see Chs 10–13 and 34). It has been hypothesised that enkephalins (see Ch. 16) are also implicated in the mediation of vomiting, acting possibly at δ (CTZ) or μ (vomiting centre) opioid receptors. Substance P (see Ch. 13) acting at neurokinin-1 receptors in the CTZ, and endocannabinoids (Ch. 15), may also be involved.

ANTIEMETIC DRUGS

Several antiemetic agents are available, and these are generally used for specific conditions, although there may be some overlap. Such drugs are of particular importance as an adjunct to cancer chemotherapy, where the nausea and vomiting produced by many cytotoxics (see Ch. 51) can be almost unendurable.[3] In using drugs to treat the morning sickness of pregnancy, the problem of potential damage to the fetus has always to be borne in mind. In general, *all* drugs should be avoided during the first 3 months of pregnancy, if possible. Details of the main categories of antiemetics are given below, and their main clinical uses are summarised in the box.

Receptor antagonists

Many H_1 (see Ch. 14), muscarinic (see Ch. 10) and 5-HT_3 (see Ch. 12) receptor antagonists exhibit clinically useful antiemetic activity. Of the H_1 antagonists, **cinnarizine**, **cyclizine**, **meclizine** and **promethazine** are the most commonly employed; they are effective against nausea and vomiting arising from many causes, including motion sickness and the presence of irritants in the stomach. None are very effective against substances that act directly on the CTZ. Promethazine has proven of particular benefit for morning sickness of pregnancy, and has been used by NASA to

---

The reflex mechanism of vomiting

- Emetic stimuli include:
  - chemicals or drugs in blood or intestine
  - neuronal input from gastrointestinal tract, labyrinth and central nervous system (CNS).
- Pathways and mediators include:
  - impulses from chemoreceptor trigger zone and various other CNS centres relayed to the vomiting centre
  - chemical transmitters such as histamine, acetylcholine, dopamine and 5-hydroxytryptamine, acting on H_1, muscarinic, D_2 and 5-HT_3 receptors, respectively.
- Antiemetic drugs include:
  - H_1 receptor antagonists (e.g. cyclizine)
  - muscarinic antagonists (e.g. hyoscine)
  - 5-HT_3 receptor antagonists (e.g. ondansetron)
  - D_2 receptor antagonists (e.g. metoclopramide)
  - cannabinoids (e.g. nabilone)
  - neurokinin-1 antagonists (e.g. aprepitant).
- Main side effects of principal antiemetics include:
  - drowsiness and antiparasympathetic effects (hyoscine, nabilone > cinnarizine)
  - dystonic reactions (thiethylperazine > metoclopramide)
  - general CNS disturbances (nabilone)
  - headache, gastrointestinal tract upsets (ondansetron).

Clinical use of antiemetic drugs

- Histamine H_1 receptor antagonists (see also clinical box in Ch. 14, p. 236):
  - **cyclizine**: motion sickness
  - **cinnarizine**: motion sickness, vestibular disorders (e.g. Ménière's disease)
  - **promethazine**: severe morning sickness of pregnancy.
- Muscarinic receptor antagonists:
  - **hyoscine**: motion sickness.
- Dopamine D_2 receptor antagonists:
  - phenothiazines (e.g. **prochlorperazine**): vomiting caused by uraemia, radiation, viral gastroenteritis, severe morning sickness of pregnancy
  - **metoclopramide**: vomiting caused by uraemia, radiation, gastrointestinal disorders, cytotoxic drugs.
- 5-Hydroxytryptamine 5-HT_3 receptor antagonists (e.g. **ondansetron**): cytotoxic drugs or radiation, postoperative vomiting.
- Cannabinoids (e.g. **nabilone**): cytotoxic drugs (see Ch. 15).

---

[3]It was reported that a young, medically qualified patient being treated by combination chemotherapy for sarcoma stated that 'the severity of vomiting at times made the thought of death seem like a welcome relief'.

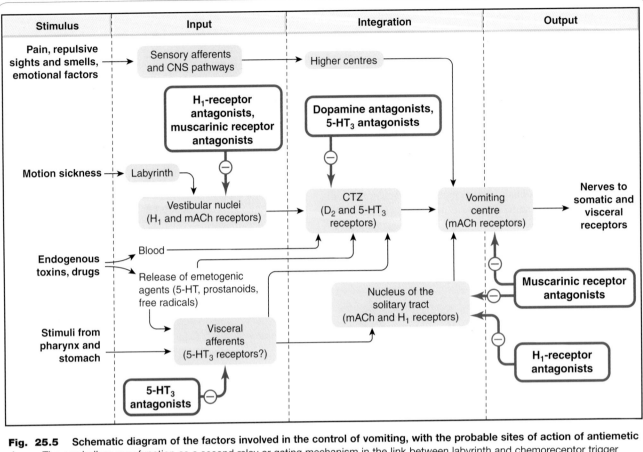

Fig. 25.5 **Schematic diagram of the factors involved in the control of vomiting, with the probable sites of action of antiemetic drugs.** The cerebellum may function as a second relay or gating mechanism in the link between labyrinth and chemoreceptor trigger zone (CTZ; not shown). 5-HT$_3$, 5-hydroxytryptamine type 3; ACh, acetylcholine; D$_2$, dopamine D$_2$; H$_1$, histamine H$_1$; M, muscarinic. (Based partly on a diagram from Borison H L et al. 1981 J Clin Pharmacol 21: 235–295.)

treat space motion sickness. Drowsiness and sedation, while possibly contributing to their clinical efficacy, are the chief unwanted effects.

Muscarinic antagonists are also good general purpose antiemetics. **Hyoscine (scopolamine)** is the most widely used example. It is employed principally for prophylaxis and treatment of motion sickness, and may be administered orally or as a transdermal patch. Dry mouth and blurred vision are the most common unwanted effects. Drowsiness also occurs, but the drug has less sedative action than the antihistamines.

Selective 5-HT$_3$ receptor antagonists, including **ondansetron**, **granisetron**, **tropisetron** and **dolasetron**, are of particular value in preventing and treating postoperative nausea and vomiting, or that caused by radiation therapy or administration of cytotoxic drugs such as **cisplatin**. The primary site of action of these drugs is the CTZ. They may be given orally or by injection (sometimes helpful if nausea is already present).

Unwanted effects such as headache and gastrointestinal upsets are relatively uncommon.

Antipsychotic drugs

Phenothiazines are dealt with in Chapter 38, and only those aspects relevant to the control of vomiting will be considered here. Anti-psychotic phenothiazines, such as **chlorpromazine**, **perphenazine**, **prochlorperazine** and **trifluoperazine**, are effective antiemetics commonly used for treating the more severe manifestations of these disorders, particularly the nausea and vomiting associated with cancer, radiation therapy, cytotoxics, opioids, anaesthetics and other drugs. They can be administered orally, intravenously or by suppository. They act mainly as antagonists of the dopamine D$_2$ receptors in the CTZ (see Fig. 25.5) but may also block histamine and muscarinic receptors.

Unwanted effects are relatively frequent and include sedation (especially chlorpromazine), hypotension, and extrapyramidal symptoms including dystonias and tardive dyskinesia (Ch. 38).

Other antipsychotics, such as **haloperidol** and **levomepromazine** (Ch. 38), also act as D$_2$ antagonists in the CTZ and can be used for acute chemotherapy-induced emesis.

Metoclopramide and domperidone

Metoclopramide is a D$_2$ receptor antagonist (Fig. 25.5), closely related to the phenothiazine group, that acts centrally on the CTZ and also has a peripheral action on the gastrointestinal tract itself, increasing the motility of the oesophagus, stomach and intestine. This not only adds to the antiemetic effect but explains its use in the treatment of gastro-oesophageal reflux (see below), and hepatic and biliary disorders. As metoclopramide also blocks dopamine receptors (see Ch. 37) elsewhere in the central nervous system (CNS), it produces a number of unwanted effects including disorders of movement (more common in children and young adults), fatigue, motor restlessness, spasmodic *torticollis* (involuntary twisting of the neck) and *occulogyric crises* (involuntary upward eye movements). It stimulates prolactin release (see Ch. 28), causing galactorrhoea and disorders of menstruation.

Domperidone is a similar drug often used to treat vomiting due to cytotoxic therapy as well as gastrointestinal symptoms. Unlike metoclopramide, it does not readily penetrate the blood–brain barrier and is consequently less prone to produce central side effects. Both drugs are given orally, have plasma half-lives of 4–5 hours and are excreted in the urine.

Cannabinoids

Anecdotal evidence originally suggested the possibility of using cannabinoids as antiemetics (see Pertwee, 2001). Since that time, synthetic cannabinol derivatives such as **nabilone** have been found to decrease vomiting caused by agents that stimulate the CTZ, and are sometimes effective where other drugs have failed (see Ch. 15, p. 253). The antiemetic effect is antagonised by **naloxone**, which implies that opioid receptors may be important in the mechanism of action. Nabilone is given orally; it is well absorbed from the gastrointestinal tract and is metabolised in many tissues. Its plasma half-life is approximately 120 minutes, and its metabolites are excreted in the urine and faeces.

Unwanted effects are common, especially drowsiness, dizziness and dry mouth. Mood changes and postural hypotension are also fairly frequent. Some patients experience hallucinations and psychotic reactions, resembling the effect of other cannabinoids (see Ch. 15).

Steroids and neurokinin antagonists

High-dose glucocorticoids (particularly **dexamethasone**; see Chs 14 and 28) can also control emesis, especially when this is caused by cytotoxics such as cisplatin. The mechanism of action is not clear. Dexamethasone can be used alone but is frequently deployed in combination with a phenothiazine, ondansetron or the neurokinin-1 antagonist **aprepitant** (Ch. 16). The rationale for investigating the last of these for this indication was based on the idea that, because substance P causes vomiting when injected intravenously and is also found both in gastrointestinal vagal afferent nerves and in the vomiting centre itself, neurokinin-1 antagonists could be effective antiemetics.

THE MOTILITY OF THE GASTROINTESTINAL TRACT

Drugs that alter the motility of the gastrointestinal tract include:

- purgatives, which accelerate the passage of food through the intestine
- agents that increase the motility of the gastrointestinal smooth muscle without causing purgation
- antidiarrhoeal drugs, which decrease motility
- antispasmodic drugs, which decrease smooth muscle tone.

PURGATIVES

The transit of food through the intestine may be hastened by several different types of drugs, including *laxatives*, *faecal softeners* and *stimulant purgatives*. These agents may be used to relieve constipation or to clear the bowel prior to surgery or examination.

Bulk and osmotic laxatives

The *bulk laxatives* include **methylcellulose** and certain plant extracts such as **sterculia**, **agar**, **bran** and **ispaghula husk**. These agents are polysaccharide polymers that are not broken down by the normal processes of digestion in the upper part of the gastrointestinal tract. They form a bulky hydrated mass in the gut lumen promoting peristalsis and improving faecal consistency. They may take several days to work but have no serious unwanted effects.

The *osmotic laxatives* consist of poorly absorbed solutes—the saline purgatives—and **lactulose**. The main salts in use are magnesium sulfate and magnesium hydroxide. By producing an osmotic load, these agents trap increased volumes of fluid in the lumen of the bowel, accelerating the transfer of the gut contents through the small intestine. This results in an abnormally large volume entering the colon, causing distension and purgation within about an hour. Abdominal cramps can occur. The amount of magnesium absorbed after an oral dose is usually too small to have adverse systemic effects, but these salts should be avoided in small children and in patients with poor renal function, in whom they can cause heart block, neuromuscular block or CNS depression. While isotonic or hypotonic solutions of saline purgatives cause purgation, hypertonic solutions can cause vomiting. Sometimes, other sodium salts of **phosphate** and **citrate** are given rectally, by suppository, to relieve constipation.

Lactulose is a semisynthetic disaccharide of fructose and galactose. It is poorly absorbed and produces an effect similar to that of the other osmotic laxatives. It takes 2–3 days to act. *Unwanted effects*, seen with high doses, include flatulence, cramps, diarrhoea and electrolyte disturbance. Tolerance can develop. Another agent, **macrogols**, which consists of inert ethylene glycol polymers, acts in the same way.

Faecal softeners

Docusate sodium is a surface-active compound that acts in the gastrointestinal tract in a manner similar to a detergent and produces softer faeces. It is also a weak stimulant laxative. Other agents that achieve the same effect include **arachis oil**, which is given as an enema, and **liquid paraffin**, although this is now seldom used.

Stimulant laxatives

The stimulant laxative drugs act mainly by increasing electrolyte and hence water secretion by the mucosa, and also by increasing peristalsis—possibly by stimulating enteric nerves. Abdominal cramping may be experienced as a side effect with almost any of these drugs.

Bisacodyl may be given by mouth but is often given by suppository. In the latter case, it stimulates the rectal mucosa, inducing defecation in 15–30 minutes. **Glycerol** suppositories act in the same manner. **Sodium picosulfate** and docusate sodium have similar actions. The former is given orally and is often used in preparation for intestinal surgery or colonoscopy.

Senna and **dantron** are anthroquinone laxatives. The active principle (after hydrolysis of glycosidic linkages in the case of the plant extract, senna) directly stimulates the myenteric plexus, resulting in increased peristalsis and thus defecation. Another member of the family is dantron. As this drug is a skin irritant and may be carcinogenic, it is generally used only in the terminally ill.

Laxatives of any type should not be used when there is obstruction of the bowel. Overuse can lead to an atonic colon where the natural propulsive activity is diminished. In these circumstances, the only way to achieve defecation is to take further amounts of laxatives, so a sort of dependency arises.

DRUGS THAT INCREASE GASTROINTESTINAL MOTILITY

Domperidone is primarily used as an antiemetic (as described above), but it also increases gastrointestinal motility (although the mechanism is unknown). Clinically, it increases lower oesophageal sphincter pressure (thus inhibiting gastro-oesophageal reflux), increases gastric emptying and enhances duodenal peristalsis. It is useful in disorders of gastric emptying and in chronic gastric reflux.

Metoclopramide (also an antiemetic; see above) stimulates gastric motility, causing a marked acceleration of gastric emptying. It is useful in gastro-oesophageal reflux and in disorders of gastric emptying, but is ineffective in paralytic ileus.

Now withdrawn (because it precipitated fatal cardiac arrhythmias), **cisapride** stimulates acetylcholine release in the myenteric plexus in the upper gastrointestinal tract through a 5-HT_4 receptor–mediated effect. This raises oesophageal sphincter pressure and increases gut motility. The drug was used for treating reflux oesophagitis and in disorders of gastric emptying.

ANTIDIARRHOEAL AGENTS

Diarrhoea is the frequent passage of liquid faeces, and this is generally accompanied by abdominal cramps and sometimes nausea and vomiting. It may be viewed as a physiological mechanism for rapidly ridding the gut of poisonous or irritating substances. There are numerous causes, including underlying disease, infection, toxins and even anxiety. It may also arise as a side effect of drug or radiation therapy. Repercussions range from mild discomfort and inconvenience to a medical emergency requiring hospitalisation and parenteral fluid and electrolyte replacement therapy. Globally, acute diarrhoeal disease is one of the principal causes of death in malnourished infants, especially in developing countries where medical care is less accessible.

During an episode of diarrhoea, there is an increase in the motility of the gastrointestinal tract, accompanied by an increased secretion coupled with a decreased absorption of fluid, which leads to a loss of electrolytes (particularly Na^+) and water. Cholera toxins and some other bacterial toxins produce a profound increase in electrolyte and fluid secretion by irreversibly activating the guanine nucleotide regulatory proteins that couple the surface receptors of the mucosal cells to adenylate cyclase (see Ch. 3).

There are three approaches to the treatment of severe acute diarrhoea:

- maintenance of fluid and electrolyte balance
- use of anti-infective agents
- use of spasmolytic or other antidiarrhoeal agents.

The maintenance of fluid and electrolyte balance by means of oral rehydration is the first priority, and wider application of this cheap and simple remedy could save the lives of many infants in the developing world. Many patients require no other treatment. In the ileum, as in parts of the nephron, there is cotransport of Na^+ and glucose across the epithelial cell. The presence of glucose (and some amino acids) therefore enhances Na^+ absorption and thus water uptake. Preparations of sodium chloride and glucose for oral rehydration are available in powder form, ready to be dissolved in water before use.

Many gastrointestinal infections are viral in origin, and because those that are bacterial generally resolve fairly rapidly, the use of anti-infective agents is usually neither necessary nor useful. Other cases may require more aggressive therapy, however. *Campylobacter* sp. is the commonest strain of bacterial organism causing gastroenteritis in the UK, and severe infections may require **erythromycin** or **ciprofloxacin** (Ch. 46). The most common bacterial organisms encountered by travellers include *Escherichia coli*, *Salmonella* and *Shigella*, as well as protozoa such as *Giardia* and *Cryptosporidium* spp. Chemotherapy may be necessary in treating these and other more serious infections.

Other types of antidiarrhoeal drug that mitigate the symptoms of the condition include spasmolytic or antimotility agents, adsorbents, and agents that modify fluid and electrolyte transport. These are dealt with below.

Traveller's diarrhoea

More than 3 million people cross international borders each year. Many travel hopefully, but some 20–50% come back ill, having encountered enterotoxin-producing *E. coli* (the most common cause) or other organisms. Most infections are mild and self-limiting, requiring only oral replacement of fluid and salt, as detailed above. General principles for the treatment of traveller's diarrhoea are detailed by Gorbach (1987), who flippantly (although accurately) observed that 'travel broadens the mind and loosens the bowels'. Up-to-date information on the condition, including the prevalence of infectious organisms around the globe as well as recommended treatment guidelines, is issued in the UK by the National Travel Health Network and Centre (see web links in the reference list).

ANTIMOTILITY AND SPASMOLYTIC AGENTS

The main pharmacological agents that decrease motility are opiates (details in Ch. 41) and muscarinic receptor antagonists (details in Ch. 10). Agents in this latter group are seldom employed as primary therapy for diarrhoea because of their actions on other systems, but small doses of **atropine** are used, combined with **diphenoxylate** (see below). The action of **morphine**, the archetypal opiate, on the alimentary tract is complex; it increases the tone and rhythmic contractions of the intestine but diminishes propulsive activity. The pyloric, ileocolic and anal sphincters are contracted, and the tone of the large intestine is markedly increased. Its overall effect is constipating.

The main opiates used for the symptomatic relief of diarrhoea are **codeine** (a morphine congener), diphenoxylate and **loperamide** (both **pethidine** congeners that do not readily penetrate the blood–brain barrier and are used only for their actions in the gut). All may have unwanted effects including constipation, abdominal cramps, drowsiness and dizziness. Paralytic ileus can also occur. They should not be used in young (< 4 years of age) children.

Loperamide is the drug of first choice for traveller's diarrhoea and is a component of several proprietary antidiarrhoeal medicines. It has a relatively selective action on the gastrointestinal tract and undergoes significant enterohepatic cycling. It reduces the frequency of abdominal cramps, decreases the passage of faeces and shortens the duration of the illness.

Diphenoxylate also lacks morphine-like activity in the CNS, although large doses (25-fold higher) produce typical opioid effects. Preparations of diphenoxylate usually contain atropine as well. Codeine and loperamide have antisecretory actions in addition to their effects on intestinal motility. Cannabinoid receptor agonists also reduce gut motility in animals, most probably by decreasing acetylcholine release from enteric nerves. There have been anecdotal reports of a beneficial effect of cannabis against dysentery and cholera.

Drugs that reduce spasm in the gut are also of value in irritable bowel syndrome and diverticular disease. Muscarinic receptor antagonists are dealt with in Chapter 10. They decrease spasm by inhibiting parasympathetic activity. Agents available include atropine, hyoscine, **propantheline** and **dicycloverine**. The last named is thought to have some additional direct relaxant action on smooth muscle. **Mebeverine**, a derivative of reserpine, has a direct relaxant action on gastrointestinal smooth muscle. Unwanted effects are few.

Adsorbents

Adsorbent agents are used extensively in the symptomatic treatment of diarrhoea, although properly controlled trials proving efficacy have not been carried out. The main preparations used contain kaolin, pectin, chalk, charcoal, methyl cellulose and activated attapulgite (magnesium aluminium silicate). It has been suggested that these agents may act by adsorbing microorganisms or toxins, by altering the intestinal flora or by coating and protecting the intestinal mucosa, but there is no hard evidence for this. They are often given as mixtures with other drugs (e.g. **kaolin and** morphine mixture BP).

DRUGS FOR CHRONIC BOWEL DISEASE

This category comprises *irritable bowel syndrome*, *ulcerative colitis* and *Crohn's disease*. The first of these is characterised by bouts of diarrhoea, constipation or abdominal pain. Approximately one-third of patients fall prey to each of these manifestations. The aetiology of the disease is uncertain, but psychological factors may play a part. Treatment is symptomatic, with loperamide or a laxative. Ulcerative colitis and Crohn's disease

> **Drugs and gastrointestinal tract motility**
>
> - Purgatives include:
>   - bulk laxatives (e.g. **ispaghula** husk, first choice for slow action)
>   - osmotic laxatives (e.g. **lactulose**)
>   - faecal softeners (e.g. **docusate**)
>   - stimulant purgatives (e.g. **senna**).
> - Drugs that can increase motility without purgation:
>   - **domperidone**, used in disorders of gastric emptying.
> - Drugs used to treat diarrhoea:
>   - oral rehydration with isotonic solutions of NaCl plus glucose or starch-based cereal (important in infants)
>   - antimotility agents, for example **loperamide** (unwanted effects: drowsiness and nausea)
>   - absorbents (e.g. **magnesium aluminium silicate**).

are inflammatory disorders, the latter being a granulomatous condition especially affecting the terminal ileum and the colon. Again, both conditions have uncertain aetiology. The following agents are used.

Glucocorticoids

Glucocorticoids are potent anti-inflammatory agents and are dealt with fully in Chapters 14 and 28. The drugs of choice are **prednisolone** or **budesonide**, given orally or locally into the bowel by suppository or enema.

Aminosalicylates

While glucocorticoids are useful for the acute attacks of inflammatory bowel diseases, they are not the ideal for the long-term treatment (because of their side effects). Maintenance of remission in both ulcerative colitis and Crohn's is generally achieved using the aminosalicylates, although they are less useful in the latter condition.

Sulfasalazine

Sulfasalazine is a combination of the sulfonamide **sulfapyridine** with **5-aminosalicylic acid**. The latter forms the active moiety when it is released in the colon. Its mechanism of action is obscure. It may reduce inflammation by scavenging free radicals, by inhibiting prostaglandin and leukotriene production, and/or by decreasing neutrophil chemotaxis and superoxide generation. Its unwanted effects are diarrhoea, salicylate sensitivity and interstitial nephritis. 5-aminosalicylic acid is not absorbed but the sulfapyridine moiety, which seems to be therapeutically inert in this instance, is absorbed, and its unwanted effects are those associated with the sulfonamides (see Ch. 46).

Newer compounds in this class, which presumably share a similar mechanism of action, include **mesalazine** (5-aminosalicylic acid itself), **olsalazine** (two molecules of 5-aminosalicylic acid linked by a diazo bond, which is hydrolysed by colonic bacteria) and **balsalazide** (4-aminosalicylic acid).

Other drugs

The immunosuppressants **azathioprine** and **6-mercaptopurine** (see Ch. 14) are also sometimes used in patients with severe disease. Recently, the cytokine inhibitor **infliximab** (see Ch. 14) has been used with success for the treatment of inflammatory bowel diseases. The drug is expensive, and in the UK its use is restricted to severe Crohn's disease that is unresponsive to glucocorticoids or immunomodulators. The antiallergy drug **sodium cromoglicate** is sometimes used for treating gastrointestinal symptoms associated with food allergies.

DRUGS AFFECTING THE BILIARY SYSTEM

Drugs used to treat cholesterol cholelithiasis

The commonest pathological condition of the biliary tract is cholesterol *cholelithiasis*, i.e. the formation of gallstones with high cholesterol content. Surgery is generally the preferred option, but there are orally active drugs that dissolve non-calcified 'radiolucent' cholesterol gallstones. The principal agent is **ursodeoxycholic acid**, a minor constituent of human bile (but the main bile acid in the bear, hence *urso*). Diarrhoea is the main unwanted effect.

Drugs affecting biliary spasm

Biliary colic, the pain produced by the passage of gallstones through the bile duct, can be very intense, and immediate relief may be required. Morphine relieves the pain effectively, but it may have an undesirable local effect because it constricts the *sphincter of Oddi* and raises the pressure in the bile duct. **Buprenorphine** may be preferable. Pethidine has similar actions, although it relaxes other smooth muscle, for example that of the ureter. Atropine is commonly employed to relieve biliary spasm because it has antispasmodic action and may be used in conjunction with morphine. The nitrates (see Ch. 17) can produce a marked fall of intrabiliary pressure and may be used to relieve biliary spasm.

REFERENCES AND FURTHER READING

Seminal and classic paper

Black J W, Duncan W A M, Durant C J et al. 1972 Definition and antagonism of histamine H$_2$-receptors. Nature 236: 385–390 (*Seminal paper outlining the pharmacological approach to inhibition of acid secretion through antagonism at an alternative histamine receptor*)

Innervation and hormones of the gastrointestinal tract

Hansen M B 2003 The enteric nervous system II: gastrointestinal functions. Pharmacol Toxicol 92: 249–257 (*Small review on the role of the enteric nervous system in the control of gastrointestinal motility, secretory activity, blood flow and immune status; easy to read*)

Sanger G J 2004 Neurokinin NK$_1$ and NK$_3$ receptors as targets for drugs to treat gastrointestinal motility disorders and pain. Br J Pharmacol 141: 1303–1312. (*Useful review that deals with the present and potential future uses of neurokinin antagonists in gastrointestinal physiology and pathology*)

Spiller R 2002 Serotonergic modulating drugs for functional gastrointestinal diseases. Br J Clin Pharmacol 54: 11–20 (*An excellent and 'easily digestible' article describing the latest thinking on the use of 5-hydroxytryptamine agonists and antagonists in gastrointestinal function; useful diagrams*)

Van Oudenhove L, Demyttenaere K, Tack J, Aziz Q 2004 Central nervous system involvement in functional gastrointestinal disorders. Best Pract Res Clin Gastroenterol 18: 663–680 (*Small review that focuses on the role of the CNS—as revealed by imaging studies—in regulating gastrointestinal function; also discusses the relationship between psychiatric disorders and gastrointestinal disorders*)

Gastric secretion

Shankley N P, Welsh N J, Black J W 1992. Histamine dependence of pentagastrin-stimulated acid secretion in rats. Yale J Biol Med 65: 613–619 (*Paper that critically examines the one-cell and two-cell hypotheses of gastric acid secretion*)

Drugs in gastric disorders

Axon A, Forman D 1997 *Helicobacter* gastroduodenitis: a serious infectious disease. Br Med J 314: 1430–1431 (*Editorial comment*)

Bateman D N 1997 Proton-pump inhibitors: three of a kind? Lancet 349: 1637–1638 (*Editorial commentary*)

Blaser M J 1996 The bacteria behind ulcers. Sci Am Feb: 92–97 (*Simple coverage, very good diagrams*)

Blaser M J 1998 *Helicobacter pylori* and gastric disease. Br Med J 316: 1507–1510 (*Succinct review; emphasis on future developments*)

Horn J H 2000 The proton-pump inhibitors: similarities and differences. Clin Ther 22: 266–280 (*Excellent overview*)

Huang J Q, Hunt R H 2001 Pharmacological and pharmacodynamic essentials of H$_2$-receptor antagonists and proton pump inhibitors for the practising physician. Baillières Best Pract Res Clin Gastroenterol 15: 355–370

Klotz U 2000 The role of aminosalicylates at the beginning of the new millennium in the treatment of chronic inflammatory bowel disease. Eur J Clin Pharmacol 56: 353–362

Pertwee R G 2001 Cannabinoids and the gastrointestinal tract. Gut 48: 859–867

Rauws E A J, van der Hulst R W M 1998 The management of *H. pylori* infection. Br Med J 316: 162–163 (*Editorial commentary*)

Yeomans N D, Tulassy Z et al. 1998 A comparison of omeprazole with ranitidine for ulcers associated with nonsteroidal antiinflammatory drugs. N Engl J Med 338: 719–726

Vomiting

American Gastroenterological Association 2001 Technical review on nausea and vomiting. Gastroenterology 120: 263–286

Hesketh P J 2001 Potential role of the NK$_1$ receptor antagonists in chemotherapy-induced nausea and vomiting. Support Care Cancer 9: 350–354

Hornby P J 2001 Central neurocircuitry associated with emesis. Am J Med 111: 106S–112S (*Comprehensive review of central control of vomiting*)

Tramèr M R, Moore R et al. 1997 A quantitative systematic review of ondansetron in treatment of established postoperative nausea and vomiting. Br Med J 314: 1088–1092

Yates B J, Miller A D, Lucot J B 1998 Physiological basis and pharmacology of motion sickness: an update. Brain Res Bull 5: 395–406 (*Good account of the mechanisms underlying motion sickness and its treatment*)

Motility of the gastrointestinal tract

De Las Casas C, Adachi J, Dupont H 1999 Travellers' diarrhoea. Aliment Pharmacol Ther 13: 1373–1378 (*Review article*)

Gorbach S L 1987 Bacterial diarrhoea and its treatment. Lancet II: 1378–1382

Huizinga J D, Thuneberg L et al. 1997 Interstitial cells of Cajal as targets for pharmacological intervention in gastrointestinal motor disorders. Trends Pharmacol Sci 18: 393–403

The biliary system

Bateson M C 1997 Bile acid research and applications. Lancet 349: 5–6

Useful web resources

http://www.nathnac.org (*This is the site for the UK Health Protection Agency's National Travel Health Network and Centre. There are two components to the site, one for lay people and one for health professionals. Click on the latter and navigate to the* Travellers' diarrhoea *article for current information and advice.*)

The endocrine pancreas and the control of blood glucose

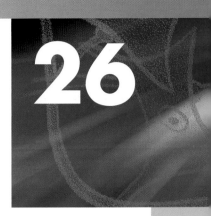

26

OVERVIEW

Insulin is the main hormone controlling intermediary metabolism. Its most obvious acute effect is to lower blood glucose. Reduced (or absent) secretion of insulin, often coupled with reduced sensitivity to its action (insulin resistance), causes diabetes mellitus, the prevalence of which is rapidly increasing to epidemic proportions. The consequences of diabetes are dire—especially complications of atherosclerosis, kidney failure and blindness.

In this chapter, we describe pancreatic hormones, emphasising insulin and the control of blood glucose. The second part of the chapter is devoted to diabetes mellitus and its treatment with drugs—insulins and the orally active hypoglycaemic agents. Oral hypoglycaemic drugs include biguanides, α-glucosidase inhibitors, sulfonylureas and other drugs that stimulate insulin secretion, and the thiazolidinediones.

PANCREATIC ISLET HORMONES

The islets of Langerhans contain four main cell types, all of which secrete peptide hormones: B (or β) cells secrete *insulin*, A cells secrete *glucagon*, D cells secrete *somatostatin* and PP cells secrete *pancreatic polypeptide* (the function of which is unknown). The core of each islet contains mainly the predominant B cells surrounded by a mantle of A cells interspersed with D cells or PP cells (see Fig. 26.1). In addition to insulin, B cells secrete a peptide known as *islet amyloid polypeptide* or *amylin*, which delays gastric emptying and opposes insulin by stimulating glycogen breakdown in striated muscle. Glucagon also opposes insulin, increasing blood glucose and stimulating protein breakdown in muscle. Somatostatin inhibits secretion of insulin and of glucagon. It is widely distributed outside the pancreas and is also released from the hypothalamus, inhibiting the release of growth hormone from the pituitary (p. 422).

INSULIN

Insulin was the first protein for which an amino acid sequence was determined (by Sanger's group in Cambridge in 1955). It consists of two peptide chains (A and B, of 21 and 30 amino acid residues, respectively).

SYNTHESIS AND SECRETION

Like other peptide hormones (see Ch. 16), insulin is synthesised as a precursor (preproinsulin) in the rough endoplasmic reticulum. Preproinsulin is transported to the Golgi apparatus, where it undergoes proteolytic cleavage first to proinsulin and then to insulin plus a fragment of uncertain function called C-peptide.[1] Insulin and C-peptide are stored in granules in B cells, and are normally cosecreted by exocytosis in equimolar amounts together with smaller and variable amounts of proinsulin. The main factor controlling the synthesis and secretion of insulin is the blood glucose concentration (Fig. 26.1). B cells respond both to the absolute glucose concentration and to the rate of change of blood glucose. Other stimuli to insulin release include amino acids (particularly arginine and leucine), fatty acids, the parasympathetic nervous system, peptide hormones for the gut (see below) and drugs that act on *sulfonylurea receptors*.

There is a steady basal release of insulin and also a response to an increase in blood glucose. This response has two phases: an initial rapid phase reflecting release of stored hormone, and a slower, delayed phase reflecting both continued release of stored hormone and new synthesis (Fig. 26.2). The response is abnormal in diabetes mellitus, as discussed later.

ATP-sensitive potassium channels (K_{ATP}; Ch. 4, pp. 63-64) determine the resting membrane potential in B cells. Glucose

---

[1]Not to be confused with C-reactive peptide, which is an acute phase reactant used clinically as a marker of inflammation (Ch. 13).

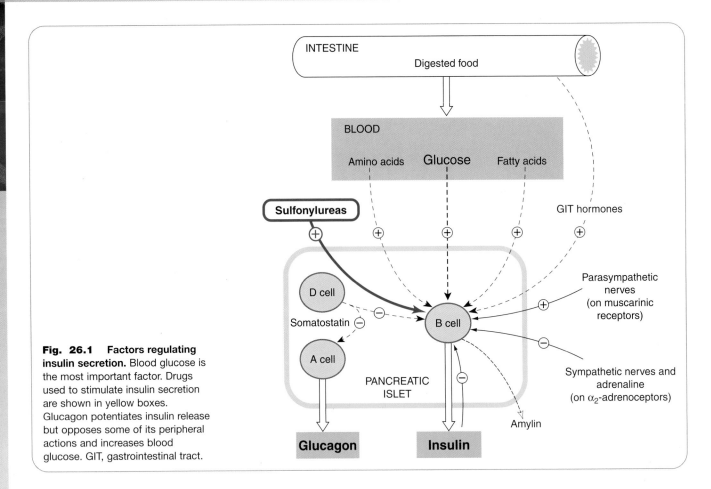

Fig. 26.1 Factors regulating insulin secretion. Blood glucose is the most important factor. Drugs used to stimulate insulin secretion are shown in yellow boxes. Glucagon potentiates insulin release but opposes some of its peripheral actions and increases blood glucose. GIT, gastrointestinal tract.

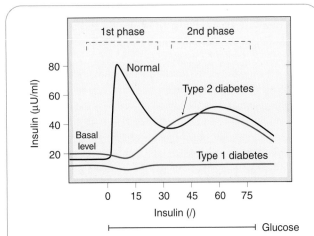

Fig. 26.2 Schematic diagram of the two-phase release of insulin in response to a constant glucose infusion. The first phase is missing in type 2 (non–insulin-dependent) diabetes mellitus, and both are missing in type 1 (insulin-dependent) diabetes mellitus. The first phase is also produced by amino acids, sulfonylureas, glucagon and gastrointestinal tract hormones. (Data from Pfeifer et al. 1981 Am J Med 70: 579–588.)

enters B cells via a membrane transporter called Glut-2, and its subsequent metabolism via glucokinase (the rate-limiting enzyme that acts as the 'glucose sensor' linking insulin secretion to extracellular glucose) and glycolysis increases intracellular ATP. This blocks K_{ATP} channels, causing membrane depolarisation and opening of voltage-dependent calcium channels, leading to Ca^{2+} influx. The resulting increase in cytoplasmic Ca^{2+} triggers insulin secretion, but only in the presence of amplifying messengers including diacylglycerol, non-esterified arachidonic acid (which facilitates further Ca^{2+} entry), and 12-lipoxygenase products of arachidonic acid (mainly *12-S-hydroxyeicosatetraenoic acid* or *12-S-HETE*; see Ch. 13). Phospholipases are commonly activated by Ca^{2+}, but free arachidonic acid is liberated in B cells by an ATP-sensitive Ca^{2+}-insensitive (ASCI) phospholipase A_2. Consequently, in B cells, Ca^{2+} entry and arachidonic acid production are both driven by ATP, linking cellular energy status to insulin secretion.

▼ Many gastrointestinal hormones influence insulin secretion, including *gastrin, secretin, cholecystokinin, gastric inhibitory polypeptide (GIP), glucagon-like peptide (GLP)* and GLP_1 (the amide of a fragment of GLP), all of which stimulate insulin secretion. They are released by eating. This explains why oral glucose causes greater insulin release than does the same amount of glucose administered intravenously. These hormones (in particular GIP and GLP_1) provide an anticipatory signal from the gastrointestinal tract to the islets, and offer some novel prospects for treating diabetes.

The GLP1 is rapidly inactivated. Continuous infusion improves diabetic control but is impractical for routine use. Alternative strategies include the use of stable analogues such as **exenatide**, a GLP$_1$ agonist that was recently approved in the USA, or of drugs that antagonise the dipeptidase enzyme (DPP-IV) that inactivates GLP1.

Insulin release is *inhibited* by the sympathetic nervous system (Fig. 26.1). *Adrenaline (epinephrine)* increases blood glucose by inhibiting insulin release (via α_2 adrenoceptors) and by promoting glycogenolysis via β_2 adrenoceptors in striated muscle and liver. Several peptides, including somatostatin, galanin (an endogenous K_{ATP} activator) and amylin, also inhibit insulin release.

About one-fifth of the insulin stored in the pancreas of the human adult is secreted daily. Circulating insulin is measured by immunoassay, but this may give an overestimate because many insulin antibodies cross-react with proinsulin and its less active degradation products. The plasma insulin concentration after an overnight fast is 20–50 pmol/l. Plasma insulin concentration is reduced in patients with type 1 (insulin-dependent) diabetes mellitus (see below), and markedly increased in patients with insulinomas (uncommon functioning tumours of B cells), as is C-peptide, with which it is coreleased.[2] It is also raised in obesity and other normoglycaemic insulin-resistant states.

ACTIONS

Insulin is the main hormone controlling intermediary metabolism, having actions on liver, muscle and fat (Table 26.1). It is an anabolic

---

[2]Insulin for injection does not contain C-peptide, which therefore provides a means of distinguishing endogenous from exogenous insulin. This is used to differentiate insulinoma (an insulin-secreting tumour causing high circulating insulin with high C-peptide) from surreptitious injection of insulin (high insulin, normal or low C-peptide). Deliberate induction of hypoglycaemia by self-injection with insulin is a well-recognised, if unusual, manifestation of psychiatric disorder, especially in health professionals—it has also been used in murder.

hormone: its overall effect is to conserve fuel by facilitating the uptake and storage of glucose, amino acids and fats after a meal. Acutely, it reduces blood sugar. Consequently, a *fall* in plasma insulin increases blood glucose. The biochemical pathways through which insulin exerts its effects are summarised in Figure 26.3, and molecular aspects of its mechanism are discussed below.

Effect of insulin on carbohydrate metabolism

Insulin influences glucose metabolism in most tissues, especially the liver, where it inhibits glycogenolysis (glycogen breakdown) and gluconeogenesis (synthesis of glucose from non-carbohydrate sources) while stimulating glycogen synthesis. It also increases glucose utilisation (glycolysis), but the overall effect is to increase hepatic glycogen stores.

In muscle, unlike liver, uptake of glucose is slow and is the rate-limiting step in carbohydrate metabolism. The main effects of insulin are to increase facilitated transport of glucose via a transporter called Glut-4, and to stimulate glycogen synthesis and glycolysis.

Insulin increases glucose uptake by Glut-4 in adipose tissue as well as in muscle, enhancing glucose metabolism. One of the main end products of glucose metabolism in adipose tissue is glycerol, which is esterified with fatty acids to form triglycerides, thereby affecting fat metabolism (see below and Table 26.1).

Effect of insulin on fat metabolism

Insulin increases synthesis of fatty acid and triglyceride in adipose tissue and in liver. It inhibits lipolysis, partly via dephosphorylation (and hence inactivation) of lipases (Table 26.1). It also inhibits the lipolytic actions of adrenaline, growth hormone and glucagon by opposing their actions on adenylate cyclase.

Effect of insulin on protein metabolism

Insulin stimulates uptake of amino acids into muscle and increases protein synthesis. It also decreases protein catabolism and inhibits oxidation of amino acids in the liver.

Table 26.1 Effects of insulin on carbohydrate, fat and protein metabolism

Type of metabolism	Liver cells	Fat cells	Muscle
Carbohydrate metabolism	↓ Gluconeogenesis	↑ Glucose uptake	↑ Glucose uptake
	↓ Glycogenolysis	↑ Glycerol synthesis	↑ Glycolysis
	↑ Glycolysis		↑ Glycogenesis
	↑ Glycogenesis		
Fat metabolism	↑ Lipogenesis	↑ Synthesis of triglycerides	–
	↓ Lipolysis	↑ Fatty acid synthesis	
		↓ Lipolysis	
Protein metabolism	↓ Protein breakdown	–	↑ Amino acid uptake
			↑ Protein synthesis

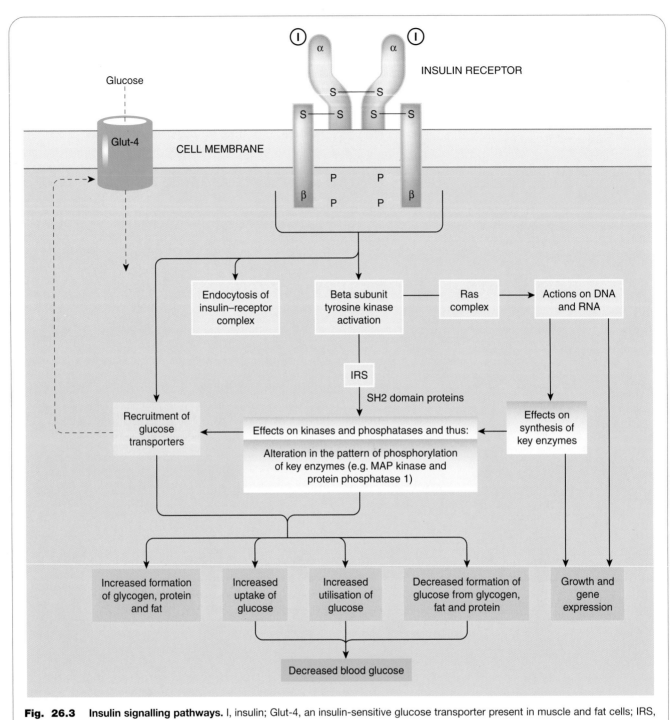

Fig. 26.3 **Insulin signalling pathways.** I, insulin; Glut-4, an insulin-sensitive glucose transporter present in muscle and fat cells; IRS, insulin receptor substrate (several forms: 1–4).

Other metabolic effects of insulin

Other metabolic effects of insulin include transport into cells of K^+,[3] Ca^{2+}, nucleosides and inorganic phosphate.

Long-term effects of insulin

In addition to its rapid effects on metabolism, exerted via altered activity of enzymes and transport proteins, insulin has long-term actions via altered enzyme synthesis. It is an important anabolic hormone during fetal development. It stimulates cell proliferation and is implicated in somatic and visceral growth and development.

▼ Mitogenic actions of insulin are of great concern in the development of insulin analogues, because these are intended for long-term use and

---

[3]This action is exploited in the emergency treatment of hyperkalaemia by intravenous glucose with insulin (see Ch. 24, p. 382).

because mammary tumours develop in rats given one long-acting insulin analogue known as B10-asp insulin.

MECHANISM OF ACTION

Insulin binds to a specific receptor on the surface of its target cells. The receptor is a large transmembrane glycoprotein complex belonging to the kinase-linked type 3 receptor superfamily (Ch. 3, pp. 43-46) and consisting of two α and two β subunits (Fig. 26.3). Occupied receptors aggregate into clusters, which are subsequently internalised in vesicles, resulting in down-regulation. Internalised insulin is degraded in lysosomes, but the receptors are recycled to the plasma membrane.

▼ The signal transduction mechanisms that link receptor binding to the biological effects of insulin are complex. Receptor autophosphorylation —the first step in signal transduction—is a consequence of dimerisation, allowing each receptor to phosphorylate the other, as explained in Chapter 3.

Insulin receptor substrate (IRS) proteins undergo rapid tyrosine phosphorylation specifically in response to insulin and insulin-like growth factor-1 but not to other growth factors. The best characterised substrate is IRS-1, which contains 22 tyrosine residues that are potential phosphorylation sites. It interacts with proteins that contain a so-called SH2 domain (see Ch. 3, Fig. 3.15), thereby passing on the insulin signal. Knockout mice lacking IRS-1 are hyporesponsive to insulin (insulin-resistant) but do not become diabetic because of robust B-cell compensation with increased insulin secretion. By contrast, mice lacking IRS-2 fail to compensate and develop overt diabetes, implicating the IRS-2 gene as a candidate for human type 2 diabetes (IRS proteins are reviewed by Lee & White, 2004). Activation of phosphatidylinositol 3-kinase by interaction of its SH2 domain with phosphorylated IRS has several important effects, including recruitment of insulin-sensitive glucose transporters (Glut-4) from the Golgi apparatus to the plasma membrane in muscle and fat cells.

The longer-term actions of insulin entail effects on DNA and RNA, mediated partly at least by the Ras signalling complex. Ras is a protein that regulates cell growth and cycles between an active GTP-bound form and an inactive GDP-bound form (see Chs 3 and 51). Insulin shifts the equilibrium in favour of the active form, and initiates a phosphorylation cascade that results in activation of mitogen-activated protein kinase, which in turn activates several nuclear transcription factors, leading to the expression of genes that are involved both with cell growth and with intermediary metabolism. Regulation of the rate of mRNA transcription by insulin provides an important means of modulating enzyme activity.

Insulin for treatment of diabetes mellitus is considered below.

GLUCAGON

Glucagon is a single-chain polypeptide of 21 amino acid residues.

SYNTHESIS AND SECRETION

Glucagon is synthesised mainly in the A cell of the islets, but also in the upper gastrointestinal tract. It has considerable structural homology with other gastrointestinal tract hormones, including *secretin, vasoactive intestinal peptide* and *GIP* (see Ch. 25).

One of the main physiological stimuli to glucagon secretion is the concentration of amino acids, in particular L-arginine, in plasma. Therefore an increase in secretion follows ingestion of a high-protein meal, but compared with insulin there is relatively little change in plasma glucagon concentrations throughout the day.

Endocrine pancreas and blood glucose

- Islets of Langerhans secrete insulin from B (or β) cells, glucagon from A cells and somatostatin from D cells.
- Many factors stimulate insulin secretion, but the main one is blood glucose.
- Insulin has essential metabolic actions as a fuel storage hormone and also affects cell growth and differentiation. It decreases blood glucose by:
  — increasing glucose uptake into muscle and fat via Glut-4
  — increasing glycogen synthesis
  — decreasing gluconeogenesis
  — decreasing glycogen breakdown.
- Glucagon is a fuel-mobilising hormone, stimulating gluconeogenesis and glycogenolysis, also lipolysis and proteolysis. It increases blood sugar and also increases the force of contraction of the heart.
- Diabetes mellitus is a chronic metabolic disorder in which there is hyperglycaemia. There are two main types:
  — type 1 (insulin-dependent) diabetes, with an absolute deficiency of insulin
  — type 2 (non–insulin-dependent) diabetes, with a relative deficiency of insulin associated with reduced sensitivity to its action (insulin resistance).

Glucagon secretion is stimulated by low and inhibited by high concentrations of glucose and fatty acids in the plasma. Sympathetic nerve activity and circulating adrenaline stimulate glucagon release via β adrenoceptors. Parasympathetic nerve activity also increases secretion, whereas somatostatin, released from D cells adjacent to the glucagon-secreting A cells in the periphery of the islets, inhibits glucagon release.[4]

ACTIONS

Glucagon increases blood glucose and causes breakdown of fat and protein. It acts on specific G-protein–coupled receptors to stimulate adenylate cyclase, and consequently its actions are somewhat similar to β adrenoceptor–mediated actions of adrenaline. Unlike adrenaline, however, its metabolic effects are more pronounced than its cardiovascular actions. Glucagon is proportionately more active on liver, while the metabolic actions of adrenaline are more pronounced on muscle and fat. Glucagon stimulates glycogen breakdown and gluconeogenesis, and inhibits glycogen synthesis and glucose oxidation. Its metabolic actions on target tissues are thus the opposite of those of insulin. Glucagon increases

---

[4]**Octreotide**, a somatostatin analogue (see p. 422), is used to treat the syndrome (which includes relatively mild hyperglycaemia but profound muscle catabolism) caused by rare glucagon-secreting tumours.

the rate and force of contraction of the heart, although less markedly than adrenaline.

Clinical uses of glucagon are summarised in the box.

SOMATOSTATIN

Somatostatin is secreted by the D cells of the islets. It is also generated in the hypothalamus, where it acts to inhibit the release of growth hormone (see Ch. 28). In the islet, it inhibits release of insulin and of glucagon. **Octreotide** is a long-acting analogue of somatostatin (see above). It inhibits release of a number of hormones, and is used clinically to relieve symptoms from several uncommon gastroenteropancreatic endocrine tumours, and for treatment of acromegaly[5] (the endocrine disorder caused by a functioning tumour of cells that secrete growth hormone from the anterior pituitary; see Ch. 28).

AMYLIN (ISLET AMYLOID POLYPEPTIDE)

▼ The term *amyloid* refers to amorphous protein deposits in different tissues that occur in a variety of diseases, including several neurodegenerative conditions (see Ch. 35). Amyloid deposits occur in the pancreas of patients with diabetes mellitus, although it is not known if this is functionally important. The major component of pancreatic amyloid is a 37–amino acid residue peptide known as islet amyloid polypeptide or amylin. This is stored with insulin in secretory granules in B cells and is cosecreted with insulin. Amylin delays gastric emptying. Supraphysiological concentrations stimulate the breakdown of glycogen to lactate in striated muscle. Amylin also inhibits insulin secretion (Fig. 26.1). It is structurally related to calcitonin (see Ch. 31) and has weak calcitonin-like actions on calcium metabolism and osteoclast activity. It is also about 50% identical with calcitonin gene–related peptide (CGRP; see Ch. 16), and large intravenous doses cause vasodilatation, presumably by an action on CGRP receptors. Whether amylin has a role in the physiological control of glucose metabolism is controversial, but there is interest in the therapeutic potential of amylin agonists (such as **pramlintide,** an analogue with three proline substitutions that reduce its tendency to aggregate into insoluble fibrils)—see Schmitz et al. (2004) for a review.

Clinical uses of glucagon

- **Glucagon** can be given intramuscularly or subcutaneously as well as intravenously.
- Treatment of *hypoglycaemia* in unconscious patients (who cannot drink); unlike intravenous glucose, it can be administered by non-medical personnel (e.g. spouses or ambulance crew). It is useful if obtaining intravenous access is difficult.
- Treatment of *acute cardiac failure* precipitated by β-adrenoceptor antagonists.

CONTROL OF BLOOD GLUCOSE

Glucose is the obligatory source of energy for the brain, and physiological control of blood glucose reflects the need to maintain adequate fuel supplies in the face of intermittent food intake and variable metabolic demands. More fuel is made available by feeding than is immediately required, and excess calories are stored as glycogen or fat. During fasting, these energy stores need to be mobilised in a regulated manner. The most important regulatory hormone is insulin, the actions of which are described above. Increased blood sugar stimulates insulin secretion, whereas reduced blood sugar reduces insulin secretion. Hypoglycaemia, caused by excessive insulin, not only reduces insulin secretion but also elicits secretion of an array of 'counter-regulatory' hormones, including *glucagon, adrenaline, glucocorticoids* and *growth hormone*, all of which increase blood glucose. Their main effects on glucose uptake and carbohydrate metabolism are summarised and contrasted with those of insulin in Table 26.2.

DIABETES MELLITUS

Diabetes mellitus is a chronic metabolic disorder characterised by a high blood glucose concentration—hyperglycaemia (fasting plasma glucose > 7.0 mmol/l, or plasma glucose > 11.1 mmol/l 2 hours after a meal)—caused by insulin deficiency, often combined with insulin resistance. Hyperglycaemia occurs because of uncontrolled hepatic glucose output and reduced uptake of glucose by skeletal muscle with reduced glycogen synthesis. When the renal threshold for glucose reabsorption is exceeded, glucose spills over into the urine (glycosuria) and causes an osmotic diuresis (polyuria), which, in turn, results in dehydration, thirst and increased drinking (polydipsia). Insulin deficiency causes wasting through increased breakdown and reduced synthesis of proteins. *Diabetic ketoacidosis* is an acute emergency. It develops in the absence of insulin because of accelerated breakdown of fat to acetyl-CoA, which, in the absence of aerobic carbohydrate metabolism, is converted to acetoacetate and β-hydroxybutyrate (which cause acidosis) and acetone (a ketone).

Various complications develop as a consequence of the metabolic derangements in diabetes, often over many years. Many of these are the result of disease of blood vessels, either large (macrovascular disease) or small (microangiopathy). Dysfunction of vascular endothelium (see Ch. 20, p. 321) is an early and critical event in the development of vascular complications. Oxygen-derived free radicals, protein kinase C and non-enzymic products of glucose and albumin (called *advanced glycation end products*) have been implicated. *Macrovascular disease* consists of accelerated atheroma (Ch. 21) and its thrombotic complications (Ch. 22), which are commoner and more severe in diabetic patients. *Microangiopathy* is a distinctive feature of diabetes mellitus and particularly affects the retina, kidney and peripheral nerves. Diabetes mellitus is the commonest cause of chronic renal failure, which itself represents a huge and rapidly increasing problem, the costs of which to society as well as to individual patients are staggering. Coexistent hypertension promotes progressive renal damage, and treatment of hypertension slows the progression of diabetic

---

[5]Octreotide is used either short term before surgery on the pituitary tumour, or while waiting for radiotherapy of the tumour to take effect, or if other treatments have been ineffective.

Table 26.2 The effect of hormones on blood glucose

Hormone	Main actions	Main stimulus for secretion	Main effect
Main regulatory hormone			
Insulin	↑ Glucose uptake ↑ Glycogen synthesis ↓ Glycogenolysis ↓ Gluconeogenesis	Acute rise in blood glucose glucose	↓ Blood glucose
Main counter-regulatory hormones			
Glucagon	↑ Glycogenolysis ↑ Glyconeogenesis	Hypoglycaemia (i.e. blood glucose < 3 mmol/l), (e.g. with exercise, stress, high protein meals), etc.	↑ Blood glucose
Adrenaline (epinephrine)	↑ Glycogenolysis		
Glucocorticoids	↓ Glucose uptake ↑ Gluconeogenesis ↓ Glucose uptake and utilisation		
Growth hormone	↓ Glucose uptake		

nephropathy and reduces myocardial infarction. *Angiotensin-converting enzyme inhibitors* or *angiotensin receptor antagonists* (Ch. 19) are more effective in preventing diabetic nephropathy than other antihypertensive drugs, perhaps because they prevent fibroproliferative actions of angiotensin II and aldosterone.

Diabetic neuropathy is associated with accumulation of osmotically active metabolites of glucose, produced by the action of aldose reductase, but *aldose reductase inhibitors* have been disappointing as therapeutic drugs (see Chung & Chung, 2005, for a review).

There are two main types of diabetes mellitus:

- type 1 diabetes (previously known as insulin-dependent diabetes mellitus—IDDM—or juvenile-onset diabetes)
- type 2 diabetes (previously known as non–insulin-dependent diabetes mellitus—NIDDM—or maturity-onset diabetes).

In type 1 diabetes, there is an absolute deficiency of insulin resulting from autoimmune destruction of B cells. Without insulin treatment, such patients will ultimately die with diabetic ketoacidosis.

▼ *Type 1* diabetic patients are usually young (children or adolescents) and not obese when they first develop symptoms. There is an inherited predisposition, with a 10-fold increased incidence in first-degree relatives of an index case, and strong associations with particular histocompatibility antigens (HLA types). Studies of identical twins have shown that genetically predisposed individuals must additionally be exposed to an environmental factor such as viral infection (e.g. with coxsackievirus or echovirus). Viral infection may damage pancreatic B cells and expose antigens that initiate a self-perpetuating autoimmune process. The patient becomes overtly diabetic only when more than 90% of the B cells have been destroyed. This natural history provides a tantalising prospect of intervening in the prediabetic stage, and a variety of strategies have been mooted, including immunosuppression, early insulin therapy, antioxidants, nicotinamide and many others, but so far these have disappointed.

Type 2 diabetes is accompanied both by insulin resistance (which precedes overt disease) and by impaired insulin secretion, each of which are important in its pathogenesis. Such patients are often obese and usually present in adult life, the incidence rising progressively with age as B-cell function declines. Treatment is initially dietary, although oral hypoglycaemic drugs usually become necessary, and about one-third of patients ultimately require insulin. Prospective studies have demonstrated a relentless deterioration in diabetic control[6] over the years.

Insulin secretion in the two main forms of diabetes is shown schematically in Figure 26.2, contrasted with the normal response.

There are many other less common forms of diabetes mellitus in addition to the two main ones described above, and hyperglycaemia can also be a clinically important adverse effect of several drugs, including glucocorticoids (Ch. 28), high doses of thiazide diuretics (Ch. 24) and several of the protease inhibitors used to treat HIV infection (Ch. 47).

TREATMENT OF DIABETES MELLITUS

Insulin is essential for the treatment of type 1 diabetes. For many years, it was assumed, as an act of faith, that normalising plasma glucose would prevent diabetic complications. The Diabetes Control and Complications Trial (American Diabetes Association, 1993) showed that this faith was well placed: type 1 diabetic patients were randomly allocated to intensive or conventional management. Mean fasting blood glucose concentration was

---

[6]Diabetic control is not easily estimated by determination of blood glucose, because this is so variable. Instead, glycated haemoglobin (haemoglobin A_{1C}) is measured. This provides an integrated measure of control over the lifespan of the red cell: approximately 120 days.

2.8 mmol/l lower in the intensively treated group, who had a substantial reduction in the occurrence and progression of retinopathy, nephropathy and neuropathy over a period of 4–9 years. These benefits outweighed a threefold increase in severe hypoglycaemic attacks and modest excess weight gain.

The UK Prospective Diabetes Study showed that lowering blood pressure markedly improves outcome in type 2 diabetes (see above). Optimal control of blood glucose was not achieved even in intensively treated patients. Better metabolic control did improve outcome, but the magnitude of the benefit was disappointing and statistically significant only for microvascular complications. Consequently, realistic goals in type 2 diabetic patients are usually less ambitious than in younger type 1 patients. Diet is the cornerstone (albeit one with a tendency to crumble), combined with increased exercise. Oral agents are used to control symptoms from hyperglycaemia, as well as to limit microvascular complications. Dietary measures and *statins* to prevent atheromatous disease (Ch. 20) are crucial. Details of dietary management and treatment for specific diabetic complications are beyond the scope of this book.

INSULIN TREATMENT

Effects of insulin and its mechanism of action are described above (pp. 399-401). Here we describe pharmacokinetic aspects and adverse effects, both of which are central to its therapeutic use. Insulin for clinical use was once either porcine or bovine but is now almost entirely human (made by recombinant DNA technology). Porcine and bovine insulins differ from human insulin in their amino acid sequence, and are liable to elicit an immune response, a problem that is avoided by the use of recombinant human insulin. Although recombinant insulin is more consistent in quality than insulins extracted from pancreases of freshly slaughtered animals, doses are still quantified in terms of units of activity, with which doctors and patients are familiar, rather than of mass.

Pharmacokinetic aspects and insulin preparations

Insulin is destroyed in the gastrointestinal tract, and must be given parenterally—usually subcutaneously, but intravenously or occasionally intramuscularly in emergencies. Intraperitoneal insulin is used in diabetic patients with end-stage renal failure treated by ambulatory peritoneal dialysis. Pulmonary absorption of insulin occurs, and inhalation of an aerosol is a promising route of administration, especially for type 2 patients. Other new approaches include incorporation of insulin into biodegradable polymer microspheres, and its encapsulation with a lectin in a glucose-permeable membrane.[7] Once absorbed, insulin has an elimination half-life of approximately 10 minutes. It is inactivated enzymically in the liver and kidney, and 10% is excreted in the urine. Renal impairment reduces insulin requirement.

One of the main problems in using insulin is to avoid wide fluctuations in plasma concentration and thus in blood glucose. Different formulations vary in the timing of their peak effect and duration of action. Soluble insulin produces a rapid and short-lived effect. Longer-acting preparations are made by precipitating insulin with protamine or zinc, thus forming finely divided amorphous solid or relatively insoluble crystals, which are injected as a suspension from which insulin is slowly absorbed. These preparations include isophane insulin and amorphous or crystalline insulin zinc suspensions. Mixtures of different forms in fixed proportions are available. **Insulin lispro** is an insulin analogue in which a lysine and a proline residue are 'switched'. It acts more rapidly but for a shorter time than natural insulin, enabling patients to inject themselves immediately before the start of a meal. **Insulin glargine** is another modified insulin analogue, designed with the opposite intention, namely to provide a constant basal insulin supply and mimic physiological postabsorptive basal insulin secretion. Insulin glargine, which is a clear solution, forms a microprecipitate at the physiological pH of subcutaneous tissue, and absorption from the subcutaneous site of injection is prolonged. Used in conjunction with short-acting insulin, it lowers postabsorptive plasma glucose.

Various dosage regimens are used. Type 1 patients commonly inject a combination of short- and intermediate-acting insulins twice daily, before breakfast and before the evening meal. Improved control of blood glucose can be achieved with multiple daily injections of short-acting insulins with meals, and a longer-acting insulin at night. Insulin pumps are used in hospital and sometimes, by specialists, in outpatients. The most sophisticated forms of pump regulate the dose by means of a sensor that continuously measures blood glucose, but these are not routinely available.

Unwanted effects

The main undesirable effect of insulin is hypoglycaemia. This is common and, if very severe, can cause brain damage. In one large clinical trial, intensive insulin therapy resulted in a threefold increase in severe hypoglycaemia compared with usual care. The treatment of hypoglycaemia is to take a sweet drink or snack or, if the patient is unconscious, to give intravenous glucose or intramuscular glucagon (see above). Rebound hyperglycaemia ('Somogyi effect') can follow insulin-induced hypoglycaemia, because of the release of counter-regulatory hormones (see above). This can cause hyperglycaemia before breakfast following an unrecognised hypoglycaemic attack during sleep in the early hours of the morning. It is essential to appreciate this possibility to avoid the mistake of increasing (rather than reducing) the evening dose of insulin in this situation.

Allergy to human insulin is unusual but can occur. It may take the form of local or systemic reactions. Insulin resistance as a consequence of antibody formation is rare.

Clinical uses of insulin are summarised in the box.

ORAL HYPOGLYCAEMIC AGENTS

The main oral hypoglycaemic agents (see the box on p. 408) are **metformin** (a biguanide), *sulfonylureas* and other drugs that

---

[7]This could, in theory, provide variable release of insulin controlled by the prevailing glucose concentration, because glucose and glycosylated insulin compete for binding sites on the lectin.

THE ENDOCRINE PANCREAS AND THE CONTROL OF BLOOD GLUCOSE

Clinical uses of insulin

- Patients with *type 1 diabetes* require long-term **insulin**:
  - an intermediate-acting preparation (e.g. **isophane insulin**) is often combined with soluble insulin taken before meals.
- **Soluble insulin** is used (intravenously) in emergency treatment of hyperglycaemic emergencies (e.g. *diabetic ketoacidosis*).
- Many patients with *type 2 diabetes* ultimately need insulin.
- Short-term treatment of patients with type 2 diabetes or impaired glucose tolerance during intercurrent events (e.g. *operations, infections, myocardial infarction*).
- During pregnancy, for gestational diabetes not controlled by diet alone.
- Emergency treatment of hyperkalaemia: insulin is given with glucose to lower extracellular K^+ via redistribution into cells.

act on the sulfonylurea receptor, and *glitazones*. **Acarbose** is an α-glucosidase inhibitor.

Biguanides

Metformin is the only drug of this class presently available in the UK.

Actions and mechanism

Biguanides lower blood glucose by mechanisms that are complex and incompletely understood. They increase glucose uptake and utilisation in skeletal muscle (thereby reducing insulin resistance) and reduce hepatic glucose production (gluconeogenesis). Metformin, while preventing hyperglycaemia, does not cause hypoglycaemia. It also reduces low-density and very low-density lipoproteins (LDL and VLDL, respectively).

Pharmacokinetic aspects

Metformin has a half-life of about 3 hours and is excreted unchanged in the urine.

Unwanted effects

The commonest unwanted effects of metformin are dose-related gastrointestinal disturbances (e.g. anorexia, diarrhoea, nausea), which are usually but not always transient. Lactic acidosis is a rare but potentially fatal toxic effect, and metformin should not be given to patients with renal or hepatic disease, hypoxic pulmonary disease, heart failure or shock. Such patients are predisposed to lactic acidosis because of reduced drug elimination or reduced tissue oxygenation. It should also be avoided in other situations that predispose to lactic acidosis, and is contraindicated in pregnancy. Long-term use may interfere with absorption of vitamin B_{12}.

Clinical use

Metformin is used to treat patients with type 2 diabetes. It does not stimulate appetite (rather the reverse; see above!) and is consequently the drug of first choice in the majority of type 2 patients who are obese and who fail treatment with diet alone. It can be combined with sulfonylureas, glitazones or insulin.

Sulfonylureas

The sulfonylureas were developed following the chance observation that a sulfonamide derivative (used to treat typhoid) caused hypoglycaemia. Numerous sulfonylureas are available. The first used therapeutically were **tolbutamide** and **chlorpropamide**. Chlorpropamide has a long duration of action and a substantial fraction is excreted in the urine. Consequently, it can cause severe hypoglycaemia, especially in elderly patients in whom renal function declines inevitably but insidiously (Ch. 24). It causes flushing after alcohol because of a disulfiram-like effect (Ch. 43), and has an action like that of antidiuretic hormone on the distal nephron, giving rise to hyponatraemia and water intoxication. Williams (1994) comments that 'time honoured but idiosyncratic chlorpropamide should now be laid to rest'—a sentiment with which we concur. Tolbutamide, however, remains useful. So-called second-generation sulfonylureas (e.g. **glibenclamide**, **glipizide**; see Table 26.3) are more potent (on a milligram basis), but their maximum hypoglycaemic effect is no greater and control of blood glucose no better than with tolbutamide. These drugs all contain the sulfonylurea moiety and act in the same way, but different substitutions result in differences in pharmacokinetics and hence in duration of action (see Table 26.3).

Mechanism of action

The principal action of sulfonylureas is on B cells (Fig. 26.1), stimulating insulin secretion (the equivalent of phase 1 in Fig. 26.2) and thus reducing plasma glucose. High-affinity receptors for sulfonylureas are present on the K_{ATP} channels (Ch. 4, p. 64) in B-cell plasma membranes, and the binding of various sulfonylureas parallels their potency in stimulating insulin release. Block by sulfonylurea drugs of K_{ATP} channel activation causes depolarisation, Ca^{2+} entry and insulin secretion. (Compare this with the physiological control of insulin scretion, see p. 398 above.)

Pharmacokinetic aspects

Sulfonylureas are well absorbed after oral administration, and most reach peak plasma concentrations within 2–4 hours. The duration of action varies (Table 26.3). All bind strongly to plasma albumin and are implicated in interactions with other drugs (e.g. salicylates and sulfonamides) that compete for these binding sites (see below and Ch. 52). Most sulfonylureas (or their active metabolites) are excreted in the urine, so their action is increased in the elderly and in patients with renal disease.

Most sulfonylureas cross the placenta and enter breast milk; as a result, use of sulfonylureas is contraindicated in pregnancy and in breast feeding when diet and, if necessary, insulin are used.

Unwanted effects

The sulfonylureas are usually well tolerated. Unwanted effects are specified in Table 26.3. The commonest adverse effect is hypoglycaemia, which can be severe and prolonged. Its

Table 26.3 Oral hypoglycaemic sulfonylurea drugs

Drug	Relative potency[a]	Duration of action and (half-life) (hours)	Pharmacokinetic aspects[b]	General comments
Tolbutamide	1	6–12 (4)	Some converted in liver to weakly active hydroxytolbutamide; some carboxylated to inactive compound. Renal excretion.	A safe drug; least likely to cause hypoglycaemia. May decrease iodide uptake by thyroid. Contraindicated in liver failure.
Glibenclamide[c]	150	18–24 (10)	Some is oxidised in the liver to moderately active products and is excreted in urine; 50% is excreted unchanged in the faeces.	May cause hypoglycaemia. The active metabolite accumulates in renal failure.
Glipizide	100	16–24 (7)	Peak plasma levels in 1 hour. Most is metabolised in the liver to inactive products, which are excreted in urine; 12% is excreted in faeces.	May cause hypoglycaemia. Has diuretic action. Only inactive products accumulate in renal failure.

[a]Relative to tolbutamide.
[b]All are highly protein-bound (90–95%).
[c]Termed *gliburide* in USA.

incidence is related to the potency and duration of action of the agent, the highest incidence occurring with chlorpropamide and glibenclamide and the lowest with tolbutamide. Glibenclamide is best avoided in the elderly and in patients with even mild renal impairment because of the risk of hypoglycaemia, because several of its metabolites are excreted in urine and are moderately active. Sulfonylureas stimulate appetite (probably via their effects on insulin secretion and blood glucose) and often cause weight gain. This is a major concern in obese diabetic patients. About 3% of patients experience gastrointestinal upsets. Allergic skin rashes can occur, and bone marrow damage (Ch. 53), although very rare, can be severe.

During and for a few days after acute myocardial infarction, insulin must be substituted for sulfonylurea treatment. This is associated with a substantial reduction in short-term mortality, although it remains unclear if this is due to a specifically beneficial effect of insulin or to a detrimental effect of sulfonylurea drugs in this setting, or both. Another vexing question is whether prolonged therapy with oral hypoglycaemic drugs has adverse effects on the cardiovascular system. A study in the USA in the 1970s found that after 4–5 years of treatment, there was an increase in cardiovascular deaths in the group treated with oral drugs compared with the groups treated with insulin or placebo. Blockade of K_{ATP} in heart and vascular tissue could theoretically have adverse effects, but evidence for an adverse cardiovascular effect is unclear.

Drug interactions
Several drugs augment the hypoglycaemic effect of the sulfonylureas. Non-steroidal anti-inflammatory drugs, coumarins, some uricosuric drugs (e.g. **sulfinpyrazone**), alcohol, monoamine oxidase inhibitors, some antibacterial drugs (including **sulfonamides**, **trimethoprim** and **chloramphenicol**) and some imidazole antifungal drugs have all been reported to produce severe hypoglycaemia when given with a sulfonylurea. The probable basis of most of these interactions is competition for metabolising enzymes, but interference with plasma protein binding or with excretion may play some part.

Agents that decrease the action of sulfonylureas on blood glucose include high doses of thiazide diuretics and corticosteroids.

Clinical use
Sulfonylureas require functional B cells, so they are useful in the early stages of type 2 diabetes. They can be combined with metformin or with thiazolidinediones.

Other drugs that stimulate insulin secretion
Several drugs that lack the sulfonylurea moiety but stimulate insulin secretion have recently been developed. These include **repaglinide** and **nateglinide**. These act, like the sulfonylureas, by blocking the sulfonylurea receptor on K_{ATP} channels in pancreatic B cells. Thus nateglinide, which is structurally derived from D-phenylalanine ('the first of a new class of insulin secretion enhancers' according to one piece of promotional literature), competes with glibenclamide for specific binding sites on B cells. Like sulfonylureas, it inhibits flux of radioactive rubidium ions (which traverse K_{ATP} channels) from B cells loaded with this isotope and blocks these channels in patch clamp experiments. It is much less potent than most sulfonylureas (with the exception of tolbutamide), and has rapid onset and offset kinetics. These features, coupled with rapid absorption (time to maximal plasma concentration approximately 55 minutes after

an oral dose) and elimination (half-life approximately 3 hours), lead to short duration of action and a low risk of hypoglycaemia.[8] These drugs are administered shortly before a meal to reduce the postprandial glucose rise in type 2 diabetic patients whose condition is inadequately controlled with diet and exercise. A potential advantage is that they may cause less weight gain than conventional sulfonylureas. Later in the course of the disease, they can be combined with other oral agents such as metformin or thiazolidinediones. Unlike glibenclamide, these drugs are relatively selective for K_{ATP} channels on B cells versus K_{ATP} channels in vascular smooth muscle.

Thiazolidinediones (glitazones)

The thiazolidinediones (or glitazones) were developed following the chance observation that a clofibrate analogue, **ciglitazone**, which was being screened for effects on lipids, unexpectedly lowered blood glucose. Ciglitazone caused liver toxicity, as did **troglitazone**, but there are only rare reports of hepatotoxicity with currently marketed thiazolidinediones (**rosiglitazone** and **pioglitazone**).

Effects

The effect of thiazolidinediones on blood glucose is slow in onset, the maximum effect being achieved after only 1–2 months of treatment. Thiazolidinediones reduce hepatic glucose output and increase glucose uptake into muscle, enhancing the effectiveness of endogenous insulin and reducing the amount of exogenous insulin needed to maintain a given level of blood glucose by approximately 30%. The reduction in blood glucose is often accompanied by reductions in circulating insulin and free fatty acids. Triglycerides may decline, while LDL and high-density lipoprotein (HDL) are either unchanged or slightly increased, with little alteration in LDL:HDL ratio. The proportion of small dense LDL particles (believed to be the most atherogenic; Ch. 20) is reduced. Weight gain of 1–4 kg is common, usually stabilising in 6–12 months. Some of this is attributable to fluid retention: there is an increase in plasma volume of up to 500 ml, with a concomitant reduction in haemoglobin concentration caused by haemodilution; there is also an increase in extravascular fluid, and increased deposition of subcutaneous (as opposed to visceral) fat.

Mechanism of action

Thiazolidinediones bind to a nuclear receptor called the *peroxisome proliferator-activated receptor-γ* (*PPARγ*), which is complexed with retinoid X receptor (RXR; see Ch. 3).[9] PPARγ occurs mainly in adipose tissue, but also in muscle and liver. It causes differentiation of adipocytes (this contributes to the unwanted effect of weight gain), increases lipogenesis and enhances uptake of fatty acids and glucose. It also promotes amiloride-sensitive sodium ion reabsorption in renal collecting ducts, explaining the adverse effect of fluid retention (Guan et al., 2005). Endogenous agonists of PPARγ include unsaturated fatty acids and various derivatives of these, including prostaglandin J_2. Thiazolidinediones are exogenous agonists, which cause the PPARγ–RXR complex to bind to DNA, promoting transcription of several genes with products that are important in insulin signalling. These include lipoprotein lipase, fatty acid transporter protein, adipocyte fatty acid–binding protein, Glut-4, phosphoenolpyruvate carboxykinase, malic enzyme and others. It remains something of a mystery that glucose homeostasis should be so responsive to drugs that bind to receptors found mainly in fat cells; it has been suggested that the explanation may lie in resetting of the glucose–fatty acid (Randle) cycle by the reduction in circulating free fatty acids.

Pharmacokinetic aspects

Both rosiglitazone and pioglitazone are rapidly and nearly completely absorbed, with time to peak plasma concentration of less than 2 hours. Both are highly (> 99%) bound to plasma proteins, both are subject to hepatic metabolism and both have a short (< 7 hours) elimination half-life for the parent drug, but substantially longer (up to 150 hours for rosiglitazone, up to 24 hours for pioglitazone) for the metabolites. Rosiglitazone is metabolised by CYP2C8 to weakly active metabolites, pioglitazone mainly by a CYP2C isozyme and CYP3A4 to active metabolites. The metabolites of rosiglitazone are eliminated mainly in urine, and those of pioglitazone mainly in bile.

Unwanted effects

The serious hepatotoxicity of ciglitazone and troglitazone was not encountered during clinical trials of rosiglitazone or pioglitazone, and reports of liver dysfunction since their general release have been rare. Regular blood tests of liver function are currently recommended. One (unproven) hypothesis is that the hepatotoxicity of troglitazone is caused by quinone metabolites of its α-tocopherol side-chain, which are not formed from the newer thiazolidinediones. The commonest unwanted effects of rosiglitazone and pioglitazone are weight gain and fluid retention (see above). Fluid retention is a substantial concern, because it can precipitate or worsen heart failure, which contraindicates their use. Symptoms of uncertain cause, including headache, fatigue and gastrointestinal disturbances, have also been reported. Thiazolidinediones are contraindicated in pregnant or breast-feeding women and in children. It is theoretically possible that these drugs could cause ovulation to resume in women who are anovulatory because of insulin resistance (e.g. with polycystic ovary syndrome).

Interactions

Thiazolidinediones are additive with other oral hypoglycaemic drugs. In Europe, both rosiglitazone and pioglitazone are contraindicated for use with insulin because of concern that these combinations increase the risk of heart failure, although in the USA thiazolidinediones are widely used in combination with insulin.

---

[8]It is ironic that these recently introduced and aggressively marketed drugs share many of the properties of tolbutamine, the oldest, least expensive and least fashionable of the sulfonylureas. Perhaps diabetologists should turn some of their investigative effort to studying how best to use this Cinderella drug!

[9]Compare with fibrates (to which thiazolidinediones are structurally related), which bind to PPARα (see Ch. 20).

Clinical use

Because insulin resistance is one important component of the pathogenesis of type 2 diabetes, and has been implicated in the excess cardiovascular mortality that accompanies the common 'metabolic syndrome' (visceral obesity, hypertension, dyslipidaemia, insulin resistance, etc.), there is a good rationale for glitazones in type 2 diabetes. This probably explains their widespread adoption into clinical practice, especially in the USA. There is, however, as yet no evidence that this optimism is justified in terms of improved clinical outcomes (see for example Gale, 2001). Clinical trial evidence to date is from short-term studies and supports their use in combination with metformin or with a sulfonylurea in patients whose condition is inadequately controlled on one of these drugs and are unsuited to addition of the other. It is hoped that evidence to support wider and more useful applications (e.g. as monotherapy or as triple therapy with both metformin and a sulfonylurea) will soon be forthcoming. Potential clinical uses unrelated to diabetes, including fatty liver and atheromatous disease, are under investigation.

α-Glucosidase inhibitors

Acarbose, an inhibitor of intestinal α-glucosidase, is used in type 2 patients whose diabetes is inadequately controlled by diet with or without other agents. It delays carbohydrate absorption, reducing the postprandial increase in blood glucose. The commonest adverse effects are related to its main action and consist of flatulence, loose stools or diarrhoea, and abdominal pain and bloating. Like metformin, it may be particularly helpful in obese type 2 patients, and it can be coadministered with metformin.

Potential new antidiabetic drugs

Several agents are currently being studied, including α₂-adrenoceptor antagonists and inhibitors of fatty acid oxidation. Lipolysis in fat cells is controlled by adrenoceptors of the β₃ subtype (see Ch. 11). The possibility of using selective β₃ agonists, currently in development, in the treatment of obese patients with

type 2 diabetes is being investigated (see Ch. 27). There is interest in inhibitors of protein kinase C, for example ruboxistaurin (LY333531), an inhibitor specific for the β isoform of PKC, because of evidence implicating activation of this pathway in the development of vascular diabetic complications (Aiello, 2005).

Drugs in diabetes

Insulin

- Human insulin is made by recombinant DNA technology. For routine use, it is given subcutaneously (by intravenous infusion in emergencies).
- Different formulations of insulin differ in their duration of action:
  - fast- and short-acting soluble insulin: peak action after subcutaneous dose 2–4 hours and duration 6–8 hours; it is the only formulation that can be given intravenously
  - intermediate-acting insulin (e.g. isophane insulin)
  - long-acting forms (e.g. insulin zinc suspension).
- The main unwanted effect is hypoglycaemia.
- Altering the amino acid sequence ('designer' insulins, e.g. **lispro** and **glargine**) can usefully alter insulin kinetics.

Oral hypoglycaemic drugs

- These are used in type 2 diabetes.
- Biguanides (e.g. **metformin**):
  - have complex peripheral actions in the presence of residual insulin, increasing glucose uptake in striated muscle and inhibiting hepatic glucose output and intestinal glucose absorption
  - cause anorexia and encourage weight loss
  - can be combined with sulfonylureas.
- Sulfonylureas and other drugs that stimulate insulin secretion (e.g. **tolbutamide**, **glibenclamide**, **nateglinide**):
  - can cause hypoglycaemia (which stimulates appetite and leads to weight gain)
  - are effective only if B cells are functional
  - block ATP-sensitive potassium channels in B cells
  - are well tolerated but promote weight gain.
- Thiazolidinediones (e.g. **rosiglitazone**, **pioglitazone**)
  - increase insulin sensitivity and lower blood glucose in type 2 diabetes
  - can cause weight gain and oedema
  - are peroxisome proliferator-activated receptor-γ (a nuclear receptor) agonists.
- α-Glucosidase inhibitor: **acarbose**
  - reduces carbohydrate absorption
  - causes flatulence and diarrhoea.

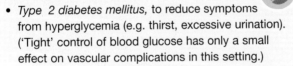

Clinical uses of oral hypoglycaemic drugs

- *Type 2 diabetes mellitus,* to reduce symptoms from hyperglycemia (e.g. thirst, excessive urination). ('Tight' control of blood glucose has only a small effect on vascular complications in this setting.)
- **Metformin** is preferred for obese patients unless contraindicated by factor(s) that predispose to lactic acidosis (renal or liver failure, heart failure, hypoxaemia).
- **Acarbose** (α-glucosidase inhibitor) reduces carbohydrate absorption; it causes flatulence and diarrhoea.
- Drugs that act on the sulfonylurea receptor (e.g. **tolbutamide**, **glibenclamide**) are well tolerated but often promote weight gain.
- Thiazolidinediones are used in patients unable to tolerate metformin/sulfonylurea combinations or where either of these classes of drugs is contra-indicated.

REFERENCES AND FURTHER READING

Several of the references below are to specific chapters of particular relevance in Pickup J C, Williams J (eds) 2002 Textbook of diabetes, 3rd edn. Blackwell Science, Oxford. This extremely readable, well-illustrated and authoritative textbook offers excellent further reading.

Physiological and pathophysiological aspects

Dunn M J 1997 Familial persistent hyperinsulinemic hypoglycemia of infancy and mutations in the sulfonylurea receptor. N Engl J Med 336: 703–706 (*A rare disease resulting from disorder of potassium channels as a result of mutation in the sulfonylurea receptor*)

Lee Y H, White M F 2004 Insulin receptor substrate proteins and diabetes. Arch Pharm Res 27: 361–370 (*Reviews the discovery of IRS proteins and their role linking cell surface receptors to intracellular signalling cascades. 'Understanding the regulation and signaling by IRS1 and IRS2 in cell growth, metabolism and survival will reveal new strategies to prevent or cure diabetes and other metabolic diseases.'*)

Maratos-Flier E, Goldstein B J, Kahn C R 2002 The insulin receptor and postreceptor mechanisms. In: Pickup J C, Williams J (eds) Textbook of diabetes, 3rd edn. Blackwell Science, Oxford

Turk J, Gross R W, Ramanadham S 1993 Perspectives in diabetes. Amplification of insulin secretion by lipid messengers. Diabetes 42: 367–374 (*Amplifying intracellular messengers include diacylglycerol, non-esterified arachidonic acid, 12-S-HETE*)

Way K J, Katai N, King G L 2001 Protein kinase C and the development of diabetic vascular complications. Diabet Med 18: 945–959 (*Reviews the considerable evidence implicating protein kinase C activation in the aetiology of diabetic vascular complications*)

Withers D J, Gutierrez J S, Towery H et al. 1998 Disruption of IRS-2 causes type 2 diabetes in mice. Nature 391: 900–904 (*Dysfunction of IRS-2 may 'contribute to the pathophysiology of human type 2 diabetes'; see also accompanying commentary by Avruch J, A signal for β-cell failure, pp. 846–847*)

Zimmet P, Alberti K G M M, Shaw J 2001 Global and societal implications of the diabetes epidemic. Nature 414: 782–787 (*Changes in human behaviour have resulted in a dramatic increase in type 2 diabetes worldwide*)

Insulins

Bolli G B, Owens D R 2000 Insulin glargine. Lancet 356: 443–445 (*Balanced, succinct commentary. 'In the 50 years since NPH insulin was devised by Hagedorn and Lente insulin by Hallas-Møller, no improved formulations of intermediate acting or long-acting insulin preparations have been introduced until now.' Insulin glargine could represent a milestone.*)

Owens D R, Zinman B, Bolli G B 2001 Insulins today and beyond. Lancet 358: 739–746 (*Reviews the physiology of glucose homeostasis, genetically engineered 'designer' insulins, and developments in insulin delivery and glucose sensing*)

Saltiel A R, Kahn C R 2001 Insulin signaling and the regulation of glucose and lipid metabolism. Nature 414: 799–806 (*Discusses insulin resistance and related hormonal and signalling events*)

Saltiel A R, Pessin J E 2002 Insulin signaling pathways in space and time. Trends Cell Biol 12: 65–70

Skyler J S, Cefalu W T, Kourides I A et al. 2001 Efficacy of inhaled human insulin in type 1 diabetes mellitus: a randomized proof-of-concept study. Lancet 357: 324–325 (*Preprandial inhaled insulin is a less invasive alternative to injection; see also a paper on type 2 patients from the same group, showing that 3 months of treatment with inhaled insulin was effective and well tolerated without adverse pulmonary effects: Ann Intern Med 2001; 134: 203–207*)

Oral hypoglycaemic drugs

de Fronzo R A, Goodman A M 1995 Efficacy of metformin in patients with non–insulin-dependent diabetes mellitus. N Engl J Med 333: 541–549 (*See also accompanying editorial on metformin by Crofford O B, pp. 588–589*)

Dornhorst A 2001 Insulinotropic meglitinide analogues. Lancet 358: 1709–1716 (*Reviews rationale for this class, which includes repaglinide and nateglinide*)

Gale E A M 2001 Lessons from the glitazones: a story of drug development. Lancet 357: 1870–1875 (*Fighting stuff: 'Troglitazone was voluntarily withdrawn in Europe, but went on to generate sales of over $2 billion in the USA and caused 90 cases of liver failure before being withdrawn. Rosiglitazone and pioglitazone reached the USA for use alone or in combination with other drugs whereas in Europe the same dossiers were used to apply for a limited licence as second-line agents. How should we use them? How did they achieve blockbuster status without any clear evidence of advantage over existing therapy?'*)

Guan Y et al. 2005 Thiazolidinediones expand body fluid volume through PPARγ stimulation of ENaC-mediated renal salt absorption. Nat Med 11: 861–865 (*Mechanism of fluid retention caused by thiazolidinediones and suggestion that amiloride may provide a specific therapy for this. Human studies will no doubt follow... See also News and Views article in the same issue: TZDs and diabetes: testing the waters by A F Semenkovich, pp. 822–824*)

Hu S et al. 2000 Pancreatic β-cell K$_{ATP}$ channel activity and membrane-binding studies with nateglinide: a comparison with sulphonylureas and repaglinide.

J Pharmacol Exp Ther 293: 444–452 (*In competition binding studies, nateglinide displaced ^{3}H-glibenclamide with lower affinity than all sulfonylureas studied except tolbutamide*)

Perfetti R, D'Amico E 2005 Rational drug design and PPAR agonists. Curr Diab Rep 5: 340–345 (*Reviews thiazolidinediones, and discusses novel drugs in development*)

Williams G 1994 Managements of non–insulin-dependent diabetes mellitus. Lancet 343: 95–100

Other drugs for diabetes, and therapeutic aspects

ACE Inhibitors in Diabetic Nephropathy Trialist Group 2001 Should all patients with type 1 diabetes mellitus and microalbuminuria receive angiotensin converting enzyme inhibitors? A meta-analysis of individual patient data. Ann Intern Med 134: 370–379 (*Either that or a sartan—see Brenner et al., 2001, below*)

Aiello L P 2005 The effect of ruboxistaurin on visual loss in patients with moderately severe to very severe nonproliferative diabetic retinopathy initial results of the Protein Kinase C Beta Inhibitor Diabetic Retinopathy Study (PKC-DRS) multicenter randomized clinical trial. Diabetes 54: 2188–2197 (*Ruboxistaurin was well tolerated and reduced the risk of visual loss but did not prevent progression of retinopathy*)

American Diabetes Association 1993 Implications of the Diabetes Control and Complications Trial. Diabetes 42: 1555–1558 (*Landmark clinical trial*)

Brenner B M et al. 2001 Effects of losartan on renal and cardiovascular outcomes in patients with type 2 diabetes and nephropathy. N Engl J Med 345: 861–869 (*Significant renal benefits from the AT$_1$ antagonist; see also two adjacent articles: Lewis E J et al., pp. 851–860, and Parving H-H et al., pp. 870–878, and an editorial on prevention of renal disease caused by type 2 diabetes by Hostetter T H, pp. 910–911*)

Chung S S M, Chung S K 2005 Aldose reductase in diabetic microvascular complications. Curr Drug Targets 6: 475–486 (*Reviews pathogenic mechanisms of the polyol pathway, and discusses possible reasons for the unimpressive effects to date of aldose reductase inhibitors; argues that renewed efforts could be warranted*)

Schmitz O, Brock B, Schmitz O 2004 Amylin agonists: a novel approach in the treatment of diabetes. Diabetes 53(suppl): S233–S238 (*Reviews actions of amylin in animal and human models, and the results from clinical trials with the amylin analogue pramlintide*)

Thompson R G, Peterson J, Gottlieb A, Mullane J 1997 Effects of pramlintide, an analog of human amylin, on plasma glucose profiles in patients with IDDM: results of a multicenter trial. Diabetes 46: 632–636 (*This amylin analogue lowered blood glucose when added to patients' usual insulin*)

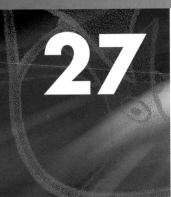

27 Obesity

OVERVIEW

Obesity is a growing health issue around the world and is reaching epidemic proportions in some nations. The problem is not restricted to the inhabitants of the affluent countries, to the adult population, or to any one socioeconomic class. Body fat represents stored energy, and obesity occurs when the homeostatic mechanisms controlling energy balance become disordered or overwhelmed. In this chapter, we explore first the endogenous regulation of appetite and body mass, and then consider the main health implications of obesity and its pathophysiology. We conclude with a discussion of the two drugs currently licensed for the treatment of obesity, and glance at the future of pharmacological treatment of this condition.

BACKGROUND

Survival requires a continuous provision of energy to maintain homeostasis even when the supply of food is intermittent. Evolution has furnished a mechanism for storing any excess energy latent in foodstuffs in adipose tissue as energy-dense triglycerides, such that these can be easily mobilised when food is absent or less abundant. This mechanism, controlled by the so-called thrifty genes, was an obvious asset to our hunter-gatherer ancestors. However, in many societies a combination of sedentary lifestyle, genetic susceptibility, cultural influences and unrestricted access to an ample supply of calorie-dense foods is leading to a global epidemic of obesity, or 'globesity' as it sometimes called.

DEFINITION OF OBESITY

If the 'ideal weight' of an individual is that which maximises life expectancy, 'obesity' may be defined as an illness where the health (and hence life expectancy) is adversely affected by excess body fat.[1] But at what point does an individual become 'obese'? The generally accepted benchmark, as proposed by the World Health Organization expert committee, is the *body mass index* (*BMI*). The BMI is calculated by dividing the body mass (in kg) by the square of the height (in metres). Although it is not a perfect index (e.g. it does not distinguish between fat and lean mass), the BMI is generally well correlated with other measurements of body fat, and it is widely employed in obesity studies. While there are problems in defining a 'healthy' weight for a particular population, it is generally agreed that people with a BMI of $< 18.5 \text{ kg/m}^2$ should be classified as 'underweight', and those with a BMI of $18.5–24.9 \text{ kg/m}^2$ are regarded as of 'acceptable' or 'normal' weight. A BMI in the range of $25.0–29.9 \text{ kg/m}^2$ signifies 'grade 1 overweight'. If the BMI is between 30.0 and 39.9 kg/m^2, the patient is deemed to be obese or 'grade 2 overweight', while those with a BMI of $> 40 \text{ kg/m}^2$ are said to be 'grade 3 overweight' or morbidly obese.

As the BMI obviously depends on the overall energy balance, another, operational, definition of obesity would be that it is a multifactorial disorder of energy balance in which calorie intake

---

[1] 'Persons who are naturally very fat are apt to die earlier than those who are slender' observed Hippocrates.

over the long term exceeds energy output, resulting in an abnormally high BMI.

THE HOMEOSTATIC MECHANISMS CONTROLLING ENERGY BALANCE

A common view, and one that is implicitly encouraged by authors of numerous dieting books as well as the enormously lucrative dieting industry in general, is that obesity is simply the result of bad diet or wilful overeating (hyperphagia). In truth, however, the situation is more complex. Many people exposed to the same dietary choices fail to become obese, and the failure rate in such diets is high (probably 90%), with most eventually returning to their original starting weight, suggesting the operation of some intrinsic homeostatic system that strives to maintain a particular set weight. This mechanism is normally exceptionally precise, and it has been calculated that it is capable of regulating energy balance to 0.17% per decade (Weigle, 1994). A truly remarkable feat considering the day-to-day variations in food intake.

Studies of obesity in monozygotic and dizygotic twins have established a strong genetic influence on the susceptibility to the disease, and studies of rare mutations in mice (and more recently in humans) have led to the discovery and elucidation of the neuroendocrine pathways that match food intake with energy expenditure, and to the concept that it is, in fact, disorders of this system that are responsible for the onset and maintenance of the disease.

THE ROLE OF LEPTIN IN BODY WEIGHT REGULATION

At the beginning of the 20th century, it was observed that patients with damage to the hypothalamus tended to gain weight. In the 1940s, it was also shown that discrete lesions in the hypothalamus of rodents caused them to become obese. As early as 1953, Kennedy proposed, on the basis of experiments on rats, that a hormone released from adipose tissue acted on the hypothalamus to regulate body fat and food intake, thus setting the stage for future discoveries in this area.

It was well established that mice can become obese as a result of mutations in certain genes. At least five of these have now been identified—including the *ob* (obesity), *tub* (tubby), *fat* and *db* (diabetes) genes. Mice that are homozygous for mutant forms of these genes—*ob/ob* mice and *db/db* mice—eat excessively and have low energy expenditure, become grossly fat, and have numerous metabolic and other abnormalities. Weight gain in an *ob/ob* mouse is suppressed if its circulation is linked to that of a normal mouse, implying that the obesity is caused by lack of a blood-borne factor.

An important breakthrough came in 1994, when Friedman and his colleagues (see Zhang et al., 1994) cloned the *ob* gene and identified its protein product—*leptin* (the word is derived from the Greek *leptos*, meaning thin). When recombinant leptin was administered to *ob/ob* mice, it strikingly reduced food intake and body weight. It had a similar effect when injected directly into the lateral or the third ventricle, implying that it acted on the regions of the brain that control food intake and energy balance. Recombinant leptin has similar effects in humans (see Fig. 27.1).

Leptin mRNA is expressed in adipocytes; its synthesis is increased by glucocorticoids, insulin and the oestrogens, and it is reduced by β-adrenoceptor agonists. In humans, the concentration of leptin in the circulation varies according to the fat stores and BMI in normal subjects; the release is pulsatile and inversely related to hydrocortisone levels. Leptin enters the central nervous system (CNS) by a saturable transport mechanism, in amounts proportional to the plasma level. It acts on hypothalamic nuclei that express specific leptin receptors. Insulin also plays an important part in regulating energy balance. It strongly stimulates leptin expression in fat cells. But its role as a fat sensor is more complex (see below, pp. 412-413), and it is accepted that leptin has the more critical role.

Today, the adipocyte is regarded not only as a storage depot for fat, but also as an important staging post on the energy information highway. These cells secrete a host of other cytokines and other autocrine, paracrine and endocrine mediators, leading some authorities to consider that adipose tissue is a dispersed endocrine organ (Ahima & Flier, 2000a; Frühbeck et al., 2001).

INTEGRATION OF INFORMATION AND EFFECT ON ENERGY BALANCE

Leptin's main targets in the hypothalamus are two groups of neurons in the *arcuate nucleus*. These have opposing actions, and energy homeostasis depends, in the first instance, on the balance between these actions. In one group, the peptides *neuropeptide Y* (*NPY*) and *agouti-related peptide* are colocalised. The other group contains the protein *prepro-opiomelanocortin* (*POMC*) and releases α-*melanocyte-stimulating hormone* (α-*MSH*), which is a proteolytic product of POMC cleavage. Both groups of neurons express specific leptin receptors.

Falling leptin levels activate the first group of neurons, resulting in increased food intake (an *orexigenic* effect), and synthesis and storage of fat (anabolism), as well as decreased energy expenditure. Conversely, rising leptin levels activate the second group of neurons, producing the opposite *anorexigenic* and catabolic effect. The signal transduction mechanisms triggered by leptin receptor activation are thought to involve the Jak/Stat pathway (Ch. 3) and activation of an ATP-sensitive potassium channel. Orexigenic neurons project into the paraventricular nucleus, and anorexigenic neurons into the lateral hypothalamic area. Interestingly, these two areas had previously been identified, using lesioning techniques, as 'hunger' and 'satiety' centres.

The integration of the information on fat stores (adiposity signals) with other nutritional information is very complex. Leptin, although apparently a crucial coordinator, is only one part of the process. Insulin receptors also occur on both groups of hypothalamic neurons, and it is thought that leptin and insulin act in concert at this important regulatory site.

Some of the existing information on energy balance and the control of body weight and fat depots is shown in Figure 27.2 (see also Friedman, 1997).

▼ Numerous factors other than those included in the figure are involved in regulating food intake and energy expenditure, including orexigenic

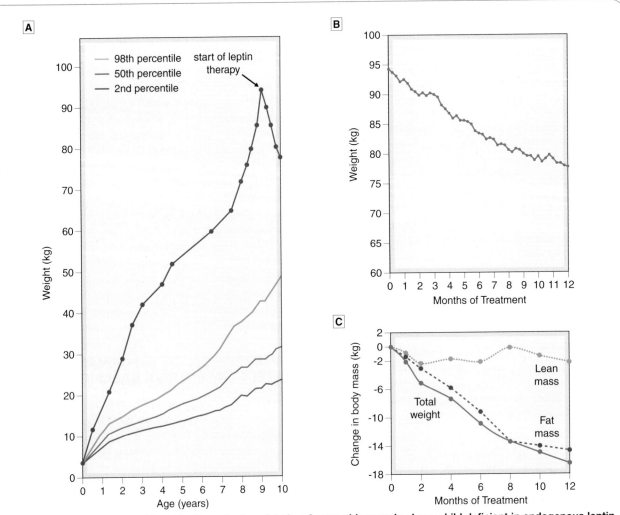

Fig. 27.1 The effect of recombinant leptin on body weight in a 9-year-old severely obese child deficient in endogenous leptin because of a frame shift mutation in the leptin gene. Although of normal birth weight, the child began gaining weight at 4 months and was constantly demanding food. When treatment was initiated, the child weighed 94.4 kg. Weight loss began after 2 weeks' treatment, and her eating pattern returned to normal. She had lost 15.6 kg of body fat after 1 year of treatment. (Data and figure adapted from, Farooqi et al. 1999 N Engl J Med 341: 879–884.)

factors such as melanin-concentrating hormone, orexins A and B, galanin, GABA, growth hormone–releasing hormone and ghrelin, as well as anorexigenic factors such as corticotrophin-releasing hormone, the 'cocaine and amphetamine-regulated transcript', neurotensin, tumour necrosis factor (TNF)-α, interleukin-1β, 5-hydroxytryptamine, glucagon-like peptides, bombesin, ciliary neurotrophic factor and the satiety factor cholecystokinin. (For more details, see Ahima & Osei, 2001.) It will come as no surprise to learn that many of these are being targeted to produce novel antiobesity drugs (see below).

REGULATION OF FOOD INTAKE AND ENERGY EXPENDITURE

Food intake is of course modified by a multitude of physiological, psychological, financial and social factors, and so the long-term regulation of energy balance by adiposity signals such as leptin and insulin must of necessity occur against a background of day-to-day variations in meal size, frequency and content. Food intake appears to be modulated by feedback loops in which signals from

the gastrointestinal tract are transmitted to the CNS, apparently converging on the *nucleus tractus solitarius*. Some of these signals arise from vagal and other spinal afferents originating in the gastro-intestinal tract. Another important endocrine afferent signal is *cholecystokinin*—a peptide secreted by the duodenum in response to the process of eating and digestion of (especially fatty) foodstuffs. Cholecystokinin acts locally on cholecystokinin A receptors in the gastrointestinal tract to stimulate vagal afferents and may, in its capacity as a neurotransmitter, also act on chole-cystokinin B receptors in the brain in order to function as a satiety factor. Studies in rodents show how these short-term satiety signals are integrated into the overall context of the body's energy economy by regulation of meal size. For example, the stimu-lation of food intake by NPY is largely attributable to larger meal sizes, whereas treatment with leptin leads to a reduction in meal size rather than frequency.

As mentioned above, insulin also has a significant role in the control of energy metabolism. It stimulates leptin release from fat

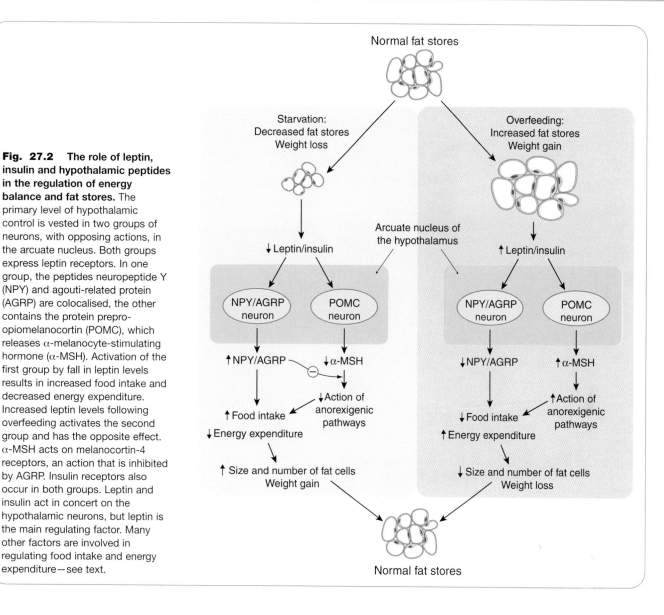

Fig. 27.2 The role of leptin, insulin and hypothalamic peptides in the regulation of energy balance and fat stores. The primary level of hypothalamic control is vested in two groups of neurons, with opposing actions, in the arcuate nucleus. Both groups express leptin receptors. In one group, the peptides neuropeptide Y (NPY) and agouti-related protein (AGRP) are colocalised, the other contains the protein prepro-opiomelanocortin (POMC), which releases α-melanocyte-stimulating hormone (α-MSH). Activation of the first group by fall in leptin levels results in increased food intake and decreased energy expenditure. Increased leptin levels following overfeeding activates the second group and has the opposite effect. α-MSH acts on melanocortin-4 receptors, an action that is inhibited by AGRP. Insulin receptors also occur in both groups. Leptin and insulin act in concert on the hypothalamic neurons, but leptin is the main regulating factor. Many other factors are involved in regulating food intake and energy expenditure—see text.

cells, and it decreases food intake by affecting the actions of NPY in the CNS (see Fig. 27.2). However, insulin may also, in some circumstances, increase food intake, presumably indirectly, by an effect on blood glucose. Thus patients with type 2 diabetes mellitus usually gain weight when treated with insulin or sulfonylureas—an effect that is of clinical importance (see Ch. 26).

Monoamines such as noradrenaline (norepinephrine), serotonin and dopamine also play a role in the modulation of satiety signals. Noradrenaline is colocalised with NPY in some neurons and greatly potentiates its hyperphagic action. Deficit of dopamine impairs feeding behaviour, as do agonists at the $5HT_{2C}$ receptor; antagonists at this receptor have the reverse effect.

Balancing food intake is the energy expenditure required to maintain metabolism, physical activity and *thermogenesis* (heat production). The metabolic aspects of energy expenditure include, among other things, cardiorespiratory work and the actions of a multitude of enzymes. Physical activity increases all these, as well as increasing energy expenditure by the skeletal muscles. Lowering the environmental temperature (e.g. exposure to cold) or feeding

also stimulates thermogenesis, and the reverse is also true. The often dramatic (20–40% increase) thermogenic effects of feeding may provide a partial protection against developing obesity.

The sympathetic nervous system (sometimes in concert with thyroid hormone) plays a significant part in the regulation of energy expenditure in cardiovascular and skeletal muscle function during physical activity, as well as in the thermogenic response of adipose tissue and the response to cold. Both 'white' and 'brown' (the colour is apparently caused by the high density of mitochondria) fat cells (but especially the latter) have a major role in thermogenesis. Brown fat, which is densely innervated by the sympathetic nervous system, is abundant in rodents and human infants, although in human adults these cells are generally to be found more interspersed with white fat cells. Because of their abundant mitochondria, they are remarkable heat generators, producing more heat and less ATP than white fat cells. The basis for this, as determined in mice, is the presence of mitochondrial uncoupling proteins (UCP). Three isoforms, UCP-1, -2 and -3, are known and have different distributions, although all are found in

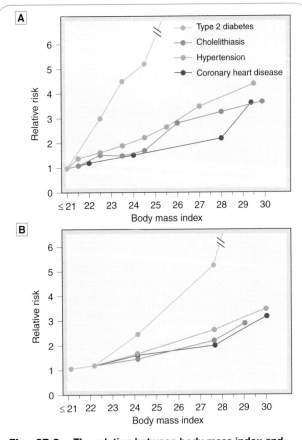

Fig. 27.3 **The relation between body mass index and the relative risk of the diseases specified.** Ⓐ The figures for women, initially 30–55 years of age, who were followed for 18 years. Ⓑ The figures for men, initially 40–65 years of age, who were followed up for 10 years. (Adapted from Kopelman P G 2000 Nature 404: 635–643; data from Willet W C, Dietz W H, Colditz G A 1999 N Engl J Med 341: 427–433.)

brown fat. These proteins 'uncouple' oxidative phosphorylation, so that mitochondria continue oxidative metabolism but produce much less ATP, thus promoting net energy loss as heat. As one might anticipate, exposure to cold or leptin administration increases both the activity and (after prolonged stimulation) the amount of UCP-1 in brown fat. Noradrenaline, acting on β adrenoceptors (mainly β_3) in brown fat, increases the activity of the peroxisome proliferator-activated receptor-γ (PPARγ) transcription factor, which, together with its coactivator PPARγ coactivator (PGC)-1, activates the gene for UCP-1. The expression of β_3 adrenoceptors is decreased in genetically obese mice.

OBESITY AS A HEALTH PROBLEM

Obesity is a growing and costly global health problem. According to the World Health Organization, there are more than 1 billion overweight adults, approximately one-third of whom are obese according to the criteria outlined above. National obesity levels vary enormously, being less than 5% in China, Japan and parts of Africa, to a staggering 75% in parts of Samoa. Obesity levels in

Energy balance

Energy balance depends on food intake, energy storage in fat, and energy expenditure. In most individuals, the process is tightly regulated by a homeostatic system that integrates inputs from a number of internal sensors and external factors. Important components of the system include the following.

- Hormones that signal the level of fat stores (e.g. leptin). Increasing fat storage leads to raised plasma leptin release from adipocytes, which signals through neuronal pathways in the central nervous system (CNS).
- Hypothalamic neurons with leptin receptors sense increased body fat and release α-melanocyte-stimulating hormone, which activates systems that decrease food intake and increase energy expenditure. Decreased leptin causes the release from other neurons of neuropeptide Y and agouti-related protein, which have the opposite effect.
- Along with leptin, insulin has a critical role in energy homeostasis, but many other factors also play a part: other hormones, cytokines, autonomic transmitters, other CNS neuropeptide transmitters, and a variety of other mediators released from adipose tissue (which is now regarded as an endocrine organ).

the USA, Europe and the UK (among others) have increased three-fold since 1980, with figures of 31% being quoted for the USA and about 25% for many other industrialised nations (Padwal et al., 2003). The disease is not confined to adults: some 22 million children under 5 years old are estimated to be overweight. In the USA, the number of overweight children has doubled, and the number of overweight adolescents has trebled, since 1980. Ironically, obesity often coexists with malnutrition in many developing countries. All socioeconomic classes are affected. In the poorest countries, it is the top socioeconomic classes in whom obesity is prevalent, but in the West it is usually the reverse.

While obesity itself is rarely fatal, it brings with it the risk of increased susceptibility to a host of metabolic and other disorders, the most important of which are type 2 diabetes, cardiovascular conditions, cancers (particularly hormone-dependent), and respiratory and digestive problems, as well as osteoarthritis. Increasingly, social stigma is suffered by obese individuals, leading to a sense of psychological isolation. One commentator (Kopelman, 2000) has remarked that obesity '...is beginning to replace under-nutrition and infectious diseases as the most significant contributor to ill health'. The total costs of obesity-related illness are hard to estimate. Figures in the range of 2–7% of the total healthcare budget are often given but are probably an underestimate.

The risk of developing type 2 diabetes (which represents 85% of all cases of the disease) rises sharply with increasing BMI. At one time, this disease was found mainly in the adult population, but it is increasingly seen in obese children, often striking even before the onset of puberty. The World Health Organization reports that 90% of those diagnosed with the disease are obese. In a study of the disease in women, the risk of developing diabetes was closely correlated with BMI, increasing fivefold when the BMI was 25 kg/m², to 93-fold when the BMI was 35 kg/m² or above (Colditz et al., 1995). Through several mechanisms, the elevated plasma fatty acids, characteristic of the obese individual, lead to inappropriate secretion of insulin and down-regulation of insulin receptors. Eventually, when the system can no longer compensate, insulin resistance supervenes (see Ch. 26 for further details of insulin actions).

Cardiovascular disease is also increased in the obese individual, partly because of the increased oxygen demand secondary to the extra tissue mass, and the increase in cardiac output that is necessary to accommodate this. Secondary structural alterations in the heart, coupled with other vascular changes including an increased peripheral resistance, may lead eventually to heart failure. The increased thoracic and abdominal adipose tissue reduces lung volume and makes respiration difficult. This is especially the case when the patient is lying down and the mass of abdominal fat presses down on the peritoneal cavity, displacing other organs, which further reduce the diaphragm and other respiratory muscles. This itself can cause serious sleep disorders secondary to changes in blood gases.

Obese subjects have an increased risk of colon, breast, prostate, gall bladder, ovarian and uterine cancer. Numerous other disorders are associated with excess body weight, including osteoarthritis, hyperuricaemia and male hypogonadism. Gross obesity (BMI over 40 kg/m²) is associated with a 12-fold increase in mortality in the group aged 25–35 years compared with those in this age group with a BMI of 20–25 kg/m².

THE PATHOPHYSIOLOGY OF HUMAN OBESITY

In most adult subjects, body fat and body weight remain more or less constant over many years, even decades, in the face of very large variations in food intake and energy expenditure—amounting to about a million calories per year. The steady-state body weight and BMI of an individual is, as has been stressed above, the result of the integration of multiple interacting factors, and perturbations— either in the direction of increase or decrease—are resisted by homeostatic mechanisms. How, then, does obesity occur? Why is it so difficult for the obese to lose weight and maintain the lower weight?

The main determinant is manifestly a disturbance of the homeostatic mechanisms that control energy balance, but genetic endowment underlies this disturbance. Other factors, such as food intake and lack of physical activity, contribute, and there are, of course, social, cultural and psychological aspects. We will deal below with the imbalance of homeostatic mechanisms and genetic endowment, and then briefly mention the role of food intake and physical activity. The role of social, cultural and psychological aspects we will leave (with a profound sigh of relief) to the psychosociologists.

OBESITY AS A DISORDER OF THE HOMEOSTATIC CONTROL OF ENERGY BALANCE

Because the homeostatic control of energy balance is extremely complex, it is not easy to determine what goes wrong in obesity. When the leptin story unfolded, it was thought that alterations in leptin kinetics might provide a simple explanation. There is a considerable interindividual variation in sensitivity to leptin, and some individuals seem to produce insufficient amounts of this hormone. Paradoxically, however, plasma leptin is often higher in obese individuals, compared with non-obese subjects, not lower as might be expected (Fig. 27.2). The reason for this is that *resistance* to leptin rather than insufficient hormone is more prevalent in obesity. Such resistance could be caused by defects in leptin synthesis, in its carriage in the circulation, in its transport into the CNS, in leptin receptors in the hypothalamus (as occurs in *db/db* mice) or in postreceptor signalling. There is some evidence that the action of a member of the family of suppressors of cytokine signalling, SOCS-3, may underlie or contribute to leptin resistance.

Dysfunction of mediators other than leptin could be implicated in obesity. For example, TNF-α, another cytokine that can relay information from fat tissue to brain, is increased in the adipose tissue of insulin-resistant obese individuals. Another pathophysiological alteration in obesity is a reduced insulin sensitivity of muscle and fat, and decreased β₃ adrenoceptor function in brown adipose tissue (see above) may also occur; alternatively, UCP-2, one of the proteins that uncouple oxidative phosphorylation in adipocytes, could be dysfunctional in obese individuals.

A further suggestion is that alterations in the function of specific nuclear receptors, such as PPARα, β and γ, may play a role in obesity. These receptors regulate gene expression of enzymes associated with lipid and glucose homeostasis, and they also promote the genesis of adipose tissue. PPARγ is expressed preferentially in fat cells and synergises with another transcription factor, C/EBPα, to convert precursor cells to fat cells (see Spiegelman & Flier, 1996). The gene for UCP (see above) in white fat cells also has regulatory sites that respond to PPARα and C/EBPα. A new class of agents, the *thiazoladinediones*, bind to and activate PPARγ (see Ch. 26). One of these, **troglitazone**, is licensed in the UK for treatment of type 2 diabetes. The pathophysiology of obesity could involve disturbance(s) in any of the multitude of other factors involved in energy balance.

GENETIC FACTORS AND OBESITY

Analyses of large-scale (> 100 000) studies in human monozygotic and dizygotic twin pairs indicate that 50–90% of the variance of BMI can be attributed to genetic factors, and suggest a relatively minor role for environmental factors (Barsh et al., 2000). This conclusion may seem surprising, but feeding studies using laboratory rodents where food intake is held constant have demonstrated the importance of genetic background to body weight regulation, and this is especially true for high-fat diets. The prevailing viewpoint is that susceptibility to obesity is largely determined by genetic factors, while environmental factors determine the expression of the disease.

The discovery that spontaneous mutations arising in single genes (e.g. the *ob/ob* genotype) produced obese phenotypes in mice led to a search for equivalent genes in humans. A recent review (Pérusse et al., 2005) reported over 170 human obesity cases that could be traced to single gene mutations in 10 different genes. Leptin receptor or POMC mutations are sometimes observed, but MC4R mutations, however, seem to be more prevalent (3–5%) in obese patients (e.g. see Barsh et al., 2000). In general, however, human obesity should be regarded as a polygenic disorder involving the interaction of many genes. At the time of writing, > 600 genes, markers and chromosomal regions are under investigation for linkage to human obesity (Pérusse et al., 2005), and all information is annually updated on the Obesity Gene Map Database (http//obesitygene.pbrc.edu).

Other genes that appear to be involved include the β_3 adrenoceptor and the glucocorticoid receptor. Decreased function of the β_3 adrenoceptor gene could be associated with impairment of lipolysis in white fat or with thermogenesis in brown fat. A mutation of this gene has been found to be associated with abdominal obesity, insulin resistance and early-onset type 2 diabetes in some subjects and a markedly increased propensity to gain weight in a separate group of morbidly obese subjects. Alterations in the function of the glucocorticoid receptor could be associated with obesity through the permissive effect of glucocorticoids on several aspects of fat metabolism and energy balance.

FOOD INTAKE AND OBESITY

As Spiegelman & Flier (1996) point out, 'one need not be a rocket scientist to notice that increased food intake tends to be associated with obesity'. A typical obese subject will usually have gained 20 kg over a decade or so. This means that there has been a daily excess of energy input over output of 30–40 kcal initially, increasing gradually to maintain the increased body weight.

The type of food eaten, as well as the quantity, can disturb energy homeostasis. Fat is an energy-dense foodstuff, and it may be that the mechanisms regulating appetite react more rapidly to carbohydrate and protein than to fat—too slowly to stop an individual consuming too much high-fat food before the satiety systems come into play.

Obese individuals diet to lose weight. However, when a subject reduces calorie intake, shifts into negative energy balance and loses weight, the resting metabolic rate decreases, and there is a concomitant reduction in energy expenditure. Thus an individual who was previously obese and is now of normal weight generally needs fewer calories to maintain that weight than an individual who has never been obese. The decrease in energy expenditure appears to be largely caused by an alteration in the conversion efficiency of chemical energy to mechanical work in the skeletal muscles. This adaptation to the caloric reduction contributes to the difficulty of maintaining weight loss by diet.

PHYSICAL EXERCISE AND OBESITY

It used to be said that the only exercise effective in combating obesity was pushing one's chair back from the table. It is now recognised that physical activity—i.e. increased energy expenditure—has a much more positive role in reducing fat storage and adjusting energy balance in the obese, particularly if associated with modification of the diet. An inadvertent, natural population study provides an example. Many years ago, a tribe of Pima Indians split into two groups. One group settled in Mexico and continued to live simply at subsistence level, eating frugally and spending most of the week in hard physical labour. They are generally lean and have a low incidence of type 2 diabetes. The other group moved to the USA—an environment with easy access to calorie-rich food and less need for hard physical work. They are, on average, 57 lbs (26 kg) heavier than the Mexican group and have a high incidence of early-onset type 2 diabetes.

PHARMACOLOGICAL APPROACHES TO THE PROBLEM OF OBESITY

The first weapons in the fight against obesity are diet and exercise. Unfortunately, these often fail or show only short-term efficacy, leaving only heroic surgical techniques (such as gastric stapling or bypass) or drug therapy as a viable alternative.

The attempt to control appetite with drugs has had a long and largely undistinguished history. Many types of 'anorectic' (e.g.

Obesity

- Obesity is a multifactorial disorder of energy balance, in which long-term calorie intake exceeds energy output.
- It is characterised by an excessive body mass index (BMI; weight in kg divided by the square of height in m).
- A subject with a BMI of 20–25 kg/m² is considered as having a healthy body weight, one with a BMI of 25–30 kg/m² as overweight, and one with a BMI > 30 kg/m² as obese.
- Obesity is a growing problem in most rich nations; the incidence—at present approximately 30% in the USA and 15–20% in Europe—is increasing.
- A BMI > 30 kg/m² significantly increases the risk of type 2 diabetes, hypercholesterolaemia, hypertension, ischaemic heart disease, gallstones and some cancers.
- The causes of obesity may include:
  - deficiencies in the genesis of and/or the response to leptin or other adiposity signals
  - defects in the hypothalamic neuronal systems responding to leptin or other adiposity signals
  - defects in the systems controlling energy expenditure (e.g. reduced sympathetic activity), decreased metabolic expenditure of energy, or decreased thermogenesis caused by a reduction in β_3 adrenoceptor-mediated tone and/or dysfunction of the proteins that uncouple oxidative phosphorylation
  - an important genetic contribution.

appetite suppressant) agents have been tested in the past, including the uncoupling agent **DNP**, **amphetamines** and **fenfluramine**. However, these are no longer used, and the only two drugs currently licensed in the UK for the treatment of obesity are **sibutramine** and **orlistat**. The two agents work in totally different ways, with sibutramine acting on the CNS to suppress appetite (a true anorectic effect), while orlistat acts within the gastrointestinal tract to prevent fat absorption. Neither should be given without other concomitant dietary and other therapy (e.g. exercise). As might be imagined, the quest for further effective antiobesity agents is the subject of a prodigious effort by the pharmaceutical industry.

SIBUTRAMINE

Sibutramine, originally intended as an antidepressant, has shown promise in the treatment of obesity. The drug inhibits the reuptake of serotonin and noradrenaline at the hypothalamic sites that regulate food intake. Its main effects are to reduce food intake and cause dose-dependent weight loss (see Fig. 27.4), the weight loss being associated with a decrease in obesity-related risk factors. Sibutramine enhances satiety and is reported to produce a reduction in waist circumference (i.e. a reduction in visceral fat), a decrease in plasma triglycerides and very low-density lipoproteins, but an increase in high-density lipoproteins. In addition, beneficial effects on hyperinsulinaemia and the rate of glucose metabolism are said to occur. There is some evidence that the weight loss is associated with higher energy expenditure, possibly through an increase in thermogenesis mediated by the sympathetic nervous system.

A recent meta-analysis of three long-term treatment studies utilising sibutramine in comparison with placebo (Padwal et al., 2003) concluded that there was a 4.6% loss of weight after 1 year's treatment with the drug. There was also a higher (15%) increase in patients who lost more than 10% of their body mass among those taking the drug.

In the UK, the drug is licensed for use in periods up to a year, and the National Institute for Health and Clinical Excellence has advised that it should not be given to people who have not already tried conscientiously to lose weight by other means.

Pharmacokinetic aspects

Sibutramine is given orally, is well absorbed and undergoes extensive first-pass metabolism. The metabolites are responsible for the pharmacological actions. Steady-state blood levels of the metabolites occur within 4 days. The active metabolites are inactivated in the liver, and 85% of the inactive residues are excreted in the urine and faeces.

Unwanted effects

Sibutramine increases heart rate and blood pressure. Regular monitoring of these parameters is essential, and the drug is contraindicated if cardiovascular disease is present or if the systolic or diastolic pressure is raised by 10 mmHg or more. Other unwanted effects include dry mouth, constipation and insomnia. Interactions with drugs that are metabolised by one of the P450 isoenzymes can occur.

ORLISTAT

Orlistat reacts with serine residues at the active sites of gastric and pancreatic lipases, irreversibly inhibiting the enzymes and thereby preventing the breakdown of dietary fat to fatty acids and glycerols. It therefore causes a dose-related decrease in fat absorption and a corresponding increase in faecal fat excretion that plateaus at some 30% of dietary fat. Given with a low-calorie diet in obese individuals, it produces a modest but consistent loss of

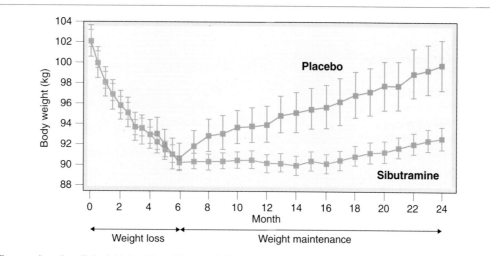

Fig. 27.4 **The results of a clinical trial of the efficacy of sibutramine in maintaining weight loss.** Patients selected for the trial had a body mass index of 30–45 kg/m² and were put on to an initial 6-month treatment programme including oral sibutramine, an individualised 600 kcal/day dietary deficit programme, and activity and behavioural advice. The results are shown in the 'weight loss' section of the graph. (Only patients who had lost 5% of their body weight are represented; 467 of the 499 who completed the 6-month programme.) These responders were then entered into a randomised, placebo-controlled, double-blind parallel group trial to evaluate the effect of sibutramine on weight maintenance. (Figure adapted from James et al. 2000 Lancet v: 2119–2125.)

weight compared with in placebo-treated control subjects. In a recent meta-analysis of 11 long-term placebo-controlled trials encompassing over 6000 patients, orlistat was found to produce a 2.9% greater reduction in body weight than in the control group, and 12% more patients lost 10% or more of their body weight compared with the controls (Padwal et al., 2003).

Orlistat is also reported to be effective in patients suffering from type 2 diabetes and other complications of obesity, to reduce leptin levels and blood pressure, to protect against weight loss–induced changes in biliary secretion, to delay gastric emptying and gastric secretion, to improve several important metabolic parameters, and not to interfere with the release or action of thyroid and other important hormones (Curran & Scott, 2004). It does not induce changes in energy expenditure.

Pharmacokinetic aspects

Virtually all (97%) of orlistat is excreted in the faeces (83% unchanged), with only negligible amounts of the drug or its metabolites being absorbed.

Unwanted effects

Abdominal cramps, flatus with discharge and faecal incontinence can occur, as can intestinal borborygmi (rumbling) and oily spotting. Surprisingly, in view of the possibility of these antisocial effects occurring, the drug is well tolerated. Supplementary therapy with fat-soluble vitamins may be needed, and there has been a report of decreased absorption of contraceptive pills.

No significant drug interactions have been noted, except in the case of **ciclosporin** (see Ch. 14), where reduced absorption of the latter drug has been reported.

PSYCHOTROPIC DRUG THERAPY IN OBESITY

While they cannot be regarded as specific therapies, a common clinical finding is that some subgroups of obese patients, such as those with concomitant depression, respond well to mood-altering drugs such as the selective serotonin uptake inhibitors (see Ch. 39). A discussion of this whole area is beyond the scope of this chapter, and the reader is referred to Appolinario et al. (2004) for further information.

NEW APPROACHES TO OBESITY THERAPY

Rare cases of leptin deficiency in patients have been successfully treated by long-term treatment with the hormone, but this is an unusual intervention and unlikely to be of more than limited use in the future. Many other approaches are being piloted; in fact, a recent review of the area estimated that there were more than 150 novel agents under development (Kaplan, 2005). Some of these aim to exploit the action or production of neuroendocrine satiety signals such as cholecystokinin to produce appetite suppression, while others aim to alter the CNS levels of neurotransmitters such as NPY or melanocortins, which transduce changes in humoral adiposity signals such as leptin (Halford, 2001). The tractability of the MC4 receptor itself as a drug target, coupled with the observation that defects in MC4 signalling are prevalent in obesity, has attracted much interest from the pharmaceutical industry.

Another approach entirely has originated from research in the cannabinoid field (see Ch. 15 for further details). From the clinical (and indeed, anecdotal) observation that marijuana and Δ^9-tetrahydrocannabinol can stimulate appetite has arisen the notion that cannabinoid receptors, especially the CB_1 receptor, may be involved in the control of energy balance (see Di Marzo & Matias, 2005; Vickers & Kennett, 2005). A selective CB_1 antagonist, **rimonabant**, has been developed (Ch. 15) and is currently undergoing phase III clinical trials for a variety of indications, including smoking cessation, obesity and metabolic syndrome (Boyd et al., 2005).

Clinical uses of antiobesity drugs

- The main treatment of obesity is a suitable diet and increased exercise.
- **Orlistat**, which causes fat malabsorption, is considered for severely obese individuals, especially with additional cardiovascular risk factors (e.g. diabetes mellitus, hypertension).

- Many centrally acting appetite suppressants have been withdrawn because of addiction, pulmonary hypertension or other serious adverse effects. **Sibutramine** is one possible adjunctive treatment of severely obese individuals.

REFERENCES AND FURTHER READING

Body weight regulation

Ahima R S, Flier J S 2000a Adipose tissue as an endocrine organ. Trends Endocrinol Metab 11: 327–332 (*Succinct article on the new view of adipose tissue*)

Ahima R S, Flier J S 2000b Leptin. Annu Rev Physiol 62: 413–437 (*Comprehensive review of leptin: its*

expression, actions in hypothalamus, role in energy homeostasis and other actions)

Ahima R S, Osei S 2001 Molecular regulation of eating behaviour: new insights and prospects for future strategies. Trends Mol Med 7: 205–213 (*Praiseworthy short review; excellent figures and useful tables of the*

mediators involved in stimulation and inhibition of feeding behaviour)

Friedman J M 1997 The alphabet of weight control. Nature 385: 119–120

Frühbeck G, Gómez-Ambrosi et al. 2001 The adipocyte: a model for integration of endocrine and metabolic signalling in energy metabolism regulation. Am J Physiol Endocrinol Metab 280: E827–E847 (*Detailed review covering receptors on and the factors secreted by the fat cell, and the role of these factors in energy homeostasis*)

Kennedy G C 1953 The role of depot fat in the hypothalamic control of food intake in the rat. Proc R Soc 140: 578–592 (*The paper that put forward the proposal, based on experiments on rats, that there was a hypothalamus-based homeostatic mechanism for controlling body fat*)

Lowell B B, Spiegelman B M 2000 Towards a molecular understanding of adaptive thermogenesis. Nature 404: 652–660 (*Detailed coverage of the role of the mitochondria, UCP-1 and PPAR in adaptive thermogenesis, emphasising the control of mitochondrial genes*)

Schwartz M W, Woods S C et al. 2000 Central nervous control of food intake. Nature 404: 661–671 (*Outlines a model that delineates the roles of hormones and neuropeptides in the control of food intake. Outstanding diagrams. Note that there are several other excellent articles in this* Nature Insight *supplement on obesity.*)

Spiegelman B M, Flier J S 1996 Adipogenesis and obesity: rounding out the big picture. Cell 87: 377–389

Spiegelman B M, Flier J S 2001 Obesity regulation and energy balance. Cell 104: 531–543 (*Excellent review with up-to-date coverage of the CNS control of energy intake/body weight, monogenic obesities, leptin physiology, central neural circuits, the melanocortin pathway, the role of insulin, and adaptive thermogenesis*)

Weigle D S 1994 Appetite and the regulation of body composition. FASEB J 8: 302–310

Obesity as a disease

Colditz G A, Willett W C, Rotnitzky A, Manson J E 1995 Weight gain as a risk factor for clinical diabetes mellitus in women. Ann Intern Med 122: 481–486

Kopelman P G 2000 Obesity as a medical problem. Nature 404: 635–643

Obesity genetics

Barsh G S, Farooqi I S, O'Rahilly S 2000 Genetics of body-weight regulation. Nature 404: 644–651

Loos R J, Rankinen T 2005 Gene–diet interactions on body weight changes. J Am Diet Assoc 105(5 suppl 1): S29–S34 (*Discusses gene–environment studies relating to obesity, drawing on data from monozygotic twins and candidate gene approaches*)

Pérusse C et al. 2005 The human obesity gene map: the 2004 update. Obes Res 13: 381–490 (*Detailed review of the genes, markers and chromosomal regions that*

have been shown to be associated with human obesity; *see also web site below*)

Zhang Y, Proenca R et al. 1994 Positional cloning of the mouse obese gene and its human homologue. Nature 372: 425–432

Drugs in obesity

Appolinario J C, Bueno J R, Coutinho W 2004 Psychotropic drugs in the treatment of obesity: what promise? CNS Drugs 18: 629–651

Bray G A, Greenway F L 1999 Current and potential drugs for treatment of obesity. Endocr Rev 20: 875–905 (*Comprehensive review of agents that affect or could affect food intake, metabolism and energy expenditure, with details of drugs in development*)

Chiesi M, Huppertz C, Hofbauer K G 2001 Pharmacotherapy of obesity: targets and perspectives. Trends Pharmacol Sci 22: 247–254 (*Commendable, succinct review; table of the potential targets, and useful, simple figures of the central and peripheral pathways of energy regulation and of the regulation of thermogenesis*)

Clapham J C, Arch J R S, Tadayyon M 2001 Anti-obesity drugs: a critical review of current therapies and future opportunities. Pharmacol Ther 89: 81–121 (*Comprehensive review covering, under energy intake; biogenic amines, cannabinoids, neuropeptides, leptin, gastrointestinal tract peptides and inhibitors of fat absorption; and under energy expenditure,* β_3-*adrenoceptor agonists and uncoupling proteins*)

Collins P, Williams G 2001 Drug treatment of obesity: from past failures to future successes? Br J Clin Pharmacol 51: 13–25 (*Overview—from a clinical perspective—of currently available antiobesity drugs and potential future drugs; well written*)

Crowley V E F, Yeo G S H, O'Rahilly S 2002 Obesity therapy: altering the energy intake-and-expenditure balance sheet. Nat Rev Drug Discov 1: 276–286 (*Review stressing that pharmacological approaches to obesity therapy necessitate altering the balance between energy intake and expenditure and/or altering the partitioning of nutrients between lean tissue and fat*)

Curran M P, Scott L J 2004 Orlistat: a review of its use in the management of patients with obesity. Drugs 64: 2845–2864

Després J-P, Lemieux I, Prud'homme D 2001 Treatment of obesity: need to focus on high risk abdominally obese patients. Br Med J 322: 716–722 (*Succinct review giving simple clear coverage of the clinical approach to obesity therapy, with simple clear diagrams*)

James W P T, Finer N, Kopelman P et al. 2000 Effect of sibutramine on weight maintenance after weight loss: a randomised trial. Lancet 256: 2119–2125 (*Report of*

the results of a multicentre randomised double-blind clinical trial*)

Padwal R, Li S K, Lau D C 2003 Long-term pharmacotherapy for overweight and obesity: a systematic review and meta-analysis of randomized controlled trials. Int J Obes Relat Metab Disord 27: 1437–1446.

Yanovski S Z, Yanovski J A 2002 Obesity. N Engl J Med 346: 591–602 (*Outlines non-pharmacological approaches to promoting weight loss and then discusses in more detail the use of antiobesity drugs*)

Future drug treatments for obesity

Boyd S T, Fremming B A 2005 Rimonabant—a selective CB$_1$ antagonist. Ann Pharmacother 39: 684–690 (*A review of the pharmacology of rimonabant based on published studies*)

Després J-P, Golay A, Sjostrom L 2005 Effects of rimonabant on metabolic risk factors in overweight patients with dyslipidemia. N Engl J Med 353: 2121–2134 (*The results of an original study, in over 1000 patients, of this novel antiobesity agent*)

Di Marzo V, Matias I 2005 Endocannabinoid control of food intake and energy balance. Nat Neurosci 8: 585–589 (*A discussion of the putative role of endocannabinoids in this complex physiological mechanism; also considers therapeutic applications arising from this area*)

Donnelly R 2003 Researching new treatments for obesity: from neuroscience to inflammation. Diabetes Obes Metab 5: 1–4

Halford J C 2001 Pharmacology of appetite suppression: implication for the treatment of obesity. Curr Drug Targets 2: 353–370

Kaplan L M 2005 Pharmacological therapies for obesity. Gastroenterol Clin North Am 34: 91–104

Lefebvre P J, Scheen A J 2001 Obesity: causes and new treatments. Exp Clin Endocrinol Diabet 109(suppl 2): S215–S224

Mertens I L, Van Gaal L F 2000 Promising new approaches to the management of obesity. Drugs 60: 1–9

Vickers S P, Kennett G A 2005 Cannabinoids and the regulation of ingestive behaviour. Curr Drug Targets 6: 215–223

Useful web resources

http://obesitygene.pbrc.edu (*This is the web site of the Obesity Gene Map Database*)

http://www.who.int (*This is the World Health Organization web page that carries data about the prevalence of 'globesity' and its distribution around the world; click on the* Health topics *link and navigate to* Obesity *in the alphabetical list of topics for further information*)

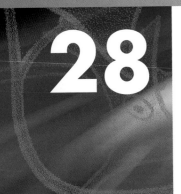

28

The pituitary and the adrenal cortex

OVERVIEW

The pituitary and adrenal glands are major sites for the synthesis and release of hormones that profoundly affect the biochemistry and physiology of almost all cells, and which are crucial to the understanding of the actions of many anti-inflammatory and other drugs. The pituitary itself is controlled by hormones released from the hypothalamus and, in turn, the hypothalamic –pituitary axis orchestrates the activity of the adrenal (and other endocrine) glands. In the first part of this chapter, we examine the control of pituitary function by hypothalamic hormones and review the physiological roles and clinical uses of both anterior and posterior pituitary hormones. The second part of the chapter concentrates on the actions of adrenal hormones and, in particular, the anti-inflammatory effect of glucocorticoids. This should be read in conjunction with the relevant sections of Chapters 3 and 14.

THE PITUITARY

The pituitary gland comprises three different structures arising from two different embryological precursors. The *anterior pituitary* and the *intermediate lobe* are derived from the endoderm of the buccal cavity, while the *posterior pituitary* is derived from neural ectoderm. The main parts of the gland, the anterior and posterior lobes, receive independent neuronal input from the hypothalamus, with which they have an intimate functional relationship.

ANTERIOR PITUITARY (ADENOHYPOPHYSIS)

The anterior pituitary (*adenohypophysis*) secretes a number of hormones crucial for normal physiological function. Within this tissue are specialised cells such as *corticotrophs*, *lactotrophs* (mammotrophs), *somatotrophs*, *thyrotrophs* and *gonadotrophs*, which secrete hormones that regulate different endocrine organs of the body (Table 28.1). Interspersed among these are other cell types, including the *folliculostellate cells* that exert a nurturing and regulatory influence on the hormone-secreting endocrine cells.

Secretion from the anterior pituitary is largely regulated by 'factors'[1]—in effect hormones—that are derived from the hypothalamus and that reach the pituitary through the bloodstream. Blood vessels to the hypothalamus divide in its tissue to form a meshwork of capillaries, the primary plexus (Fig. 28.1), which drains into the hypophyseal *portal vessels*. These pass through the pituitary stalk to feed a secondary plexus of capillaries in the anterior pituitary. Peptidergic neurons in the hypothalamus secrete a variety of releasing or inhibitory hormones directly into the capillaries of the primary plexus (Table 28.1 and Fig. 28.1). Most of these regulate the secretion of hormones from the anterior lobe, although the melanocyte-stimulating hormones (MSHs) are secreted mainly from the intermediate lobe.

Negative feedback pathways between the hormones of the hypothalamus, the anterior pituitary and the peripheral endocrine glands regulate the release of stimulatory hormones and integrate the functions of individual components of the endocrine system into a functional whole. In *long negative feedback* pathways, hormones secreted from the peripheral glands exert regulatory actions on both the hypothalamus and the anterior pituitary. The mediators of the *short negative feedback* pathways are anterior pituitary hormones that act directly on the hypothalamus.

The peptidergic neurons in the hypothalamus are themselves influenced by other centres within the central nervous system (CNS). This action is mediated through pathways that release dopamine, noradrenaline (norepinephrine), 5-hydroxytryptamine

---

[1] The word 'factor' was originally coined at a time when their structure and function were not known. These are blood-borne messengers, and as such are clearly hormones. Nevertheless, the term *factor*, however irrational, lingers on.

Table 28.1 Hormones secreted by the hypothalamus and the anterior pituitary

Hypothalamic factor/hormone (and related drugs)	Hormone affected in anterior pituitary (and related drugs)	Main effects of anterior pituitary hormone
Corticotrophin-releasing factor	Adrenocorticotrophic hormone (corticotrophin, tetracosactide)	Stimulates secretion of adrenal cortical hormones (mainly glucocorticoids); maintains integrity of adrenal cortex
Thyrotrophin-releasing hormone (TRH, protirelin)	Thyroid-stimulating hormone (thyrotrophin)	Stimulates synthesis and secretion of thyroid hormones, thyroxine and triiodothyronine; maintains integrity of thyroid gland
Growth hormone–releasing factor	Growth hormone (somatotrophin)	Regulates growth, partly directly, partly through evoking the release of somatomedins from the liver and elsewhere; increases protein synthesis, increases blood glucose, stimulates lipolysis
Growth hormone release–inhibiting factor (somatostatin, octreotide)	Growth hormone	As above
Gonadotrophin-releasing hormone (GnRH, somatorelin, sermorelin)	Follicle-stimulating hormone (FSH; see Ch. 30)	Stimulates the growth of the ovum and the Graafian follicle in the female, and gametogenesis in the male; with LH, stimulates the secretion of oestrogen throughout the menstrual cycle and progesterone in the second half
	Luteinising hormone (LH) or interstitial cell–stimulating hormone (see Ch. 30)	Stimulates ovulation and the development of the corpus luteum; with FSH, stimulates secretion of oestrogen and progesterone in menstrual cycle; in male, regulates testosterone secretion
Prolactin release–inhibiting factor (probably dopamine)	Prolactin	Together with other hormones, prolactin, promotes development of mammary tissue during pregnancy; stimulates milk production in the postpartum period
Prolactin-releasing factor	Prolactin	As above
Melanocyte-stimulating hormone (MSH) releasing factor	α-, β- and γ-MSH	Promotes formation of melanin, which causes darkening of skin; MSH is anti-inflammatory and helps to regulate feeding
MSH release–inhibiting factor	α-, β- and γ-MSH	As above

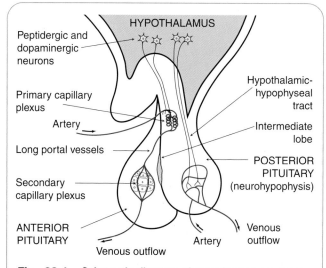

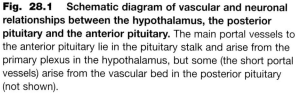

Fig. 28.1 **Schematic diagram of vascular and neuronal relationships between the hypothalamus, the posterior pituitary and the anterior pituitary.** The main portal vessels to the anterior pituitary lie in the pituitary stalk and arise from the primary plexus in the hypothalamus, but some (the short portal vessels) arise from the vascular bed in the posterior pituitary (not shown).

and the opioid peptides, the last of these being found in very high density in the hypothalamus (see Ch. 16). Hypothalamic control of the anterior pituitary is also exerted through the *tuberohypophyseal dopaminergic pathway*, the neurons of which lie in close apposition to the primary capillary plexus (see Ch. 32). Dopamine secreted directly into the hypophyseal portal circulation reaches the anterior pituitary in the blood.

HYPOTHALAMIC HORMONES

The secretion of anterior pituitary hormones is regulated by some six sets of *releasing factors* that originate in the hypothalamus. These are listed in Table 28.1 and are described in more detail below. Some are used clinically for diagnosis or treatment, whereas others are useful research tools. Many of these releasing factor hormones also function as neurotransmitters or neuromodulators elsewhere in the CNS (Ch. 32).

GROWTH HORMONE–RELEASING FACTOR (SOMATORELIN)

Growth hormone–releasing factor (GHRF) is a peptide with 40–44 amino acid residues. An analogue, **sermorelin**, has been introduced as a diagnostic test for growth hormone secretion. The main action of GHRF is summarised in Figure 28.2. Given intravenously, subcutaneously or intranasally (generally the former), it causes secretion of growth hormone within minutes and peak concentrations in 60 minutes. The action is selective for the somatotrophs in the anterior pituitary, and no other pituitary hormones are affected. *Unwanted effects* are rare.

SOMATOSTATIN

Somatostatin is a peptide of 14 amino acid residues. It inhibits the release of growth hormone and thyroid-stimulating hormone (TSH, thyrotrophin) from the anterior pituitary (Fig. 28.2), and insulin and glucagon from the pancreas; it also decreases the release of most gastrointestinal hormones, and reduces gastric acid and pancreatic secretion.

Octreotide is a long-acting analogue of somatostatin (see also Ch. 26 and Ch. 51). It is used for the treatment of tumours secreting vasoactive intestinal peptide, carcinoid tumours (Ch. 12), glucagonomas and various pituitary adenomas. It also has a place in the therapy of acromegaly (a condition in which there is oversecretion of growth hormone in an adult) and of bleeding oesophageal varices. Octreotide is generally given subcutaneously. The peak action is at 2 hours, and the suppressant effect lasts for up to 8 hours.

Unwanted effects include pain at the injection site and gastrointestinal disturbances. Gallstones and postprandial hyperglycaemia have also been reported, and acute hepatitis has occurred in a few cases.

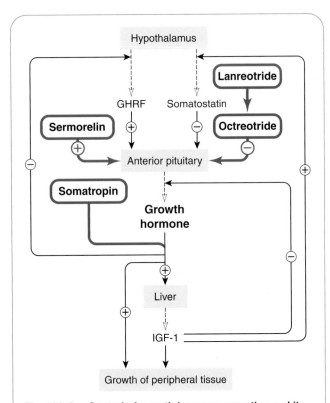

Fig. 28.2 Control of growth hormone secretion and its actions. Drugs are shown in yellow boxes. GHRF, growth hormone–releasing factor; IGF-1, insulin-like growth factor-1.

Lanreotide has similar effects but is also used in the treatment of thyroid tumours.

THYROTROPHIN-RELEASING HORMONE (PROTIRELIN)

Thyrotrophin-releasing hormone (TRH) from the hypothalamus releases TSH from the anterior pituitary. **Protirelin** is a synthetic TSH used for the diagnosis of thyroid disorders (see Ch. 29). Given intravenously in normal subjects, it causes an increase in plasma TSH concentration, whereas in patients with *hyper*thyroidism there is a blunted response because the raised blood thyroxine concentration has a negative feedback effect on the anterior pituitary. The opposite occurs with *hypo*thyroidism, where there is an intrinsic defect in the thyroid itself.

CORTICOTROPHIN-RELEASING FACTOR

Corticotrophin-releasing factor (CRF) is a peptide that releases **adrenocorticotrophic hormone** (**ACTH**, corticotrophin) and β-endorphin from the anterior pituitary. CRF acts synergistically with *antidiuretic hormone* (*ADH*; arginine-**vasopressin**), and both its action and its release are inhibited by *glucocorticoids* (see Fig. 28.4, below). Synthetic preparations have been used to test the ability of the pituitary to secrete ACTH, and to assess whether ACTH deficiency is caused by a pituitary or a hypothalamic defect. It has also been used to evaluate hypothalamic pituitary function after therapy for Cushing's syndrome (see Fig. 28.7, below).

GONADOTROPHIN-RELEASING HORMONE

Gonadotrophin- (or luteinising hormone–) releasing hormone is a decapeptide that releases both *follicle-stimulating hormone* and *luteinising hormone*. It is also available as a preparation called **gonadorelin**. Its primary clinical utility is in the treatment of infertility, and its actions are described in Chapter 30.

ANTERIOR PITUITARY HORMONES

The main hormones of the anterior pituitary are listed in Table 28.1. The gonadotrophins are dealt with in Chapter 30, and TSH in Chapter 29. The remainder are dealt with below.

GROWTH HORMONE (SOMATOTROPHIN)

Growth hormone is secreted by the somatotroph cells and is the most abundant pituitary hormone. Secretion is high in the newborn, decreasing at 4 years to an intermediate level, which is then maintained until after puberty, after which there is a further decline. Several recombinant preparations of growth hormone, or **somatropin**, are available for treating growth defects and other developmental problems (see below).

Regulation of secretion

Secretion of growth hormone is regulated by the action of hypothalamic GHRF modulated by somatostatin, as described above and outlined in Figure 28.2. One of the mediators of growth hormone action, *insulin-like growth factor (IGF)-1*, which is released from the liver (see below), has an inhibitory effect on growth hormone secretion by stimulating somatostatin release from the hypothalamus.

Growth hormone release, like other anterior pituitary secretions, is pulsatile, and its plasma concentration may fluctuate 10- to 100-fold. These surges occur repeatedly during the day and night, and reflect the dynamics of hypothalamic control. Deep sleep is a potent stimulus to growth hormone secretion, particularly in children.

Actions

The main effect of growth hormone (and its analogues) is to stimulate normal growth and, in doing this, it affects many tissues, acting in conjunction with other hormones secreted from the thyroid, the gonads and the adrenal cortex. It stimulates hepatic production of the IGFs—also termed *somatomedins*—which mediate most of its anabolic actions. Receptors for IGF-1 (the principal mediator) exist on many cell types, including liver cells and fat cells.

Growth hormone stimulates the uptake of amino acids and protein synthesis, especially in skeletal muscle. IGF-1 mediates many of these anabolic effects, acting on skeletal muscle and also on the cartilage at the epiphyses of long bones, thus influencing bone growth.

Disorders of production and clinical use

Deficiency of growth hormone results in *pituitary dwarfism*. In this condition, which may result from lack of GHRF or a failure of IGF generation or action, the normal proportions of the body are maintained. Growth hormone is used therapeutically in patients (often children) with growth hormone deficiency and with the short stature associated with *Turner's syndrome*. It may also be used to correct chronic renal insufficiency in children. Satisfactory linear growth can be achieved by giving somatropin subcutaneously, six to seven times per week, and therapy is most successful when started early. Humans are insensitive to growth hormone of other species, so human growth hormone must be used clinically. This used to be obtained from human cadavers, leading to the spread of Creutzfeldt–Jakob disease, a prion-mediated neurodegenerative disorder (Ch. 35). Human growth hormone is now prepared by recombinant DNA technology, which avoids the risk of prion contamination.

An excessive production of growth hormone in children results in *gigantism*. An excessive production in adults, which is usually the result of a benign pituitary tumour, results in *acromegaly*, in which there is enlargement mainly of facial structures and of the hands and feet. The dopamine agonist **bromocriptine** and octreotide may mitigate the condition, but effective treatment demands removal or irradiation of the tumour.

PROLACTIN

Prolactin is secreted from the anterior pituitary by *lactotroph* (mammotroph) cells. These are abundant in the gland and increase in number during pregnancy, probably under the influence of oestrogen.

Regulation of secretion

Prolactin secretion is under tonic inhibitory control by the hypothalamus (Fig. 28.3 and Table 28.1), the inhibitory mediator being dopamine (acting on D_2 receptors on the lactotrophs). The main stimulus for release is suckling; in rats, both the smell and the sounds of hungry pups are also effective triggers. Neural reflexes from the breast may stimulate the secretion from the hypothalamus of prolactin-releasing factor(s), possible candidates for which include TRH and **oxytocin**. Oestrogens increase both prolactin secretion and the proliferation of lactotrophs through release, from a subset of lactotrophs, of the neuropeptide galanin. Dopamine antagonists (used mainly as antipsychotic drugs; see Ch. 38) are potent stimulants of prolactin release, whereas agonists such as bromocriptine (see below and also Chs 12, 35 and 38) suppress prolactin release. Bromocriptine is also used in parkinsonism.

Actions

There are at least three specific receptor subtypes that bind prolactin, and these are not only found in the mammary gland but are widely distributed throughout the body, including the brain, ovary, heart and lungs. The main function of prolactin in women is the control of milk production. At parturition, when the blood level of oestrogen falls, the prolactin concentration rises and lactation is initiated. Maintenance of lactation depends on suckling, which stimulates a reflex secretion of prolactin by neural pathways, causing a 10- to 100-fold increase within 30 minutes.

Together with other hormones, prolactin is responsible for the proliferation and differentiation of mammary tissue during pregnancy. It inhibits gonadotrophin release and/or the response of the ovaries to these trophic hormones. This is one of the reasons

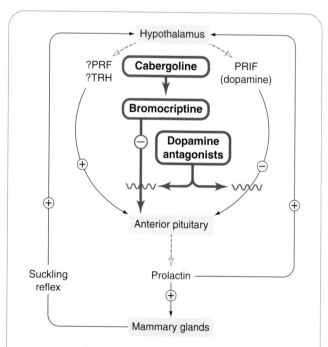

Fig. 28.3 **Control of prolactin secretion.** Drugs are shown in yellow boxes. PRF, prolactin-releasing factor; PRIF, prolactin release–inhibiting factor; TRH, thyrotrophin-releasing hormone.

why ovulation does not usually occur during breast feeding, and it is believed to constitute a natural contraceptive mechanism.

▼ According to one rather appealing hypothesis, the high postpartum concentration of prolactin reflects its biological function as a 'parental' hormone. Certainly broodiness and nest-building activity can be induced in birds, mice and rabbits by prolactin injections. It is rather attractive to think that it might have a similar action in humans, although this is conjectural. Prolactin also exerts other, apparently unrelated, actions, including stimulating mitogenesis in lymphocytes. There is some evidence that it may play a part in regulating immune responses.

Modification of prolactin secretion

Prolactin itself is not used clinically. Bromocriptine, which stimulates dopamine receptors, is used to decrease excessive prolactin secretion (e.g. that results from *prolactinomas*). It is well absorbed orally, and peak concentrations occur after 2 hours. Unwanted reactions include nausea and vomiting. Dizziness, constipation and postural hypotension may also occur. **Cabergoline** is a related compound with similar effects, and **quinagolide**, having actions similar to those of ergot-derived dopamine agonists, may also be used for *hyperprolactinaemia*.

ADRENOCORTICOTROPHIC HORMONE

Adrenocorticotrophic hormone (corticotrophin) is the anterior pituitary secretion that controls the synthesis and release of the glucocorticoids of the adrenal cortex (see Table 28.1 and p. 427). It is a polypeptide hormone with 39 amino acid residues derived from the precursor pro-opiomelanocortin by sequential proteolytic processing. Detail of the regulation of ACTH secretion is shown in Figure 28.4.

▼ This hormone occupies (together with *cortisone*) an important place in the history of inflammation therapy because of the work of Hench and his colleagues in the 1940s, who first observed that both substances had anti-inflammatory effects in patients with rheumatoid disease. The effect of ACTH was thought to be secondary to stimulation of the adrenal cortex but, interestingly, the hormone also has anti-inflammatory actions in its own right, through activation of macrophage (melanocortin) MC$_3$ receptors (Getting et al., 2002).

Adrenocorticotrophic hormone itself is not often used in therapy today, because its action is less predictable than that of the corticosteroids and it may provokes antibody formation. **Tetracosactide**, a synthetic polypeptide that consists of the first 24 N-terminal residues of human ACTH, has the same drawbacks but is now

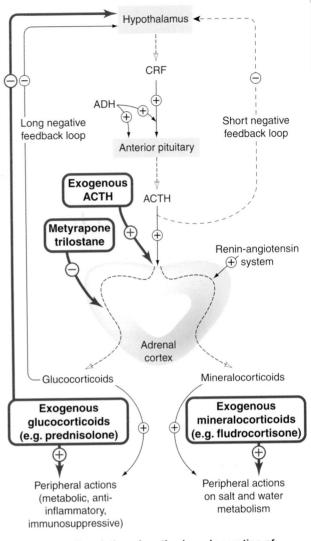

Fig. 28.4 Regulation of synthesis and secretion of adrenal corticosteroids. The long negative feedback loop is more important than the short loop (dashed lines). Adrenocorticotrophic hormone (ACTH, corticotrophin) has only a minimal effect on mineralocorticoid production. Drugs are shown in yellow boxes. ADH, antidiuretic hormone (vasopressin); CRF, corticotrophin-releasing factor.

widely used in its stead for assessing the competency of the adrenal cortex (see below).

The concentration of ACTH in the blood is reduced by glucocorticoids, forming the basis of the **dexamethasone** *suppression test* (see p. 433).

Actions

Tetracosactide and ACTH have two actions on the adrenal cortex.

- Stimulation of the synthesis and release of glucocorticoids. This action occurs within minutes of injection, and the main biological actions are those of the steroids released.
- A trophic action on adrenal cortical cells, and regulation of the levels of key mitochondrial steroidogenic enzymes. The

---

Clinical use of bromocriptine

- To prevent lactation
- To treat galactorrhoea (i.e. non-puerperal lactation in either sex), owing to excessive prolactin secretion.
- To treat prolactin-secreting pituitary tumours (prolactinomas).
- In the treatment of parkinsonism (Ch. 35) and of acromegaly.

loss of this effect accounts for the adrenal atrophy that results from chronic glucocorticoid administration (see p. 429), which suppresses ACTH secretion.

The main use of tetracosactide is in the diagnosis of adrenal cortical insufficiency. The drug is given intramuscularly, and the concentration of **hydrocortisone** in the plasma is measured by radioimmunoassay.

MELANOCYTE-STIMULATING HORMONE

The MSH peptides, α-, β- and γ-MSH, are peptide hormones with structural similarity to ACTH and are derived from the same precursor. Together, these peptides are referred to as *melanocortins*, because their first recognised action was to stimulate the production of melanin by specialised skin cells called *melanocytes*. As such, they play an important part in determining hair coloration, skin colour and reaction to ultraviolet light.

Melanocyte-stimulating hormone acts on melanocortin receptors, of which five (MC_{1-5}) have been cloned. These are G-protein–coupled receptors that activate cAMP synthesis. Melanin formation is under the control of the MC_1 receptor, and excessive α-MSH production can provoke abnormal proliferation of melanocytes and may predispose to melanoma.

▼ Melanocortins exhibit numerous other biological effects. For example, α-MSH inhibits cytokine (interleukin [IL]-1β and tumour necrosis factor-α [TNF]) release, reduces neutrophil infiltration, and exhibits anti-inflammatory and antipyretic activity. Levels of α-MSH are increased in synovial fluid of patients with rheumatoid arthritis. MC_1 and MC_3 receptors mediate the immunomodulatory effect of MSH. Agonists at these receptors with potential anti-inflammatory activity are being sought.

γ-Melanocyte–stimulating hormone increases blood pressure, heart rate and cerebral blood flow following intracerebroventricular or intravenous injection. These effects are likely mediated by the MC_4 receptor. Central injection of α-MSH also causes changes in animal behaviour, such as increased grooming and sexual activity as well as reduced feeding.

Two naturally occurring ligands for melanocortin receptors (*agouti-signalling protein* and *agouti-related peptide*, together called the *agouti*) have been discovered in human tissues. These are proteins that competitively antagonise the effect of MSH at melanocortin receptors. Their precise role in the body is not known.

Adrenocorticotrophic hormone (corticotrophin) and the adrenal steroids

- Adrenocorticotrophic hormone (ACTH) stimulates synthesis and release of glucocorticoids (e.g. hydrocortisone), and also some androgens, from the adrenal cortex.
- Corticotrophin-releasing factor from the hypothalamus regulates ACTH release, and is regulated in turn by neural factors and negative feedback effects of plasma glucocorticoids.
- Mineralocorticoid (e.g. aldosterone) release from the adrenal cortex is controlled by the renin–angiotensin system.

The anterior pituitary gland and hypothalamus

- The anterior pituitary gland secretes hormones that regulate:
  - the release of *glucocorticoids* from adrenal cortex
  - the release of *thyroid hormones*
  - *ovulation* in the female and spermatogenesis in the male, and the *release of sex hormones*
  - *growth*
  - *mammary gland* structure and function.
- Each anterior pituitary hormone is regulated by a specific hypothalamic releasing factor. Feedback mechanisms govern the release of these factors. Substances available for clinical use include:
  - *growth hormone–releasing factor* (sermorelin) and analogues of growth hormone (somatrem, somatropin)
  - *thyrotrophin-releasing factor* (protirelin) and *thyroid-stimulating hormone* (thyrotrophin; used to test thyroid function)
  - octreotide and lanreotide, *analogues of somatostatin*, which inhibit growth hormone release
  - corticotrophin-releasing factor, used in diagnosis
  - gonadotrophin-releasing factor.

POSTERIOR PITUITARY (NEUROHYPOPHYSIS)

The posterior pituitary gland consists largely of the terminals of nerve cells that lie in the *supraoptic* and *paraventricular* nuclei of the hypothalamus. Their axons form the *hypothalamic-hypophyseal tract*, and the fibres terminate in dilated nerve endings in close association with capillaries in the posterior pituitary gland (Fig. 28.1). Peptides, synthesised in the hypothalamic nuclei, pass down these axons into the posterior pituitary, where they are stored and eventually secreted into the bloodstream.

The two main hormones of the posterior pituitary are oxytocin (which contracts the smooth muscle of the uterus; see Ch. 30) and ADH (also called vasopressin; see Chs 19 and 24). Several similar peptides have been synthesised that vary in their antidiuretic, vasopressor and oxytocic (uterine stimulant) properties.

ANTIDIURETIC HORMONE

Regulation of secretion and physiological role

Antidiuretic hormone released from the posterior pituitary has a crucial role in the control of the water content of the body through its action on the cells of the distal part of the nephron and the collecting tubules in the kidney (see Ch. 24). The hypothalamic nuclei that control fluid balance lie close to the nuclei that synthesise and secrete ADH.

One of the main stimuli to ADH release is an increase in plasma osmolality (which produces a sensation of thirst). A decrease in circulating blood volume (*hypovolaemia*) is another, and here the stimuli arise from baroreceptors in the cardiovascular system or from angiotensin release. *Diabetes insipidus* is a condition in which large volumes of dilute urine are produced because ADH secretion is reduced or absent, or because of a reduced sensitivity of the kidney to the hormone.

Antidiuretic hormone receptors

There are three classes of receptor for ADH: V_1, V_2 and V_3. V_2 receptors, which are coupled to adenylate cyclase, mediate its main physiological actions in the kidney, whereas the V_1 and V_3 receptors are coupled to the phospholipase C/inositol trisphosphate system.

Actions

Renal actions

Antidiuretic hormone binds to V_2 receptors in the basolateral membrane of the cells of the distal tubule and collecting ducts of the nephron. Its main effect in the collecting duct is to increase the rate of insertion of water channels into the lumenal membrane, thus increasing the permeability of the membrane to water (see Ch. 24). It also activates urea transporters and transiently increases Na^+ absorption, particularly in the distal tubule.

Several drugs affect the action of ADH. Non-steroidal anti-inflammatory drugs and **carbamazepine** increase, and **lithium**, **colchicine** and **vinca alkaloids** decrease, ADH effects. The effects of the last two agents are secondary to their action on the microtubules required for translocation of water channels. **Demeclocycline** counteracts the action of ADH and can be used to treat patients with *hyponatraemia* (and thus water retention) caused by excessive secretion of ADH.

Other non-renal actions

Antidiuretic hormone causes contraction of smooth muscle, particularly in the cardiovascular system, by acting on V_1 receptors (see Ch. 19). The affinity of these receptors for ADH is lower than that of the V_2 receptors, and smooth muscle effects are seen only with doses larger than those affecting the kidney. ADH also stimulates blood platelet aggregation and mobilisation of coagulation factors. In the CNS, ADH acts as a neuromodulator and neurotransmitter. When released into the pituitary 'portal circulation', it promotes the release of ACTH from the anterior pituitary by an action on V_3 receptors (Fig. 28.4).

Pharmacokinetic aspects

Antidiuretic hormone, as well as various analogues, is used clinically either for the treatment of *diabetes insipidus* or as a vasoconstrictor. The analogues have been developed to (a) increase the duration of action and (b) shift the potency between V_1 and V_2 receptors.

The main substances used are vasopressin (ADH itself: short duration of action, weak selectivity for V_2 receptors, given by subcutaneous or intramuscular injection, or by intravenous infusion), **desmopressin** (increased duration of action, V_2-selective and usually given as a nasal spray), **terlipressin** (increased duration of action, low but protracted vasopressor action and minimal antidiuretic properties) and **felypressin** (short duration

of action, vasoconstrictor effect is used with local anaesthetics such as **prilocaine** to prolong its action; see Ch. 44).

Vasopressin is rapidly eliminated, with a plasma half-life of 10 minutes and a short duration of action. Metabolism is by tissue peptidases, and 33% is removed by the kidney. Desmopressin is less subject to degradation by peptidases, and its plasma half-life is 75 minutes.

▼ Various synthetic non-peptide agonists and antagonists of ADH have been synthesised and are used as experimental tools. Several orally active V_1 receptor antagonists are under study for the treatment of dysmenorrhoea (for a review of ADH receptor antagonists and their possible clinical uses, see Thibonnier et al., 2001).

Unwanted effects

There are few unwanted effects if the antidiuretic peptides are administered intranasally in therapeutic doses, although intravenous vasopressin may cause spasm of the coronary arteries, with resultant angina.

OXYTOCIN

Oxytocin is discussed in Chapter 30.

> **Posterior pituitary**
>
> - The posterior pituitary secretes:
>   — oxytocin (see Ch. 30)
>   — antidiuretic hormone (vasopressin), which acts on V_2 receptors in the distal kidney tubule to increase water reabsorption and, in higher concentrations, on V_1 receptors to cause vasoconstriction. It also stimulates adrenocorticotrophic hormone secretion.
> - Substances available for clinical use are vasopressin and the analogues desmopressin and terlipressin.

> **Clinical use of antidiuretic hormone (vasopressin) and analogues**
>
> - *Diabetes insipidus*: **lypressin, desmopressin**.
> - Initial treatment of bleeding *oesophageal varices*: **vasopressin, terlipressin, lypressin**. (**Octreotide**—a somatostatin analogue—is also used, but direct injection of sclerosant via an endoscope is the main treatment.)
> - Prophylaxis against bleeding in *haemophilia* (e.g. before tooth extraction): **vasopressin, desmopressin** (by increasing the concentration of factor VIII).
> - **Felypressin** is used as a vasoconstrictor with local anaesthetics (see Ch. 44).
> - **Desmopressin** is used for persistent nocturnal *enuresis* in older children and adults.

THE ADRENAL CORTEX

ADRENAL STEROIDS

The adrenal glands are situated above the kidneys, and for this reason they are sometimes referred to as the suprarenal glands. At a gross level, the gland comprises two components: the *medulla*, which secretes catecholamines (see Ch. 9), and the *cortex*, which secretes adrenal steroids. The latter structure, which concerns us in this section, may be divided further on a histological basis into three concentric zones: the *zona glomerulosa* (the outermost layer) that elaborates mineralocorticoids, the *zona fasciculata* that elaborates glucocorticoids, and the innermost *zona reticularis*. While the principal adrenal steroids are those with mineralocorticoid and glucocorticoid activity, some sex steroids (mainly androgens) are also secreted by the gland but will not be considered further in this chapter.

The mineralocorticoids regulate water and electrolyte balance, and the main endogenous hormone is *aldosterone*. The glucocorticoids have widespread actions on intermediate metabolism, affecting carbohydrate and protein metabolism, as well as a potent regulatory effect on our endogenous 'defence' reactions such as the innate and acquired immune response. The adrenal secretes a mixture of glucocorticoids, but the main hormone in humans is *hydrocortisone* (also, confusingly, called *cortisol*), but in rodents *corticosterone* predominates. The mineralocorticoid and glucocorticoid actions are not completely separated in naturally occurring steroids, some glucocorticoids having quite substantial effects on water and electrolyte balance. In fact, hydrocortisone and aldosterone are equiactive on mineralocorticoid receptors, but, in mineralocorticoid-sensitive tissues such as the kidney, the action of *11β-hydroxysteroid dehydrogenase* converts hydrocortisone to an inactive metabolite *cortisone*,[2] thereby protecting the receptor from inappropriate activation. With the exception of *replacement therapy* (see below), glucocorticoids are most commonly employed for their anti-inflammatory and immunosuppressive properties. Under these circumstances, all their metabolic and other actions are seen as unwanted side effects. Synthetic steroids have been developed in which it has been possible to separate, to some degree, the glucocorticoid from the mineralocorticoid actions (see Table 28.2), but it has not been possible to separate the anti-inflammatory actions from the other actions of the glucocorticoids.

The adrenal gland is essential to life, and animals deprived of these glands are able to survive only under rigorously controlled conditions. In humans, a deficiency in corticosteroid production, termed *Addison's disease*, is characterised by muscular weakness, low blood pressure, depression, anorexia, loss of weight and hypoglycaemia. Addison's disease may have an autoimmune aetiology, or it may result from destruction of the gland by

chronic inflammatory conditions such as tuberculosis. Because of the negative feedback effects that glucocorticoids exert on ACTH release, a decreased production of endogenous corticoids also occurs when glucocorticoids are given therapeutically for prolonged periods. This can result in deficiency when treatment is discontinued, and is the reason why glucocorticoid therapy is usually tapered off to allow recovery of anterior pituitary function.

When corticosteroids are produced in excess, the clinical picture depends on which of the steroids predominates. Excessive glucocorticoid activity results in *Cushing's syndrome*, the manifestations of which are outlined in Figure 28.7. This can be caused by hypersecretion from the adrenal glands or by prolonged therapeutic glucocorticoid regimens. An excessive production of mineralocorticoids results in disturbances of Na^+ and K^+ balance. This may occur with hyperactivity of the adrenals or tumours of the glands (*primary hyperaldosteronism*, or *Conn's syndrome*, an uncommon but important cause of hypertension; see Ch. 19), or with excessive renin–angiotensin action such as occurs in kidney disease, cirrhosis of the liver or congestive cardiac failure (*secondary hyperaldosteronism*).

GLUCOCORTICOIDS

Synthesis and release

Adrenal steroids are synthesised and released as required, under the influence of circulating ACTH secreted from the anterior pituitary gland (see p. 424 and Fig. 28.4). ACTH secretion is (positively) regulated by CRF released from the hypothalamus and vasopressin from the posterior gland, and (negatively) by blood glucocorticoids. The release of CRF, in turn, is inhibited by the level of glucocorticoids in the blood, and is influenced by input from the CNS. This functional hypothalamic–pituitary–adrenal unit is referred to as the *HPA axis*.

Glucocorticoids are always present in the blood, but in healthy humans there is a well-defined circadian rhythm in the secretion, with the blood concentration being highest early in the morning, gradually diminishing throughout the day and reaching a low point in the evening or night. Opioid peptides also exercise a tonic inhibitory control on the secretion of CRF, and psychological factors can affect the release of vasopressin and CRF, as can stimuli such as excessive heat or cold, injury or infections. This is the principal mechanism whereby the HPA axis is activated in response to a threatening environment.

The precursor of glucocorticoids is cholesterol (Fig. 28.5). The initial step, the conversion of cholesterol to *pregnenolone*, is the rate-limiting step and is itself regulated by ACTH. Some of the reactions in the biosynthetic pathway can be inhibited by drugs. **Metyrapone** prevents the β-hydroxylation at C11, and thus the formation of hydrocortisone and corticosterone. Synthesis is blocked at the 11-deoxycorticosteroid stage, and as these substances have no negative feedback effects on the hypothalamus and pituitary, there is a marked increase in ACTH in the blood. Metyrapone can therefore be used to test ACTH production, and may also be used to treat patients with Cushing's syndrome. **Trilostane** (also of use in Cushing's syndrome and primary hyperaldosteronism) blocks an earlier step in the pathway—the 3β-dehydrogenase.

---

[2] Oddly, it was *cortisone* that was originally demonstrated to have potent anti-inflammatory activity in the classic studies by Hench and his colleagues in 1949. The reason for this apparent anomaly is that an isoform of 11β-hydroxysteroid dehydrogenase present in some tissues can transform this steroid back into cortisol (i.e. hydrocortisone), thus restoring biological activity.

Glucocorticoids

Common drugs used include hydrocortisone, prednisolone and dexamethasone.

Metabolic actions

- *Carbohydrates*: decreased uptake and utilisation of glucose accompanied by increased gluconeogenesis; this causes a tendency to hyperglycaemia.
- *Proteins*: increased catabolism, reduced anabolism.
- *Lipids*: a permissive effect on lipolytic hormones and a redistribution of fat, as observed in Cushing's syndrome.

Regulatory actions

- *Hypothalamus and anterior pituitary gland*: a negative feedback action resulting in reduced release of endogenous glucocorticoids.
- *Cardiovascular system*: reduced vasodilatation, decreased fluid exudation.
- *Musculoskeletal*: decreasing osteoblast and increasing osteoclast activity.
- *Inflammation and immunity*:
  - *acute inflammation*: decreased influx and activity of leucocytes
  - *chronic inflammation*: decreased activity of mononuclear cells, decreased angiogenesis, less fibrosis
  - *lymphoid tissues*: decreased clonal expansion of T and B cells, and decreased action of cytokine-secreting T cells.
- *Mediators*:
  - decreased production and action of cytokines, including interleukins, tumour necrosis factor-α and granulocyte macrophage colony-stimulating factor
  - reduced generation of eicosanoids
  - decreased generation of IgG
  - decrease in complement components in the blood
  - increased release of anti-inflammatory factors such as interleukin-10 and annexin 1.
- *Overall effects*: reduction in the activity of the innate and acquired immune systems, but also decreased healing and diminution in the protective aspects of the inflammatory response.

Aminoglutethimide inhibits the initial step in the biosynthetic pathway and has the same overall effect as metyrapone. **Ketoconazole**, an antifungal agent (Ch. 48), used in higher doses also inhibits steroidogenesis and may be of value in the specialised treatment of Cushing's syndrome.

Mechanism of action

The glucocorticoid effects relevant to this discussion are initiated by interaction of the drugs with specific intracellular glucocorticoid receptors belonging to the *nuclear receptor superfamily*

(although there may be other binding proteins or sites; see Norman et al., 2004). This superfamily (see Ch. 3 for structural details) also includes the receptors for mineralocorticoids, the sex steroids, thyroid hormones, vitamin D_3 and retinoic acid.

After entering cells (probably by passive diffusion), the glucocorticoids bind to specific receptors in the cytoplasm. Two receptors have been described, termed *GRα* and *GRβ* (highly homologous but lacking part of the C terminal). Although it may modulate signalling through the GRα receptor under some circumstances, GRβ does not appear to function as a glucocorticoid receptor in vivo and will not be discussed further. GRα has been cloned and contains 777 amino acid residues. It has a high affinity for glucocorticoids and is found in virtually all tissues at a density of between 3000 and 30 000 copies per cell, the number varying between different tissues.

In its 'resting', unliganded state, the receptor dwells in the cytoplasm as part of a complex of proteins that include *heat shock proteins* (*HSPs*) 56 and 90. After binding the steroid, the receptor dissociates from the HSPs and undergoes a conformational change that exposes a DNA-binding domain (see Figs 28.6 and 3.3). Subsequent events have yet to be fully delineated; in the best characterised example, steroid–receptor complexes form homodimers (and possibly heterodimers with the mineralocorticoid receptor too), then translocate to the nucleus possibly using the cytoskeleton. Here, they bind to positive or negative glucocorticoid response elements present in the promoters of target genes, thus bringing about corresponding changes (induction or repression) in transcription. The receptor is eventually recycled in an ATP-dependent process and combined again with HSPs in the cytoplasm to complete the cycle.

Several molecular mechanisms by which changes in gene transcription are accomplished have been identified, and these are shown in Figure 28.6. Regulation, particularly repression, is generally achieved in concert with various transcription factors, such as AP1 and nuclear factor κB. Induction stimulates the fresh formation of specific mRNAs, which then direct the synthesis of specific proteins. It is estimated that approximately 1% of nuclear genes can be regulated by glucocorticoids using such pathways.

In addition to these 'nuclear' events, it has become evident in recent years that the liganded receptor itself, in either a monomeric or a dimeric form, may trigger signal transduction events while still in the cytosolic compartment. One of these effects, germane to the anti-inflammatory profile of these drugs, is the release, following phosphorylation, of the protein *annexin-1* (formerly *lipocortin*), which has potent effects on leucocyte trafficking and other biological actions. The significance of such 'receptor-mediated, non-genomic' actions is that they can happen rapidly (within a few minutes), as they do not entail changes in mRNA/protein synthesis that occur over a longer timeframe.

Actions

General metabolic and systemic effects

The main metabolic effects are on carbohydrate and protein metabolism. The hormones and their synthetic congeners cause both a decrease in the uptake and utilisation of glucose and an increase in gluconeogenesis, resulting in a tendency to hyperglycaemia

Table 28.2 Comparison of the main corticosteroid agents used for systemic therapy (using hydrocortisone as a standard)

Compound	Relative affinity for glucocorticoid receptors[a]	Approximate relative potency in clinical use		Duration of action after oral dose[b]	Comments
		Anti-inflammatory	Sodium retaining		
Hydrocortisone (cortisol)	1	1	1	Short	Drug of choice for replacement therapy
Cortisone	0.01	0.8	0.8	Short	Cheap; inactive until converted to hydrocortisone; not used as anti-inflammatory because of mineralocorticoid effects
Corticosterone	0.85	0.3	15	Short	–
Prednisolone	2.2	4	0.8	Intermediate	Drug of choice for systemic anti-inflammatory and immunosuppressive effects
Prednisone	0.05	4	0.8	Intermediate	Inactive until converted to prednisolone
Methylprednisolone	11.9	5	Minimal	Intermediate	Anti-inflammatory and immunosuppressive
Triamcinolone	1.9	5	None	Intermediate	Relatively more toxic than others
Dexamethasone	7.1	30	Minimal	Long	Anti-inflammatory and immunosuppressive, used especially where water retention is undesirable (e.g. cerebral oedema); drug of choice for suppression of adrenocorticotrophic hormone production
Betamethasone	5.4	30	Negligible	Long	Anti-inflammatory and immunosuppressive, used especially when water retention is undesirable
Deoxycortone	0.19	Negligible	50	–	–
Fludrocortisone	3.5	15	150	Short	Drug of choice for mineralocorticoid effects
Aldosterone	0.38	None	500	–	Endogenous mineralocorticoid

[a]Human fetal lung cells.
[b]Duration of action (half-lives in hours): short, 8–12; intermediate, 12–36; long, 36–72.
(Data for relative affinity obtained from Baxter J D, Rousseau G G (eds) 1979 Glucocorticoid hormone action. Monographs on endocrinology, vol 12. Springer-Verlag, Berlin.)

(see Ch. 26). There is a concomitant increase in glycogen storage, which may be a result of insulin secretion in response to the increase in blood sugar. Overall, there is decreased protein synthesis and increased protein breakdown, particularly in muscle, and this can lead to wasting. Glucocorticoids also have a 'permissive' effect on the cAMP-dependent lipolytic response to catecholamines and other hormones. Such hormones cause lipase activation through a cAMP-dependent kinase, the synthesis of which requires the presence of glucocorticoids (see below). Large doses of glucocorticoids given over a long period result in the redistribution of body fat characteristic of Cushing's syndrome (Fig. 28.7).

Glucocorticoids tend to produce a negative calcium balance by decreasing Ca^{2+} absorption in the gastrointestinal tract and increasing its excretion by the kidney. This may result in osteoporosis (see below). In non-physiological concentrations, the glucocorticoids have some mineralocorticoid actions (see below), causing Na^+ retention and K^+ loss—possibly by swamping the protective 11β-hydroxysteroid dehydrogenase and acting at mineralocorticoid receptors.

Negative feedback effects on the anterior pituitary and hypothalamus

Both endogenous and exogenous glucocorticoids have a negative feedback effect on the secretion of CRF and ACTH (see Fig. 28.4). Administration of exogenous glucocorticoids depresses the secretion of CRF and ACTH, thus inhibiting the secretion of endogenous glucocorticoids and potentially causing atrophy of

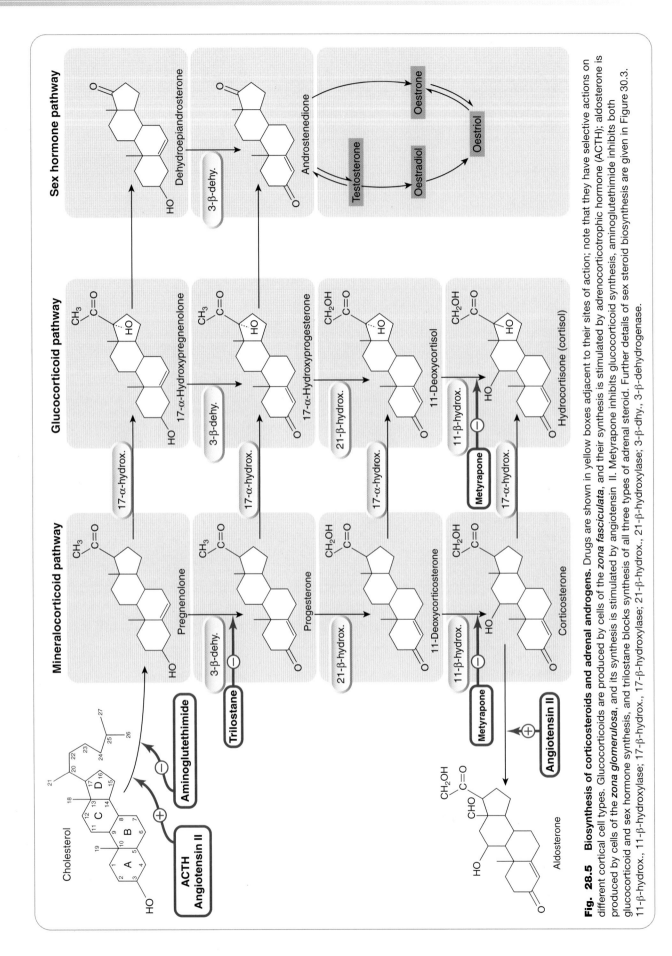

Fig. 28.5 **Biosynthesis of corticosteroids and adrenal androgens.** Drugs are shown in yellow boxes adjacent to their sites of action; note that they have selective actions on different cortical cell types. Glucocorticoids are produced by cells of the *zona fasciculata*, and their synthesis is stimulated by adrenocorticotrophic hormone (ACTH); aldosterone is produced by cells of the *zona glomerulosa*, and its synthesis is stimulated by angiotensin II. Metyrapone inhibits glucocorticoid synthesis, aminoglutethimide inhibits both glucocorticoid and sex hormone synthesis, and trilostane blocks synthesis of all three types of adrenal steroid. Further details of sex steroid biosynthesis are given in Figure 30.3. 11-β-hydrox., 11-β-hydroxylase; 17-β-hydrox., 17-β-hydroxylase; 21-β-hydrox., 21-β-hydroxylase; 3-β-dhy., 3-β-dehydrogenase.

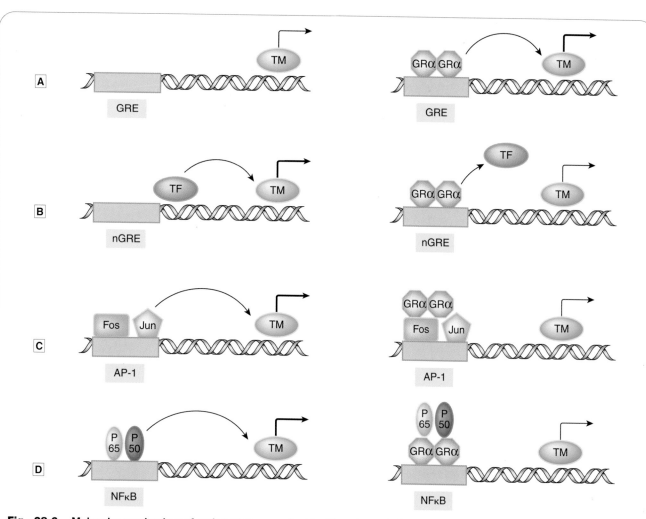

Fig. 28.6 Molecular mechanism of action of glucocorticoids. The schematic figure shows three possible ways by which the liganded glucocorticoid receptor can control gene expression following translocation to the nucleus. **A** *Basic transactivation mechanism.* Here, the transcriptional machinery (TM) is presumed to be operating at a low level. The liganded glucocorticoid receptor (GR) dimer binds to one or more 'positive' glucocorticoid response elements (GREs) within the promoter sequence (shaded zone) and up-regulates transcription. **B** *Basic transrepression mechanism.* The transcriptional machinery is constitutively driven by transcription factors (TF). In binding to the 'negative' GRE (nGRE), the receptor complex displaces these factors and expression falls. **C** *Fos/Jun mechanism.* Transcription is driven at a high level by Fos/Jun transcription factors binding to their AP-1 regulatory site. This effect is reduced in the presence of the GR. **D** *Nuclear factor κB mechanism.* The transcription factors P65 and P50 bind to the NFκB site, promoting gene expression. This is prevented by the presence of the GR, which binds the transcription factors, preventing their action (this may occur in the cytoplasm also). For further details of the structure of GR, see Chapter 3. (Modified from Oakley R H, Cidlowski J A in Gorlding N J, Flower R J (eds) 2001 Glucocorticoids. Birkhauser Verl.)

the adrenal cortex. If therapy is prolonged, it may take many months to return to normal function when the drugs are stopped.

Anti-inflammatory and immunosuppressive effects

Endogenous glucocorticoids maintain a low-level anti-inflammatory tonus that can be readily demonstrated by observing the heightened response of adrenalectomised animals to even mild inflammatory stimuli. A failure of appropriate secretion in response to injury or infection may underlie certain chronic inflammatory pathologies. Glucocorticoids are the anti-inflammatory drugs *par excellence*, and when given therapeutically have powerful anti-inflammatory and immunosuppressive effects. They inhibit both the early and the late manifestations of inflammation, i.e. not only

the initial redness, heat, pain and swelling, but also the later stages of wound healing and repair, and the proliferative reactions seen in chronic inflammation (Ch. 13). They reverse virtually all types of inflammatory reaction, whether caused by invading pathogens, by chemical or physical stimuli, or by inappropriately deployed immune responses such as are seen in hypersensitivity or auto-immune disease. When used clinically to suppress graft rejection, glucocorticoids suppress the initiation and generation of an immune response mounted against this new 'invader' more efficiently than an established response in which clonal proliferation has already occurred. Given that the glucocorticoids are able to modify the expression of so many genes, and that the extent and direction of regulation varies between tissues and even at different times

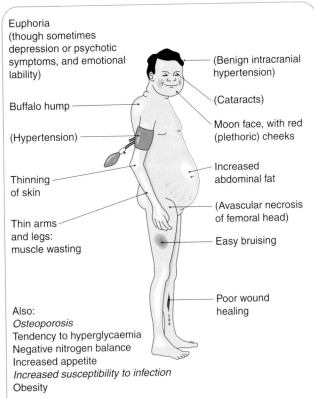

Euphoria
(though sometimes depression or psychotic symptoms, and emotional lability)

Buffalo hump

(Hypertension)

Thinning of skin

Thin arms and legs: muscle wasting

(Benign intracranial hypertension)

(Cataracts)

Moon face, with red (plethoric) cheeks

Increased abdominal fat

(Avascular necrosis of femoral head)

Easy bruising

Poor wound healing

Also:
Osteoporosis
Tendency to hyperglycaemia
Negative nitrogen balance
Increased appetite
Increased susceptibility to infection
Obesity

Fig. 28.7 **Cushing's syndrome.** This is caused by excessive exposure to glucocorticoids, and may be caused by disease (e.g. an adrenocorticotrophic hormone–secreting tumour) or by prolonged administration of glucocorticoid drugs (iatrogenic Cushing's). Italicised effects are particularly common. Less frequent effects, related to dose and duration of therapy, are shown in parentheses. (Adapted from Baxter JD, Rousseau GG (eds) 1979 Glucocorticoid hormone action. Monographs on endocrinology, vol 12. Springer-Verlag, Berlin.)

- decreased generation of many cytokines, including IL-1, IL-2, IL-3, IL-4, IL-5, IL-6, IL-8, tumour necrosis factor-α, cell adhesion factors and granulocyte macrophage colony-stimulating factor, secondary to inhibition of gene transcription
- reduction in the concentration of complement components in the plasma
- decreased generation of induced nitric oxide
- decreased histamine release from basophils
- decreased IgG production
- increased synthesis of anti-inflammatory factors such as IL-10, IL-1–soluble receptor and annexin-1.

Inflammation is an important protective response designed to ensure the survival of an infected or injured host. It therefore strikes many as odd that we should not only have potent anti-inflammatory hormones circulating constantly in the blood, but that these should be dramatically increased during such threatening episodes. A useful explanatory paradigm is that of Munck et al. (1984); according to this idea, the anti-inflammatory and immunosuppressive actions may play a crucial counter-regulatory role, in that they prevent excessive activation of inflammation and other powerful defence reactions, which might, if unchecked, themselves threaten homeostasis. Certainly, this view is borne out by experimental work with adrenalectomised animals. While these drugs are of great value in treating conditions characterised by

during disease, you will not be surprised to learn that their anti-inflammatory effects are fearsomely complex. Some prominent actions may be highlighted, but these should not be considered a complete list.

Actions on inflammatory cells include:

- decreased egress of neutrophils from blood vessels and reduced activation of neutrophils and macrophages secondary to decreased transcription of the genes for cell adhesion factors and cytokines
- decreased activation of T-helper cells and reduced clonal proliferation of T cells, secondary to decreased transcription of genes for IL-2 and its receptor (see below)
- decreased fibroblast function, less production of collagen and glycosaminoglycans, and thus reduced healing and repair
- reduced activity of osteoblasts but increased activation of osteoclasts and therefore a tendency to develop osteoporosis.

Action on the mediators of inflammatory and immune responses include:

- decreased production of prostanoids owing to decreased expression of cyclo-oxygenase-2

Mechanism of action of the glucocorticoids

- Glucocorticoids bind intracellular receptors that then dimerise, migrate to the nucleus, and interact with DNA to modify gene transcription, inducing synthesis of some proteins and inhibiting synthesis of others.
- *Metabolic actions*: most mediator proteins are enzymes, for example cAMP-dependent kinase, but not all actions on genes are known.
- *Anti-inflammatory and immunosuppressive actions*: known actions include:
  - inhibition of transcription of the genes for cyclo-oxygenase-2, cytokines and interleukins, cell adhesion molecules, and the inducible form of nitric oxide synthase
  - block of vitamin D₃-mediated induction of the osteocalcin gene in osteoblasts, and modification of transcription of the collagenase genes
  - increased synthesis and release of annexin-1, which has potent anti-inflammatory effects on cells and mediator release, and may also mediate negative feedback at the level of the hypothalamus and anterior pituitary gland.
- Some rapid non-genomic effects of glucocorticoids have also been observed.

hypersensitivity and unwanted inflammation, they carry the hazard that they are able to suppress the same defence reactions that provide protection to infection and promote healing.

Unwanted effects

Unwanted effects are likely to occur with large doses or prolonged administration rather than replacement therapy. Possible unwanted effects include suppression of the response to infection or injury; an opportunistic infection can be potentially very serious unless quickly treated with antimicrobial agents along with an increase in the dose of steroid. Wound healing may be impaired, and peptic ulceration may also occur.

Sudden withdrawal of the drugs after prolonged therapy may result in acute adrenal insufficiency through suppression of the patient's capacity to synthesise corticosteroids.[3] Careful procedures for phased withdrawal should be followed. Recovery of full adrenal function usually takes about 2 months, although it can take 18 months or more.

When the drugs are used in anti-inflammatory and immuno-suppressive therapy, the metabolic actions and the effects on water and electrolyte balance and on organ systems are considered unwanted side effects, and Cushing's syndrome may occur (see Fig. 28.7). Osteoporosis, with the attendant hazard of fractures, is probably one of the main limitations to long-term glucocorticoid therapy. These drugs influence bone density by regulation of calcium and phosphate metabolism and through effects on collagen turnover. Given over a long term, glucocorticoids reduce the function of osteoblasts (which lay down bone matrix) and increase the activity of osteoclasts (which digest bone matrix). An effect on the blood supply to bone can result in avascular necrosis of the head of the femur (see Ch. 31).

The tendency to hyperglycaemia that occurs with exogenous glucocorticoids may develop into actual diabetes. Another limitation is the development of muscle wasting and weakness. In children, the inhibitory metabolic (particularly those on protein metabolism) and hormonal effects may result in inhibition of growth if drug treatment is continued for more than 6 months or so, even if fairly low doses are used.

Reports of central effects are quite common; some patients experience euphoria, but others may become depressed or develop psychotic symptoms. In fact, the circadian secretion of hydro-cortisone may be disturbed in some depressed patients, and the *dexamethasone suppression test* can be used to identify these individuals. Other toxic effects that have been reported include glaucoma, raised intracranial pressure, hypercoagulability of the blood, fever and disorders of menstruation, and an increased incidence of cataracts. Oral thrush (candidiasis, a fungal infection; see Ch. 48) frequently occurs when glucocorticoids are taken by inhalation, because of suppression of local anti-infective mechanisms.

Pharmacokinetic aspects

Glucocorticoids may be administered by a variety of routes. Most are active when given orally, and all can be given systemically, either intramuscularly or intravenously. Most may also be given topically—injected intra-articularly, given by aerosol into the respiratory tract, administered as drops into the eye or the nose, or applied in creams or ointments to the skin. Topical administration diminishes the likelihood of systemic toxic effects unless large quantities are used. When prolonged use of systemic glucocorticoids is necessary, therapy on alternate days may decrease the unwanted effects. Inhaled or intranasal glucocorticoids are listed in Table 28.3.

Endogenous glucocorticoids are transported in the plasma bound to corticosteroid-binding globulin (CBG) and to albumin. CBG accounts for about 77% of bound hydrocortisone, but many synthetic glucocorticoids are not bound at all. Albumin has a lower affinity for hydrocortisone but binds both natural and synthetic steroids. Both CBG-bound and albumin-bound steroids are biologically inactive.

As small lipophilic molecules, glucocorticoids probably enter their target cells by simple diffusion. Hydrocortisone has a plasma half-life of 90 minutes, although its main biological effects have 2–8 hours' latency. Biological inactivation, which occurs in liver cells and elsewhere, is initiated by reduction of the C4–C5 double bond. Cortisone and **prednisone** are inactive until converted in vivo to hydrocortisone and **prednisolone**, respectively.

The clinical use of the glucocorticoids is given in the clinical box. Dexamethasone can be used to test HPA axis function in the dexamethasone suppression test. A low dose, usually given at night, should suppress the hypothalamus and pituitary, and result in reduced ACTH secretion and hydrocortisone output, as measured in the plasma about 9 hours later. Failure of suppression implies hypersecretion of ACTH or of glucocorticoids (Cushing's syndrome).

MINERALOCORTICOIDS

The main endogenous mineralocorticoid is aldosterone. Its chief action is to increase Na^+ reabsorption by the distal tubules in the

Table 28.3 Inhaled or intranasal glucocorticoids

Compound	Approximate potency[a]
Beclomethasone	0.59
Budesonide	0.78
Flunisolide	2
Fluticasone	1
Mometasone	1
Triamcinolone	0.45

[a]Fluticasone = 1.

[3]Patients on long-term glucocorticoid theraphy are advised to carry a card stating, 'I am a patient on STEROID TREATMENT which must not be stopped abruptly'.

kidney, with concomitant increased excretion of K$^+$ and H$^+$ (see Ch. 24). An excessive secretion of mineralocorticoids, as in Conn's syndrome, causes marked Na$^+$ and water retention, with a resultant increase in the volume of extracellular fluid, hypokalaemia, alkalosis and hypertension. A decreased secretion, as in Addison's disease, causes net Na$^+$ loss, which is relatively more pronounced than water loss. The osmotic pressure of the extracellular fluid is thus reduced, resulting in a shift of fluid into the intracellular

compartment and a marked decrease in extracellular fluid volume. There is a concomitant decrease in the excretion of K$^+$, resulting in hyperkalaemia.

Regulation of aldosterone synthesis and release

The regulation of the synthesis and release of aldosterone is complex. Control depends mainly on the electrolyte composition of the plasma and on the angiotensin II system (Fig. 28.4 and Chs 19 and 24). Low plasma Na$^+$ or high plasma K$^+$ concentrations affect the *zona glomerulosa* cells of the adrenal directly, stimulating aldosterone release. Depletion of body Na$^+$ also activates the renin-angiotensin system (see Fig. 19.4). One of the effects of angiotensin II is to increase the synthesis and release of aldosterone.

Mechanism of action

Like other steroid hormones, aldosterone acts through specific intracellular receptors of the nuclear receptor family. Unlike the glucocorticoid receptor, which occurs in most tissues, the *mineralocorticoid receptor* is largely restricted to a few tissues, such as the kidney and the transporting epithelia of the colon and bladder. Cells containing mineralocorticoid receptors also contain the 11β-hydroxysteroid dehydrogenase enzyme (see above), which converts glucocorticoids into metabolites with low affinity for the mineralocorticoid receptors, thus ensuring that the cells are affected only by bona fide mineralocorticoid hormone. Interestingly, this enzyme is inhibited by **carbenoxolone** (used to treat ulcers; see Ch. 25) and liquorice. If this inhibition is marked, it allows corticosterone to act on the mineralocorticoid receptor, producing a syndrome similar to Conn's syndrome (primary hyperaldosteronism).

As with the glucocorticoids, the interaction of aldosterone with its receptor initiates transcription and translation of specific proteins, resulting in an increase in the number of sodium channels in the apical membrane of the cell, and subsequently an increase in the number of Na$^+$/K$^+$ ATPase molecules in the basolateral membrane (see Fig. 24.9). The ensuing increased K$^+$ excretion into the tubule results from an influx of K$^+$ into the cell by the action of the basal Na$^+$/K$^+$ ATPase, coupled with an increased efflux of K$^+$ through apical potassium channels. In addition to the genomic effects, there is evidence for a rapid non-genomic effect of aldosterone on Na$^+$ influx, through an action on the Na$^+$–H$^+$ exchanger in the apical membrane.

Clinical use of mineralocorticoids and antagonists

The main clinical use of mineralocorticoids is in replacement therapy. The most commonly used drug is **fludrocortisone** (Table 28.2 and Fig. 28.4), which can be taken orally. **Spironolactone** is a competitive antagonist of aldosterone, and it also prevents the mineralocorticoid effects of other adrenal steroids on the renal tubule (Ch. 24). Side effects include gynaecomastia and impotence, because spironolactone also has some blocking action on androgen and progesterone receptors. It is used in conjunction with other diuretics in the treatment of oedema. **Eplerenone** has a similar indication and mechanism of action, although fewer side effects.

> ### Clinical use of glucocorticoids
>
> - Replacement therapy for patients with adrenal failure (*Addison's disease*).
> - Anti-inflammatory/immunosuppressive therapy (see also Ch. 14):
>   — in *asthma* (Ch. 23; clinical box on p. 364)
>   — topically in various inflammatory conditions of skin, eye, ear or nose (e.g. *eczema, allergic conjunctivitis* or *rhinitis*)
>   — *hypersensitivity states* (e.g. severe allergic reactions)
>   — in miscellaneous diseases with autoimmune and inflammatory components (e.g. *rheumatoid arthritis* and other 'connective tissue' diseases, *inflammatory bowel diseases*, some forms of *haemolytic anaemia, idiopathic thrombocytopenic purpura*)
>   — to prevent *graft-versus-host disease* following organ or bone marrow transplantation.
> - In *neoplastic* disease (Ch. 51):
>   — in combination with cytotoxic drugs in treatment of specific malignancies (e.g. *Hodgkin's disease, acute lymphocytic leukaemia*)
>   — to reduce cerebral oedema in patients with metastatic or primary *brain tumours* (**dexamethasone**)

> ### Pharmacokinetics and unwanted actions of the glucocorticoids
>
> - Administration can be oral, topical or parenteral. The drugs are transported in the blood by corticosteroid-binding globulin and enter cells by diffusion. They are metabolised in the liver.
> - Unwanted effects are seen mainly after prolonged systemic use as anti-inflammatory or immunosuppressive agents but not usually with replacement therapy. The most important are:
>   — suppression of response to infection
>   — suppression of endogenous glucocorticoid synthesis
>   — metabolic actions (see above)
>   — osteoporosis
>   — iatrogenic Cushing's syndrome (see Fig. 28.7).

Mineralocorticoids

🔑

- Fludrocortisone is given orally to produce a mineralocorticoid effect. This drug:
  - increases Na^+ reabsorption in distal tubules and increases K^+ and H^+ efflux into the tubules
  - acts on intracellular receptors that modulate DNA transcription, causing synthesis of protein mediators
  - is used together with a glucocorticoid in replacement therapy.

NEW DIRECTIONS IN GLUCOCORTICOID THERAPY

Glucocorticoids are so effective that any further development in anti-inflammatories would scarcely be required if it wasn't for one thing—the side effects. While these are seldom a problem with topical administration or short (1–2 weeks) courses of oral therapy, they severely limit the use of these agents in chronic disease. The Holy Grail would be a glucocorticoid possessing the anti-inflammatory but not the unwanted metabolic or other effects. For many years, the pharmaceutical industry pursued simple strategies based on the development of structural analogues of hydrocortisone. While this yielded many new active and interesting compounds (several of which are in clinical use today), they never achieved 'separation' of these actions. An alternative idea was to develop drugs that were topically applied (e.g. by inhalation for asthmatics) and that were preferably metabolically unstable, such that any leakage from the site of topical administration caused minimal systemic effects. While these ideas bore fruit, it still was not an ideal solution.

Recently, investigators have taken another tack. As glucocorticoids function as anti-inflammatories largely by *down-regulating* genes (e.g. cytokines) that promote the inflammatory response, and many of the side effects are caused by *over-expression* of metabolic and other genes (causing, for example, diabetes), and because these effects are brought about through different pathways, researchers have sought steroids that may have one set of actions without the other. At the time of writing, modest successes have been achieved with these 'dissociated' steroids (see Schacke et al., 2002; Schacke & Rehwinkel, 2004), but it is too early to tell whether they will really make a difference in the clinic.

Another approach has been to focus on the actual mechanism of receptor activation. It is clear that not all glucocorticoids bind to the receptor in the same way, and the dynamics of the resulting liganded complex may vary (Adcock, 2003). This could alter the ability of the steroid–receptor complex to initiate transcriptional and other changes in a way that could be beneficial to the profile of the drug.

Yet another idea has been to manipulate the *histone deacetylase* enzymes that are responsible for facilitating the transcriptional regulation of genes following nuclear receptor binding to response elements (Hayashi et al., 2004). One current notion is that there may be a specific isoform of this enzyme that deals with gene up-regulation, and that if this could be inhibited, it would lessen the possibility of those unwanted effects.

REFERENCES AND FURTHER READING

The hypothalamus and pituitary

Birnbaumer M 2000 Vasopressin receptors. Trends Endocrinol Metab 11: 406–410

Clark R G, Robinson C A F 1996 Up and down the growth hormone cascade. Cytokine Growth Factor Rev 1: 65–80 (*A review covering the cascade that controls the primary regulators of growth and metabolism, namely growth hormone and the insulin-like growth factors*)

Drolet G, Rivest S 2001 Corticotropin-releasing hormone and its receptors; an evaluation at the transcription level in vivo. Peptides 22: 761–767

Freeman M E, Kanyicska B, Lerant A, Nagy G 2000 Prolactin: structure, function and regulation of secretion. Physiol Res 80: 1524–1585 (*Comprehensive review of prolactin and its receptors*)

Jørgensen J O L, Christiansen J S 1993 Growth hormone therapy. Lancet 341: 1247–1248

Lamberts S W J, van der Lely A-J et al. 1996 Octreotide. N Engl J Med 334: 246–254 (*A review covering somatostatin receptors, somatostatin analogues, and treatment of tumours expressing somatostatin receptors with octreotide*)

Okada S, Kopchick J J 2001 Biological effects of growth hormone and its antagonist. Trends Mol Med 7: 126–132

Thibonnier M, Coles P, Thibonnier A et al. 2001 The basic and clinical pharmacology of nonpeptide vasopressin receptor antagonists. Annu Rev Pharmacol 41: 175–202 (*Authoritative account of ADH receptors and the search for new antagonists*)

Vance M L 1994 Hypopituitarism. N Engl J Med 330: 1651–1662 (*Review of causes, clinical features and hormone replacement therapy of hypopituitarism*)

Wikberg J E S, Muceniece R, Mandrika I et al. 2000 New aspects on the melanocortins and their receptors. Pharmacol Res 42: 393–420 (*Detailed review of the varied biological roles of melanocortins and their receptors*)

ACTH and the adrenal corticosteroids

Mechanism of action

Adcock I M 2003 Glucocorticoids: new mechanisms and future agents. Curr Allergy Asthma Rep 3: 249–257 (*Excellent review of advances in glucocorticoid pharmacology*)

Bastl C, Hayslett J P 1992 The cellular action of aldosterone in target epithelia. Kidney Int 42: 250–264 (*A detailed review covering the aldosterone receptor and regulation of gene expression, aldosterone action on electrogenic and electroneutral Na^+ transport, and on K^+ and H^+ secretion*)

Borski R J 2000 Nongenomic membrane actions of glucocorticoids in vertebrates. Trends Endocrinol Metab 11: 427–436 (*A thought-provoking account of the non-genomic effects of glucocorticoids*)

Falkenstein E, Tillmann H C, Christ M et al. 2000 Multiple actions of steroid hormones—a focus on rapid, nongenomic effects. Pharmacol Rev 52: 513–556

Funder J W 1997 Glucocorticoid and mineralocorticoid receptors: biology and clinical relevance. Annu Rev Med 48: 231–240 (*Succinct review of glucocorticoid and mineralocorticoid receptors, differences in glucocorticoid receptor– and mineralocorticoid receptor–mediated transcription and responses, and steroid resistance*)

Getting S J, Christian H C, Flower R J, Perretti M 2002 Activation of melanocortin type 3 receptor as a molecular mechanism for adrenocorticotropic hormone efficacy in gouty arthritis. Arthritis Rheum 46: 2765–2775 (*Original paper that demonstrates that ACTH has intrinsic anti-inflammatory actions that are independent of the adrenals*)

Hayashi R, Wada H, Ito K, Adcock I M 2004 Effects of glucocorticoids on gene transcription. Eur J Pharmacol 500: 51–62 (*Good basic review of glucocorticoid action; easy to read*)

Norman A W, Mizwicki M T, Norman D P 2004 Steroid-hormone rapid actions, membrane receptors and a conformational ensemble model. Nat Rev Drug Discov 3: 27–41 (*Fairly advanced reading but contains many useful tables and excellent diagrams; well worth the effort if this subject interests you*)

Rhodes D, Klug A 1993 Zinc fingers. Sci Am Feb: 32–39 (*Clear discussion of the role of zinc fingers, such as those utilised by nuclear receptors, in regulating gene transcription; excellent diagrams, of course*)

Roviezzo F, Getting S J, Paul-Clark M J et al. 2002 The annexin-1 knockout mouse: what it tells us about the inflammatory response. J Physiol Pharmacol 53: 541–553 (*Short and easy-to-read review on the role of the protein annexin 1 in the inflammatory response and the action of glucocorticoids*)

Tak P P, Firestein G S 2001 NF-kappaB: a key role in inflammatory diseases. J Clin Invest 107: 7–11 (*Succinct and very readable account of the role of nuclear factor κB in inflammation*)

Tsai M-J, O'Malley B W 1994 Molecular mechanisms of action of steroid/thyroid receptor superfamily members. Annu Rev Biochem 63: 451–486 (*Detailed review, by one of the pioneers of the field, of the molecular biology of these receptors, including gene activation and gene silencing*)

Physiological and pharmacological actions

Buckingham J C 1998 Stress and the hypothalamo–pituitary–immune axis. Int J Tissue React 20: 23–34 (*Clear review of the complexities of the effect of stress on HPA axis function*)

Buckingham J C, Flower R J 1997 Lipocortin 1: a second messenger of glucocorticoid action in the hypothalamic–pituitary–adrenocortical axis. Mol Med Today 3: 296–302 (*Outline of HPA axis function, glucocorticoid action, and the possible role of lipocortin-1 (now known as annexin-1) in both*)

de Kloet E R 2000 Stress in the brain. Eur J Pharmacol 405: 187–198

Munck A, Guyre P M, Holbrook N J 1984 Physiological functions of glucocorticoids in stress and their relation to pharmacological actions. Endocr Rev 5: 25–44 (*Seminal review suggesting that the anti-inflammatory/immunosuppressive actions of the glucocorticoids have a physiological function; required reading if you want to understand glucocorticoid physiology and pharmacology*)

Clinical and therapeutic aspects

Lamberts S W J, Bruining H A, de Jong F S 1997 Corticosteroid therapy in severe illness. N Engl J Med 337: 1285–1292 (*Review with succinct coverage of normal response of adrenal to illness, followed by more detail on clinical therapy*)

Schacke H, Docke W D, Asadullah K 2002 Mechanisms involved in the side effects of glucocorticoids. Pharmacol Ther 96: 23–43 (*Useful review dealing with side effects and 'dissociated steroids'*)

Schacke H, Rehwinkel H 2004 Dissociated glucocorticoid receptor ligands. Curr Opin Investig Drugs 5: 524–528

Schacke H, Rehwinkel H, Asadullah K 2005 Dissociated glucocorticoid receptor ligands: compounds with an improved therapeutic index. Curr Opin Investig Drugs 6: 503–507 (*More details about the dissociated steroid concept, with several examples*)

Wilckens T 1995 Glucocorticoids and immune dysfunction: physiological relevance and pathogenic potential of hormonal dysfunction. Trends Pharmacol Sci 16: 193–197 (*Covers glucocorticoid interaction with their receptors, heat shock protein 90, AP-1 and nuclear factor κB transcription factors; clear diagram*)

Books

Buckingham J C, Gillies G E, Cowell A M (eds) 1997 Stress, stress hormones and the immune system. John Wiley, Chichester (*Another excellent source book for information that covers the concepts of stress, the release of cortisol and its subsequent physiological actions*)

Goulding N J, Flower R J (eds) 2001 Milestones in drug therapy: glucocorticoids. Birkhauser Verlag, Basel (*A useful source of information on all aspects of glucocorticoid biology and pharmacology, containing chapters by some of the leaders in the field*)

The thyroid 29

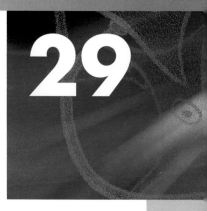

OVERVIEW

Diseases of the thyroid gland are prevalent, and in this chapter we deal with drug therapy used to mitigate these disorders. We set the scene by briefly outlining the structure, regulation and physiology of the thyroid, and highlight the most common abnormalities of thyroid function. We then go on to consider the drugs that replace the thyroid hormones when these cease to function adequately, and the drugs that decrease thyroid function when this is excessive.

SYNTHESIS, STORAGE AND SECRETION OF THYROID HORMONES

The thyroid gland secretes three main hormones: *thyroxine* (T_4), *triiodothyronine* (T_3) and *calcitonin*. T_4 and T_3 are critically important for normal growth and development and for energy metabolism. Calcitonin is involved in the control of plasma Ca^{2+} and is dealt with in Chapter 31. The term *thyroid hormone* will be used here solely to refer to T_4 and T_3.

The functional unit of the thyroid is the follicle or *acinus*. Each follicle consists of a single layer of epithelial cells around a cavity, the follicle lumen, which is filled with a thick colloid containing *thyroglobulin*. Thyroglobulin is a large glycoprotein, each molecule of which contains about 115 tyrosine residues. It is synthesised, glycosylated and then secreted into the lumen of the follicle, where iodination of the tyrosine residues occurs. Surrounding the follicles is a dense capillary network, and the rate of blood flow through the gland is very high in comparison with other tissues. The main steps in the synthesis, storage and secretion of thyroid hormone (Fig. 29.1) are as follow:

- uptake of plasma iodide by the follicle cells
- oxidation of iodide and iodination of tyrosine residues of thyroglobulin
- secretion of thyroid hormone.

Uptake of plasma iodide by the follicle cells

Iodide uptake is an energy-dependent process occurring against a gradient, which is normally about 25:1. Iodide is captured from the blood and moved to the lumen by two transporters: the Na^+/I^- symporter (NIS) located at the basolateral surface of the thyrocytes (the energy being provided by the Na^+/K^+ ATPase), and *pendrin*[1] (*PDS*), an I^-/Cl^- porter in the apical membranes (Nilsson, 2001; Yoshida et al., 2004). Numerous mutations have been discovered in the *NIS* and *PDS* genes, and these contribute to thyroid disease in some patients.

Oxidation of iodide and iodination of tyrosine residues

The oxidation of iodide and its incorporation into thyroglobulin (termed the *organification* of iodide) is catalysed by *thyroperoxidase*, an enzyme situated at the inner surface of the cell at the interface with the colloid. The reaction requires the presence of hydrogen peroxide (H_2O_2) as an oxidising agent. The process is very rapid: labelled iodide (^{125}I) is found in the lumen within 40 seconds of intravenous injection. Iodination occurs after the tyrosine has been incorporated into thyroglobulin. The process believed to occur is shown in Figure 29.2.

Tyrosine residues are iodinated first at position 3 on the ring, forming *monoiodotyrosine* (*MIT*) and then, in some molecules, on position 5 as well, forming *diiodotyrosine* (*DIT*). While still incorporated into thyroglobulin, these molecules are then coupled in pairs, either MIT with DIT to form T_3, or two DIT molecules to form T_4 (Fig. 29.3). The mechanism for coupling is believed to

---

[1]So called because it is implicated in the pathophysiology of *Pendred's* syndrome, named after the eponymous English physician who first described this form of familial goitre.

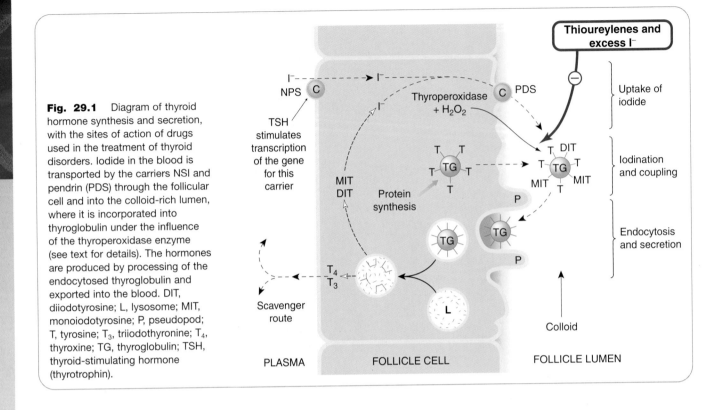

Fig. 29.1 Diagram of thyroid hormone synthesis and secretion, with the sites of action of drugs used in the treatment of thyroid disorders. Iodide in the blood is transported by the carriers NSI and pendrin (PDS) through the follicular cell and into the colloid-rich lumen, where it is incorporated into thyroglobulin under the influence of the thyroperoxidase enzyme (see text for details). The hormones are produced by processing of the endocytosed thyroglobulin and exported into the blood. DIT, diiodotyrosine; L, lysosome; MIT, monoiodotyrosine; P, pseudopod; T, tyrosine; T_3, triiodothyronine; T_4, thyroxine; TG, thyroglobulin; TSH, thyroid-stimulating hormone (thyrotrophin).

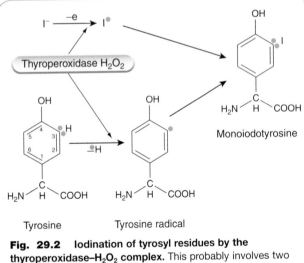

Fig. 29.2 **Iodination of tyrosyl residues by the thyroperoxidase–H_2O_2 complex.** This probably involves two sites on the enzyme, one of which removes an electron from iodide to give the free radical I•; another removes an electron from tyrosine to give the tyrosyl radical (shown by orange dot). Monoiodotyrosine results from the addition of the two radicals.

involve a peroxidase system similar to that involved in iodination. About one-fifth of the tyrosine residues in thyroglobulin are iodinated in this way.

The iodinated thyroglobulin of the thyroid forms a large store of thyroid hormone with a relatively slow turnover. This is in contrast to some other endocrine secretions (e.g. the hormones of the adrenal cortex), which are not stored but synthesised and released as required.

Secretion of thyroid hormone

The thyroglobulin molecule is taken up into the follicle cell by endocytosis (Fig. 29.1). The endocytotic vesicles then fuse with lysosomes, and proteolytic enzymes act on thyroglobulin, releasing T_4 and T_3 to be secreted into the plasma. The surplus MIT and DIT, which are released at the same time, are scavenged by the cell, where the iodide is removed enzymatically and reused.

REGULATION OF THYROID FUNCTION

Thyrotrophin-releasing hormone (TRH), released from the hypothalamus in response to various stimuli, releases *thyroid-stimulating hormone (TSH;* thyrotrophin) from the anterior pituitary (Fig. 29.4), as does the synthetic tripeptide **protirelin** (pyroglutamyl–histidyl–proline amide), which is used in this way for diagnostic purposes (see p. 439). TSH acts on receptors on the membrane of thyroid follicle cells through a mechanism that involves cAMP and phosphatidylinositol 3-kinase. It controls all aspects of thyroid hormone synthesis, including:

- the uptake of iodide by follicle cells, by stimulating transcription of the iodide transporter genes; this is the main mechanism by which it regulates thyroid function
- the synthesis and secretion of thyroglobulin
- the generation of H_2O_2 and the iodination of tyrosine
- the endocytosis and proteolysis of thyroglobulin
- the actual secretion of T_3 and T_4
- the blood flow through the gland.

Thyroid-stimulating hormone also has a trophic action on the thyroid cells; it stimulates the transcription of the genes for thyroglobulin and thyroperoxidase, as well as the I⁻ transporters.

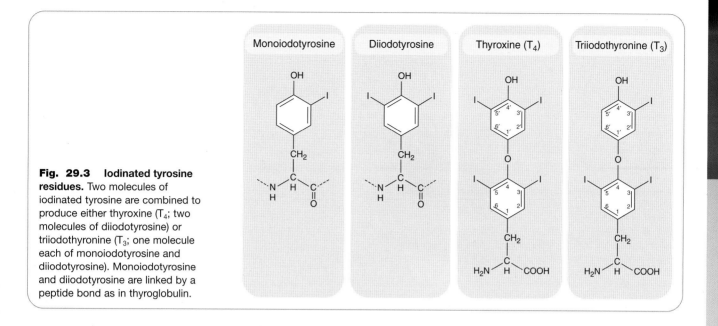

Fig. 29.3 Iodinated tyrosine residues. Two molecules of iodinated tyrosine are combined to produce either thyroxine (T$_4$; two molecules of diiodotyrosine) or triiodothyronine (T$_3$; one molecule each of monoiodotyrosine and diiodotyrosine). Monoiodotyrosine and diiodotyrosine are linked by a peptide bond as in thyroglobulin.

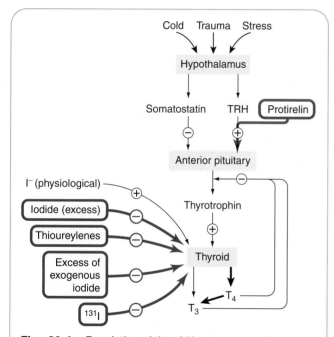

Fig. 29.4 Regulation of thyroid hormone secretion. Iodide (I$^-$) is essential for thyroid hormone synthesis, but excess of endogenous or exogenous iodide (30 times the daily requirement of iodine) actually inhibits the increased thyroid hormone production, which occurs in thyrotoxicosis. Protirelin as well as recombinant thyrotrophin-releasing hormone (TSH) is sometimes used to stimulate the system for diagnostic purposes, as is the administration of ^{131}I (see text for details). T$_3$, triiodothyronine; T$_4$, thyroxine.

actions of T$_4$ and TRH (and probably also somatostatin) on the pituitary, although even high concentrations of thyroid hormone do not totally inhibit TSH secretion.

The other main factor influencing thyroid function is the plasma iodide concentration. About 100 nmol of T$_4$ is synthesised daily, necessitating uptake by the gland of approximately 500 nmol of iodide each day (equivalent to about 70 mg of iodine). A *reduced* iodine intake, with *reduced* plasma iodide concentration, will result in a decrease of hormone production and an increase in TSH secretion. An *increased* plasma iodide has the opposite effect, although this may be modified by other factors (see below). The overall feedback mechanism responds to changes of iodide slowly over fairly long periods of days or weeks, because there is a large reserve capacity for the binding and uptake of iodide in the thyroid. The size and vascularity of the thyroid are reduced by an increase in plasma iodide. Diets deficient in iodine eventually result in a continuous excessive compensatory secretion of TSH, and eventually in an increase in vascularity and (sometimes gross) hypertrophy of the gland. 'Derbyshire neck' was the name given to this condition in a part of the UK where sources of dietary iodine were once scarce.

ACTIONS OF THE THYROID HORMONES

The physiological actions of the thyroid hormones fall into two categories: those affecting metabolism and those affecting growth and development.

EFFECTS ON METABOLISM

The thyroid hormones produce a general increase in the metabolism of carbohydrates, fats and proteins, and regulate these processes in most tissues, T$_3$ being three to five times more active than T$_4$ in this respect (Fig. 29.5). Although the thyroid hormones directly control the activity of some of the enzymes of

The production of TSH is also regulated by a negative feedback effect of thyroid hormones on the anterior pituitary gland, T$_3$ being more active than T$_4$ in this respect. The peptide *somatostatin* (see p. 421) also reduces basal TSH release. The control of the secretion of TSH thus depends on a balance between the

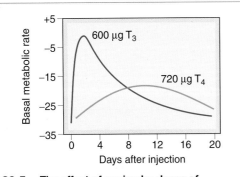

Fig. 29.5 The effect of equimolar doses of triiodothyronine (T₃) and thyroxine (T₄) on basal metabolic rate in a hypothyroid subject. Note that this figure is meant only to illustrate overall differences in effect; thyroxine is not given clinically in a single bolus dose as here, but in regular daily doses so that the effect builds up to a plateau. The apparent differences in potency really represent differences in kinetics, reflecting the prehormone role of T₄. (From Blackburn C M et al. 1954 J Clin Invest 33: 819.)

carbohydrate metabolism, most effects are brought about in conjunction with other hormones, such as insulin, glucagon, the glucocorticoids and the catecholamines. There is an increase in oxygen consumption and heat production, which is manifested as an increase in the measured basal metabolic rate. This reflects action of these hormones on tissues such as heart, kidney, liver and muscle, although not on others, such as the gonads, brain or spleen. The calorigenic action is important as part of the response to a cold environment. Administration of thyroid hormone results in augmented cardiac rate and output, and increased tendency to dysrhythmias such as atrial fibrillation.

EFFECTS ON GROWTH AND DEVELOPMENT

The thyroid hormones have a critical effect on growth, partly by a direct action on cells, and also indirectly by influencing growth hormone production and potentiating its effects on its target tissues. The hormones are important for a normal response to parathormone and calcitonin as well as for skeletal development; they are also essential for normal growth and maturation of the central nervous system.

MECHANISM OF ACTION

While there is some evidence for non-genomic actions (see Bassett et al., 2003; Lazar, 2003), these hormones act mainly through a mechanism dependent on occupation of a member of the nuclear receptor family, TR (Ch. 3 and Fig. 3.17). Two distinct genes, TRα and TRβ, code for several receptor isoforms that have distinct functions. T₄ may be regarded as a prohormone, because when it enters the cell, it is first converted to T₃, which then binds with high affinity to a member of the TR family. This interaction is likely to take place in the nucleus, where TR isoforms generally act as a repressor of target genes. When T₃ is bound, the receptors change conformation, the corepressor complex

is released and a coactivator complex is recruited, which then activates transcription—resulting in generation of mRNA and protein synthesis.

TRANSPORT AND METABOLISM

Both hormones are transported in the blood bound mainly to *thyroxine-binding globulin* (*TBG*). Plasma concentrations of these hormones can be measured by radioimmunoassay, and normally fall into the range 1×10^{-7} mol/l (T₄) and 2×10^{-9} mol/l for T₃. Both are eventually metabolised in their target tissues by deiodination, deamination, decarboxylation, and conjugation with glucuronic and sulfuric acids. The liver is a major site of metabolism, and the free and conjugated forms are excreted partly in the bile and partly in the urine. The metabolic clearance of T₃ is 20 times faster than that of T₄ (which is about 6 days). The long half-life of T₄ is a consequence of its strong binding to TBG. Abnormalities in the metabolism of these hormones may occur naturally or be induced by drugs or heavy metals, and this may give rise to a variety of (uncommon) clinical conditions such as the 'low T₃ syndrome'.

ABNORMALITIES OF THYROID FUNCTION

Thyroid disorders are among the most common endocrine diseases, and subclinical thyroid disease is particularly prevalent in the middle-aged and elderly. They are accompanied by many extrathyroidal symptoms, particularly in the heart and skin. One cause of organ dysfunction is thyroid cancer. Depending on where it is located, this can affect all aspects of glandular function including iodide uptake, TSH expression and thyroglobulin synthesis. Many other thyroid disorders have an autoimmune basis; the ultimate reason for this is not clear, although it may be linked to polymorphisms in the *PDS, TNF-α* or other genes. Regardless of causation, there are two principal manifestations of the disease.

HYPERTHYROIDISM (THYROTOXICOSIS)

In thyrotoxicosis, there is excessive activity of the thyroid hormones, resulting in a high metabolic rate, an increase in skin temperature and sweating, and a marked sensitivity to heat. Nervousness, tremor, tachycardia, heat sensitivity and increased appetite associated with loss of weight occur. There are several types of hyperthyroidism, but only two are common: diffuse toxic goitre (also called *Graves' disease* or *exophthalmic* goitre) and *toxic nodular goitre.*

Diffuse toxic goitre is an organ-specific autoimmune disease caused by thyroid-stimulating immunoglobulins directed at the TSH receptor. Constitutively active mutations of the TRH receptor may also be involved. As is indicated by the name, patients with exophthalmic goitre have protrusion of the eyeballs. The pathogenesis of this condition is not fully understood, but it is thought to be caused by the presence of TSH receptor-like proteins in orbital tissues. There is also an enhanced sensitivity to catecholamines. Toxic nodular goitre is caused by a benign neoplasm or adenoma, and may develop in patients with long-standing simple goitre (see below). This condition does not usually have concomitant exophthalmos. The antidysrhythmic drug **amiodarone** (Ch. 18) is rich in iodine and can cause either hyperthyroidism or hypothyroidism. Some other iodine-containing drugs, such as **iopanoic acid** and its congeners, which are used as imaging agents used to visualise the gall bladder, may also interfere with thyroid function but may have some clinical utility in treating hyperthyroidism,

SIMPLE, NON-TOXIC GOITRE

A dietary deficiency of iodine, if prolonged, causes a rise in plasma TRH and eventually an increase in the size of the gland. This condition is known as simple or non-toxic goitre. Another cause is ingestion of *goitrogens* (e.g. from cassava root). The enlarged thyroid usually manages to produce normal amounts of thyroid hormone, although if the iodine deficiency is very severe, hypothyroidism may supervene.

HYPOTHYROIDISM

A decreased activity of the thyroid results in hypothyroidism, and in severe cases *myxoedema*. Once again, this disease is immunological in origin, and the manifestations include low metabolic rate, slow speech, deep hoarse voice, lethargy, bradycardia, sensitivity to cold, and mental impairment. Patients also develop a characteristic thickening of the skin (caused by the subcutaneous deposition of glycosaminoglycans), which gives myxoedema its name. *Hashimoto's thyroiditis*, a chronic autoimmune disease in which there is an immune reaction against thyroglobulin or some other component of thyroid tissue, can lead to hypothyroidism and myxoedema. Therapy of thyroid tumours with **radioiodine** (see below) is another cause of hypothyroidism.

Thyroid deficiency during development, caused by congenital absence or incomplete development of the thyroid, which is the most prevalent endocrine disorder in the newborn (1 in 3000–4000 births) causes *cretinism*, characterised by gross retardation of growth and mental deficiency. *Pendred's syndrome*, an autosomal recessive disorder caused by mutations in the PDS transporter gene, may cause goitre as well as deafness and other symptoms (see Hadj Kacem et al., 2003).

DRUGS USED IN DISEASES OF THE THYROID

HYPERTHYROIDISM

Hyperthyroidism may be treated pharmacologically or surgically. In general, surgery is used only when there are mechanical problems resulting from compression of the trachea, and it is usual to remove only part of the organ. Although the condition of hyperthyroidism can be controlled with antithyroid drugs, the disease is not 'cured', because the drugs do not alter the underlying autoimmune mechanisms. Furthermore, there is little evidence that these drugs affect the course of the exophthalmos associated with Graves' disease.

> **The thyroid**
>
> - Thyroid hormones, triiodothyronine (T_3) and thyroxine (T_4), are synthesised by iodination of tyrosine residues on thyroglobulin within the lumen of the thyroid follicle.
> - Hormone synthesis and secretion are regulated by thyroid-stimulating hormone (thyrotrophin) and influenced by plasma iodide.
> - There is a large pool of T_4 in the body; it has a low turnover rate and is found mainly in the circulation.
> - There is a small pool of T_3 in the body; it has a fast turnover rate and is found mainly intracellularly.
> - Within cells, the T_4 is converted to T_3, which interacts with a nuclear receptor to regulate gene transcription.
> - T_3 and T_4 actions:
>   - stimulation of metabolism, causing increased oxygen consumption and increased metabolic rate
>   - regulation of growth and development.
> - Abnormalities of thyroid function include:
>   - hyperthyroidism (thyrotoxicosis); either diffuse toxic goitre or toxic nodular goitre
>   - hypothyroidism; in adults this causes myxoedema, in infants cretinism
>   - simple non-toxic goitre caused by dietary iodine deficiency, usually with normal thyroid function.

RADIOIODINE

Radioiodine is a first-line treatment for hyperthyroidism (particularly in the USA). The isotope used is [131]I (usually as the sodium salt), and the dose generally 5–15 millicuries. Given orally, it is taken up and processed by the thyroid in the same way as the stable form of iodide, eventually becoming incorporated into thyroglobulin. The isotope emits both β radiation and γ rays. The γ rays pass through the tissue without causing damage, but the β particles have a very short range; they are absorbed by the tissue and exert a powerful cytotoxic action that is restricted to the cells of the thyroid follicles, resulting in significant destruction of the tissue. [131]I has a half-life of 8 days, so by 2 months its radioactivity has effectively disappeared. It is given as one single dose, but its cytotoxic effect on the gland is delayed for 1–2 months and does not reach its maximum for a further 2 months.

Hypothyroidism will eventually occur after treatment with radioiodine, particularly in patients with Graves' disease, but is easily managed by replacement therapy with T_4. Radioiodine is best avoided in children and also in pregnant patients because of potential damage to the fetus. There is a theoretical risk of thyroid cancer following the treatment.

The uptake of ^{131}I and other isotopes of iodine may also be used diagnostically as a test of thyroid function. A tracer dose of the isotope is given orally or intravenously, and the amount accumulated by the thyroid is measured by a γ-scintillation counter placed over the gland. Another use for this drug is the treatment of thyroid cancer.

THIOUREYLENES

The thioureylene group of drugs comprises **carbimazole**, **methimazole** and **propylthiouracil**. Chemically, they are related to thiourea, and the thiocarbamide (S–C–N) group is essential for antithyroid activity.

Mechanism of action

Thioureylenes decrease the output of thyroid hormones from the gland, and cause a gradual reduction in the signs and symptoms of thyrotoxicosis, the basal metabolic rate and pulse rate returning to normal over a period of 3–4 weeks. Their mode of action is not completely understood, but there is evidence that they inhibit the iodination of tyrosyl residues in thyroglobulin (see Figs 29.1 and 29.2). It is thought that they inhibit the thyroperoxidase-catalysed oxidation reactions by acting as substrates for the postulated peroxidase–iodinium complex, thus competitively inhibiting the interaction with tyrosine. Propyl-thiouracil has the additional effect of reducing the deiodination of T_4 to T_3 in peripheral tissues.

Pharmacokinetic aspects

Thioureylenes are given orally. Carbimazole is rapidly converted to methimazole, which is distributed throughout the body water and has a plasma half-life of 6–15 hours. An average dose of carbimazole produces more than 90% inhibition of thyroid incorporation of iodine within 12 hours. The clinical response to this and other antithyroid drugs, however, may take several weeks (Fig. 29.6). This is not only because T_4 has a long half-life, but also because the thyroid may have large stores of hormone, which need to be depleted before the drug's action can be fully manifest. Propylthiouracil is thought to act somewhat more rapidly because of its additional effect as an inhibitor of the peripheral conversion of T_4 to T_3.

Both methimazole and propylthiouracil cross the placenta and also appear in the milk, but this effect is less pronounced with propylthiouracil, because it is more strongly bound to plasma protein. After degradation, the metabolites are excreted in the urine, propylthiouracil being excreted more rapidly than methimazole. The thioureylenes may be concentrated in the thyroid.

Unwanted effects

The most important unwanted effect is granulocytopenia (see Ch. 22). This is relatively rare, having an incidence of 0.1–1.2%, and is reversible on cessation of treatment. Rashes are more common (2–25%), and other symptoms, such as headaches, nausea, jaundice and pain in the joints, can occur.

IODINE/IODIDE

Iodine is converted in vivo to iodide (I^-), which temporarily inhibits the release of thyroid hormones. When high doses of iodine are given to thyrotoxic patients, the symptoms subside within 1–2 days. There is inhibition of the secretion of thyroid hormones and, over a period of 10–14 days, a marked reduction in vascularity of the gland, which becomes smaller and firmer. Iodine is often given orally in a solution with potassium iodide ('Lugol's iodine'). With continuous administration, its effect reaches maximum within 10–15 days and then decreases. The mechanism of action is not entirely clear; it may inhibit iodination of thyroglobulin, possibly by reducing the H_2O_2 generation that is necessary for this process.

The main uses of iodine/iodide are for the preparation of hyperthyroid subjects for surgical resection of the gland, and as part of the treatment of severe thyrotoxic crisis (*thyroid storm*). Allergic reactions can occur; these include angio-oedema, rashes, drug fever, lacrimation, conjunctivitis, pain in the salivary glands and a cold-like syndrome.

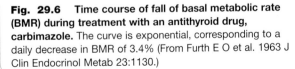

Fig. 29.6 **Time course of fall of basal metabolic rate (BMR) during treatment with an antithyroid drug, carbimazole.** The curve is exponential, corresponding to a daily decrease in BMR of 3.4% (From Furth E O et al. 1963 J Clin Endocrinol Metab 23:1130.)

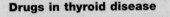

Drugs in thyroid disease

Drugs for hyperthyroidism
- *Radioiodine*, given orally, is selectively taken up by thyroid and damages cells; it emits short-range β radiation, which affects only thyroid follicle cells. Hypothyroidism will eventually occur.
- *Thioureylenes* (e.g. propylthiouracil) decrease the synthesis of thyroid hormones; the mechanism is through inhibition of thyroperoxidase, thus reducing iodination of thyroglobulin. They are given orally.
- *Iodine*, given orally in high doses, transiently reduces thyroid hormone secretion and decreases vascularity of the gland.

Drugs for hypothyroidism
- *Thyroxine* has all the actions of endogenous thyroxine; it is given orally.
- *Liothyronine* has all the actions of endogenous triiodothyronine; it is given intravenously.

OTHER DRUGS USED

The *β-adrenoceptor antagonists*, for example **propranolol** (Ch. 11), are not antithyroid agents as such, but they are useful for decreasing many of the signs and symptoms of hyperthyroidism—the tachycardia, dysrhythmias, tremor and agitation. They are used during the preparation of thyrotoxic patients for surgery, as well as in most hyperthyroid patients during the initial treatment period while the thioureylenes or radioiodine take effect, and as part of the treatment of acute hyperthyroid crisis. **Guanethidine**, a noradrenergic-blocking agent (Ch. 11), is used in eye drops to ameliorate the exophthalmos of hyperthyroidism (which is not relieved by antithyroid drugs); it acts by relaxing the sympathetically innervated smooth muscle that causes eyelid retraction. Glucocorticoids (e.g. **prednisolone**) or surgical decompression may be needed to mitigate severe exophthalmia in Graves' disease. Some other drugs (e.g. cholecystographic agents) or pesticides/environmental contaminant (e.g. polychlorinated biphenyls) may interfere with the normal production of thyroid hormones.

HYPOTHYROIDISM

There are no drugs that specifically augment the synthesis or release of thyroid hormones. The only effective treatment for hypothyroidism, unless it is caused by iodine deficiency (which is treated with iodide; see above), is to administer the thyroid hormones themselves as replacement therapy. **Thyroxine** and **triiodothyronine** (**liothyronine**) are available and are given orally. Thyroxine as the sodium salt in doses of 50–100 micrograms/day is the usual first-line drug of choice. Liothyronine has a faster onset but a shorter duration of action, and is generally reserved for acute emergencies such as the rare condition of myxoedema coma, where these properties are an advantage.

Unwanted effects may occur with overdose, and in addition to the signs and symptoms of hyperthyroidism there is a risk of precipitating angina pectoris, cardiac dysrhythmias or even cardiac failure. The effects of less severe overdose are more insidious; the patient feels well but bone resorption is increased, leading to osteoporosis.

The use of drugs acting on the thyroid is summarised in the clinical box.

> **Clinical use of drugs acting on the thyroid**
>
> **Radioiodine**
> - Hyperthyroidism (Graves' disease, multinodular toxic goitre).
> - Relapse of hyperthyroidism after failed medical or surgical treatment.
>
> **Carbimazole or propylthiouracil**
> - Hyperthyroidism (diffuse toxic goitre); at least 1 year of treatment is needed.
> - Preliminary to surgery for toxic goitre.
> - Part of the treatment of *thyroid storm* (very severe hyperthyroidism); **propylthiouracil** is preferred. The β-adrenoceptor antagonists (e.g. **propranolol**) are also used.
>
> **Thyroid hormones and iodine**
> - **Thyroxine (T$_4$)** is the standard replacement therapy for *hypothyroidism*.
> - **Liothyronine (T$_3$)** is the treatment of choice for *myxoedema coma*.
> - Iodine dissolved in aqueous potassium iodide (**'Lugol's iodine'**) is used short-term to control thyrotoxicosis *preoperatively*. It reduces the vascularity of the gland.

REFERENCES AND FURTHER READING

Bassett J H D, Harvey C B, Williams G R 2003 Mechanisms of thyroid hormone receptor–specific nuclear and extra nuclear actions. Mol Cell Endocrinol 213: 1–11 (*An excellent and comprehensive review dealing with the actions of thyroid hormones through the nuclear receptor mechanism as well as other actions through G-protein–coupled receptors and other pathways*)

Braga M, Cooper D S 2001 Clinical review 129. Oral cholecystographic agents and the thyroid. J Clin Endocrinol Metab 86: 1853–1860 (*Discusses the effect of imaging agents on thyroid function*)

Braga-Basaria M, Ringel M D 2003 Clinical review 158. Beyond radioiodine: a review of potential new therapeutic approaches for thyroid cancer. J Clin Endocrinol Metab 88: 1947–1960 (*Discusses some new strategies that might be used to control thyroid carcinoma*)

Franklin J A 1995 The management of hyperthyroidism.

N Engl J Med 330: 1731–1738 (*An excellent review of the drug treatment of hyperthyroidism*)

Hadj Kacem H, Rebai A, Kaffel N et al. 2003. PDS is a new susceptibility gene to autoimmune thyroid diseases: association and linkage study. J Clin Endocrinol Metab 88: 2274–2280 (*Interesting article on the PDS transporter protein and its contribution to disease susceptibility*)

Kahaly G J, Dillmann W H 2005 Thyroid hormone action in the heart. Endocr Rev 26: 704–728 (*A very interesting review focusing on the cardiac actions of thyroid hormones; much historical detail*)

Kelly G S 2000 Peripheral metabolism of thyroid hormones: a review. Altern Med Rev 5: 306–333 (*This review focuses on the role of peripheral metabolism in thyroid hormone action*)

Lazar M A 2003 Thyroid hormone action: a binding contract. J Clin Invest 112: 497–499 (*A short and accessible article dealing with the main nuclear receptor–mediated effects of thyroid hormones as well as some other potential mechanisms of action*)

Lazarus J H 1997 Hyperthyroidism. Lancet 349: 339–343 (*A 'seminar' covering aetiology, clinical features, pathophysiology, diagnosis and treatment*)

Lindsay R S 1997 Hypothyroidism. Lancet 349: 413–417 (*A 'seminar' emphasising the management of hypothyroidism*)

Niepomniszcze H, Amad R H 2001 Skin disorders and thyroid diseases. J Endocrinol Invest 24: 628–638 (*Another review of the extrathyroidal effects and their link to various skin pathologies*)

Nilsson M 2001 Iodide handling by the thyroid epithelial cell. Exp Clin Endocrinol Diabetes 109: 13–17 (*Useful and readable review of iodide handling by the thyroid gland*)

Paschke R, Ludgate M 1997 The thyrotropin receptor and its diseases. N Engl J Med 337: 1675–1679 (*Reviews aspects of TSH biology and disease*)

Roberts C G, Ladenson P W 2004 Hypothyroidism. Lancet 363: 793–803 (*Authoritative and accessible review dealing with this thyroid pathology*)

Schmutzler C, Kohrle J 1998 Implications of the molecular characterization of the sodium–iodide symporter (NIS). Exp Clin Endocrinol Diabetes 106: S1–S10 (*Discusses the diagnostic and therapeutic implications of the information now available as a result of the cloning of NIS*)

Suh J M, Song J H, Kim D W et al. 2003 Regulation of the phosphatidylinositol 3-kinase, Akt/protein kinase B, FRAP/mammalian target of rapamycin, and ribosomal S6 kinase 1 signaling pathways by thyroid-stimulating hormone (TSH) and stimulating type TSH receptor antibodies in the thyroid gland. J Biol Chem 278: 21960–21971 (*A research paper dealing with the signalling at the TSH receptor*)

Surks M I, Ortiz E, Daniels G H et al. 2004 Subclinical thyroid disease: scientific review and guidelines for diagnosis and management. JAMA 291: 228–238 (*Discusses and reviews the treatment of subclinical thyroid disease in detail; primarily of interest to clinical students*)

Yen P M 2001 Physiological and molecular basis of thyroid hormone action. Physiol Rev 81: 1097–1142 (*Comprehensive review of thyroid hormone–receptor interaction and the effects of thyroid hormone on target tissues*)

Yoshida A, Hisatome I, Taniguchi S et al. 2004 Mechanism of iodide/chloride exchange by pendrin. Endocrinology 145: 4301–4308 (*An original research article that takes an electrophysiological approach to understanding of the PDS transporter and its relationship to Pendred's syndrome*)

Zhang J, Lazar M 2000 The mechanism of action of thyroid hormones. Annu Rev Physiol 62: 439–466 (*Detailed review of the molecular aspects of thyroid hormone/receptor interaction*)

The reproductive system

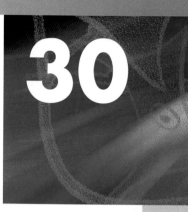

30

OVERVIEW

Drugs that affect reproduction (both by preventing conception and more recently for treating infertility) have had profound consequences for individuals and for society. In this chapter, we describe the endocrine control of the female and male reproductive systems, because this forms the basis for understanding many important drugs. The principle of negative feedback, which is stressed, is central to understanding how hormones interact to control reproduction,[1] and many drugs, including agents used to prevent or assist conception, work by influencing negative feedback mechanisms. Oestrogen replacement therapy prevents postmenopausal bone loss as well as treating symptoms of oestrogen deficiency, benefits that are offset by effects on the breast and endometrium, and by an increase in thromboembolism. There is a separate section on drugs that alter the contractile state of the uterus, which are important in obstetrics: drugs that stimulate uterine contraction—'oxytocic' drugs—are used to induce labour or abortion and to prevent postpartum haemorrhage, whereas uterine relaxants are used, much less effectively, to delay labour. There is a section on drugs for erectile dysfunction, which have made a remarkable transition from below-the-counter charlatanry to medical orthodoxy.

ENDOCRINE CONTROL OF REPRODUCTION AND DRUGS THAT INFLUENCE THIS

Hormonal control of the reproductive systems in men and women involves sex steroids from the gonads, hypothalamic peptides, and glycoprotein gonadotrophins from the anterior pituitary.

NEUROHORMONAL CONTROL OF THE FEMALE REPRODUCTIVE SYSTEM

At puberty, an increased output of the hormones of the hypothalamus and anterior pituitary stimulates secretion of oestrogenic sex steroids. These are responsible for the maturation of the reproductive organs and the development of the secondary sexual characteristics, and also for a phase of accelerated growth followed by closure of the epiphyses of the long bones. Sex steroids are thereafter involved in the regulation of the cyclic changes

---

[1]Recognition that negative feedback is central to endocrine control was a profound insight, made in 1930 by Dorothy Price, a laboratory assistant in the University of Chicago experimenting on effects of testosterone in rats. She referred to it as 'reciprocal influence'.

expressed in the menstrual cycle, and are important in pregnancy. A simplified outline of the inter-relationship of these substances in the physiological control of the menstrual cycle is given in Figures 30.1 and 30.2.

The menstrual cycle begins with *menstruation*, which lasts for 3–6 days, during which the superficial layer of uterine endometrium is shed. The endometrium regenerates during the *follicular phase* of the cycle after menstrual flow has stopped. A releasing factor, the *gonadotrophin-releasing hormone (GnRH)*, is secreted from peptidergic neurons in the hypothalamus in a pulsatile fashion, the frequency being about one burst of discharges per hour. GnRH stimulates the anterior pituitary to release gonadotrophic hormones (Fig. 30.1)—*follicle-stimulating hormone (FSH)* and *luteinising hormone (LH)*. These act on the ovaries (Fig. 30.2A) to promote development of small groups of follicles, each of which contains an ovum. One follicle develops faster than the others and forms the Graafian follicle (Figs 30.1 and 30.2E), and the rest degenerate. The ripening Graafian follicle consists of thecal and granulosa cells surrounding a fluid-filled centre, within which lies an ovum. Oestrogens are produced by the granulosa cells stimulated by FSH, from androgen precursor molecules derived from thecal cells stimulated by LH. Oestrogens are responsible for the proliferative phase of endometrial regeneration, which occurs from day 5 or 6 until mid-cycle (Fig. 30.2B,F). During this phase, the endometrium increases in thickness and

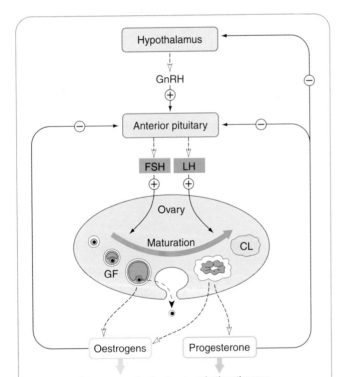

Fig. 30.1 Hormonal control of the female reproductive system. The Graafian follicle (GF) is shown developing on the left, then involuting to form the corpus luteum (CL) on the right, after the ovum (•) has been released. FSH, follicle-stimulating hormone; GnRH, gonadotrophin-releasing hormone; LH, luteinising hormone.

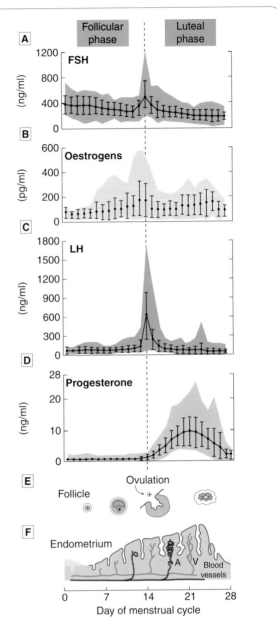

Fig. 30.2 Plasma concentrations of ovarian hormones and gonadotrophins in women during normal menstrual cycles. Values are the mean ± standard deviation of 40 women. The shaded areas indicate the entire range of observations. Day 1 is the onset of menstruation. E and F show diagrammatically the changes in the ovarian follicle and the endometrium during the cycle. Ovulation on day 14 of the menstrual cycle occurs with the mid-cycle peak of luteinising hormone (LH), represented by the vertical dashed line. A, arterioles; FSH, follicle-stimulating hormone; V, venules. (After van de Wiele R L, Dyrenfurth I 1974 Pharmacol Rev 25: 189–217.)

vascularity, and at the peak of oestrogen secretion there is a prolific cervical secretion of mucus of pH 8–9, rich in protein and carbohydrate, which facilitates entry of spermatozoa. Oestrogen has a negative feedback effect on the anterior pituitary, decreasing gonadotrophin release during chronic administration of oestrogen as oral contraception (see below). In contrast, the high endogenous oestrogen secretion just before mid-cycle sensitises LH-releasing cells of the pituitary to the action of the GnRH and causes the mid-cycle surge of LH secretion (Fig. 30.2C). This, in turn, causes rapid swelling and rupture of the Graafian follicle, resulting in ovulation. If fertilisation occurs, the fertilised ovum passes down the fallopian tubes to the uterus, starting to divide as it goes.

Stimulated by LH, cells of the ruptured follicle proliferate and develop into the corpus luteum, which secretes progesterone. Progesterone acts, in turn, on oestrogen-primed endometrium, stimulating the *secretory phase* of the cycle, which renders the endometrium suitable for the implantation of a fertilised ovum. During this phase, cervical mucus becomes more viscous, less alkaline, less copious and in general less welcoming for sperm. Progesterone exerts negative feedback on hypothalamus and pituitary, decreasing the release of LH. It also has a thermogenic effect, causing a rise in body temperature of about 0.5°C at ovulation, which is maintained until the end of the cycle.

If implantation of the ovum does not occur, progesterone secretion stops, triggering menstruation. If implantation does occur, the corpus luteum continues to secrete progesterone, which, by its effect on the hypothalamus and anterior pituitary, prevents further ovulation. The chorion (an antecedent of the placenta) secretes *human chorionic gonadotrophin* (HCG), which maintains the lining of the womb during pregnancy. For reasons that are not physiologically obvious, HCG has an additional pharmacological action in stimulating ovulation. As pregnancy proceeds, the placenta develops further hormonal functions and secretes a gamut of hormone variants (often with post-translational modifications), including *gonadotrophins* as well as *progesterone* and *oestrogens*. Progesterone secreted during pregnancy controls the development of the secretory alveoli in the mammary gland, while oestrogen stimulates the lactiferous ducts. After parturition, oestrogens, along with *prolactin* (see Ch. 28, pp. 423-424), are responsible for stimulating and maintaining lactation, whereas high doses of exogenous oestrogen suppress this.

Oestrogens are dealt with below, progestogens (progesterone-like drugs) on page 449, androgens on page 451, and the gonadotrophins on page 454.

BEHAVIOURAL EFFECTS OF SEX HORMONES

As well as controlling the menstrual cycle, sex steroids affect sexual behaviour. Two types of control are recognised: *organisational* and *activational*. The former refers to the fact that sexual differentiation of the brain can be permanently altered by the presence or absence of sex steroids at key stages in development.

In rats, administration of androgens to females within a few days of birth results in long-term virilisation of behaviour. Conversely, neonatal castration of male rats causes them to develop behaviourally as females. Brain development in the absence of sex steroids follows female lines, but is switched to the male pattern by exposure of the hypothalamus to androgen at a key stage of development. Similar but less complete behavioural virilisation of female offspring has been demonstrated following androgen administration in non-human primates, and probably also occurs in humans if pregnant women are exposed to excessive androgen.

> **Hormonal control of the female reproductive system** 🔑
>
> - The menstrual cycle starts with menstruation.
> - Gonadotrophin-releasing hormone, released from the hypothalamus, acts on the anterior pituitary to release follicle-stimulating hormone (FSH) and luteinising hormone (LH).
> - FSH and LH stimulate follicle development in the ovary. FSH is the main hormone stimulating oestrogen release. LH stimulates ovulation at mid-cycle and is the main hormone controlling subsequent progesterone secretion from the corpus luteum.
> - Oestrogen controls the proliferative phase of the endometrium and has negative feedback effects on the anterior pituitary. Progesterone controls the later secretory phase, and has negative feedback effects on both hypothalamus and anterior pituitary.
> - If a fertilised ovum is implanted, the corpus luteum continues to secrete progesterone.
> - After implantation, human chorionic gonadotrophin from the chorion becomes important, and later in pregnancy progesterone and other hormones are secreted by the placenta.

The activational effect of sex steroids refers to their ability to modify sexual behaviour after brain development is complete. In general, oestrogens and androgens increase sexual activity in the appropriate sex. *Oxytocin*, which is important during parturition (see below), also has roles in mating and parenting behaviours, its action in the central nervous system being regulated by oestrogen (see Ch. 28).

OESTROGENS

Oestrogens are synthesised by the ovary and placenta, and in small amounts by the testis and adrenal cortex. As for other steroids, the starting substance for oestrogen synthesis is cholesterol. The immediate precursors to the oestrogens are androgenic substances—androstenedione or testosterone (Fig. 30.3). There are three main endogenous oestrogens in humans: *oestradiol*, *oestrone* and *oestriol* (Fig. 30.3). Oestradiol is the most potent and is the principal oestrogen secreted by the ovary. At the beginning of the menstrual cycle, the plasma concentration is 0.2 nmol/l, rising to ~2.2 nmol/l in mid-cycle.

Actions

Oestrogen acts in concert with progesterone, and induces synthesis of progesterone receptors in uterus, vagina, anterior pituitary and hypothalamus. Conversely, progesterone *decreases* oestrogen receptor expression in the reproductive tract. Prolactin (see Ch. 28) also influences oestrogen action by increasing the numbers of oestrogen receptors in the mammary gland, but has no effect on oestrogen receptor expression in the uterus.

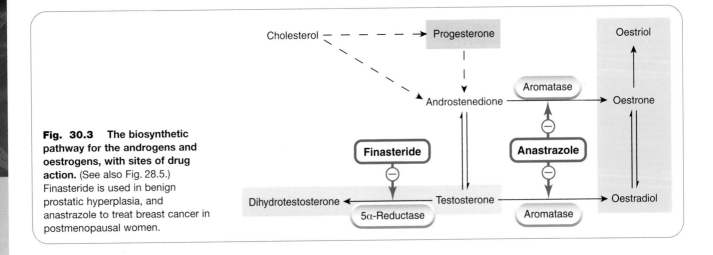

Fig. 30.3 The biosynthetic pathway for the androgens and oestrogens, with sites of drug action. (See also Fig. 28.5.) Finasteride is used in benign prostatic hyperplasia, and anastrazole to treat breast cancer in postmenopausal women.

Effects of exogenous oestrogen depend on the state of sexual maturity when the oestrogen is administered:

- in primary hypogonadism: oestrogen stimulates development of secondary sexual characteristics and accelerates growth
- in adults with primary amenorrhoea: oestrogen, given cyclically with a progestogen, induces an artificial cycle
- in sexually mature women: oestrogen (with a progestogen) is contraceptive
- at or after the menopause: oestrogen replacement prevents menopausal symptoms and bone loss.

Oestrogens have several metabolic actions, including mineralo-corticoid (retention of salt and water) and mild anabolic actions. They increase plasma concentrations of high-density lipoproteins, a potentially beneficial effect (Ch. 20) that may contribute to the relatively low risk of atheromatous disease in premenopausal women compared with men of the same age. Oestrogens increase the coagulability of blood, and increase the risk of thromboembolism. This effect is dose-related.

Mechanism of action

As with other steroids, oestrogen binds to type 4 nuclear receptors (Ch. 3, pp. 46-48). There are at least two types of oestrogen receptor, termed *ERα* and *ERβ*, the roles of which are currently being investigated using mice in which the gene coding one or other of these has been 'knocked out' (Ch. 6, p. 92). Binding is followed by interaction of the resultant complexes with nuclear sites and subsequent genomic effects—either gene transcription (i.e. DNA-directed RNA and protein synthesis) or gene repression (inhibition of transcription). More details are given in Chapters 3 and 28. In addition to these 'classic' intracellular receptors, some oestrogen effects, in particular its rapid vascular actions, may be initiated by interaction with membrane receptors (e.g. Chen et al., 1999). Acute vasodilatation caused by 17-β-oestradiol is mediated by nitric oxide, and a plant-derived (*phyto-*) oestrogen called **genistein** (which is selective for ERβ, as well as having quite distinct effects from inhibition of protein kinase C) is as potent as 17-β-oestradiol in this regard. Oestrogen receptor modulators (receptor-selective oestrogen agonists or antagonists) are mentioned briefly immediately below this section.

Preparations

Many preparations (oral, transdermal, intramuscular, implantable and topical) of oestrogens are available for a wide range of indications. These preparations include natural (e.g. **estradiol**, **estriol**) and synthetic (e.g. **mestranol**, **ethinylestradiol**, **stilbestrol**) oestrogens. Oestrogens are presented either as single agents or combined with progestogen.

The clinical use of oestrogens and antioestrogens is given in the box.

Pharmacokinetic aspects

Natural as well as synthetic oestrogens are well absorbed in the gastrointestinal tract, but after absorption the natural oestrogens are rapidly metabolised in the liver, whereas synthetic oestrogens are degraded less rapidly. There is a variable amount of entero-hepatic cycling, which forms the basis for drug interaction, because broad-spectrum antibiotic use alters bowel flora and can thereby render oral contraception ineffective (Ch. 52). Most oestrogens are readily absorbed from skin and mucous membranes. They may be given topically in the vagina as creams or pessaries for local effect. In the plasma, natural oestrogens are bound to albumin

---

> **Clinical use of oestrogens and antioestrogens**
>
> **Oestrogens**
> - Replacement therapy:
>   - primary ovarian failure (e.g. Turner's syndrome)
>   - secondary ovarian failure (menopause) for flushing, vaginal dryness and to preserve bone mass.
> - Contraception.
> - Prostate and breast cancer (these uses have largely been superseded by other hormonal manipulations; see Ch. 51)
>
> **Antioestrogens**
> - To treat oestrogen-sensitive breast cancer (tamoxifen).
> - To induce ovulation (clomiphene) in treating infertility.

and to a sex steroid–binding globulin. Natural oestrogens are excreted in the urine as glucuronides and sulfates.

Unwanted effects

Unwanted effects of oestrogens include tenderness in the breasts, nausea, vomiting, anorexia, retention of salt and water with resultant oedema, and increased risk of thromboembolism. More details of the unwanted effects of oral contraceptives are given on page 455.

Used intermittently for postmenopausal replacement therapy, oestrogens cause menstruation-like bleeding. Oestrogen causes endometrial hyperplasia unless given cyclically with a progestogen. When administered to males, oestrogens result in feminisation.

Oestrogen administration to pregnant women can cause genital abnormalities in their offspring. Carcinoma of the vagina was more common in young women whose mothers were given stilbestrol in early pregnancy in a misguided attempt to prevent miscarriage (see Ch. 53).

Clinical use

Clinical uses of oestrogens are given in the box on page 448. In addition, see the section below (pp. 450-451) on postmenopausal hormone replacement therapy (HRT).

OESTROGEN RECEPTOR MODULATOR

Raloxifene, a 'selective oestrogen receptor modulator', has anti-oestrogenic effects on breast and uterus but oestrogenic effects on bone, lipid metabolism and blood coagulation. It is used for prevention and treatment of postmenopausal osteoporosis (Ch. 31, p. 467) and reduces the incidence of oestrogen receptor–positive breast cancer, although its role in therapy of breast cancer is undefined. Unlike oestrogen, it does not prevent menopausal flushes.

ANTIOESTROGENS

Antioestrogens compete with natural oestrogens for receptors in target organs. **Tamoxifen** has antioestrogenic action on mammary tissue but oestrogenic actions on plasma lipids, endometrium and bone. It produces mild oestrogen-like adverse effects consistent with partial agonist activity. The tamoxifen–oestrogen receptor complex does not readily dissociate, so there is interference with the recycling of receptors.

Tamoxifen up-regulates transforming growth factor-β, decreased function of which is associated with the progression of malignancy, and which has a role in controlling the balance between bone-producing osteoblasts and bone-resorbing osteoclasts (Ch. 31).

Tamoxifen is discussed further in Chapter 51.

Clomiphene inhibits oestrogen binding in the anterior pituitary, so preventing the normal modulation by negative feedback and causing increased secretion of GnRH and gonadotrophins. This results in a marked stimulation and enlargement of the ovaries and increased oestrogen secretion. The main effect of their antioestrogen action in the pituitary is that they induce ovulation. It is used in treating infertility caused by lack of ovulation. Twins are common, but multiple pregnancy is unusual.

PROGESTOGENS

The natural progestational hormone (*progestogen*) is progesterone (see Figs 30.2 and 30.3). This is secreted by the corpus luteum in the second part of the menstrual cycle, and by the placenta during pregnancy. Small amounts are also secreted by testis and adrenal cortex.

Mechanism of action

Progestogens act, as do other steroid hormones, on nuclear receptors. The density of progesterone receptors is controlled by oestrogens (see above).

Preparations

There are two main groups of progestogens.

- The naturally occurring hormone and its derivatives (e.g. **hydroxyprogesterone**, **medroxyprogesterone**, **dyhydrogesterone**). Progesterone itself is virtually inactive orally, because after absorption it is metabolised in the liver, and hepatic extraction is nearly complete. Other preparations are available for oral administration, intramuscular injection, or administration via the vagina or rectum.

Oestrogens and antioestrogens

- The endogenous oestrogens are oestradiol (the most potent), oestrone and oestriol; there are numerous exogenous synthetic forms (e.g. ethinylestradiol).
- Mechanism of action involves interaction with nuclear receptors (termed ERα or ERβ) in target tissues, resulting in modification of gene transcription.
- Their pharmacological effects depend on the sexual maturity of the recipient:
  - before puberty, they stimulate development of secondary sexual characteristics
  - given cyclically in the female adult, they induce an artificial menstrual cycle and are used for contraception
  - given at or after the menopause, they prevent menopausal symptoms and protect against osteoporosis, but increase thromboembolism.
- Antioestrogens are competitive antagonists or partial agonists. **Tamoxifen** is used in oestrogen-dependent breast cancer. **Clomiphene** induces ovulation by inhibiting the negative feedback effects on the hypothalamus and anterior pituitary.
- Selective drugs that are oestrogen agonists in some tissues but antagonists in others are being developed. **Raloxifene** (one such drug) is used to treat and prevent osteoporosis.

- Testosterone derivatives (e.g. **norethisterone**, **norgestrel** and **ethynodiol**) can be given orally. The first two have some androgenic activity and are metabolised to give oestrogenic products. Newer progestogens used in contraception include **desogestrel** and **gestodene**; they may have less adverse effects on lipids than ethynodiol and may be considered for women who experience side effects such as acne, depression or breakthrough bleeding with the older drugs. However, these newer drugs have been associated with higher risks of venous thromboembolic disease (see below).

Actions

The pharmacological actions of the progestogens are in essence the same as the physiological actions of progesterone described above. Specific effects relevant to contraception are detailed on pages 454-456.

Pharmacokinetic aspects

Injected progesterone is bound to albumin, not to the sex steroid–binding globulin. Some is stored in adipose tissue. It is metabolised in the liver, and the products, pregnanolone and pregnanediol, are conjugated with glucuronic acid and excreted in the urine.

Unwanted effects

Unwanted effects of progestogens include weak androgenic actions. Other unwanted effects include acne, fluid retention, weight change, depression, change in libido, breast discomfort, premenstrual symptoms, irregular menstrual cycles and breakthrough bleeding. There is an increased incidence of thromboembolism.

Clinical use

Clinical uses are summarised in the box on this page.

> **Clinical use of progestogens and antiprogestogens**
>
> **Progestogens**
> - Contraception:
>   - with oestrogen in *combined oral contraceptive pill*
>   - as *progesterone-only contraceptive pill*
>   - as injectable or implantable progesterone-only contraception
>   - as part of an intrauterine contraceptive system.
> - Combined with oestrogen for *oestrogen replacement therapy* in women with an intact uterus, to prevent endometrial hyperplasia and carcinoma.
> - For *endometriosis*.
> - In *endometrial carcinoma*; use in breast and renal cancer has declined.
> - Poorly validated uses have included various menstrual disorders.
>
> **Antiprogestogens**
> - Medical termination of pregnancy: **mifepristone** (partial agonist) combined with a prostaglandin (e.g. **gemeprost**).

ANTIPROGESTOGENS

Mifepristone is a partial agonist at progesterone receptors. It sensitises the uterus to the action of prostaglandins. It is given orally and has a plasma half-life of 21 hours. Mifepristone is used, in combination with a prostaglandin (e.g. **gemeprost**; see below), as a medical alternative to surgical termination of pregnancy (see clinical box).

POSTMENOPAUSAL HORMONE REPLACEMENT THERAPY

At the menopause, whether natural or surgically induced, ovarian function decreases and oestrogen levels fall. There is a long history of disagreement regarding the pros and cons of hormone replacement therapy (HRT) in this context, with the prevailing wisdom undergoing several revisions over the years (see Davis et al., 2005). Short-term HRT has some clear-cut benefits:

- improvement of symptoms caused by reduced oestrogen, for example hot flushes and vaginal dryness
- prevention and treatment of osteoporosis, but other drugs are often preferable for this (Ch. 31).

Oestrogen replacement does *not* reduce the risk of coronary heart disease, despite earlier hopes, nor is there evidence that it reduces age-related decline in cognitive function (indeed, some trials suggest the reverse). Drawbacks include:

- cyclical withdrawal bleeding
- adverse effects related to progestogen (see above)
- increased risk of endometrial cancer if oestrogen is given unopposed by progestogen

---

> **Progestogens and antiprogestogens**
>
>
>
> - The endogenous hormone is progesterone. Examples of synthetic drugs are the progesterone derivative **medroxyprogesterone** and the testosterone derivative **norethisterone**.
> - Mechanism of action involves intracellular receptor/altered gene expression, as for other steroid hormones. Oestrogen stimulates synthesis of progesterone receptors, whereas progesterone inhibits synthesis of oestrogen receptors.
> - Main therapeutic uses are in oral contraception and oestrogen replacement regimens, and to treat endometriosis.
> - The antiprogestogen **mifepristone**, in combination with prostaglandin analogues, is an effective medical alternative to surgical termination of early pregnancy.

- increased risk of breast cancer, related to the duration of HRT use and disappearing within 5 years of stopping; in women using combined HRT for 5 years, breast cancer is diagnosed in about 4 extra cases in 1000 (British Medical Association and Royal Pharmaceutical Society of Great Britain, 2005)
- increased risk of venous thromboembolism (risk approximately doubled in women using combined HRT for 5 years).

Oestrogens used in HRT can be given orally (conjugated estrogens, estradiol, estriol), vaginally (estriol), by transdermal patch (estradiol) or by subcutaneous implant (estradiol). **Tibolone** is marketed for the short-term treatment of symptoms of oestrogen deficiency. It has oestrogenic, progestogenic and weak androgenic activity, and can be used continuously without cyclical progesterone (avoiding the inconvenience of withdrawal bleeding).

NEUROHORMONAL CONTROL OF THE MALE REPRODUCTIVE SYSTEM

As in the female, endocrine secretions from the hypothalamus, anterior pituitary and gonads control the male reproductive system. A simplified outline of the inter-relationship of these factors is given in Figure 30.4. GnRH controls the secretion of gonadotrophins by the anterior pituitary. This secretion is not cyclical as in menstruating women; in both sexes, it is pulsatile (see below). FSH is responsible for the integrity of the seminiferous tubules, and after puberty is important in gametogenesis through an action

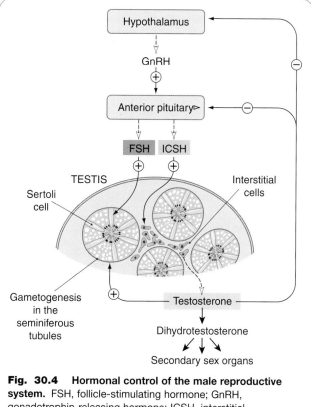

Fig. 30.4 Hormonal control of the male reproductive system. FSH, follicle-stimulating hormone; GnRH, gonadotrophin-releasing hormone; ICSH, interstitial cell–stimulating hormone.

on *Sertoli cells*, which nourish and support developing spermatozoa. LH, which in the male is also called interstitial cell–stimulating hormone (ICSH), stimulates the interstitial cells (*Leydig cells*) to secrete androgens—in particular *testosterone*. LH/ICSH secretion begins at puberty, and the consequent secretion of testosterone causes maturation of the reproductive organs and development of secondary sexual characteristics. Thereafter, the primary function of testosterone is the maintenance of spermatogenesis and hence fertility—an action mediated by Sertoli cells. Testosterone is also important in the maturation of spermatozoa as they pass through the epididymis and vas deferens. A further action is a feedback effect on the anterior pituitary, modulating its sensitivity to GnRH and thus influencing secretion of LH/ICSH. Testosterone has marked anabolic effects, causing development of the musculature and increased bone growth, resulting in a rapid increase in height (the pubertal growth spurt) at puberty, followed by closure of the epiphyses of the long bones.

Secretion of testosterone is mainly controlled by LH/ICSH, but FSH also plays a part, possibly by releasing a factor similar to GnRH from the Sertoli cells (which are its primary target). The interstitial cells that synthesise testosterone also have receptors for prolactin, which may influence testosterone production by increasing the number of receptors for LH/ICSH.

ANDROGENS

Testosterone is the main natural androgen. It is synthesised mainly by the interstitial cells of the testis, and in smaller amounts by the ovaries and adrenal cortex. Adrenal production of androgens is under the control of adrenocorticotrophic hormone (corticotrophin). As for other steroid hormones, cholesterol is the starting substance. Dehydroepiandrosterone and androstenedione are important intermediates. They are released from the gonads and the adrenal cortex, and converted to testosterone in the liver (see Fig. 30.3).

Actions

In general, the effects of exogenous androgens are the same as those of testosterone, and depend on the age and sex of the recipient. If administered to boys at the age of puberty, there is rapid development of secondary sexual characteristics, maturation of the reproductive organs and a marked increase in muscular strength. Height increases more gradually. The anabolic effects can be accompanied by retention of salt and water. The skin thickens and may darken, and sebaceous glands become more active (which can result in acne). There is growth of hair on the face and on pubic and axillary regions. The vocal cords hypertrophy, resulting in a lower pitch to the voice. Androgens cause a feeling of well-being and an increase in physical vigour, and may increase libido. Whether they are responsible for sexual behaviour as such is controversial, as is their contribution to aggressive behaviour.

If given to prepubertal males, the individuals concerned do not reach their full predicted height because of premature closure of the epiphyses of the long bones.

Administration of 'male' doses to women results in masculinisation, but lower doses (e.g. 300 µg/day testosterone patches) restore plasma testosterone to normal female concentrations and improve sexual dysfunction in women following ovariectomy, without adverse effects (Shifren et al., 2000; Braunstein et al., 2005).

Mechanism of action

In most target cells, testosterone works through an active metabolite, *dihydrotestosterone*, to which it is converted locally by a 5α-reductase enzyme. In contrast, testosterone itself causes virilisation of the genital tract in the male embryo and regulates LH/ICSH production in anterior pituitary cells. Testosterone and dihydrotestosterone modify gene transcription by interacting with intracellular receptors.

Preparations

Testosterone itself can be given by subcutaneous implantation or by transdermal patches. Various esters (e.g. enanthate and propionate) are given by intramuscular depot injection. Testosterone undecanoate and mesterolone can be given orally.

Pharmacokinetic aspects

If given orally, testosterone is rapidly metabolised in the liver. It is therefore usually injected. Virtually all testosterone in the circulation is bound to plasma protein—mainly to the sex steroid-binding globulin. The elimination half-life of free testosterone is short (10–20 minutes). It is inactivated in the liver by conversion to androstenedione (see Fig. 30.3). This has weak androgenic activity in its own right and can be reconverted to testosterone, although approximately 90% of testosterone is eliminated as metabolites rather than the parent compound. Synthetic androgens are less rapidly metabolised, and some are excreted in the urine unchanged.

Unwanted effects

Unwanted effects of androgens include eventual decrease of gonadotrophin release, with resultant infertility, and salt and water retention leading to oedema. Adenocarcinoma of the liver has been reported. Androgens impair growth in children (via premature fusion of epiphyses), cause acne, and lead to masculinisation in girls. Adverse effects of testosterone replacement and monitoring for these are reviewed by Rhoden & Morgentaler (2004).

Clinical use

The clinical use of androgens is given in the box.

ANABOLIC STEROIDS

Androgens can be modified chemically to alter the balance of anabolic and other effects. Such 'anabolic steroids' (e.g. **nandrolone**) increase protein synthesis and muscle development, but clinical use (e.g. in debilitating disease) has been disappointing. They are used in the therapy of aplastic anaemia, and (notoriously) abused by some athletes. Unwanted effects are described above, under *Androgens*. In addition, cholestatic jaundice, liver tumours and increased risk of coronary heart disease are recognised adverse effects of high-dose anabolic steroids.

> **Androgens and the hormonal control of the male reproductive system**
>
> - Gonadotrophin-releasing hormone from the hypothalamus acts on the anterior pituitary to release both follicle-stimulating hormone, which stimulates gametogenesis, and luteinising hormone (also called interstitial cell–stimulating hormone), which stimulates androgen secretion.
> - The endogenous hormone is testosterone; intramuscular depot injections of testosterone esters are used for replacement therapy.
> - Mechanism of action is via intracellular receptors.
> - Effects depend on age/sex, and include development of male secondary sexual characteristics in prepubertal boys and masculinisation in women.

> **Clinical use of androgens and antiandrogens**
>
> - Androgens (**testosterone** preparations) as hormone replacement in:
>   - male *hypogonadism* due to pituitary or testicular disease (e.g. 2.5 mg/day patches)
>   - hyposexuality following ovariectomy (e.g. 300 μg/day patches).
> - Antiandrogens (e.g. **flutamide, cyproterone**) are used as part of the treatment of *prostatic cancer*.
> - 5α-Reductase inhibitors (e.g. **finasteride**) are used in benign prostatic hypertrophy.

ANTIANDROGENS

Both *oestrogens* and *progestogens* have antiandrogen activity, oestrogens mainly by inhibiting gonadotrophin secretion and progestogens by competing with androgens in target organs. **Cyproterone** is a derivative of progesterone and has weak progestational activity. It is a partial agonist at androgen receptors, competing with dihydrotestosterone for receptors in androgen-sensitive target tissues. Through its effect in the hypothalamus, it depresses the synthesis of gonadotrophins. It is used as an adjunct in the treatment of prostatic cancer during initiation of GnRH treatment (see below). It is also used in the therapy of precocious puberty in males, and of masculinisation and acne in women. It also has a central nervous system effect, decreasing libido, and has been used to treat hypersexuality in male sexual offenders.[2]

---

[2]As with the oestrogens, very different doses are used for these different conditions, for example 2 mg/day for acne, 100 mg/day for hypersexuality, and 300 mg/day for prostatic cancer.

Flutamide is a non-steroidal antiandrogen used with GnRH in the treatment of prostate cancer.

Drugs can have antiandrogen action by inhibiting synthetic enzymes. **Finasteride** inhibits the enzyme (5α-reductase) that converts testosterone to dihydrotestosterone (Fig. 30.3), which has greater affinity than testosterone for androgen receptors in the prostate gland. Finasteride is well absorbed after oral administration, has a half-life of about 7 hours, and is excreted in the urine and faeces. It is used to treat benign prostatic hyperplasia, although α_1-adrenoceptor antagonists, **terazosin** or **tamsulosin** (Ch. 11, p. 179), are more effective (working by the entirely different mechanism of relaxing smooth muscle in the capsule of the prostate gland). Surgery is the preferred option (especially by surgeons).

GONADOTROPHIN-RELEASING HORMONE: AGONISTS AND ANTAGONISTS

Gonadotrophin-releasing hormone (GnRH) is a decapeptide that controls the secretion of FSH and LH by the anterior pituitary. Secretion of GnRH is controlled by neural input from other parts of the brain, and through negative feedback by the sex steroids (Figs 30.1 and 30.5). Exogenous androgens, oestrogens and progestogens all inhibit GnRH secretion, but only progestogens exert this effect at doses that do not have marked hormonal actions on peripheral tissues, presumably because progesterone receptors in the reproductive tract are sparse unless they have been induced by previous exposure to oestrogen. **Danazol** (see below) is a synthetic steroid that inhibits release of GnRH and, consequently, of gonadotrophins (FSH and LH). **Clomiphene** is an oestrogen antagonist that stimulates gonadotrophin release by inhibiting the negative feedback effects of endogenous oestrogen; it is used to treat infertility (see above and Fig. 30.5).

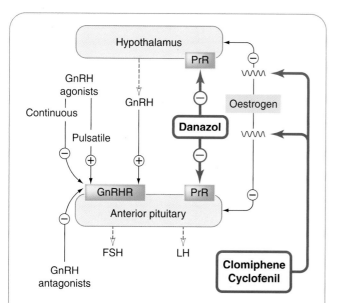

Fig. 30.5 **Regulation of gonadotrophin (follicle-stimulating hormone, FSH; luteinising hormone, LH) release from the anterior pituitary.** GnRHR, GnRH receptor; PrR, progestogen receptor.

Synthetic GnRH is termed **gonadorelin**. Numerous analogues of GnRH, both agonists and antagonists, have been synthesised. **Buserelin**, **leuprorelin**, **goserelin** and **nafarelin** are agonists, the last being 200 times more potent than endogenous GnRH.

Pharmacokinetics and clinical use

Gonadotrophin-releasing hormone agonists, given by subcutaneous infusion in pulses to mimic physiological secretion of GnRH, stimulate gonadotrophin release (Fig. 30.5) and induce ovulation. They are absorbed intact following nasal administration (Ch. 7). Continuous use, by nasal spray or as depot preparations, stimulates gonadotrophin release transiently, but then paradoxically *inhibits* gonadotrophin release (Fig. 30.5) because of down-regulation (desensitisation) of GnRH receptors in the pituitary. GnRH analogues are given in this fashion to cause gonadal suppression in various sex hormone–dependent conditions, including prostate and breast cancers, endometriosis (endometrial tissue outside the uterine cavity) and large uterine fibroids. Continuous, non-pulsatile administration inhibits spermatogenesis and ovulation, raising the possibility (which is under investigation) that GnRH analogues could be useful as contraceptives. GnRH agonists are used by specialists in infertility treatment, not to stimulate ovulation (which is achieved using gonadotrophin preparations) but to suppress the pituitary before administration of FSH or HCG (see below). It was originally hoped that GnRH *antagonists* would be useful for contraception, but this has not been realised.

Unwanted effects of GnRH analogues

Unwanted effects of GnRH agonists in women, for example flushing, vaginal dryness and bone loss, result from hypo-oestrogenism. The initial stimulation of gonadotrophin secretion on starting treatment can cause transient worsening of pain from bone metastases in men with prostate cancer, so treatment is started only after the patient has received an androgen receptor antagonist such as **flutamide** (see above and Ch. 51).

DANAZOL

Actions and pharmacokinetics

Danazol inhibits gonadotrophin secretion (especially the mid-cycle surge), and consequently reduces oestrogen synthesis in the ovary (Fig. 30.5). In men, it reduces androgen synthesis and spermatogenesis. It has androgenic activity. It is orally active and metabolised in the liver.

Clinical uses

Danazol is used in sex hormone–dependent conditions including endometriosis, breast dysplasia and gynaecomastia. An additional specialist use is to reduce attacks of swelling in hereditary angio-oedema (Ch. 23, p. 365).

Unwanted effects

Unwanted effects are common, and include gastrointestinal disturbances, weight gain, fluid retention, dizziness, menopausal symptoms, muscle cramps and headache. Danazol has a virilising action in females.

GONADOTROPHINS AND ANALOGUES

Gonadotrophins (FSH, LH and HCG) are glycoproteins produced and secreted by the anterior pituitary (see Ch. 28) or chorion and placenta. Large amounts of gonadotrophins are present in the urine of women following the menopause, in whom oestrogen no longer exerts feedback inhibition on the pituitary, which consequently secretes large amounts of FSH and LH.[3] The chorion and placenta secrete HCG.

Preparations

Gonadotrophins are extracted from urine of pregnant (HCG) or postmenopausal women (human menopausal gonadotrophin, which contains a mixture of FSH and LH). Recombinant FSH (**follitrophin**) is also available.

Pharmacokinetics and clinical use

Gonadotrophin preparations are given by injection. They are used to treat infertility caused by lack of ovulation as a result of hypopituitarism, or following failure of treatment with **clomiphene**; they are also used by specialists to induce ovulation to enable eggs to be collected[4] for in vitro fertilisation and reimplantation into the uterine cavity in women whose infertility is caused by mechanical obstruction of their fallopian tubes. For this use, gonadotrophin is usually administered after endogenous secretion of FSH and LH has been suppressed using a continuously administered GnRH agonist (see above). Gonadotrophins are also sometimes used in men with infertility caused by a low sperm count as a result of hypogonadotrophic hypogonadism (a disorder that is sometimes accompanied by lifelong anosmia, i.e. lack of sense of smell). (Gonadotrophins do not, of course, work for patients whose low sperm count is the result of primary testicular failure.) HCG has been used to stimulate testosterone synthesis in boys with delayed puberty, but testosterone is usually preferred.

DRUGS USED FOR CONTRACEPTION

ORAL CONTRACEPTIVES

There are two main types of oral contraceptives:

- combinations of an oestrogen with a progestogen (the combined pill)
- progestogen alone (the progestogen-only pill).

The combined pill

The combined oral contraceptive pill is extremely effective, at least in the absence of intercurrent illness and of treatment with potentially interacting drugs (see below). The oestrogen in most

> **Gonadotrophin-releasing hormone and gonadotrophins**
>
> - Gonadotrophin-releasing hormone is a decapeptide; **gonadorelin** is the synthetic form. **Nafarelin** is a potent analogue.
> - Given in pulsatile fashion, they stimulate gonadotrophin release; given continuously, they inhibit it.
> - The gonadotrophins, follicle-stimulating hormone and luteinising hormone, are glycoproteins.
> - Preparations of gonadotrophins (e.g. chorionic gonadotrophin) are used to treat infertility caused by lack of ovulation.
> - **Danazol** is a modified progestogen that inhibits gonadotrophin production by an action on the hypothalamus and anterior pituitary.

combined preparations (second-generation pills)[5] is **ethinylestradiol**, although a few preparations contain **mestranol** instead. The progestogen may be **norethisterone**, **levonorgestrel**, **ethynodiol**, or—in 'third-generation' pills—**desogestrel** or **gestodene**, which are more potent, have less androgenic action and cause less change in lipoprotein metabolism, but which probably cause a greater risk of thromboembolism than do second-generation preparations. The oestrogen content is generally 20–50 μg of ethinylestradiol or its equivalent, and a preparation is chosen with the lowest oestrogen and progestogen content that is well tolerated and gives good cycle control in the individual woman. This combined pill is taken for 21 consecutive days followed by 7 pill-free days, which causes a withdrawal bleed. Normal cycles of menstruation usually commence fairly soon after discontinuing treatment, and permanent loss of fertility (which may be a result of early menopause rather than a long-term consequence of the contraceptive pill) is rare.

The mode of action is as follows:

- oestrogen inhibits secretion of FSH via negative feedback on the anterior pituitary, and thus suppresses development of the ovarian follicle
- progestogen inhibits secretion of LH and thus prevents ovulation; it also makes the cervical mucus less suitable for the passage of sperm
- oestrogen and progestogen act in concert to alter the endometrium in such a way as to discourage implantation.

They may also interfere with the coordinated contractions of cervix, uterus and fallopian tubes that facilitate fertilisation and implantation.

---

[3]This forms the basis for the standard blood test, estimation of plasma LH/FSH concentrations, to confirm whether a woman is postmenopausal.

[4]The eggs are harvested using laparoscopy, a technique whereby a flexible fibre-optic instrument is inserted under anaesthesia just below the umbilicus, the ovaries inspected at the predicted time of ovulation, and eggs retrieved.

[5]The first-generation pills, containing more than 50 μg of oestrogen, were shown in the 1970s to be associated with an increased risk of deep vein thrombosis and pulmonary embolism.

Potential unwanted and beneficial effects of the combined pill

More than 200 million women worldwide have used this method since the 1960s, and in general the combined pill constitutes a safe and effective method of contraception. There are distinct health benefits from taking the pill (see below), and serious adverse effects are rare. However, minor unwanted effects constitute drawbacks to its use, and several important questions need to be considered.

Common adverse effects

The common effects are:

- weight gain, owing to fluid retention or an anabolic effect, or both
- mild nausea, flushing, dizziness, depression or irritability
- skin changes (e.g. acne and/or an increase in pigmentation)
- amenorrhoea of variable duration on cessation of taking the pill.

Questions that need to be considered

Is there an increased risk of cardiovascular disease (venous thromboembolism, myocardial infarction, stroke)? With second-generation pills (oestrogen content less than 50 μg), the risk of thromboembolism is small (incidence approximately 15 per 100 000 users per year, compared with 5 per 100 000 non-pregnant non-users per year or 60 per 100 000 pregnancies). The risk is greatest in subgroups with additional factors, such as smoking (which increases risk substantially) and long-continued use of the pill, especially in women over 35 years of age. For preparations containing the third-generation progestogens **desogestrel** or **gestodene**, the incidence of thromboembolic disease is approximately 25 per 100 000 users per year, which is still a small absolute risk that is substantially less than that caused by a pregnancy. In general, as stated by Baird & Glasier (1993), 'the evidence suggests that after risk factors (e.g. smoking, hypertension, and obesity) have been identified, combined oral contraceptives are safe for most women for most of their reproductive lives'.

Is there an increase in the risk of cancer? One large epidemiological study suggests that there may be a duration-related increase in the risk of breast cancer, the risk being 0.5 excess cancers per 10 000 women aged 16–19, and 4.7 excess cancers per 10 000 women at age 25–29. The cancers were less advanced in pill users, and thus potentially more treatable (see Hemminki, 1996).

Does the pill increase blood pressure? A marked increase in arterial blood pressure occurs in a small percentage of women shortly after starting the combined oral contraceptive pill. This is associated with increased circulating angiotensinogen, and disappears when treatment is stopped. Blood pressure is therefore monitored carefully when oral contraceptive treatment is started, and an alternative method substituted if necessary.

Is there an impairment in glucose tolerance? Older progestogen preparations impaired glucose tolerance, but this is not a problem with the newer compounds.

Beneficial effects

The combined pill markedly decreases menstrual symptoms such as irregular periods and intermenstrual bleeding. Iron deficiency anaemia and premenstrual tension are reduced, as are benign breast disease, uterine fibroids and functional cysts of the ovaries.

Unwanted pregnancy, carrying a maternal mortality ranging from 1 in 10 000 in developed countries to 1 in 150 in Africa, is avoided.

The progestogen-only pill

The drugs used in progestogen-only pills include **norethisterone**, **levonorgestrel** or **ethynodiol**. The pill is taken daily without interruption. The mode of action is primarily on the cervical mucus, which is made inhospitable to sperm. The progestogen probably also hinders implantation through its effect on the endometrium and on the motility and secretions of the fallopian tubes (see above).

Potential beneficial and unwanted effects of the progestogen-only pill

Progestogen-only contraceptives offer a suitable alternative to the combined pill for some women in whom oestrogen is contraindicated, and are suitable for women whose blood pressure increases unacceptably during treatment with oestrogen. However, their contraceptive effect is less reliable than that of the combination pill, and missing a dose may result in conception. Disturbances of menstruation (especially irregular bleeding) are common. Only a small proportion of women use this form of contraception, so long-term safety data are less reliable than for the combined pill.

Pharmacokinetics of oral contraceptives: drug interactions

Combined and progestogen-only oral contraceptives are metabolised by hepatic cytochrome P450 enzymes. Because the minimum effective dose of oestrogen is used (in order to avoid excess risk of thromboembolism), any increase in its clearance may result in contraceptive failure, and indeed enzyme-inducing drugs can have this effect not only for combined but also for progesterone-only pills. Such drugs include (par excellence) **rifampicin** and **rifabutin**, as well as **carbamazepine**, **phenytoin**, **griseofulvin** and others. Enterohepatic recycling of oestrogen is mentioned above (p. 448). Broad-spectrum antibiotics such as **amoxicillin** can disturb this by altering the intestinal flora, and cause failure of the combined pill. This does not occur with progesterone-only pills.

OTHER DRUG REGIMENS USED FOR CONTRACEPTION

POSTCOITAL (EMERGENCY) CONTRACEPTION

Oral administration of **levonorgestrel**, alone or combined with oestrogen, is effective if taken within 72 hours of unprotected intercourse, repeated 12 hours later. Nausea and vomiting are common (and the pills may then be lost: replacement tablets can be taken with an antiemetic such as **domperidone**). Insertion of an intrauterine device is more effective than hormonal methods, and works up to 5 days after intercourse.

LONG-ACTING PROGESTOGEN-ONLY CONTRACEPTION

Medroxyprogesterone can be given intramuscularly as a contraceptive. This is effective and safe. However, menstrual irregularities

---

Oral contraceptives 🔑

The combined pill

- The combined pill contains an oestrogen and a progestogen. It is taken for 21 consecutive days out of 28.
- Mode of action: the oestrogen inhibits follicle-stimulating hormone release and therefore follicle development; the progestogen inhibits luteinising hormone release and therefore ovulation, and makes cervical mucus inhospitable for sperm; together, they render the endometrium unsuitable for implantation.
- Drawbacks: weight gain, nausea, mood changes and skin pigmentation can occur.
- Serious unwanted effects are rare. A small proportion of women develop reversible hypertension; there is evidence both for and against an increased risk of breast cancer. There is a small increased risk of thromboembolism with third-generation pills.
- There are several beneficial effects, not least the avoidance of unwanted pregnancy, which itself carries risks to health.

The progestogen-only pill

- The progestogen-only pill is taken continuously. It differs from the combined pill in that the contraceptive effect is less reliable and is mainly a result of the alteration of cervical mucus. Irregular bleeding is common.

---

are common, and infertility may persist for many months after cessation of treatment.

Levonorgestrel implanted subcutaneously in non-biodegradable capsules is used by approximately 3 million women worldwide. This route of administration bypasses the liver, thus avoiding first-pass metabolism. The tubes release their progestogen content slowly over 5 years. Irregular bleeding and headache are common.

A levonorgestrel-impregnated intrauterine device has contraceptive action for 3–5 years.

THE UTERUS

The physiological and pharmacological responses of the uterus vary at different stages of the menstrual cycle and during pregnancy.

THE MOTILITY OF THE UTERUS

Uterine muscle contracts rhythmically both in vitro and in vivo, the contractions originating in the muscle itself. Myometrial cells in the fundus act as pacemakers and give rise to conducted action potentials. The electrophysiological activity of these pacemaker cells is regulated by the sex hormones.

The non-pregnant human uterus contracts spontaneously but weakly during the first part of the cycle, and more strongly during the luteal phase and during menstruation. Uterine movements are depressed in early pregnancy because oestrogen, potentiated by progesterone, hyperpolarises myometrial cells. This suppresses spontaneous contractions. Towards the end of gestation, however, contractions recommence; these increase in force and frequency, and become fully coordinated during parturition. The nerve supply to the uterus includes both excitatory and inhibitory sympathetic components: adrenaline, acting on β_2-adrenoceptors, inhibits uterine contraction, whereas noradrenaline, acting on α-adrenoceptors, stimulates contraction.

DRUGS THAT STIMULATE THE UTERUS

Drugs that stimulate the pregnant uterus and are important in obstetrics include oxytocin, ergometrine and prostaglandins.

OXYTOCIN

As explained in Chapter 28, the neurohypophyseal hormone oxytocin (an octapeptide) regulates myometrial activity. Oxytocin release is stimulated by cervical dilatation, and by suckling, but its role in parturition is incompletely understood. Oxytocin for clinical use is prepared synthetically.

Actions

On the uterus. Oxytocin contracts the uterus. Oestrogen induces oxytocin receptor synthesis and, consequently, the uterus at term is highly sensitive to this hormone. Given by slow intravenous infusion to induce labour, oxytocin causes regular coordinated contractions that travel from fundus to cervix. Both amplitude and frequency of these contractions are related to dose, the uterus relaxing completely between contractions during low-dose infusion. Larger doses further increase the frequency of the contractions, and there is incomplete relaxation between them. Still higher doses cause sustained contractions that interfere with blood flow through the placenta and cause fetal distress or death.

Other actions.[6] Oxytocin contracts myoepithelial cells in the mammary gland, which causes 'milk let-down'—the expression of milk from the alveoli and ducts. It also has a vasodilator action. A weak antidiuretic action can result in water retention, which can be problematic in patients with cardiac or renal disease, or preeclampsia.[7]

Clinical use

The clinical use of oxytocin is given in the box on page 457.

---

[6]Oxytocin receptors are found not only in the uterus but also in the brain, particularly in the limbic system. Animal experiments have shown that oxytocin is important in mating and parenting behaviour.

[7]Eclampsia is a pathological condition (involving, among other things, high blood pressure, swelling and seizures) that occurs in pregnant women.

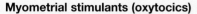

Pharmacokinetic aspects

Oxytocin can be given by intravenous injection or intramuscularly, but is most often given by intravenous infusion. It is inactivated in the liver and kidneys, and by circulating placental oxytocinase.

Unwanted effects of oxytocin

Unwanted effects of oxytocin include dose-related hypotension (arising from its vasodilator action), with associated reflex tachycardia. Its antidiuretic hormone-like effect on water excretion by the kidney causes water retention and, unless water intake is curtailed, consequent hyponatraemia.

ERGOMETRINE

Ergot (*Claviceps purpurea*) is a fungus that grows on rye and contains a surprising variety of pharmacologically active substances (see Ch. 12). Ergot poisoning, which was once common, was often associated with abortion. In 1935, **ergometrine** was isolated and was recognised as the oxytocic principle in ergot.

Actions

Ergometrine contracts the human uterus. This action depends partly on the contractile state of the organ. On a contracted uterus (the normal state following delivery), ergometrine has relatively little effect. However, if the uterus is inappropriately relaxed, ergometrine initiates strong contraction, thus reducing bleeding from the placental bed (the raw surface from which the placenta has detached). Ergometrine also has a moderate degree of vasoconstrictor action per se.

The mechanism of action of ergometrine on smooth muscle is not understood. It is possible that it acts partly on α adrenoceptors, like the related alkaloid ergotamine (see Ch. 9), and partly on 5-hydroxytryptamine receptors.

The clinical use of ergometrine is given in the box on this page.

Pharmacokinetic aspects and unwanted effects

Ergometrine can be given orally, intramuscularly or intravenously. It has a very rapid onset of action and its effect lasts for 3–6 hours.

Ergometrine can produce vomiting, probably by an effect on dopamine D_2 receptors in the chemoreceptor trigger zone (see Fig. 25.5). Vasoconstriction with an increase in blood pressure associated with nausea, blurred vision and headache can occur, as can vasospasm of the coronary arteries, resulting in angina.

PROSTAGLANDINS

Endogenous prostaglandins

Prostaglandins are discussed in detail in Chapter 13. The endometrium and myometrium have substantial prostaglandin-synthesising capacity, particularly in the second, proliferative phase of the menstrual cycle. Prostaglandin (PG) $F_{2\alpha}$ is generated in large amounts, and has been implicated in the ischaemic necrosis of the endometrium that precedes menstruation (although it has relatively little vasoconstrictor action on many human blood vessels, in contrast to some other mammalian species). Vasodilator prostaglandins, PGE_2 and PGI_2 (prostacyclin), are also generated by the uterus.

In addition to their vasoactive properties, the E and F prostaglandins contract the non-pregnant as well as the pregnant uterus. The sensitivity of uterine muscle to prostaglandins increases during gestation. Their role in parturition is not fully understood, but as cyclo-oxygenase inhibitors can delay labour (see below), they probably play some part in this.

Prostaglandins also play a part in two of the main disorders of menstruation: dysmenorrhoea (painful menstruation) and menorrhagia (excessive blood loss). Dysmenorrhoea is associated with increased production of PGE_2 and $PGF_{2\alpha}$; *non-steroidal anti-inflammatory drugs*, which inhibit prostaglandin biosynthesis (see Ch. 14), are used to treat dysmenorrhoea. Menorrhagia, in the absence of uterine pathology, may be caused by a combination of increased vasodilatation and reduced haemostasis. Increased generation by the uterus of PGI_2 (which inhibits platelet aggregation) could impair haemostasis as well as causing vasodilatation. Non-steroidal anti-inflammatory drugs (e.g. **mefenamic acid**) are used to treat menorrhagia as well as dysmenorrhoea.

Prostaglandin preparations

Prostaglandins of the E and F series promote coordinated contractions of the body of the pregnant uterus, while relaxing the cervix. E and F prostaglandins reliably cause abortion in early and middle pregnancy, unlike oxytocin, which generally does not cause expulsion of the uterine contents at this stage. The prostaglandins used in obstetrics are **dinoprostone** (PGE$_2$), **carboprost** (15-methyl PGF$_{2\alpha}$) and **gemeprost** or **misoprostol** (PGE$_1$ analogues). Dinoprostone can be given intravaginally as a gel or as tablets, or by the extra-amniotic route as a solution. Carboprost is given by deep intramuscular injection. Gemeprost or misoprostol are given intravaginally.

Unwanted effects

Unwanted effects include uterine pain, nausea and vomiting, which occur in about 50% of patients when the drugs are used as abortifacients. Dinoprost may cause cardiovascular collapse if it escapes into the circulation after intra-amniotic injection. Phlebitis can occur at the site of intravenous infusion. When combined with mifepristone, a progestogen antagonist (see p. 450) that sensitises the uterus to prostaglandins, lower doses of the prostaglandins (e.g. misoprostol) can be used to terminate pregnancy and side effects are reduced.

Clinical use

The clinical use of prostaglandin analogues is given on page 457.

DRUGS THAT INHIBIT UTERINE CONTRACTION

Selective β$_2$-adrenoceptor agonists, such as **ritodrine** or **salbutamol**, inhibit spontaneous or oxytocin-induced contractions of the pregnant uterus. These uterine relaxants are used in selected patients to prevent premature labour occurring between 22 and 33 weeks of gestation in otherwise uncomplicated pregnancies. They can delay delivery by 48 hours, time that can be used to administer glucocorticoid therapy to the mother so as to mature the lungs of the baby and reduce neonatal respiratory distress, and to optimise logistics such as making sure the baby is born in a facility with neonatal intensive care. It has been difficult to

demonstrate that any of the drugs used to delay labour improve the outcome for the baby. Risks to the mother, especially pulmonary oedema, increase after 48 hours, and myometrial response is reduced, so prolonged treatment is avoided. Cyclo-oxygenase inhibitors (e.g. **indometacin**) inhibit labour, but their use could cause problems in the baby, including renal dysfunction and delayed closure of the ductus arteriosus, both of which are influenced by endogenous prostaglandins.

An oxytocin receptor antagonist, **atosiban**, provides an alternative to a β$_2$-adrenoceptor agonist. It is given as an intravenous bolus followed by an intravenous infusion for not more than 48 hours. Adverse effects include symptoms of vasodilation, nausea, vomiting, and hyperglycaemia.

ERECTILE DYSFUNCTION

Erectile function depends on complex interactions between physiological and psychological factors. Erection is caused by vasorelaxation in the arteries and arterioles supplying the erectile tissue. This increases penile blood flow. Relaxation of trabecular smooth muscle causes filling of the sinusoids. This compresses the plexuses of subtunical venules between the trabeculae and the tunica albuginea, occluding venous outflow and causing erection. During sexual intercourse, reflex contraction of the ischiocavernosus muscles compresses the base of the corpora cavernosa, and the intracavernosal pressure can reach several hundred millimetres of mercury during this phase of rigid erection. Innervation of the penis includes autonomic and somatic nerves. Nitric oxide is probably the main mediator of erection and is released both from nitrergic nerves and from endothelium (Ch. 17; Fig. 17.6).

Erectile function is adversely affected by several therapeutic drugs (including many antipsychotic, antidepressant and antihypertensive agents), but in long-term randomised controlled trials an appreciable percentage of men who discontinue treatment because of erectile dysfunction had been receiving placebo, and psychiatric and vascular disease can themselves cause sexual dysfunction. Furthermore, erectile dysfunction is common in middle-aged and older men, even if they have no psychiatric or cardiovascular problems. There are several organic causes, including hypogonadism (see above), hyperprolactinaemia (see Ch. 28), arterial disease and various causes of neuropathy (most commonly diabetes), but often no organic cause is identified, or the problem is a result of a combination of organic and psychological factors, notably anxiety relating to sexual performance, which can establish a vicious circle.

Over the centuries, there has been a huge trade in parts of various creatures that have the misfortune to bear some fancied resemblance to human genitalia, in the pathetic belief that consuming these will restore virility or act as an aphrodisiac (i.e. a drug that stimulates libido). Alcohol (Ch. 43) 'provokes the desire but takes away the performance', and cannabis (Ch. 15) can also release inhibitions and probably does the same. **Yohimbine** (an α$_2$ antagonist; Ch. 11) may have some positive effect in this regard, but even with meta-analysis the number of subjects randomised is not very impressive, and efficacy somewhat unconvincing. **Apomorphine** (a dopamine agonist;

> **Drugs acting on the uterus** 🔑
>
> - At parturition, oxytocin causes regular coordinated uterine contractions, each followed by relaxation; **ergometrine**, an ergot alkaloid, causes uterine contractions with an increase in basal tone. **Atosiban**, an antagonist of oxytocin, delays labour.
> - Prostaglandin (PG) analogues, for example **dinoprostone** (PGE$_2$) and **dinoprost** (PGF$_{2\alpha}$), contract the pregnant uterus but relax the cervix. Cyclo-oxygenase inhibitors inhibit PG synthesis and delay labour. They also alleviate symptoms of dysmenorrhoea and menorrhagia.
> - The β$_2$-adrenoceptor agonists (e.g. **ritodrine**) inhibit spontaneous and oxytocin-induced contractions of the pregnant uterus.

Ch. 35) causes erections in humans as well as in rodents when injected subcutaneously, but it is a powerful emetic, an effect that is usually regarded as socially unacceptable in this context. Despite this rather obvious disadvantage, a sublingual preparation is licensed for erectile dysfunction.[8] Nausea is said to subside with continued use—but really!

The generally negative picture picked up somewhat when it was found that injecting vasodilator drugs directly into the corpora cavernosa causes penile erection. **Papaverine** (Ch. 19), if necessary with the addition of **phentolamine**, was used in this way. The route of administration is not acceptable to most men, but diabetics in particular are often not needle-shy, and this approach was a real boon to many such patients. **PGE₁ (alprostadil)** is often combined with other vasodilators when given intracavernosally. It can also be given transurethrally as an alternative (albeit still a somewhat unromantic one) to injection. Adverse effects of all these drugs include priapism, which is no joke. Treatment consists of aspiration of blood (using sterile technique) and, if necessary, cautious intracavernosal administration of a vasoconstrictor such as **phenylephrine**. Intracavernosal and transurethral preparations are still available, but orally active *phosphodiesterase inhibitors* are now generally the drugs of choice.

PHOSPHODIESTERASE TYPE V INHIBITORS

Sildenafil, the first selective phosphodiesterase type V inhibitor (see also Chs 17 and 19), was found incidentally to influence erectile function. **Tadalafil** and **vardenafil** are also phosphodiesterase type V inhibitors licensed to treat erectile dysfunction. Tadalafil is longer acting than sildenafil. In contrast to intracavernosal vasodilators, phosphodiesterase type V inhibitors are not sufficient to cause erection independent of sexual desire, but enhance the erectile response to sexual stimulation. They have transformed the treatment of erectile dysfunction.

---

[8]Ironically so, because apomorphine was used as 'aversion therapy' in a misguided attempt to 'cure' homosexuality by conditioning individuals to associate homoerotic stimuli with nausea and vomiting, during the not-so-very-far-off time when homosexuality was classified as a psychiatric disease ('only apomorphine cures'–William Burroughs, *Naked Lunch*. Grove Press, 1966).

Mechanism of action

Phosphodiesterase V is the isoform that inactivates cGMP. Nitrergic nerves release nitric oxide (or a related nitrosothiol), which diffuses into smooth muscle cells, where it activates guanylate cyclase. The resulting increase in cytoplasmic cGMP mediates vasodilation via activation of protein kinase G (Ch. 17). Consequently, inhibition of phosphodiesterase V potentiates the effect on penile vascular smooth muscle of endothelium-derived nitric oxide and of nitrergic nerves that are activated by sexual stimulation. Other vascular beds are also affected, suggesting other possible uses, notably in pulmonary hypertension (Ch. 19, p. 317).

Pharmacokinetic aspects and drug interactions

Peak plasma concentrations of sildenafil occur approximately 30–120 minutes after an oral dose and are delayed by eating, so it is taken an hour or more before sexual activity. It is given as a single dose as needed. It is metabolised by the 3A4 isoenzyme of cytochrome P450, which is induced by **carbamazepine**, **rifampicin** and barbiturates, and inhibited by **cimetidine**, macrolide antibiotics, antifungal imidazolines, some antiviral drugs (such as **ritonavir**) and also by grapefruit juice (Ch. 8). These drugs can potentially interact with sildenafil in consequence. Tadalafil has a longer half-life than sildenafil, so can be taken longer before sexual activity. A clinically important pharmacodynamic interaction occurs with *organic nitrates*, which work through increasing cGMP (Ch. 17) and are therefore markedly potentiated by sildenafil. Consequently, concurrent nitrate use, including use of **nicorandil**, contraindicates the use of any phosphodiesterase type V inhibitor.

Unwanted effects

Many of the unwanted effects of phosphodiesterase type V inhibitors are caused by vasodilation in other vascular beds; these effects include hypotension, flushing and headache. Visual disturbances have occasionally been reported and are of concern because sildenafil has some action on phosphodiesterase VI, which is present in retina and important in vision. The manufacturers advise that sildenafil should not be used in patients with hereditary retinal degenerative diseases (such as retinitis pigmentosa) because of the theoretical risk posed by this. Vardenafil is more selective for the type V isozyme than is sildenafil (reviewed by Doggrell, 2005), but is also contraindicated in patients with hereditary retinal disorders.

REFERENCES AND FURTHER READING

Sex hormones and their control

Bagatelle C J, Bremner W J 1996 Androgens in men— uses and abuses. N Engl J Med 334: 707–714 (*A review of the biology, pharmacology and use of androgens*)

British Medical Association and Royal Pharmaceutical Society of Great Britain 2005 Sex hormones. In: British National Formulary 50. BMA and RPSGB, London, pp. 366–381

Chen Z et al. 1999 Estrogen receptor α mediates the nongenomic activation of endothelial nitric oxide synthase by estrogen. J Clin Invest 103: 401–406 (*Acute vasodilator action of oestrogen may involve membrane ERα rather than the classic intracellular receptor pathway*)

Gruber C J, Tschugguel W, Schneeberger C, Huber J C 2002 Production and actions of estrogens. N Engl J Med 346: 340–352 (*Review focusing on the new biochemical aspects of the action of oestrogen— including phyto-oestrogens and selective oestrogen receptor modulators—as well as physiological and clinical aspects*)

Huirne J A F, Lambalk C B 2001 Gonadotrophin- releasing hormone receptor antagonists. Lancet 358: 1793–1803 (*Review discussing the clinical potential of this relatively new class of drugs*)

Olive D L, Pritts E A 2001 Treatment of endometriosis. N Engl J Med 34: 266–275 (*Critical review of existing evidence—which is thin—forms the basis for sensible recommendations regarding treatment of pelvic pain or infertility from endometriosis using oral contraceptives and GnRH agonist therapy with oestrogen–progestin add-back*)

Rhoden E L, Morgentaler A 2004 Risks of testosterone- replacement therapy and recommendations for monitoring. N Engl J Med 350: 482–492 (*Review*)

Contraceptives

Baird D T, Glasier A F 1999 Science, medicine and the future: contraception. Br Med J 319: 969–972 (*Predicts that antiprogestins will replace progestogen- only pills and lead to 'once-a-month' pills, and that pills for men will become available in 10–15 years, orally active non-peptide GnRH antagonists*)

Djerassi C 2001 This man's pill: reflections on the 50th birthday of the pill. Oxford University Press, New York (*Scientific and autobiographical memoir by polymath steroid chemist who worked on 'the pill' at its inception under Syntex in Mexico, and has continued thinking about human reproduction in a broad biological and biosocial sense ever since*)

Hemminki E 1996 Oral contraceptives and breast cancer. Br Med J 313: 63–64

Postmenopausal aspects

Braunstein G D et al. 2005 Safety and efficacy of a testosterone patch for the treatment of hypoactive sexual desire disorder in surgically menopausal women—a randomized, placebo-controlled trial. Arch Intern Med 165: 1582–1589 (*A 300 μg/day testosterone patch increased sexual desire and frequency of satisfying sexual activity and was well tolerated in women who developed hypoactive sexual desire disorder after surgical menopause*)

Cummings S R et al. 1999 The effect of raloxifene on risk of breast cancer in postmenopausal women: results of the MORE randomized trial. JAMA 281: 2189–2197 (*A total of 7705 postmenopausal women with osteoporosis randomised to raloxifene or placebo and observed for a median of 40 months; raloxifene reduced the incidence of oestrogen receptor–positive breast cancer by 90%*)

Davis S R, Dinatale I, Rivera-Woll L, Davison S 2005 Postmenopausal hormone therapy: from monkey glands to transdermal patches. J Endocrinol 185: 207–222 (*Reviews the history of knowledge of the menopause and the development of hormonal therapy for climacteric complaints, and summarises current evidence for specific benefits and risks of hormone treatment*)

Grodstein F, Clarkson T B, Manson J E 2003 Understanding the divergent data on postmenopausal hormone therapy. N Engl J Med 348: 645–650 (*Commentary*)

Hulley S et al. 1998 Randomized trial of estrogen plus progestin for secondary prevention of coronary heart disease in postmenopausal women. JAMA 280: 605–613 (*A total of 2763 postmenopausal women who had suffered a previous coronary event randomised to active or placebo and observed for a mean of 4.1 years. The incidence of fatal myocardial infarction was similar in the two groups, despite favourable changes in low- and high-density lipoproteins cholesterol in the HRT group. Venous thromboembolism was increased by a factor of 2.89 in the active group.*)

Khaw K-T 1998 Hormone replacement therapy again: risk–benefit relation differs between population and individuals. Br Med J 316: 1842–1843 (*Emphasises concerns over the risk–benefit balance of long-term use of HRT in healthy women*)

Pedersen A T, Lidegaard Ø et al. 1997 Hormone replacement therapy and risk of non-fatal stroke. Lancet 350: 1277–1283

Rosing J et al. 1997 Oral contraceptives and venous thromboembolism: different sensitivities to activated protein C in women using second- and third- generation oral contraceptives. Br J Haematol 97: 233–238 (*A proposed explanation for the thrombogenic potential of third-generation pills*)

Shifren J L et al. 2000 Transdermal testosterone treatment in women with impaired sexual function after oophorectomy. N Engl J Med 343: 682–688 (*Transdermal testosterone improves sexual function and psychological well-being in women who have undergone oophorectomy and hysterectomy*)

The uterus

Norwitz E R, Robinson J N, Challis J R 1999 The control of labor. N Engl J Med 341: 660–666 (*Review*)

Thornton S, Vatish M, Slater D 2001 Oxytocin antagonists: clinical and scientific considerations. Exp Physiol 86: 297–302 (*Reviews rationale for uterine relaxants in preterm labour; evidence for administering atosiban; and the role of oxytocin, vasopressin and their receptors in the onset of labour*)

Wray S 1993 Uterine contraction and physiological mechanisms of modulation. Am J Physiol 264 (Cell Physiol 33): C1–C18 (*A review on uterine function*)

Erectile dysfunction

Andersson K-E 2001 Pharmacology of penile erection. Pharmacol Rev 53: 417–450 (*Scholarly review covering central and peripheral regulation, and a very wide-ranging coverage of the pharmacology of possible future as well as of current therapies*)

Doggrell S A 2005 Comparison of clinical trials with sildenafil, vardenafil and tadalafil in erectile dysfunction. Expert Opin Pharmacother 6: 75–84 (*Vardenafil is similarly effective to sildenafil. Its only advantage is that it does not inhibit phosphodiesterase VI to alter colour perception, a rare side effect that sometimes occurs with sildenafil. Tadalafil has a longer duration of action.*)

Edwards G (ed) 2002 The pharmacokinetics and pharmacodynamics of sildenafil citrate. Br J Clin Pharmacol 53(suppl 1) (*Articles on this selective phosphodiesterase type V inhibitor, which has revolutionised treatment of erectile dysfunction*)

Lue T F 2000 Drug therapy: erectile dysfunction. N Engl J Med 342: 1802–1813 (*Excellent review succinctly covering the physiology of penile erection, pathophysiology and diagnosis of erectile dysfunction, and drug therapy*)

Bone metabolism

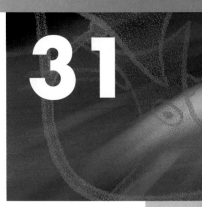

31

OVERVIEW

The human skeleton undergoes a continuous process of remodelling throughout life—some bone being resorbed and new bone being laid down. With advancing age, there is an increasing possibility of structural deterioration and decreased bone mass (osteoporosis). This constitutes a major health problem throughout the world, and there are, in addition, various other conditions that can lead to pathological changes in bone that require therapy. In the past decade, there have been significant advances in the understanding of bone biology, which have led to new drugs and may yet lead to further new drugs. In this chapter, we consider first the processes involved in bone remodelling and then go on to describe the pharmacological agents used to treat disorders of bone.

BONE STRUCTURE AND COMPOSITION

The human skeleton consists of 80% cortical bone and 20% trabecular bone. Cortical bone is the dense, compact outer part, and trabecular bone the inner meshwork. The former predominates in the shafts of long bones, the latter in the vertebrae, the epiphyses of long bones and the iliac crest. Trabecular bone, having a large surface area, is metabolically more active and more affected by factors that lead to bone loss (see below).

The main minerals in bone are calcium and phosphates. More than 99% of the calcium in the body is in the skeleton, mostly as crystalline hydroxyapatite but some as non-crystalline phosphates and carbonates; together, these make up half the bone mass.

The main cells in bone homeostasis are osteoblasts, osteoclasts and osteocytes.

- Osteoblasts, which are derived from precursor cells in the bone marrow and the periosteum, secrete important components of the extracellular matrix—the osteoid, particularly the collagen. They also have a role in the activation of osteoclasts (see below).
- Osteoclasts are multinucleated bone-resorbing cells derived from precursor cells of the macrophage/monocyte lineage.
- Osteocytes are derived from the osteoblasts, which, during the formation of new bone, become embedded in the bony matrix and differentiate into osteocytes. These cells form a connected cellular network that, along with the nerve fibres in bone, is thought to have a role in the response to mechanical loading.
- Other cells of importance are monocytes/macrophages, lymphocytes and vascular endothelial cells; these secrete cytokines and other mediators necessary for bone remodelling (see below).

The organic matrix of bone is termed *osteoid* (as mentioned above), the principal component of which is collagen. But there are also other components such as proteoglycans, osteocalcin and various phosphoproteins, one of which, osteonectin, binds to both calcium and collagen and thus links these two major constituents of bone matrix.

Calcium phosphate crystals in the form of hydroxyapatite $[Ca_{10}(PO_4)_6(OH)_2]$ are deposited in the osteoid, converting it into hard bone matrix.

Bone plays a major role in overall calcium homeostasis in the body (see below).

461

BONE REMODELLING

The process of remodelling involves the following:

- the activity of two main cell types: osteoblasts that secrete new bone matrix and osteoclasts that break it down (Fig. 31.1).
- the actions of a variety of cytokines; see Figs 31.1 and 31.2
- the turnover of bone minerals—particularly calcium and phosphate
- the actions of several hormones: parathyroid hormone (PTH), the vitamin D family, oestrogens, growth hormone, steroids, calcitonin and various cytokines.

Diet, drugs and physical factors (exercise, loading) also affect remodelling. Bone loss—of 0.5–1% per year—starts in the 35–40 age group in both sexes. The rate accelerates by as much as 10-fold during the menopause in women (or with castration in men), and then gradually settles at 1–3% per year. The loss during the menopause is due to increased osteoclast activity (see below) and affects mainly trabecular bone; the later loss in both sexes with increasing age is due to decreased osteoblast numbers (see below) and affects mainly cortical bone.

THE ACTION OF CELLS AND CYTOKINES

A cycle of remodelling starts with recruitment of the cells that give rise to osteoclast precursors, and their differentiation to mature multinuceated osteoclasts by cytokines (Fig. 31.1). The osteoclasts adhere to an area of trabecular bone, developing a ruffled border at the attachment site. They move along the bone, digging a pit by secreting hydrogen ions and proteolytic enzymes. This process gradually liberates cytokines such as insulin-like growth factor (IGF)-1 and transforming growth factor (TGF)-β, which have been embedded in the osteoid (Fig. 31.1); these in turn recruit

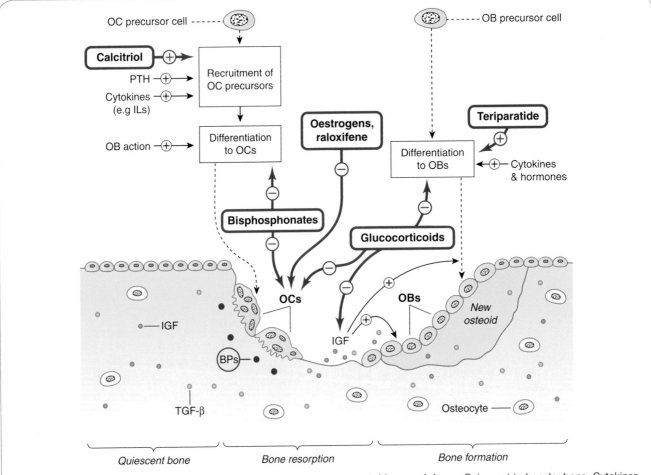

Fig. 31.1 **The bone-remodelling cycle and the action of hormones, cytokines and drugs.** Quiescent trabecular bone. Cytokines such as insulin-like growth factor (IGF) and transforming growth factor (TGF)-β, shown as dots, are embedded in the bone matrix. Bone resorption. Osteoclast (OC) precursor cells, recruited by cytokines and hormones, are activated by osteoblasts (OBs) to form mobile multinuclear OCs (see Fig. 31.2) that move along the bone surface, resorbing bone and releasing the embedded cytokines. Bone formation. The released cytokines recruit OBs, which lay down osteoid and embed cytokines IGF and TGF-β in it. Some OBs also become embedded, forming terminal osteocytes. The osteoid then becomes mineralised, and lining cells cover the area (not shown). Oestrogens cause apoptosis (programmed cell death) of OCs. Note that pharmacological concentrations of glucocorticoids have the effects specified above, but physiological concentrations are required for OB differentiation. BPs, embedded bisphosphonates—these are ingested by OCs when bone is resorbed (not shown); IL, interleukin; PTH, parathyroid hormone.

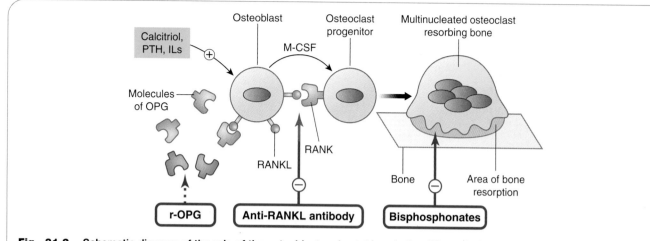

Fig. 31.2 **Schematic diagram of the role of the osteoblast and cytokines in the differentiation and activation of the osteoclast and the action of antiresorptive drugs.** The osteoblast is stimulated by calcitriol, parathyroid hormone (PTH) and interleukins (ILs) to express a surface ligand, the RANK ligand (RANKL). RANKL expression is increased by various interleukins, parathormone, tumour necrosis factor (TNF)-α, prostaglandin E2 and glucocorticoids. RANKL interacts with a receptor on the osteoclast—an osteoclast differentiation and activation receptor termed RANK (<u>r</u>eceptor <u>a</u>ctivator of <u>n</u>uclear factor <u>k</u>appa B). This, with macrophage colony-stimulating factor (M-CSF) released by the osteoblast, causes differentiation and activation of the osteoclast progenitors to form mature osteoclasts (not shown). Fusion of osteoclasts occurs to give giant multinucleated bone-resorbing cells, which are polarised with a ruffled border on the bone-resorbing side (shown). Bisphosphonates inhibit bone resorption by osteoclasts. Anti-RANKL antibodies (e.g. denosumab) bind RANKL and prevent the RANK–RANKL interaction. The osteoblast also releases 'decoy' molecules of osteoprotegerin (OPG), which can bind RANKL and prevent activation of the RANK receptor. Recombinant OPG (r-OPG)—which has this effect—is in clinical trial. Stromal cells may also function in the manner shown above for osteoblasts.

and activate successive teams of osteoblasts that have been stimulated to develop from precursor cells and are awaiting the call to duty (see Fig. 31.1 and below). The osteoblasts invade the site, synthesising and secreting the organic matrix of bone, the osteoid, and secreting IGF-1 and TGF-β (which become embedded in the osteoid; see above). Some osteoblasts become embedded in the osteoid, forming terminal osteocytes; others interact with and activate osteoclast precursors—and we are back to the beginning of the cycle.

Cytokines involved in bone remodelling other than IGF-1 and TGF-β include other members of the TGF-β family, such as the bone morphogenic proteins, a range of interleukins, prostaglandins, various hormones, and members of the tumour necrosis factor family. A member of this last family—a ligand for a receptor on the osteoclast precursor cell—is of particular importance. The receptor is termed (wait for it—biological terminology has fallen over its own feet here) *RANK*, which stands for <u>r</u>eceptor <u>a</u>ctivator of <u>n</u>uclear factor <u>k</u>appa B (NFκB)—NFκB being the principal transduction factor involved in osteoclast differentiation and activation. And the ligand is termed, unsurprisingly, *RANK ligand (RANKL)*.

The stromal cell and the osteoblast synthesise and release a molecule termed *osteoprotegerin (OPG)*, identical with RANK, which functions as a decoy receptor. In a sibling-undermining process by the two cells (osteoblast/stromal cell and osteoclast precursor), OPG can bind to RANKL[1] (generated by the very cell

that OPG itself is generated by) and inhibit RANKL's binding to its intended receptor, RANK, on the osteoclast precursor cell (Fig. 31.2). (See Hofbauer & Schoppet, 2004; Roodman, 2004; Theoleyre et al., 2004; Kostenuik, 2005.)

The ratio of RANKL to OPG is critical in the formation and activity of osteoclasts.

THE TURNOVER OF BONE MINERALS

The main bone minerals are calcium and phosphates.

CALCIUM METABOLISM

The daily turnover of bone minerals during remodelling involves about 700 mg of calcium. Calcium has numerous roles in physiological functioning. Intracellular Ca^{2+} constitutes only a small proportion of body calcium, but it has a major role in cellular function (see Ch. 3). An influx of Ca^{2+} with increase of Ca^{2+} in the cytosol is part of the signal transduction mechanism of many cells, so the concentration of Ca^{2+} in the extracellular fluid and the plasma needs to be controlled with great precision. The concentration of Ca^{2+} in the cytoplasm of cells is about 100 nmol/l, whereas in the plasma it is about 2.5 mmol/l. The plasma Ca^{2+} concentration is regulated by complex interactions between PTH and various forms of vitamin D (Figs 31.3 and 31.4); calcitonin also plays a part.

Calcium absorption in the intestine involves a Ca^{2+}-binding protein whose synthesis is regulated by calcitriol (see Fig. 31.3 and below). It is probable that the overall calcium content of the body is regulated largely by this absorption mechanism, because

---

[1]RANKL is also sometimes confusingly termed *OPG ligand*.

urinary Ca^{2+} excretion normally remains more or less constant. However, with high blood Ca^{2+} concentrations, urinary excretion increases, and with low blood concentrations urinary excretion can be reduced by PTH and calcitriol, both of which enhance Ca^{2+} reabsorption in the renal tubules (Fig. 31.3).

PHOSPHATE METABOLISM

Phosphates are important constituents of bone, and are also critically important in the structure and function of all the cells of the body. They play a significant part in enzymic reactions in the cell; they have roles as intracellular buffers and in the excretion of hydrogen ions in the kidney.

Phosphate absorption is an energy-requiring process regulated by calcitriol (see below). Phosphate deposition in bone, as hydroxyapatite, depends on the plasma concentration of PTH, which, with calcitriol, tends to mobilise both Ca^{2+} and phosphate from the bone matrix. Phosphate is excreted by the kidney; here PTH inhibits reabsorption and thus increases excretion.

HORMONES INVOLVED IN BONE METABOLISM AND REMODELLING

The main hormones involved in bone metabolism and remodelling are PTH, members of the vitamin D family, oestrogens and calcitonin. Glucocorticoids and thyroid hormone[2] also affect bone.

PARATHYROID HORMONE

Parathyroid hormone, which consists of a single-chain polypeptide of 84 amino acids, is an important physiological regulator of Ca^{2+} metabolism. It maintains the plasma Ca^{2+} concentration by mobilising Ca^{2+} from bone, by promoting its reabsorption by the kidney, and in particular by stimulating the synthesis of calcitriol,

---

[2]Over-replacement of thyroxine in hypothyroidism results in osteoporosis; see Roberts & Ladenson (2004).

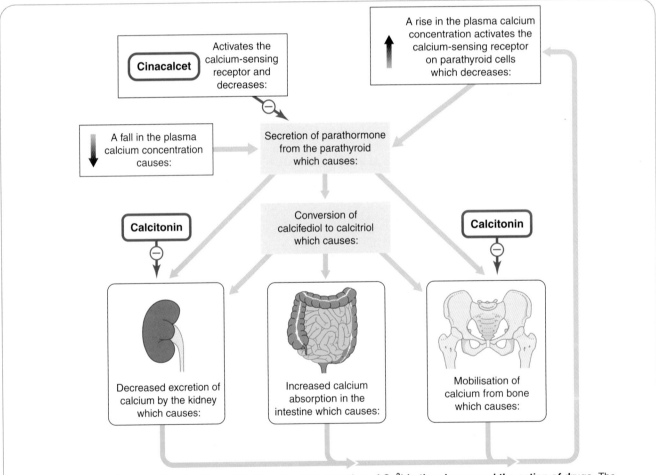

Fig. 31.3 The main factors involved in maintaining the concentration of Ca^{2+} in the plasma and the action of drugs. The calcium receptor on the parathyroid cell is a G-protein–coupled receptor. Calcifediol and calcitriol are metabolites of vitamin D_3 and constitute the 'hormones' 25-hydroxy-vitamin D_3 and 1,25-dihydroxy-vitamin D_3, respectively. Endogenous calcitonin, secreted by the thyroid, inhibits Ca^{2+} mobilisation from bone and decreases its resorption in the kidney, thus reducing blood Ca^{2+}. Calcitonin is also used therapeutically in osteoporosis.

which in turn increases Ca^{2+} absorption from the intestine and synergises with PTH in mobilising bone Ca^{2+} (Figs. 31.3 and 31.4). PTH promotes phosphate excretion, and thus its net effect is to increase the concentration of Ca^{2+} in the plasma and lower that of phosphate.

The mobilisation of Ca^{2+} from bone by PTH is mediated, at least in part, by stimulation of the recruitment and activation of osteoclasts. Pathological oversecretion of PTH (hyperparathyroidism) inhibits osteoblast activity (not shown in Fig. 31.1). But given therapeutically in a low intermittent dose, PTH and fragments of PTH paradoxically stimulate osteoblast activity and enhance bone formation (see below).

Parathyroid hormone is synthesised in the cells of the parathyroid glands and stored in vesicles. The principal factor controlling secretion is the concentration of ionised calcium in the plasma, low plasma Ca^{2+} stimulating secretion, high plasma Ca^{2+} decreasing it by binding to and activating a Ca^{2+}-sensing G-protein–coupled surface receptor (Fig. 31.3). (See Stewart, 2004.)

VITAMIN D

Vitamin D is a prehormone that is converted in the body into a number of biologically active metabolites that function as true hormones, circulating in the blood and regulating the activities of various cell types (see Reichel et al., 1989). Their main action is the maintenance of plasma Ca^{2+} by increasing Ca^{2+} absorption in the intestine, mobilising Ca^{2+} from bone and decreasing its renal excretion (see Fig. 31.3). Vitamin D is really a family of hormones (see below) which act on receptors belonging to the superfamily of steroid hormone *nuclear* receptors (see p. 428 top of right column and p. 45 for details). In humans, there are two sources of vitamin D:

- dietary ergocalciferol (D_2), derived from ergosterol in plants
- cholecalciferol (D_3) generated in the skin from 7-dehydrocholesterol by the action of ultraviolet irradiation, the 7-dehydrocholesterol having been formed from cholesterol in the wall of the intestine.

Cholecalciferol (vitamin D_3) is converted to 25-hydroxy-vitamin D_3 (calcifediol) in the liver, and this is converted to a series of other metabolites of varying activity in the kidney, the most potent of which is 1,25-dihydroxy-vitamin D_3 (calcitriol) (see Fig. 31.4).

The synthesis of calcitriol from calcifediol is regulated by PTH, and is also influenced by the phosphate concentration in the plasma and by the calcitriol concentration itself through a negative feedback mechanism (Fig. 31.4). Receptors for calcitriol have been identified in virtually every tissue except liver, and it

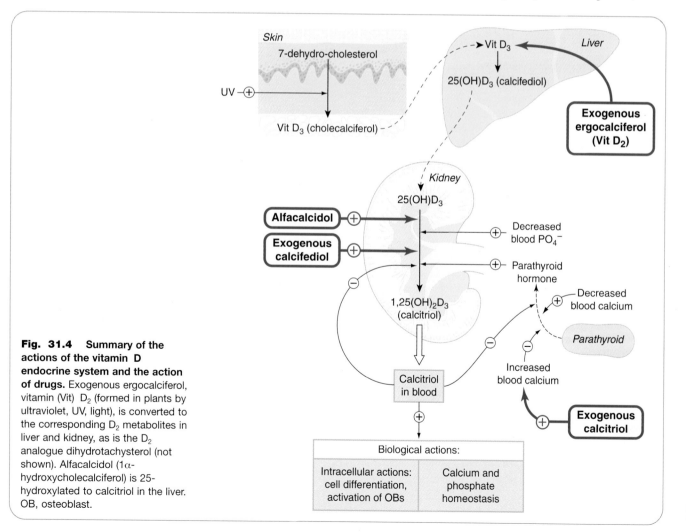

Fig. 31.4 Summary of the actions of the vitamin D endocrine system and the action of drugs. Exogenous ergocalciferol, vitamin (Vit) D_2 (formed in plants by ultraviolet, UV, light), is converted to the corresponding D_2 metabolites in liver and kidney, as is the D_2 analogue dihydrotachysterol (not shown). Alfacalcidol (1α-hydroxycholecalciferol) is 25-hydroxylated to calcitriol in the liver. OB, osteoblast.

is now considered that calcitriol may be important in the functioning of many cell types.

The main actions of calcitriol are the stimulation of absorption of Ca^{2+} and phosphate in the intestine, and the mobilisation of Ca^{2+} from bone, but it also increases Ca^{2+} reabsorption in the kidney tubules (Fig. 31.3). Its effect on bone involves promotion of maturation of osteoclasts and indirect stimulation of their activity (Figs 31.1 and 31.3). It decreases collagen synthesis by osteoblasts, and its effect on these cells is by the classic steroid pathway, involving intracellular receptors and an effect on the DNA. However, the effect on bone is complex and is clearly not confined to mobilising Ca^{2+}, because in clinical vitamin D deficiency (see below), in which the mineralisation of bone is impaired, administration of vitamin D restores bone formation. One explanation may lie in the fact that calcitriol stimulates synthesis of osteocalcin, the vitamin K–dependent, Ca^{2+}-binding protein of bone matrix.

OESTROGENS

During reproductive life in the female, oestrogens have an important role in maintenance of bone integrity. They inhibit the cytokines that recruit osteoclasts, and oppose the bone-resorbing, Ca^{2+}-mobilising action of PTH. Withdrawal of oestrogen, as happens at the menopause, can lead to osteoporosis.

CALCITONIN

Calcitonin is a hormone secreted by the specialised 'C' cells found in the thyroid follicles.

The main action of calcitonin is on bone; it inhibits bone resorption by binding to a specific receptor on osteoclasts, inhibiting their action. In the kidney, it decreases the reabsorption of both Ca^{2+} and phosphate in the proximal tubules. Its overall effect is to decrease the plasma Ca^{2+} concentration. See Figures 31.3 and 31.4.

Secretion is determined mainly by the plasma Ca^{2+} concentration.

GLUCOCORTICOIDS

Physiological concentrations of glucocorticoids are required for osteoblast differentiation. Excessive pharmacological concentrations inhibit bone formation by inhibiting osteoblast differentiation and activity, and may stimulate osteoclast action—leading to osteoporosis. This latter effect is also evident when pathological concentrations of endogenous glucocorticoids are present, as in Cushing's syndrome (see Fig. 28.7).

DISORDERS OF BONE

DISORDERS OF THE STRUCTURE OF BONE

The reduction of bone mass with distortion of the microarchitecture is termed *osteoporosis*; a reduction in the mineral content is termed *osteopenia*. Osteoporotic bone can fracture easily after minimal trauma—and frequently does. The commonest causes of

osteoporosis are postmenopausal deficiency of oestrogen and age-related deterioration in bone homeostasis. It is calculated that, in England and Wales, one in two women and one in five men over the age of 50 will have a fracture due to osteoporosis (Van Staa et al., 2001), while in the USA a 50-year-old woman is estimated to have a 40% lifetime risk of an osteoporotic fracture (Strewler, 2005). But osteoporosis can also occur secondary to conditions such as rheumatoid arthritis, and can result from other factors, such as excessive thyroxine or glucocorticoid administration. Up to half the patients on long-term oral glucocorticoid therapy can suffer fractures due to excessive bone loss. Because life expectancy has increased significantly in the developed world, osteoporosis is now regarded as being of epidemic proportions, and has become an important public health problem. Drugs that prevent its development are being actively sought. The treatment of osteoporosis involves either antiresorptive (anticatabolic) drugs (e.g. the bisphosphonates, raloxifene) or anabolic drugs that stimulate bone formation (PTH, teriparatide) (see Riggs & Parfitt, 2005). Newer compounds (e.g. strontium ranelate; see below) have both actions.

Other diseases of bone requiring drug therapy are osteomalacia and rickets (the juvenile form of osteomalacia), in which there are defects in bone mineralisation due to vitamin D deficiency, and Paget's disease, in which there is distortion of the processes of bone resorption and remodelling.

DISORDERS OF BONE MINERAL METABOLISM

Hypocalcaemia occurs with hypoparathyroidism, vitamin D deficiencies, congenital rickets and some kidney diseases; hypercalcaemia with hyperparathyroidism and some malignancies, also sarcoidosis.

Bone remodelling

- Bone is continuously remodelled throughout life. The events of the remodelling cycle are as follow:
  - *osteoclasts,* having been activated by osteoblasts, resorb bone by digging pits in trabecular bone. Into these pits the bone-forming *osteoblasts* secrete osteoid (bone matrix), which consists mainly of collagen but also contains osteocalcin, osteonectin, phosphoproteins and the cytokines insulin growth factor (IGF) and transforming growth factor (TGF)-β
  - the osteoid is then mineralised, i.e. complex calcium phosphate crystals (hydroxyapatites) are deposited.
- Bone metabolism and mineralisation involve the action of parathyroid hormone, the vitamin D family, calcitonin and various cytokines (e.g. IGF, the TGF-β family and interleukins). Declining physiological levels of oestrogens and therapeutic levels of glucocorticoids can result in bone resorption not balanced by bone formation—leading to osteoporosis.

Phosphate deficiency and hypophosphataemia can occur in nutritional deficiency states (e.g. in alcoholic individuals and patients receiving parenteral nutrition).

Hyperphosphataemia is a common problem in patients with renal failure, and is treated with phosphate-bonding compounds such as the anion exchange resin sevelamer (Ch. 25).

DRUGS USED IN BONE DISORDERS

BISPHOSPHONATES

Bisphosphonates are enzyme-resistant analogues of pyrophosphate that inhibit bone resorption by an action mainly on the osteoclasts. After administration, they are bound to bone minerals in the matrix and are released slowly as bone is resorbed by the osteoclasts, which are thus exposed to high concentrations of the drugs.

The main bisphosphonates available for clinical use are **alendronate** and **risedronate**. Others are disodium pamidronate and sodium clodronate. A newer compound, zoledronic acid, which is given only once in a single intravenous infusion, is now used for malignancy and is in clinical trial for Paget's disease and osteoporosis.

Mechanism of action

In terms of their molecular mechanism of action, the bisphosphonates can be grouped into two classes.

- The simple compounds that are very similar to pyrophosphate are incorporated into ATP analogues that accumulate within the osteoclasts and promote their apoptosis.
- The potent, nitrogen-containing bisphosphonates—such as alendronate and ibandronate—interfere with the formation of the ruffled border at the attachment site of the cell to bone, preventing bone resorption (see Fig. 31.2).

▼ The nitrogen-containing bisphosphonates appear to inhibit farnesyl diphosphate synthase, an enzyme in the mevalonate pathway. Inhibition of this enzyme prevents the synthesis of certain lipids that are essential for the activity of small GTPase signalling proteins necessary in the formation of the ruffled border (Rogers, 2003; Strewler, 2005).

It is now known that bisphosphonates are incorporated into the bone matrix and ingested by osteoclasts when these resorb bone.

Pharmacokinetic aspects

Bisphosphonates are usually given orally and are poorly absorbed. They may be given intravenously in malignancy. About 50% of a dose accumulates at sites of bone mineralisation, where it remains, potentially for months or years, until the bone is resorbed. The free drug is excreted unchanged by the kidney.

Absorption is impaired by food, particularly milk, so the drugs must be taken on an empty stomach.

Unwanted effects include gastrointestinal disturbances, which can be severe, and occasionally bone pain. Peptic ulcers have occurred. Alendronate can cause oesophagitis.

Disodium etidronate can increase the risk of fractures due to reduced calcification of bone; this is less likely if it is given cyclically.

> **Clinical uses of bisphosphonates (e.g. alendronate, pamidronate)**
>
> - Paget's disease of bone.
> - *Hypercalcaemia* caused by malignant disease.
> - Prevention or treatment of *postmenopausal osteoporosis* (as an alternative or addition to oestrogens).
> - Prevention or treatment of *glucocorticoid-induced osteoporosis*.
> - They are under investigation for the treatment of cancer metastases in bone.

OESTROGENS AND RELATED COMPOUNDS

The decline in oestrogen levels is a major factor in postmenopausal osteoporosis, and there is evidence that giving hormone replacement therapy (HRT; see Ch. 30) can ameliorate this condition. But HRT has actions on many systems, and newer non-hormonal agents have now been developed that exhibit agonist actions on some tissues and antagonist actions on others. These are termed *selective oestrogen receptor modulators* (*SERMS*). Raloxifene is a SERM that has agonist activity on bone and the cardiovascular system, and antagonist activity on mammary tissue and the uterus.

RALOXIFENE

Actions and mechanism of action

Raloxifene produces a dose-dependent increase in osteoblast activity and reduction in osteoclast action.

It is well absorbed in the gastrointestinal tract, and undergoes extensive first-pass metabolism in the liver to give the glucuronide. (Colestyramine, given with it, reduces the enterohepatic cycling of raloxifene by 60%.)

Thus bioavailability is only about 2%. It is widely distributed in the tissues, and is converted to an active metabolite in liver, lungs, bone, spleen, uterus and kidneys. Its half-life averages 32 hours. It is excreted mainly in the faeces.

Unwanted effects

Hot flushes and leg cramps are common. In a recent clinical trial, raloxifene was found to be associated with venous thromboembolism; however, other authorities state that there is less risk of this adverse effect in younger patients.

PARATHYROID HORMONE

Until recently, there had been little or no clinical use for PTH as such, but then it was realised that PTH and fragments of PTH paradoxically stimulate osteoblast activity and enhance bone formation, and they are now considered to be important compounds in the treatment of osteoporosis (see below). The main compound used is **teriparatide**—the peptide fragment (1–34) of recombinant parathormone.

Actions and mechanism of action

Teriparatide has anabolic effects on bone. It increases bone mass, structural integrity and bone strength by increasing the number of osteoblasts and by activating those osteoblasts already in bone. It also reduces osteoblast apoptosis.

It acts on the G-protein–dependent PTH receptor-1 in the membrane of target cells, and its effects are mediated through adenylate cyclase, phospholipases A, C and D, and increases in intracellular Ca^{2+} and cyclic AMP.

(See Brixen et al., 2004; Cappuzzo & Delafuente, 2004; Dobnig, 2004; Quattrocchi & Kourlas, 2004.)

Pharmacokinetic aspects

Given subcutaneously once daily, peak concentrations occur after 30 minutes. The serum distribution half-life is 10 minutes after intravenous injection and 1 hour after subcutaneous injection.

Unwanted effects

Teriparatide is well tolerated, and serious adverse effects are few. Nausea, dizziness, headache and arthralgias can occur. Mild hypercalcaemia, transient orthostatic hypotension, nausea, dizziness, headache and leg cramps have been reported.

Clinical use

The clinical use of teriparatide is given on page 466. Note that there is controversy as to whether or not this drug should be given sequentially or in combination with one of the bisphosphonates (Heaney & Recker, 2005); however, a bisphosphonate should be given at the end of a course of teriparatide to prevent teriparatide withdrawal bone loss.

STRONTIUM RANELATE

This compound, newly introduced for treatment of osteoporosis, is composed of two atoms of strontium combined with organic ranelic acid, the latter being a carrier for the active strontium component. It inhibits bone resorption and also stimulates bone formation. In recent trials, it has been shown to be effective in preventing vertebral and non-vertebral fractures in older women (see Fogelman & Blake, 2005).

The precise mechanism of action is not clear. Strontium is similar to calcium as regards its absorption in the gastrointestinal tract, its incorporation into bone and its renal elimination. Strontium atoms are adsorbed on to the hydroxyapatite crystals, but eventually they exchange for calcium in the bone minerals and remain in the bone for many years.

The drug is well tolerated; a low incidence of nausea and diarrhoea is reported.

VITAMIN D PREPARATIONS

Vitamin D preparations are used in the treatment of vitamin D deficiencies, bone problems associated with renal failure, and hypoparathyroidism—acute hypoparathyroidism necessitating the use of intravenous calcium and injectable vitamin D preparations.

The main vitamin D preparation used clinically is **ergocalciferol**; also available for clinical use are alfacalcidol and calcitriol. All can be given orally and are well absorbed from the intestine. Vitamin D preparations are fat-soluble, and bile salts are necessary for absorption. Injectable forms of calciferol are available. Newer vitamin D analogues with less potential to cause hypercalcaemia are the vitamin D sterols 19-nor-paracalcitol and doxercalciferol (Salusky, 2005).

Pharmacokinetic aspects

Given orally, vitamin D is bound to a specific α-globulin in the blood. The plasma half-life is about 22 hours, but vitamin D can be found in the fat for many months. The main route of elimination is in the faeces.

The clinical use of vitamin D preparations is given in the box on this page.

Unwanted effects

Excessive intake of vitamin D causes hypercalcaemia, the manifestations of which include constipation, depression, weakness and fatigue. There is a reduced ability to concentrate the urine, resulting in polyuria and polydipsia. If hypercalcaemia persists, calcium salts are deposited in the kidney and urine, causing renal failure and kidney stones.

Some anticonvulsant drugs (e.g. phenytoin; see Ch. 40) increase the requirement for vitamin D.

CALCITONIN

The main preparation available for clinical use (see the clinical box on p. 469) is **salcatonin** (synthetic salmon calcitonin). Synthetic human **calcitonin** is now also available. Calcitonin is given by subcutaneous or intramuscular injection, and there may be a local inflammatory action at the injection site. It can also be given intranasally. Its plasma half-life is 4–12 minutes, but its action lasts for several hours.

Unwanted effects include nausea and vomiting. Facial flushing may occur, as may a tingling sensation in the hands and an unpleasant taste in the mouth.

The clinical uses of calcitonin are given on page 466.

Clinical uses of vitamin D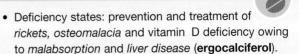

- Deficiency states: prevention and treatment of *rickets, osteomalacia* and vitamin D deficiency owing to *malabsorption* and *liver disease* (**ergocalciferol**).
- Hypocalcaemia caused by *hypoparathyroidism* (**ergocalciferol**).
- *Osteodystrophy* of *chronic renal failure*, which is the consequence of decreased calcitriol generation (**calcitriol** or **alphacalcidol**).
- Plasma Ca^{2+} levels should be monitored during therapy with vitamin D.

CALCIUM SALTS

Calcium salts used therapeutically include calcium gluconate and calcium lactate, given orally. Calcium gluconate is also used for intravenous injection in emergency treatment of hyperkalaemia (Ch. 24); intramuscular injection is not used, because it causes local necrosis.

Calcium carbonate, an antacid, is poorly absorbed in the gut, but there is concern about systemic absorption and the potential to cause arterial calcification. An oral preparation of hydroxyapatite is available.

Unwanted effects: oral calcium salts can cause gastrointestinal disturbance. Intravenous administration requires care, especially in patients on cardiac glycosides (see Ch. 18).

The clinical use of the calcium salts is given on this page.

CALCIMIMETIC COMPOUNDS

Calcimimetics enhance the sensitivity of the parathyroid Ca^{2+}-sensing receptor to the concentration of blood Ca^{2+}. The effect is to decrease the secretion of PTH and reduce the serum Ca^{2+} concentration. There are two types of calcimimetics.

- Type I are agonists, and include inorganic and organic polycations.
- Type II are allosteric activators that activate the receptor by altering its conformation. One such compound is cinacalcet, which is in clinical trial for the treatment of hyperparathyroidism (Nemeth et al., 2004; Peacock et al., 2005).

POTENTIAL NEW THERAPIES

NEW DRUGS FOR OSTEOPOROSIS

There is growing interest in the possible value of anabolic compounds that *stimulate bone formation*—for use alone or in combination with the *antiresorptive drugs* (see Rosen & Bilezekian, 2001). Teriparatide, the first anabolic compound licensed for osteoporosis, is already available for use. A new antiresorptive compound, an anti-RANKL antibody named denosumab, is now available; this specifically blocks RANKL binding to RANK and is in phase III trial (Bekker et al. 2004; Kostenuik, 2005).

Other potential anabolic agents being considered for future development are IGF-1 and insulin-like growth hormone (see Fig. 31.1) and the statins. These last, commonly given to reduce blood cholesterol (Ch. 20), have been shown to increase the gene expression of bone morphogenic protein-2, and to increase bone formation in vitro. Thiazides (Ch. 24) have a small effect in slowing bone loss and might be of value in combination therapy.

Possible new antiresorptive agents on the horizon include agents related to OPG—a physiological inhibitor of bone resorption.

POTENTIAL NEW THERAPIES FOR BONE DISEASES

Recombinant OPG has been tried in juvenile Paget's disease, with promising results (Cundy et al., 2005; Deftos, 2005).

Clinical uses of calcium salts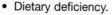

- Dietary deficiency.
- Hypocalcaemia caused by *hypoparathyroidism* or *malabsorption* (intravenous for acute tetany).
- Calcium carbonate is an antacid; it is poorly absorbed and binds phosphate in the gut. It is used to treat hyperphosphataemia (Ch. 24, p. 382).
- Prevention and treatment of osteoporosis (often with oestrogen, bisphosphonate, vitamin D or calcitonin).
- Cardiac dysrhythmias caused by severe hyperkalaemia (intravenous; see Ch. 18).

Parathyroid, vitamin D and bone mineral homeostasis

- The vitamin D family are true hormones; precursors are converted to calcifediol in the liver, then to the main hormone, calcitriol, in kidney.
- Calcitriol increases plasma Ca^{2+} by mobilising it from bone, increasing its absorption in the intestine and decreasing its excretion by the kidney.
- Parathyroid hormone (PTH) increases blood Ca^{2+} by increasing calcitriol synthesis, mobilising Ca^{2+} from bone and reducing renal Ca^{2+} excretion. (But, paradoxically, small doses of PTH given intermittently increase bone formation.)
- Calcitonin (secreted from the thyroid) reduces Ca^{2+} resorption from bone by inhibiting osteoclast activity.

Clinical uses of calcitonin/salcatonin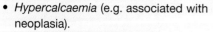

- *Hypercalcaemia* (e.g. associated with neoplasia).
- *Paget's disease* of bone (to relieve pain and reduce neurological complications).
- Postmenopausal and corticosteroid-induced *osteoporosis* (with other agents).

REFERENCES AND FURTHER READING

Bekker P J, Holloway D L, Rasmussen A S et al. 2004 A single-dose placebo-controlled study of AMG 162, a fully human monoclonal antibody to RANKL, in postmenopausal women. J Bone Miner Res 19: 1059–1066 (*A phase III trial of an anti-RANKL antibody shows promise*)

Brixen K T, Christensen P M et al. 2004 Teriparatide (biosynthetic human parathyroid hormone 1–34): a new paradigm in the treatment of osteoporosis. Basic Clin Pharmacol Toxicol 94: 260–270 (*A minireview of the action, mechanism of action, clinical studies and adverse effects*)

Bushinskey D A, Monk R D 1998 Calcium. Lancet 352: 306–311 (*Calcium homeostasis, its disorders and the treatment thereof*)

Cappuzzo K A, Delafuente J C 2004 Teriparatide for severe osteoporosis. Ann Pharmacother 38: 294–302

Clemett D, Spenser C M 2000 Raloxifene: a review of its use in postmenopausal osteoporosis. Drugs 60: 379–411 (*Comprehensive review covering the mechanism of action, pharmacology, pharmacokinetic aspects, therapeutic use and adverse effects of raloxifene*)

Compston J E 2001 Sex steroids and bone. Physiol Rev 81: 419–447 (*Excellent, comprehensive review of steroid actions and mechanisms of action on bone, starting with bone structure; clear coverage of remodelling*)

Cundy T, Davidson J, Rutland M D 2005 Recombinant osteoprotegerin for juvenile Paget's disease. N Engl Med J 353: 918–923

Deftos L J 2005 Treatment of Paget's disease—taming the wild osteoclast. N Engl Med J 353: 872–875 (Editorial covering the use of OPG and zoledronic acid for Paget's disease; excellent diagram. See also article by Cundy et al. in the same issue, pp. 918–923.)

Dobnig H 2004 A review of teriparatide and its clinical efficacy in the treatment of osteoporosis. Expert Opin Pharmacother 5: 1153–1162 (*A general outline of the topic specified*)

Fogelman I, Blake G M 2005 Strontium ranelate for the treatment of osteoporosis. Br Med J 330: 1400–1401 (*Crisp editorial analysis*)

Heaney R P, Recker R R 2005 Combination and sequential therapy for osteoporosis. N Engl J Med 353: 624–625 (*Editorial*)

Hofbauer L C, Schoppet M 2004 Clinical implications of the osteoprotegerin/RANK/RANKL system for bone and vascular diseases. JAMA 292: 490–495 (*Worthwhile coverage; good diagrams of the role of the OPG–RANK–RANKL system in the immune, skeletal and vascular systems*)

Horowitz M C, Xi Y et al. 2001 Control of osteoclastogenesis and bone resorption by members of the TNF family of receptors and ligands. Cytokine Growth Factor Rev 12: 9–18 (*Worthwhile minireview, good diagram*)

Khosia S 2003 Parathyroid hormone plus alendronate: a combination that does not add up. N Engl J Med 349: 1277–1279 (*Editorial warning*)

Kleerekoper M, Schein J R 2001 Comparative safety of bone remodeling agents with a focus on osteoporosis therapies. J Clin Pharmacol 41: 239–250 (*Covers briefly the epidemiology of osteoporosis; outlines the various bone remodelling agents available and gives a good summary table of their benefits*)

Kostenuik P J 2005 Osteoprotegerin and RANKL regulate bone resorption, density, geometry and strength. Curr Opin Pharmacol 5: 618–625 (*Up-to-date coverage of the OPG–RANKL system, with mention of the new anti-RANKL antibody, denosumab*)

Kostenuik P J, Shalhoub V 2001 Osteoprotegerin: a physiological and pharmacological inhibitor of bone resorption. Curr Pharm Des 7: 613–635 (*Detailed coverage of the role of OPG–RANK–OPGK in bone remodelling; states that the OPG pathway 'represents a potential goldmine of therapeutic targets'*)

Lufkin E G, Wong M, Deal C 2001 The role of selective oestrogen receptor modulators in the prevention and treatment of osteoporosis. Rheum Dis Clin North Am 27: 163–184 (*Good description of the pathogenesis of osteoporosis, with outline of main current therapies; gives details of clinical trials with raloxifene and considers combination therapies*)

Manolagas S C 2000 Birth and death of bone cells: basic regulatory mechanisms and implications for the pathogenesis and treatment of osteoporosis. Endocr Rev 21: 115–137 (*Outstanding, comprehensive review*)

Nemeth E F, Heaton W H et al. 2004 Pharmacodynamics of the type II calcimimetic compound cinacalcet HCl. J Pharmacol Exp Ther 398: 627–635 (*Detailed study of pharmacokinetics aspects and the pharmacological action of cinacalcet hydrochloride*)

Peacock M, Bilezikian J P, Klassen P S et al. 2005 Cinacalcet hydrochloride maintains long-term normocalcaemia in patients with primary hyperparathyroidism. J Clin Endocrinol Metab 90: 135–141

Quattrocchi E, Kourlas H 2004 New drugs. Teriparatide: a review. Clin Ther 26: 841–854 (*Excellent review*)

Reginster J-V 2005 Treatment of postmenopausal osteoporosis. Br Med J 330: 859–860 (*Editorial on the main drugs used*)

Reichel H, Koeftler H P, Norman A W 1989 The role of the vitamin D endocrine system in health and disease. N Engl J Med 320: 980–991 (*Good comprehensive early review*)

Reid I R, Ames R W et al. 2000 Hydrochlorothiazide reduces loss of cortical bone in normal postmenopausal women: a randomized controlled trial. Am J Med 109: 362–370 (*The results suggest that thiazides may possibly be useful in prevention but not treatment of postmenopausal osteoporosis*)

Riggs B L, Parfitt A M 2005 Drugs used to treat osteoporosis: the critical need for a uniform nomenclature based on their action on bone remodeling. J Bone Miner Res 20: 177–184

Salusky I B 2005 Are new vitamin D analogues in renal bone disease superior to calcitriol? Pediatr Nephrol 20: 393–398

van Staa T P, Dennison E M, Leufkens H G, Cooper C 2001 Epidemiology of fractures in England and Wales. Bone 29: 517–522

Whyte M P 2006 The long and the short of bone therapy. N Engl J Med 354: 860–863 (*Succinct article on the present status of and future possibilities for bone therapy. Exellent diagram.*)

Remodelling

Roberts C G, Ladenson P W 2004 Hypothyroidism. Lancet 363: 793–803

Rogers M J 2003 New insights into the mechanisms of action of the bisphosphonates. Curr Pharm Des 9: 2643–2658 (*Covers the different mechanisms of action of the simple bisphosphonates, for example etidronate, and the nitrogen-containing bisphosphonates, for example zoledronate*)

Roodman G D 2004 Mechanisms of bone metastasis. N Engl Med J 350: 1655–1664 (*Has excellent section on bone remodelling, with good diagrams*)

Rosen C J, Bilezekian J P 2001 Anabolic therapy for osteoporosis. J Clin Endocrinol Metab 86: 957–964 (*Well-written article clarifying the potential role of non-resorptive agents in the therapy of osteoporosis; neat figure of the interaction between osteoblasts and osteoclasts*)

Stewart J F 2004 Translational implications of the parathyroid calcium receptor. N Engl J Med 351: 324–326 (*Succinct article with useful diagram*)

Strewler G J 2005 Decimal point—osteoporosis therapy at the 10-year mark. N Engl J Med 350: 1172–1174 (*Crisp article concentrating mainly on bisphosphonates; excellent diagram of bisphosphonate action*)

Theoleyre S, Wittrant Y et al. 2004 The molecular triad of OPG/RANK/RANKL: involvement in the orchestration of pathophysiological bone modeling. Cytokine Growth Factor Rev 15: 49–60 (*Comprehensive review*)

Tolar J, Teitelbaum S L, Orchard P J 2004 Osteopetrosis. N Engl J Med 351: 2839–2849 (*Very good review; has excellent section on the biology of osteoclasts, with very good diagrams*)

Whitfield J F, Morley P 1995 Small bone-building fragments of parathyroid hormone: new therapeutic agents for osteoporosis. Trends Pharmacol Sci 16: 382–385 (*Useful review with cheerful diagram of bone remodelling*)

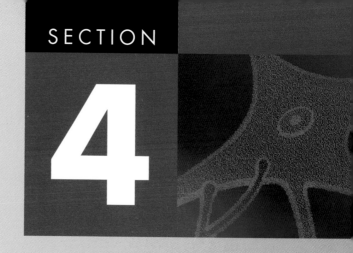

THE NERVOUS SYSTEM

Chemical transmission and drug action in the central nervous system

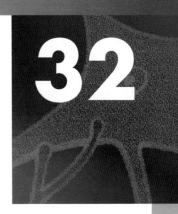

32

OVERVIEW

Brain function is the single most important aspect of physiology that defines the difference between humans and other species. Disorders of brain function, whether primary or secondary to malfunction of other systems, are a major concern of human society, and a field in which pharmacological intervention plays a key role. In this chapter, we introduce some basic principles of neuropharmacology that underlie much of the material in the rest of this section.

INTRODUCTION

There are two reasons why understanding the action of drugs on the central nervous system (CNS) presents a particularly challenging problem. The first is that centrally acting drugs are of special significance to humankind. Not only are they of major therapeutic importance,[1] but they are also the drugs that humans most commonly administer to themselves for non-medical reasons (e.g. alcohol, tea and coffee, cannabis, nicotine, opiates, amphetamines and so on). The second reason is that the CNS is functionally far more complex than any other system in the body, and this

makes the understanding of drug effects very much more difficult. The relationship between the behaviour of individual cells and that of the organ as a whole is far less direct in the brain than, for example, in the heart or kidney. In these latter organs, a detailed understanding of how a drug affects the cells gives us a fairly clear idea of what effect it will produce on the organ (and on the animal) as a whole. In the brain, this is simply not true. Thus we may know that a drug mimics the action of 5-hydroxytryptamine in its effect on nerve cells, and we know empirically that such drugs often cause hallucinations. However, other drugs that enhance the action of 5-hydroxytryptamine, such as antidepressants (Ch. 39) affect mood and behaviour in a quite different way. Currently, the link between a drug's action at the biochemical and cellular level and its effects on high-level brain function remain largely mysterious. Functional brain imaging is beginning to reveal relationships between brain activity in specific regions and mental function, and this tool is being used increasingly to probe drug effects. Nevertheless, the fairly gross (millimetre scale) resolution currently achievable with imaging methods is far from being able to reveal events at the level of individual neurons and synapses. Despite sustained progress in understanding the cellular and biochemical effects produced by centrally acting drugs, and the increasing use of brain imaging to study brain function and drug effects, the gulf between our understanding of drug action at the cellular level and at the functional and behavioural level remains, for the most part, very wide. Attempts to bridge it seem, at times, like throwing candy floss into the Grand Canyon.

A few bridge-heads have nonetheless been established, some more firmly than others. Thus the relationship between dopaminergic pathways in the extrapyramidal system and the effects of drugs in alleviating or exacerbating the symptoms of Parkinson's disease (see Ch. 35) is clear-cut. Also reasonably firm is the link between the functions of noradrenaline (norepinephrine) and 5-hydroxytryptamine in certain parts of the brain and the symptoms of depression (see Ch. 39), and that between GABA and anxiety (Ch. 37). Less well established is the connection between hyperactivity in dopaminergic pathways and schizophrenia (see Ch. 38). On the other hand, attempts to relate the condition of epilepsy to an identifiable cellular disturbance (see Ch. 40) have been very disappointing, even though the abnormal neuronal discharge pattern in epilepsy seems, on the face of it, a much simpler kind of disturbance than, for example, the altered mood of a depressed patient. Many CNS drugs are used to treat psychiatric disorders that are defined according to their symptomatology rather than on the basis of causative factors or clinical signs

---

[1] In Britain in 2003, 118 million prescriptions (about 20% of all prescriptions), costing £1.3 billion, were for CNS drugs as defined by the British National Formulary. This amounted to nearly two per person across the whole population.

and investigations. What is called 'schizophrenia' or 'depression' on the basis of particular symptoms is likely to consist of several distinct disorders caused by different mechanisms and responding to drugs in different ways. Much effort is going into pinning down the biological basis of psychiatric disorders—a necessary step to improve the design of better drugs for clinical use—but the task is daunting and progress is slow.

In this chapter, we outline the general principles governing the action of drugs on the CNS. Most neuroactive drugs work by interfering with the chemical signals that underlie brain function, and the next two chapters discuss the major CNS transmitter systems and the ways in which drugs affect them. In Chapter 35, we focus on neurodegenerative diseases, and the remaining chapters in this section deal with the main classes of neuroactive drugs that are currently in use.

Background information will be found in neurobiology textbooks such as Kandel et al. (2000), and in texts on neuropharmacology such as Nestler et al. (2001) and Cooper et al. (2004). For exhaustive coverage, see Davis et al. (2002).

CHEMICAL SIGNALLING IN THE NERVOUS SYSTEM

The brain (like every other organ in the body!) is basically a chemical machine; it controls the main functions of a higher animal across timescales ranging from milliseconds (e.g. returning a 100 mph tennis serve) to years (e.g. remembering how to ride a bicycle).[2] The chemical signalling mechanisms cover a correspondingly wide dynamic range, as summarised, in a very general way, in Figure 32.1. Currently, we understand much about drug effects on events at the fast end of the spectrum—synaptic transmission and neuromodulation—but much less about long-term adaptive processes, although it is quite evident that the latter are of great importance for the neurological and psychiatric disorders that are susceptible to drug treatment.

---

[2]Memory of the basic facts of pharmacology seems to come somewhere in the middle of this range (skewed towards the short end).

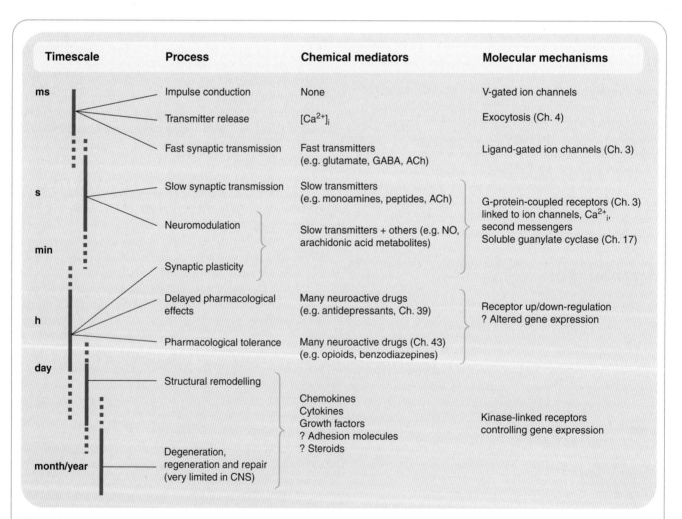

Fig. 32.1 Chemical signalling in the nervous system. Knowledge of the mediators and mechanisms becomes sparser as we move from the rapid events of synaptic transmission to the slower ones involving remodelling and alterations of gene expression. ACh, acetylcholine; CNS, central nervous system; NO, nitric oxide.

The original concept of neurotransmission envisaged a substance released by one neuron and acting rapidly, briefly and at short range on the membrane of an adjacent (postsynaptic) neuron, causing excitation or inhibition. The principles outlined in Chapter 9 apply to the central as well as the peripheral nervous system. It is now clear that chemical mediators within the brain can produce slow and long-lasting effects; that they can act rather diffusely, at a considerable distance from their site of release; and that they can produce diverse effects, for example on transmitter synthesis, on the expression of neurotransmitter receptors and on neuronal morphology, in addition to affecting the ionic conductance of the postsynaptic cell membrane. This form of signalling has been termed *non-synaptic communication* (see Vizi, 2000). The term *neuromodulator* is often used to denote a mediator, the actions of which do not conform to the original neurotransmitter concept. The term is not clearly defined, and it covers not only the diffusely acting neuropeptide mediators, but also mediators such as nitric oxide and arachidonic acid metabolites, which are not stored and released like conventional neurotransmitters, and may come from non-neuronal cells, particularly glia, as well as neurons. In general, neuromodulation relates to *synaptic plasticity*, including short-term physiological events such as the regulation of presynaptic transmitter release or postsynaptic excitability. Longer term *neurotrophic* effects are involved in regulating the growth and morphology of neurons, as well as their functional properties. Table 32.1 summarises the types of chemical mediator that operate in the CNS.

Glial cells, particularly astrocytes, which are the main non-neuronal cells in the CNS and outnumber neurons by 10 to 1, also play an important signalling role. Once thought of mainly as housekeeping cells, whose function was merely to look after the fastidious neurons, they are increasingly seen as 'inexcitable neurons' with a major communications role to play (see Bezzi & Volterra, 2001; Fields & Stevens-Graham, 2002), albeit on a slower timescale than that of neuronal communication. These cells express a range of receptors and transporters similar to those present in neurons, and also release a wide variety of mediators, including glutamate, lipid mediators and growth factors. They respond to chemical signals from neurons, and also from neighbouring astrocytes and microglial cells (the CNS equivalent of macrophages, which function much like inflammatory cells in peripheral tissues). Electrical coupling between astrocytes causes them often to respond in concert in a particular brain region, thus controlling the chemical environment in which the neurons operate. Although they do not conduct action potentials, and do not send signals to other parts of the body, astrocytes are otherwise very similar to neurons and play a crucial communication role within the brain. Because they are difficult to study in situ, however, our knowledge of how they function, and how they respond to drugs, is still fragmentary. It is an area to watch closely.

TARGETS FOR DRUG ACTION

To recapitulate what was discussed in Chapters 2 and 3, neuro-active drugs act on one of four types of target proteins, namely ion channels, receptors, enzymes and transport proteins. Of the four main receptor families—ionotropic receptors, G–protein–coupled receptors, kinase-linked receptors and nuclear receptors—current drugs target mainly the first two.

In the last two or three decades, knowledge about these targets in the CNS has accumulated rapidly, particularly as follows.

- As well as 40 or more small-molecule and peptide mediators, the importance of other 'non-classical' mediators—nitric oxide, eicosanoids, growth factors, etc.—has become apparent (see Barañano et al., 2001).
- Considerable molecular diversity of known receptor molecules and ion channels (see Ch. 3) has been revealed.

Table 32.1 Types of chemical mediators in the central nervous system

Mediator type[a]	Examples	Targets	Main functional role
Conventional small-molecule mediators	Glutamate, GABA, acetylcholine, dopamine, 5-hydroxytryptamine, etc.	Ligand-gated ion channels G-protein–coupled receptors	Fast synaptic neurotransmission Neuromodulation
Neuropeptides	Substance P, neuropeptide Y, corticotrophin-releasing factor, etc.	G-protein–coupled receptors	Neuromodulation
Lipid mediators	Prostaglandins, endocannabinoids	G-protein–coupled receptors	Neuromodulation
Nitric oxide	–	Guanylate cyclase	Neuromodulation
Neurotrophins, cytokines	Nerve growth factor, brain-derived neurotrophic factor, interleukin-1	Kinase-linked receptors	Neuronal growth, survival and functional plasticity
Steroids	Androgens, oestrogens	Nuclear receptors (also membrane receptors)	Functional plasticity

[a]Most central nervous system pharmacology is currently centred on small-molecule mediators and, less commonly, neuropeptides. Other mediator types have yet to be targeted for therapeutic purposes.

Chemical transmission in the central nervous system

- The basic processes of synaptic transmission in the central nervous system are essentially similar to those operating in the periphery (Ch. 9).
- Glial cells, particularly astrocytes, participate actively in chemical signalling, functioning essentially as 'inexcitable neurons'.
- The terms *neurotransmitter, neuromodulator* and *neurotrophic factor* refer to chemical mediators that operate over different timescales. In general:
  - neurotransmitters are released by presynaptic terminals and produce rapid excitatory or inhibitory responses in postsynaptic neurons
  - neuromodulators are released by neurons and by astrocytes, and produce slower pre- or postsynaptic responses
  - neurotrophic factors are released mainly by non-neuronal cells and act on tyrosine kinase–linked receptors that regulate gene expression and control neuronal growth and phenotypic characteristics
  - fast neurotransmitters (e.g. glutamate, GABA) operate through ligand-gated ion channels
  - slow neurotransmitters and neuromodulators (e.g. dopamine, neuropeptides, prostanoids) operate mainly through G-protein–coupled receptors.
- The same agent (e.g. glutamate, 5-hydroxytryptamine, acetylcholine) may act through both ligand-gated channels and G-protein–coupled receptors and function as both neurotransmitter and neuromodulator.
- Many chemical mediators, including glutamate, nitric oxide and arachidonic acid metabolites, are produced by glia as well as neurons.
- Many mediators (e.g. cytokines, chemokines, growth factors, steroids) control long-term changes in the brain (e.g. synaptic plasticity and remodelling), mainly by affecting gene transcription.

- All the receptors and channels are expressed in at least three or four (often more) subtypes, with quite characteristic distributions in different brain areas. In most cases, we have little clear idea of what this diversity means at a functional level, although the study of transgenic 'gene knockouts' is beginning to provide some clues. From the pharmacological standpoint, the molecular diversity of such targets raises the possibility that drugs with improved selectivity of action—blocking one kind of sodium channel without affecting others, for example—may be discovered. So far, however, the potential of these new approaches in terms of improved drugs for neurological and psychiatric diseases remains largely unrealised. Hope, however (and certainly hype), springs eternal.

- The pathophysiology of neurodegeneration in conditions such as Alzheimer's disease and stroke is beginning to be understood (see Ch. 35), and progress is being made in understanding the mechanisms underlying drug dependence (see Ch. 43). These advances are suggesting new strategies for treating these disabling conditions. Other areas of brain research (e.g. the neurobiology of epilepsy, schizophrenia and depressive illnesses) are advancing less rapidly, but there is still progress to report.

DRUG ACTION IN THE CENTRAL NERVOUS SYSTEM

As we have already emphasised, the molecular and cellular mechanisms underlying drug action in the CNS and in the periphery are essentially similar. Understanding how drugs affect brain function is, however, made difficult by several factors. One is the complexity of neuronal interconnections in the brain—the wiring diagram. Figure 32.2 illustrates in a schematic way the kind of interconnections that typically exist for, say, a noradrenergic neuron in the locus coeruleus (see Ch. 34), shown as **neuron 1** in the diagram, releasing **transmitter *a*** at its terminals. Release of *a* affects **neuron 2** (which releases **transmitter *b***), and also affects neuron 1 by direct feedback and, indirectly, by affecting presynaptic inputs impinging on neuron 1. The firing pattern of neuron 2 also affects the system, partly through interneuronal connections (**neuron 3**, releasing **transmitter *c***). Even at this grossly oversimplified level, the effects on the system of blocking or enhancing the release or actions of one or other of the transmitters are difficult to predict, and will depend greatly on the relative strength of the various excitatory and inhibitory synaptic connections, and on external inputs (*x* and *y* in the diagram). Added to this complexity at the level of neuronal interconnections is the influence of the glial cells, mentioned above. A further important complicating factor is that a range of secondary, adaptive responses is generally set in train by any drug-induced perturbation of the system. Typically, an increase in transmitter release, or interference with transmitter reuptake, is countered by inhibition of transmitter synthesis, enhanced transporter expression or decreased receptor expression. These changes, which involve altered gene expression, generally take time (hours, days or weeks) to develop and are not evident in acute pharmacological experiments.

In the clinical situation, the effects of psychotropic drugs often take weeks to develop, so it is likely that they reflect the adaptive responses rather than the immediate pharmacodynamic effects of the drug. This is well documented for antidepressant drugs (Ch. 39) and some antipsychotic drugs (Ch. 38). The development of dependence on drugs such as opiates, benzodiazepines and psychostimulants is similarly gradual (Ch. 43). Thus one has to take into account not only the primary interaction of the drug with its target, but also the secondary response of the brain to this primary effect; it is often the secondary response, rather than the primary effect, which leads to clinical benefit.

A further important factor in CNS pharmacology is the existence of the blood–brain barrier (see Ch. 4), penetration of which requires molecules to traverse the vascular endothelial cells

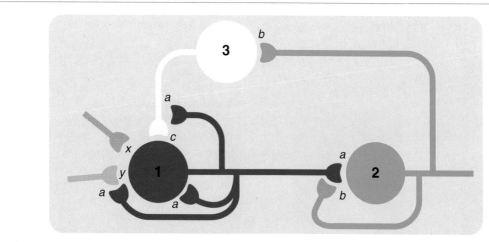
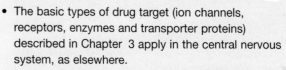

Fig. 32.2 **Simplified scheme of neuronal interconnections in the central nervous system.** Neurons 1, 2 and 3 are shown releasing transmitters *a*, *b* and *c*, respectively, which may be excitatory or inhibitory. Boutons of neuron 1 terminate on neuron 2, but also on neuron 1 itself, and on presynaptic terminals of other neurons that make synaptic connections with neuron 1. Neuron 2 also feeds back on neuron 1 via interneuron 3. Transmitters (*x* and *y*) released by other neurons are also shown impinging on neuron 1. Even with such a simple network, the effects of drug-induced interference with specific transmitter systems can be difficult to predict.

rather than going between them. In general, only small non-polar molecules can diffuse passively across cell membranes. Some neuroactive drugs penetrate the blood–brain barrier in this way, but many do so via transporters, which either facilitate entry into the brain or diminish it by pumping the compound from the endothelial cell interior back into the bloodstream. Drugs that gain entry in this way include L-dopa (Ch. 35), valproate (Ch. 40) and various sedative histamine antagonists (Ch. 14). Drugs that are excluded include many antibacterial and anticancer drugs that are substrates for the P-glycoprotein transporter (see Chs 4 and 45). Several such transporters have been identified, and their importance in relation to drug action in the brain is becoming increasingly apparent (see review by Tamai & Tsuji, 2000).

THE CLASSIFICATION OF PSYCHOTROPIC DRUGS

Psychotropic drugs are defined as those that affect mood and behaviour. Because these indices of brain function are difficult to define and measure, there is no consistent basis for classifying psychotropic drugs. Instead, we find a confusing mêlée of terms relating to chemical structure (**benzodiazepines, butyrophenones,** etc.), biochemical target (**monoamine oxidase inhibitors, serotonin reuptake inhibitors, opiates,** etc.), behavioural effect (**hallucinogens, psychomotor stimulants**) or clinical use (**antidepressants, antipsychotic agents, antiepileptic drugs,** etc.), together with a number of indefinable rogue categories (**atypical antipsychotic drugs, nootropic drugs**) thrown in for good measure.

However, grumbling about terminology is fruitless. The following classification is based on that suggested in 1967 by the World Health Organization; although flawed, it provides a basis for the material presented later (Chs 37–43).

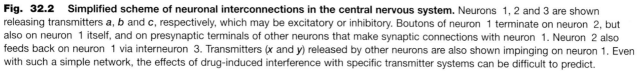

Drug action in the central nervous system

- The basic types of drug target (ion channels, receptors, enzymes and transporter proteins) described in Chapter 3 apply in the central nervous system, as elsewhere.
- Most of these targets occur in several different molecular isoforms, the functional significance of which is, in most cases, unclear.
- Many of the currently available neuroactive drugs are relatively non-specific, affecting several different targets, the principal ones being receptors, ion channels and transporters.
- The relationship between the pharmacological profile and the therapeutic effect of neuroactive drugs is often unclear.
- Slowly–developing secondary responses to the primary interaction of the drug with its target are often important (e.g. the delayed efficacy of antidepressant drugs, and tolerance and dependence with opiates).

- **Anaesthetic agents**
  Definition: drugs used to produce surgical anaesthesia
  Examples: halothane, propofol
  See Chapter 36
- **Anxiolytics and sedatives**
  Synonyms: hypnotics, sedatives, minor tranquillisers
  Definition: drugs that cause sleep and reduce anxiety
  Examples: barbiturates, benzodiazepines
  See Chapter 37

- **Antipsychotic drugs**
  Synonyms: neuroleptic[3] drugs, antischizophrenic drugs, major tranquillisers
  Definition: drugs that are effective in relieving the symptoms of schizophrenic illness
  Examples: clozapine, chlorpromazine, haloperidol
  See Chapter 38
- **Antidepressant drugs**
  Definition: drugs that alleviate the symptoms of depressive illness
  Examples: monoamine oxidase inhibitors, tricyclic antidepressants, selective serotonin reuptake inhibitors
  See Chapter 39
- **Analgesic drugs**
  Definition: drugs used clinically for controlling pain
  Examples: opiates, carbamazepine
  See Chapter 41
- **Psychomotor stimulants**
  Synonym: psychostimulants
  Definition: drugs that cause wakefulness and euphoria
  Examples: amphetamine, cocaine and caffeine
  See Chapter 42
- **Psychotomimetic drugs**
  Synonyms: hallucinogens, psychodysleptics[3]
  Definition: drugs that cause disturbance of perception

(particularly visual hallucinations) and of behaviour in ways that cannot be simply characterised as sedative or stimulant effects
  Examples: lysergic acid diethylamide, mescaline and phencyclidine
  See Chapter 43
- **Cognition enhancers**
  Synonyms: nootropic drugs
  Definition: drugs that improve memory and cognitive performance
  Examples: acetylcholinesterase inhibitors (e.g. **donepezil**, **galantamine**, **rivastigmine** (Ch. 10), NMDA receptor antagonists (e.g. **memantine**, Ch. 33), **piracetam** (improves cognitive function in animal tests, but not proven in humans). This is something of a wishful category, in that several classes of drugs that improve learning and memory in animal tests have not been shown to do so in humans.

Some drugs defy classification in this scheme, for example **lithium** (see Ch. 39), which is used in the treatment of manic–depressive psychosis, and **ketamine** (see Ch. 36), which is classed as a dissociative anaesthetic but produces psychotropic effects rather similar to those produced by phencyclidine.

In practice, the use of drugs in psychiatric illness frequently cuts across the specific therapeutic categories listed above. For example, it is common for antipsychotic drugs to be used as 'tranquillisers' to control extremely anxious or unruly patients, or to treat severe depression. Antidepressant drugs are often used to treat neuropathic pain (Ch. 41), and certain psychostimulants are of proven efficacy for treating hyperactive children. The simple-minded pharmacologist, confronted with the realities of clinical practice, may find this confusing. Here we will adhere to the conventional pharmacological categories, but it needs to be emphasised that in clinical use these distinctions are often disregarded.

---

[3]These strange terms are the remnants of a classification proposed by Javet in 1903, who distinguished psycholeptics (depressants of mental function), psychoanaleptics (stimulants of mental function) and psychodysleptics (drugs that produce disturbed mental function). The term *neuroleptic* (literally 'nerve seizing') was coined 50 years later to describe chlorpromazine-like drugs (see Ch. 38). It gained favour, presumably by virtue of its brevity rather than its literal meaning.

REFERENCES AND FURTHER READING

Barañano D E, Ferris C D, Snyder S H 2001 Atypical neural messengers. Trends Neurosci 24: 99–106 (*Short trendy review on some established mediators, such as nitric oxide, and some speculative ones, such as carbon monoxide and D-serine*]

Bezzi P, Volterra A 2001 A neuron–glia signalling network in the active brain. Curr Opin Neurobiol 11: 387–394 (*Good short review emphasising the intercommunication between glial cells and neurons—a topic still poorly understood but of growing importance*)

Cooper J R, Bloom F E, Roth R H 2004 Biochemical basis of neuropharmacology. Oxford University Press, New York (*Excellent and readable account focusing on basic rather than clinical aspects*)

Davis K L, Charney D, Coyle J T, Nemeroff C (eds) 2002 Neuropsychopharmacology: the fifth generation of progress. Lippincott, Williams & Wilkins, Philadelphia (*A 2000-page monster with excellent and authoritative articles on basic and clinical aspects*)

De Boer A G, van der Sandt I C J, Gaillard P J 2003 The role of drug transporters at the blood–brain barrier. Annu Rev Pharmacol Toxicol 43: 626–629 (*Comprehensive review of the molecular nature of blood–brain barrier transporters and their pharmacological significance*)

Fields R D, Stevens-Graham B 2002 New insights into neuron–glia communication. Science 298: 556–562

Kandel E, Schwartz J H, Jessell T M 2000 Principles of neural science, 4th edn. Elsevier, New York (*Excellent

and detailed standard text on neurobiology—little emphasis on pharmacology*)

Nestler E J, Hyman S E, Malenka R C 2001 Molecular neuropharmacology. McGraw-Hill, New York (*Good modern textbook*)

Tamai I, Tsuji A 2000 Transporter-mediated permeation of drugs across the blood–brain barrier. J Pharm Sci 89: 1372–1388 (*Good review of the role of transport mechanisms in determining transfer of drugs and endogenous molecules into and out of the brain*)

Vizi E S 2000 Role of high affinity receptors and membrane transporters in nonsynaptic communication and drug action in the central nervous system. Pharm Rev 52: 63–89 (*Comprehensive review of neuromodulatory mechanisms in the CNS*)

Amino acid transmitters

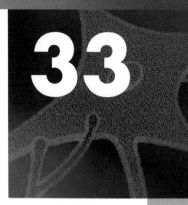

33

OVERVIEW

In this chapter, we discuss the major neurotransmitters in the central nervous system (CNS), namely the excitatory transmitter, glutamate, and the inhibitory transmitters, GABA and glycine. It is an area in which scientific interest has been intense in recent years, producing a prolific literature and, for many of us, a stiff measure of information overload. Unravelling some of the complexities of amino acid receptors and signalling mechanisms has thrown considerable light on their role in brain function and their likely involvement in CNS disease. Drugs that target specific receptors and transporters have been developed, but translating this knowledge into drugs for therapeutic use has been very slow-going. Here, we present the pharmacological principles and include recent references for those seeking more detail.

EXCITATORY AMINO ACIDS

EXCITATORY AMINO ACIDS AS CNS TRANSMITTERS

L-**glutamate** is the principal and ubiquitous excitatory transmitter in the CNS (see Cotman et al., 1995, for general review). **Aspartate** plays a similar role in certain brain regions, and possibly also **homocysteate**, but this is controversial. The realisation of glutamate's importance came slowly (see Watkins & Jane, 2006). By the 1950s (in the words of Krnjevic, one of the glutamate pioneers, the 'era of Prehistory'), work on the peripheral nervous system had highlighted the transmitter roles of acetylcholine and catecholamines, and as the brain also contained these substances, there seemed little reason to look further. The presence of **γ-aminobutyric acid** (**GABA**; see below) in the brain, and its powerful inhibitory effect on neurons, were discovered in the 1950s, and its transmitter role was postulated. At the same time, work by Curtis's group in Canberra showed that glutamate and various other acidic amino acids produced a strong excitatory effect, but it seemed inconceivable that such workaday metabolites could actually be transmitters. Through the 1960s (the 'Dark Ages'), GABA and excitatory amino acids (EAAs) were thought, even by their discoverers, to be mere pharmacological curiosities. In the 1970s (the 'Renaissance'), the humblest amino acid, **glycine**, was established as an inhibitory transmitter in the spinal cord, giving the lie to the idea that transmitters had to be exotic molecules, too beautiful for any role but to sink into the arms of a receptor. Once glycine had been accepted, the rest quickly followed (the 'Baroque era', an apt phrase to describe the intricate detail that has since been added to the basic discovery). A major advance was the discovery of EAA antagonists, based on the work of Watkins in Bristol, which enabled the physiological role of glutamate to be established unequivocally, and also led to the realisation that EAA receptors are heterogeneous.

To do justice to the wealth of discovery in this field in the past two decades is beyond the range of this book; for recent reviews giving more detail, see Conn & Pin (1997), Dingledine et al. (1999) and Javitt (2004). Here we concentrate on pharmacological aspects. Disappointingly, hardly any therapeutic drugs have yet been introduced on the basis of EAA mechanisms,[1] despite the many

---

[1]Memantine, an NMDA antagonist, is licensed for the treatment of moderate to severe Alzheimer's disease (Ch. 35) but is no magic wand!

METABOLISM AND RELEASE OF AMINO ACIDS

Glutamate is widely and fairly uniformly distributed in the CNS, where its concentration is much higher than in other tissues. It has an important metabolic role, the metabolic and neurotransmitter pools being linked by *transaminase* enzymes that catalyse the interconversion of glutamate and α-oxoglutarate (Fig. 33.1). Glutamate in the CNS comes mainly from either *glucose*, via the Krebs cycle, or *glutamine*, which is synthesised by glial cells and taken up by the neurons; very little comes from the periphery. The interconnection between the pathways for the synthesis of EAAs and inhibitory amino acids (GABA and glycine), shown in Figure 33.1, makes it difficult to use experimental manipulations of transmitter synthesis to study the functional role of individual amino acids, because disturbance of any one step will affect both excitatory and inhibitory mediators.

In common with other transmitters, glutamate is stored in synaptic vesicles and released by Ca^{2+}-dependent exocytosis; specific transporter proteins account for its uptake by neurons and other cells, and for its accumulation by synaptic vesicles (see Ch. 9). Released glutamate is taken up by cells in exchange for Na^+ (cf. monoamine transporters—Ch. 9), and transported into synaptic vesicles, by a different transporter driven by the proton gradient across the vesicle membrane. In contrast to the situation with monoamine synthesis and transport (Chs 11 and 34), few drugs (none in clinical use) are known that interfere specifically with glutamate metabolism.

The action of glutamate is terminated mainly by carrier-mediated reuptake into the nerve terminals and neighbouring astrocytes (Fig. 33.2). This transport can, under some circumstances (e.g. depolarisation by increased extracellular K^+), operate in reverse and constitute a source of glutamate release (see Takahashi et al., 1997), a process that may occur under pathological conditions such as brain ischaemia (see Ch. 35). Glutamate taken up by astrocytes is converted to *glutamine* and recycled, via transporters, back to the neurons, which convert the glutamine back to glutamate. Glutamine, which lacks the pharmacological activity of glutamate, thus serves as a pool of inactive transmitter under the regulatory control of the astrocytes, which act as ball boys, returning the ammunition in harmless form in order to rearm the neurons.

Glutamate uptake is coupled to Na^+ entry, and several transporters have been cloned and characterised in detail (see Shigeri et al., 2004).

GLUTAMATE

GLUTAMATE RECEPTOR SUBTYPES

On the basis of studies with selective agonists and antagonists (Fig. 33.3), four main subtypes of EAA receptors can be distinguished, namely **NMDA**, **AMPA**, **kainate** and **metabotropic** receptors (Table 33.1), all of which have been cloned and studied in great detail (see Conn & Pin, 1997; Dingledine et al., 1999). The first three are *ionotropic receptors*, named according to their specific agonists.[2] The channel consists of four subunits,

---

[2]AMPA and kainate receptors are pharmacologically similar and are often lumped together as *AMPA/kainate* or *non-NMDA* receptors.

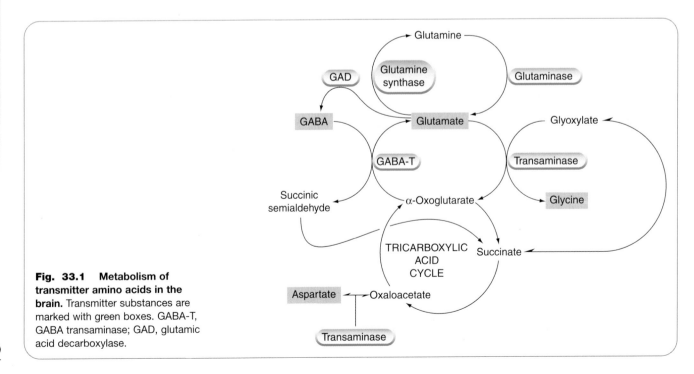

Fig. 33.1 Metabolism of transmitter amino acids in the brain. Transmitter substances are marked with green boxes. GABA-T, GABA transaminase; GAD, glutamic acid decarboxylase.

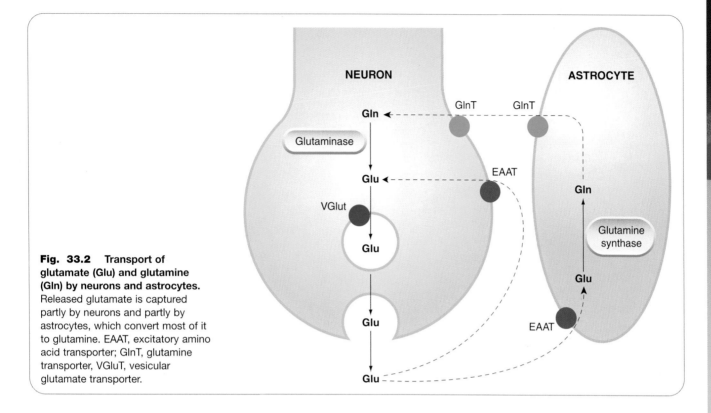

Fig. 33.2 **Transport of glutamate (Glu) and glutamine (Gln) by neurons and astrocytes.** Released glutamate is captured partly by neurons and partly by astrocytes, which convert most of it to glutamine. EAAT, excitatory amino acid transporter; GlnT, glutamine transporter, VGluT, vesicular glutamate transporter.

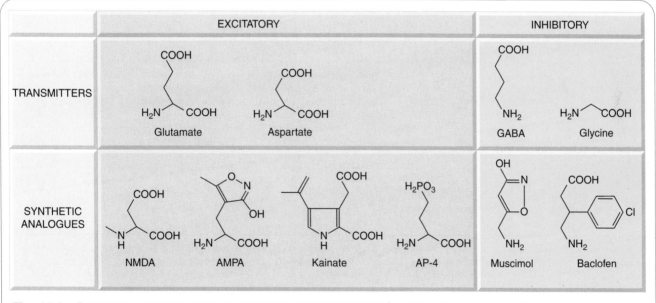

Fig. 33.3 **Structures of agonists acting on glutamate, GABA and glycine receptors.** The receptor specificity of these compounds is shown in Tables 33.1 and 33.2. AP-4, 3-amino-4-phosphonopentanoic acid. AMPA, α amino-3-hydroxy-5-methylisoxazole-4-propianic acid; NMDA, N-methyl-D-asparatic acid.

each with the 'pore loop' structure shown in Figure 3.18. NMDA receptors are assembled from two types of subunit, NR₁ and NR₂, each of which can exist in different isoforms and splice variants, giving rise to many different receptor isoforms in the brain, whose significance is not yet understood—a scenario by now familiar to our readers. The subunits comprising AMPA and kainate receptors, termed $GluR_{1-7}$ and $KA_{1,2}$, are closely related to, but

distinct from, NR subunits. AMPA receptors consist of combinations of $GluR_{1-4}$.[3] AMPA receptors lacking the $GluR_2$ subunit

[3]AMPA receptor subunits are also subject to other kinds of variation, namely alternative splicing, giving rise to the engagingly named *flip* and *flop* variants, and RNA editing at the single amino acid level, both of which contribute yet more functional diversity to this motley family.

Table 33.1 Properties of excitatory amino acid receptors

	NMDA		AMPA	Kainate	Metabotropic
Subunit composition	Tetramers consisting of NR_1 and NR_2 subunits		Tetramers consisting of $GluR_{1-4}$ subunits (variants associated with alternative splicing and RNA editing)	Tetramers consisting of $GluR_{5-7}$ subunits plus $KA_{1,2}$	Dimeric G-protein–coupled receptors
	Receptor site	**Modulatory site (glycine)**			
Endogenous agonist(s)	Glutamate Aspartate	Glycine D-Serine	Glutamate	Glutamate	Glutamate
Other agonist(s)[a]	NMDA	Cycloserine	AMPA Quisqualate	Kainate Domoate	D-AP4 ACPD
Antagonist(s)[a]	AP-5, AP-7 CGS 19755 (selfotel) CPP LY 235959	7-Chloro-kynurenic acid ACEA 1021 HA-466	NBQX CNQX LY 293558	NBQX LY 377770	MCPG
Other modulators	Polyamines (e.g. spermine, spermidine) Mg^{2+}, Zn^{2+}		Cyclothiazide Aniracetam Ampakines[b] Piracetam	–	–
Channel blockers	Dizocilpine (MK801) Phencyclidine Ketamine Remacemide Memantine Mg^{2+}		–	–	Not applicable
Effector mechanism	Ligand-gated cation channel (slow kinetics, high Ca^{2+} permeability)		Ligand-gated cation channel (fast kinetics; channels possessing $GluR_2$ subunits show low Ca^{2+} permeability)	Ligand-gated cation channel (fast kinetics, low Ca^{2+} permeability)	G-protein–coupled (inositol trisphosphate formation and release of Ca^{2+})
Location	Postsynaptic (also glial) Wide distribution		Postsynaptic	Pre- and postsynaptic	Pre- and postsynaptic
Function	Slow epsp Synaptic plasticity (long-term potentiation, long-term depression) Excitotoxicity		Fast epsp Wide distribution	Fast epsp ? Presynaptic inhibition Limited distribution	Synaptic modulation Excitotoxicity

ACPD, 1-aminocyclopentane-1,3-dicarboxylic acid; AP-5, 2-amino-5-phosphonopentanoic acid; AP-7, 2-amino-7-phosphonoheptanoic acid; CNQX, 6-cyano-7-nitroquinoxaline-2,3-dione; CPP, 3-(2-carboxypirazin-4-yl)-propyl-1-phosphonic acid; epsp, excitatory postsynaptic potential; MCPG, α-methyl-4-carboxyphenylglycine; NBQX, 2,3-dihydro-6-nitro-7-sulfamoyl-benzoquinoxaline. (Other structures are shown in Figure 33.3.)

[a]Structures of experimental compounds can be found in Brauner-Osborne et al. (J Med Chem 43: 2609–2645, 2002).

[b]Ampakine is a term invented to describe a number of compounds that appear to enhance the action of AMPA receptor agonists.

have much higher permeability to Ca^{2+} than the others, which has important functional consequences (see Ch. 4). The metabotropic receptors are G-protein–coupled receptors linked to intracellular second messenger systems (see Ch. 3; Conn & Pin, 1997), and comprise eight subtypes in three main classes (Table 33.1). They are unusual in showing no sequence homology with other G-protein–coupled receptors. They possess a very large extracellular N-terminal tail (class C; see Table 3.2), which contains the glutamate-binding site, in contrast to most amine receptors (class A), in which the agonist binding site is buried among the transmembrane helices (Ch. 3).

Binding studies show that glutamate receptors are most abundant in the cortex, basal ganglia and sensory pathways. NMDA and AMPA receptors are generally colocalised, but kainate receptors have a much more restricted distribution. Expression of the many different receptor subtypes in the brain also shows distinct regional differences, but we have hardly begun to understand the significance of this extreme organisational complexity.

SPECIAL FEATURES OF NMDA RECEPTORS

The NMDA receptors and their associated channels have been studied in more detail than the other types and show special pharmacological properties, summarised in Figure 33.4, which are postulated to play a role in pathophysiological mechanisms.

- They are highly permeable to Ca^{2+}, as well as to other cations, so activation of NMDA receptors is particularly effective in promoting Ca^{2+} entry.
- They are readily blocked by Mg^{2+}, and this block shows marked voltage dependence. It occurs at physiological Mg^{2+} concentrations when the cell is normally polarised, but disappears if the cell is depolarised.
- Activation of NMDA receptors requires **glycine** as well as glutamate (Fig. 33.5). The binding site for glycine is distinct

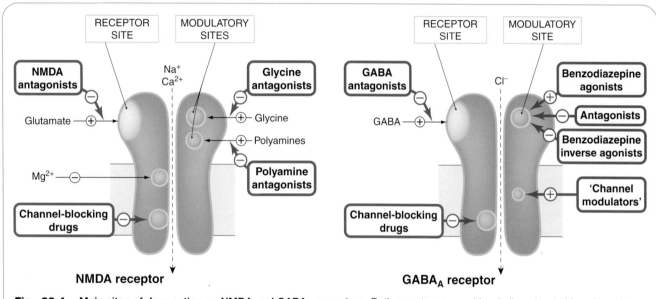

Fig. 33.4   Main sites of drug action on NMDA and GABA$_A$ receptors. Both receptors are multimeric ligand-gated ion channels. Drugs can act as agonists or antagonists at the neurotransmitter receptor site or at modulatory sites associated with the receptor. They can also act to block the ion channel at one or more distinct sites. In the case of the GABA$_A$ receptor, the mechanism by which 'channel modulators' (e.g. ethanol, anaesthetic agents) facilitate channel opening is uncertain; they may affect both ligand binding and channel sites. The location of the different binding sites shown in the figure is largely imaginary, although study of mutated receptors is beginning to reveal where they actually reside. Examples of the different drug classes are given in Tables 33.1 and 33.2.

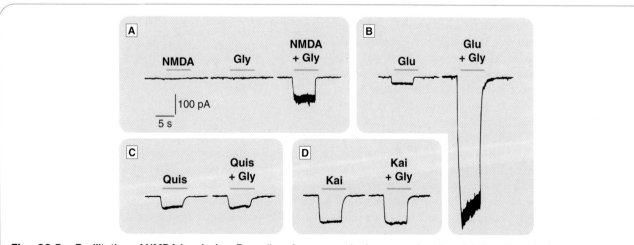

Fig. 33.5   Facilitation of NMDA by glycine. Recordings from mouse brain neurons in culture (whole-cell patch clamp technique). Downward deflections represent inward current through excitatory amino acid–activated ion channels. **A** NMDA (10 μmol/l) or glycine (1 μmol/l) applied separately had little or no effect, but together produced a response. **B** The response to glutamate (10 μmol/l, Glu) was strongly potentiated by glycine (1 μmol/l, Gly). C and D. Responses of AMPA and kainate receptors to quisqualate (Quis) and kainate (Kai) were unaffected by glycine. (From Johnson J W, Ascher P 1987 Nature 325: 529–531.)

from the glutamate-binding site, and both have to be occupied for the channel to open. This discovery caused a stir, because glycine had hitherto been recognised as an inhibitory transmitter (see below), so to find it facilitating excitation ran counter to the prevailing doctrine. The concentration of glycine required depends on the subunit composition of the NMDA receptor; for some NMDA receptor subtypes, physiological variation of the glycine concentration may serve as a regulatory mechanism, whereas others are fully activated at all physiological glycine concentrations. Competitive antagonists at the glycine site (see Table 33.1) indirectly inhibit the action of glutamate. Recently (see Miller, 2004), a surprising molecule,[4] namely **D-serine**, has been found to activate the NMDA receptor via the glycine site and to be released from astrocytes.

- Certain well-known anaesthetic and psychotomimetic agents, such as **ketamine** (Ch. 36) and **phencyclidine** (Ch. 42), are selective blocking agents for NMDA-operated channels. The experimental compound **dizocilpine** (codename MK801) shares this property.
- Certain endogenous polyamines (e.g. **spermine**, **spermidine**) act on a different accessory site to facilitate channel opening. The experimental drugs **ifenprodil** and **eliprodil** block their action.

FUNCTIONAL ROLE OF GLUTAMATE RECEPTORS

The AMPA receptors, and in certain brain regions kainate receptors (see Bleakman & Lodge, 1998), serve to mediate fast excitatory synaptic transmission in the CNS—absolutely essential for our brains to function. Kainate receptors also have a presynaptic role (see Huettner, 2003). AMPA receptors occur on astrocytes as well as on neurons, and these cells (see Ch. 32) play an important role in communication in the brain. NMDA receptors (which often coexist with AMPA receptors) contribute a slow component to the excitatory synaptic potential (Fig. 33.6), the magnitude of which varies in different pathways. Metabotropic glutamate receptors are linked either to inositol trisphosphate production and release of intracellular Ca^{2+}, or to inhibition of adenylyl cyclase (see Ch. 3). They are located both pre- and postsynaptically, like other glutamate receptors, and also occur on astrocytes. Their effects on transmission are modulatory rather than direct, comprising mainly postsynaptic excitatory effects (by inhibition of potassium channels) and presynaptic inhibition (by inhibition of calcium channels).

In general, it appears that NMDA and metabotropic receptors play a particular role in long-term adaptive and pathological changes in the brain, and are of particular interest as potential drug targets. AMPA/kainate receptors, on the other hand, are mainly responsible for fast excitatory transmission, and if they are fully

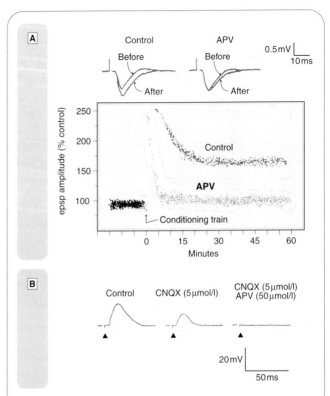

Fig. 33.6 **Effects of excitatory amino acid receptor antagonists on synaptic transmission.** Ⓐ APV (NMDA antagonist) prevents long-term potentiation (LTP) in the rat hippocampus without affecting the fast excitatory postsynaptic potential (epsp). Top records show the extracellularly recorded fast epsp (downward deflection) before, and 50 minutes after, a conditioning train of stimuli (100 Hz for 2 s). The presence of LTP in the control preparation is indicated by the increase in epsp amplitude. In the presence of APV (50 μmol/l), the normal epsp is unchanged, but LTP does not occur. Lower trace shows epsp amplitude as a function of time. The conditioning train produces a short-lasting increase in epsp amplitude, which still occurs in the presence of APV, but the long-lasting effect is prevented. Ⓑ Block of fast and slow components of epsp by CNQX (6-cyano-7-nitroquinoxaline-2,3-dione; AMPA receptor antagonist) and APV (NMDA receptor antagonist). The epsp (upward deflection) in a hippocampal neuron recorded with intracellular electrode is partly blocked by CNQX (5 μmol/l), leaving behind a slow component, which is blocked by APV (50 μmol/l). (From: (A) Malinow R, Madison D, Tsien R W 1988 Nature 335: 821; (B) Andreasen M, Lambert J D, Jensen M S 1989 J Physiol 414: 317–336.)

blocked, brain function shuts down entirely; nevertheless, they too are involved in synaptic plasticity.

Two aspects of glutamate receptor function are of particular pathophysiological importance, namely *synaptic plasticity*, discussed here, and *excitotoxicity* (discussed in Ch. 35).

SYNAPTIC PLASTICITY AND LONG-TERM POTENTIATION

Synaptic plasticity is a general term to describe long-term changes in synaptic connectivity and efficacy, either following physiological

---

[4]Surprising, because it is the 'wrong' enantiomer for amino acids of higher organisms. Nevertheless, vertebrates possess specific enzymes and transporters for this D amino acid, which is abundant in the brain.

alterations in neuronal activity (as in learning and memory), or resulting from pathological disturbances (as in epilepsy, chronic pain or drug dependence). Synaptic plasticity underlies much of what we call 'brain function', and understanding it has been a Holy Grail for neurobiologists for decades. Needless to say, no single mechanism is responsible; however, one significant and much-studied[5] component is *long-term potentiation* (*LTP*), a phenomenon in which glutamate and NMDA receptors play a central role.

Long-term potentiation (see Malenka & Nicoll, 1999; Bennett, 2000) is a long-lasting (hours in vitro, days or weeks in vivo) enhancement of synaptic transmission that occurs at various CNS synapses following a short (conditioning) burst of high-frequency presynaptic stimulation. Its counterpart is *long-term depression*, which is produced by a longer train of stimuli at lower frequency. These phenomena have been studied in great detail in the hippocampus (Fig. 33.6), which plays a central role in learning and memory. It has been argued that 'learning', in the synaptic sense, can occur if synaptic strength is enhanced following *simultaneous* activity in both pre- and postsynaptic neurons. LTP shows this characteristic; it does not occur if presynaptic activity fails to excite the postsynaptic neuron, or if the latter is activated independently, for instance by a different presynaptic input. Thus LTP initiation involves both the presynaptic and postsynaptic components, and it results from enhanced activation of AMPA receptors at EAA synapses. The facilitatory process also appears to involve both pre- and postsynaptic elements (although the small-print argument rumbles on about whether increased transmitter release does or does not occur in LTP); the response of postsynaptic AMPA receptors to glutamate is increased, and so (probably) is glutamate release. Increased expression and trafficking of AMPA receptors to synaptic sites also occurs. The following experimental results have led to the model shown in Figure 33.7, in which activation of NMDA receptors and metabotropic glutamate receptors indirectly sensitises AMPA receptors.

- NMDA antagonists prevent LTP, without affecting normal, non-potentiated transmission (which depends on AMPA receptors). Disruption of the NMDA receptor gene has the same effect.
- LTP occurs only if the postsynaptic cell is depolarised at the time when the conditioning burst of stimulation is delivered. Blocking AMPA receptors prevents this, and prevents LTP.
- Antagonists at metabotropic glutamate receptors reduce the duration of LTP; LTP is also impaired in transgenic mice lacking the mGluR$_1$ receptor.
- Ca^{2+} entry into the postsynaptic cell is required, and there is evidence that activation of protein kinase C (see Ch. 3), resulting in phosphorylation of AMPA receptors, is involved in the mechanism of potentiation.
- LTP is reduced by agents that block the synthesis or effects of *nitric oxide* or *arachidonic acid*. One or both of these mediators may be the hitherto elusive 'retrograde messenger' through which events in the postsynaptic cell are able to

influence the presynaptic nerve terminal. *Anandamide*, released by the postsynaptic cell, may also play a role by reducing the release of GABA from inhibitory nerve endings (see Ch. 15).

▼ Two special properties of the NMDA receptor and channel underlie its involvement in LTP, namely voltage-dependent channel block by Mg^{2+} and its high Ca^{2+} permeability. At normal membrane potentials, the NMDA channel is blocked by Mg^{2+}; a sustained postsynaptic depolarisation produced by glutamate acting repeatedly on AMPA receptors, however, removes the Mg^{2+} block, and NMDA receptor activation then allows Ca^{2+} to enter the cell. The metabotropic EAA receptor also contributes to the increase in [Ca^{2+}]$_i$. This rise in [Ca^{2+}]$_i$ in the postsynaptic cell activates protein kinases, phospholipases and nitric oxide synthase, which act jointly (by mechanisms that are not fully understood) to facilitate transmission via AMPA receptors. Initially, during the *induction phase* of LTP, phosphorylation of AMPA receptors increases their responsiveness to glutamate. Later, during the *maintenance phase*, more AMPA receptors are recruited to the postsynaptic membrane as a result of altered receptor trafficking; later still, various other mediators and signalling pathways are activated, causing structural changes and leading to a permanent increase in the number of synaptic contacts.

Although LTP is well established as a synaptic phenomenon, its relationship to learning and memory remains controversial (although the evidence is suggestive). For example, NMDA receptor antagonists applied to the hippocampus impair learning in rats; also, 'saturation' of LTP by electrical stimulation of the hippocampus has been found to impair the ability of rats to learn how to navigate a maze. Furthermore, LTP-like changes have been detected after learning has taken place. Thus there is hope that drugs capable of enhancing LTP may improve learning and memory.

Long-term potentiation is just one manifestation of synaptic plasticity, whereby neuronal connections respond to changes in the activity of the nervous system. Other phenomena, including short-term potentiation and long-term depression, also occur, and they too appear to involve glutamate receptors (see Malenka & Nicoll, 1993). LTP and long-term depression are not confined to hippocampal regions involved in learning and memory, but occur throughout the CNS. Glutamate receptors play a central role in all cases so far studied, but other mediators, such as endocannabinoids, may also be involved (see Malenka & Bear, 2004).

DRUGS ACTING ON GLUTAMATE RECEPTORS

ANTAGONISTS

Much effort, based on the work of Watkins and his colleagues, has gone into the search for selective glutamate antagonists, partly to provide tools for better understanding the physiological roles of the different types of EAA receptor, and partly as potential therapeutic agents with which to treat, for example, epilepsy, psychiatric and neurodegenerative disorders.

The main types of EAA antagonists are shown in Table 33.1. They are selective for the main receptor types but generally not for specific subtypes. Many of these compounds, although very useful as experimental tools in vitro, are unable to penetrate the blood–brain barrier, so they are not effective when given systemically.

NMDA receptors, as discussed above, require glycine as well as NMDA to activate them, so blocking of the glycine site is an alternative way to produce antagonism. **Kynurenic acid** and the more potent analogue **7-chloro-kynurenic acid** act in this way, as do various compounds currently in development.

Another site of block is the channel itself, where various substances act, for example **ketamine** and **phencyclidine**. **Dizocilpine**, **remacemide** and **memantine** are more recent

---

[5]A recent review noted that over 3000 papers on LTP were published during the 1990s, nearly one per day. Which is a lot!

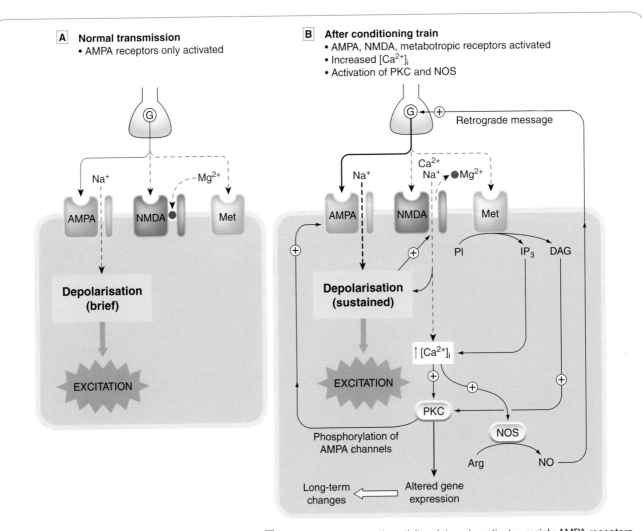

Fig. 33.7 Mechanisms of long-term potentiation. **A** With infrequent synaptic activity, glutamate activates mainly AMPA receptors. There is insufficient glutamate to activate metabotropic receptors, and NMDA receptor channels are blocked by Mg^{2+}. **B** After a conditioning train of stimuli, enough glutamate is released to activate metabotropic receptors, and NMDA channels are unblocked by the sustained depolarisation. The resulting increase in $[Ca^{2+}]_i$ activates various enzymes, including the following.

- Protein kinase C (PKC) phosphorylates various proteins, including AMPA receptors (causing facilitation of transmitter action) and other signal transduction molecules controlling gene transcription (not shown) in the postsynaptic cell.
- Nitric oxide synthase (NOS). Release of nitric oxide (NO) facilitates glutamate release (retrograde signalling, otherwise known as NO turning back).
- Phospholipase A_2 (not shown) catalyses the formation of arachidonic acid (Ch. 13), a retrograde messenger that increases presynaptic glutamate release.
- A phospholipase (NAPE-PLD, not shown) that catalyses production of the endocannabinoid, anandamide (Ch. 15). Anandamide appears to act on GABAergic inhibitory nerve terminals, enhancing transmission by suppressing GABA release. A, AMPA receptor; DAG, diacylglycerol; G, glutamate; IP_3, inositol (1,4,5) triphosphate; Met, metabotropic receptor; N, NMDA receptor; PI, phosphatidylinositol.

examples. These agents are lipid-soluble and thus able to cross the blood–brain barrier.

The potential therapeutic interest in glutamate antagonists lies mainly in the reduction of brain damage following strokes and head injury (Ch. 35), as well as in the treatment of epilepsy (Ch. 40) and of Alzheimer's disease (Ch. 35). They have also been considered for indications, such as drug dependence (Ch. 43) and schizophrenia (Ch. 38), where the rationale is less clear. Trials with NMDA antagonists and channel blockers have so far proved disappointing, and a serious drawback of these agents is their tendency to cause hallucinatory and other disturbances (also a

feature of phencyclidine; Ch. 42). Only two NMDA receptor antagonists, ketamine (anaesthesia and analgesia; see Chs 36 and 41) and memantine (Alzheimer's disease; Ch. 35) are in clinical use. Glycine site antagonists may have fewer unwanted effects, and experimental compounds have been tested in clinical trials for conditions such as stroke and epilepsy (see Jansen & Dannhart, 2003); the results have been inconclusive. AMPA receptor antagonists seem unpromising as therapeutic agents, because the available agents (as might be expected) produce overall CNS depression, including respiratory depression and motor incoordination, with little margin of safety. Only if subtype selectivity can be achieved is this approach likely to succeed. Against this unpromising background, antagonists at metabotropic receptors may offer the best hope (see Nicoletti et al., 1996), but such compounds are not yet available for clinical use.

Overall, the promise foreseen for glutamate receptor ligands in the clinic has simply not, so far, been fulfilled. The problem may be that glutamate is such a ubiquitous and multifunctional mediator—involved, it seems, in almost every aspect of brain function—that attempting to improve specific malfunction by flooding the brain with a compound that affects the glutamate system in some way is just too crude a strategy.

AGONISTS AND POSITIVE MODULATORS

Various agonists at EAA receptors that are used experimentally are shown in Table 33.1. From the clinical perspective, interest centres on the theory that positive AMPA receptor modulators, which act by reducing receptor desensitisation, may improve memory and cognitive performance. **Cyclothiazide**, a compound related to **thiazide diuretics** (Ch. 24), acts in this way but is toxic; drugs such as **piracetam** and **aniracetam**, which are used in dementia (not routinely, at least in the UK) (Ch. 35) also sensitise AMPA receptors, although it is not certain that this accounts for their psychotropic effects. Other so-called ampakines are in development as possible drugs for improving cognitive performance.

γ-AMINOBUTYRIC ACID

GABA is the main inhibitory transmitter in the brain. In the spinal cord and brain stem, glycine is also important.

SYNTHESIS, STORAGE AND FUNCTION

GABA occurs in brain tissue but not in other mammalian tissues, except in trace amounts. It is particularly abundant (about 10 μmol/g tissue) in the nigrostriatal system, but occurs at lower concentrations (2–5 μmol/g) throughout the grey matter.

GABA is formed from glutamate (Fig. 33.1) by the action of *glutamic acid decarboxylase (GAD)*, an enzyme found only in GABA-synthesising neurons in the brain. Immunohistochemical labelling of GAD is used to map the GABA pathways in the brain. GABA is destroyed by a transamination reaction in which the amino group is transferred to α-oxoglutaric acid (to yield glutamate), with the production of succinic semialdehyde and then succinic acid. This reaction is catalysed by *GABA transaminase*, which is inhibited by **vigabatrine**, a compound used to treat epilepsy (Ch. 40). GABAergic neurons and astrocytes take up GABA via specific transporters, and it is this, rather than GABA transaminase, which removes the GABA after it has been released. GABA transport is inhibited by **guvacine** and **nipecotic acid**.

GABA functions as an inhibitory transmitter in many different CNS pathways. About 20% of CNS neurons are GABAergic; most are short interneurons, but long GABAergic tracts run to the cerebellum and striatum. The widespread distribution of GABA, and the fact that virtually all neurons are sensitive to its

---

Excitatory amino acids

- Excitatory amino acids (EAAs), namely glutamate, aspartate, and possibly homocysteate, are the main fast excitatory transmitters in the central nervous system.
- Glutamate is formed mainly from the Krebs cycle intermediate α-oxoglutarate by the action of GABA transaminase.
- There are four main EAA receptor subtypes:
  — NMDA
  — AMPA
  — kainate
  — metabotropic.
- NMDA, AMPA and kainate receptors are ionotropic receptors regulating cation channels; metabotropic receptors are G-protein–coupled receptors and act through intracellular second messengers. There are many molecular subtypes within each class.
- The channels controlled by NMDA receptors are highly permeable to Ca^{2+} and are blocked by Mg^{2+}.
- AMPA and kainate receptors are involved in fast excitatory transmission; NMDA receptors mediate slower excitatory responses and, through their effect in controlling Ca^{2+} entry, play a more complex role in controlling synaptic plasticity (e.g. long-term potentiation).
- Competitive NMDA receptor antagonists include AP-5 (2-amino-5-phosphonopentanoic acid) and CPP (3-(2-carboxypirazin-4-yl)-propyl-1-phosphonic acid); the NMDA-operated ion channel is blocked by dizocilpine, as well as by the psychotomimetic drugs ketamine and phencyclidine.
- CNQX (6-cyano-7-nitroquinoxaline-2,3-dione) is a selective AMPA receptor antagonist.
- NMDA receptors require low concentrations of glycine as a coagonist, in addition to glutamate; 7-chlorokynurenate blocks this action of glycine.
- NMDA receptor activation is increased by endogenous polyamines, such as spermine, acting on a modulatory site that is blocked by ifenprodil.
- The entry of excessive amounts of Ca^{2+} produced by NMDA receptor activation can result in cell death—excitotoxicity (see Ch. 35).
- Metabotropic receptors are dimeric G-protein–coupled receptors linked to inositol trisphosphate formation and intracellular Ca^{2+} release. They play a part in glutamate-mediated synaptic plasticity and excitotoxicity. Specific agonists and antagonists are known.
- EAA receptor antagonists have yet to be developed for clinical use.

inhibitory effect, suggests that its function is ubiquitous in the brain. GABA serves as a transmitter at about 30% of all the synapses in the CNS.

GABA RECEPTORS: STRUCTURE AND PHARMACOLOGY

GABA acts on two distinct types of receptor, one (the *GABA_A receptor*) being a ligand-gated channel, the other (*GABA_B*) being a G-protein–coupled receptor.[6] GABA_A receptors (see Barnard, 2000) belong to the same structural class as nicotinic acetylcholine receptors (see Fig. 3.18). They are pentamers, most of them composed of three different subunits (α, β, γ), each of which can exist in three to six molecular subtypes. There are a great many possible permutations, of which one ($\alpha_1\beta_2\gamma_2$) is by far the most abundant overall, although dozens of other functional variants are expressed in specific regions—a familiar pattern of heterogeneity typical of neurotransmitter receptors. We so far have only a rudimentary understanding of their functional roles (see Mody & Pearce, 2004).

GABA_A receptors located postsynaptically mediate fast postsynaptic inhibition, the channel being selectively permeable to Cl⁻. GABA_A receptors located perisynaptically are responsible for slow inhibitory effects produced by GABA diffusing further from its site of release. Thus GABA produces inhibition by acting both as a fast 'point-to-point' transmitter and as an 'action-at-a-distance' neuromodulator. It is possible that different GABA_A receptor subtypes are involved in these two modes. Because the equilibrium membrane potential for Cl⁻ is usually negative to the resting potential, increasing Cl⁻ permeability hyperpolarises the cell, thereby reducing its excitability.[7]

GABA_B receptors (see Bettler et al., 2004) are located pre- and postsynaptically, and they are typical G-protein–coupled receptors, but unusual in that the functional receptor is a dimer consisting of two different subunits (see Ch. 3). Apart from minor splice variants, only a single isoform is known—also unusual among G-protein–coupled receptors. GABA_B receptors exert their effects by inhibiting voltage-gated calcium channels (thus reducing transmitter release) and by opening potassium channels (thus reducing postsynaptic excitability), these actions resulting from inhibition of adenylyl cyclase.

It is believed that glutamate and GABA, and their receptors, evolved very early, so these receptors probably represent the venerable aristocrats from which upstarts such as the neuropeptide receptors evolved much later.

DRUGS ACTING ON GABA RECEPTORS
GABA_A RECEPTORS

GABA_A receptors resemble NMDA receptors in that drugs may act at several different sites (Fig. 33.4; see Johnston, 1996). These include:

- the GABA-binding site
- several modulatory sites
- the ion channel.

There is growing evidence that the different receptor subtypes differ in their pharmacological properties but, with the exception of benzodiazepines (see below), the picture is far from clear.

GABA_A receptors are the target for several important centrally acting drugs, notably **benzodiazepines**, **barbiturates** and **neurosteroids** (see below). **General anaesthetics** (Ch. 36) also act on GABA_A receptors, as well as on other targets. The main agonists, antagonists and modulatory substances that act on GABA receptors are shown in Table 33.2.

Muscimol, derived from a hallucinogenic mushroom, resembles GABA chemically and is a powerful GABA_A receptor agonist. A synthetic analogue, **gaboxadol** (previously known as THIP from its chemical structure) is a partial agonist in development as a hypnotic drug (Ch. 37). **Bicuculline**, a naturally occurring convulsant compound, is a specific antagonist that blocks the fast inhibitory synaptic potential in most CNS synapses. **Gabazine**, a synthetic GABA analogue, is similar. These compounds are useful experimental tools but have no therapeutic uses.

Benzodiazepines, which have powerful sedative and anxiolytic effects (see Ch. 37), selectively potentiate the effects of GABA on GABA_A receptors. They bind with high affinity to an accessory site (the 'benzodiazepine receptor') on the GABA_A receptor, in such a way that the binding of GABA is facilitated and its agonist effect is enhanced. Studies on recombinant GABA_A receptors have shown that a small region of the γ subunit confers benzodiazepine sensitivity, and mutations in this region affect the level of constitutive activity (see Ch. 2) at this site, and its sensitivity to benzodiazepines.[8] Association with particular α subunits is also required. Thus not all GABA_A receptors are affected by benzodiazepines. Sedative benzodiazepines, such as **diazepam**, are agonists (enhancing the action of GABA), whereas convulsant analogues, such as **flumazenil** (Ch. 37) are antagonists or inverse agonists.

Modulators that also enhance the action of GABA, but whose site of action is less well defined than that of benzodiazepines (shown as 'channel modulators' in Fig. 33.4), include other CNS depressants such as **barbiturates** (see Ch. 37), anaesthetic agents (Ch. 36) and neurosteroids. Neurosteroids (see Lambert et al., 2003) are compounds that are related to steroid hormones but

---

[6]A third class, GABA_C, has recently been proposed (see Bormann, 2000). Closely resembling GABA_A receptors in their structure and function, GABA_C receptors are constructed from a different family of subunits (termed *p*), and have slightly different pharmacological properties. Their functional significance remains unknown.

[7]During early brain development (in which GABA plays an important role), and also in some regions of the adult brain, GABA has an excitatory rather than an inhibitory effect, because the intracellular Cl⁻ concentration is relatively high, so that the equilibrium potential is positive to the resting membrane potential.

[8]Interestingly, there is evidence from transgenic animals, in which specific GABA_A receptor subunits were knocked out, that the anxiolytic and sedative effects of benzodiazepines are separable in terms of their molecular targets (see Rudolph et al., 2001), a discovery with important implications for the development of improved anxiolytic drugs.

Table 33.2 Properties of inhibitory amino acid receptors

	GABA$_A$			GABA$_B$	Glycine
	Receptor site	*Modulatory site (benzodiazepine)*	*Modulatory site (others)*		
Endogenous agonist(s)	GABA	?Diazepam-binding inhibitor	Various neurosteroids (e.g. progesterone metabolites)	GABA	Glycine β-Alanine Taurine
Other agonist(s)	Muscimol Gaboxadol (THIP^a, partial agonist)	Anxiolytic benzodiazepines (e.g. diazepam)	Barbiturates Steroid anaesthetics (e.g. alphaxolone)	Baclofen	–
Antagonist(s)	Bicuculline Gabazine	Flumazenil	–	Phaclofen CGP 35348 and others	Strychnine
Channel blocker	Picrotoxin			Not applicable	–
Effector mechanism(s)	Ligand-gated chloride channel			G-protein–coupled receptor; inhibition of adenylyl cyclase	Ligand-gated chloride channel
Location	Widespread; mainly GABAergic interneurons			Pre- and postsynaptic Widespread	Postsynaptic Mainly in brain stem and spinal cord
Function	Postsynaptic inhibition (fast ipsp)			Presynaptic inhibition (decreased Ca^{2+} entry) Postsynaptic inhibition (increased K$^+$ permeability)	Postsynaptic inhibition (fast ipsp)

ipsp, inhibitory postsynaptic potential.
^{a}THIP is an abbreviation of the chemical name of gaboxadol.

that act (like benzodiazepines) to enhance activation of GABA$_A$ receptors as well as on conventional intracellular steroid receptors. Interestingly, they include metabolites of progesterone and androgens that are formed in the nervous system, and are believed to have a physiological role. Synthetic neurosteroids include **alphaxolone**, developed as an anaesthetic agent (Ch. 36). Another putative endogenous modulator of GABA-mediated transmission is a peptide, *diazepam binding inhibitor*, which occurs in the brain and elsewhere but whose physiological role is unclear.

Picrotoxin (Ch. 42) is a convulsant that acts by blocking the chloride channel associated with the GABA$_A$ receptor, thus blocking the postsynaptic inhibitory effect of GABA. It has no therapeutic uses.

GABA$_B$ RECEPTORS

When the importance of GABA as an inhibitory transmitter was recognised, it was thought that a GABA-like substance might prove to be effective in controlling epilepsy and other convulsive states; because GABA itself fails to penetrate the blood–brain barrier, more lipophilic GABA analogues were sought, one of which, **baclofen**, was introduced in 1972. Unlike GABA, baclofen has little postsynaptic inhibitory effect, and its actions are not blocked by bicuculline. These findings led to the recognition

of the GABA$_B$ receptor, for which baclofen is a selective agonist (see Bowery, 1993). Baclofen is used to treat spasticity and related motor disorders (Ch. 37).

Competitive antagonists for the GABA$_B$ receptor include a number of experimental compounds (e.g. **saclofen** and more potent compounds with improved brain penetration, such as **CGP 35348**). Tests in animals have shown that these compounds produce only slight effects on CNS function (in contrast to the powerful convulsant effects of GABA$_A$ antagonists). The main effect observed, paradoxically, was an antiepileptic action, specifically in an animal model of absence seizures (see Ch. 37), together with enhanced cognitive performance. Whether such compounds will prove to have therapeutic uses remains to be seen.

γ-HYDROXYBUTYRATE

▼ γ-Hydroxybutyrate (see Wong et al., 2004) occurs naturally in the brain as a side product of GABA synthesis. As a synthetic drug from 1960 onwards, it has found favour with bodybuilders, based on its ability to evoke the release of growth hormone, and with party-goers, based on its euphoric and disinhibitory effects. In common with many abused drugs (see Ch. 43), it activates 'reward pathways' in the brain, and its use is now illegal in most countries. The pharmacological properties of GHB are not well understood, although it is believed to activate GABA$_B$ receptors, partly through conversion to GABA, and may also bind to specific GHB receptor sites, of which little is known.

GLYCINE

▼ Glycine is present in particularly high concentration (5 µmol/g) in the grey matter of the spinal cord. Applied ionophoretically to motor neurons or interneurons, it produces an inhibitory hyperpolarisation that is indistinguishable from the inhibitory synaptic response. **Strychnine** (see Ch. 42), a convulsant poison that acts mainly on the spinal cord, blocks both the synaptic inhibitory response and the response to glycine. This, together with direct measurements of glycine release in response to nerve stimulation, provides strong evidence for its physiological transmitter role. β-**Alanine** has pharmacological effects and a pattern of distribution very similar to those of glycine, but its action is not blocked by strychnine.

The inhibitory effect of glycine is quite distinct from its role in facilitating activation of NMDA receptors (see p. 483).

The glycine receptor (see Laube et al., 2002) resembles the GABA$_A$ receptor; it is a multimeric ligand-gated chloride channel, of which a number of subtypes have been identified by cloning, and mutations of the receptor have been identified in some inherited neurological disorders associated with muscle spasm and reflex hyperexcitability. There are no therapeutic drugs that act specifically by modifying glycinergic transmission, although it turns out that many of the compounds (such as benzodiazepines and anaesthetic agents) that enhance GABA$_A$ receptor activation act similarly on glycine receptors. **Tetanus toxin**, a bacterial toxin resembling **botulinum toxin** (Ch. 10), acts selectively to prevent glycine release from inhibitory interneurons in the spinal cord, causing excessive reflex hyperexcitability and violent muscle spasms (lockjaw).

CONCLUDING REMARKS

The study of amino acids and their receptors in the brain has been one of the most active fields of research in the past two decades, and the amount of information available is prodigious. These signalling systems have been speculatively implicated in almost every kind of neurological and psychiatric disorder, and the pharmaceutical industry has put a great deal of effort into identifying specific ligands—agonists, antagonists, modulators, enzyme inhibitors, transport inhibitors—designed to influence them. However, despite a large number of pharmacologically unimpeachable compounds having emerged, and many clinical trials having been undertaken, there have been no major therapeutic breakthroughs. The optimistic view is that a better understanding of the particular functions of the many molecular subtypes of these targets, and the design of more subtype-specific ligands, will lead to future breakthroughs. Expectations have, however, undoubtedly dimmed in recent years.

Inhibitory amino acids: GABA and glycine

- GABA is the main inhibitory transmitter in the brain.
- It is present fairly uniformly throughout the brain; there is very little in peripheral tissues.
- GABA is formed from glutamate by the action of glutamic acid decarboxylase. Its action is terminated mainly by reuptake, but also by deamination, catalysed by GABA transaminase.
- There are two types of GABA receptor: GABA$_A$ and GABA$_B$.
- GABA$_A$ receptors, which occur mainly postsynaptically, are directly coupled to chloride channels, the opening of which reduces membrane excitability. Muscimol is a specific GABA$_A$ agonist, and the convulsant bicuculline is an antagonist.
- Other drugs that interact with GABA$_A$ receptors and channels include:
  - benzodiazepine tranquillisers, which act at an accessory binding site to facilitate the action of GABA
  - convulsants such as picrotoxin, which block the anion channel
  - neurosteroids, including endogenous progesterone metabolites, and other CNS depressants, such as barbiturates and some general anaesthetic agents, which facilitate the action of GABA.
- GABA$_B$ receptors are G-protein–coupled receptors linked to inhibition of cAMP formation. They cause pre- and postsynaptic inhibition by inhibiting calcium channel opening and increasing K$^+$ conductance. Baclofen is a GABA$_B$ receptor agonist used to treat spasticity. GABA$_B$ antagonists are not yet in clinical use.
- Glycine is an inhibitory transmitter mainly in the spinal cord, acting on its own receptor, structurally and functionally similar to the GABA$_A$ receptor.
- The convulsant drug strychnine is a competitive glycine antagonist. Tetanus toxin acts mainly by interfering with glycine release.

REFERENCES AND FURTHER READING

Excitatory amino acids

Bleakman D, Lodge D 1998 Neuropharmacology of AMPA and kainate receptors. Neuropharmacology 37: 187–204 (*Review giving molecular and functional information on these receptors*)

Conn P J, Pin J-P 1997 Pharmacology and functions of metabotropic glutamate receptors. Annu Rev Pharmacol 37: 205–237

Cotman C W, Kahle J S, Miller S E et al. 1995 Excitatory amino acid transmission. In: Bloom F E,

Kupfer D J (eds) Psychopharmacology: a fourth generation of progress. Raven Press, New York, pp. 75–85

Dingledine R, Borges K, Bowie D, Traynelis S F 1999 The glutamate receptor ion channels. Pharmacol Rev 51: 8–61 (*Comprehensive review focusing on molecular aspects, with section on potential therapeutic applications*)

Huettner J E 2003 Kainate receptors and synaptic transmission. Prog Neurobiol 70: 387–407. (*Review of

the role of pre- and postsynaptic kainate receptors at CNS synapses*)

Jansen M, Dannhart G 2003 Antagonists and agonists at the glycine site of the NMDA receptor for therapeutic applications. Eur J Med Chem 38: 661–670 (*Update on efforts to develop glycine site ligands for clinical use*)

Javitt D C 2004 Glutamate as a therapeutic target in psychiatric disorders. Mol Psychiatry 9: 984–997 (*Summary of glutamate receptor subtypes, with *speculation about their possible relevance to psychiatric disorders*)

Nicoletti F, Bruno V, Copani A et al. 1996 Metabotropic glutamate receptors: a new target for the therapy of neurodegenerative disorders? Trends Neurosci 19: 267–271

Shigeri Y, Seal R P, Shimamoto K 2004 Molecular pharmacology of glutamate transporters. Brain Res Rev 45: 250–265

Takahashi M, Billups B, Rossi D et al. 1997 The role of glutamate transporters in glutamate homeostasis in the brain. J Exp Biol 200: 401–409

Watkins J C, Jane D E 2006 The glutamate story. Br J Pharmacol 147(suppl 1): S100–S108 (*A brief and engaging history by one of the pioneers in the discovery of glutamate as a CNS transmitter*)

Inhibitory amino acids

Barnard E A 2000 The molecular architecture of $GABA_A$ receptors. In: Möhler H (ed) Pharmacology of GABA and glycine neurotransmission. Handbook of experimental pharmacology 150. Springer-Verlag, Berlin, pp. 79–100 (*Authoritative review on the molecular subtypes of $GABA_A$ receptors*)

Bettler B, Kaupmann K, Mosbacher J, Gassmann M 2004 Molecular structure and function of $GABA_B$ receptors. Physiol Rev 84: 835–867 (*Comprehensive*

review article by the team that first cloned the $GABA_B$ receptor and discovered its unusual heterodimeric structure)

Bormann J 2000 The ABC of GABA receptors. Trends Pharmacol Sci 21: 16–19 (*Discussion about the putative $GABA_C$ receptor, mainly a taxonomic dispute at this stage*)

Bowery N G 1993 $GABA_B$ receptor pharmacology. Annu Rev Pharmacol Toxicol 33: 109–147

Johnston G A R 1996 $GABA_A$-receptor pharmacology. Pharmacol Ther 69: 173–198

Lambert J J, Belelli D, Peden D R et al. 2003 Neurosteroid modulation of $GABA_A$ receptors. Prog Neurobiol 71: 67–80

Laube B, Maksay G, Schemm R, Betz H 2002 Modulation of glycine receptor function: a novel approach for therapeutic intervention at inhibitory synapses? Trends Pharmacol Sci 23: 519–527 (*Short review that focuses on pharmacological properties of glycine receptors*)

Mody I, Pearce R A 2004 Diversity of inhibitory transmission through $GABA_A$ receptors. Trends Neurosci 27: 569–575 (*An update on what we know about the functional roles of the many $GABA_A$ receptor subtypes in the brain*)

Rudolph U, Crestani F, Möhler H 2001 $GABA_A$ receptor subtypes: dissecting their pharmacological functions.

Trends Pharmacol Sci 22: 188–194 (*Recent data on transgenic mice with altered $GABA_A$ receptors giving rise to changes in benzodiazepine effects*)

Wong C G T, Gibson K M, Snead O C 2004 From street to brain: neurobiology of the recreational drug γ-hydroxybutyric acid. Trends Pharmacol Sci 25: 29–34 (*Short review article*)

Physiological aspects

Bennett M R 2000 The concept of long term potentiation of transmission at synapses. Prog Neurobiol 60: 109–137 (*An excellent and not overlong review of this complex phenomenon*)

Malenka R C, Bear M F 2004 LTP and LTD: an embarrassment of riches. Neuron 44: 5–21 (*Useful summary of some key experimental data; not for those who want the simple story*)

Malenka R C, Nicoll R A 1993 NMDA-receptor–dependent synaptic plasticity: multiple forms and mechanisms. Trends Neurosci 16: 521–527

Malenka R C, Nicoll R A 1999 Long-term potentiation—a decade of progress? Science 285: 1870–1874 (*A useful update that presents a simple unifying hypothesis*)

Miller R F 2004 D-serine as a glial modulator of nerve cells. Glia 47: 275–283 (*Review of the role of glial-derived D-serine in brain function*)

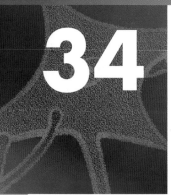

34

Other transmitters and modulators

OVERVIEW

The principal 'amine' transmitters in the central nervous system (CNS), namely noradrenaline dopamine, 5-hydroxytryptamine (5-HT, serotonin) and acetylcholine (ACh), are described in this chapter, with briefer coverage of other mediators, including histamine, melatonin and purines. The monoamines were the first CNS transmitters to be identified, and during the 1960s a combination of neurochemistry and neuropharmacology led to many important discoveries about their role, and

about the ability of drugs to influence these systems. Many of the drugs that are discussed in later chapters owe their effects to mechanisms that are related to these mediators. Amine mediators differ from the amino acid transmitters discussed in Chapter 33 in being localised to small populations of neurons with cell bodies in the brain stem and basal forebrain, which project diffusely to cortical and other areas. These amine-containing neurons function as 'modulatory aerosols', and they are broadly associated with high-level behaviours (e.g. the stereotypic behaviour associated with enhanced dopamine activity; see below), rather than with localised synaptic excitation or inhibition.[1] More recently, some 'atypical' chemical mediators, such as nitric oxide (NO; Ch. 17) and endocannabinoids (Ch. 15) have come on the scene, and they are discussed at the end of the chapter. The other major class of CNS mediators, the neuropeptides, are described in Chapter 16, and information on specific neuropeptides appears in later chapters in this section.

INTRODUCTION

Although we know much about the many different mediators, their cognate receptors, and signalling mechanisms at the cellular level, when describing their effects on brain function we fall back on relatively crude terms—psychopharmacologists will be at our throats for so underrating the sophistication of their measurements—such as 'motor coordination', 'arousal', 'cognitive impairment' and 'exploratory behaviour'. The gap between these two levels of understanding (the Grand Canyon referred to in Ch. 32) still frustrates the best efforts to link drug action at the molecular level to drug action at the therapeutic level. Modern approaches, such as the use of transgenic animal technology (see Ch. 6) and non-invasive imaging techniques, are helping to forge links, but there is still a long way to go.

---

[1]They are, if you like, voices from the nether regions, which make you happy or sad, sleepy or alert, cautious or adventurous, energetic or lazy, although you do not quite know why—very much the stuff of mental illness.

More detail on the content of this chapter can be found in Davis et al. (2002) and Cooper et al. (2003).

NORADRENALINE

The basic processes responsible for the synthesis, storage, release and reuptake of noradrenaline are the same in the brain as in the periphery (Ch. 11), and the same types of adrenoceptor are also found in pre- and postsynaptic locations in the brain.

NORADRENERGIC PATHWAYS IN THE CNS

Although the transmitter role of noradrenaline in the brain was suspected in the 1950s, detailed analysis of its neuronal distribution became possible only when the fluorescence technique, based on the formation of a fluorescent derivative of catecholamines when tissues are exposed to formaldehyde, was devised by Falck and Hillarp. Detailed maps of the pathway of noradrenergic, dopaminergic and serotonergic neurons in laboratory animals were produced and later confirmed in human brains. The cell bodies of noradrenergic neurons occur in small clusters in the pons and medulla, and they send extensively branching axons to many other parts of the brain and spinal cord (Fig. 34.1). The most prominent cluster is the *locus coeruleus (LC)*, located in the pons. Although it contains only about 10 000 neurons in humans, the axons, running in a discrete *medial forebrain bundle,* give rise to many millions of noradrenergic nerve terminals throughout the cortex, hippo-

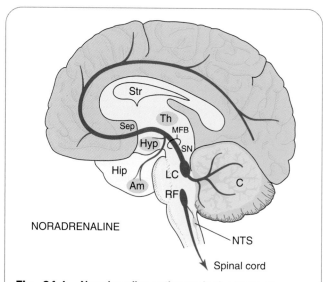

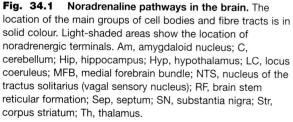

Fig. 34.1 Noradrenaline pathways in the brain. The location of the main groups of cell bodies and fibre tracts is in solid colour. Light-shaded areas show the location of noradrenergic terminals. Am, amygdaloid nucleus; C, cerebellum; Hip, hippocampus; Hyp, hypothalamus; LC, locus coeruleus; MFB, medial forebrain bundle; NTS, nucleus of the tractus solitarius (vagal sensory nucleus); RF, brain stem reticular formation; Sep, septum; SN, substantia nigra; Str, corpus striatum; Th, thalamus.

campus and cerebellum. These nerve terminals do not form distinct synaptic contacts but appear to release transmitter diffusely—justifying the aerosol analogy. The LC is involved in the descending control of pain pathways (Ch. 41, Fig. 41.5).

Other noradrenergic neurons lie close to the LC in the pons and medulla, and project to the hypothalamus, hippocampus and other parts of the forebrain, as well as to the cerebellum and spinal cord. A small cluster of *adrenergic* neurons, which release adrenaline rather than noradrenaline, lies more ventrally in the brain stem, projecting mainly to the pons, medulla and hypothalamus. Rather little is known about them, but they are believed to be important in cardiovascular control.

FUNCTIONAL ASPECTS

Noradrenaline applied to individual neurons usually causes inhibition, and in most cases this is produced by activation of β-adrenoceptors linked to cAMP accumulation. In some situations, however, noradrenaline has an excitatory effect, which is mediated by either α– or β-adrenoceptors and involves other signal transduction pathways (see Chs 3 and 4). See Ashton-Jones (2002) for a recent review.

Arousal and mood

Attention has focused mainly on the LC, which is the source of most of the noradrenaline released in the brain, and from which neuronal activity can be measured by implanted electrodes. LC neurons are silent during sleep, and their activity increases with behavioural arousal. 'Wake-up' stimuli of an unfamiliar or threatening kind excite these neurons much more effectively than familiar stimuli. Amphetamine-like drugs, which release catecholamines in the brain, increase wakefulness, alertness and exploratory activity (although, in this case, firing of LC neurons is actually reduced, by feedback mechanisms; see Ch. 42).

There is a close relationship between mood and state of arousal; depressed individuals are usually lethargic and unresponsive to external stimuli. The catecholamine hypothesis of affective disorders (see Ch. 39) suggested that depression results from a functional deficiency of noradrenaline in certain parts of the brain, while mania results from an excess. This remains controversial, and subsequent findings suggest that 5-HT may be more important than noradrenaline in relation to mood.

Blood pressure regulation

The role of central, as well as peripheral, noradrenergic synapses in blood pressure control is shown by the action of hypotensive drugs such as **clonidine** and **methyldopa** (see Chs 11 and 19), which decrease the discharge of sympathetic nerves emerging from the CNS. They cause hypotension when injected locally into the medulla or fourth ventricle, in much smaller amounts than are required when the drugs are given systemically. Noradrenaline and other α$_2$-adrenoceptor agonists have the same effect when injected locally. Noradrenergic synapses in the medulla probably form part of the baroreceptor reflex pathway, because stimulation or antagonism of α$_2$-adrenoceptors in this part of the brain has a powerful effect on the activity of baroreceptor reflexes.

Ascending noradrenergic fibres run to the hypothalamus, and descending fibres run to the lateral horn region of the spinal cord, acting to increase sympathetic discharge in the periphery. It has been suggested that these regulatory neurons may release adrenaline rather than noradrenaline. Some catecholamine-containing cells in the brain stem contain phenylethanolamine *N*-methyl transferase (the enzyme that converts noradrenaline to adrenaline; see Ch. 11), and inhibition of this enzyme interferes with the baroreceptor reflex.

DOPAMINE

Dopamine is particularly important in relation to neuropharmacology, because it is involved in several common disorders of brain function, notably Parkinson's disease, schizophrenia and attention deficit disorder, as well as in drug dependence and certain endocrine disorders. Many of the drugs used clinically to treat these conditions work by influencing dopamine transmission.

The distribution of dopamine in the brain is more restricted than that of noradrenaline. Dopamine is most abundant in the *corpus striatum*, a part of the extrapyramidal motor system concerned with the coordination of movement (see Ch. 35), and high concentrations also occur in certain parts of the *limbic system* and *hypothalamus* (where its release into the pituitary blood supply inhibits secretion of prolactin; Ch. 28).

The synthesis of dopamine follows the same route as that of noradrenaline (see Fig. 11.2), namely conversion of tyrosine to dopa (the rate-limiting step), followed by decarboxylation to form dopamine. Dopaminergic neurons lack dopamine β-hydroxylase, and thus do not produce noradrenaline.

Dopamine is largely recaptured, following its release from nerve terminals, by a specific dopamine transporter, one of the large family of monoamine transporters (see Ch. 4). It is metabolised by monoamine oxidase and catechol-*O*-methyl transferase (Fig. 34.2), the main products being dihydroxyphenylacetic acid (DOPAC) and homovanillic acid (HVA, the methoxy derivative of DOPAC). The brain content of HVA is often used as an index of dopamine turnover. Drugs that cause the release of dopamine increase HVA, often without changing the concentration of dopamine. DOPAC and HVA, and their sulfate conjugates, are excreted in the urine, which provides an index of dopamine release in human subjects.

6-hydroxydopamine, which selectively destroys dopaminergic nerve terminals, is commonly used as a research tool. It is taken up by the dopamine transporter and converted to a reactive metabolite that causes oxidative cytotoxicity.

DOPAMINERGIC PATHWAYS IN THE CNS

Dopaminergic neurons form three main systems (Fig. 34.3).

- The **nigrostriatal pathway**, accounting for about 75% of the dopamine in the brain, consists of cell bodies in the *substantia nigra* whose axons terminate in the *corpus striatum*. These fibres run in the *medial forebrain bundle* along with other

> **Noradrenaline in the CNS**
>
> - Mechanisms for synthesis, storage, release and reuptake of noradrenaline in the central nervous system (CNS) are essentially the same as in the periphery, as are the receptors (Ch. 11).
> - Noradrenergic cell bodies occur in discrete clusters, mainly in the pons and medulla, one important such cell group being the locus coeruleus.
> - Noradrenergic pathways, running mainly in the medial forebrain bundle and descending spinal tracts, terminate diffusely in the cortex, hippocampus, hypothalamus, cerebellum and spinal cord.
> - The actions of noradrenaline are mainly inhibitory (β-receptors), but some are excitatory (α- or β-receptors).
> - Noradrenergic transmission is believed to be important in:
>   - the 'arousal' system, controlling wakefulness and alertness
>   - blood pressure regulation
>   - control of mood (functional deficiency contributing to depression).
> - Psychotropic drugs that act partly or mainly on noradrenergic transmission in the CNS include antidepressants, cocaine and amphetamine. Some antihypertensive drugs (e.g. clonidine, methyldopa) act mainly on noradrenergic transmission in the CNS.

monoamine-containing fibres. The abundance of dopamine-containing neurons in the human striatum can be appreciated from the image shown in Figure 34.4, which was obtained by injecting a dopa derivative containing radioactive fluorine, and scanning for radioactivity 3 hours later by positron emission tomography.

- The **mesolimbic/mesocortical pathways**, whose cell bodies occur in groups in the midbrain and whose fibres project, also via the medial forebrain bundle, to parts of the limbic system, especially the *nucleus accumbens* and the *amygdaloid nucleus* and to the frontal cortex.
- The **tuberohypophyseal system** is a group of short neurons running from the ventral hypothalamus to the median eminence and pituitary gland, the secretions of which they regulate.

The functions of these systems are discussed below. There are also many local dopaminergic interneurons in other brain regions and in the retina.

DOPAMINE RECEPTORS

Two types of receptor, D_1 and D_2 (linked, respectively, to activation and inhibition of adenylyl cyclase), were originally distinguished on pharmacological and biochemical grounds. Gene cloning revealed further subgroups, D_1 to D_5 (for review, see Missale et al., 1998). The original D_1 family now includes D_1 and D_5, while

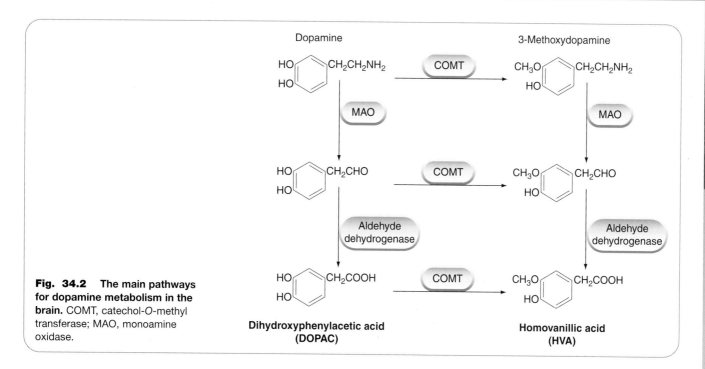

Fig. 34.2 **The main pathways for dopamine metabolism in the brain.** COMT, catechol-*O*-methyl transferase; MAO, monoamine oxidase.

Dopamine

3-Methoxydopamine

Dihydroxyphenylacetic acid (DOPAC)

Homovanillic acid (HVA)

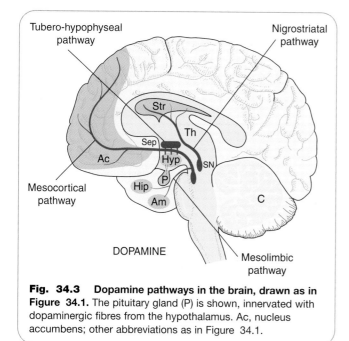

Fig. 34.3 **Dopamine pathways in the brain, drawn as in Figure 34.1.** The pituitary gland (P) is shown, innervated with dopaminergic fibres from the hypothalamus. Ac, nucleus accumbens; other abbreviations as in Figure 34.1.

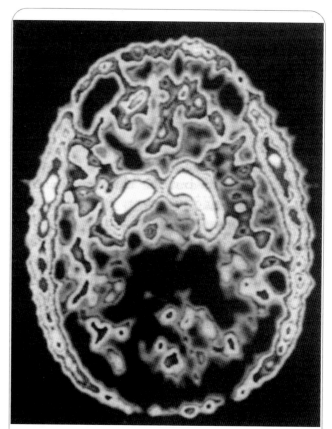

Fig. 34.4 **Dopamine in the basal ganglia of a human subject.** The subject was injected with 5-fluoro-dopa labelled with the positron-emitting isotope ^{18}F, which was localised 3 hours later by the technique of positron emission tomography. The isotope is accumulated (white areas) by the dopa uptake system of the neurons of the basal ganglia, and to a smaller extent in the frontal cortex. It is also seen in the scalp and temporalis muscles. (From Garnett E S et al. Nature 305: 137.)

the D_2 family, which is pharmacologically more important in the CNS, consists of D_2, D_3 and D_4 (see Table 34.1). Splice variants, leading to long and short forms of D_2, and genetic polymorphisms, particularly of D_4 (see below), have subsequently been identified.

▼All belong to the family of G-protein–coupled transmembrane receptors described in Chapter 3, and their signal transduction mechanisms—linked via adenylyl cyclase and/or phospholipid hydrolysis to the control of potassium and calcium channels, arachidonic acid release, etc.—are similar to those of other such receptors. A key component in the signal transduction pathway is the protein DARPP-32 (32-kDa dopamine- and cAMP-regulated phosphoprotein; see Girault & Greengard, 2004). When intracellular cAMP is increased through

Table 34.1 Dopamine receptors

	Functional role	D₁ type		D₂ type		
		D_1	D_5	D_2	D_3	D_4
Distribution						
Cortex	Arousal, mood	+++	–	++	–	+
Limbic system	Emotion, stereotypic behaviour	+++	+	++	+	+
Striatum	Motor control	+++	+	++	+	+
Ventral hypothalamus and anterior pituitary	Prolactin secretion	–	–	++	+	–
Agonists						
Dopamine		+ (low potency)		+ (high potency)		
Apomorphine		PA (low potency)		+ (high potency)		
Bromocriptine		PA (low potency)		+ (high potency)		
Antagonists						
Chlorpromazine		+	+	+++	+++	+
Haloperidol		++	+	+++	+++	+++
Spiperone		–	–	+++	+++	+++
Sulpiride		–	–	+++	++	–
Clozapine		+	+	+	+	++
Ariprazole		–	–	++ (PA)	+	–
Signal transduction		Increase cAMP		Decrease cAMP and/or increase inositol trisphosphate		
Effect		Mainly postsynaptic inhibition		Pre- and postsynaptic inhibition Stimulation/inhibition of hormone release		

PA, partial agonist.

activation of D_1 receptors, and protein kinase A, DARPP-32 is phosphorylated (Fig. 34.5). Phosphorylated DARPP-32 acts as an inhibitor of protein phosphatases such as protein phosphatase-1 and calcineurin, thus acting in concert with protein kinases and favouring protein phosphorylation—effectively an amplifying mechanism. Activation of D_2 receptors opposes the effect of D_1 receptor activation.

Dopamine receptors are expressed in the brain in distinct but overlapping areas. D_1 receptors are the most abundant and widespread in areas receiving a dopaminergic innervation (namely the striatum, limbic system, thalamus and hypothalamus; Fig. 34.3), as are D_2 receptors, which also occur in the pituitary gland. D_3 receptors occur in the limbic system but not in the striatum. Because dopamine antagonists used as antipsychotic drugs (Ch. 38) owe their actions to effects in the mesolimbic system but often cause motor side effects by blocking receptors in the striatum, there is interest in targeting the D_3 and D_4 receptors as a means of avoiding these side effects. The D_4 receptor is much more weakly expressed, mainly in the cortex and limbic systems, but is a focus of interest because of its possible relationship to the mechanism of schizophrenia (Ch. 38) and drug dependence (Ch. 43).

▼ The D_4 receptor displays an unexpected polymorphism in humans, with a varying number (from 2 to 10) of 16 amino acid repeat sequences being expressed in the third intracellular loop, which participates in

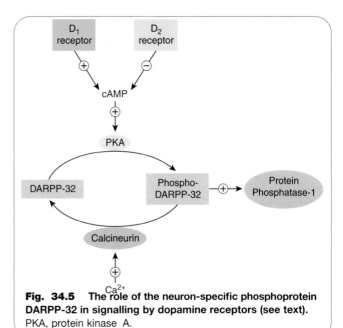

Fig. 34.5 The role of the neuron-specific phosphoprotein DARPP-32 in signalling by dopamine receptors (see text). PKA, protein kinase A.

G-protein coupling (Ch. 3). However, neither this polymorphism nor the long/short splice variants in the D_2 receptor are associated with significant changes in receptor function. Expectations that D_4 receptor polymorphism might be related to the occurrence of schizophrenia in humans were disappointed after several studies failed to find any correlation. There may be a connection with attention deficit hyperactivity disorder (see Tarazi et al., 2004).

Dopamine, like many other transmitters and modulators, acts presynaptically as well as postsynaptically. Presynaptic D_3 receptors occur mainly on dopaminergic neurons, for example those in the striatum and limbic system, where they act to inhibit dopamine synthesis and release. Dopamine antagonists, by blocking these receptors, increase dopamine synthesis and release, and cause accumulation of dopamine metabolites in these parts of the brain. They also cause an increase in the rate of firing of dopaminergic neurons (see Cooper et al., 2003), probably by blocking a neuronal feedback pathway.

Dopamine receptors also mediate various effects in the periphery (mediated by D_1 receptors), notably renal vasodilatation and increased myocardial contractility (dopamine itself has been used clinically in the treatment of circulatory shock; see Ch. 19), although its efficacy and safety are questionable.

FUNCTIONAL ASPECTS

The functions of dopaminergic pathways divide broadly into:

* motor control (nigrostriatal system)
* behavioural effects (mesolimbic and mesocortical systems)
* endocrine control (tuberohypophyseal system).

Dopamine and motor systems

Ungerstedt showed, in 1968, that bilateral ablation of the substantia nigra in rats, which destroys the nigrostriatal neurons, causes profound catalepsy, the animals becoming so inactive that they die of starvation unless artificially fed. Unilateral lesions produced by 6-hydroxydopamine injection caused the animal to turn in circles *towards* the lesioned side, because of an imbalance of dopamine action in the corpus striatum between the two sides of the brain. Conversely, unilateral injection of **apomorphine** (a dopamine receptor agonist) into the striatum causes circling *away* from the injected side. If apomorphine is given systemically to normal rats, it causes, as one would expect, no asymmetrical pattern of locomotion, but if given systemically to animals with unilateral lesions of the substantia nigra made days or weeks earlier, apomorphine causes circling away from the lesioned side. This is because denervation supersensitivity (see Ch. 9) on one side, following the destruction of dopaminergic terminals, results in an asymmetric response to apomorphine. In these animals, administration of drugs that act by releasing dopamine (e.g. **amphetamine**) causes turning *towards* the lesioned side, because the dopaminergic nerve terminals are present only on the normal side. This 'turning model' has been extremely useful in investigating the action of drugs on dopaminergic neurons and dopamine receptors.

Parkinson's disease (Ch. 35) is a disorder of motor control, associated with a deficiency of dopamine in the nigrostriatal pathway.

Many antipsychotic drugs (see Ch. 38) are D_2 receptor antagonists, whose major side effect is to cause movement disorders, probably associated with block of D_2 receptors in the nigrostriatal pathway.

Transgenic mice lacking D_2 receptors show greatly reduced spontaneous movement, resembling Parkinson's disease.

Behavioural effects

Administration of amphetamine to rats, which releases both dopamine and noradrenaline, causes a cessation of normal 'ratty' behaviour (exploration and grooming), and the appearance of repeated 'stereotyped' behaviour (rearing, gnawing and so on) unrelated to external stimuli. These effects are prevented by dopamine antagonists and by destruction of dopamine-containing cell bodies in the midbrain, but not by drugs that inhibit the noradrenergic system. These amphetamine-induced motor disturbances in rats probably reflect hyperactivity in the nigrostriatal dopaminergic system.

Amphetamine also causes a general increase in motor activity, which can be measured, for example, by counting electronically the frequency at which a rat crosses from one part of its enclosure to another. This effect, in contrast to stereotypy, appears to be related to the mesolimbic and mesocortical dopaminergic pathways. There is some evidence (see Ch. 38) that schizophrenia in humans is associated with dopaminergic hyperactivity. Chronic administration of amphetamine to a few rats in a large colony produces various types of abnormal social interaction, including withdrawal and aggressive behaviour, but it is difficult to quantify such effects or to establish their relationship to schizophrenia in humans.

Amphetamine, cocaine (which acts by inhibiting the dopamine transporter; Ch. 9) and also other addictive drugs (Ch. 43) activate mesocortical dopaminergic 'reward' pathways, which play a key role in drug dependence. The main receptor involved appears to be D_1, and transgenic mice lacking D_1 receptors behave as though generally demotivated, with reduced food intake and insensitivity to amphetamine and cocaine (see Sibley, 1999).

Neuroendocrine function

The tuberohypophyseal dopaminergic pathway (see Fig. 34.3) is involved in the control of prolactin secretion. The hypothalamus secretes various mediators (mostly small peptides; see Ch. 28), which control the secretion of different hormones from the pituitary gland. One of these mediators, which has an inhibitory effect on prolactin release, is dopamine. This system is of clinical importance. Many antipsychotic drugs (see Ch. 38), by blocking D_2 receptors, increase prolactin secretion and can cause breast development and lactation, even in males. **Bromocriptine**, a dopamine receptor agonist derived from ergot, is used clinically to suppress prolactin secretion by tumours of the pituitary gland.

Growth hormone production is increased in normal subjects by dopamine, but bromocriptine paradoxically *inhibits* the excessive secretion responsible for acromegaly (probably because it desensitises dopamine receptors, in contrast to the physiological release of dopamine, which is pulsatile) and has a useful therapeutic effect, provided it is given before excessive

Dopamine in the CNS

- Dopamine is a neurotransmitter as well as being the precursor for noradrenaline. It is degraded in a similar fashion to noradrenaline, giving rise mainly to dihydroxyphenylacetic acid and homovanillic acid, which are excreted in the urine.
- There are three main dopaminergic pathways:
  — nigrostriatal pathway, important in motor control
  — mesolimbic/mesocortical pathways, running from groups of cells in the midbrain to parts of the limbic system, especially the nucleus accumbens, and to the cortex; they are involved in emotion and drug-induced reward systems
  — tuberohypophyseal neurons running from the hypothalamus to the pituitary gland, whose secretions they regulate.
- There are five dopamine receptor subtypes. D_1 and D_5 receptors are linked to stimulation of adenylyl cyclase. D_2, D_3 and D_4 receptors are linked to inhibition of adenylyl cyclase. Most known functions of dopamine appear to be mediated mainly by receptors of the D_2 family.
- Receptors of the D_2 family may be implicated in schizophrenia. The D_4 receptor shows marked polymorphism in humans, but no clear relationship with disease has been established.
- Parkinson's disease is associated with a deficiency of nigrostriatal dopaminergic neurons.
- Behavioural effects of an excess of dopamine activity consist of stereotyped behaviour patterns and can be produced by dopamine-releasing agents (e.g. amphetamine) and dopamine agonists (e.g. apomorphine).
- Hormone release from the anterior pituitary gland is regulated by dopamine, especially prolactin release (inhibited) and growth hormone release (stimulated).
- Dopamine acts on the chemoreceptor trigger zone to cause nausea and vomiting.

growth has taken place. It is now rarely used, as other agents are more effective (see Ch. 28).

Vomiting

Pharmacological evidence strongly suggests that dopaminergic neurons have a role in the production of nausea and vomiting. Thus nearly all dopamine receptor agonists (e.g. bromocriptine) and other drugs that increase dopamine release in the brain (e.g. **levodopa**; Ch. 35) cause nausea and vomiting as side effects, while many dopamine antagonists (e.g. **phenothiazines, metoclopramide**; Ch. 25) have antiemetic activity. D_2 receptors occur in the area of the medulla (chemoreceptor trigger zone) associated with the initiation of vomiting (Ch. 25), and are assumed to mediate this effect.

5-HYDROXYTRYPTAMINE

The occurrence and functions of 5-HT in the periphery are described in Chapter 12. Interest in 5-HT as a possible CNS transmitter dates from 1953, when Gaddum found that **lysergic acid diethylamide (LSD)**, a drug known to be a powerful hallucinogen (see Ch. 42), acted as a 5-HT antagonist on peripheral tissues, and suggested that its central effects might also be related to this action. The presence of 5-HT in the brain was demonstrated a few years later. Even though brain accounts for only about 1% of the total body content, 5-HT is an important CNS transmitter (see Cooper et al., 2003).

In its formation, storage and release, 5-HT resembles noradrenaline (see Fig. 12.1). Its precursor is tryptophan, an amino acid derived from dietary protein, the plasma content of which varies considerably according to food intake and time of day. Tryptophan is actively taken up into neurons, converted by tryptophan hydroxylase to 5-hydroxytryptophan, and then decarboxylated by a non-specific amino acid decarboxylase to 5-HT. Tryptophan hydroxylase can be selectively and irreversibly inhibited by **p-chlorophenylalanine** (**PCPA**). Availability of tryptophan and the activity of tryptophan hydroxylase are thought to be the main factors that regulate 5-HT synthesis. The decarboxylase is very similar, if not identical, to dopa decarboxylase, and does not play any role in regulating 5-HT synthesis. Following release, 5-HT is largely recovered by neuronal uptake, this mechanism being inhibited by many of the same drugs (e.g. **tricyclic antidepressants**) that inhibit catecholamine uptake. The carrier is not identical, however, and inhibitors show varying degrees of specificity between the two. **Selective serotonin reuptake inhibitors** (see Ch. 39) constitute an important group of antidepressant drugs. 5-HT is degraded almost entirely by monoamine oxidase (Fig. 12.1), which converts it to 5-hydroxyindole acetaldehyde, most of which is dehydrogenated to form 5-hydroxyindole acetic acid, which is excreted in the urine.

5-HT PATHWAYS IN THE CNS

The distribution of 5-HT-containing neurons (Fig. 34.6) resembles that of noradrenergic neurons. The cell bodies are grouped in the pons and upper medulla, close to the midline (raphe), and are often referred to as *raphe nuclei*. The rostrally situated nuclei project, via the medial forebrain bundle, to many parts of the cortex, hippocampus, basal ganglia, limbic system and hypothalamus. The caudally situated cells project to the cerebellum, medulla and spinal cord.

5-HT RECEPTORS IN THE CNS

The main 5-HT receptor types are shown in Table 12.1. All are G-protein–coupled receptors except for 5-HT$_3$, which is a ligand-gated cation channel. All are expressed in the CNS, and their functional roles have been extensively analysed. With 14 identified subtypes, and a large number of pharmacological tools of relatively low specificity, assigning clear-cut functions to 5-HT receptors is not simple. A detailed account of our present

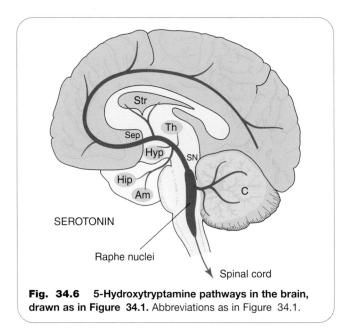

Fig. 34.6 **5-Hydroxytryptamine pathways in the brain, drawn as in Figure 34.1.** Abbreviations as in Figure 34.1.

state of knowledge is given by Barnes & Sharp (1999). Knowledge about the newer members of the family (5-HT$_{5-7}$ receptors) is summarised in recent reviews by Woolley et al. (2004) and Hedlund & Sutcliffe (2005).

Certain generalisations can be made.

- 5-HT$_1$ receptors are predominantly inhibitory in their effects. 5-HT$_{1A}$ receptors are expressed as autoreceptors by the 5-HT neurons in the raphe nuclei, and their autoinhibitory effect tends to limit the rate of firing of these cells. They are also widely distributed in the limbic system, and are believed to be the main target of drugs used to treat anxiety and depression (see Chs 37 and 39). 5-HT$_{1B}$ and 5-HT$_{1D}$ receptors are found mainly as presynaptic inhibitory receptors in the basal ganglia. Agonists acting on peripheral 5-HT$_{1D}$ receptors are used to treat migraine (see Ch. 12).
- 5-HT$_2$ receptors (mostly 5-HT$_{2A}$ in the brain) exert an excitatory postsynaptic effect, and are abundant in the cortex and limbic system. They are believed to be the target of various hallucinogenic drugs (see Ch. 42). The use of 5-HT$_2$ receptor antagonists such as **methysergide** in treating migraine is discussed in Chapter 12.
- 5-HT$_3$ receptors are found chiefly in the *area postrema* (a region of the medulla involved in vomiting; see Ch. 25) and other parts of the brain stem, extending to the dorsal horn of the spinal cord. They are also present in certain parts of the cortex, as well as in the peripheral nervous system. They are excitatory ionotropic receptors, and specific antagonists (e.g. **ondansetron**; see Chs 12 and 25) are used to treat nausea and vomiting. They may also have anxiolytic affects, but this is less clear.
- 5-HT$_4$ receptors are important in the gastrointestinal tract (see Chs 12 and 25), and are also expressed in the brain, particularly in the striatum. They exert a presynaptic facilitatory effect, particularly on ACh release, thus enhancing cognitive performance.

- 5-HT$_6$ receptors occur only in the CNS, particularly in the hippocampus, cortex and limbic system. They are considered potential targets for drugs to improve cognition or relieve symptoms of schizophrenia, although no such drugs are yet available.
- 5-HT$_7$ receptors occur in the hippocampus, cortex, thalamus and hypothalamus, and also in blood vessels and the gastrointestinal tract. Likely CNS functions include thermoregulation and endocrine regulation, as well as suspected involvement in mood, cognitive function, and sleep. Selective antagonists are being developed for clinical use in a variety of potential indications.

FUNCTIONAL ASPECTS

The precise localisation of 5-HT neurons in the brain stem has allowed their electrical activity to be studied in detail and correlated with behavioural and other effects produced by drugs thought to affect 5-HT-mediated transmission. 5-HT cells show an unusual, highly regular, slow discharge pattern, and are strongly inhibited by 5-HT$_1$ receptor agonists, suggesting a local inhibitory feedback mechanism.

In vertebrates, certain physiological and behavioural functions relate particularly to 5-HT pathways (see Barnes & Sharp, 1999), namely:

- hallucinations and behavioural changes
- sleep, wakefulness and mood
- feeding behaviour
- control of sensory transmission (especially pain pathways; see Ch. 41).

Hallucinatory effects

Many hallucinogenic drugs (e.g. LSD, Ch. 42) are agonists at 5-HT$_{2A}$ receptors and depress the firing of brain-stem 5-HT neurons. These neurons exert an inhibitory influence on cortical neurons, and it is suggested that a loss of cortical inhibition underlies the hallucinogenic effect, as well as certain behavioural effects in experimental animals, such as the 'wet dog shakes' that occur in rats when the 5-HT precursor 5-hydroxytryptophan is administered. Many antipsychotic drugs (Ch. 38) are antagonists at 5-HT$_{2A}$ receptors in addition to blocking dopamine D$_2$ receptors.

Sleep, wakefulness and mood

Lesions of the raphe nuclei, or depletion of 5-HT by PCPA administration, abolish sleep in experimental animals, whereas microinjection of 5-HT at specific points in the brain stem induces sleep. Attempts to cure insomnia in humans by giving 5-HT precursors (tryptophan or 5-hydroxytryptophan) have, however, proved unsuccessful. There is evidence that 5-HT, as well as noradrenaline, may be involved in the control of mood (see Ch. 39), and the use of tryptophan to enhance 5-HT synthesis has been tried in depression, with equivocal results.

Feeding and appetite

In experimental animals, 5-HT$_{1A}$ agonists such as 8-hydroxy-2-(di-n-propylamino)tetralin (8-OH-DPAT) cause hyperphagia, leading to obesity. Antagonists acting on 5-HT$_2$ receptors, including several antipsychotic drugs used clinically, also increase appetite and cause weight gain. On the other hand, antidepressant drugs that inhibit 5-HT uptake (serotonin reuptake inhibitors; see Ch. 39) cause loss of appetite.

Sensory transmission

After lesions of the raphe nuclei or administration of PCPA, animals show exaggerated responses to many forms of sensory stimulus. They are startled much more easily, and also quickly develop avoidance responses to stimuli that would not normally bother them. It appears that the normal ability to disregard irrelevant forms of sensory input requires intact 5-HT pathways. The 'sensory enhancement' produced by hallucinogenic drugs may be partly due to loss of this gatekeeper function of 5-HT. 5-HT also exerts an inhibitory effect on transmission in the pain pathway, both in the spinal cord and in the brain, and there is a synergistic effect between 5-HT and analgesics such as morphine (see Ch. 38). Thus depletion of 5-HT by PCPA, or selective lesions to the descending 5-HT-containing neurons that run to the dorsal horn, antagonise the analgesic effect of morphine, while inhibitors of 5-HT uptake have the opposite effect.

Other possible roles

Other putative roles of 5-HT include various autonomic and endocrine functions, such as the regulation of body temperature, blood pressure and sexual function. Further information can be found in Azmitia & Whitaker-Azmitia (1995) and Cooper et al. (2003).

Several classes of drugs used clinically influence 5-HT-mediated transmission. They include:

- serotonin reuptake inhibitors, such as **fluoxetine**, used as antidepressants (Ch. 39)
- 5-HT$_{1D}$ receptor agonists, such as **sumatriptan** (Ch. 12), used to treat migraine
- **buspirone**, a 5-HT$_{1A}$ receptor agonist used in treating anxiety (Ch. 37)
- 5-HT$_3$ receptor antagonists, such as **ondansetron**, used as antiemetic agents (see Ch. 25), which are also active in animal models of anxiety
- antipsychotic drugs (e.g. **clozapine**, Ch. 38), which owe their efficacy partly to an action on 5-HT receptors.

Efforts are being made to identify drugs that selectively target other 5-HT receptor subtypes in the hope of discovering improved drugs for use in different CNS indications. As a result, many code-numbered compounds have been characterised experimentally, but very few have been registered for clinical use in recent years.

ACETYLCHOLINE

There are numerous cholinergic neurons in the CNS, and the basic processes by which ACh is synthesised, stored and released are the same as in the periphery (see Ch. 10). Various biochemical markers have been used to locate cholinergic neurons in the brain, the most useful being choline acetyltransferase, the enzyme responsible for ACh synthesis, and the transporters that capture choline and package ACh, which can be labelled by immunofluorescence. Biochemical studies on ACh precursors and metabolites are generally more difficult than corresponding studies on other amine transmitters, because the relevant substances, choline and acetate, are involved in many processes other than ACh metabolism.

5-Hydroxytryptamine in the CNS

- The processes of synthesis, storage, release, reuptake and degradation of 5-hydroxytryptamine (5-HT) in the brain are very similar to events in the periphery (Ch. 12).
- Availability of tryptophan is the main factor regulating synthesis.
- Urinary excretion of 5-hydroxyindole acetic acid provides a measure of 5-HT turnover.
- 5-HT neurons are concentrated in the midline raphe nuclei in the pons and medulla, projecting diffusely to the cortex, limbic system, hypothalamus and spinal cord, similar to the noradrenergic projections.
- Functions associated with 5-HT pathways include:
  - various behavioural responses (e.g. hallucinatory behaviour, 'wet dog shakes')
  - feeding behaviour
  - control of mood and emotion
  - control of sleep/wakefulness
  - control of sensory pathways, including nociception
  - control of body temperature
  - vomiting.
- 5-HT can exert inhibitory or excitatory effects on individual neurons, acting either presynaptically or postsynaptically.
- The main receptor subtypes (see Table 12.1) in the CNS are 5-HT$_{1A}$, 5-HT$_{1B}$, 5-HT$_{1D}$, 5-HT$_2$ and 5-HT$_3$. Associations of behavioural and physiological functions with these receptors have been partly worked out. Other receptor types (5-HT$_{4-7}$) also occur in the central nervous system, but less is known about their function.
- Drugs acting selectively on 5-HT receptors or transporters include:
  - 'triptans' (e.g. sumatriptan), 5-HT$_{1D}$ agonists used to treat migraine (See Ch. 12)
  - 5-HT$_2$ antagonists (e.g. ketanserin) used for migraine prophylaxis (see Ch. 12)
  - selective serotonin uptake inhibitors (e.g. fluoxetine) used to treat depression (see Ch. 39)
  - ondansetron, 5-HT$_3$ antagonist, used to treat chemotherapy-induced emesis (see Ch. 12).

CHOLINERGIC PATHWAYS IN THE CNS

Acetylcholine is very widely distributed in the brain, occurring in all parts of the forebrain (including the cortex), midbrain and brain stem, although there is little in the cerebellum. Some of the main cholinergic pathways in the brain are shown in Figure 34.7. Cholinergic neurons in the forebrain and brain stem send diffuse projections to many parts of the cortex and hippocampus—a pattern similar to that of the amine pathways described above. These neurons lie in a discrete area of the basal forebrain, forming the *magnocellular forebrain nuclei* (so called because the cell bodies are conspicuously large). Degeneration of one of these, the *nucleus basalis of Meynert*, which projects mainly to the cortex, is associated with Alzheimer's disease (Ch. 35). Another cluster, the *septohippocampal nucleus*, provides the main cholinergic input to the hippocampus, and is involved in memory. In addition, there are—in contrast to the monoamine pathways—many local cholinergic interneurons, particularly in the corpus striatum, these being important in relation to Parkinson's disease and Huntington's chorea (Ch. 35).

ACETYLCHOLINE RECEPTORS

Acetylcholine has mainly excitatory effects, which are mediated by various subtypes of either nicotinic (ionotropic) or muscarinic (G-protein–coupled) receptors (see Ch. 10). Some muscarinic ACh receptors (mAChRs) are inhibitory.

The mAChRs in the brain are predominantly of the M_1 class (i.e. M_1, M_3 and M_5 subtypes; see Ch. 10), and the central actions of muscarinic antagonists and anticholinesterases depend on block and stimulation of these receptors, respectively. mAChRs act presynaptically to inhibit ACh release from cholinergic neurons, and muscarinic antagonists, by blocking this inhibition, markedly increase ACh release. Many of the behavioural effects associated with cholinergic pathways seem to be produced by ACh acting on mAChRs.

Nicotinic ACh receptors (nAChRs) are also widespread in the brain but much sparser than mAChRs. They are typical pentameric ionotropic receptors (Ch. 3; see Hogg et al., 2003), assembled from α and β subunits, each of which come in several isoforms (Table 10.1). The main ones occurring in the brain are the heteropentameric $\alpha_4\beta_2$ subtype (occurring mainly in the cortex) and the homomeric α_7 subtype (mainly in the hippocampus). Other isoforms occur at lower densities in many brain regions. For the most part, nAChRs are located presynaptically and act to facilitate the release of other transmitters, such as glutamate and dopamine, although in a few situations they function postsynaptically to mediate fast excitatory transmission, as in the periphery. Nicotine (see Ch. 43) exerts its central effects by agonist action on nAChRs of the $\alpha_4\beta_2$ subtype.

Many of the drugs that block nAChRs (e.g. **tubocurarine**; see Ch. 10) do not cross the blood–brain barrier, and even those that do (e.g. **mecamylamine**) produce only modest CNS effects. Various nAChR knockout mouse strains have been produced and studied. Deletion of the various CNS-specific nAChR subtypes generally has rather little effect, although some cognitive impairment can be detected.

FUNCTIONAL ASPECTS

The functional roles of cholinergic pathways have been deduced mainly from studies of the action of drugs that mimic, accentuate or block the actions of ACh, and recently from studies of transgenic animals in which particular nAChRs were deleted or mutated (see Cordero-Erausquin et al., 2000; Hogg et al., 2003).

The main functions ascribed to cholinergic pathways are related to arousal, learning and memory, and motor control. Electroencephalography (EEG) recording can be used to monitor the state of arousal in humans or in experimental animals. A drowsy, inattentive state is associated with a large-amplitude, low-frequency EEG record, which switches to a low-amplitude, high-frequency pattern on arousal by any sensory stimulus. Administration of **physostigmine** (an anticholinesterase that crosses the blood–brain barrier) produces EEG arousal, whereas **atropine** has the opposite effect. It is presumed that the cholinergic projection from the ventral forebrain to the cortex mediates this response. The relationship of this response to behaviour is confusing, however, for physostigmine in humans causes a state of lethargy and anxiety, and in rats it depresses exploratory activity, whereas atropine often causes excitement and agitation in humans and increases exploratory activity in rats, effects opposite to what one might expect. In contrast to atropine, **hyoscine** causes sedation in humans and animals; the reason for the difference is not known.

▼ There is evidence that cholinergic pathways, in particular the septohippocampal pathway, are involved in learning and short-term memory (see Hagan & Morris, 1988). For example (Fig. 34.8), mice may be trained to execute a maze-running manoeuvre in response to a buzzer, and many will remember the correct response when retested 7 days later. Intracerebral injection of a muscarinic agonist, **arecoline**, immediately after the training session reduces the percentage of animals that forget the correct response when retested, whereas an injection of the muscarinic antagonist **hyoscine** has the opposite effect. In the experiment shown in Figure 34.8, a deliberate bias was introduced, in that the mice selected for the arecoline test were particularly dim (the fast learners having been

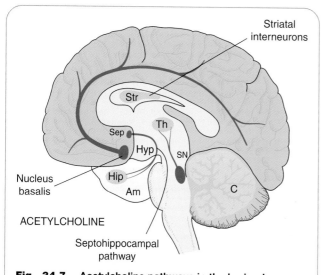

Fig. 34.7 Acetylcholine pathways in the brain, drawn as in **Figure 34.1**. Abbreviations as in Figure 34.1.

Striatal interneurons

Str

Th

Sep

Hyp

SN

Hip

C

Am

Nucleus basalis

ACETYLCHOLINE

Septohippocampal pathway

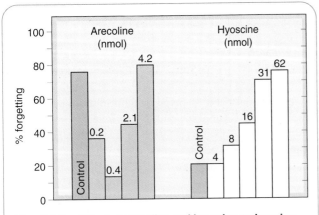

Fig. 34.8   Effect of arecoline and hyoscine on learning.
Mice were trained to perform a behavioural feat in order to avoid
an electric shock, and tested for their ability to remember it
7 days later. Mice in the group that performed least well (left)
were given the cholinergic agonist arecoline by
intracerebroventricular injection; at low doses, their
performance improved markedly, but at higher doses their
performance declined. Animals in the group that performed
best in the initial test were given the muscarinic receptor
antagonist hyoscine, which caused a deterioration of their
performance. (From Flood J F, Landry D W, Jarvik M E et al.
1981 Brain Res 215: 177–185.)

Acetylcholine in the CNS

- Synthesis, storage and release of acetylcholine
  (ACh) in the central nervous system (CNS) are
  essentially the same as in the periphery (Ch. 10).
- ACh is widely distributed in the CNS, important
  pathways being:
  — basal forebrain (magnocellular) nuclei, which send
    a diffuse projection to most forebrain structures,
    including the cortex
  — septohippocampal projection
  — short interneurons in the striatum and nucleus
    accumbens.
- Certain neurodegenerative diseases, especially
  dementia and Parkinson's disease (see Ch. 35), are
  associated with abnormalities in cholinergic pathways.
- Both nicotinic and muscarinic ACh receptors occur in
  the CNS. The former mediate the central effects of
  nicotine. Nicotinic receptors are mainly located
  presynaptically; there are few examples of transmission
  mediated by postsynaptic nicotinic receptors.
- Muscarinic receptors appear to mediate the main
  behavioural effects associated with ACh, namely effects
  on arousal and on learning and short-term memory.
- Muscarinic antagonists (e.g. hyoscine) cause
  amnesia.
- Acetylcholinesterase released from neurons may have
  functional effects distinct from its effects on cholinergic
  transmission.

excluded), and the training was brief, so that the forgetting rate in the control group was about 70%; an optimal dose of arecoline reduced this to about 15%. The scopolamine test was done on the cleverest mice (the no hopers being excluded), and the training was more thorough, so the forgetting rate in the control group was only about 20%, and this was increased by scopolamine. More recently, synthetic muscarinic agonists have been shown partially to restore learning and memory deficits induced in experimental animals by lesions of the septohippocampal cholinergic pathway. Scopolamine also impairs memory in human subjects and causes amnesia when used as preanaesthetic medication. M_1 mAChR knockout mice, however, show only slight impairment of learning and memory (see Wess, 2004).

Nicotine increases alertness and also enhances learning and memory, as can various synthetic agonists at neuronal nAChRs. Conversely, CNS-active nAChR antagonists such as mecamylamine cause detectable, although slight, impairment of learning and memory. Transgenic mice with disruption of brain nAChRs are only slightly impaired in spatial learning tasks. In conclusion, both nAChRs and mAChRs may play a role in learning and memory, while nAChRs also mediate behavioural arousal. Receptor knockout mice are surprisingly little affected, suggesting that alternative mechanisms may be able to compensate for the loss of ACh receptor signalling.

Transgenic mice that overexpress acetylcholinesterase (and hence show impaired cholinergic transmission) behave normally but develop a learning deficit after a few months (Beeri et al., 1995). The interpretation is not simple, however, because these mice also respond poorly to muscarinic and nicotinic agonists, suggesting that more complex secondary effects were produced.

Involvement of neuronal nAChRs in pain transmission is suggested by the recent finding that **epibatidine**, a compound extracted from frog skin, which is a selective agonist at these receptors, has powerful analgesic properties in animals (Ch. 41), as does nicotine itself.

The significance of cholinergic neurons in neurodegenerative conditions such as dementia and Parkinson's disease is discussed in Chapter 35.

Acetylcholinesterase may have, in addition to its primary role of disposing quickly of released ACh, various trophic functions—not necessarily related to its enzymic activity—in the regulation of neuronal growth and synapse formation (see Soreq & Sediman, 2001), about which we know very little at present.

PURINES

Both adenosine and ATP act as transmitters and/or modulators in the CNS (for review, see Dunwiddie & Masino, 2001; Robertson et al., 2001) as they do in the periphery (Ch. 12). Mapping the pathways is difficult, because purinergic neurons are not easily identifiable histochemically, but it is likely that adenosine serves as a very widespread neuromodulator, while ATP has more specific synaptic functions as a fast transmitter and as a local modulator.

Adenosine is produced intracellularly from ATP (see Fig. 12.4). It is not packaged into vesicles but is released mainly by carrier-mediated transport. Because the intracellular concentration of ATP (several mM) greatly exceeds that of adenosine, conversion of a small proportion of ATP results in a large increase in adenosine. ATP is packaged into vesicles and released by exocytosis as a conventional transmitter, but can also leak out of cells in large amounts under conditions of tissue damage. In high concentrations,

ATP can act as an excitotoxin (like glutamate, see Ch. 33) and cause further neuronal damage. It is also quickly converted to adenosine (Fig. 12.4), which exerts a protective effect. These special characteristics of adenosine metabolism suggest that it serves mainly as a safety mechanism, protecting the neurons from damage when their viability is threatened, for example by ischaemia or seizure activity.

As discussed in Chapter 12, adenosine produces its effects through G-protein–coupled receptors (A_1, A_{2A}, A_{2B} and A_3), while ATP acts on P_2 receptors, P_{2X} being ligand-gated cation channels, P_{2Y} being G-protein–coupled. P_{2Y} receptors produce mainly inhibitory effects, while the P_{2X} receptors are excitatory, producing both pre- and postsynaptic effects in much the same way as nAChRs. All these receptors are more or less widely distributed in the brain.

The overall effect of adenosine, or of various A receptor agonists, is inhibitory, leading to effects such as drowsiness, motor incoordination, analgesia and anticonvulsant activity. Xanthines, such as **caffeine** (Ch. 42), which are antagonists at A_2 receptors, produce arousal and alertness. Many synthetic adenosine agonists have been developed, because such drugs could be useful in treating conditions such as epilepsy, pain and sleep disorders. A further possible use is in neuroprotection, because the inhibitory effect of adenosine on neuronal excitability and glutamate release is able, in experimental models, to protect the brain against ischaemic damage (see Ch. 35). No such drugs are yet available for clinical use.

Little is known about the function of ATP as a chemical mediator in the brain. Because it is quickly metabolised to ADP and adenosine, its pharmacological actions are difficult to unravel, and there are few selective agonists or antagonists for ATP receptors. It may play a role in nociception, because ATP is released by tissue damage and causes pain by stimulating unmyelinated afferent nerve terminals, which express P_{2X} receptors.

HISTAMINE

▼ Histamine is present in the brain in much smaller amounts than in other tissues, such as skin and lung, but undoubtedly serves a neurotransmitter role (see Brown et al., 2001). The cell bodies of histaminergic neurons, which also synthesise and release a variety of other transmitters, are restricted to a small part of the hypothalamus, and their axons run to virtually all parts of the brain—an 'aerosol' arrangement similar to that of other monoamines. Unusually, no uptake mechanism for histamine is present, its action being terminated instead by enzymic methylation.

Histamine acts on three types of receptor (H_{1-3}; Ch. 13), all of which are G-protein–coupled receptors and occur in most brain regions. H_1 receptors are mainly located postsynaptically and cause excitation; H_2 and H_3 receptors are inhibitory, respectively post- and presynaptic, H_3 receptors being inhibitory autoreceptors on histamine-releasing neurons.

Like other monoamine transmitters, histamine is involved in many different CNS functions. Histamine release follows a distinct circadian pattern, the neurons being active by day and silent by night. H_1 receptors in the cortex and reticular activating system contribute to arousal and wakefulness, and H_1 receptor antagonists produce sedation (see Ch. 13). Other functions ascribed to histamine include control of food and water intake, and thermoregulation, but these are less well characterised. Antihistamines are widely used to control nausea and vomiting, for example in motion sickness and middle ear disorders, suggesting a role for histamine in these reflexes.

OTHER CNS MEDIATORS

We now move from the familiar neuropharmacological territory of the 'classic' monoamines to some of the frontier towns, bordering on the Wild West. Useful drugs are still few and far between in this area, and if applied pharmacology is your main concern, you can safely skip the next part and wait a few years for law and order to be established.

MELATONIN

▼ Melatonin (reviewed by Brzezinski, 1997) is something of a mystery. It is synthesised exclusively in the pineal, an endocrine gland that plays a role in establishing circadian rhythms. The gland contains two enzymes, not found elsewhere, which convert 5-HT by acetylation and O-methylation to melatonin, its hormonal product. Melatonin secretion (in all animals, whether diurnal or nocturnal in their habits) is high at night and low by day. This rhythm is controlled by input from the retina, via a noradrenergic retinohypothalamic tract that terminates in the suprachiasmatic nucleus in the hypothalamus, a structure often termed the 'biological clock', which generates the circadian rhythm. The suprachiasmatic nucleus controls the pineal, not directly, but via sympathetic fibres supplying the gland. This retinal control system serves to inhibit melatonin secretion when the light intensity is high. It does not itself generate the circadian rhythm, but rather 'entrains' it to the light–dark cycle. Circadian rhythms, including the rhythmic secretion of melatonin, continue even in the absence of light–dark cues, but usually with a periodicity rather longer than 24 hours.

Melatonin receptors (as you will have guessed) are widespread, and come in different types. The main ones are typical G-protein–coupled receptors, found mainly in the brain and retina but also in peripheral tissues. Another type has been identified as one of the previous 'orphan receptors' (see Ch. 3), a member of the retinoic acid intracellular receptor family that regulates gene transcription. We currently know very little about the physiological processes that are controlled by melatonin, although there is intense research activity in this area.

The use of melatonin for medicinal purposes has become something of an 'alternative medicine' fad, although there are few properly controlled trials of its efficacy. Given orally, melatonin is well absorbed but quickly metabolised, its plasma half-life being a few minutes. It has been promoted as a means of controlling jet lag, or of improving the performance of night shift workers, based on its ability to reset the circadian clock, and controlled studies have confirmed that melatonin given in the evening can alleviate the effects of jet lag. A single dose appears to have the effect of resynchronising the physiological secretory cycle, although it is not clear how this occurs. It causes sleepiness, and there is some disagreement about whether its actions are distinguishable from those of conventional hypnotic drugs (see Ch. 37). Claims that melatonin produces other effects (e.g. on mood and immune function) have yet to be confirmed. Synthetic agonists and antagonists have been produced and are being tested in a range of indications, mainly sleep disorders.

NITRIC OXIDE

Nitric oxide as a peripheral mediator is discussed in Chapter 17. Its significance as an important chemical mediator in the nervous system became apparent only about 15 years ago, and demanded a considerable readjustment of our views about neurotransmission and neuromodulation (for review, see Dawson & Snyder, 1994). The main defining criteria for transmitter substances—namely that neurons should possess machinery for synthesising and storing the substance, that it should be released from neurons by exocytosis,

Other transmitters and modulators

Purines

- ATP functions as a neurotransmitter, being stored in vesicles and released by exocytosis. It acts, via ionotropic receptors, as a fast excitatory transmitter in certain pathways and, via metabotropic receptors, as a neuromodulator.
- Cytosolic ATP is present at relatively high concentration and can be released directly if neuronal viability is compromised (e.g. in stroke). Excessive release may be neurotoxic.
- Released ATP is rapidly converted to ADP, AMP and adenosine.
- Adenosine is not stored in vesicles but is released by carrier mechanisms or generated from released ATP, mainly under pathological conditions.
- Adenosine exerts mainly inhibitory effects, through A_1 and A_2 receptors, resulting in sedative, anticonvulsant and neuroprotective effects, and acting as a safety mechanism.
- Methylxanthines (e.g. caffeine) are antagonists at A_2 receptors and increase wakefulness.

Histamine

- Histamine fulfils the criteria for a neurotransmitter. Histaminergic neurons originate in a small area of the hypothalamus and have a widespread distribution.
- H_1, H_2 and H_3 receptors are widespread in the brain. H_1 and H_3 receptors are mainly excitatory; H_2 receptors are inhibitory.
- The functions of histamine are not well understood, the main clues being that histaminergic neurons are active during waking hours, and H_1 receptor antagonists are strongly sedative.
- H_1 receptor antagonists are antiemetic.

Melatonin

- Melatonin is synthesised from 5-hydroxytryptamine, mainly in the pineal gland, from which it is released as a circulating hormone.
- Secretion is controlled by light intensity, being low by day and high by night. Fibres from the retina run to the suprachiasmatic nucleus ('biological clock'), which controls the pineal gland via its sympathetic innervation.
- Melatonin acts on several types of receptor in the brain and periphery. Given orally, it causes sedation and also 'resets' the biological clock, being used for this purpose to counter jet lag.
- Other claimed actions of melatonin (e.g. on mood and immune function) are controversial.

Nitric oxide (see Ch. 17)

- Neuronal nitric oxide synthase (nNOS) is present in many central nervous system neurons, and nitric oxide (NO) production is increased by mechanisms (e.g. transmitter action) that raise intracellular Ca^{2+}.
- NO affects neuronal function by increasing cGMP formation, producing both inhibitory and excitatory effects on neurons.
- In larger amounts, NO forms peroxynitrite, which contributes to neurotoxicity.
- Inhibition of nNOS reduces long-term potentiation and long-term depression, probably because NO functions as a retrograde messenger. Inhibition of nNOS also protects against ischaemic brain damage in animal models.
- Carbon monoxide shares many properties with NO and may also be a neural mediator.

Lipid mediators

- Arachidonic acid is produced in neurons by receptor-mediated hydrolysis of phospholipid. It is converted to various eicosanoids and to anandamide.
- Arachidonic acid itself, as well as its active products, can produce rapid and slow effects by regulation of ion channels and protein kinase cascades. Such effects can occur in the donor cell or in adjacent cells and nerve terminals.
- Anandamide is an endogenous activator of cannabinoid receptors (Ch. 15) and also of the vanilloid receptor (Ch. 41).
- The functional role of lipid mediators in the central nervous system is still poorly understood.

that it should interact with specific membrane receptors, and that there should be mechanisms for its inactivation—do not apply to NO. Moreover, it is an inorganic toxic gas, not at all like the kind of molecule we are used to. The mediator function of NO, and probably also carbon monoxide (CO), is now well established, however (see Bredt & Snyder, 1992; Vincent, 1995; Barañano et al., 2001). NO diffuses rapidly through cell membranes, and its action is not highly localised. Its half-life depends greatly on the chemical environment, ranging from seconds in blood to several minutes in normal tissues. The rate of inactivation of

NO (see Ch. 17, reaction 17.1) increases disproportionately with NO concentration, so low levels of NO are relatively stable. The presence of superoxide, with which NO reacts (see below), shortens its half-life considerably.

Nitric oxide in the nervous system is produced mainly by the constitutive neuronal form of *nitric oxide synthase (nNOS*; see Ch. 17), which can be detected either histochemically or by immunolabelling. This enzyme is present in roughly 2% of neurons, both short interneurons and long-tract neurons, in virtually all brain areas, with particular concentrations in the cerebellum and hippocampus. It occurs in cell bodies and dendrites, as well as in axon terminals, suggesting (because NO is not stored, but released as it is made) that the release of NO is not restricted to conventional neurotransmitter release sites. nNOS is calmodulin-dependent and is activated by a rise in intracellular Ca^{2+} concentration, which can occur by many mechanisms, including action potential conduction and neurotransmitter action. Many studies have shown that NO production is increased by activation of synaptic pathways, or by other events, such as brain ischaemia (see Ch. 35).

Nitric oxide exerts its effects in two main ways.

- By activation of soluble guanylate cyclase, leading to the production of cGMP, leading to various phosphorylation cascades (Ch. 3). This 'physiological' control mechanism operates at low NO concentrations of about $0.1\,\mu M$.
- By reacting with the superoxide free radical to generate peroxynitrite, a highly toxic anion that acts by oxidising various intracellular proteins. This requires concentrations of $1-10\,\mu M$, which are achieved in brain ischaemia.

There is good evidence that NO plays a role in long-term potentiation and depression (see Ch. 33), because these phenomena are reduced or prevented by NOS inhibitors and are absent in transgenic mice in which the *nNOS* gene has been disrupted.

Based on the same kind of evidence, NO is also believed to play an important part in the mechanisms by which ischaemia causes neuronal death (see Ch. 35). There is also speculation that it may be involved in other processes, including neurodegeneration in Parkinson's disease, senile dementia and amyotrophic lateral sclerosis, and the local control of blood flow linked to neuronal activity. If substantiated, these theories will open up major new therapeutic possibilities in some hitherto intractable disease areas.

▼ **Carbon monoxide** is best known as a poisonous gas present in vehicle exhaust, which binds strongly to haemoglobin, causing tissue anoxia. However, it is also formed endogenously and has many features in common with NO (see Verma et al., 1993; Barañano et al., 2001). Neurons and other cells contain a CO-generating enzyme, *haem oxygenase,* and CO, like NO, activates guanylate cyclase.

The role of CO as a CNS mediator is not well established, but there is some evidence that it plays a role in the cerebellum and also in olfactory neurons, where cGMP-sensitive ion channels are involved in the transduction process.

Undoubtedly, further functions of NO and CO in the brain remain to be identified, and novel therapeutic approaches may come from targeting the different steps in the synthetic and signal transduction pathways for these surprising mediators. We may have to endure the ponderous whimsy of many 'NO' puns, but it should be worth it in the end.

LIPID MEDIATORS

▼ The formation of arachidonic acid, and its conversion to **eicosanoids** (mainly prostaglandins, leukotrienes and hydroxyeicosatetraenoic acids [HETEs]; see Ch. 13) and to the endogenous cannabinoid receptor ligand **anandamide** (see Ch. 15) are known to take place in the CNS. They doubtless play an important role, although our knowledge in this area is still fragmentary (for reviews, see Piomelli, 1995; Piomelli et al., 2000), partly because there are few selective inhibitors that can be used to probe the various steps in the rather lengthy biochemical pathways through which the mediators are formed and exert their effects. Figure 34.9 shows a schematic view of the different possibilities, but it should be

realised that evidence as to the functional importance of these pathways is still very limited.

Phospholipid cleavage, leading to arachidonic acid production, occurs in neurons in response to receptor activation by many different mediators, including neurotransmitters. The arachidonic acid so formed can act directly as an intracellular messenger, controlling both ion channels and various parts of the protein kinase cascade (see Ch. 3), producing both rapid and delayed effects on neuronal function. Arachidonic acid can also be metabolised to anandamide and to eicosanoids, some of which (principally the HETEs) can also act as intracellular messengers acting in the same cell. Eicosanoids can also exert an autocrine effect via membrane receptors expressed by the cell. Both arachidonic acid itself and its products escape readily from the cell of origin and can affect neighbouring structures, including presynaptic terminals (retrograde signalling) and adjacent cells (paracrine signalling), by acting on receptors or by acting directly as intracellular messengers. Theoretically, the possibilities are numerous, but there are so far only a few instances where this system is known to play a significant role. These include our old friend long-term potentiation (Ch. 33), one component of which is prevented by inhibition of phospholipase A_2, where arachidonic acid is believed to serve as a retrograde messenger causing facilitation of transmitter release by the presynaptic nerve terminal. A second well-studied system is the *Aplysia* sensory neuron, where the effects of various inhibitory mediators, acting on membrane receptors, are exerted through the intracellular actions of arachidonic acid and its products.

One surprise in this field has been the discovery that anandamide, besides being an agonist at cannabinoid receptors, also activates vanilloid receptors (see Ch. 41), which are involved in the response of peripheral sensory nerve terminals to painful stimuli. What role, if any, anandamide has in pain transmission remains to be seen.

A FINAL MESSAGE

In the last two chapters, we have taken a long and tortuous tour through the brain and its chemistry, with two questions at the back of our minds: What mediators and what receptors play a key role in what brain functions? How does the information relate to existing and future drugs that aim to correct malfunctions? Despite the efforts of a huge army of researchers deploying an arsenal of powerful new techniques, the answers to these questions seem to remain as elusive as ever. Although transgenic techniques allow specific gene products (i.e. proteins) to be modified in a much more precise and controllable way than can be achieved pharmacologically, behavioural analysis of transgenic animals has failed to clear the air very much. The array of potential CNS targets—comprising multiple receptor subtypes, many with the added complexity of heteromeric assemblies, splice variants, etc., along with regulatory mechanisms that control their expression and localisation—continues to grow in complexity. Speculation about the best target to aim at in order to ameliorate the effect of a particular brain malfunction, such as stroke or schizophrenia, has become less focused, even if better informed, than it was two decades ago. In the ensuing chapters in this section, we shall find that most of the therapeutic successes have come from chance discoveries that were followed up empirically; few have followed a logical, mechanism-based route to success. The optimistic view is that this is changing, and that future therapeutic discoveries will depend less on luck and more on molecular logic. But the revolution is slow in coming. One of the key problems, perhaps, is that the brain puts cells, organelles and molecules exactly

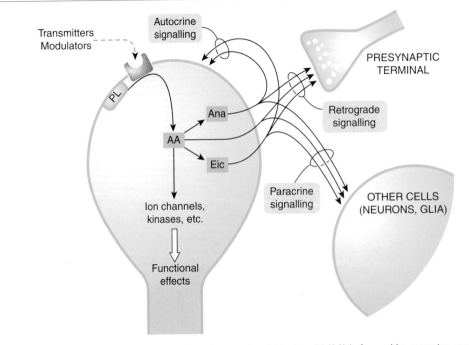

Fig. 34.9 Postulated modes of signalling by lipid mediators. Arachidonic acid (AA) is formed by receptor-mediated cleavage of membrane phospholipid. It can act directly as an intracellular messenger on ion channels or components of different kinase cascades, producing various long- and short-term effects. It can also be converted to eicosanoids (prostaglandins, leukotrienes or hydroxyeicosatetraenoic acids [HETEs]) or to anandamide (Ana). HETEs can also act directly as intracellular messengers. All these mediators diffuse out of the cell, and exert effects on presynaptic terminals and neighbouring cells, acting either on extracellular receptors or intracellularly. There are examples of most of these modes of signalling but only limited information about their functional significance in the nervous system. Eic, eicosanoids; PL, membrane phospholipid.

where they are needed, and uses the same molecules to perform different functions in different locations. Drug discovery scientists are getting quite good at devising molecule-specific ligands (see Ch. 56), but we lack delivery systems able to target them anatomically even to macroscopic brain regions, let alone to specific cells and subcellular structures.

REFERENCES AND FURTHER READING

General references

Cooper J R, Bloom F E, Roth R H 2003 Biochemical basis of neuropharmacology. Oxford University Press, New York (*Clear and well-written textbook giving more detailed information on many topics covered in this chapter*)

Davis K L, Charney D, Coyle J T, Nemeroff C (eds) 2002 Neuropsychopharmacology: the fifth generation of progress. Lippincott, Williams & Wilkins, Philadelphia (*A 2000-page monster with excellent and authoritative articles on basic and clinical aspects*)

Nestler E J, Hyman S E, Malenka R C 2001 Molecular neuropharmacology. McGraw-Hill, New York (*Good modern textbook*)

Noradrenaline

Ashton-Jones G 2002 Noradrenaline. In: Davis K L, Charney D, Coyle J T, Nemeroff C (eds) 2002 Neuropsychopharmacology: the fifth generation of progress. Lippincott, Williams & Wilkins, Philadelphia

Dopamine

Girault J-A, Greengard P 2004 The neurobiology of dopamine signalling. Arch Neurol 61: 641–644 (*Short review article*)

Missale C, Nash S R, Robinson S W et al. 1998 Dopamine receptors: from structure to function. Physiol Rev 78: 198–225 (*Comprehensive review article*)

Seeman P, Van Tol H H M 1994 Dopamine receptor pharmacology. Trends Pharmacol Sci 15: 264–270 (*Introductory review article*)

Sibley D R 1999 New insights into dopaminergic receptor function using antisense and genetically altered animals. Annu Rev Pharmacol Toxicol 39: 313–341

Svenningsson P, Nishi A, Fisone G et al. 2004 DARPP-32: an integrator of neurotransmission Annu Rev Pharmacol Toxicol 44: 269–296 (*Review article describing the multiple roles of this component of the dopamine signalling pathway*)

Tarazi F I, Zhang K, Baldessarini R J 2004 Dopamine D$_4$ receptors: beyond schizophrenia. J Recept Signal Transduct 24: 131–147 (*Dismisses link between D$_4$ receptor polymorphism and schizophrenia, suggesting possible link with attention deficit hyperactivity disorder, impulsivity and cognitive function*)

5-Hydroxytryptamine

Azmitia E C, Whitaker-Azmitia P M 1995 Anatomy, cell biology and plasticity of the serotonergic system. In:

Bloom F E, Kupfer D J (eds) Psychopharmacology: a fourth generation of progress. Raven Press, New York (*General review article*)

Barnes N M, Sharp T 1999 A review of central 5-HT receptors and their function. Neuropharmacology 38: 1083–1152 (*Detailed compilation of data relating to distribution, pharmacology and function of 5-HT receptors in the CNS; useful information source but not particularly illuminating*)

Hedlund P B, Sutcliffe J G 2004 Functional, molecular and pharmacological advances in 5-HT$_7$ receptor research. Trends Pharmacol Sci 25: 481–486 (*Reviews current understanding of role of 5-HT$_7$ receptors, including data from receptor knockout mice*)

Woolley M L, Marsden C A, Fone K C 2004 5-HT$_6$ receptors. Curr Drug Targets CNS Neurol Disord 3: 59–79 (*General review article focusing on the many possible clinical applications of 5-HT$_6$ receptor agonists and antagonists*)

Acetylcholine

Beeri R, Andres C, Lev-Lehman E et al. 1995 Transgenic expression of human acetylcholinesterase induces progressive cognitive deterioration in mice. Curr Biol

5: 1063–1071 (*Describes a transgenic mouse model with impaired cholinergic transmission leading to cognitive changes*)

Cordero-Erausquin M, Marubio L M, Klink R, Changeux J-P 2000 Nicotinic receptor function: new perspectives from knockout mice. Trends Pharmacol Sci 21: 211–217 (*Short review article*)

Hagan J J, Morris R G M 1988 The cholinergic hypothesis of memory: a review of animal experiments. In: Iversen L L, Iversen S, Snyder S H (eds) Handbook of psychopharmacology, vol 20. Plenum, New York, pp 237–323 (*Useful summary, now rather dated, of evidence implicating ACh in learning and memory*)

Hogg R C, Raggenbass M, Bertrand D 2003 Nicotinic acetylcholine receptors: from structure to brain function. Rev Physiol Biochem Pharmacol 147: 1–46 (*General review of molecular and functional properties of brain nAChRs*)

Soreq H, Sediman S 2001 Acetylcholinesterase—new roles for an old actor. Nat Rev Neurosci 2: 294–302 (*Speculative review of evidence suggesting functions for acetylcholinesterase other than ACh hydrolysis*)

Wess J 2004 Muscarinic acetylcholine receptor knockout mice: novel phenotypes and clinical implications. Annu Rev Pharmacol Toxicol 44: 423–450 (*Description of functional effects of deleting various peripheral and central mAChR isoforms*)

Other messengers

Barañano D E, Ferris C D, Snyder S H 2001 Atypical neural messengers. Trends Neurosci 24: 99–106 (*Short trendy review on some established mediators, such as NO, and some speculative ones, such as CO and D-serine*)

Bredt D S, Snyder S H 1992 Nitric oxide, a novel neuronal messenger. Neuron 8: 3–11 (*Widely quoted review article that anticipates many later discoveries*)

Brown R E, Stevens D R, Haas H L 2001 The physiology of brain histamine. Prog Neurobiol 63: 637–672 (*Useful review article*)

Brzezinski A 1997 Melatonin in humans. New Engl J Med 336: 186–195 (*Clear and well-referenced review article; recommended as an introduction*)

Dawson T M, Snyder S H 1994 Gases as biological messengers: nitric oxide and carbon monoxide in the brain. J Neurosci 14: 5147–5159 (*Excellent introductory review summarising ideas in a new area*)

Dunwiddie T V, Masino S A 2001 The role and regulation of adenosine in the central nervous system. Annu Rev Neurosci 24: 31–55 (*Good short review emphasising the protective role of adenosine*)

Piomelli D 1995 Arachidonic acid. In: Bloom F E, Kupfer D J (eds) Psychopharmacology: a fourth generation of progress. Raven Press, New York (*Excellent review article*)

Piomelli D, Giuffrida A, Calignano A, Fonseca F R 2000 The endocannabinoid system as a target for therapeutic drugs. Trends Pharmacol Sci 21: 218–224 (*Short review article on role of anandamide in CNS*)

Robertson S J, Ennion S J, Evans R J, Edwards F A 2001 Synaptic P2X receptors. Curr Opin Neurobiol 11: 378–386 (*Review on transmitter role of ATP, focusing on receptor pharmacology*)

Verma A, Hirsch D J, Glatt C E et al. 1993 Carbon monoxide: a putative neural messenger. Science 259: 381–384 (*Speculative review that points out similarities with NO*)

Vincent S R (ed) 1995 Nitric oxide in the nervous system. Academic Press, London (*Useful compendium of review articles on all aspects of NO in the nervous system*)

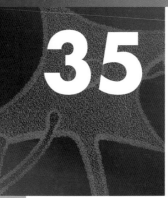

35

Neurodegenerative diseases

OVERVIEW

As a rule, dead neurons in the adult central nervous system (CNS) are not replaced,[1] nor can their terminals regenerate when their axons are interrupted. Therefore any pathological process causing neuronal death generally has irreversible consequences. At first sight, this appears to be very unpromising territory for pharmacological intervention, and indeed drug therapy is currently very limited, except in the case of Parkinson's disease (PD) (see below). Nevertheless, the

incidence and social impact of neurodegenerative brain disorders in ageing populations has resulted in a massive research effort in recent years.

In this chapter, we focus mainly on three common neurodegenerative conditions: *Alzheimer's disease* (*AD*), *PD* and *ischaemic brain damage* (*stroke*). AD and PD are the commonest examples of a group of chronic, slowly developing conditions that include various *prion diseases* (e.g. Creutzfeldt–Jakob disease, CJD, see below). They have a common aetiology in that they are caused by the aggregation of misfolded variants of normal physiological proteins (see reviews by Forman et al., 2004; Mallucci & Collinge, 2005). This new understanding has suggested a range of potential new therapeutic strategies in this important area. To date, though, the available therapeutic interventions are aimed at compensating for, rather than preventing or reversing, the neuronal loss.

Stroke, which is also a common disorder of enormous socioeconomic importance, results from acute ischaemic brain damage, quite different from the aetiology of chronic neurodegenerative diseases, requiring different but equally challenging therapeutic approaches. The main topics discussed are:

- mechanisms responsible for neuronal death, focusing on protein aggregation (e.g. amyloidosis), excitotoxicity, oxidative stress and apoptosis
- pharmacological approaches to *neuroprotection*, based on the above mechanisms
- pharmacological approaches to compensation for neuronal loss (applicable mainly to AD and PD).

PROTEIN MISFOLDING AND AGGREGATION IN CHRONIC NEURODEGENERATIVE DISEASES

Misfolding means the adoption of abnormal conformations, by certain normally expressed proteins such that they tend to form large insoluble aggregates (Fig. 35.1). The conversion of the linear amino acid chain produced by the ribosome into a functional protein requires it to be folded correctly into a compact conformation with specific amino acids correctly located on its surface.

---

[1]It is recognised that new neurons are formed from progenitor cells in certain regions of the adult brain, even in primates. Whether this occurs in the cortex, and whether it plays any role in learning and memory, is a matter of dispute (see Gross, 2000; Rakic, 2002). Certainly, it plays little if any role in brain repair. However, learning how to harness the inherent ability of neuronal progenitors (stem cells) to form new neurons is seen as an obvious approach to treating neurodegenerative disorders.

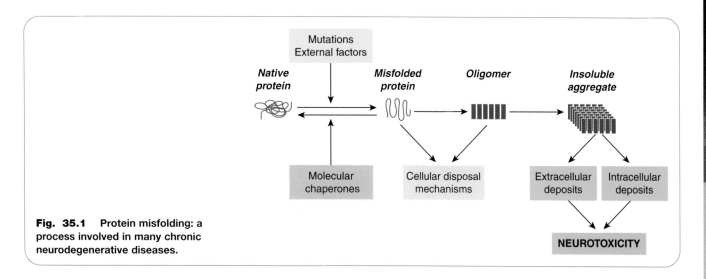

Fig. 35.1 Protein misfolding: a process involved in many chronic neurodegenerative diseases.

This complicated stepwise sequence can easily go wrong and lead to misfolded variants that are unable to find a way back to the correct 'native' conformation. The misfolded molecules are non-functional with respect to the normal function of the protein, but can nonetheless make mischief within the cell. The misfolding often means that hydrophobic residues that would normally be buried in the core of the protein are exposed on its surface, which gives the molecules a strong tendency to aggregate, initially as oligomers, and then as insoluble microscopic aggregates (Fig. 35.1). They also tend to stick to cell membranes. The tendency to adopt such conformations may be favoured by specific mutations of the protein in question, or by infection with prions (see below).

Misfolded conformations can be generated spontaneously at a low rate throughout life, so that aggregates accumulate gradually with age. In the nervous system, the aggregates often form distinct structures, generally known as *amyloid deposits,* that are visible under the microscope and are characteristic of neurodegenerative disease. Although the mechanisms are not clear, such aggregates, or the misfolded protein precursors, lead to neuronal death. Examples of neurodegenerative diseases that are caused by such protein misfolding and aggregation are shown in Table 35.1.

The brain possesses a variety of protective mechanisms that limit the accumulation of such protein aggregates. The main ones are the production of 'chaperone' proteins, which bind to newly synthesised or misfolded proteins and encourage them to fold correctly, and the 'ubiquitination' reaction, which prepares proteins for destruction within the cell. Accumulation of protein deposits occurs when these protective mechanisms are unable to cope. For reviews of these mechanisms, see Stefani & Dobson (2003) and Selkoe (2004).

MECHANISMS OF NEURONAL DEATH

Acute injury to cells causes them to undergo *necrosis,* recognised pathologically by cell swelling, vacuolisation and lysis, and associated with Ca^{2+} overload of the cells and membrane damage (see below). Necrotic cells typically spill their contents into the

Protein misfolding

- Many chronic neurodegenerative diseases involve the misfolding of normal or mutated forms of physiological proteins. Examples include Alzheimer's disease, Parkinson's disease, amyotrophic lateral sclerosis and many less common diseases.
- Misfolded proteins are normally removed by intracellular degradation pathways, which may be altered in neurodegenerative disorders.
- Misfolded proteins tend to aggregate, initially as soluble oligomers, later as large insoluble aggregates that accumulate intracellularly or extracellularly as microscopic deposits, which are stable and resistant to proteolysis.
- Misfolded proteins often present hydrophobic surface residues that promote aggregation and association with membranes.
- The mechanisms responsible for neuronal death are unclear, but there is evidence that both the soluble aggregates and the microscopic deposits may be neurotoxic.

surrounding tissue, evoking an inflammatory response. Cells can also die by *apoptosis* or programmed cell death (see Ch. 5), a slower process that is essential for many processes throughout life, including development, immune regulation and tissue remodelling. Apoptosis, as well as necrosis, occurs in many neurodegenerative disorders (including acute conditions such as stroke and head injury; for review, see Jellinger, 2001). The distinction between necrosis and apoptosis as processes leading to neurodegeneration is not absolute, for challenges such as excitotoxicity and oxidative stress may be enough to kill cells directly by necrosis or, if less intense, may induce them to undergo apoptosis. Both processes therefore represent possible targets for putative neuroprotective drug therapy. Pharmacological interference with the apoptotic pathway may become possible in the future, but for the present most efforts

Table 35.1 Examples of neurodegenerative diseases associated with protein misfolding and aggregation[a]

Disease	Protein	Characteristic pathology	Notes
Alzheimer's disease	β-Amyloid (Aβ)	Amyloid plaques	Aβ mutations occur in rare familial forms of Alzheimer's disease
	Tau	Neurofibrillary tangles	Implicated in other pathologies ('tauopathies'} as well as Alzheimer's disease
Parkinson's disease	α-Synuclein	Lewy bodies	α-Synuclein mutations occur in some types of familial Parkinson's disease
Creutzfeldt–Jakob disease	Prion protein	Insoluble aggregates of prion protein	Transmitted by infection with prion protein in its misfolded state
Huntington's disease	Huntingtin	No gross lesions	One of several genetic 'polyglutamine repeat' disorders
Amyotrophic lateral sclerosis (motor neuron disease)	Superoxide dismutase	Loss of motor neurons	Mutated superoxide dismutase tends to form aggregates; loss of enzyme function increases susceptibility to oxidative stress

[a]Protein aggregation disorders are often collectively known as *amyloidoses* and commonly affect organs other than the brain.

are directed at the processes involved in cell necrosis, and at compensating pharmacologically for the neuronal loss.

EXCITOTOXICITY

Despite its ubiquitous role as a neurotransmitter, **glutamate** is highly toxic to neurons, a phenomenon dubbed *excitotoxicity* (see Ch. 33). A low concentration of glutamate applied to neurons in culture kills the cells, and the finding in the 1970s that glutamate given orally produces neurodegeneration in vivo caused considerable alarm because of the widespread use of glutamate as a 'taste-enhancing' food additive. The 'Chinese restaurant syndrome'—an acute attack of neck stiffness and chest pain—is well known, but so far the possibility of more serious neurotoxicity is only hypothetical.

Local injection of **kainic acid** is used experimentally to produce neurotoxic lesions. It acts by excitation of local glutamate-releasing neurons, and the release of glutamate, acting on NMDA and also metabotropic receptors (Ch. 33), leads to neuronal death.

Calcium overload is the essential factor in excitotoxicity. The mechanisms by which this occurs and leads to cell death are as follows (Fig. 35.2).

- Glutamate activates NMDA, AMPA and metabotropic receptors (sites 1, 2 and 3). Activation of AMPA receptors depolarises the cell, which unblocks the NMDA channels (see Ch. 33), permitting Ca^{2+} entry. Depolarisation also opens voltage-activated calcium channels (site 4), releasing more glutamate. Metabotropic receptors cause the release of intracellular Ca^{2+} from the endoplasmic reticulum. Na^+ entry further contributes to Ca^{2+} entry by stimulating Ca^{2+}/Na^+ exchange (site 5). Depolarisation inhibits or reverses glutamate uptake (site 6), thus increasing the extracellular glutamate concentration.
- The mechanisms that normally operate to counteract the rise in $[Ca^{2+}]_i$ include the Ca^{2+} efflux pump (site 7) and, indirectly, the Na^+ pump (site 8).

- The mitochondria and endoplasmic reticulum act as capacious sinks for Ca^{2+} and normally keep $[Ca^{2+}]_i$ under control. Loading of the mitochondrial stores beyond a certain point, however, disrupts mitochondrial function, reducing ATP synthesis, thus reducing the energy available for the membrane pumps and for Ca^{2+} accumulation by the endoplasmic reticulum. Formation of reactive oxygen species is also enhanced. This represents the danger point at which positive feedback exaggerates the process.
- Raised $[Ca^{2+}]_i$ affects many processes, the chief ones relevant to neurotoxicity being:
  —increased glutamate release
  —activation of proteases (calpains) and lipases, causing membrane damage
  —activation of nitric oxide synthase; while low concentrations of nitric oxide are neuroprotective, high concentrations in the presence of reactive oxygen species generate peroxynitrite and hydroxyl free radicals, which damage many important biomolecules, including membrane lipids, proteins and DNA
  —increased arachidonic acid release, which increases free radical production and also inhibits glutamate uptake (site 6).

Glutamate and Ca^{2+} are arguably the two most ubiquitous chemical signals, extracellular and intracellular, respectively, underlying brain function, so it is disconcerting that such cytotoxic mayhem can be unleashed when they get out of control. Both are stored in dangerous amounts in subcellular organelles, like hand grenades in an ammunition store. Defence against excitotoxicity is clearly essential if our brains are to have any chance of staying alive. Mitochondrial energy metabolism provides one line of defence (see above), and impaired mitochondrial function, by rendering neurons vulnerable to excitotoxic damage, may be a factor in various neurodegenerative conditions, including PD.

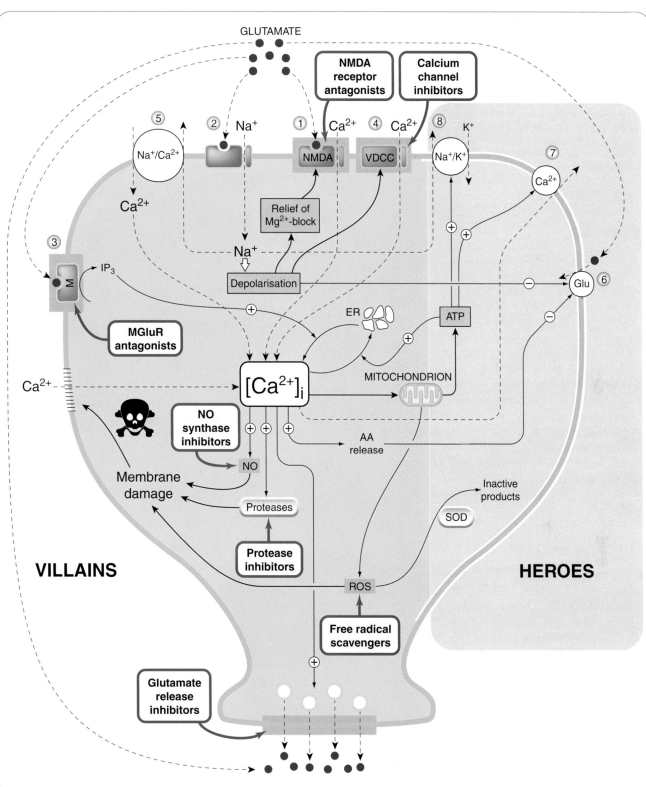

Fig. 35.2 Mechanisms of excitotoxicity. Membrane receptors, ion channels and transporters, identified by numbers 1–8, are discussed in the text. Possible sites of action of neuroprotective drugs (not yet of proven clinical value) are highlighted. Mechanisms on the left (villains) are those that favour cell death, while those on the right (heroes) are protective. See text for details. AA, arachidonic acid; ER, endoplasmic reticulum; Glu, glutamate uptake; IP$_3$, inositol trisphosphate; M, MGluR, metabotropic glutamate receptor; NO, nitric oxide; ROS, reactive oxygen species; SOD, superoxide dismutase; VDCC, voltage-dependent calcium channel.

The role of excitotoxicity in ischaemic brain damage is well established (see below), and it is also believed to be a factor in other neurodegenerative diseases, such as those discussed below (see Lipton & Rosenberg, 1994).

▼ There are several examples of neurodegenerative conditions caused by environmental toxins acting as agonists on glutamate receptors. **Domoic acid** is a glutamate analogue produced by mussels, which was identified as the cause of an epidemic of severe mental and neurological deterioration in a group of Newfoundlanders in 1987. On the island of Guam, a syndrome combining the features of dementia, paralysis and PD was traced to an excitotoxic amino acid, β-methylamino-alanine, in the seeds of a local plant. Discouraging the consumption of these seeds has largely eliminated the disease.

APOPTOSIS

Apoptosis can be initiated by various cell surface signals (see Ch. 5). The cell is systematically dismantled, and the shrunken remnants are removed by macrophages without causing inflammation. Apoptotic cells can be identified by a staining technique that detects the characteristic DNA breaks. Many different signalling pathways can result in apoptosis, but in all cases the final pathway resulting in cell death is the activation of a family of proteases (*caspases*), which inactivate various intracellular proteins. Neural apoptosis is normally prevented by neuronal growth factors, including nerve growth factor and brain-derived neurotrophic factor, secreted proteins that are required for the survival of different populations of neurons in the CNS. These growth factors regulate the expression of the two gene products Bax and Bcl-2, Bax being proapoptotic and Bcl-2 being antiapoptotic (see Ch. 5). Blocking apoptosis by interfering at specific points on these pathways represents an attractive strategy for developing neuroprotective drugs, but one that has yet to bear fruit.

OXIDATIVE STRESS

The brain has high energy needs, which are met almost entirely by mitochondrial oxidative phosphorylation, generating ATP at the same time as reducing molecular O_2 to H_2O. Under certain conditions, highly reactive oxygen species, for example oxygen and hydroxyl free radicals and H_2O_2, may be generated as side products of this process (see Coyle & Puttfarken, 1993). Oxidative stress is the result of excessive production of these reactive species. They can also be produced as a by-product of other biochemical pathways, including nitric oxide synthesis and arachidonic acid metabolism (which are implicated in excitotoxicity; see above), as well as the mixed function oxidase system (see Ch. 8). Unchecked, reactive oxygen radicals attack many key molecules, including enzymes, membrane lipids and DNA. Not surprisingly, defence mechanisms are provided, in the form of enzymes such as *superoxide dismutase* (*SOD*) and *catalase*, as well as antioxidants such as *ascorbic acid, glutathione* and *α-tocopherol* (vitamin E), which normally keep these reactive species in check. Some cytokines, especially tumour necrosis factor (TNF-α), which is produced in conditions of brain ischaemia or inflammation (Ch. 13), exert a protective effect, partly by increasing the expression of SOD. Transgenic animals lacking TNF receptors show enhanced susceptibility to brain ischaemia. Mutations of the gene encoding

SOD (Fig. 35.2) are associated with a progressive form of motor neuron disease known as *amyotrophic lateral sclerosis*, a fatal paralytic disease resulting from progressive degeneration of motor neurons, and transgenic mice expressing mutated SOD develop a similar condition.[2] Accumulation of aggregates of misfolded mutated SOD (see above) may also contribute to neurodegeneration. It is possible that accumulated or inherited mutations in enzymes such as those of the mitochondrial respiratory chain lead to a congenital or age-related increase in susceptibility to oxidative stress, which is manifest in different kinds of inherited neurodegenerative disorders (such as Huntington's disease), and in age-related neurodegeneration.

Several possible targets for therapeutic intervention with neuroprotective drugs are shown in Figure 35.2. Disappointingly, intense effort to find effective drugs for a range of neurodegenerative disorders in which excitotoxicity is believed to play a part has had very limited success. **Riluzole**, a compound that inhibits both the release and the postsynaptic action of glutamate, retards to some degree the deterioration of patients with amyotrophic lateral sclerosis. **Memantine**, a compound first described 40 years ago, is a weak NMDA receptor antagonist that produces slight improvement in moderate-to-severe cases of AD, and was recently approved for clinical use.

ISCHAEMIC BRAIN DAMAGE

After heart disease and cancer, strokes are the commonest cause of death in Europe and North America, and the 70% that are non-fatal are the commonest cause of disability. Approximately 85% of strokes are ischaemic, usually due to thrombosis of a major cerebral artery. The remainder are haemorrhagic, due to rupture of a cerebral artery.

PATHOPHYSIOLOGY

Interruption of blood supply to the brain initiates the cascade of neuronal events shown in Figure 35.2, which lead in turn to later consequences, including cerebral oedema and inflammation, which can also contribute to brain damage (see Dirnagl et al., 1999). Further damage can occur following reperfusion, because of the production of reactive oxygen species when the oxygenation is restored. Reperfusion injury may be an important component in stroke patients. These secondary processes often take hours to develop, providing a window of opportunity for therapeutic intervention. The lesion produced by occlusion of a major cerebral artery consists of a central core in which the neurons quickly undergo irreversible necrosis, surrounded by a *penumbra* of compromised tissue in which inflammation and apoptotic cell death develop over a period of several hours. It is assumed that neuroprotective therapies, given within a few hours, might inhibit this secondary penumbral damage.

---

[2]Surprisingly, the SOD mutation responsible is more, rather than less, active than the normal enzyme. The mechanism by which it causes neurodegeneration is not clear.

- Excitatory amino acids (e.g. glutamate) can cause neuronal death.
- Excitotoxicity is associated mainly with activation of NMDA receptors, but other types of excitatory amino acid receptors also contribute.
- Excitotoxicity results from a sustained rise in intracellular Ca^{2+} concentration (Ca^{2+} overload).
- Excitotoxicity can occur under pathological conditions (e.g. cerebral ischaemia, epilepsy) in which excessive glutamate release occurs. It can also occur when chemicals such as kainic acid are administered.
- Raised intracellular Ca^{2+} causes cell death by various mechanisms, including activation of proteases, formation of free radicals, and lipid peroxidation. Formation of nitric oxide and arachidonic acid are also involved.
- Various mechanisms act normally to protect neurons against excitotoxicity, the main ones being Ca^{2+} transport systems, mitochondrial function and the production of free radical scavengers.
- Oxidative stress refers to conditions (e.g. hypoxia) in which the protective mechanisms are compromised, reactive oxygen species accumulate, and neurons become more susceptible to excitotoxic damage.
- Excitotoxicity due to environmental chemicals may contribute to some neurodegenerative disorders.
- Measures designed to reduce excitotoxicity include the use of glutamate antagonists, calcium channel–blocking drugs and free radical scavengers; none are yet proven for clinical use.

Glutamate excitotoxicity plays a critical role in brain ischaemia. Ischaemia causes depolarisation of neurons, and the release of large amounts of glutamate. Ca^{2+} accumulation occurs, partly as a result of glutamate acting on NMDA receptors, for both Ca^{2+} entry and cell death following cerebral ischaemia are inhibited by drugs that block NMDA receptors or channels (see Ch. 33). Nitric oxide is also produced in amounts much greater than result from normal neuronal activity (i.e. to levels that are toxic rather than modulatory).

THERAPEUTIC APPROACHES

The only drug currently approved for treating strokes is recombinant **tissue plasminogen activator** (**tPA**), given intravenously, which helps to restore blood flow by dispersing the thrombus (see Ch. 21). It gives significant, but slight, functional benefit to patients who survive. To be effective, it must be given within about 3 hours of the thrombotic episode. Also, it should not be given in the 15% of cases where the cause is haemorrhage rather than thrombosis. Because this can be determined only by brain scanning, tPA is actually given to only 1–2% of stroke victims.

A preferable approach would be to use neuroprotective agents aimed at rescuing cells in the penumbral region of the lesion,

which are otherwise likely to die. In animal models involving cerebral artery occlusion, many drugs targeted at the mechanisms shown in Figure 35.2 (not to mention many others that have been tested on the basis of more far-flung theories) act in this way to reduce the size of the infarct. These include glutamate antagonists, calcium and sodium channel inhibitors, free radical scavengers, anti-inflammatory drugs, protease inhibitors and others. It seems that almost anything works. Altogether, Green et al. (2003) reported that more than 37 such agents had been tested in more than 114 clinical trials, and all had failed to show efficacy. The dispiriting list of failures includes calcium and sodium channel blockers (e.g. **nimodipine, fosphenytoin**), NMDA receptor antagonists (**selfotel, eliprodil, dextromethorphan**), drugs that inhibit glutamate release (**adenosine analogues, lobeluzole**), drugs that enhance GABA effects (e.g. **chlormethiazole**), and various free radical scavengers (e.g. **tirilazad**). Green et al (2003) argue, reasonably enough, that the animal models in use fail to replicate the clinical situation, and urge the use of more rigorous experimental protocols to make animal models more predictive, but a success rate of zero among 37 compounds suggests that the models are more deeply flawed.

Controlled clinical trials on stroke patients are problematic and very expensive, partly because of the large variability of outcome in terms of functional recovery, which means that large groups of patients (typically several hundred) need to be observed for several months. The need to start therapy within hours of the attack is an additional problem.

Stroke treatment is certainly not—so far at least—one of pharmacology's success stories, and medical hopes rest more on prevention (e.g. by controlling blood pressure,[3] taking **aspirin** and preventing atherosclerosis) than on treatment.

- Associated with intracerebral thrombosis or haemorrhage (less common), resulting in rapid death of neurons by necrosis in the centre of the lesion, followed by more gradual (hours) degeneration of cells in penumbra due to excitotoxicity and inflammation.
- Spontaneous functional recovery occurs to a highly variable degree.
- Although many types of drug that interfere with excitotoxicity (*see Protein misfolding box*) are able to reduce infarct size in experimental animals, none of these have so far proved efficacious in humans.
- Tissue plasminogen activator, which disperses blood clots, is beneficial if it is given within 3 hours.
- None of the many neuroprotective drugs that are effective in animal models are efficacious in the clinical trials.

---

[3]It is not obvious why hypertension should predispose to thrombotic as opposed to haemorrhagic stroke, yet studies have shown that normalising blood pressure effectively eliminates the increased risk of stroke.

ALZHEIMER'S DISEASE

Loss of cognitive ability with age is considered to be a normal process whose rate and extent is very variable. AD was originally defined as *presenile dementia*, but it now appears that the same pathology underlies the dementia irrespective of the age of onset. AD refers to dementia that does not have an antecedent cause, such as stroke, brain trauma or alcohol. Its prevalence rises sharply with age, from about 5% at 65 to 90% or more at 95. Until recently, age-related dementia was considered to result from the steady loss of neurons that normally goes on throughout life, possibly accelerated by a failing blood supply associated with atherosclerosis. Studies over the past three decades have, however, revealed specific genetic and molecular mechanisms underlying AD (reviewed by Selkoe, 1997; Bossy-Wetzel et al., 2004), which have opened potential new therapeutic opportunities (see Yamada & Nabeshima, 2000).

PATHOGENESIS OF ALZHEIMER'S DISEASE

Alzheimer's disease is associated with brain shrinkage and localised loss of neurons, mainly in the hippocampus and basal forebrain. The loss of cholinergic neurons in the hippocampus and frontal cortex is a feature of the disease, and is thought to underlie the cognitive deficit and loss of short-term memory that occur in AD. Two microscopic features are characteristic of the disease, namely extracellular *amyloid plaques*, consisting of amorphous extracellular deposits of β-amyloid protein (known as Aβ), and intraneuronal *neurofibrillary tangles*, comprising filaments of a phosphorylated form of a microtubule-associated protein (Tau). Both of these deposits are protein aggregates that result from misfolding of native proteins, as discussed above. They appear also in normal brains, although in smaller numbers. The early appearance of amyloid deposits presages the development of AD, although symptoms may not develop for many years. Altered processing of amyloid protein from its precursor (amyloid precursor protein, APP; see Bossy-Wetzel et al., 2004) is now recognised as the key to the pathogenesis of AD. This conclusion is based on several lines of evidence, particularly the genetic analysis of certain, relatively rare, types of familial AD, in which mutations of the APP gene, or of other genes that control amyloid processing, have been discovered. The APP gene resides on chromosome 21, which is duplicated in Down's syndrome, in which early AD-like dementia occurs in association with overexpression of APP.

▼ Amyloid deposits consist of aggregates of Aβ (Fig. 35.3) containing 40 or 42 residues. Aβ40 is produced normally in small amounts, whereas Aβ42 is overproduced as a result of the genetic mutations mentioned above. Both proteins aggregate to form amyloid plaques, but Aβ42 shows a stronger tendency than Aβ40 to do so, and appears to be the main culprit in amyloid formation. Aβ40 and 42 are produced by proteolytic cleavage of a much larger (770 amino acid) APP, a membrane protein normally expressed by many cells, including CNS neurons. The proteases that cut out the Aβ sequence are known as *secretases*. Normally, *α-secretase* acts to release the large extracellular domain as soluble APP, which serves various poorly understood trophic functions. Formation of Aβ involves cleavage at two different points, including one in the intramembrane domain of APP, by β- and *γ-secretases* (Fig. 35.3). *γ*-Secretase is a clumsy enzyme—actually a large intramembrane complex of several proteins—

that lacks precision and cuts APP at different points in the transmembrane domain, generating Aβ fragments of different lengths, including Aβ40 and 42. Mutations in this region of the APP gene affect the preferred cleavage point, tending to favour formation of Aβ42. Mutations of the unrelated *presenilin* genes result in increased activity of *γ-secretase*, because the *presenilin* proteins form part of the *γ*-secretase complex. These different AD-related mutations increase the ratio of Aβ42:Aβ40, which can be detected in plasma, serving as a marker for familial AD. Mutations in another gene, that for the lipid transport protein ApoE4, also predispose to AD, probably because of expression of abnormal ApoE4 proteins that facilitate the aggregation of Aβ.

It is uncertain exactly how Aβ accumulation causes neurodegeneration, and whether the damage is done by soluble Aβ monomers or oligomers, or by amyloid plaques. There is some evidence that the cells die by apoptosis, although an inflammatory response is also evident. Expression of Alzheimer mutations in transgenic animals causes plaque formation and neurodegeneration, and also increases the susceptibility of CNS neurons to other challenges, such as ischaemia, excitotoxicity and oxidative stress, and this increased vulnerability may be the cause of the progressive neurodegeneration in AD. These transgenic models will be of great value in testing potential drug therapies aimed at retarding the neurodegenerative process.

The other main player on the biochemical stage is *Tau*, the protein of which the neurofibrillary tangles are composed (Fig. 35.3). Their role in neurodegeneration is unclear, although similar 'tauopathies' occur in many neurodegenerative conditions (see Lee et al., 2001). Tau is a normal constituent of neurons, being associated with intracellular microtubules. In AD and other tauopathies, it becomes abnormally phosphorylated and is deposited intracellularly as *paired helical filaments* with a characteristic microscopic appearance. When the cells die, these filaments aggregate as extracellular neurofibrillary tangles. It is possible, but not proven, that Tau phosphorylation is enhanced by the presence of Aβ plaques. Whether hyperphosphorylation and intracellular deposition of Tau harms the cell is not certain, although it is known that Tau phosphorylation impairs fast axonal transport, a process that depends on microtubules.

Alzheimer's disease

- Alzheimer's disease (AD) is a common age-related dementia distinct from vascular dementia associated with brain infarction.
- The main pathological features of AD comprise amyloid plaques, neurofibrillary tangles and a loss of neurons (particularly cholinergic neurons of the basal forebrain).
- Amyloid plaques consist of aggregates of the Aβ fragment of amyloid precursor protein (APP), a normal neuronal membrane protein, produced by the action of β- and γ-secretases. AD is associated with excessive Aβ formation, resulting in neurotoxicity.
- Familial AD (rare) results from mutations in the *APP* gene, or in *presenilin* genes (involved in γ-secretase function), both of which cause increased Aβ formation.
- Neurofibrillary tangles comprise intracellular aggregates of a highly phosphorylated form of a normal neuronal protein (Tau). The relationship of these structures to neurodegeneration is not known.
- Loss of cholinergic neurons is believed to account for much of the learning and memory deficit in AD.

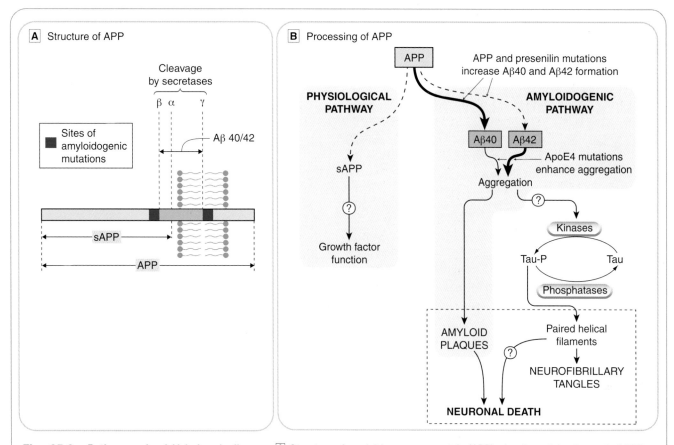

Fig. 35.3 **Pathogenesis of Alzheimer's disease.** **A** Structure of amyloid precursor protein (APP), showing origin of secreted APP (sAPP) and Aβ amyloid protein. The regions involved in amyloidogenic mutations discovered in some cases of familial Alzheimer's disease are shown flanking the Aβ sequence. APP cleavage involves three proteases: secretases α, β and γ. α-Secretase produces soluble APP, whereas β- and γ-secretases generate Aβ amyloid protein. γ-Secretase can cut at different points, generating Aβ peptides of varying lengths, including Aβ40 and Aβ42, the latter having a high tendency to aggregate as amyloid plaques. **B** Processing of APP. The main 'physiological' pathway gives rise to sAPP, which exerts a number of trophic functions. Cleavage of APP at different sites gives rise to Aβ, the predominant form normally being Aβ40, which is weakly amyloidogenic. Mutations in APP or presenilins increase the proportion of APP, which is degraded via the amyloidogenic pathway, and also increase the proportion converted to the much more strongly amyloidogenic form Aβ42. Aggregation of Aβ is favoured by mutations in the *apoE4* gene.

Loss of cholinergic neurons

Although changes in many transmitter systems have been observed, mainly from measurements on post-mortem AD brain tissue, a relatively selective loss of cholinergic neurons in the basal forebrain nuclei (Ch. 34) is characteristic. This discovery, made in 1976, implied that pharmacological approaches to restoring cholinergic function might be feasible, leading to the use of cholinesterase inhibitors to treat AD (see below).

Choline acetyl transferase activity, acetylcholine content, and acetylcholinesterase and choline transport in the cortex and hippocampus are all reduced considerably in AD but not in other disorders, such as depression or schizophrenia. Muscarinic receptor density, determined by binding studies, is not affected, but nicotinic receptors, particularly in the cortex, are reduced. The reason for the selective loss of cholinergic neurons resulting from Aβ formation is not known.

THERAPEUTIC APPROACHES

Recent advances in understanding the process of neurodegeneration in AD have yet to result in therapies able to retard it. Currently, cholinesterase inhibitors (see Ch.10) and memantine (see above) are the only drugs approved for treating AD, although many drugs have been claimed to improve cognitive performance and several new approaches are being explored (see Citron, 2004).

Cholinesterase inhibitors

Tacrine, the first drug approved for treating AD, was investigated on the basis that enhancement of cholinergic transmission might compensate for the cholinergic deficit. Trials showed modest improvements in tests of memory and cognition in about 40% of AD patients, but no improvement in other functional measures that affect quality of life. Tacrine has to be given four times daily and produces cholinergic side effects such as nausea and abdominal cramps, as well as hepatotoxicity in some patients, so it is far from an ideal drug. Later compounds, which also have limited efficacy but are more effective than tacrine in improving quality of life, include **donepezil, rivastigmine** and **galantamine** (Table 35.2). These drugs produce a measurable, although slight, improvement of cognitive function in AD patients, but this may be too small to be significant in terms of everyday life.

There is some evidence from laboratory studies that cholinesterase inhibitors may act somehow to reduce the formation or neurotoxicity of Aβ, and therefore retard the progression of AD as well as producing symptomatic benefit. Clinical trials, however, have shown only a small improvement in cognitive function, with no effect on disease progression.

Other drugs aimed at improving cholinergic function that are being investigated include other cholinesterase inhibitors and a variety of muscarinic and nicotinic receptor agonists, none of which look promising on the basis of early clinical results.

Other drugs

▼ **Dihydroergotamuine** was used for many years to treat dementia. It acts as a cerebral vasodilator, but trials showed it to produce little if any cognitive improvement. 'Nootropic' drugs such as **piracetam** and **aniracetam** improve memory in animal tests, possibly by enhancing glutamate release, but are probably ineffective in AD.

Inhibiting neurodegeneration

▼ For most of the disorders discussed in this chapter, including AD, the Holy Grail, which so far eludes us, would be a drug that retards neurodegeneration. Now that we have several well-characterised targets, such as Aβ formation by the β- and γ-secretases, and Aβ neurotoxicity, together with a range of transgenic animal models of AD on which compounds can be tested, the prospects certainly look brighter than

they did a decade ago. Particular developments are worth mentioning (see Selkoe & Schenk, 2003, and Citron, 2004, for more details).

Inhibitors of β- and γ-secretase have been identified and are undergoing clinical trials. Unfortunately, γ-secretase plays a role in other signalling pathways besides Aβ formation, so inhibitors are likely to produce unwanted as well as beneficial effects.

An ingenious new approach was taken by Schenk et al. (1999), who immunised AD transgenic mice with Aβ protein, and found that this not only prevented but also reversed plaque formation. Initial trials in humans had to be terminated because of neuroinflammatory complications, but work on developing better immunisation strategies is continuing,

Epidemiological studies reveal that some non-steroidal anti-inflammatory drugs (NSAIDs; see Ch. 14) used routinely to treat arthritis reduce the likelihood of developing AD. **Ibuprofen** and **indometacin** have this effect, although other NSAIDs, such as **aspirin**, do not, nor do anti-inflammatory steroids such as **prednisolone**. Recent work (see De Strooper & König, 2001) suggests that NSAIDs may reduce Aβ42 formation by regulating γ-secretase, an effect unrelated to cyclo-oxygenase inhibition, by which NSAIDs reduce inflammation. It may therefore be possible to find compounds that target γ-secretase selectively without inhibiting cyclo-oxygenase, thus avoiding the side effects associated with current NSAIDs. Disappointingly, clinical trials with various NSAIDs have so far failed to show any effect on cognitive performance or disease progression in AD patients (see Townsend & Pratico, 2005).

Aβ plaques bind copper and zinc, and removal of these metal ions promotes dissolution of the plaques. The amoebicidal drug **clioquinol** is a metal-chelating agent that causes regression of amyloid deposits in animal models of AD, and showed some benefit in initial clinical trials. Clioquinol itself has known toxic effects in humans, which preclude its routine clinical use, but less toxic metal-chelating agents are under investigation.

Shortage of growth factors (particularly **nerve growth factor**) may contribute to the loss of forebrain cholinergic neurons in AD. Administering growth factors into the brain is not realistic for routine therapy, but alternative approaches, such as implanting cells engineered to secrete nerve growth factor, are under investigation.

Table 35.2 Cholinesterase inhibitors used in the treatment of Alzheimer's disease[a]

Drug	Type of inhibition	Duration of action	Main side effects	Notes
Tacrine	Short acting, reversible Affects both AChE and BuChE	~ 6 h	Few cholinergic side effects Can cause hepatotoxicity	The first anticholinesterase shown to be effective in Alzheimer's disease Monitoring for hepatotoxicity needed
Donepezil	Short-acting, reversible AChE-selective	~ 24 h	Slight cholinergic side effects	–
Rivastigmine	Slowly reversible Affects both AChE and BuChE	~ 8 h	Cholinergic side effects that tend to subside with continuing treatment	Gradual dose escalation to minimise side effects
Galantamine	Reversible, non-selective Also enhances nicotinic acetylcholine receptor activation by allosteric mechanism	~ 8 h	Few side effects	Dual mechanism of action postulated

AChE, acetylcholinesterase; BuChE, butyryl cholinesterase.
[a]Similar level of limited clinical benefit for all drugs. No clinical evidence for retardation of disease process, although animal tests suggest diminution of Aβ and plaque formation by a mechanism not related to cholinesterase inhibition.

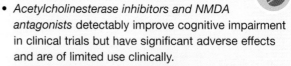

Currently, the only drugs approved for the treatment of AD are various cholinesterase inhibitors (Table 35.2) and **memantine**, an NMDA receptor antagonist believed to work by inhibiting glutamate-induced excitotoxicity. It has only mild side effects, and clinical trials data show it to produce a slight but significant improvement in cognitive function in moderate-to-severe AD.

PARKINSON'S DISEASE

FEATURES OF PARKINSON'S DISEASE

Parkinson's disease is a progressive disorder of movement that occurs mainly in the elderly. The chief symptoms are:

- tremor at rest, usually starting in the hands ('pill-rolling' tremor), which tends to diminish during voluntary activity
- muscle rigidity, detectable as an increased resistance in passive limb movement
- suppression of voluntary movements (hypokinesis), due partly to muscle rigidity and partly to an inherent inertia of the motor system, which means that motor activity is difficult to stop as well as to initiate.

Parkinsonian patients walk with a characteristic shuffling gait. They find it hard to start, and once in progress they cannot quickly stop or change direction. PD is commonly associated with dementia, probably because the degenerative process is not confined to the basal ganglia but also affects other parts of the brain.

Parkinson's disease often occurs with no obvious underlying cause, but it may be the result of cerebral ischaemia, viral encephalitis or other types of pathological damage. The symptoms can also be drug-induced, the main drugs involved being those that reduce the amount of dopamine in the brain (e.g. **reserpine;** see Ch. 11) or block dopamine receptors (e.g. antipsychotic drugs such as **chlorpromazine;** see Ch. 38). There are rare instances of early-onset PD that runs in families, and several gene mutations have been identified, the most important being *synuclein* and *parkin*. Study of these gene mutations has given some clues about the mechanism underlying the neurodegenerative process (see below).

NEUROCHEMICAL CHANGES

Parkinson's disease affects the basal ganglia, and its neurochemical origin was discovered in 1960 by Hornykiewicz, who showed that the dopamine content of the substantia nigra and corpus striatum (see Ch. 34) in post-mortem brains of PD patients was extremely low (usually less than 10% of normal), associated with a loss of dopaminergic neurons in the substantia nigra and degeneration of nerve terminals in the striatum. Other monoamines, such as noradrenaline and 5-hydroxytryptamine, were much less affected than dopamine. Later studies (e.g. with positron emission tomography scanning to reveal dopamine transport in the striatum) have shown a loss of dopamine over several years, with symptoms of PD appearing only when the striatal dopamine content has fallen to 20–40% of normal. Lesions of the nigrostriatal tract or chemically induced depletion of dopamine in experimental animals also produce symptoms of PD. The symptom most clearly related to dopamine deficiency is hypokinesia, which occurs immediately and invariably in lesioned animals. Rigidity and tremor involve

more complex neurochemical disturbances of other transmitters (particularly acetylcholine, noradrenaline, 5-hydroxytryptamine and GABA) as well as dopamine. In experimental lesions, two secondary consequences follow damage to the nigrostriatal tract, namely a hyperactivity of the remaining dopaminergic neurons, which show an increased rate of transmitter turnover, and an increase in the number of dopamine receptors, which produces a state of denervation hypersensitivity (see Ch. 9). The striatum expresses mainly D_1 (excitatory) and D_2 (inhibitory) receptors (see Ch. 34), but fewer D_3 and D_4 receptors. A simplified diagram of the neuronal circuitry involved, and the pathways primarily affected in PD and Huntington's disease, is shown in Figure 35.4.

Cholinergic interneurons of the corpus striatum (not shown in Fig. 35.4) are also involved in PD and Huntington's disease. Acetylcholine release from the striatum is strongly inhibited by dopamine, and it is suggested that hyperactivity of these cholinergic neurons contributes to the symptoms of PD. The opposite happens in Huntington's disease, and in both conditions therapies aimed at redressing the balance between the dopaminergic and cholinergic neurons are, up to a point, beneficial.

PATHOGENESIS OF PARKINSON'S DISEASE

Parkinson's disease is believed to be caused mainly by environmental factors, although the rare types of hereditary PD have provided some valuable clues about the mechanism. As with other neurodegenerative disorders, the damage is caused by protein misfolding and aggregation, aided and abetted by three familiar villains, namely excitotoxicity, oxidative stress and apoptosis (see Lotharius & Brundin, 2002; Vila & Przedhorski, 2004). Aspects of the pathogenesis and animal models of PD are described by Beal (2001).

> **Clinical use of drugs in dementia**
>
> - *Acetylcholinesterase inhibitors and NMDA antagonists* detectably improve cognitive impairment in clinical trials but have significant adverse effects and are of limited use clinically.
> - Efficacy is monitored periodically in individual patients, and administration continued only if the drugs are believed to be working and their effect in slowing functional and behavioural deterioration is judged to outweigh adverse effects.
>
> - **Acetylcholinesterase inhibitors:**
>   — examples include **donepezil, galantamine, rivastigmine**
>   — used in mild to moderate Alzheimer's disease.
> - **NMDA receptor antagonists:**
>   — for example **memantine** (see Ch. 33, p. 485)
>   — used in moderate to severe Alzheimer's disease.

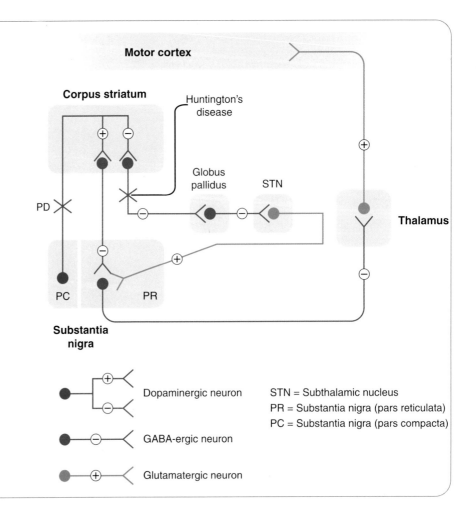

Fig. 35.4   Simplified diagram of the organisation of the extrapyramidal motor system and the defects that occur in Parkinson's disease (PD) and Huntington's disease. Normally, activity in nigrostriatal dopamine neurons causes excitation of striatonigral neurons and inhibition of striatal neurons that project to the globus pallidus. In either case, because of the different pathways involved, the activity of GABAergic neurons in the substantia nigra is suppressed, releasing the restraint on the thalamus and cortex, causing motor stimulation. In PD, the dopaminergic pathway from the substantia nigra (pars compacta) to the striatum is impaired. In Huntington's disease, the GABAergic striatopallidal pathway is impaired, producing effects opposite to the changes in PD. PC, substantia nigra (pars compacta); PR, substantia nigra (pars reticulata); STN, subthalamic nucleus.

Neurotoxins

New light was thrown on the possible aetiology of PD by a chance event. In 1982, a group of young drug addicts in California suddenly developed an exceptionally severe form of PD (known as the 'frozen addict' syndrome), and the cause was traced to the compound **1-methyl-4-phenyl-1,2,3,6-tetrahydropyridine** (**MPTP**), which was a contaminant in a preparation used as a heroin substitute (see Langston, 1985). MPTP causes irreversible destruction of nigrostriatal dopaminergic neurons in various species, and produces a PD-like state in primates. MPTP acts by being converted to a toxic metabolite, MPP^+, by the enzyme *monoamine oxidase* (*MAO*, specifically by the MAO-B subtype; see Ch. 39). MPP^+ is taken up by the dopamine transport system, and thus acts selectively on dopaminergic neurons; it inhibits mitochondrial oxidation reactions, producing oxidative stress (see above). MPTP appears to be selective in destroying nigrostriatal neurons and does not affect dopaminergic neurons elsewhere—the reason for this is unknown. **Selegiline**, a selective MAO-B inhibitor (see below), prevents MPTP-induced neurotoxicity by blocking its conversion to MPP^+. Selegiline is also used in treating PD (see below); as well as inhibiting dopamine breakdown, it might also work by blocking the metabolic activation of a putative endogenous, or environmental, MPTP-like substance, which is involved in the causation of PD. It is possible that dopamine itself could be the culprit, because

oxidation of dopamine gives rise to potentially toxic metabolites. Whether or not the action of MPTP reflects the natural pathogenesis of PD, the MPTP model is a very useful experimental tool for testing possible therapies.

Various herbicides, such as **rotenone**, that selectively inhibit mitochondrial function cause a PD-like syndrome in animals, suggesting that environmental toxins could be a factor in human PD, because impaired mitochondrial function is a feature of the disease in humans.

Molecular aspects

▼ Parkinson's disease, as well as several other neurodegenerative disorders, is associated with the development of intracellular protein aggregates known as *Lewy bodies* in various parts of the brain. They consist largely of α-synuclein, a synaptic protein present in large amounts in normal brains. Mutations occur in rare types of hereditary PD (see above), and it is believed that such mutations render the protein resistant to degradation within cells, causing it to pile up in Lewy bodies. It is possible (see Lotharius & Brundin, 2002) that the normal function of α-synuclein is related to synaptic vesicle recycling, and that the mutated form loses this functionality, with the result that vesicular storage of dopamine is impaired. This may lead to an increase in cytosolic dopamine, degradation of which produces reactive oxygen species and hence neurotoxicity. Consistent with the α-synuclein hypothesis, the other mutation associated with PD (*parkin*) also involves a protein that participates in the intracellular degradation of rogue proteins. Other gene mutations that have been identified as risk factors for early-onset PD code for proteins involved in mitochondrial function, making cells more susceptible to oxidative stress.

Thus, a picture similar to AD pathogenesis is slowly emerging. Misfolded α-synuclein, facilitated by genetic mutations or possibly by environmental factors, builds up in the cell as a result of impaired protein degradation (resulting from defective parkin) in the form of Lewy bodies, which, by unknown mechanisms, compromise cell survival. If oxidative stress is increased, as a result of ischaemia, mitochondrial poisons or mutations of certain mitochondrial proteins, the result is cell death.

DRUG TREATMENT OF PARKINSON'S DISEASE

Despite past optimism, none of the drugs used to treat PD affect the progression of the disease. For general reviews of current and future approaches, see Hagan et al. (1997) and Olanow (2004). Currently, the main drugs used are **levodopa** and various dopamine agonists. Of less importance are:

- MAO-B inhibitors (e.g. **selegiline**)
- drugs that release dopamine (e.g. **amantadine**)
- muscarinic acetylcholine receptor antagonists (e.g. **benztropine**).

LEVODOPA

Levodopa is the first-line treatment for PD and is combined with a peripheral dopa decarboxylase inhibitor, either **carbidopa** or **benserazide**, which reduces the dose needed by about 10-fold and diminishes the peripheral side effects. It is well absorbed from the small intestine, a process that relies on active transport, although much of it is inactivated by MAO in the wall of the intestine. The plasma half-life is short (about 2 hours). Conversion to dopamine in the periphery, which would otherwise account for about 95%

of the levodopa dose and cause troublesome side effects, is largely prevented by the decarboxylase inhibitor. Decarboxylation occurs rapidly within the brain, because the decarboxylase inhibitors do not penetrate the blood–brain barrier. It is not certain whether the effect depends on an increased release of dopamine from the few surviving dopaminergic neurons or on a 'flooding' of the synapse with exogenous dopamine. Because synthetic dopamine agonists (see below) are equally effective, the latter explanation is more likely, and animal studies suggest that levodopa can act even when no dopaminergic nerve terminals are present. On the other hand, the therapeutic effectiveness of levodopa decreases as the disease advances, so part of its action may rely on the presence of functional dopaminergic neurons. Combination of levodopa plus dopa decarboxylase inhibitor with **entacapone**, an inhibitor of catechol-*O*-methyl transferase (COMT; see Ch. 11) to inhibit its degradation, is used in patients troubled by 'end of dose' motor fluctuations.

Therapeutic effectiveness and unwanted effects of levodopa

About 80% of patients show initial improvement with levodopa, particularly of rigidity and hypokinesia, and about 20% are restored virtually to normal motor function. As time progresses, the effectiveness of levodopa gradually declines (Fig. 35.5). In a typical study

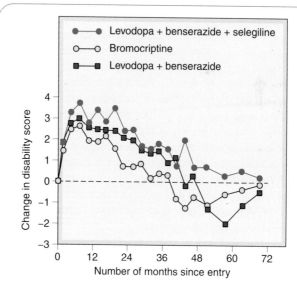

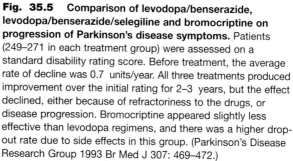

Fig. 35.5 Comparison of levodopa/benserazide, levodopa/benserazide/selegiline and bromocriptine on progression of Parkinson's disease symptoms. Patients (249–271 in each treatment group) were assessed on a standard disability rating score. Before treatment, the average rate of decline was 0.7 units/year. All three treatments produced improvement over the initial rating for 2–3 years, but the effect declined, either because of refractoriness to the drugs, or disease progression. Bromocriptine appeared slightly less effective than levodopa regimens, and there was a higher drop-out rate due to side effects in this group. (Parkinson's Disease Research Group 1993 Br Med J 307: 469–472.)

> **Parkinson's disease**
>
> - Degenerative disease of the basal ganglia causing tremor at rest, muscle rigidity hypokinesia, often with dementia.
> - Associated with aggregation of α-synuclein (a protein normally involved in vesicle recycling) in the form of characteristic Lewy bodies.
> - Often idiopathic but may follow stroke or virus infection; can be drug-induced (neuroleptic drugs). Rare familial forms also occur, associated with various gene mutations, including α-synuclein.
> - Associated with early degeneration of dopaminergic nigrostriatal neurons, followed by more general neurodegeneration.
> - Can be induced by 1-methyl-4-phenyl-1,2,3,6-tetrahydropyridine (MPTP), a neurotoxin affecting dopamine neurons. Similar environmental neurotoxins, as well as genetic factors, may be involved in human Parkinson's disease.

of 100 patients treated with levodopa for 5 years, only 34 were better than they had been at the beginning of the trial, 32 patients having died and 21 having withdrawn from the trial. It is likely that the loss of effectiveness of levodopa mainly reflects the natural progression of the disease, but receptor down-regulation and other compensatory mechanisms may also contribute. There is no evidence that levodopa can actually accelerate the neurodegenerative process through overproduction of dopamine, as was suspected on theoretical grounds (see above). Overall, levodopa increases the life expectancy of PD patients, probably as a result of improved motor function, although some symptoms (e.g. dysphagia, cognitive decline) are not improved.

Unwanted effects

There are two main types of unwanted effect.

- Involuntary writhing movements (dyskinesia), which do not appear initially but develop in the majority of patients within 2 years of starting levodopa therapy. These movements usually affect the face and limbs, and can become very severe. They occur at the time of the peak therapeutic effect, and the margin between the beneficial and the dyskinetic effect becomes progressively narrower. Levodopa is short acting, and the fluctuating plasma concentration of the drug may favour the development of dyskinesias, as longer-acting dopamine agonists may be less problematic in this regard.
- Rapid fluctuations in clinical state, where hypokinesia and rigidity may suddenly worsen for anything from a few minutes to a few hours, and then improve again. This 'on–off effect' is not seen in untreated PD patients or with other anti-PD drugs. The 'off effect' can be so sudden that the patient stops while walking and feels rooted to the spot, or is unable to rise from a chair in which he or she had sat down normally a few moments earlier. As with the dyskinesias, the problem seems to reflect the fluctuating plasma concentration of levodopa, and it is suggested that as the disease advances, the ability of neurons to store dopamine is lost, so the therapeutic benefit of levodopa depends increasingly on the continuous formation of extraneuronal dopamine, which requires a continuous supply of levodopa. The use of sustained-release preparations, or coadministration of COMT inhibitors such as entacapone (see above), may be used to counteract the fluctuations in plasma concentration of levodopa.

In addition to these slowly developing side effects, levodopa produces several acute effects, which are experienced by most patients at first but tend to disappear after a few weeks. The main ones are as follow.

- Nausea and anorexia. **Domperidone**, a dopamine antagonist that works in the chemoreceptor trigger zone (where the blood–brain barrier is leaky) but does not gain access to the basal ganglia, may be useful in preventing this effect.
- Hypotension: postural hypotension is a problem in a few patients.
- Psychological effects. Levodopa, by increasing dopamine activity in the brain, can produce a schizophrenia-like syndrome (see Ch. 38) with delusions and hallucinations. More commonly,

in about 20% of patients, it causes confusion, disorientation, insomnia or nightmares.

SELEGILINE

Selegiline is a MAO inhibitor that is selective for MAO-B, which predominates in dopamine-containing regions of the CNS. It therefore lacks the unwanted peripheral effects of non-selective MAO inhibitors used to treat depression (Ch. 37) and, in contrast to them, does not provoke the 'cheese reaction' or interact so frequently with other drugs. Inhibition of MAO-B protects dopamine from intraneuronal degradation and was initially used as an adjunct to levodopa. Long-term trials showed that the combination of selegiline and levodopa was more effective than levodopa alone in relieving symptoms and prolonging life. Recognition of the role of MAO-B in neurotoxicity (see above) suggested that selegiline might be neuroprotective rather than merely enhancing the action of levodopa, but clinical studies do not support this. A large-scale trial (Fig. 35.5) showed no difference when selegiline was added to levodopa/benserazide treatment.

OTHER DRUGS USED IN PARKINSON'S DISEASE

Dopamine receptor agonists

Bromocriptine, derived from the ergot alkaloids (see Ch. 12), is a potent agonist at dopamine (D_2) receptors in the CNS. It inhibits the release of prolactin from the anterior pituitary gland, and was first introduced for the treatment of galactorrhoea and gynaecomastia (Ch. 28), but is effective also in PD (Fig. 35.5). Its duration of action is longer (plasma half-life 6–8 hours) than that of levodopa, so that it does not need to be given so frequently. It was hoped that bromocriptine might be effective in patients who had become refractory to levodopa through loss of dopaminergic neurons, but this has not been clearly established. The main side effects of bromocriptine are nausea and vomiting, and (rarely but seriously) peritoneal fibrosis, as seen with other ergot derivatives (see Ch. 12). Newer dopamine receptor agonists include **lisuride, pergolide, ropinirole, cabergoline** and **pramipexole.** They are longer acting than levodopa and need to be given only once or twice daily, with less tendency to cause dyskinesias and on–off effects. Their main side effects are confusion and occasionally delusions, and sleep disturbances. Pramipexole may have antioxidant effects, as well as a protective effect on mitochondria. Whether these potentially neuroprotective properties are significant clinically remains to be discovered. Clinical trials have shown little difference between these drugs.

Amantadine

▼ Amantadine was introduced as an antiviral drug and discovered by accident in 1969 to be beneficial in PD. Many possible mechanisms for its action have been suggested based on neurochemical evidence of increased dopamine release, inhibition of amine uptake, or a direct action on dopamine receptors. Most authors now suggest, although not with much conviction, that increased dopamine release is primarily responsible for the clinical effects.

Amantadine is less effective than levodopa or bromocriptine, and its action declines with time. Its side effects are considerably less severe, although qualitatively similar to those of levodopa.

Drugs used in Parkinson's disease

- Drugs act by counteracting deficiency of dopamine in basal ganglia or by blocking muscarinic receptors. None of the available drugs affect the underlying neurodegeneration.
- Drugs include:
  - **levodopa** (dopamine precursor; Ch. 11), given with an inhibitor of peripheral dopa decarboxylase (e.g. **carbidopa**) to minimise side effects; sometimes a catechol-*O*-methyltransferase inhibitor

  (e.g. **entacapone**) is also given, especially to patients with 'end of dose' motor fluctuations
  - **bromocriptine** (dopamine agonist; Ch. 28)
  - **selegiline** (monoamine oxidase B inhibitor)
  - **amantadine** (which may enhance dopamine release)
  - **benzatropine** (muscarinic receptor antagonist used for parkinsonism caused by antipsychotic drugs).
- Neurotransplantation, still in an experimental phase, may be effective but results are variable.

Acetylcholine antagonists

▼ For more than a century, until levodopa was discovered, atropine and related drugs were the main form of treatment for PD. Muscarinic acetylcholine receptors exert an inhibitory effect on dopaminergic nerve terminals, suppression of which compensates for a lack of dopamine. The side effects of muscarinic antagonists—dry mouth, constipation, impaired vision, urinary retention—are troublesome, and they are now rarely used, except to treat parkinsonian symptoms in patients receiving antipsychotic drugs (which are dopamine antagonists and thus nullify the effect of L-dopa; see Ch. 38).

NEURAL TRANSPLANTATION

▼ Parkinson's disease is the first neurodegenerative disease for which neural transplantation was attempted in 1982, amid much publicity. Various transplantation approaches have been tried, based on the injection of dissociated fetal cells directly into the striatum. Trials in patients with PD (see Bjorklund & Lindvall, 2000; Barker & Rosser, 2001) have mainly involved injection of midbrain neurons from aborted human fetuses. It has been shown that such transplants are able to survive and establish synaptic connections but, despite reports of miracle cures, controlled studies so far have shown little clinical benefit. Some patients have gone on to develop serious dyskinesias, possibly due to dopamine overproduction. The use of fetal material is, of course, fraught with difficulties (usually cells from five or more fetuses are needed for one transplant). Hopes for the future rest mainly on the possibility of developing preparations of immortalised neuronal precursor cells that can be multiplied in culture, and that will differentiate into functional postmitotic neurons after transplantation. Efforts are continuing to develop transplantation as a means of treating other conditions, such as Huntington's disease, stroke and epilepsy, as well as PD, but the field remains highly controversial (see Bjorklund & Lindvall, 2000; Barker & Rosser, 2001).

HUNTINGTON'S DISEASE

▼ Huntington's disease is an inherited (autosomal dominant) disorder resulting in progressive brain degeneration, starting in adulthood and causing rapid deterioration and death. As well as dementia, it causes severe motor symptoms in the form of involuntary writhing movements, which are highly disabling. It is the commonest of a group of so-called trinucleotide repeat neurodegenerative diseases, associated with the expansion of the number of repeats of the CAG sequence in specific genes, and hence the number (50 or more) of consecutive glutamine residues in the expressed protein (see Gusella & MacDonald, 2000). The larger the number of repeats, the earlier the appearance of symptoms. The protein coded by the Huntington's disease gene, *huntingtin*, interacts with various regulatory proteins, including one of the caspases (see above), which participates in excitotoxicity and apoptosis. Some of these interactions are

enhanced by the poly-Gln repeat in the mutant protein, and this may account for the neuronal loss, which affects mainly the cortex and the striatum, resulting in progressive dementia and severe involuntary jerky (choreiform) movements. The mutant protein is also prone to misfolding and aggregation, as described above. Studies on post-mortem brains showed that the dopamine content of the striatum was normal or slightly increased, while there was a 75% reduction in the activity of *glutamic acid decarboxylase*, the enzyme responsible for GABA synthesis (Ch. 34). It is believed that the loss of GABA-mediated inhibition in the basal ganglia produces a hyperactivity of dopaminergic synapses, so the syndrome is in some senses a mirror image of PD (Fig. 35.4). The effects of drugs that influence dopaminergic transmission are correspondingly the opposite of those that are observed in PD, dopamine antagonists being effective in reducing the involuntary movements, while drugs such as levodopa and bromocriptine make them worse. Drugs used to alleviate the motor symptoms include dopamine antagonists, such as **chlorpromazine** (Ch. 38), and the GABA agonist **baclofen** (Ch. 33). These do not affect dementia or retard the course of the disease, and it is possible that drugs that inhibit excitotoxicity, or possibly neural transplantation procedures when these become available (see above), may prove useful.

NEURODEGENERATIVE PRION DISEASES

▼ A group of human and animal diseases associated with a characteristic type of neurodegeneration, known as *spongiform encephalopathy* because of the vacuolated appearance of the affected brain, has recently been the focus of intense research activity (see Collinge, 2001; Prusiner, 2001). A key feature of these diseases is that they are transmissible through an infective agent, although not, in general, across species. The recent upsurge of interest has been spurred mainly by the discovery that the bovine form of the disease, bovine spongiform encephalopathy (BSE), is transmissible to humans. Different human forms of spongiform encephalopathy include CJD (which is unrelated to BSE) and the new variant form (vCJD), as yet very rare, which results from eating, or close contact with, infected beef or human tissue. Another human form is *kuru*, a neurodegenerative disease affecting cannibalistic tribes in Papua New Guinea. These diseases cause a progressive, and sometimes rapid, dementia and loss of motor coordination, for which no therapies currently exist. *Scrapie*, a common disease of domestic sheep, is another example, and it may have been the practice of feeding sheep offal to domestic cattle that initiated an epidemic of BSE in Britain during the 1980s, leading to the appearance of vCJD in humans in the mid-1990s. Although the BSE epidemic has been controlled, there is concern that more human cases may develop in its wake, because the incubation period—known to be long—is uncertain.

Prion diseases are examples of protein misfolding diseases (see above) in which the prion protein adopts a misfolded conformation that forms insoluble aggregates. The infectious agent responsible for transmissible spongiform encephalopathies such as vCJD is, unusually, a protein, known as a prion. The protein involved (PrP^C) is a normal cytosolic constituent of the brain and other tissues, whose functions are not known. As a result of altered glycosylation, the protein can become misfolded, forming the insoluble PrP^{Sc} form, which has the ability to recruit normal PrP^C molecules to the misfolded PrP^{Sc}, thus starting a chain reaction. PrP^{Sc}—the infective agent—accumulates and aggregates as insoluble fibrils, and is responsible for the progressive neurodegeneration. In support of this unusual form of infectivity, it has been shown that injection of PrP^{Sc} into normal mice causes spongiform encephalopathy, whereas PrP knockout mice, which are otherwise fairly normal, are resistant because they lack the substrate for the autocatalytic generation of PrP^{Sc}. Fortunately, the infection does not easily cross between species, because there are differences between the *PrP* genes of different species. It is possible that a mutation of the *PrP* gene in either sheep or cattle produced the variant form that became infective in humans.

This chain of events bears some similarity to that of AD, in that the brain accumulates an abnormal form of a normally expressed protein.

There is as yet no known treatment for this type of encephalopathy, but laboratory experiments suggest that two very familiar drugs, namely **quinacrine** (an antimalarial drug) and **chlorpromazine** (a widely used antipsychotic drug; Ch. 38), can inhibit PrP^{Sc} aggregation in mouse models. Both are under investigation for treating human CJD. Other possible strategies, none yet tested in patients, are discussed by Mallucci & Collinge (2005).

REFERENCES AND FURTHER READING

Pathogenesis

Bossy-Wetzel E, Schwarzenbacher R, Lipton S A 2004 Molecular pathways to neurodegeneration. Nat Med 10(suppl): S2–S9 (*Review of molecular mechanisms underlying various chronic neurodegenerative diseases, including those discussed in the chapter*)

Coyle J T, Puttfarken P 1993 Oxidative stress, glutamate and neurodegenerative disorders. Science 262: 689–695 (*Good review article*)

Forman M S, Trojanowski J G, Lee V M-Y 2004 Neurodegenerative diseases: a decade of discoveries paves the way for therapeutic breakthroughs. Nat Med 10: 1055–1063 (*General review on pathogenesis of neurodegenerative diseases—not much on therapeutic approaches, despite the title*)

Gusella J F, MacDonald M E 2000 Molecular genetics: unmasking polyglutamine triggers in neurodegenerative disease. Nat Rev Neurosci 1: 109–115 (*General review on trinucleotide repeat disorders and how the brain damage is produced*)

Jellinger K A 2001 Cell death mechanisms in neurodegeneration. J Cell Mol Med 5: 1–17 (*Useful review article covering acute as well as chronic disorders leading to neurodegeneration*)

Lee V M-Y, Goedert M, Trojanowski J Q 2001 Neurodegenerative tauopathies. Annu Rev Neurosci 24: 1121–1159 (*Detailed review of the uncertain role of Tau proteins in neurodegeneration*)

Selkoe D J 2004 Cell biology of protein misfolding: the examples of Alzheimer's and Parkinson's diseases. Nat Cell Biol 6: 1054–1061 (*Good review article by one of the pioneers in identifying the amyloid hypothesis*)

Stefani M, Dobson C M 2003 Protein aggregation and aggregate toxicity: new insights into protein folding, misfolding diseases and biological evolution. J Mol Med 81: 678–699 (*Excellent review article on protein misfolding as the underlying cause of chronic neurodegenerative disease*)

Yamada K, Nabeshima T 2000 Animal models of Alzheimer's disease and evaluation of anti-dementia drugs. Pharmacol Ther 88: 93–113 (*Describes pathology of AD, transgenic and other animal models, and therapeutic approaches*)

Alzheimer's disease

Citron M 2004 Strategies for disease modification in Alzheimer's disease. Nat Rev Neurosci 5: 677–685 (*A review—generally optimistic—of the status of new therapeutic strategies for treating AD*)

Schenk D et al. 1999 Immunization with amyloid-beta attenuates Alzheimer-disease–like pathology in the PDAPP mouse. Nature 400: 173–177 (*Report of an ingenious experiment that could have implications for AD treatment in humans*)

Selkoe D J 1997 Alzheimer's disease: genotypes, phenotype and treatments. Science 275: 630–631 (*Short but informative summary of recent advances in Alzheimer genetics*)

Selkoe D J, Schenk D 2003 Alzheimer's disease: molecular understanding predicts amyloid-based therapeutics. Annu Rev Pharmacol Toxicol 43: 545–584 (*Comprehensive review article*)

Parkinson's disease

Beal F W 2001 Experimental models of Parkinson's disease. Nat Rev Neurosci 2: 325–332 (*Useful review article covering many aspects of PD pathogenesis*)

Hagan J J, Middlemiss D N, Sharpe P C, Poste G H 1997 Parkinson's disease: prospects for improved therapy. Trends Pharmacol Sci 18: 156–163 (*Excellent review of current trends*)

Langston W J 1985 MPTP and Parkinson's disease. Trends Neurosci 8: 79–83 (*Readable account of the MPTP story by its discoverer*)

Lipton S A, Rosenberg P A 1994 Excitatory amino acids as a final common pathway for neurologic disorders. New Engl J Med 330: 613–622 (*Review emphasising central role of glutamate in neurodegeneration*)

Lotharius J, Brundin P 2002 Pathogenesis of Parkinson's disease: dopamine, vesicles and α-synuclein. Nat Rev Neurosci 3: 833–842. (*Review of PD pathogenesis, emphasising the possible role of dopamine itself as a likely source of neurotoxic metabolites*)

Olanow C W 2004 The scientific basis for the current treatment of Parkinson's disease. Annu Rev Med 55: 41–60 (*Detailed review of current PD therapeutics, based on knowledge of pathophysiology*)

Vila M, Przedhorski S 2004 Genetic clues to the pathogenesis of Parkinson's disease. Nat Med 10(suppl): S58–S62 (*Account of the various mutations associated with PD, and how they may contribute to pathogenesis*)

Stroke

Dirnagl U, Iadecola C, Moskowitz M A 1999 Pathobiology of ischaemic stroke: an integrated view. Trends Neurosci 22: 391–397 (*Useful review of mechanisms underlying neuronal damage in stroke*)

Green A R, Odergren T, Ashwood T 2003 Animal models of stroke: do they have value for discovering neuroprotective agents? Trends Pharmacol Sci 24: 402–408 (*Article suggesting reasons why drug efficacy in animal models does not predict success in the clinic*)

Prion diseases

Collinge J 2001 Prion diseases of humans and animals: their causes and molecular basis. Annu Rev Neurosci 24: 519–550 (*Useful review article*)

Prusiner S B 2001 Neurodegenerative disease and prions. New Engl J Med 344: 1544–1551 (*General review article by the discoverer of prions*)

Therapeutic strategies

Barker R A, Rosser A E 2001 Neural transplantation therapies for Parkinson's and Huntington's diseases. Drug Discov Today 6: 575–582 (*Informative and balanced review article on a controversial topic*)

Bjorklund A, Lindvall O 2000 Cell replacement therapies for central nervous system disorders. Nat Neurosci 3: 537–544 (*Upbeat review by pioneers in the field of neural transplantation*)

Citron M 2004 Strategies for disease modification in Alzheimer's disease. Nat Rev Neurosci 5: 677–685 (*A review—generally optimistic—of the status of new therapeutic strategies for treating AD*)

De Strooper B, König G 2001 An inflammatory drug prospect. Nature 414: 159–160 (*Informative commentary on publication by Weggen et al. in the same issue, describing effects of NSAIDs on APP cleavage*)

Gross C G 2000 Neurogenesis in the adult brain: death of a dogma. Nat Rev Neurosci 1: 67–73

Mallucci G, Collinge J 2005 Rational targeting for prion therapeutics. Nat Rev Neurosci 6: 23–34 (*Realistic review of possible approaches to treating prion diseases; a very difficult problem with nothing really in sight yet*)

Rakic P 2002 Neurogenesis in the adult primate cortex: an evaluation of the evidence. Nat Rev Neurosci 3: 65–71

Townsend K P, Pratico D 2005 Novel therapeutic opportunities for Alzheimer's disease: focus on nonsteroidal antiinflammatory drugs. FASEB J 19: 1592–1601 (*Discussion of possible drug targets for treatment of AD, including animal studies and clinical trials data—largely negative, so far*)

General anaesthetic agents

36

In this chapter, we describe the pharmacology of the main agents in current use, which fall into two main groups: inhalation agents and intravenous agents. Detailed information on the clinical pharmacology and use of anaesthetic agents can be found in specialised textbooks (e.g. Evers & Maze, 2004).

OVERVIEW

General anaesthetics are used to render patients unaware of, and unresponsive to, painful stimulation during surgical procedures. They are given systemically and exert their main effects on the central nervous system (CNS), in contrast to local anaesthetics (see Ch. 44), which work by blocking conduction of impulses in peripheral sensory nerves. Although we now take them for granted, general anaesthetics are the drugs that paved the way for modern surgery. Without them, much of modern medicine would be impossible.

INTRODUCTION

Many drugs, including, for example, **ethanol** and **morphine**, can produce a state of insensibility and obliviousness to pain but are not used as anaesthetics. For a drug to be useful as an anaesthetic, it must be readily controllable, so that induction and recovery are rapid, allowing the level of anaesthesia to be adjusted as required during the course of the operation. For this reason, it was only when inhalation anaesthetics were first discovered, in 1846, that most surgical operations became a practical possibility. Until that time, surgeons relied on being able to operate on struggling patients at lightning speed, and most operations were amputations. Inhalation is still the commonest route of administration for anaesthetics, although induction is usually carried out with intravenous agents.

▼ The use of **nitrous oxide** to relieve the pain of surgery was suggested by Humphrey Davy in 1800. He was the first person to make nitrous oxide, and he tested its effects on several people, including himself and the Prime Minister, noting that it caused euphoria, analgesia and loss of consciousness. The use of nitrous oxide, billed as 'laughing gas', became a popular fairground entertainment and came to the notice of an American dentist, Horace Wells, who had a tooth extracted under its influence, while he himself squeezed the inhalation bag. **Ether** also first gained publicity in a disreputable way, through the spread of 'ether frolics', at which it was used to produce euphoria among the guests (explosions, too, one might have thought). William Morton, also a dentist and a student at Harvard Medical School, used it successfully to extract a tooth in 1846 and then suggested to Warren, the illustrious chief surgeon at Massachusetts General Hospital, that he should administer it for one of Warren's operations. Warren grudgingly agreed, and on 16 October 1846 a large audience was gathered in the main operating theatre;[1] after some preliminary fumbling, Morton's demonstration was a spectacular success. 'Gentlemen, this is no humbug' was the most gracious comment that Warren could bring himself to make to the assembled audience. A more wordy appreciation came later from Oliver Wendell Holmes

---

[1]Now preserved as the ether dome, a museum piece at Massachusetts General Hospital.

(1847), the neurologist-poet-philosopher who first coined the word 'anaesthesia':

'The knife is searching for disease, the pulleys are dragging back dislocated limbs—Nature herself is working out the primal curse which doomed the tenderest of her creatures to the sharpest of her trials, but the fierce extremity of suffering has been steeped in the waters of forgetfulness, and the deepest furrow in the knotted brow of agony has been smoothed forever.'

Morton subsequently sank into an endless and bitter dispute over the patent rights, and contributed nothing more to medical science. In the same year, James Simpson, professor of obstetrics in Glasgow, used chloroform to relieve the pain of childbirth, bringing on himself fierce denunciation from the clergy, one of whom wrote:

'Chloroform is a decoy of Satan, apparently offering itself to bless women; but in the end it will harden society and rob God of the deep, earnest cries which arise in time of trouble, for help.'

Opposition was effectively silenced in 1853, when Queen Victoria gave birth to her seventh child under the influence of chloroform, and the procedure became known as *anaesthésie à la reine*.

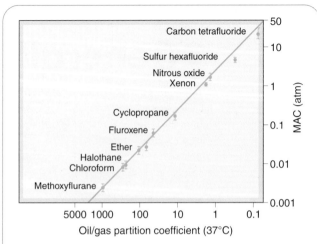

Fig. 36.1 **Correlation of anaesthetic potency with oil:gas partition coefficient.** Anaesthetic potency in humans is expressed as minimum alveolar partial pressure (MAC) required to produce surgical anaesthesia. There is a close correlation with lipid solubility, expressed as the oil:gas partition coefficient. (From: Halsey, 1989.)

MECHANISM OF ACTION OF ANAESTHETIC DRUGS

Unlike most drugs, inhalation anaesthetics, which include substances as diverse as **halothane**, **nitrous oxide** and xenon, belong to no recognisable chemical class. The shape and electronic configuration of the molecule is relatively unimportant, and the pharmacological action seems to require only that the molecule has certain physicochemical properties. Early theories, particularly the lipid theory (see below), were therefore based on rather general physicochemical ideas. Because we now know much more about the functional components of cell membranes—the principal structures affected by anaesthetic drugs—the emphasis has shifted towards identifying specific protein targets.

Accounts of the different theories of anaesthesia are given by Halsey (1989), Little (1996) and Franks & Lieb (1994).

LIPID THEORY

Overton and Meyer, at the turn of the 20th century, showed a close correlation between anaesthetic potency and lipid solubility in a diverse group of simple and unreactive organic compounds that were tested for their ability to immobilise tadpoles. This led to a bold theory, formulated by Meyer in 1937: 'Narcosis commences when any chemically indifferent substance has attained a certain molar concentration in the lipids of the cell'.

The relationship between anaesthetic activity and lipid solubility has been repeatedly confirmed. Anaesthetic potency in humans is usually expressed as the *minimal alveolar concentration (MAC)* required to abolish the response to surgical incision in 50% of subjects. Figure 36.1 shows the correlation between MAC (inversely proportional to potency) and lipid solubility, expressed as oil:water partition coefficient, for a wide range of inhalation anaesthetics. The Overton–Meyer studies did not suggest any particular mechanism, but revealed an impressive correlation, for which any theory of anaesthesia needs to account. Oil:water partition was assumed to predict partition into membrane lipids, consistent with the suggestion that anaesthesia results from an alteration of membrane function.

How the simple introduction of inert foreign molecules into the lipid bilayer could cause a functional disturbance is not explained by the lipid theory. Two possible mechanisms, namely *volume expansion* and *increased membrane fluidity*, have been suggested and tested experimentally, but both are now largely discredited (see Halsey, 1989; Little, 1996), and attention has swung from lipids to proteins, the correlation of potency with lipid solubility being explained by the effect of lipid solubility on the concentration of anaesthetic adjacent to its supposed protein target in the hydrophobic region of neuronal cell membranes.

EFFECTS ON ION CHANNELS

Following early studies that showed that anaesthetics can bind to various proteins as well as lipids, it was found that anaesthetics affect many ligand-gated ion channels (see Franks & Lieb 1994; Rudolph & Antkowiak, 2004). Many anaesthetic agents are able, at concentrations reached during anaesthesia, to inhibit the function of excitatory receptors, such as the ionotropic glutamate, acetylcholine or 5-hydroxytryptamine receptors, as well as enhancing the function of inhibitory receptors such as $GABA_A$ and glycine. The $GABA_A$ receptor is the sole target for benzodiazepines (see Ch. 37) and also appears to be a major target for intravenous anaesthetics, such as **thiopental, propofol** and **etomidate** (see below), that act at a site on the receptor different from the benzodiazepine binding site. Studies of experimentally mutated receptors (see Rudolph & Antkowiak, 2004) have confirmed this and succeeded in identifying the specific 'modulatory sites' through which the anaesthetic drugs exert their effects on channel function. The 'two-pore domain' potassium channel known as TREK (see Ch. 4) is another specifically anaesthetic-sensitive channel. It is activated, thus reducing membrane excitability, by low concentrations of volatile anaesthetics (see Franks & Lieb, 1999).

In summary, general anaesthetics inhibit excitatory channels (especially glutamate receptors) and facilitate inhibitory channels (particularly GABA$_A$ but also glycine and certain potassium channels), and these interactions are targeted at specific hydrophobic domains of the channel proteins. This is probably a serious oversimplification: as Little (1996) emphasises, individual anaesthetics differ in their actions and affect cellular function in several different ways, so a unitary theory is unlikely to be sufficient, but it does provide a useful starting point.

EFFECTS OF ANAESTHETICS ON THE NERVOUS SYSTEM

At the cellular level, the effect of anaesthetics is mainly to inhibit synaptic transmission, any effects on axonal conduction probably being relatively unimportant.

Inhibition of synaptic transmission could be due to reduction of transmitter release, inhibition of the action of the transmitter, or reduction of the excitability of the postsynaptic cell. Although all three effects have been described, most studies suggest that reduced transmitter release and reduced postsynaptic response are the main factors. Reduced acetylcholine release occurs at peripheral synapses, and reduced sensitivity to excitatory transmitters (due to inhibition of ligand-gated ion channels; see above) occurs at both peripheral and central synapses.

Inhibitory synaptic transmission is usually potentiated by general anaesthetics, particularly barbiturates, volatile anaesthetics having similar but less strong actions (see Rudolph & Antkowiak, 2004).

The anaesthetic state comprises several components, including unconsciousness, loss of reflexes (muscle relaxation) and analgesia. Much effort has gone into identifying the brain regions on which anaesthetics act to produce these effects. The most sensitive regions appear to be the midbrain reticular formation and thalamic sensory relay nuclei, inhibition of which results in unconsciousness and analgesia, respectively. Some anaesthetics cause inhibition at spinal level, producing a loss of reflex responses to painful stimuli, although, in practice, neuromuscular-blocking drugs (Ch. 10) are used to produce muscle relaxation rather than relying on the anaesthetic alone. Anaesthetics, even in low concentrations, cause short-term amnesia, i.e. experiences occurring during the influence of the drug are not recalled later, even though the subject was responsive at the time.[2] It is likely that interference with hippocampal function produces this effect, because the hippocampus is involved in short-term memory, and certain hippocampal synapses are highly susceptible to inhibition by anaesthetics.

As the anaesthetic concentration is increased, all brain functions are affected, including motor control and reflex activity,

---

[2]The benzodiazepine flunitrazepam, Rohypnol, has achieved a nasty notoriety because its amnesia-producing and tranquillising effect led to its use as a rapists' aid along with compounds such as ketamine (Ch. 43) and γ-hydroxy butyric acid.

Theories of anaesthesia

- Many simple, unreactive compounds produce narcotic effects, the extreme example being the inert gas xenon.
- Anaesthetic potency is closely correlated with lipid solubility (Overton–Meyer correlation), not with chemical structure.
- Earlier theories of anaesthesia postulate interaction with the lipid membrane bilayer. Recent work favours interaction with ligand-gated membrane ion channels.
- Most anaesthetics enhance the activity of inhibitory GABA$_A$ receptors, and many inhibit activation of excitatory receptors such as glutamate and nicotinic acetylcholine receptors.

respiration and autonomic regulation. Therefore it is not possible to identify a critical 'target site' in the brain responsible for all the phenomena of anaesthesia.

High concentrations of any general anaesthetic affect all parts of the CNS, causing complete shut-down and, in the absence of artificial respiration, death from respiratory failure. The margin between surgical anaesthesia and potentially fatal respiratory and circulatory depression is quite narrow, requiring careful monitoring by the anaesthetist and rapid adjustment of the level of anaesthesia, as required.

EFFECTS ON THE CARDIOVASCULAR AND RESPIRATORY SYSTEMS

All anaesthetics decrease cardiac contractility, but their effects on cardiac output and blood pressure vary because of concomitant actions on the sympathetic nervous system and vascular smooth muscle. **Nitrous oxide** increases sympathetic discharge and plasma noradrenaline concentration, and if used alone increases heart rate and blood pressure. **Halothane** and other halogenated anaesthetics have the opposite effect.

Many anaesthetics, especially **halothane**, cause ventricular extrasystoles. The mechanism involves sensitisation to adrenaline. Electrocardiogram monitoring shows that extrasystolic beats occur very commonly in patients under halothane anaesthesia, with no harm coming to the patient. If catecholamine secretion is excessive, however (par excellence in phaeochromocytoma; see Ch. 11), there is a risk of precipitating ventricular fibrillation.

With the exception of **nitrous oxide** and **ketamine**, all anaesthetics depress respiration markedly and increase arterial $P\text{co}_2$. Nitrous oxide has much less effect, mainly because its low potency prevents very deep anaesthesia from being produced with this drug (see below). Some inhalation anaesthetics, particularly **desflurane** among agents commonly used nowadays, are pungent and liable to cause laryngospasm and bronchospasm, so desflurane is not used for inducing anaesthesia but only for maintaining it.

Pharmacological effects of anaesthetic agents

- Anaesthesia involves three main neurophysiological changes: unconsciousness, loss of response to painful stimulation and loss of reflexes.
- At supra-anaesthetic doses, all anaesthetic agents can cause death by loss of cardiovascular reflexes and respiratory paralysis.
- At the cellular level, anaesthetic agents affect synaptic transmission rather than axonal conduction. The release of excitatory transmitters and the response of the postsynaptic receptors are both inhibited. GABA-mediated inhibitory transmission is enhanced by most anaesthetics.
- Although all parts of the nervous system are affected by anaesthetic agents, the main targets appear to be the thalamus, cortex and hippocampus.
- Most anaesthetic agents (with exceptions, such as ketamine and benzodiazepines) produce similar neurophysiological effects and differ mainly in respect of their pharmacokinetic properties and toxicity.
- Most anaesthetic agents cause cardiovascular depression by effects on the myocardium and blood vessels, as well as on the nervous system. Halogenated anaesthetic agents are likely to cause cardiac dysrhythmias, accentuated by circulating catecholamines.

Clinical uses of general anaesthetics

- *Intravenous anaesthetics* are used for:
  - induction of anaesthesia (e.g. **thiopental, etomidate**)
  - maintenance of anaesthesia throughout surgery ('total intravenous anaesthesia', e.g. **propofol** given in combination with muscle relaxants and analgesics).
- *Inhalational anaesthetics* (gases or volatile liquids) are used for maintenance of anaesthesia. Points to note are that:
  - volatile liquids (e.g. **halothane, sevoflurane**) are vaporised with air, oxygen or oxygen–nitrous oxide mixtures as the carrier gas
  - **halothane** hepatotoxicity (see Ch. 53) occurs more often after repeated exposure
  - all inhalational anaesthetics can trigger *malignant hyperthermia* in susceptible individuals (Ch. 10).

INHALATION ANAESTHETICS

We next consider the pharmacological properties of general anaesthetics; it should be remembered that these are rarely used alone. The anaesthetic state consists of three main components, namely *loss of consciousness, analgesia* and *muscle relaxation*. In practice, these effects are produced with a combination of drugs. A common approach for a major surgical operation would be to produce unconsciousness rapidly with an intravenous induction agent (e.g. **propofol**); to maintain unconsciousness and produce analgesia with one or more inhalation agents (e.g. **nitrous oxide** and **halothane**), which might be supplemented with an intravenous analgesic agent (e.g. an opiate; see Ch. 41); and to produce muscle paralysis with a neuromuscular-blocking drug (e.g. **atracurium**; see Ch. 10). Such a procedure results in much faster induction and recovery, avoiding long (and hazardous) periods of semiconsciousness, and it enables surgery to be carried out with relatively little impairment of homeostatic reflexes.

Most inhalation anaesthetics that were once widely used, such as **ether, chloroform, trichloroethylene, cyclopropane** and **methoxyflurane**, have now been replaced in clinical practice, particularly by the 'flurane' series (**enflurane, isoflurane, sevoflurane, desflurane**), which have improved pharmacokinetic properties, fewer side effects and are non-flammable. Of the older agents, **nitrous oxide** is still used widely (especially in obstetric practice), and **halothane** occasionally.

Anaesthetics, like many other CNS depressants, are potentially addictive (see Ch. 43).

PHARMACOKINETIC ASPECTS

An important characteristic of an inhalation anaesthetic is the speed at which the arterial blood concentration, which governs the pharmacological effect, follows changes in the concentration of the drug in the inspired air. Ideally, the blood concentration should follow as quickly as possible, so that the depth of anaesthesia can be controlled rapidly. In particular, the blood concentration should fall to a subanaesthetic level rapidly when administration is stopped, so that the patient recovers consciousness with minimal delay. A prolonged semicomatose state, in which respiratory reflexes are weak or absent, is particularly hazardous.

The lungs are the only quantitatively important route by which inhalation anaesthetics enter and leave the body. Metabolic degradation of anaesthetics (see below), although important in relation to their toxicity, is generally insignificant in determining their duration of action. Anaesthetics are all small, lipid-soluble molecules that readily cross alveolar membranes. It is therefore the rates of delivery of drug to and from the lungs, via (respectively) the inspired air and bloodstream, that determine the overall kinetic behaviour of an anaesthetic. The reason that anaesthetics vary in their kinetic behaviour is that their relative solubilities in blood, and in body fat, vary between one drug and another.

The main factors that determine the speed of induction and recovery can be summarised as follow.

- Properties of the anaesthetic:
  —blood:gas partition coefficient (i.e. solubility in blood)
  —oil:gas partition coefficient (i.e. solubility in fat).

- Physiological factors:
  —alveolar ventilation rate
  —cardiac output.

THE SOLUBILITY OF ANAESTHETICS

Anaesthetics can be regarded physicochemically as ideal gases: their solubility in different media is expressed as *partition coefficients*, defined as the ratio of the concentration of the agent in two phases at equilibrium.

The *blood:gas partition coefficient* is the main factor that determines the rate of induction and recovery of an inhalation anaesthetic, and the lower the blood:gas partition coefficient the faster is induction and recovery.

The *oil:gas partition coefficient*, a measure of fat solubility, determines the potency of an anaesthetic (as already discussed) and also influences the kinetics of its distribution in the body, the main effect being that high lipid solubility delays recovery from anaesthesia. Values of blood:gas and oil:gas partition coefficients for some anaesthetics are given in Table 36.1.

Table 36.1   Characteristics of inhalation anaesthetics

Drug	Partition coefficient		Minimum alveolar concentration (% v/v)	Induction/recovery	Main adverse effect(s) and disadvantage(s)	Notes
	Blood:gas	*Oil:gas*				
Ether	12.0	65	1.9	Slow	Respiratory irritation Nausea and vomiting Explosion risk	Now obsolete, except where modern facilities are lacking
Halothane	2.4	220	0.8	Medium	Hypotension Cardiac arrhythmias Hepatotoxicity (with repeated use) Malignant hyperthermia (rare)	In common use but declining in favour of newer agents Significant metabolism to trifluoracetate
Nitrous oxide	0.5	1.4	100[a]	Fast	Few adverse effects Risk of anaemia (with prolonged or repeated use) Accumulation in gaseous cavities	Good analgesic effect Low potency precludes use as sole anaesthetic agent—normally combined with other inhalation agents
Enflurane	1.9	98	0.7	Medium	Risk of convulsions (slight) Malignant hyperthermia (rare)	Widely used Similar characteristics to halothane, with less risk of hepatic toxicity
Isoflurane	1.4	91	1.2	Medium	Few adverse effects Possible risk of coronary ischemia in susceptible patients	Widely used as alternative to halothane
Desflurane	0.4	23	6.1	Fast	Respiratory tract irritation, cough, bronchospasm	Used for day case surgery because of fast onset and recovery (comparable with nitrous oxide)
Sevoflurane	0.6	53	2.1	Fast	Few reported Theoretical risk of renal toxicity owing to fluoride	Recently introduced Similar to desflurane

[a]Theoretical value based on experiments under hyperbaric conditions.

INDUCTION AND RECOVERY

Cerebral blood flow is a substantial fraction of cardiac output, and the blood–brain barrier is freely permeable to anaesthetics, so the concentration of anaesthetic in the brain closely tracks that in the arterial blood. The kinetics of transfer of anaesthetic between the inspired air and the arterial blood therefore determine the kinetics of the pharmacological effect.

If an anaesthetic is added to the inspired air at a concentration that, at equilibrium, will produce surgical anaesthesia, the rate at which this equilibrium is approached depends mainly on the blood:gas partition coefficient. Contrary to what one might intuitively suppose, the *lower* the solubility in blood, the *faster* is the process of equilibration. This is because less drug has to be absorbed via the lungs in order to achieve a given partial pressure in the blood. Thus a single lungful of air containing a low-solubility agent will bring the partial pressure in the blood closer to that of the inspired air than is the case for a high-solubility agent, and a smaller number of breaths (i.e. a shorter time) will be needed to reach equilibrium. The same principle applies in reverse for wash out of the drug, recovery being faster with a low-solubility agent. Figure 36.2 shows the much faster equilibration for **nitrous oxide**, a low-solubility agent, than for **ether**, a high solubility agent.

The transfer of anaesthetic between blood and tissues also affects the kinetics of equilibration. Figure 36.3 shows a very simple model of the circulation, in which two tissue compartments are included. Body fat has a low blood flow and

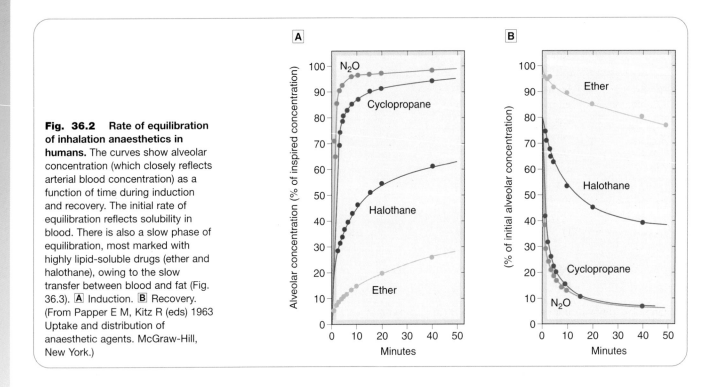

Fig. 36.2 Rate of equilibration of inhalation anaesthetics in humans. The curves show alveolar concentration (which closely reflects arterial blood concentration) as a function of time during induction and recovery. The initial rate of equilibration reflects solubility in blood. There is also a slow phase of equilibration, most marked with highly lipid-soluble drugs (ether and halothane), owing to the slow transfer between blood and fat (Fig. 36.3). **A** Induction. **B** Recovery. (From Papper E M, Kitz R (eds) 1963 Uptake and distribution of anaesthetic agents. McGraw-Hill, New York.)

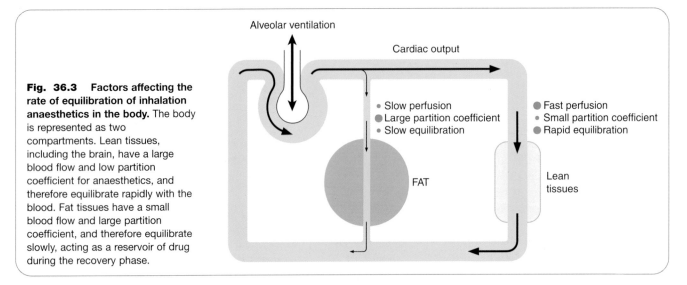

Fig. 36.3 Factors affecting the rate of equilibration of inhalation anaesthetics in the body. The body is represented as two compartments. Lean tissues, including the brain, have a large blood flow and low partition coefficient for anaesthetics, and therefore equilibrate rapidly with the blood. Fat tissues have a small blood flow and large partition coefficient, and therefore equilibrate slowly, acting as a reservoir of drug during the recovery phase.

often a high anaesthetic solubility (see Table 36.1), and constitutes about 20% of the volume of a representative man. Therefore, for a drug such as **halothane**, which is about 100 times more soluble in fat than in water, the amount present in fat after complete equilibration would be roughly 95% of the total amount in the body. Because of the low blood flow to adipose tissue, it takes many hours for the drug to enter and leave the fat, which results in a pronounced slow phase of equilibration following the rapid phase associated with the blood–gas exchanges (Fig. 36.2). The more fat-soluble the anaesthetic and the fatter the patient, the more pronounced this slow phase becomes.

Of the physiological factors affecting the rate of equilibration of inhalation anaesthetics, alveolar ventilation is the most important. The greater the ventilation rate, the faster is equilibration, particularly for drugs that have high blood:gas partition coefficients. Respiratory depressant drugs, such as **morphine** (see Ch. 41), can thus retard recovery from anaesthesia.

Recovery from anaesthesia involves the same processes as induction but in reverse (Fig. 36.2), the rapid phase of recovery being followed by a slow 'hangover'. If anaesthesia with a highly fat-soluble drug has been maintained for a long time, so that the fat has had time to accumulate a substantial amount of the anaesthetic, this hangover can become very pronounced and the patient may remain drowsy for some hours. Because of these kinetic factors, the search for improved inhalation anaesthetics has focused on agents with low blood and tissue solubility. Newer drugs, which show kinetic properties similar to those of **nitrous oxide** but have higher potency, include **sevoflurane** and **desflurane** (Table 36.1).

METABOLISM AND TOXICITY OF INHALATION ANAESTHETICS

Metabolism, although not quantitatively important as a route of elimination of inhalation anaesthetics, can generate toxic metabolites. **Chloroform** (now obsolete) causes hepatotoxicity associated with free radical formation in liver cells. **Methoxyflurane**, a halogenated ether, is no longer used because about 50% is metabolised to fluoride and oxalate, which cause renal toxicity. **Enflurane** and **sevoflurane** also generate fluoride, but at much lower (non-toxic) concentrations (Table 36.1). **Halothane** is the only volatile anaesthetic in current use that undergoes substantial metabolism, about 30% being converted to bromide, trifluoroacetic acid and other metabolites that are implicated in rare instances of liver toxicity (see below).

The problem of toxicity of low concentrations of anaesthetics inhaled over long periods by operating theatre staff causes much concern, following the demonstration that such chronic low-level exposure (and associated metabolite formation) leads to liver toxicity in experimental animals. Epidemiological studies of operating theatre staff have shown increased incidence of liver disease and of certain types of leukaemia, and of spontaneous abortion and congenital malformations, compared with control groups not exposed to anaesthetic agents. Although causation has not been clearly established, strict measures are used to minimise the escape of anaesthetics into the air of operating theatres.

INDIVIDUAL INHALATION ANAESTHETICS

The inhalation anaesthetics currently used in developed countries are **halothane**, **nitrous oxide**, **enflurane** and **isoflurane**. **Ether**, now largely obsolete, is still used in some parts of the world. It is explosive and highly irritant, and commonly causes postoperative nausea and respiratory complications. **Methoxyflurane** (see above) is no longer used because of its renal toxicity. **Desflurane** and **sevoflurane** have gained popularity because they overcome many of the problems of the earlier drugs. The newer compounds are all halogen-substituted hydrocarbons of very similar 'spot the difference' structure. After 50 years of this kind of musical chairs chemistry, there is a sense that we may have reached the end of the line with sevoflurane. **Xenon**, an inert gas shown many years ago to have anaesthetic properties, is making something of a comeback in the clinic because—not surprisingly for an inert gas—it lacks toxicity, but its relatively low potency and high cost are disadvantages.

HALOTHANE

Halothane is a widely used inhalation anaesthetic, but its use is now declining in favour of **isoflurane** and other drugs (see below). It is non-explosive and non-irritant; induction and recovery are relatively fast; and it is highly potent and can easily produce respiratory and cardiovascular failure, so the concentration administered needs to be controlled accurately. Even in normal anaesthetic concentrations, halothane causes a fall in blood pressure, partly due to myocardial depression and partly to vasodilatation.

> **Pharmacokinetic properties of inhalation anaesthetics**
>
> - Rapid induction and recovery are important properties of an anaesthetic agent, allowing flexible control over the depth of anaesthesia.
> - Speed of induction and recovery are determined by two properties of the anaesthetic: solubility in blood (blood:gas partition coefficient) and solubility in fat (lipid solubility).
> - Agents with low blood:gas partition coefficients produce rapid induction and recovery (e.g. nitrous oxide, desflurane); agents with high blood:gas partition coefficients show slow induction and recovery (e.g. halothane).
> - Agents with high lipid solubility (e.g. halothane) accumulate gradually in body fat and may produce a prolonged 'hangover' if used for a long operation.
> - Some halogenated anaesthetics (especially halothane and methoxyflurane) are metabolised. This is not very important in determining their duration of action, but contributes to toxicity (e.g. renal toxicity associated with fluoride production with methoxyflurane—no longer used).

Halothane is not analgesic and has a relaxant effect on the uterus, which limits its usefulness for obstetric purposes.

Adverse effects

In common with many halogenated anaesthetics, halothane sensitises the heart to adrenaline, predisposing to cardiac dysrhythmia. This may be important, notably in operations for phaeochromocytoma (see Ch. 11 and above). Two rare but serious adverse reactions associated with halothane are *hepatotoxicity* and *malignant hyperthermia*.

Halothane hepatitis. One major study of 850 000 anaesthetic administrations identified nine deaths from otherwise unexplained liver failure. Seven of the nine patients had received halothane. Subsequent reports suggest that hepatotoxicity is associated with *repeated* administration of halothane. A study of 62 cases of unexplained serious liver disease in the UK showed that 66% were associated with repeated halothane administration, consistent with an immune mechanism. Halothane metabolism yields *trifluoroacetic acid* (see above), which reacts covalently with protein, especially in liver cells where halothane metabolism occurs. Fluoroacetylated liver proteins are believed to initiate an immune response (Ch. 53).

Malignant hyperthermia. This is caused by heat production in skeletal muscle, due to excessive release of Ca^{2+} from the sarcoplasmic reticulum. The result is muscle contracture, acidosis, increased metabolism, and an associated dramatic rise in body temperature that can be fatal unless treated promptly. Triggers include other halogenated anaesthetics and neuromuscular-blocking drugs (see Ch. 10), as well as **halothane**. Susceptibility has a genetic basis, being associated with mutations in the gene encoding the *ryanodine receptor*, which controls Ca^{2+} release from the sarcoplasmic reticulum (Ch. 4). Why such mutations induce sensitivity of the channel to anaesthetics and other drugs is not clear. Malignant hyperthermia is treated with **dantrolene**, a muscle relaxant drug that blocks these calcium channels.

NITROUS OXIDE

Nitrous oxide (N_2O, not to be confused with nitric oxide, NO) is an odourless gas with many advantageous features for anaesthesia, and is in widespread use. It is rapid in action because of its low blood:gas partition coefficient (Table 36.1), and is an effective *analgesic* in concentrations too low to cause unconsciousness. It is used in this way to reduce pain during childbirth. Its potency is low; even at 80% in the inspired gas mixture, nitrous oxide does not produce surgical anaesthesia. It is not therefore used on its own as an anaesthetic, but is very often used (as 70% nitrous oxide in oxygen) as an adjunct to volatile anaesthetics, allowing them to be used at lower concentrations. During recovery from nitrous oxide anaesthesia, the transfer of the gas from the blood into the alveoli can be sufficient to reduce, by dilution, the alveolar partial pressure of oxygen, producing transient hypoxia (known as diffusional hypoxia). This is important for patients with respiratory disease.

Given for brief periods, nitrous oxide is devoid of any serious toxic effects, but prolonged exposure (> 6 hours) causes inactivation of *methionine synthase*, an enzyme required for DNA and protein synthesis, resulting in bone marrow depression that may cause anaemia and leucopenia, so its use should be avoided in patients with anaemia related to vitamin B_{12} deficiency. Bone marrow depression does not occur with brief exposure to nitrous oxide, but prolonged or repeated use should be avoided. Nitrous oxide 'sniffers' are subject to this danger.

Nitrous oxide tends to enter gaseous cavities in the body, causing them to expand. This can be dangerous if a pneumothorax or vascular air embolus is present, or if the intestine is obstructed.

Prolonged exposure to very low concentrations of nitrous oxide, far below the level causing anaesthesia, may affect protein and DNA synthesis very markedly, and nitrous oxide has been suspected to be a cause of the increased frequency of abortion and fetal abnormality among operating theatre staff.

ENFLURANE

Enflurane is a halogenated ether similar to halothane in its potency and moderate speed of induction. It was introduced as an alternative to **methoxyflurane**, its advantages being that at therapeutic levels it produces less fluoride (and hence less renal toxicity) than methoxyflurane and is less fat-soluble so that onset and recovery are faster. Its main drawback is that it can cause seizures, either during induction or following recovery from anaesthesia. In this connection, it is interesting that a related substance, the fluorine-substituted diethyl-ether hexafluoroether, is a powerful convulsant agent, although the mechanism is not understood. Enflurane can induce malignant hyperthermia.

ISOFLURANE, DESFLURANE AND SEVOFLURANE

Isoflurane is now the most widely used volatile anaesthetic. It is broadly similar to enflurane, but is not appreciably metabolised and lacks the proconvulsive property of enflurane. It is expensive to manufacture because of the difficulty in separating isomers formed during synthesis. It can cause hypotension and is a powerful coronary vasodilator. This can exacerbate cardiac ischaemia in patients with coronary disease, because of the 'steal' phenomenon (see Ch. 18).

Desflurane is chemically similar to isoflurane, but its lower solubility in blood and fat means that induction and recovery are faster, so it is increasingly used as an anaesthetic for day case surgery. It is not appreciably metabolised. It is less potent than the drugs described above, the MAC being about 6%. At the concentrations used for induction (about 10%), desflurane causes some respiratory tract irritation, which can lead to coughing and bronchospasm.

Sevoflurane resembles desflurane but is more potent and does not cause respiratory irritation. It is partially (about 3%) metabolised, and detectable levels of fluoride are produced, although this does not appear to be sufficient to cause toxicity. Like other halogenated anaesthetics, sevoflurane can cause malignant hyperthermia in genetically susceptible individuals.

Many inhalation anaesthetics have been introduced and gradually superseded, mainly because of their inflammable nature or because of toxicity. They include **chloroform** (hepatotoxicity and cardiac dysrhythmias), **diethyl ether** (explosive and highly irritant to the respiratory tract, leading to postoperative complications), **vinyl ether** (explosive), **cyclopropane** (explosive, strongly depressant to respiration, and hypotensive), **trichloroethylene** (chemically unstable, no special advantages), and **methoxyflurane** (slow recovery and renal toxicity).

Further information is available in many excellent textbooks of anaesthesia (e.g. Miller, 1999).

INTRAVENOUS ANAESTHETIC AGENTS

Even the fastest-acting inhalation anaesthetics, such as **nitrous oxide**, take a few minutes to act and cause a period of excitement before anaesthesia is produced. Intravenous anaesthetics act much more rapidly, producing unconsciousness in about 20 seconds, as soon as the drug reaches the brain from its site of injection. These drugs (e.g. **thiopental, etomidate, propofol**; see below) are normally used for induction of anaesthesia. They are preferred by patients because injection generally lacks the menacing quality associated with a face mask in an apprehensive individual.

Other drugs used as intravenous induction agents include certain benzodiazepines (see Ch. 37), such as **diazepam** and **midazolam**, which act rather less rapidly than the drugs listed above. Although intravenous anaesthetics on their own are generally unsatisfactory for producing maintained anaesthesia because their elimination from the body is relatively slow compared with that of inhalation agents, **propofol** can be used in this way, and the duration of action of **ketamine** is sufficient that it can be used for short operations without the need for an inhalation agent.

The combined use of **droperidol**, a dopamine antagonist related to antipsychotic drugs (Ch. 38), and an opiate analgesic such as **fentanyl** (Ch. 41) can produce a state of deep sedation and analgesia (known as *neuroleptanalgesia*) in which the patient remains responsive to simple commands and questions, but does not respond to painful stimuli or retain any memory of the procedure. This is used for minor procedures such as endoscopy.

The properties of the main intravenous anaesthetics are summarised in Table 36.2. **Propanidid** and **althesin** were withdrawn because of allergic reactions including hypotension and bronchoconstriction.

THIOPENTAL

Thiopental (Ch. 37) is the only remaining barbiturate used as an anaesthetic. It has very high lipid solubility, and this accounts for the speed and transience of its effect when it is injected intravenously (see below). The free acid is insoluble in water, so thiopental is given as the sodium salt. This solution is strongly alkaline and is unstable, so the drug must be dissolved immediately before it is used.

Pharmacokinetic aspects

On intravenous injection, thiopental causes unconsciousness within about 20 seconds and lasts for 5–10 minutes. The anaesthetic

Individual inhalation anaesthetics

- The main agents in current use in developed countries are halothane, nitrous oxide, isoflurane, enflurane, desflurane and sevoflurane. Ether is largely obsolete.
- As a rare but serious hazard, inhalation anaesthetics (especially halothane) can cause malignant hyperthermia.
- **Halothane:**
  - widely used agent
  - potent, non-explosive and non-irritant, hypotensive; may cause dysrhythmias; about 30% metabolised
  - 'hangover' likely, due to high lipid solubility
  - risk of liver damage if used repeatedly.
- **Nitrous oxide:**
  - low potency, therefore must be combined with other agents
  - rapid induction and recovery
  - good analgesic properties
  - risk of bone marrow depression with prolonged administration
  - accumulates in gaseous cavities.
- **Enflurane:**
  - halogenated anaesthetic similar to halothane
  - less metabolism than halothane, therefore less risk of toxicity
  - faster induction and recovery than halothane (less accumulation in fat)
  - some risk of epilepsy-like seizures.
- **Isoflurane:**
  - similar to enflurane but lacks epileptogenic property
  - may precipitate myocardial ischaemia in patients with coronary disease
  - irritant to respiratory tract.
- **Desflurane:**
  - similar to isoflurane but with faster onset and recovery
  - respiratory irritant, so liable to cause coughing and laryngospasm
  - useful for day case surgery.
- **Sevoflurane:**
  - similar to desflurane, with lack of respiratory irritation.
- **Ether:**
  - obsolete except where modern facilities are not available
  - easy to administer and control
  - slow onset and recovery, with postoperative nausea and vomiting
  - analgesic and muscle relaxant properties
  - highly explosive
  - irritant to respiratory tract.

Table 36.2   Properties of intravenous anaesthetic agents

Drug	Speed of induction and recovery	Main unwanted effect(s)	Notes
Thiopental	Fast (cumulation occurs, giving slow recovery) 'Hangover'	Cardiovascular and respiratory depression	Widely used as induction agent for routine purposes
Etomidate	Fast onset, fairly fast recovery	Excitatory effects during induction and recovery Adrenocortical suppression	Less cardiovascular and respiratory depression than with thiopental Causes pain at injection site
Propofol	Fast onset, very fast recovery	Cardiovascular and respiratory depression	Rapidly metabolised Possible to use as continuous infusion Causes pain at injection site
Ketamine	Slow onset, after-effects common during recovery	Psychotomimetic effects following recovery Postoperative nausea, vomiting and salivation Raised intracranial pressure	Produces good analgesia and amnesia
Midazolam	Slower than other agents	–	Little respiratory or cardiovascular depression

effect closely parallels the concentration of thiopental in the blood reaching the brain, because its high lipid solubility allows it to cross the blood–brain barrier without noticeable delay.

The blood concentration of thiopental declines rapidly, by about 80% within 1–2 minutes, following the initial peak after intravenous injection, because the drug is redistributed, first to tissues with a large blood flow (liver, kidneys, brain, etc.) and more slowly to muscle. Uptake into body fat, although favoured by the high lipid solubility of thiopental, occurs only slowly, because of the low blood flow to this tissue. After several hours, however, most of the thiopental present in the body will have accumulated in body fat, the rest having been metabolised. Recovery from the anaesthetic effect occurs within about 5 minutes, governed entirely by redistribution of the drug to well-perfused tissues; very little is metabolised in this time. After the initial rapid decline, the blood concentration drops more slowly, over several hours, as the drug is taken up by body fat and metabolised. Consequently, thiopental produces a long-lasting hangover; furthermore, repeated intravenous doses cause progressively longer periods of anaesthesia, because the plateau in blood concentration becomes progressively more elevated as more drug accumulates in the body. For this reason, thiopental is *not* used to *maintain* surgical anaesthesia but only as an induction agent.

Thiopental binds to plasma albumin (roughly 85% of the blood content normally being bound). The fraction bound is less in states of malnutrition, liver disease or renal disease, which affect the concentration and drug-binding properties of plasma albumin, and this can appreciably reduce the dose needed for induction of anaesthesia.

Actions and side effects

The actions of thiopental on the nervous system are very similar to those of inhalation anaesthetics, although it has no analgesic effect and can cause profound respiratory depression even in amounts that fail to abolish reflex responses to painful stimuli.

Its long after-effect, associated with a slowly declining plasma concentration, means that drowsiness and some degree of respiratory depression persist for some hours.

Accidental injection of thiopental around, rather than into, the vein, or into an artery, can cause local tissue necrosis and ulceration or severe arterial spasm that can result in gangrene. Immediate injection of **procaine**, through the same needle, is the recommended procedure if this accident occurs. The risk is small now that lower concentrations of thiopental are used for intravenous injection. Thiopental, like other barbiturates, can precipitate an attack of *porphyria* in susceptible individuals (see Ch. 53).

ETOMIDATE

Etomidate has gained favour over thiopental on account of the larger margin between the anaesthetic dose and the dose needed to produce respiratory and cardiovascular depression. It is also more rapidly metabolised than thiopental, and thus less likely to cause a prolonged hangover. In other respects, etomidate is very similar to thiopental, although it appears more likely to cause involuntary movements during induction, postoperative nausea and vomiting, and pain at the injection site. Etomidate, particularly with prolonged use, suppresses the production of adrenal steroids, an effect that has been associated with an increase in mortality in severely ill patients. It should therefore not be used in patients with adrenal insufficiency. It is preferable to thiopental in patients at risk of circulatory failure.

PROPOFOL

Propofol, introduced in 1983, is also similar in its properties to thiopental, but it has the advantage of being very rapidly metabolised and therefore giving rapid recovery without any hangover effect. This enables it to be used as a continuous infusion to maintain surgical anaesthesia without the need for any inhalation agent. Propofol lacks the tendency to cause involuntary movement and adrenocortical suppression seen with etomidate. It is particularly useful for *day case surgery*.

OTHER INDUCTION AGENTS

KETAMINE

▼ Ketamine closely resembles, both chemically and pharmacologically, **phencyclidine**, which is a 'street drug' with a pronounced effect on sensory perception (see Ch. 43). Both drugs produce a similar anaesthesia-like state and profound analgesia, but ketamine produces considerably less euphoria and sensory distortion than phencyclidine and is thus more useful in anaesthesia. Both drugs are believed to act by blocking activation of one type of excitatory amino acid receptor (the NMDA receptor; see Ch. 33).

Given intravenously, ketamine takes effect more slowly (2–5 minutes) than thiopental, and produces a different effect, known as 'dissociative anaesthesia', in which there is a marked sensory loss and analgesia, as well as amnesia and paralysis of movement, without actual loss of consciousness. During induction and recovery, involuntary movements and peculiar sensory experiences often occur. Ketamine does not act simply as a depressant, and it produces cardiovascular and respiratory effects quite different from those of most anaesthetics. Blood pressure and heart rate are usually *increased*, and respiration is unaffected by effective anaesthetic doses. Ketamine, unlike other intravenous anaesthetic drugs, increases intracranial pressure, so it should not be given to patients with raised intracranial pressure or at risk of cerebral ischaemia. The main drawback of ketamine, despite the safety associated with a lack of overall depressant activity, is that hallucinations, and sometimes delirium and irrational behaviour, are common during recovery. These after-effects limit the usefulness of ketamine but are said to be less marked in children,[3] therefore ketamine, often in conjunction with a benzodiazepine, is sometimes still used for minor procedures in paediatrics.

MIDAZOLAM

Midazolam, a benzodiazepine (Ch. 37), is slower in the onset and offset of its action than the drugs discussed above but, like

ketamine, does not cause respiratory or cardiovascular depression. It is often used as a preoperative sedative and during procedures such as endoscopy, where full anaesthesia is not required.

> **Intravenous anaesthetic agents**
>
> - Most commonly used for induction of anaesthesia, followed by inhalation agent. Propofol is also used to maintain anaesthesia during surgery.
> - Thiopental, etomidate and propofol are most commonly used; all act within 20–30 seconds if given intravenously.
> - **Thiopental**:
>   - barbiturate with very high lipid solubility
>   - rapid action due to rapid transfer across blood–brain barrier; short duration (about 5 minutes) due to redistribution, mainly to muscle
>   - slowly metabolised and liable to accumulate in body fat, therefore may cause prolonged effect if given repeatedly
>   - no analgesic effect
>   - narrow margin between anaesthetic dose and dose causing cardiovascular depression
>   - risk of severe vasospasm if accidentally injected into artery.
> - **Etomidate**:
>   - similar to thiopental but more quickly metabolised
>   - less risk of cardiovascular depression
>   - may cause involuntary movements during induction
>   - possible risk of adrenocortical suppression.
> - **Propofol**:
>   - rapidly metabolised
>   - very rapid recovery; no cumulative effect
>   - useful for day case surgery.
> - **Ketamine**:
>   - analogue of phencyclidine, with similar properties
>   - action differs from other agents, probably related to effect on NMDA-type glutamate receptors
>   - onset of effect is relatively slow (2–5 minutes)
>   - produces 'dissociative' anaesthesia, in which patient may remain conscious although amnesic and insensitive to pain
>   - high incidence of dysphoria, hallucinations, etc. during recovery; used mainly for minor procedures in children
>   - raises intracranial pressure.

---

[3]A cautionary note: many adverse effects are claimed to be less marked in children, perhaps because they cannot verbalise their experiences. Until recently, muscle relaxants alone were used without anaesthesia during cardiac surgery in neonates. The babies did not complain of pain, but their circulating catecholamines reached extreme levels.

REFERENCES AND FURTHER READING

Evers A S, Maze M 2004 Anesthetic pharmacology. Churchill Livingstone, Philadelphia (*Comprehensive textbook covering basic and clinical pharmacology of anaesthetic agents*)

Franks N P, Lieb W J, 1999 Background K⁺ channels: an important target for volatile anesthetics? Nat Neurosci 2: 395–396 (*Short commentary on recent evidence suggesting that anaesthetics can activate TREK channels*)

Franks N P, Lieb W R 1994 Molecular and cellular mechanisms of general anaesthesia. Nature 367: 607–614 (*Good discussion of the opposing 'lipid' and 'protein' theories by pioneers from the protein camp*)

Halsey M J 1989 Physicochemical properties of inhalation anaesthetics. In: Nunn J F, Utting J E, Brown B R (eds) General anaesthesia. Butterworth, London (*Good summary of evidence supporting lipid theories of anaesthesia*)

Hemmings H C, Akabas M H, Goldstein P A et al. 2005 Emerging molecular mechanisms of general anaesthetic action. Trends Pharmacol Sci 26: 503–510 (*Describes effects of anaesthetics on ligand-gated and voltage-gated ion channels, particularly GABA$_A$ receptors*)

Little H J 1996 How has molecular pharmacology contributed to our understanding of the molecular mechanism(s) of general anaesthesia? Pharmacol Ther 69: 37–58 (*Balanced account of the strengths and shortcomings of current theories*)

Miller R D (ed) 1999 Anaesthesia. Churchill Livingstone, New York (*Comprehensive textbook*)

Rudolph U, Antkowiak B 2004 Molecular and neuronal substrates for general anaesthetics. Nat Rev Neurosci 5: 709–720 (*Useful review article covering both the interaction of general anaesthetic agents with different ion channels, and the neuronal pathways that are affected*)

Anxiolytic and hypnotic drugs

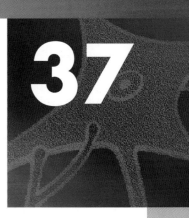

37

OVERVIEW

In this chapter, we discuss the nature of anxiety and the drugs used to treat it (anxiolytic drugs), as well as drugs used to treat insomnia (hypnotic drugs). Although the clinical objectives are different, there is some overlap between these two groups, reflecting the fact that anxiolytic drugs commonly cause a degree of sedation and drowsiness. There are, however, many sedative and hypnotic drugs that lack specific anxiolytic effects. In high doses, all these drugs cause unconsciousness and eventually death from respiratory and cardiovascular depression. Benzodiazepines form the most important group, although anxiolytic and hypnotic drugs from an earlier era are still in use. In recent years, a number of drugs acting on 5-hydroxytryptamine (5-HT) receptors in the brain, which do not have

strong sedative activity, have been introduced as anxiolytic agents. Possible new approaches, based on neuropeptide mediators, are also discussed briefly.

THE NATURE OF ANXIETY AND MEASUREMENT OF ANXIOLYTIC ACTIVITY

The normal *fear response* to threatening stimuli comprises several components, including defensive behaviours, autonomic reflexes, arousal and alertness, corticosteroid secretion and negative emotions. In *anxiety states*, these reactions occur in an anticipatory manner, independently of external events. The distinction between a 'pathological' and a 'normal' state of anxiety is not clear-cut but represents the point at which the symptoms interfere with normal productive activities. Despite (or perhaps because of) this loose distinction, anxiolytic drugs were until recently among the most widely used drugs in general practice. They have fallen out of favour as their uncertain benefit and definite risks have become evident.

Anxiety disorders as recognised clinically include:

- *generalised anxiety disorder* (an ongoing state of excessive anxiety lacking any clear reason or focus)
- *panic disorder* (sudden attacks of overwhelming fear occur in association with marked somatic symptoms, such as sweating, tachycardia, chest pains, trembling and choking). Such attacks can be induced even in normal individuals by infusion of sodium lactate, and the condition appears to have a genetic component)
- *phobias* (strong fears of specific objects or situations, e.g. snakes, open spaces, flying, social interactions)
- *post-traumatic stress disorder* (anxiety triggered by recall of past stressful experiences)
- *obsessive compulsive disorder* (compulsive ritualistic behaviour driven by irrational anxiety, e.g. fear of contamination).

It should be stressed that the treatment of such disorders generally involves psychological approaches as well as drug treatment. Furthermore, other types of drug, particularly antidepressants (Ch. 39) and sometimes antipsychotic drugs (Ch. 38), are often used to treat anxiety disorders, in addition to the anxiolytic drugs described here.

ANIMAL MODELS OF ANXIETY

▼ In addition to the subjective (emotional) component of human anxiety, there are measurable behavioural and physiological effects that also occur in experimental animals. In biological terms, anxiety induces a particular form of behavioural inhibition that occurs in response to novel environmental events that are non-rewarding (under conditions where reward is expected), threatening or painful. In animals, this behavioural inhibition may take the form of immobility or suppression of a behavioural response such as bar pressing to obtain food (see below). To develop new anxiolytic drugs, it is important to have animal tests that give a good guide to efficacy in humans, and much ingenuity has gone into developing and validating such tests.

For example, a rat placed in an unfamiliar environment normally responds by remaining immobile although alert (behavioural suppression) for a time, which may represent 'anxiety' produced by the strange environment. This immobility is reduced if anxiolytic drugs are administered. The 'elevated cross maze' is a widely used test model. Two arms of the raised horizontal cross are closed in, and the others are open. Normally, rats spend most of their time in the closed arms and avoid the open arms (afraid, possibly, of falling off). Administration of anxiolytic drugs increases the time spent in the open arms and also increases the activity of the rats as judged by the frequency of crossing the intersection.

Conflict tests can also be used. For example, a rat trained to press a bar repeatedly to obtain a food pellet normally achieves a high and consistent response rate. A conflict element is then introduced: at intervals, indicated by an auditory signal, bar pressing results in an occasional 'punishment' in the form of an electric shock in addition to the reward of a food pellet. Normally, the rat ceases pressing the bar (behavioural inhibition), and thus avoids the shock, while the signal is sounding. The effect of an anxiolytic drug is to relieve this suppressive effect, so that the rats continue bar pressing for reward despite the 'punishment'. Other types of psychotropic drug are not effective, nor are analgesic drugs. Other evidence confirms that anxiolytic drugs affect the level of behavioural inhibition produced by the 'conflict situation', rather than simply raising the pain threshold.

In other tests, aggressive behaviour is produced experimentally by lesions of the midbrain septum, or by housing mice in individual cages and then introducing a stranger. Anxiolytic drugs reduce the amount of aggressive behaviour displayed. They also increase the amount of 'social' interaction occurring between pairs of rats placed in an unfamiliar environment, this being a situation in which social interaction is greatly decreased in control animals. In many of these tests, the response is an increase in behavioural activity, so it is clear that the anxiolytic drugs are producing something more than a non-specific sedation.

TESTS ON HUMANS

▼ Various subjective 'anxiety scale' tests have been devised based on standard patient questionnaires. These have confirmed the efficacy of many anxiolytic drugs, but placebo treatment often also produces highly significant responses.

Other tests rely on measurement of the somatic and autonomic effects associated with anxiety. An example is the galvanic skin response, in which the electrical conductivity of the skin is used as a measure of sweat production. Any novel stimulus, whether pleasant or unpleasant, causes a response. This forms the basis of the lie detector test. If an innocuous stimulus is repeated at intervals, the magnitude of the response decreases (habituation). The rate of habituation is less in anxious patients than in normal subjects, and is increased by anxiolytic drugs.

A human version of the conflict test described above involves the substitution of money for food pellets, and the use of graded electric shocks as punishment. As with rats, administration of diazepam increases the rate of button pressing for money during the periods when the punishment was in operation, although the subjects reported no change in the painfulness of the electric shock. Subtler forms of torment and reward are not hard to imagine.

CLASSIFICATION OF ANXIOLYTIC AND HYPNOTIC DRUGS

The main groups of drugs (see review by Argyropoulos et al., 2000) are as follows.

- **Benzodiazepines.** This is the most important group, used as anxiolytic and hypnotic agents.
- **Buspirone.** This 5-HT$_{1A}$ receptor agonist is anxiolytic but not appreciably sedative.
- **β-Adrenoceptor antagonists** (e.g. **propranolol**; Ch. 11). These are used to treat some forms of anxiety, particularly where physical symptoms such as sweating, tremor and tachycardia are troublesome. Their effectiveness depends on block of peripheral sympathetic responses rather than on any central effects. They are sometimes used by actors and musicians to reduce the symptoms of stage fright, but their use by snooker players to minimise tremor is banned as unsportsmanlike.
- **Zolpidem.** This hypnotic acts similarly to benzodiazepines, although chemically distinct, but lacks appreciable anxiolytic activity.
- **Barbiturates.** These are now largely obsolete, superseded by benzodiazepines. Their use is now confined to anaesthesia (Ch. 36) and the treatment of epilepsy (Ch. 40).
- Miscellaneous other drugs (e.g. **chloral hydrate**, **meprobamate** and **methaqualone**). They are no longer recommended, but therapeutic habits die hard and they are occasionally used. Sedative antihistamines (see Ch. 13), such as **diphenhydramine**, are sometimes used as sleeping pills, particularly for wakeful children. They are included in various over-the-counter preparations intended to improve children's sleep patterns.

BENZODIAZEPINES

The first benzodiazepine, **chlordiazepoxide**, was synthesised by accident in 1961, the unusual seven-membered ring having been

---

Measurement of anxiolytic activity

- Behavioural tests in animals are based on measurements of the behavioural inhibition (considered to reflect 'anxiety') in response to conflict or novelty.
- Human tests for anxiolytic drugs employ psychiatric rating scales or measures of autonomic responses such as the galvanic skin response.
- Tests such as these can distinguish between anxiolytic drugs (benzodiazepines, buspirone, etc.) and sedatives (e.g. barbiturates).

produced as a result of a reaction that went wrong in the laboratories of Hoffman-la Roche. Its unexpected pharmacological activity was recognised in a routine screening procedure, and benzodiazepines quite soon became the most widely prescribed drugs in the pharmacopoeia.

CHEMISTRY AND STRUCTURE–ACTIVITY RELATIONSHIPS

The basic chemical structure of benzodiazepines consists of a seven-membered ring fused to an aromatic ring, with four main substituent groups that can be modified without loss of activity. Thousands of compounds have been made and tested, and about 20 are available for clinical use, the most important ones being listed in Table 37.1. They are basically similar in their pharmacological actions, although some degree of selectivity has been reported. For example, some, such as **clonazepam**, show anticonvulsant activity with less marked sedative effects. From a clinical point of view, differences in pharmacokinetic behaviour among different benzodiazepines (see below) are more important than differences in profile of activity. Drugs with a similar structure have been discovered that specifically antagonise the effects of the benzodiazepines, for example flumazenil (see below).

MECHANISM OF ACTION

Benzodiazepines (once thought to be acting as 'non-specific depressants') act selectively on GABA$_A$ receptors (Ch. 33),

Table 37.1 Characteristics of benzodiazepines in humans

Drug(s)	Half-life of parent compound (h)	Active metabolite	Half-life of metabolite (h)	Overall duration of action	Main use(s)
Triazolam,[a] midazolam	2–4	Hydroxylated derivative	2	Ultrashort (< 6 h)	Hypnotic Midazolam used as intravenous anaesthetic
Zolpidem[b]	2	No	–	Ultrashort (~ 4 h)	Hypnotic
Lorazepam, oxazepam, temazepam, lormetazepam	8–12	No	–	Short (12–18 h)	Anxiolytic, hypnotic
Alprazolam	6–12	Hydroxylated derivative	6	Medium (24 h)	Anxiolytic, antidepressant
Nitrazepam	16–40	No	–	Medium	Hypnotic, anxiolytic
Diazepam, chlordiazepoxide	20–40	Nordazepam	60	Long (24–48 h)	Anxiolytic, muscle relaxant Diazepam used intravenously as anticonvulsant
Flurazepam	1	Desmethyl-flurazepam	60	Long	Anxiolytic
Clonazepam	50	No	–	Long	Anticonvulsant, anxiolytic (especially mania)

[a]Triazolam has been withdrawn from use in the UK on account of side effects.
[b]Zolpidem is not a benzodiazepine but acts at the same site. Zopiclone is similar.

which mediate fast inhibitory synaptic transmission throughout the central nervous system (CNS). Benzodiazepines enhance the response to GABA by facilitating the opening of GABA-activated chloride channels (Fig. 37.1). They bind specifically to a regulatory site of the receptor, distinct from the GABA-binding site, and act allosterically to increase the affinity of GABA for the receptor. Single-channel recordings show an increase in the frequency of channel opening by a given concentration of GABA, but no change in the conductance or mean open time, consistent with an effect on GABA binding rather than the channel-gating mechanism. Benzodiazepines do not affect receptors for other amino acids, such as glycine or glutamate (Fig. 37.1).

▼ The GABA$_A$ receptor is a ligand-gated ion channel (see Ch. 3) consisting of a pentameric assembly of different subunits, the main ones being α, β and γ, each of which occurs in three or more isoforms. The potential number of combinations is therefore huge, but three combinations predominate in the adult brain, namely $\alpha_1\beta_2\gamma_2$, $\alpha_2\beta_3\gamma_2$ and $\alpha_3\beta_3\gamma_2$. The various combinations occur in different parts of the brain, and linking this diversity with physiological function and pharmacological specificity presents a difficult, although familiar, problem (see Whiting, 2003). Progress has recently been made, however, in understanding the effects of benzodiazepines at the molecular level (see Rudolph et al., 2001; Rudolph & Möhler, 2004), which may point the way to novel drugs with more specific actions. Sensitivity to benzodiazepines requires the presence of both α and β subunits, and mutation of a single amino acid (histidine 101) in the α subunit eliminates benzodiazepine sensitivity. This has been used in an ingenious series of experiments on transgenic mice in which this residue has been mutated in different α subunits. The animals were then tested to determine which benzodiazepine effects were

eliminated in these different mutants, with the interesting result that mutation of the most widely expressed variant eliminated the sedative and amnesia-producing actions of benzodiazepines, as well as diminishing the anticonvulsant effect, whereas mutation of α_2 (expressed mainly in the limbic system) eliminated the anxiolytic effect but left the sedative effect unaltered. The conclusions from this kind of study suggest that GABA$_A$ receptors containing the α_1 subunit account for sedative, amnesic and anticonvulsant effects of benzodiazepines, whereas those containing the α_2 subunit account for the anxiolytic and muscle relaxant effects. This suggests the possibility of developing novel drugs with more selective effects than existing benzodiazepines, which are non-selective with respect to different α subunits (see Whiting, 2003). To this end, an experimental α_1-selective benzodiazepine, L 838417, has been discovered, which has anxiolytic but not sedative actions in laboratory animals, as predicted from the transgenic animal data. Whether or not this will hold true in humans remains to be seen.

Peripheral benzodiazepine-binding sites, not associated with GABA receptors, are known to exist in many tissues, but their function and pharmacological significance are unknown.

PHARMACOLOGICAL EFFECTS AND USES

The main effects of benzodiazepines are:

- reduction of anxiety and aggression
- sedation and induction of sleep
- reduction of muscle tone and coordination
- anticonvulsant effect
- anterograde amnesia.

Reduction of anxiety and aggression

Benzodiazepines show anxiolytic effects in animal tests, as described above, and also exert a marked 'taming' effect, allowing animals to be handled more easily.[1] If given to the dominant member of a pair of animals (e.g. mice or monkeys) housed in the same cage, benzodiazepines reduce the number of attacks by the dominant individual and increase the number of attacks made on him. With the possible exception of **alprazolam** (Table 37.1), benzodiazepines do not have antidepressant effects. Benzodiazepines may paradoxically produce an increase in irritability and aggression in some individuals. This appears to be particularly pronounced with the ultrashort-acting drug **triazolam** (and led to its withdrawal in the UK and some other countries), and is generally more common with short-acting compounds. It is probably a manifestation of the benzodiazepine withdrawal syndrome, which occurs with all these drugs (see below) but is more acute with drugs whose action wears off rapidly.

Benzodiazepines are used mainly for treating acute anxiety states, but their use is declining in favour of antidepressants (Ch. 39), coupled with behavioural therapies in more severe cases.

The use of benzodiazepines as anxiolytic agents is reviewed by Shader & Greenblatt (1993).

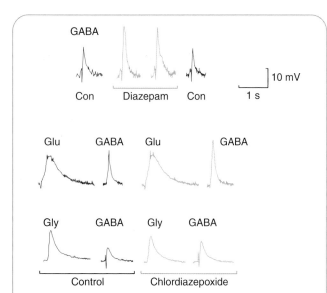

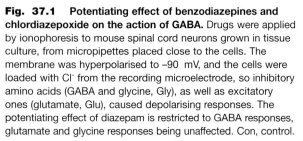

Fig. 37.1 Potentiating effect of benzodiazepines and chlordiazepoxide on the action of GABA. Drugs were applied by ionophoresis to mouse spinal cord neurons grown in tissue culture, from micropipettes placed close to the cells. The membrane was hyperpolarised to −90 mV, and the cells were loaded with Cl⁻ from the recording microelectrode, so inhibitory amino acids (GABA and glycine, Gly), as well as excitatory ones (glutamate, Glu), caused depolarising responses. The potentiating effect of diazepam is restricted to GABA responses, glutamate and glycine responses being unaffected. Con, control.

[1]This depends on the species. Cats actually become more excitable, as a colleague of one of the authors discovered to his cost when attempting to sedate a tiger in the Baltimore zoo.

Sedation and induction of sleep

Benzodiazepines decrease the time taken to get to sleep, and increase the total duration of sleep, although the latter effect occurs only in subjects who normally sleep for less than about 6 hours each night. Both effects tend to decline when benzodiazepines are taken regularly for 1–2 weeks.

On the basis of electroencephalography measurements, several levels of sleep can be recognised. Of particular psychological importance are rapid eye movement (REM) sleep, which is associated with dreaming, and slow-wave sleep, which corresponds to the deepest level of sleep when the metabolic rate and adrenal steroid secretion are at their lowest and the secretion of growth hormone is at its highest (see Ch. 28). Most hypnotic drugs reduce the proportion of REM sleep, although benzodiazepines affect it less than other hypnotics, and zolpidem (see below) least of all. Artificial interruption of REM sleep causes irritability and anxiety, even if the total amount of sleep is not reduced, and the lost REM sleep is made up for at the end of such an experiment by a rebound increase. The same rebound in REM sleep is seen at the end of a period of administration of benzodiazepines or other hypnotics. It is therefore assumed that REM sleep has a function, and that the relatively slight reduction of REM sleep by benzodiazepines is a point in their favour.

The proportion of slow-wave sleep is significantly reduced by benzodiazepines, although growth hormone secretion is unaffected.

Figure 37.2 shows the improvement of subjective ratings of sleep quality produced by a benzodiazepine, and the rebound decrease at the end of a 32-week period of drug treatment. It is notable that, although tolerance to objective effects such as reduced sleep latency occurs within a few days, this is not obvious in the subjective ratings.

Although long-term use of benzodiazepines as sleeping pills is undesirable, owing to tolerance, dependence and 'hangover' effects, occasional use (e.g. by shift workers, plane travellers, etc.) is effective.

Reduction of muscle tone and coordination

Benzodiazepines reduce muscle tone by a central action that is independent of their sedative effect. Cats are particularly sensitive to this action, and some benzodiazepines (e.g. **clonazepam, flunitrazepam**) reduce decerebrate rigidity in doses that are much smaller than those needed to produce behavioural effects. In other species, the difference is less clear. Coordination can be tested by measuring the length of time for which mice can stay on a slowly rotating horizontal plastic rod, or the time taken for them to escape from confinement by climbing up the inside of a tubular chimney. Performance in these acrobatic tricks is impaired by benzodiazepines and other sedatives, but it is not clear that particular drugs show selectivity in this respect in species other than the cat. Studies in humans have failed to show differences between benzodiazepines.

Increased muscle tone is a common feature of anxiety states in humans and may contribute to the aches and pains, including headache, which often trouble anxious patients. The relaxant effect of benzodiazepines may therefore be clinically useful. A reduction of muscle tone appears to be possible without

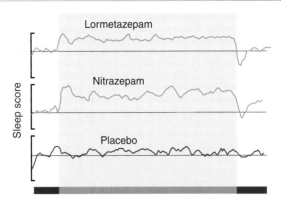

Fig. 37.2   Effects of long-term benzodiazepine treatment on sleep quality. A group of 100 poor sleepers were given, under double-blind conditions, lormetazepam 5 mg, nitrazepam 2 mg or placebo nightly for 24 weeks, the test period being preceded and followed by 4 weeks of placebo treatment. They were asked to assess, on a subjective rating scale, the quality of sleep during each night, and the results are expressed as a 5-day rolling average of these scores. The improvement in sleep quality was maintained during the 24-week test period, and was followed by a 'rebound' worsening of sleep when the test period ended. (From Oswald I et al. 1982 Br Med J 284: 860–864.)

appreciable loss of coordination. Other clinical uses of muscle relaxants are discussed in Chapter 40.

Anticonvulsant effects

All the benzodiazepines have anticonvulsant activity in experimental animal tests. They are highly effective against chemically induced convulsions caused by **pentylenetetrazol**, **bicuculline** and similar drugs (see Chs 40 and 42) but less so against electrically induced convulsions. Benzodiazepines do not affect strychnine-induced convulsions in experimental animals. This is because strychnine causes convulsions by blocking inhibitory glycine receptors (see Ch. 42), whereas bicuculline and several other chemical convulsant agents act on $GABA_A$ receptors (Ch. 30). Benzodiazepines enhance the action of GABA but not glycine, so the selectivity of their anticonvulsant action is explicable. **Clonazepam** (see above), because of its selective anticonvulsant action, is used to treat epilepsy (Ch. 40), as is **diazepam**, which is given intravenously to control life-threatening seizures in status epilepticus.

Anterograde amnesia

Benzodiazepines obliterate memory of events experienced while under their influence, an effect not seen with other CNS depressants. Minor surgical procedures can thus be performed without leaving unpleasant memories.

IS THERE AN ENDOGENOUS BENZODIAZEPINE-LIKE MEDIATOR?

▼ Whether there are endogenous ligands for the benzodiazepine receptors, whose function is to regulate the action of GABA, is still uncertain. The main candidate is a 10-kDa peptide, diazepam-binding inhibitor, isolated from rat brain. This peptide binds strongly to the benzodiazepine-binding site of the GABA$_A$ receptor, and has the opposite effect to benzodiazepines, i.e. it inhibits chloride channel opening by GABA, and when injected into the brain has an anxiogenic and proconvulsant effect. Other possible endogenous modulators of GABA$_A$ receptors include steroid metabolites (see Ch. 33). There is also evidence that benzodiazepines themselves may occur naturally in the brain. At present, there is no general agreement on the identity and function of endogenous ligands.

BENZODIAZEPINE INVERSE AGONISTS AND ANTAGONISTS

▼ The term *inverse agonist* (Ch. 2) is applied to drugs that bind to benzodiazepine receptors and exert the opposite effect to that of conventional benzodiazepines, producing signs of increased anxiety and convulsions. Diazepam-binding inhibitor is an example, and some benzodiazepine analogues act similarly. It is possible (see Fig. 37.3) to explain these complexities in terms of the two-state model discussed in Chapter 2, by postulating that the benzodiazepine receptor exists in two distinct conformations, only one of which (A) can bind a GABA molecule and open the chloride channel. The other conformation (B) cannot bind GABA. Normally, with no benzodiazepine receptor ligand present, there is an equilibrium between these two conformations; sensitivity to GABA is present but submaximal. Benzodiazepine agonists (e.g. diazepam) are postulated to bind preferentially to conformation A, thus shifting the equilibrium in favour of A and enhancing GABA sensitivity. Inverse agonists bind selectively to B and have the opposite effect. Competitive antagonists such as **flumazenil** (see below) bind equally to A and B, and consequently do not disturb the conformational equilibrium but antagonise the effect of both agonists and inverse agonists. Some of the molecular variants of the GABA$_A$ receptor (see above) seem to show different relative affinities for agonists, antagonists and inverse agonists, and it is possible that this reflects differences in the equilibrium between the A and B states as a function of the subunit composition of the receptor.

PHARMACOKINETIC ASPECTS

Benzodiazepines are well absorbed when given orally, usually giving a peak plasma concentration in about 1 hour. Some (e.g. **oxazepam**, **lorazepam**) are absorbed more slowly. They bind strongly to plasma protein, and their high lipid solubility causes many of them to accumulate gradually in body fat. They are normally given by mouth but can be given intravenously (e.g. **diazepam** in status epilepticus, **midazolam** in anaesthesia). Intramuscular injection often results in slow absorption.

Benzodiazepines are all metabolised and eventually excreted as glucuronide conjugates in the urine. They vary greatly in duration of action and can be roughly divided into short-, medium- and long-acting compounds (Table 37.1). Several are converted to active metabolites such as *N*-desmethyldiazepam (nordazepam), which has a half-life of about 60 hours, and which accounts for the tendency of many benzodiazepines to produce cumulative effects and long hangovers when they are given repeatedly. The short-acting compounds are those that are metabolised directly by conjugation with glucuronide. The main pathways are shown in Figure 37.4. Figure 37.5 shows the gradual build-up and slow disappearance of nordazepam from the plasma of a human subject given diazepam daily for 15 days.

▼ Advancing age affects the rate of oxidative reactions more than that of conjugation reactions. Thus the effect of the long-acting

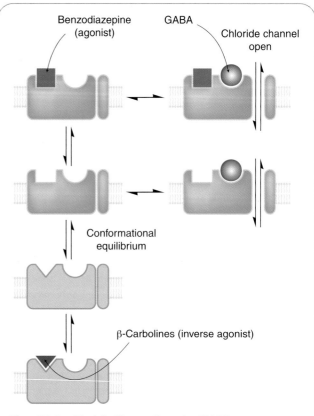

Fig. 37.3 **Model of benzodiazepine/GABA receptor interaction.** Benzodiazepine agonists (e.g. diazepam) and antagonists (e.g. flumazenil) are believed to bind to a site on the GABA receptor distinct from the GABA-binding site. A conformational equilibrium exists between states in which the benzodiazepine receptor exists in its agonist-binding conformation (above), and in its antagonist-binding conformation (below). In the latter state, the GABA receptor has a much reduced affinity for GABA; consequently, the chloride channel remains closed.

benzodiazepines, which may be used regularly as hypnotics or anxiolytic agents for many years, tends to increase with age, and it is common for drowsiness and confusion to develop insidiously for this reason.[2]

UNWANTED EFFECTS

These may be divided into:

- toxic effects resulting from acute overdosage
- unwanted effects occurring during normal therapeutic use
- tolerance and dependence.

---

[2]At the age of 91, the grandmother of one of the authors was growing increasingly forgetful and mildly dotty, having been taking nitrazepam for insomnia regularly for years. To the author's lasting shame, it took a canny general practitioner to diagnose the problem. Cancellation of the nitrazepam prescription produced a dramatic improvement.

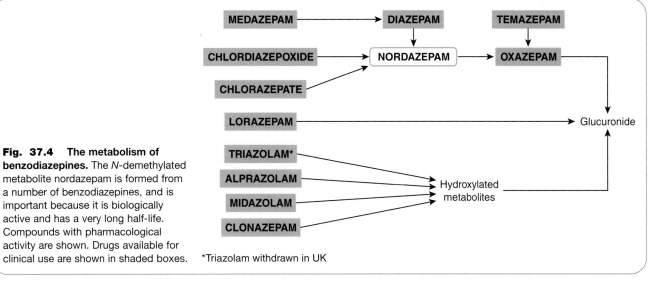

Fig. 37.4 The metabolism of benzodiazepines. The *N*-demethylated metabolite nordazepam is formed from a number of benzodiazepines, and is important because it is biologically active and has a very long half-life. Compounds with pharmacological activity are shown. Drugs available for clinical use are shown in shaded boxes.

*Triazolam withdrawn in UK

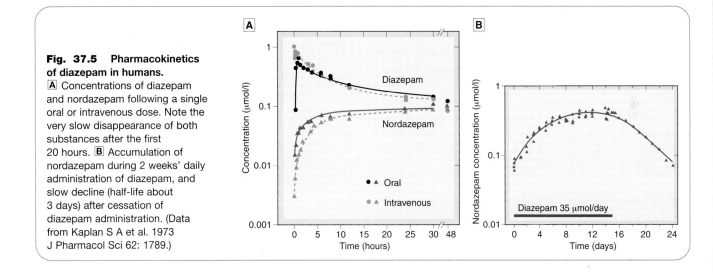

Fig. 37.5 Pharmacokinetics of diazepam in humans.
A Concentrations of diazepam and nordazepam following a single oral or intravenous dose. Note the very slow disappearance of both substances after the first 20 hours. **B** Accumulation of nordazepam during 2 weeks' daily administration of diazepam, and slow decline (half-life about 3 days) after cessation of diazepam administration. (Data from Kaplan S A et al. 1973 J Pharmacol Sci 62: 1789.)

Acute toxicity

Benzodiazepines in acute overdose are considerably less dangerous than other anxiolytic/hypnotic drugs. Because such agents are often used in attempted suicide, this is an important advantage. In overdose, benzodiazepines cause prolonged sleep, without serious depression of respiration or cardiovascular function. However, in the presence of other CNS depressants, particularly alcohol, benzodiazepines can cause severe, even life-threatening, respiratory depression. The availability of an effective antagonist, **flumazenil**, means that the effects of an acute overdose can be counteracted,[3] which is not possible for most CNS depressants.

Side effects during therapeutic use

The main side effects of benzodiazepines are drowsiness, confusion, amnesia and impaired coordination, which considerably affects manual skills such as driving performance. Benzodiazepines enhance the depressant effect of other drugs, including alcohol, in a more than additive way. The long and unpredictable duration of action of many benzodiazepines is important in relation to side effects. Long-acting drugs such as nitrazepam are no longer used as hypnotics, and even shorter-acting compounds such as lorazepam can produce a substantial day-after impairment of job performance and driving skill.

Tolerance and dependence

Tolerance (i.e. a gradual escalation of dose needed to produce the required effect) occurs with all benzodiazepines, as does *dependence*, which is their main drawback. They share these properties with other hypnotics and sedatives. Tolerance is less marked than it is with barbiturates, which produce pharmacokinetic tolerance because of induction of hepatic drug-metabolising

---

[3]In practice, patients are usually left to sleep it off, because there is a risk of seizures with flumazenil; however, flumazenil may be useful diagnostically to rule out coma of other causes.

enzymes (Ch. 8)–this does not occur with benzodiazepines. Such tolerance as does occur appears to represent a change at the receptor level, but the mechanism is not well understood.

The sleep-inducing effect shows relatively little tolerance (Fig. 37.2). In a study with intravenous diazepam given to normal subjects, its euphoric effect was not present in those taking oral diazepam daily. It is not clear whether tolerance to the anxiolytic effect is significant.

Benzodiazepines produce dependence, and this is a major problem. In human subjects and patients, stopping benzodiazepine treatment after weeks or months causes an increase in symptoms of anxiety, together with tremor and dizziness. Although animals show only a weak tendency to self-administration of benzodiazepines, withdrawal after chronic administration causes physical symptoms similar to those that follow opiate withdrawal (see Ch. 43), namely nervousness, tremor, loss of appetite and sometimes convulsions.[4] The withdrawal syndrome, in both animals and humans, is slower in onset than with barbiturates, probably because of the long plasma half-life of most benzodiazepines. Short-acting benzodiazepines cause more abrupt withdrawal effects. With **triazolam**, a very short-acting drug and no longer in use, the withdrawal effect occurred within a few hours, even after a single dose, producing early-morning insomnia and daytime anxiety when the drug was used as a hypnotic.

The physical and psychological withdrawal symptoms make it difficult for patients to give up taking benzodiazepines, but *addiction* (i.e. severe psychological dependence that outlasts the physical withdrawal syndrome), which occurs with many drugs of abuse (Ch. 43), is not a major problem.

BENZODIAZEPINE ANTAGONISTS

Competitive antagonists of benzodiazepines were first discovered in 1981. The best-known compound is **flumazenil**. This compound was originally reported to lack effects on behaviour or on drug-induced convulsions when given on its own, although it was later found to possess some 'anxiogenic' and pro-convulsant activity. Flumazenil can be used to reverse the effect of benzodiazepine overdosage (normally used only if respiration is severely depressed), or to reverse the effect of benzodiazepines such as **midazolam** used for minor surgical procedures. Flumazenil acts quickly and effectively when given by injection, but its action lasts for only about 2 hours, so drowsiness tends to return. It is often used in treating comatose patients suspected of having overdosed with benzodiazepines even before the diagnosis is confirmed on the basis of a blood sample. Convulsions may rarely occur in patients treated with

> **Benzodiazepines**
>
> - Act by binding to a specific regulatory site on the $GABA_A$ receptor, thus enhancing the inhibitory effect of GABA. Subtypes of the $GABA_A$ receptor exist in different regions of the brain and differ in their functional effects.
> - Anxiolytic benzodiazepines are agonists at this regulatory site. Other benzodiazepines (e.g. flumazenil) are antagonists and prevent the actions of the anxiolytic benzodiazepines. A further class of inverse agonists is recognised, which reduce the effectiveness of GABA and are anxiogenic; they are not used clinically.
> - Anxiolytic effects are mediated by $GABA_A$ receptors containing the α_2 subunit, while sedation occurs through those with the α_1 subunit.
> - Endogenous ligands for the benzodiazepine-binding site are believed to exist. They include peptide and steroid molecules, but their physiological function is not yet understood.
> - Benzodiazepines cause:
>   - reduction of anxiety and aggression
>   - sedation, leading to improvement of insomnia
>   - muscle relaxation and loss of motor coordination
>   - suppression of convulsions (antiepileptic effect)
>   - anterograde amnesia.
> - Differences in the pharmacological profile of different benzodiazepines are minor; clonazepam appears to have more anticonvulsant action in relation to its other effects.
> - Benzodiazepines are active orally and differ mainly in respect of their duration of action. Short-acting agents (e.g. lorazepam and temazepam, half-lives 8–12 hours) are metabolised to inactive compounds and are used mainly as sleeping pills. Some long-acting agents (e.g. diazepam and chlordiazepoxide) are converted to a long-lasting active metabolite (nordazepam).
> - Some are used intravenously, for example diazepam in status epilepticus, midazolam in anaesthesia.
> - Zolpidem is a short-acting drug that is not a benzodiazepine but acts similarly and is used as a hypnotic.
> - Benzodiazepines are relatively safe in overdose. Their main disadvantages are interaction with alcohol, long-lasting 'hangover' effects, withdrawal symptoms and the development of dependence.

---

[4]Withdrawal symptoms can be more severe. A relative of one of the authors, advised to stop taking benzodiazepines after 20 years, suffered hallucinations and one day tore down all the curtains, convinced that they were on fire.

flumazenil, and this is more common in patients receiving tricyclic antidepressants (Ch. 39). Reports that flumazenil improves the mental state of patients with severe liver disease (hepatic encephalopathy) and alcohol intoxication have not been confirmed in controlled trials.

BUSPIRONE

Buspirone is a partial agonist at 5-HT$_{1A}$ receptors (Ch. 12) and is used to treat various anxiety disorders. It also binds to dopamine receptors, but it is likely that its 5-HT-related actions are important in relation to anxiety suppression, because related compounds (e.g. **ipsapirone** and **gepirone**, neither of which are approved for clinical use, which are highly specific for 5-HT$_{1A}$ receptors; see Traber & Glaser, 1987) show similar anxiolytic activity in experimental animals. 5-HT$_{1A}$ receptors are inhibitory autoreceptors that reduce the release of 5-HT and other mediators. They also inhibit the activity of noradrenergic locus coeruleus neurons (Ch. 34) and thus interfere with arousal reactions. However, buspirone takes days or weeks to produce its effect in humans, suggesting a more complex indirect mechanism of action. Buspirone is ineffective in controlling panic attacks or severe anxiety states.

Buspirone has side effects quite different from those of benzodiazepines. It does not cause sedation or motor incoordination, nor have withdrawal effects been reported. Its main side effects are nausea, dizziness, headache and restlessness, which generally seem to be less troublesome than the side effects of benzodiazepines.

BARBITURATES

The sleep-inducing properties of barbiturates were discovered early in the 20th century, and hundreds of compounds were made and tested. Until the 1960s, they formed the largest group of hypnotics and sedatives in clinical use. Barbiturates all have depressant activity on the CNS, producing effects similar to those of inhalation anaesthetics. They cause death from respiratory and cardiovascular depression if given in large doses, which is one of the main reasons that they are now little used as anxiolytic and hypnotic agents. **Pentobarbital** and similar typical barbiturates with durations of action of 6–12 hours are still very occasionally used as sleeping pills and anxiolytic drugs, but they are less safe than benzodiazepines. Pentobarbital is often used as an anaesthetic for laboratory animals.

Barbiturates that remain in clinical use include **phenobarbital**, still occasionally used to treat epilepsy (see Ch. 40), and **thiopental**, which is widely used as an intravenous anaesthetic agent (see Ch. 36).

Barbiturates share with benzodiazepines the ability to enhance the action of GABA, but they bind to a different site on the GABA$_A$ receptor/chloride channel, and their action is less specific.

As well as being dangerous in overdose, barbiturates induce a high degree of tolerance and dependence. They also strongly induce the synthesis of hepatic cytochrome P450 and conjugating enzymes, and thus increase the rate of metabolic degradation of many other drugs, giving rise to a number of potentially troublesome drug interactions (Ch. 52). Because of enzyme induction, barbiturates are also dangerous to patients suffering from the metabolic disease porphyria.

OTHER POTENTIAL ANXIOLYTIC DRUGS

Selective serotonin reuptake inhibitors (see Ch. 39) such as **fluoxetine**, **paroxetine** and **sertraline** are used to treat certain anxiety disorders, including obsessive compulsive disorder and panic. Their action in this context appears to be independent of their antidepressant effects.

▼ Besides the GABA$_A$ and 5-HT$_{1A}$ receptor mechanisms discussed above, many other transmitters and receptors have been implicated in anxiety and panic disorders (see Sandford et al., 2000), particularly noradrenaline, and neuropeptides such as cholecystokinin (CCK) and substance P. Anxiolytic drugs aimed at these targets are in development, but none are so far available for clinical use. Various drugs that enhance the effects of GABA, developed primarily as antiepileptic drugs (see Ch. 40), may also be effective in treating anxiety disorders (see Nemeroff, 2003). They include **gabapentin**, **vigabatrin**, **tiagabine** and **valproate**.

5-HT$_3$ receptor antagonists such as **ondansetron** (Ch. 12) show anxiolytic activity in animal models but have not proved efficacious in controlled human trials. As mentioned earlier, 5-HT uptake inhibitors, such as **fluoxetine**, and mixed 5-HT/noradrenaline uptake inhibitors, which are used as antidepressant drugs (Ch. 39), also show efficacy in anxiety disorders.

> **5-HT$_{1A}$ agonists as anxiolytic drugs**
>
> - Buspirone is a potent (although non-selective) agonist at 5-HT$_{1A}$ receptors.
> - Anxiolytic effects take days or weeks to develop.
> - Side effects appear less troublesome than with benzodiazepines; they include dizziness, nausea, headache, but not sedation or loss of coordination.

> **Barbiturates**
>
> - Non-selective central nervous system depressants that produce effects ranging from sedation and reduction of anxiety to unconsciousness and death from respiratory and cardiovascular failure—therefore dangerous in overdose.
> - Act partly by enhancing action of GABA, but less specific than benzodiazepines.
> - Mainly used in anaesthesia and treatment of epilepsy; use as sedative/hypnotic agents is no longer recommended.
> - Potent inducers of hepatic drug-metabolising enzymes, especially cytochrome P450 system, so liable to cause drug interactions. Also precipitate attacks of acute porphyria in susceptible individuals.
> - Tolerance and dependence occur.

Antagonists of the neuropeptide CCK (see Ch. 16) have been tested as anxiolytic drugs. CCK, which is expressed in many areas of the brain stem and midbrain that are involved in arousal, mood and emotion, has been considered as a possible mediator of panic attacks, but non-peptide CCK antagonists have proved ineffective in clinical trials.

Clinical use of drugs as anxiolytics

- Many anxiolytic drugs (e.g. *benzodiazepines*) are also hypnotic. These should be used only for short-term (< 4 weeks) relief of severe and disabling anxiety.
- **Buspirone** (5-HT$_{1A}$ agonist; p. 544) has a different pattern of adverse effects from benzodiazepines and much lower abuse potential. Its effect is slow in onset (> 2 weeks).

Clinical use of hypnotics ('sleeping tablets')

- The cause of insomnia should be established before administering hypnotic drugs. Common causes include alcohol or other drug misuse (see Ch. 43) and physical or psychiatric disorder (especially depression).
- *Tricyclic antidepressants* (Ch. 39) cause drowsiness, so can kill two birds with one stone if taken at night by depressed patients with sleep disturbance.
- Optimal treatment of chronic insomnia is often by changing behaviour (e.g. increasing exercise, staying awake during the day) rather than with drugs.
- Most hypnotics act on specific modulatory sites on GABA$_A$ receptors (Ch. 33, Fig. 33.4) and cause dependence; they should be used only for short periods (< 4 weeks) and for severe insomnia. They can be useful for a few nights when transient factors such as admission to hospital, jet lag or an impending procedure cause insomnia.
- Hypnotic drugs include:
  - benzodiazepines (e.g. **temazepam, nitrazepam**) and related drugs (e.g. **zolpidem, zopiclone**, which also work on the benzodiazepine receptor)
  - **chloral** and **triclofos**, which were used formerly in children, but this is seldom justified
  - sedating antihistamines (e.g. **promethazine**), which cause drowsiness (see Ch. 14, and clinical box on p. 236) and are on general sale for occasional insomnia. They can impair performance the day after they are used.

REFERENCES AND FURTHER READING

Argyropoulos S V, Sandford J J, Nutt D J 2000 The psychobiology of anxiolytic drugs. Part 2: pharmacological treatments of anxiety. Pharmacol Ther 88: 213–227 (*General review article on clinically used anxiolytic drugs*)

Nemeroff C B 2003 The role of GABA in the pathophysiology and treatment of anxiety disorders. Psychopharmacol Bull 37: 133–146 (*Review article discussing the potential of various GABA-enhancing drugs as anxiolytics*)

Rudolph U, Crestani F, Möhler H 2001 GABA$_A$ receptor subtypes: dissecting their pharmacological functions.

Trends Pharmacol Sci 22: 188–194 (*Describes recent work with transgenic mice expressing mutated GABA$_A$ receptors, suggesting that anxiolytic and sedative actions of benzodiazepines may be separable*)

Rudolph U, Möhler H 2004 Analysis of GABA$_A$ receptor function and dissection of the pharmacology of benzodiazepines and general anaesthetics through mouse genetics. Annu Rev Pharmacol Toxicol 44: 475–498 (*Detailed review of extensive data relating to GABA$_A$ receptor mutations in transgenic mice*)

Sandford J J, Argyropoulos S V, Nutt D J 2000 The psychobiology of anxiolytic drugs. Part 1: basic

neurobiology. Pharmacol Ther 88: 197–212 (*Explains brain mechanisms thought to underlie actions of anxiolytic drugs*)

Shader R I, Greenblatt D J 1993 Use of benzodiazepines in anxiety disorders. New Engl J Med 328: 1398–1405

Traber J, Glaser T 1987 5-HT$_{1A}$ receptor-related anxiolytics. Trends Pharmacol Sci 8: 432–437

Whiting P 2003 GABA-A receptor subtypes in the brain: a paradigm for CNS drug discovery? Drug Discov Today 8: 445–450 (*Useful summary of the extensive data relating to GABA$_A$ receptor subtypes in relation to benzodiazepine and anaesthetic pharmacology*)

Antipsychotic drugs

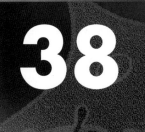

38

OVERVIEW

In this chapter, we focus on schizophrenia and the drugs used to treat it. We start by describing the illness and what is known of its pathogenesis, including the various neurochemical hypotheses and their relation to the actions of the main types of antipsychotic drugs that are in use or in development.

Psychotic illnesses include various disorders, but the term *antipsychotic drugs*—previously known as neuroleptic drugs, antischizophrenic drugs or major tranquillisers—conventionally refers to those used to treat schizophrenia, one of the most common and debilitating forms of mental illness. Pharmacologically, they are characterised as dopamine receptor antagonists, although many of them also act on other targets, particularly 5-hydroxytryptamine (5-HT) receptors, which may contribute to their clinical efficacy. Existing drugs have many drawbacks in terms of their efficacy and side effects. Gradual improvements are being achieved as new drugs are developed, but radical new approaches will probably have to wait until we have a better understanding of the biological nature of the disease, which is still poorly understood.[1]

THE NATURE OF SCHIZOPHRENIA

Schizophrenia (see Lewis & Lieberman, 2000) affects about 1% of the population. It is one of the most important forms of psychiatric illness, because it affects young people, is often chronic and is usually highly disabling. There is a strong hereditary factor in its aetiology, and evidence suggestive of a fundamental biological disorder (see below). The main clinical features of the disease are as follow.

- **Positive symptoms:**
  —delusions (often paranoid in nature)
  —hallucinations, usually in the form of voices which are often exhortatory in their message
  —thought disorder, comprising wild trains of thought, garbled sentences and irrational conclusions, sometimes associated with the feeling that thoughts are inserted or withdrawn by an outside agency
  —abnormal behaviours, such as stereotyped movements and occasionally aggressive behaviours.

- **Negative symptoms:**
  —withdrawal from social contacts
  —flattening of emotional responses.

In addition, deficits in cognitive function (e.g. attention, memory) are often present,[2] together with anxiety and depression, leading to suicide in about 10% of cases. The clinical phenotype varies greatly, particularly with respect to the balance between negative and positive symptoms, and this may have a bearing on the

---

[1]In this respect, the study of schizophrenia lags some years behind that of Alzheimer's disease (Ch. 35), where understanding of the pathogenesis has progressed rapidly to the point where promising new drug targets can be identified. On the other hand, pragmatists can argue that drugs against Alzheimer's disease are so far only marginally effective, whereas current antipsychotic drugs deliver great benefits, even though we do not quite know how they work.

[2]Kraepelin, who first described the condition, used the term *dementia praecox* (premature dementia) to describe the cognitive impairment associated with schizophrenia.

545

efficacy of antipsychotic drugs in individual cases. Schizophrenia can present dramatically, usually in young people, with predominantly positive features such as hallucinations, delusions and uncontrollable behaviour, or more insidiously in older patients with negative features such as flat mood and social withdrawal. The latter may be more debilitated than those with a florid presentation, and the prognosis is generally worse.

▼ A characteristic feature of schizophrenia is a defect in 'selective attention'. Whereas a normal individual quickly accommodates to stimuli of a familiar or inconsequential nature, and responds only to stimuli that are unexpected or significant, the ability of schizophrenic patients to discriminate between significant and insignificant stimuli seems to be impaired. Thus, the ticking of a clock may command as much attention as the words of a companion; a chance thought, which a normal person would dismiss as inconsequential, may become an irresistible imperative. 'Latent inhibition' is a form of behavioural testing in animals, which can be used as a model for this type of sensory habituation. If a rat is exposed to a 'conditioned' stimulus (such as a bell), followed by an 'unconditioned' stimulus (e.g. a foot shock) that it can avoid (e.g. by pressing a bar), it will quickly learn to press the bar as soon as it hears the bell—the conditioned response. But if it has previously heard the bell several times without any ensuing foot shock, it will learn the conditioned response less quickly, having learned to disregard the bell. Latent inhibition is a measure of the inhibitory effect of pre-exposure to the conditioned stimulus on acquisition of the conditioned response. It is often impaired in schizophrenic subjects and in animals treated with amphetamine or psychotomimetic drugs such as lysergic acid diethylamide (LSD), and is restored by many antipsychotic drugs.

Schizophrenia can follow a relapsing and remitting course, or be chronic and progressive, particularly in cases with a later onset. Chronic schizophrenia used to account for most of the patients in long-stay psychiatric hospitals; following the closure of many of these in the UK, it now accounts for many of society's outcasts.

AETIOLOGY AND PATHOGENESIS OF SCHIZOPHRENIA

GENETIC AND ENVIRONMENTAL FACTORS

The cause of schizophrenia remains unclear but involves a combination of genetic and environmental factors (see Lewis & Lieberman, 2000). The disease shows a strong, but incomplete, hereditary tendency. In first-degree relatives, the risk is about 10%, but even in monozygotic twins, one of whom has schizophrenia, the probability of the other being affected is only about 50%, pointing towards the likely importance of environmental factors. Genetic linkage studies have identified a number of susceptibility genes (see Harrison & Owen, 2003), but it is clear that no single gene is responsible. There are significant associations between polymorphisms in individual genes and the likelihood of an individual developing schizophrenia, but many are quite weak, and there appears to be no single gene that has an overriding influence.

▼ The first, and most robust, association found was with the gene for *neuregulin-1*, a gene involved with synaptic development and plasticity, with effects on NMDA receptor expression. Transgenic mice that underexpress neuregulin-1 show a phenotype resembling human schizophrenia in certain respects. This discovery was followed by the identification of about eight other susceptibility genes, several of which were involved in one way or another with glutamate-mediated transmission. They include the gene for d-amino acid oxidase (DAAO),

the enzyme responsible for making D-serine, an allosteric modulator of NMDA receptors (see Ch. 33), and G72, an activator of DAAO. Among the other genes involved, some are thought to affect monoamine transmission. Apart from focusing attention on glutamate (see Moghaddam, 2003) and confirming the likely involvement of amines such as dopamine, genetic studies have not so far pointed to any specific neurochemical abnormality underlying the schizophrenic phenotype.

Some environmental influences early in development have been identified as possible predisposing factors, particularly maternal virus infections. This and other evidence suggests that schizophrenia is associated with a neurodevelopmental disorder affecting mainly the cerebral cortex and occurring in the first few months of prenatal development (see Harrison, 1997). This view is supported by brain-imaging studies showing cortical atrophy, with enlargement of the cerebral ventricles. These structural changes are present in schizophrenic patients presenting for the first time, and are probably not progressive, suggesting that they represent an early irreversible aberration in brain development rather than a gradual neurodegeneration. Studies of post-mortem schizophrenic brains show evidence of misplaced cortical neurons with abnormal morphology. It appears to be through a combination of such genetic and developmental factors with social and environmental factors that schizophrenia becomes manifest in particular individuals. One of the environmental factors now thought to play a significant role is consumption of cannabis (see Ch. 42).

NEUROCHEMICAL THEORIES

Current ideas about the neurochemical mechanisms in schizophrenia came mainly from analysing the effects of antipsychotic and propsychotic drugs—from pharmacology rather than from neurochemistry. Instead of neurochemical theory providing the basis for rational drug treatment, the opposite occurred: drugs found by chance to be effective have provided the main clues about the nature of the disorder. Indeed, an intensive search for neurochemical abnormalities in schizophrenia proved frustrating for many years, no biochemical markers being found either in post-mortem brain material or in other samples from living patients. More recently (see below), imaging studies have succeeded in detecting neurochemical abnormalities.

The main neurochemical theories centre on dopamine and glutamate, although other mediators, particularly 5-HT, are also receiving attention (see Mortimer, 2004).

Dopamine theory

The dopamine theory was proposed by Carlson—awarded a Nobel Prize in 2000—on the basis of indirect pharmacological evidence in humans and experimental animals. **Amphetamine** releases dopamine in the brain and can produce in humans a behavioural syndrome indistinguishable from an acute schizophrenic episode—very familiar to doctors who treat drug users. In animals, dopamine release causes a specific pattern of stereotyped behaviour that resembles the repetitive behaviours sometimes seen in schizophrenic patients. Potent D_2-receptor agonists (e.g. **apomorphine** and **bromocriptine**; Ch. 34) produce similar effects in animals, and these drugs, like amphetamine, exacerbate the symptoms of schizophrenic patients. Furthermore, dopamine antagonists and drugs that block neuronal dopamine storage (e.g. **reserpine**) are effective in controlling the positive symptoms of schizophrenia, and in preventing amphetamine-induced behavioural changes. There is a strong correlation between clinical antipsychotic potency and activity in blocking D_2-receptors (Fig. 38.1), and receptor-imaging studies have shown that clinical efficacy of antipsychotic drugs is consistently achieved when D_2-receptor occupancy reaches about 80%.[3]

▼ There is no consistent biochemical evidence for excessive dopamine synthesis or release in schizophrenia. Furthermore, the production of prolactin, which might be expected to be abnormally low if dopaminergic transmission was facilitated, is normal in schizophrenic patients. One difficulty in interpreting such studies is that nearly all schizophrenic patients are treated with drugs that are known to affect dopamine metabolism, whereas the non-schizophrenic control group are not. Even where it has been possible to allow for this factor, however, most findings have proved negative. The best evidence for increased dopamine release in schizophrenic patients comes from imaging studies (Laruelle et al., 1999). A radioligand imaging technique was used to measure binding of a specific antagonist (**raclopride**) to D_2-receptors in the striatum. Injection of amphetamine caused dopamine release and thus displacement of raclopride, measured as a reduction of the signal intensity. This reduction was greater by a factor of 2 or more in schizophrenic subjects compared with in control subjects, implying a greater amphetamine-induced release of dopamine. The effect was greatest in schizophrenic individuals during acute attacks, and absent during spontaneous remissions—clear evidence linking dopamine release to the symptomatology.

An increase in dopamine receptor density in schizophrenia has been reported in some studies, but not consistently, and the interpretation is complicated by the fact that antipsychotic drug treatment is known to increase dopamine receptor expression.

The D_4-receptor has also attracted attention on account of the high degree of genetic polymorphism that it shows in human subjects, and because some of the newer antipsychotic drugs (e.g. **clozapine**; see below) turn out to have a high affinity for this receptor subtype. Genetic studies have, however, failed to show any relationship between schizophrenia and D_4-receptor polymorphism. Moreover, a specific D_4-receptor antagonist proved ineffective in clinical trials.

Another variant of the dopamine hypothesis (see Abi-Dargham & Laruelle, 2005) suggests that schizophrenia reflects an imbalance between excessive activation of D_2-receptors in subcortical regions (causing positive symptoms) and deficient activation of cortical D_1-receptors (causing negative symptoms). It is fair to say that, although dopamine is undoubtedly involved, the details remain far from clear.

Glutamate theory

Another transmitter implicated in the pathophysiology of schizophrenia is—you will not be surprised to learn—glutamate (see Goff & Coyle, 2001; Moghaddam, 2003). NMDA receptor antagonists such as **phencyclidine**, **ketamine** and **dizocilpine** (Ch. 33) produce psychotic symptoms (e.g. hallucinations, thought disorder) in humans, and reduced glutamate concentrations and glutamate receptor densities have been reported in post-mortem schizophrenic brains—one of the few fairly consistent findings.

▼ Although schizophrenia is difficult to diagnose in a mouse, transgenic mice in which NMDA receptor expression is reduced (not abolished,

---

[3]There are, however, exceptions to this simple rule. Up to one-third of schizophrenic patients fail to respond even when D_2 receptor blockade exceeds 90%, and clozapine (see Table 38.1) can be effective at much lower levels of block.

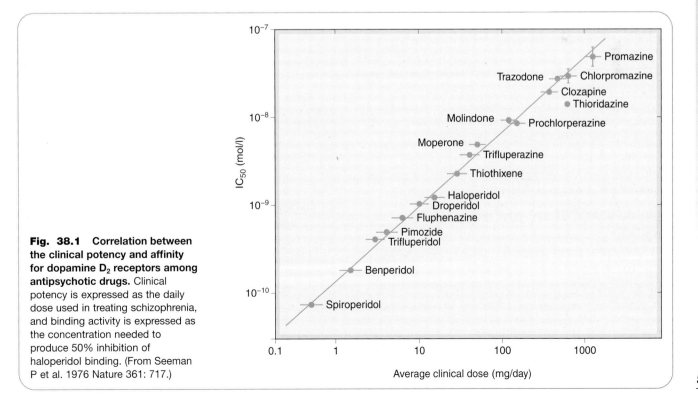

Fig. 38.1 Correlation between the clinical potency and affinity for dopamine D_2 receptors among antipsychotic drugs. Clinical potency is expressed as the daily dose used in treating schizophrenia, and binding activity is expressed as the concentration needed to produce 50% inhibition of haloperidol binding. (From Seeman P et al. 1976 Nature 361: 717.)

because this is fatal) show stereotypic behaviours and reduced social interaction that are suggestive of schizophrenia and that respond to antipsychotic drugs—evidence that supports the glutamate hypothesis. According to this view, glutamate and dopamine exert excitatory and inhibitory effects, respectively, on GABAergic striatal neurons, which project to the thalamus and constitute a sensory 'gate' (see below). Too little glutamate, or too much dopamine, disables the gate, allowing uninhibited sensory input to reach the cortex. It is also suggested that abnormal glutamate function—specifically reduced NMDA-receptor activation—could account for the cognitive deficit that is increasingly recognised as a central feature of schizophrenia, responsible in part for the negative symptoms of the disorder. One possibility is therefore that excess dopamine receptor activation is mainly responsible for positive symptoms, deficient NMDA-receptor activation for the negative symptoms. Although undoubtedly too simple, this idea is driving current efforts to develop novel antipsychotic drugs that increase NMDA-receptor activation.

Other theories

Other transmitters that may be important include 5-HT and noradrenaline (norepinephrine). The idea that 5-HT dysfunction could be involved in schizophrenia was based on the fact that LSD (see Ch. 42) produces schizophrenia-like symptoms, and has drifted in and out of favour many times (see Busatto & Kerwin, 1997).

Many effective antipsychotic drugs, in addition to blocking dopamine receptors (see below), also act as 5-HT-receptor antagonists. 5-HT modulates dopamine pathways, so the two theories are not incompatible. Many 'atypical' antipsychotic drugs (see below) produce fewer extrapyramidal side effects than dopamine-selective compounds, and combine with $5-HT_{2A}$-receptors. Whether $5-HT_{2A}$-receptor blockade accounts directly for their antipsychotic effects, or merely reduces undesirable side effects associated with D_2-receptor antagonists, remains controversial.

In conclusion, the dopamine hyperactivity theory of schizophrenia remains attractive. It is undoubtedly an oversimplification, and relates only to the positive symptoms, but it provides the best framework for understanding the action of antipsychotic drugs, although effects on 5-HT and other receptors may contribute significantly to the clinical profile of some of the newer drugs. The glutamate hypothesis is, however, gaining ground, and there are reasonable hopes that it will lead to the next generation of antipsychotic drugs (see Javitt, 2004).

ANTIPSYCHOTIC DRUGS

CLASSIFICATION OF ANTIPSYCHOTIC DRUGS

More than 20 different antipsychotic drugs are available for clinical use, but with certain exceptions the differences between them are minor.

A distinction is drawn between the drugs that were originally developed (e.g. **chlorpromazine**, **haloperidol** and many similar compounds), often referred to as *first-generation* or *typical* antipsychotic drugs, and more recently developed agents (e.g. **clozapine**, **risperidone**), which are termed *atypical* antipsychotic drugs. The term *atypical* is widely used but not clearly defined,

and experts argue endlessly about what it actually means (see Remington, 2003). Most often, it refers to the diminished tendency of the newer compounds to cause unwanted motor side effects (see below), but it is also used to describe compounds with a different pharmacological profile from first-generation compounds; several of these newer compounds improve the negative as well as the positive symptoms. In practice, however, it often serves—not very usefully—to distinguish the large group of similar first-generation dopamine antagonists from the more diverse group of newer compounds described below.

Table 38.1 summarises the main drugs that are in clinical use.

Table 38.1 Characteristics of antipsychotic drugs

Drug	Receptor affinity						Main side effects				Notes
	D_1	D_2	α adr	H_1	mACh	$5\text{-}HT_2$	EPS	Sed	Hypo	Other	
First generation											
Chlorpromazine	++	+++	+++	++	++	++	++	++	++	Increased prolactin (gynaecomastia) Hypothermia Anticholinergic effects Hypersensitivity reactions Obstructive jaundice	Phenothiazine class **Fluphenazine, trifluperazine** are similar but: • do not cause jaundice • cause less hypotension • cause more EPS Fluphenazine available as depot preparation
Thioridazine	+	++	+++	+	++	++	+	++	++	As chlorpromazine but does not cause jaundice	Phenothiazine class First drug with lower EPS tendency Withdrawn because of cardiac side effects
Haloperidol	+	+++	++	–	±	+	+++	–	++	As chlorpromazine but does not cause jaundice Fewer anticholinergic side effects	Butyrophenone class Widely used antipsychotic drug Strong EPS tendency
Flupentixol	++	+++	++	++	–	+++	++	+	+	Increased prolactin (gynaecomastia) Restlessness	**Clopentixol** is similar Available as depot preparations
Second generation (atypical)											
Sulpiride	–	+++	–	–	–	–	+	+	–	Increased prolactin (gynaecomastia)	Benzamide class Selective D_2/D_3 antagonist Less EPS than haloperidol Poorly absorbed **Amisulpride** and **pimozide** (long acting) are similar
Clozapine	++	++	++	++	++	+++	–	++	+	Risk of agranulocytosis (~1%): regular blood counts required Seizures Sedation Salivation Anticholinergic side effects Weight gain	Dibenzodiazepine class Potent antagonist at D_4-receptors No EPS Shows efficacy in 'treatment-resistant' patients Effective against negative and positive symptoms **Olanzapine** is similar, without risk of agranulocytosis, but questionable efficacy in treatment-resistant patients

Table 38.1 (cont'd) Characteristics of antipsychotic drugs

Drug	Receptor affinity						Main side effects				Notes
	D_1	D_2	α adr	H_1	mACh	$5\text{-}HT_2$	EPS	Sed	Hypo	Other	
Risperidone	–	++	++	++	++	+++	+	++	+	Weight gain EPS at high doses Hypotension	Significant risk of EPS ?Effective against negative symptoms Potent on D_4 receptors
Sertindole	–	++	++	–	–	+++	+	+	++	Ventricular arrhythmias (ECG checks advisable) Weight gain Nasal congestion	Long plasma half-life (~3 days) ?Effective against negative symptoms
Quetiapine	–	+	+++	–	+	+	+	++	++	Tachycardia Agitation Dry mouth Weight gain	Novel type acting mainly on α adrenoceptors Not yet fully evaluated
Aripiprazole	–	+++ (PA)	+	+	–	++	–	+	–	–	Recently approved drug Long acting (plasma half-life ~3 days) Unusual D_2 PA profile may account for paucity of side effects No effect on prolactin secretion No weight gain
Zotepine	++	++	+	+	+	+	–	+	–	Weight gain Hypotension Cardiac dysrhythmias	–

$5\text{-}HT_2$, 5-hydroxytryptamine type 2 receptor; adr, adrenoceptor; D_1, D_2, D_3, D_4, dopamine types 1, 2, 3 and 4 receptor, respectively; ECG, electrocardiograph; EPS, extrapyramidal side effects; H_1, histamine type 1 receptor; Hypo, hypotension; mACh, muscarinic acetylcholine receptor; PA, partial agonist; Sed, sedation.

GENERAL PROPERTIES OF ANTIPSYCHOTIC DRUGS

The therapeutic activity of the prototype drug, **chlorpromazine**, in schizophrenic patients was discovered through the acute observations of a French surgeon, Laborit, in 1947. He tested various substances, including **promethazine**, for their ability to alleviate signs of stress in patients undergoing surgery, and concluded that promethazine had a calming effect that was different from mere sedation. Elaboration of the phenothiazine structure led to chlorpromazine, the antipsychotic effect of which was demonstrated, at Laborit's instigation, by Delay and Deniker in 1953. This drug was unique in controlling the symptoms of psychotic patients without excessively sedating them. The clinical efficacy of phenothiazines was discovered long before their mechanism was guessed at (let alone understood).

Pharmacological investigation showed that phenothiazines block many different mediators, including *histamine*, *catecholamines*, *acetylcholine* and *5-HT*, and this multiplicity of actions led to the trade name Largactil for chlorpromazine. It is now clear (see Fig. 38.1) that antagonism of *dopamine* is the main determinant of antipsychotic action.

MECHANISM OF ACTION

DOPAMINE RECEPTORS AND DOPAMINERGIC NEURONS

The classification of dopamine receptors in the central nervous system is discussed in Chapter 34 (see Table 34.1). There are five subtypes, which fall into two functional classes: the D_1 type, comprising D_1 and D_5, and the D_2 type, comprising D_2, D_3 and D_4. Antipsychotic drugs owe their therapeutic effects mainly to blockade of D_2-receptors. As stated above, antipsychotic effects require about 80% block of D_2-receptors. In experimental animals, antagonism at D_2-receptors is reflected in inhibition of **amphetamine**-induced stereotypic behaviour, and of **apomorphine**-induced turning behaviour, in animals with unilateral striatal lesions (see Ch. 34). These in vivo effects are paralleled, in vitro, by inhibition of binding of a radioactive D_2 antagonist (e.g. **spiroperidol**) to brain membrane fragments. The first-generation compounds show some preference for D_2 over D_1-receptors, whereas some of the newer agents (e.g. **sulpiride**, **amisulpride**, **remoxipride**) are highly selective for D_2-receptors. **Clozapine** is relatively non-selective between D_1- and D_2-, but has high affinity for D_4.

In animal tests, all antipsychotic drugs initially *increase* and later *decrease* the electrical activity of midbrain dopaminergic neurons in the substantia nigra and ventral tegmentum, and also the release of dopamine in regions containing dopaminergic nerve terminals (see O'Donnell & Grace, 1996). These changes are possibly associated with changes in dopamine receptor expression (see later). Effects on the mesolimbic/mesocortical dopamine pathways are believed to correlate with antipsychotic effects, whereas effects on the nigrostriatal pathways are responsible for the unwanted motor effects produced by antipsychotic drugs (see below). Thus **haloperidol**, a first-generation drug with marked

unwanted motor effects, acts on both sets of dopamine neurons, whereas **clozapine** and other drugs (see Table 38.1) that have much less tendency to cause adverse motor effects affect mainly the ventral tegmental neurons.

Antipsychotic drugs, like many neuroactive compounds, take several weeks to take effect, even though their receptor-blocking action is immediate.[4] When antipsychotic drugs are administered chronically, the increase in activity of dopaminergic neurons is transient and gives way after about 3 weeks to inhibition (Fig. 38.2), at which time both the biochemical and electrophysiological markers of activity decline.

Another delayed effect of chronic administration of antipsychotic drugs is proliferation of dopamine receptors, detectable as an increase in haloperidol binding (see Seeman, 1987), with a pharmacological supersensitivity to dopamine reminiscent of the phenomenon of denervation supersensitivity (Ch. 9). The mechanism(s) of these delayed effects and their relationships to the clinical response are poorly understood.

Antipsychotic drugs show varying patterns of selectivity in their receptor-blocking effects (Table 38.1), some having high affinity for $5\text{-}HT_2$ and/or D_4-receptors. The connection between their receptor specificity and their functional and therapeutic effects, despite a wealth of fine argument, remains hidden. Were it understood, we might not have to resort to words like 'atypical' to hide our uncertainty.

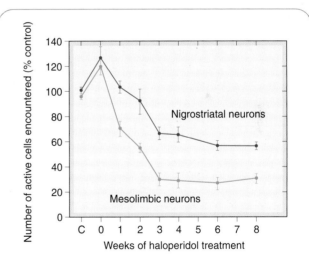

Fig. 38.2 Effect of chronic haloperidol treatment on the activity of dopaminergic neurons in the rat brain. In both regions, the activity of dopaminergic neurons, recorded with microelectrodes from anaesthetised animals, initially increases and then declines, reaching a steady level after 3 weeks. (From White F J, Wang R Y 1983 Life Sci 32: 983.)

---

[4]Their sedating effect is also immediate, allowing them to be used in acute behavioural emergencies.

Mechanism of action of antipsychotic drugs

- All antipsychotic drugs are antagonists at dopamine D_2-receptors, but most also block other monoamine receptors, especially 5-HT$_2$. Clozapine also blocks D_4-receptors.
- Antipsychotic potency generally runs parallel to activity on D_2-receptors, but other activities may determine side effect profile.
- Imaging studies suggest that therapeutic effect requires about 80% occupancy of D_2-receptors.
- Antipsychotics take days or weeks to work, suggesting that secondary effects (e.g. increase in number of D_2-receptors in limbic structure) may be more important than direct effect of D_2-receptor block.

PHARMACOLOGICAL EFFECTS OF ANTIPSYCHOTIC DRUGS

BEHAVIOURAL EFFECTS

Antipsychotic drugs produce many behavioural effects in experimental animals (see Ögren, 1996), but no single test distinguishes them clearly from other types of psychotropic drug. Antipsychotic drugs reduce spontaneous motor activity and in larger doses cause *catalepsy*, a state in which the animal remains immobile even when placed in an unnatural position. Inhibition of the hyperactivity induced by **amphetamine** parallels antipsychotic actions of these drugs, whereas their tendency to induce catalepsy parallels extrapyramidal symptoms (see below). Antipsychotic effects probably reflect D_2-receptor antagonism in the mesocortical/mesolimbic pathway, while extrapyramidal actions relate to dopamine inhibition in the striatonigral pathways.

▼ Other tests reveal effects distinct from motor inhibition. For example, in a conditioned avoidance model, a rat may be trained to respond to a conditioned stimulus, such as a buzzer, by remaining immobile and thereby avoiding a painful shock; chlorpromazine impairs performance in this test, as well as in tests that demand active motor responses. In doses too small to reduce spontaneous motor activity, chlorpromazine reduces social interactions (grooming, mating, fighting, etc.) and also impairs performance in discriminant tests (e.g. requiring the animal to respond differently to red and green lights).

All first-generation antipsychotic drugs inhibit **amphetamine**-induced behavioural changes, reflecting their action on D_2-receptors. Some atypical drugs have less activity on D_2-receptors and are less active in such models, and also in the catalepsy model. They are, however, as efficacious as the older drugs in conditioned avoidance tests. Both classic and atypical drugs, moreover, reduce the hyperactivity caused by **phencyclidine** (a glutamate antagonist; Ch. 33), which causes a schizophrenia-like syndrome in humans. Conditioned avoidance and phencyclidine tests in animals are therefore used as guides to antipsychotic activity in humans.

In humans, antipsychotic drugs produce a state of apathy and reduced initiative. The recipient displays few emotions, is slow to respond to external stimuli and tends to drowse off. The subject

is, however, easily aroused and can respond to questions accurately, with no marked loss of intellectual function. Aggressive tendencies are strongly inhibited. Effects differ from those of hypnotic and anxiolytic drugs, which also cause drowsiness and confusion but with euphoria rather than apathy.

Many antipsychotic drugs are antiemetic (see Ch. 24), reflecting antagonism at dopamine, muscarinic, histamine and possibly 5-HT receptors.

UNWANTED EFFECTS

Extrapyramidal motor disturbances and tardive dyskinesia

Antipsychotic drugs produce two main kinds of motor disturbance in humans: *acute dystonias* and *tardive dyskinesias*, collectively termed *extrapyramidal side effects*. These all result directly or indirectly from D_2-receptor blockade. Extrapyramidal side effects constitute one of the main disadvantages of first-generation antipsychotic drugs. The term *atypical* was originally applied to some of the newer compounds that show much less tendency to produce extrapyramidal side effects.

Acute dystonias are involuntary movements (restlessness, muscle spasms, protruding tongue, fixed upward gaze, torticollis, i.e. involuntary spasm of neck muscles resulting in turning of the head, etc.), often accompanied by symptoms of Parkinson's disease (Ch. 35). They occur commonly in the first few weeks, often declining with time, and are reversible on stopping drug treatment. The timing is consistent with block of the dopaminergic nigrostriatal pathway, and the relative selectivity of atypical antipsychotic drugs for the mesolimbic/mesocortical pathway could account for the diminished risk of acute dystonias with these drugs. Concomitant block of muscarinic acetylcholine receptors may also mitigate the motor effects of dopamine receptor antagonists, because these two receptor systems oppose one another (Ch. 35).

Tardive dyskinesia (see Klawans et al., 1988) develops after months or years (hence 'tardive') in 20–40% of patients treated with first-generation antipsychotic drugs, and is one of the main problems of antipsychotic therapy. Its seriousness lies in the fact that it is a disabling and often irreversible condition, which often gets worse when antipsychotic therapy is stopped and is resistant to treatment. The syndrome consists of involuntary movements, often of the face and tongue, but also of the trunk and limbs, which can be severely disabling. It resembles that seen after prolonged treatment of Parkinson's disease with levodopa. The incidence depends greatly on drug, dose and age (being commonest in patients over 50).

▼ There are several theories about the mechanism of tardive dyskinesia (see Casey, 1995). One is that it is associated with a gradual increase in the number of D_2-receptors in the striatum, which is less marked during treatment with the atypical than with the first generation of antipsychotic drugs. Another possibility is that chronic block of inhibitory dopamine receptors enhances catecholamine and/or glutamate release in the striatum, leading to excitotoxic neurodegeneration (Ch. 35). The reason why atypical antipsychotic drugs (e.g. **clozapine, olanzapine, sertindole**) are better in this regard is not clear. One possible explanation (see Kapur & Seeman, 2001) lies in differences in the *rate* at which compounds dissociate from D_2-receptors. With a rapidly dissociating compound, a

Antipsychotic-induced motor disturbances

- Major problem of antipsychotic drug treatment.
- Two main types of disturbance occur:
  - acute, reversible dystonias and Parkinson-like symptoms
  - slowly developing tardive dyskinesia, often irreversible.
- Acute symptoms comprise involuntary movements, tremor and rigidity, and are probably the direct consequence of block of nigrostriatal dopamine receptors.
- Tardive dyskinesia comprises mainly involuntary movements of face and limbs, appearing after months or years of antipsychotic treatment. It may be associated with proliferation of dopamine receptors (possibly presynaptic) in corpus striatum. Treatment is generally unsuccessful.
- Incidence of acute dystonias and tardive dyskinesia is less with atypical antipsychotics, and particularly low with clozapine, aripiprazole and zotepine. This may reflect relatively strong muscarinic receptor block with these drugs, or a degree of selectivity for the mesolimbic, as opposed to the nigrostriatal, dopamine pathways.

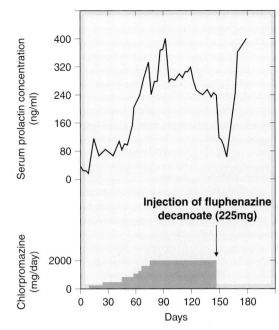

Fig. 38.3 Effects of antipsychotic drugs on prolactin secretion in a schizophrenic patient. When daily dosage with chlorpromazine was replaced with a depot injection of fluphenazine, the plasma prolactin initally dropped, because of the delay in absorption, and then returned to a high level. (From Meltzer H Y et al. 1978 In: Lipton et al. (eds) Psychopharmacology. A generation in progress. Raven Press, New York.)

brief surge of dopamine can effectively overcome the block by competition (Ch. 2), whereas with a slowly dissociating compound the level of block takes a long time to respond to the presence of endogenous dopamine, and is in practice non-competitive. Adverse motor effects may be avoided if fractional receptor occupation falls during physiological surges of dopamine—an attractive kinetic explanation that remains to be confirmed. **Clozapine** has relatively high affinity for D_1 and D_4 compared with D_2-receptors, and also has marked antimuscarinic activity. Appreciable affinity for muscarinic receptors is shared by some other antipsychotic drugs, such as **thioridazine**.[5] This pharmacological property could counteract its adverse motor effects (cf. the use of **benztropine** to reduce extrapyramidal effects of antipsychotic drugs).

Endocrine effects

Dopamine, released in the median eminence by neurons of the tuberohypophyseal pathway (see Chs 27 and 33), acts physiologically to inhibit prolactin secretion via D_2-receptors. Blocking D_2-receptors by antipsychotic drugs can therefore increase the plasma prolactin concentration (Fig. 38.3), resulting in breast swelling, pain and lactation, which can occur in men as well as in women. As can be seen from Figure 38.3, the effect is maintained during chronic antipsychotic administration, without any habituation. Other less pronounced endocrine changes have also been reported, including a decrease of growth hormone secretion, but these, unlike the prolactin response, are believed to be unimportant clinically.

Other unwanted effects

Sedation, which tends to decrease with continued use, occurs with many antipsychotic drugs. Antihistamine (H_1) activity is a property of phenothiazines and contributes to their sedative and antiemetic properties (Ch. 25), but not to their antipsychotic action.

Phenothiazines and, to a variable extent, other antipsychotic drugs, block a variety of receptors, particularly acetylcholine (muscarinic), histamine (H_1), noradrenaline (α) and 5-HT (Table 38.1).

Blocking muscarinic receptors produces a variety of peripheral effects, including blurring of vision and increased intraocular pressure, dry mouth and eyes, constipation and urinary retention (see Ch. 10). It may, however, also be beneficial in relation to extrapyramidal side effects. Acetylcholine opposes dopamine in the basal ganglia (see Ch. 35), and it is possible that the relative lack of extrapyramidal side effects with **clozapine** and **thioridazine** is due to their high antimuscarinic potency (see above).

Blocking α-adrenoceptors causes *orthostatic hypotension* (see Ch. 19) but does not seem to be important for their antipsychotic action.

Weight gain is a common and troublesome side effect, particularly associated with some of the atypical drugs, and probably related to 5-HT antagonism.

---

[5]Now withdrawn, because of a tendency to cause ventricular dysrhythmias by blocking cardiac potassium channels (see Ch. 18).

Unwanted effects of antipsychotic drugs

- Important side effects common to most drugs are extrapyramidal motor disturbances (see *Antipsychotic-induced motor disturbances* box) and endocrine disturbances (increased prolactin release); these are secondary to dopamine receptor block. Sedation, hypotension and weight gain are also common.
- Obstructive jaundice sometimes occurs with phenothiazines.
- Other side effects (dry mouth, blurred vision, hypotension, etc.) are due to block of other receptors, particularly α-adrenoceptors and muscarinic acetylcholine receptors.
- Some antipsychotic drugs cause agranulocytosis as a rare and serious idiosyncratic reaction. With clozapine, leucopenia is common and requires routine monitoring.
- Antipsychotic malignant syndrome is a rare but potentially dangerous idiosyncratic reaction.

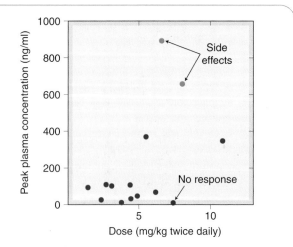

Fig. 38.4 Individual variation in the relation between dose and plasma concentration of chlorpromazine in a group of schizophrenic patients. (Data from Curry S H et al. 1970 Arch Gen Psychiatry 22: 289.)

Various idiosyncratic and hypersensitivity reactions can occur, the most important being the following.

- Jaundice, which occurs with older phenothiazines such as **chlorpromazine**. The jaundice is usually mild, associated with elevated serum alkaline phosphatase activity (an 'obstructive' pattern), and disappears quickly when the drug is stopped or substituted by a chemically unrelated antipsychotic.
- *Leucopenia* and *agranulocytosis* are rare but potentially fatal, and occur in the first few weeks of treatment. The incidence of leucopenia (usually reversible) is less than 1 in 10 000 for most antipsychotic drugs, but much higher (1–2%) with clozapine, whose use therefore requires regular monitoring of blood cell counts. Provided the drug is stopped at the first sign of leucopenia or anaemia, the effect is reversible. **Olanzapine** appears to be free of this disadvantage.
- Urticarial skin reactions are common but usually mild. Excessive sensitivity to ultraviolet light may also occur.
- *Antipsychotic malignant syndrome* is a rare but serious complication similar to the malignant hyperthermia syndrome seen with certain anaesthetics (see Ch. 36). Muscle rigidity is accompanied by a rapid rise in body temperature and mental confusion. It is usually reversible, but death from renal or cardiovascular failure occurs in 10–20% of cases.

PHARMACOKINETIC ASPECTS

Chlorpromazine, in common with many other phenothiazines, is erratically absorbed after oral administration. Figure 38.4 shows the wide range of variation of the peak plasma concentration as a function of dosage in 14 patients. Among four patients treated at the high dosage level of 6–8 mg/kg, the variation in peak plasma concentration was nearly 90-fold; two

showed marked side effects, one was well controlled and one showed no clinical response.

The relationship between the plasma concentration and the clinical effect of antipsychotic drugs is highly variable, and the dosage has to be adjusted on a trial-and-error basis. This is made even more difficult by the fact that at least 40% of schizophrenic patients fail to take drugs as prescribed. It is remarkably fortunate that the acute toxicity of antipsychotic drugs is slight, given the unpredictability of the clinical response.

The plasma half-life of most antipsychotic drugs is 15–30 hours, clearance depending entirely on hepatic transformation by a combination of oxidative and conjugative reactions.

Most antipsychotic drugs can be given orally or by intramuscular injection once or twice a day. Slow-release (depot) preparations of many are available, in which the active drug is esterified with heptanoic or decanoic acid and dissolved in oil. Given as an intramuscular injection, the drug acts for 2–4 weeks, but initially may produce acute side effects. These preparations are widely used to minimise compliance problems.

CLINICAL USE AND CLINICAL EFFICACY

The major use of antipsychotic drugs is in the treatment of *schizophrenia* and *acute behavioural emergencies*, but they are also widely used as adjunct therapy in the treatment of other illnesses, such as psychotic depression and mania. Some of the newer antipsychotic drugs (e.g. **sulpiride**) have been claimed to have specific antidepressant actions. **Phenothiazines** and related drugs are also useful as antiemetics (see Ch. 25). Minor uses include the treatment of *Huntington's chorea* (mainly **haloperidol**; see Ch. 35).

The clinical efficacy of antipsychotic drugs in enabling schizophrenic patients to lead more normal lives has been demonstrated in many controlled trials. The in-patient population (mainly chronic schizophrenics) of mental hospitals declined sharply in the 1950s and 1960s. The efficacy of the newly introduced antipsychotic drugs was a significant enabling factor, as well as the changing public and professional attitudes towards hospitalisation of the mentally ill.

Antipsychotic drugs, apart from their side effects, have two main shortcomings.

- They are effective in only about 70% of schizophrenic patients; for any single drug, the success rate is lower. The remaining 30% are classed as 'treatment-resistant' and present a major therapeutic problem. The reason for the difference between responsive and unresponsive patients is unknown at present, although there is some evidence (not conclusive) that polymorphism within the family of dopamine and 5-HT receptors may be involved (see Basile et al., 2002).
- While they control the positive symptoms (thought disorder, hallucinations, delusions, etc.) effectively, they are ineffective in relieving the negative symptoms (emotional flattening, social isolation).

The newer atypical antipsychotic drugs may overcome these shortcomings to some degree, showing efficacy in treatment-resistant patients and improving negative as well as positive symptoms. However, a recent meta-analysis (Geddes et al., 2000) suggests that while these newer drugs reduce the risk of adverse motor effects, they are not significantly better in terms of efficacy or other side effects. The older drugs, Geddes et al. suggest, may have gained a bad name for causing troublesome side effects because of the common practice of overdosing beyond the useful therapeutic range. Following a detailed review of the available clinical evidence, the National Institute for Clinical Excellence (2002) recommend the use of atypical antipsychotic drugs as first-line treatment for newly diagnosed schizophrenic patients, because of the low level of motor side effects that they produce, although—apart from the use of **clozapine** for treatment-resistant schizophrenia—there is no evidence that they are more effective than first-generation drugs in controlling symptoms.

Clinical uses of antipsychotic drugs

- *Behavioural emergencies* (e.g. violent patients with a range of psychopathologies including *mania, toxic delirium, schizophrenia* and others):
  - classic antipsychotic drugs (e.g. **chlorpromazine, haloperidol**) can rapidly control hyperactive psychotic states
  - note that the intramuscular dose is lower than the oral dose of the same drug because of presystemic metabolism.
- *Schizophrenia*
  - Many chronic schizophrenic patients are treated with first generation antipsychotic drugs. Depot injections (e.g. **flupentixol decanoate**) may be useful for maintenance treatment when

compliance with oral treatment is a problem. **Flupentixol** has *antidepressant* properties distinct from its antipsychotic action.
  - *Atypical antipsychotic drugs* (e.g. **amisulpride, olanzapine, risperidone**) are used if extrapyramidal symptoms are troublesome, if symptom control is inadequate, or for newly diagnosed patients.
  - **Clozapine** can cause *agranocytosis* but is distinctively effective against 'negative' features of schizophrenia. It is reserved for patients whose condition remains inadequately controlled despite previous use of two or more antipsychotic drugs, of which at least one is atypical. Blood count is monitored weekly for the first 18 weeks, and less frequently thereafter.

REFERENCES AND FURTHER READING

Pathogenesis of schizophrenia
Busatto G F, Kerwin R W 1997 Perspectives on the role of serotonergic mechanisms in the pharmacology of schizophrenia. J Psychopharmacol 11: 3–12 (*Assesses the evidence implicating 5-HT as well as dopamine in the action of antipsychotic drugs*)
Goff D C, Coyle J T 2001 The emerging role of glutamate in the pathophysiology and treatment of schizophrenia. Am J Psychiatry 158: 1367–1377 (*Good review article on pathophysiology, although referring to role in treatment is premature*)
Harrison P J 1997 Schizophrenia: a disorder of development. Curr Opin Neurobiol 7: 285–289 (*Reviews persuasively the evidence favouring abnormal early brain development as the basis of schizophrenia*)
Harrison P J, Owen M J 2003 Genes for schizophrenia? Recent findings and their pathophysiological implications. Lancet 361: 417–419 (*Recently identified

schizophrenia-associated genes point to possible involvement of glutamate transmission*)
Laruelle M, Abi-Dargham A, Gil R et al. 1999 Increased dopamine transmission in schizophrenia: relationship to illness phases. Biol Psychiatry 46: 56–72 (*The first direct evidence for increased dopamine function as a cause of symptoms in schizophrenia*)
Lewis D A, Lieberman J A 2000 Catching up on schizophrenia: natural history and neurobiology. Neuron 28: 325–334 (*Useful review summarising present understanding of the nature of schizophrenia*)
Moghaddam B 2003 Bringing order to the glutamate chaos in schizophrenia. Neuron 40: 861–864 (*Reviews evidence from recent genetic findings, suggesting the abnormalities in glutamate transmission may play a key role in schizophrenia*)
Mortimer A M 2004 Novel antipsychotics in schizophrenia. Expert Opin Investig Drugs 13:

315–329 (*A misleading title for a review dealing mainly with current ideas about the neurochemical abnormalities underlying schizophrenia*)
Seeman P 1987 Dopamine receptors and the dopamine hypothesis of schizophrenia. Synapse 1: 133–152 (*Convincing and widely quoted review of role of dopamine receptors in schizophrenia*)

Antipsychotic drugs
Abi-Dargham A, Laruelle M 2005 Mechanisms of action of second generation antipsychotic drugs in schizophrenia: insights from brain imaging studies. Eur Psychiatry 20: 15–27 (*Reviews recent evidence favouring imbalance between cortical and subcortical dopamine transmission in schizophrenia*)
Basile V S, Masellis M, Potkin S G, Kennedy J L 2002 Pharmacogenomics in schizophrenia: the quest for individualized therapy. Hum Mol Genet 11: 2517–2530 (*Review of inconclusive evidence for*

association between clozapine responsiveness and gene polymorphisms)

Geddes J, Freemantle N, Harrison P, Bebbington P 2000 Atypical antipsychotics in the treatment of schizophrenia: systematic overview and meta-regression analysis. Br Med J 321: 1371–1376 (*Survey of trials comparing atypical and classic drugs, showing few clear-cut differences apart from motor side effects*)

Javitt D C 2004 Glutamate as a therapeutic target in psychiatric disorders. Mol Psychiatry 9: 984–997 (*Summarises the evidence favouring disturbed glutamate function in schizophrenia, including data from recent clinical trials*)

Kapur S, Seeman P 2001 Does fast dissociation from the dopamine D_2 receptor explain the action of atypical antipsychotics? A new hypothesis. Am J Psychiatry 158: 360–369 (*Suggests that differences in dissociation rates, rather than receptor selectivity profiles, may account for differing tendency of drugs to cause motor side effects*)

National Institute for Clinical Excellence 2002 Guideline 43. Guidance for the use of newer (atypical) antipsychotic drugs for the treatment of schizophrenia. http://www.nice.org.uk (*Official UK guidance on the use of atypical antipsychotic drugs*)

O'Donnell P, Grace A A 1996 Basic neurophysiology of antipsychotic drug action. In: Chernansky J G (ed) Antipsychotics. Handbook of experimental pharmacology, vol 120. Springer, Berlin (*Review of effects of antipsychotic drugs at the neurophysiological level, emphasising distinction between acute and chronic effects*)

Ögren S O 1996 The behavioural pharmacology of typical and atypical antipsychotic drugs. In: Csernasky J G (ed) Antipsychotics. Handbook of experimental pharmacology, vol 120. Springer, Berlin

Remington G 2003 Understanding antipsychotic 'atypicality': a clinical and pharmacological moving target. J Psychiatry Neurosci 28: 275–284 (*An informative critique of the basis on which antipsychotic drugs are classified*)

Extrapyramidal side effects

Casey D E 1995 Tardive dyskinesia: pathophysiology. In: Bloom F E, Kupfer D J (eds) Psychopharmacology: a fourth generation of progress. Raven Press, New York

Klawans H L, Tanner C M, Goetz C G 1988 Epidemiology and pathophysiology of tardive dyskinesias. Adv Neurol 49: 185–197

Antidepressant drugs

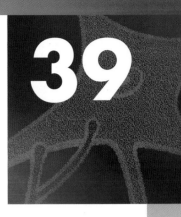

39

OVERVIEW

Depression is an extremely common psychiatric condition, about which a variety of neurochemical theories exist, and for which a corresponding variety of different types of drug are used in treatment. It is a field in which therapeutic empiricism has led the way, with mechanistic understanding tending to lag behind, part of the difficulty being that animal models cannot address the mood change that defines the human condition. In this chapter, we discuss the current understanding of the nature of the disorder, and describe the major drugs that are used to treat it. A good summary of our present state of knowledge is given by Wong & Licinio (2001)

THE NATURE OF DEPRESSION

Depression is the most common of the affective disorders (defined as disorders of mood rather than disturbances of thought or cognition); it may range from a very mild condition, bordering on normality, to severe (psychotic) depression accompanied by hallucinations and delusions. Worldwide, depression is a major cause of disability and premature death. In addition to the significant suicide risk, depressed individuals are more likely to die from other causes, such as heart disease or cancer.

The symptoms of depression include emotional and biological components.

- Emotional symptoms:
  —misery, apathy and pessimism
  —low self-esteem: feelings of guilt, inadequacy and ugliness
  —indecisiveness, loss of motivation.
- Biological symptoms:
  —retardation of thought and action
  —loss of libido
  —sleep disturbance and loss of appetite.

There are two distinct types of depressive syndrome, namely *unipolar depression*, in which the mood swings are always in the same direction, and *bipolar affective disorder*, in which depression alternates with mania. Mania is in most respects exactly the opposite, with excessive exuberance, enthusiasm and self-confidence, accompanied by impulsive actions, these signs often being combined with irritability, impatience and aggression, and sometimes with grandiose delusions of the Napoleonic kind. As with depression, the mood and actions are inappropriate to the circumstances.

Unipolar depression is commonly (about 75% of cases) non-familial, clearly associated with stressful life events, and accompanied by symptoms of anxiety and agitation; this type is sometimes termed *reactive depression*. Other cases (about 25%, sometimes termed *endogenous depression*) show a familial pattern, unrelated to external stresses, and with a somewhat different symptomatology. This distinction is made clinically, but there is little evidence that antidepressant drugs show significant selectivity between these conditions.

Bipolar depression, which usually appears in early adult life, is less common and results in oscillating depression and mania over a period of a few weeks. There is a strong hereditary tendency, but no specific susceptibility genes have been identified either by genetic linkage studies of affected families, or by comparison of affected and non-affected individuals.

THEORIES OF DEPRESSION

THE MONOAMINE THEORY

The main biochemical theory of depression is the *monoamine hypothesis*, proposed by Schildkraut in 1965, which states that depression is caused by a functional deficit of monoamine transmitters at certain sites in the brain, while mania results from a functional excess. For reviews of the evolving status of the theory, see Baker & Dewhurst (1985), Maes & Meltzer (1995) and Manji et al. (2001).

The monoamine hypothesis grew originally out of associations between the clinical effects of various drugs that cause or alleviate symptoms of depression and their known neurochemical effects on monoaminergic transmission in the brain. Initially, the hypothesis was formulated in terms of noradrenaline (norepinephrine), but subsequent work showed that most of the observations were equally consistent with 5-hydroxytryptamine (5-HT) being the key mediator. This pharmacological evidence, which is summarised below, gives general support to the monoamine hypothesis, although there are several anomalies. Attempts to obtain more direct evidence, by studying monoamine metabolism in depressed patients or by measuring changes in the number of monoamine receptors in post-mortem brain tissue, have tended to give inconsistent and equivocal results, and the interpretation of these studies is often problematic, because the changes described are not specific to depression. Similarly, investigation by functional tests of the activity of known monoaminergic pathways (e.g. those controlling pituitary hormone release) in depressed patients have also given equivocal results.

PHARMACOLOGICAL EVIDENCE

Table 39.1 summarises the main pharmacological evidence supporting the monoamine hypothesis. Although it provides reasonable support, there are several examples of drugs that might have been predicted to improve or worsen depressive symptoms, but fail to do so convincingly. It has to be recognised that the basis for predicting the effects of drugs on mood is, at best, very simple-minded. Thus supplying a transmitter precursor will not necessarily increase the release of transmitter unless availability of the precursor is rate-limiting. Similarly, a drug that releases monoamines from normal nerve terminals may fail to do so if the nerve terminals are functionally defective. The pharmacological evidence does not enable a clear distinction to be drawn between the noradrenaline and 5-HT theories of depression. Clinically, it seems that inhibitors of noradrenaline reuptake and of 5-HT reuptake are equally effective as antidepressants (see below), although individual patients may respond better to one or the other.

Any theory of depression has to take account of the fact that the direct biochemical effects of antidepressant drugs appear very rapidly, whereas their antidepressant effects take weeks to develop. A similar situation exists in relation to antipsychotic drugs (Ch. 38) and some anxiolytic drugs (Ch. 37), suggesting that the secondary, adaptive changes in the brain, rather than the primary drug effect, are responsible for the clinical improvement. Rather than thinking of the monoamine deficiency as causing direct changes in the activity of putative 'happy' or 'sad' neurons in the brain, we should think of the monoamines as regulators of longer-term trophic effects, whose time course is paralleled by mood changes (see below, p. 559).

BIOCHEMICAL STUDIES

Many studies have sought to test the amine hypothesis by looking for biochemical abnormalities in cerebrospinal fluid, blood or urine, or in post-mortem brain tissue, from depressed or manic patients. They have included studies of monoamine metabolites, receptors, enzymes and transporters, largely with negative results. The major metabolites of noradrenaline and 5-HT, respectively, are 3-methoxy-4-hydroxyphenylglycol (MHPG) and 5-hydroxyindoleacetic acid (5-HIAA). These appear in the cerebrospinal fluid, blood and

Table 39.1 Pharmacological evidence supporting the monoamine hypothesis of depression

Drug(s)	Principal action	Effect in depressed patients
Tricyclic antidepressants	Block NA and 5-HT reuptake	Mood ↑
Monoamine oxidase (MAO) inhibitors	Increase stores of NA and 5-HT	Mood ↑
Reserpine	Inhibits NA and 5-HT storage	Mood ↓
α-Methyltyrosine	Inhibits NA synthesis	Mood ↓ (calming of manic patients)
Methyldopa	Inhibits NA synthesis	Mood ↓
Electroconvulsive therapy	?Increases central nervous system responses to NA and 5-HT	Mood ↑
Tryptophan (5-hydroxytryptophan)	Increases 5-HT synthesis	Mood ? ↑ in some studies

urine (see Chs 11, 12 and 34). There are two fundamental problems in relating changes in the concentration of these metabolites in body fluids to changes in transmitter function in the brain. One is that many secondary factors can affect their concentration, such as diet; transport between cerebrospinal fluid, blood and urine; or release of monoamines from non-cerebral sites. The second is that many patients receive drug treatment, which affects the metabolite concentrations markedly.

Studies of urinary MHPG excretion in normal and depressed subjects have shown convincingly that the level is reduced in bipolar depressive patients, and is lower during the depressive than during the manic phase. In unipolar depression, however, MHPG excretion, although highly variable between patients, is not significantly lower than in control subjects, so support for the monoamine theory is at best equivocal. Plasma noradrenaline actually tends to be higher in depressed than in normal subjects, possibly because it reflects peripheral sympathetic activity, which increases with the anxiety that often accompanies depression. It too shows a cyclic variation in bipolar depressive patients.

Results pertaining to altered 5-HT metabolism are also highly variable (see Maes & Meltzer, 1995). Studies of 5-HIAA in cerebrospinal fluid and urine have generally failed to find any clear correlation with depression. Low levels of 5-HIAA occur in the brain and cerebrospinal fluid of suicide victims but may be associated with violent behaviour rather than with depression. More consistent changes have been reported in the plasma concentration of L-tryptophan (the precursor of 5-HT). Although the resting levels are not significantly different in depressed patients, the rise in plasma L-tryptophan following an intravenous or oral dose is reduced, implying lower 'L-tryptophan availability'.

Other evidence in support of the monoamine theory is that agents known to block noradrenaline or 5-HT synthesis consistently reverse the therapeutic effects of antidepressant drugs that act selectively on these two transmitter systems (see below).

In summary, there is considerable circumstantial evidence to support the monoamine hypothesis, although there are some inconsistencies, of which the most obvious are the following.

- Neither amphetamine nor cocaine has antidepressant actions, despite their ability to enhance monoamine transmission.
- Some clinically effective antidepressants seem to lack any actions that could enhance monoamine transmission.
- The biochemical changes associated with depression have, in several studies, been identical with changes observed in manic patients.

With improved neuroimaging methods for studying neurotransmitter function in the living human brain, as described in Chapter 38, some of the gaps and inconsistencies may be resolved.

NEUROENDOCRINE MECHANISMS

Various attempts have been made to test for a functional deficit of monoamine pathways in depression. Hypothalamic neurons controlling pituitary function receive noradrenergic and 5-HT inputs, which control the discharge of these cells. Hypothalamic cells release **corticotrophin-releasing hormone (CRH)**, which stimulates pituitary cells to secrete adrenocorticotrophic hormone (ACTH), leading in turn to cortisol secretion. The plasma cortisol concentration is usually high in depressed patients, and it fails to respond with the normal fall when a synthetic steroid, such as dexamethasone, is given. This formed the basis of a clinical test, the *dexamethasone suppression test* (also used in the diagnosis of Cushing's syndrome; see Ch. 28). Other hormones in plasma are also affected, for example growth hormone concentration is reduced and prolactin is increased. In general, these changes are consistent with deficient monoamine transmission, but they are not specific to depressive syndromes.

Corticotrophin-releasing hormone is widely distributed in the brain and has behavioural effects that are distinct from its endocrine functions. Injected into the brain of experimental animals, CRH mimics some effects of depression in humans, such as diminished activity, loss of appetite, and increased signs of anxiety. Furthermore, CRH concentrations in the brain and cerebrospinal fluid of depressed patients are increased. Therefore CRH hyperfunction, as well as monoamine hypofunction, may be associated with depression (see Holsboer, 1999).

NEUROPLASTICITY AND TROPHIC EFFECTS

▼ Recently (see reviews by Duman, 2004; Charney & Manji, 2004) a new idea has emerged, namely that major depression is associated with *neuronal loss in the hippocampus and prefrontal cortex*, and that antidepressant therapies of different kinds act by inhibiting or actually reversing this loss by stimulating neurogenesis.[1] This surprising idea is supported by various lines of evidence.

- Imaging and post-mortem studies show shrinkage of the hippocampus and prefrontal cortex of depressed patients, with loss of neurons and glia. Functional imaging reveals reduced neuronal activity in these regions.
- In animals, the same effect is produced by chronic stress of various kinds, or by administration of glucocorticoids, mimicking the increased cortisol secretion in human depression. Excessive glucocorticoid secretion in humans (Cushing's syndrome; see Ch. 28) often causes depression.
- Antidepressant drugs, or other treatments such as electroconvulsions (see below), promote neurogenesis in these regions, and (as in humans) restore functional activity. Preventing hippocampal neurogenesis prevents the behavioural effects of antidepressants in rats (Santarelli et al., 2003).
- 5-HT, whose action is enhanced by many antidepressants (see below), promotes neurogenesis during development, this effect being mediated by brain-derived neurotrophic factor (BDNF). Antidepressants also increase BDNF production.

▼ Figure 39.1 summarises the possible mechanisms involved. It should be stressed that these hypotheses are far from proven, but the diagram emphasises the way in which the field has moved on since

---

[1]Neurogenesis (see Ch. 35)—the formation of new neurons from stem cell precursors—occurs to a significant degree in the adult hippocampus, and possibly elsewhere in the brain, contradicting the old dogma that it occurs only during brain development.

the formulation of the monoamine hypothesis, suggesting a range of possible targets for the next generation of antidepressant drugs.[2]

For now, although it clearly needs to be modified and elaborated, Schildkraut's basic hypothesis remains the best basis for understanding the actions of current antidepressant drugs.

ANIMAL MODELS OF DEPRESSION

▼ Progress in unravelling the neurochemical mechanisms is, as in so many areas of psychopharmacology, limited by the lack of good animal models of the clinical condition. There is no known animal condition corresponding to the inherited condition of depression in humans, but various procedures have been described that produce in animals behavioural states (withdrawal from social interaction, loss of appetite, reduced motor activity, etc.) typical of human depression (see review by Porsolt, 1985). For example, the delivery of repeated inescapable painful stimuli leads to a state of 'learned helplessness', in which even when the animal is free to escape it fails to do so. Mother–infant separation in monkeys, and administration of amine-depleting drugs such as **reserpine**, also produce states that superficially resemble human depression. As well as being inherently distasteful, these experiments often require elaborate and expensive experimental protocols, and the similarity of these states to human depression is questionable. However, the learned helplessness state and the effect of mother–infant separation can be reversed by tricyclic antidepressants (TCAs) and increased by small doses of α-methyl-*p*-tyrosine (which inhibits noradrenaline synthesis), suggesting a basic similarity to depressive illness in humans.

ANTIDEPRESSANT DRUGS

TYPES OF ANTIDEPRESSANT DRUG

Antidepressant drugs fall into the following categories (Table 39.2).

- Inhibitors of monoamine uptake:
  —non-selective (noradrenaline/serotonin) uptake inhibitors; these include tricyclic antidepressants (TCAs) (e.g. **imipramine, amitriptyline**) and more recent antidepressants such as venlafaxine (somewhat selective for serotonin, although less so than selective serotonin uptake inhibitors) and **duloxetine**, which have fewer side effects than TCAs.
  —selective serotonin reuptake inhibitors (SSRIs) (e.g. **fluoxetine, fluvoxamine, paroxetine** and **sertraline**).
  —selective noradrenaline uptake inhibitors (e.g. **maprotiline, reboxetine**).

- Monoamine oxidase (MAO) inhibitors (MAOIs):
  —irreversible, non-competitive inhibitors (e.g. **phenelzine, tranylcypromine**), which are non-selective with respect to the MAO-A and -B subtypes (see below)
  —reversible, MAO-A-selective inhibitors (e.g. **moclobemide**).
- Miscellaneous (atypical) receptor-blocking compounds whose antidepressant actions are poorly understood (e.g. **mianserin, trazodone, mirtazapine**). The herbal preparation St John's wort, whose main active ingredient is **hyperforin**, has similar clinical efficacy to most of the prescribed antidepressants. It is a weak uptake inhibitor but also has other actions.[3]

Monoamine theory of depression

- The monoamine theory, proposed in 1965, suggests that depression results from functionally deficient monoaminergic (noradrenaline and/or 5-hydroxytryptamine) transmission in the central nervous system.
- The theory was based on the ability of known antidepressant drugs (tricyclic antidepressants and monoamine oxidase inhibitors) to facilitate monoaminergic transmission, and of drugs such as reserpine to cause depression.
- Biochemical studies on depressed patients do not clearly support the monoamine hypothesis in its simple form.
- An abnormally weak response of plasma cortisol to exogenous steroid (dexamethasone suppression test) is common in depression and may reflect defective monoamine transmission in the hypothalamus.
- Recent evidence suggests that depression may be associated with neurodegeneration and reduced neurogenesis in the hippocampus.
- Although the monoamine hypothesis in its simple form is insufficient as an explanation of depression, pharmacological manipulation of monoamine transmission remains the most successful therapeutic approach.
- Current approaches focus on other mediators (e.g. corticotrophin-releasing hormone), signal transduction pathways, growth factors, etc., but theories remain imprecise.

---

[2]Cynics may feel that these mechanisms, in which glutamate, neurotrophic factors, monoamines and steroids all interact to control neuronal death, survival and plasticity, are being invoked just as enthusiastically to account for almost every neurological and psychiatric disorder that you can think of, from stroke and Parkinson's disease to schizophrenia. 'Are we missing something,' they may feel, 'or are all these diseases basically the same? If so, why are their effects so different? Is this just a scientific bandwagon, or does this mechanistic convergence point to some fundamental principles of neural organisation?' We do not have the answers, of course, but it is a field worth watching.

[3]Although relatively free of acute side effects, hyperforin activates cytochrome P450, resulting in loss of efficacy, with serious consequences, of several important drugs, including ciclosporin, oral contraceptives, some anti-HIV and anticancer drugs, and oral anticoagulants—underlining the principle that herbal remedies need to be used with the same degree of informed caution as any other drug.

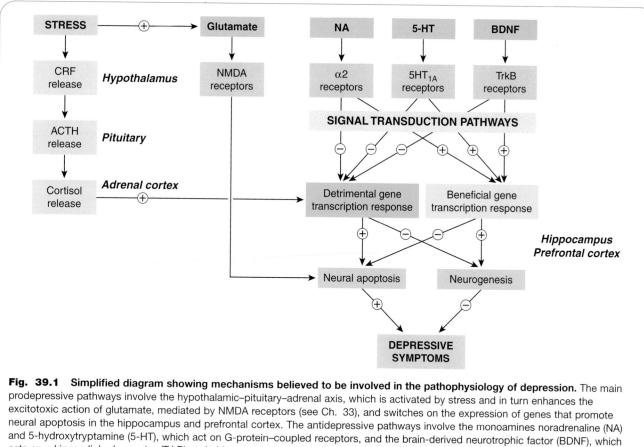

Fig. 39.1 **Simplified diagram showing mechanisms believed to be involved in the pathophysiology of depression.** The main prodepressive pathways involve the hypothalamic–pituitary–adrenal axis, which is activated by stress and in turn enhances the excitotoxic action of glutamate, mediated by NMDA receptors (see Ch. 33), and switches on the expression of genes that promote neural apoptosis in the hippocampus and prefrontal cortex. The antidepressive pathways involve the monoamines noradrenaline (NA) and 5-hydroxytryptamine (5-HT), which act on G-protein–coupled receptors, and the brain-derived neurotrophic factor (BDNF), which acts on a kinase-linked receptor (TrkB), switching on genes that protect neurons against apoptosis and also promote neurogenesis. For further detail, see Charney & Manji (2004). ACTH, adrenocorticotrophic hormone; CRF, corticotrophin-releasing factor.

Table 39.4 summarises the main features of these types of drug. Recent updates (Bosker et al., 2004; Pacher & Kecsemeti, 2004) provide more detail. Mention should also be made of electroconvulsive therapy (ECT), which is effective and usually acts more rapidly than antidepressant drugs (see later section).

MEASUREMENT OF ANTIDEPRESSANT ACTIVITY

▼ The clinical effectiveness of the first MAOI and TCA drugs was discovered by chance when these drugs were given to patients for other reasons. **Iproniazid**, the first MAOI, was originally used to treat tuberculosis, being chemically related to **isoniazid** (see Ch. 46); **imipramine**, the first TCA, resembles **chlorpromazine** (see Ch. 38) and was first tried as an antipsychotic drug. Later, the monoamine hypothesis of depression produced a biochemical rationale for their antidepressant actions, and hence ways of testing new compounds as a preliminary to clinical trials. The results of such biochemical tests are successful in predicting clinical efficacy for conventional TCAs and MAOIs, but fail to predict efficacy with many newer antidepressant drugs. Various behavioural tests have also been used (see above), although there is no animal model that satisfactorily resembles depressive illness in humans. Some of the most useful tests are the following.

• *Potentiation of noradrenaline effects in the periphery.* Stimulation of sympathetic nerves or administration of noradrenaline causes contraction of smooth muscle, which is enhanced if the noradrenaline

reuptake mechanism of the nerve terminal is blocked (see Ch. 11). This test gives positive results with monoamine uptake inhibitors but does not reveal MAOI or atypical antidepressant activity.

• *Potentiation of the central effects of* **amphetamine**. Amphetamine works partly by releasing noradrenaline in the brain, and its actions are enhanced both by MAOIs and by uptake inhibitors. Some atypical antidepressants also give a positive response, making it a useful test for predicting activity in humans.

• *Antagonism of* **reserpine**-*induced depression*. Reserpine depletes the brain of both noradrenaline and 5-HT, causing various measurable effects (hypothermia, bradycardia, reduced motor activity, etc.) that are reduced by antidepressant drugs. This test also reveals activity among the atypical antidepressants.

• *Block of amine uptake in vitro.* Among TCAs, there is a fairly good correlation between antidepressant activity and potency in inhibiting noradrenaline or 5-HT uptake, but MAOIs and many other antidepressants have no effect.

A general point that has to be borne in mind when using in vitro tests to assess potential antidepressants is that many drugs (particularly TCAs) are metabolised to pharmacologically active substances in vivo, and it is often unclear whether the parent drug or the metabolite is actually responsible for the clinical effect.

Clinically, the effect of antidepressant drugs is usually measured by a subjective rating scale such as the 17-item *Hamilton Rating Scale*. Clinical depression takes many forms, and the symptoms vary between patients and over time. Quantitation is therefore difficult, and the many clinical trials of antidepressants have generally shown rather weak effects,

- Main types are:
  — monoamine uptake inhibitors (tricyclic antidepressants, selective serotonin reuptake inhibitors and others)
  — monoamine oxidase (MAO) inhibitors
  — miscellaneous ('atypical') antidepressants, mainly non-selective receptor antagonists (e.g. trazodone, mirtazepine).
- Tricyclic antidepressants and selective serotonin reuptake inhibitors act by inhibiting uptake of noradrenaline and/or 5-HT by monoaminergic nerve terminals, thus acutely facilitating transmission.
- MAO inhibitors inhibit one or both forms of brain MAO, thus increasing the cytosolic stores of noradrenaline and 5-HT in nerve terminals. Inhibition of type A MAO correlates with antidepressant activity. Most are non-selective; moclobemide is specific for MAO-A.
- Mode of action of 'atypical' antidepressants is poorly understood.
- All types of antidepressant drug take at least 2 weeks to produce any beneficial effects, even though their pharmacological effects are produced immediately, indicating that secondary adaptive changes are important.
- The most consistent adaptive change seen with different types of antidepressant drugs is down-regulation of β and α_2-adrenoceptors, as well as 5-HT$_2$ receptors. How this is related to therapeutic effect is not clear.
- Recent evidence suggests that antidepressants may act by increasing neurogenesis in the hippocampus.

after allowance for quite large placebo responses. There is also a high degree of individual variation, with 30–40% of patients failing to show any improvement, possibly due to genetic factors (see below).

MECHANISM OF ACTION OF ANTIDEPRESSANT DRUGS

In the absence of a simple mechanistic theory to account for antidepressant action (see above), it is useful to look for pharmacological effects that the various drugs have in common, concentrating more on the slow adaptive changes that follow a similar time course to the therapeutic effect. This approach has led to the discovery that certain monoamine receptors, in particular β_1 and α_2-adrenoceptors, are consistently down-regulated following chronic antidepressant treatment. This can be demonstrated in experimental animals as a reduction in the number of binding sites, as well as by a reduction in the functional response to agonists (e.g. stimulation of cAMP formation by β-adrenoceptor agonists). Receptor down-regulation probably also occurs in humans, because endocrine

responses to **clonidine**, an α_2-adrenoceptor agonist, are reduced by long-term antidepressant treatment. Other receptors have also been studied; α_1-adrenoceptors are not consistently affected, but 5-HT$_2$-receptors are also down-regulated.

How these findings relate to the monoamine hypothesis is unclear. Loss of β-adrenoceptors as a factor in alleviating depression does not fit comfortably with theory, because β-adrenoceptor antagonists are not antidepressant, although it is the most consistent change reported. Impaired presynaptic inhibition secondary to down-regulation of α_2-adrenoceptors might, it is argued, facilitate monoamine release and thus facilitate transmission. Consistent with this possibility is the fact that some newer antidepressant drugs, such as **mirtazapine** (Table 39.4), are antagonists at various inhibitory presynaptic receptors, including α_2-adrenoceptors.

As described above, several antidepressant drugs appear to promote neurogenesis in the hippocampus, a mechanism that could account for the slow development of the therapeutic effect.

TRICYCLIC ANTIDEPRESSANT DRUGS

Tricyclic antidepressants are still widely used. They are, however, far from ideal in practice, and it was the need for drugs that act more quickly and reliably, produce fewer side effects and are less hazardous in overdose that led to the introduction of newer 5-HT reuptake inhibitors and other antidepressants.

Chemical aspects

Tricyclic antidepressants are closely related in structure to the phenothiazines (Ch. 38) and were initially synthesised (in 1949) as potential antipsychotic drugs. **Imipramine** was found to be of no use in schizophrenia but effective in depression, so related compounds, such as **clomipramine**, were synthesised. They differ from phenothiazines principally in the incorporation of an extra atom into the central ring (Fig. 39.2), which twists the structure so that the molecule is no longer planar as in phenothiazines.

Similar changes to the structure of thioxanthene-type antipsychotic drugs resulted in drugs such as **amitriptyline**. All these compounds are tertiary amines, with two methyl groups attached

- Animal models of depression include:
  — learned helplessness model
  — reversal of reserpine-induced behavioural syndrome
  — mother–infant separation in primates.
- None is a good model for human depressive illness, but they are the best available for testing new drugs.
- Biochemical and pharmacological measures include inhibition of monoamine uptake, receptor-blocking activity, enhancement of peripheral noradrenergic transmission.
- Clinical testing of antidepressant drugs necessitates allowance for large placebo effects.

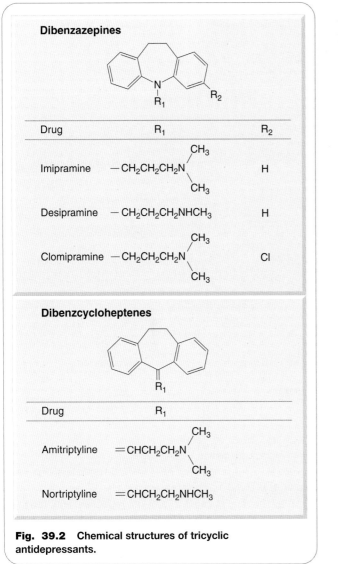

Dibenzazepines

Drug	R_1	R_2
Imipramine	$-CH_2CH_2CH_2N\begin{smallmatrix}CH_3\\CH_3\end{smallmatrix}$	H
Desipramine	$-CH_2CH_2CH_2NHCH_3$	H
Clomipramine	$-CH_2CH_2CH_2N\begin{smallmatrix}CH_3\\CH_3\end{smallmatrix}$	Cl

Dibenzcycloheptenes

Drug	R_1
Amitriptyline	$=CHCH_2CH_2N\begin{smallmatrix}CH_3\\CH_3\end{smallmatrix}$
Nortriptyline	$=CHCH_2CH_2NHCH_3$

Fig. 39.2 Chemical structures of tricyclic antidepressants.

to the basic nitrogen atom. They are quite rapidly demethylated in vivo (Fig. 39.3) to the corresponding secondary amines (**desipramine**, **nortriptyline**, etc.), which are themselves active and may be administered as drugs in their own right. Other tricyclic derivatives with slightly modified bridge structures include **doxepin**. The pharmacological differences between these drugs are not very great and relate mainly to their side effects, which are discussed below.

Mechanism of action

As discussed above, the main immediate effect of TCAs is to block the uptake of amines by nerve terminals, by competition for the binding site of the amine transporter (Ch. 11). Synthesis of amines, storage in synaptic vesicles, and release are not directly affected, although some TCAs appear to increase transmitter release indirectly by blocking presynaptic α_2-adrenoceptors. Most TCAs inhibit noradrenaline and 5-HT uptake by brain synaptosomes to a similar degree (Fig. 39.4) but have much less effect on dopamine uptake. It has been suggested that improvement of emotional symptoms reflects mainly an enhancement of 5-HT-mediated transmission, whereas relief of biological symptoms results from facilitation of noradrenergic transmission. Interpretation is made difficult by the fact that the major metabolites of TCAs have considerable pharmacological activity (in some cases greater than that of the parent drug) and often differ from the parent drug in respect of their noradrenaline/5-HT selectivity (Table 39.2).

In addition to their effects on amine uptake, most TCAs affect one or more types of neurotransmitter receptor, including muscarinic acetylcholine receptors, histamine receptors and 5-HT receptors. The antimuscarinic effects of TCAs do not contribute to their antidepressant effects but are responsible for various troublesome side effects (see below).

Actions and unwanted effects

In non-depressed human subjects, TCAs cause sedation, confusion and motor incoordination. These effects occur also in depressed patients in the first few days of treatment, but tend to wear off in 1–2 weeks as the antidepressant effect develops. In experimental animals, TCAs produce sedation, but they are able to reverse the depressant effect of **reserpine** treatment. TCAs are also used to treat *neuropathic pain* (see Ch. 41).

Unwanted effects with normal clinical dosage

Tricyclic antidepressants produce a number of troublesome side effects, mainly due to interference with autonomic control.

Atropine-like effects include dry mouth, blurred vision, constipation and urinary retention. These effects are strong with **amitriptyline** and much weaker with **desipramine**. Postural hypotension occurs with TCAs. This may seem anomalous for drugs that enhance noradrenergic transmission, and possibly results from an effect on adrenergic transmission in the medullary vasomotor centre. The other common side effect is sedation (see above), and the long duration of action means that daytime performance is often affected by drowsiness and difficulty in concentrating.

Tricyclic antidepressants, particularly in overdose, may cause ventricular dysrhythmias associated with prolongation of the QT interval (see Ch. 18). Usual therapeutic doses of TCAs increase the risk of sudden cardiac death slightly but significantly.

Interactions with other drugs

Tricyclic antidepressants are particularly likely to cause adverse effects when given in conjunction with other drugs (see Ch. 52). They rely on hepatic microsomal metabolism for elimination, and this may be inhibited by competing drugs (e.g. antipsychotic drugs and some steroids).

Tricyclic antidepressants potentiate the effects of *alcohol* and anesthetic agents, for reasons that are not well understood, and deaths have occurred as a result of this, when severe respiratory depression has followed a bout of drinking. TCAs also interfere with the action of various antihypertensive drugs (see Ch. 19), with potentially dangerous consequences, so their use in hypertensive patients requires close monitoring.

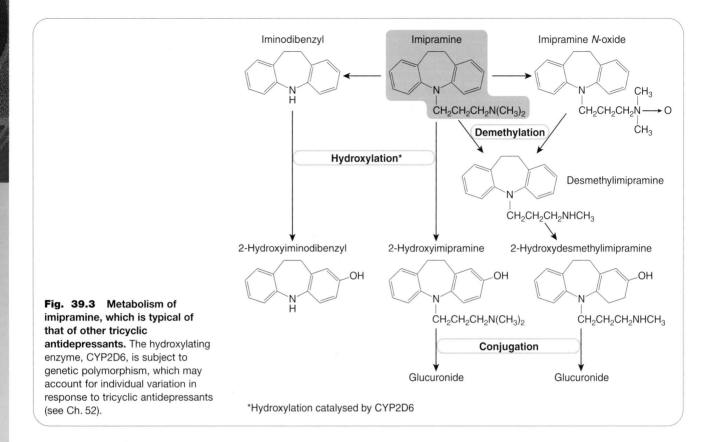

Fig. 39.3 Metabolism of imipramine, which is typical of that of other tricyclic antidepressants. The hydroxylating enzyme, CYP2D6, is subject to genetic polymorphism, which may account for individual variation in response to tricyclic antidepressants (see Ch. 52).

*Hydroxylation catalysed by CYP2D6

Acute toxicity

Tricyclic antidepressants are dangerous in overdose, and were at one time commonly used for suicide attempts, which was an important factor prompting the introduction of safer antidepressants. The main effects are on the central nervous system and the heart. The initial effect of TCA overdosage is to cause *excitement* and *delirium*, which may be accompanied by *convulsions*. This is followed by coma and respiratory depression lasting for some days. Atropine-like effects are pronounced, including flushing, dry mouth and skin, mydriasis, and inhibition of gut and bladder. Anticholinesterase drugs have been used to counter atropine-like effects but are no longer recommended. Cardiac dysrhythmias (see above) are common, and sudden death (rare) may occur from ventricular fibrillation.

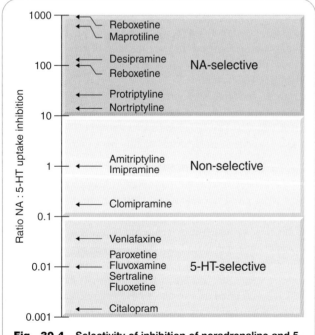

Fig. 39.4 Selectivity of inhibition of noradrenaline and 5-hydroxytryptamine uptake by various antidepressants.

Table 39.2 Inhibition of neuronal noradrenaline and 5-HT uptake by tricyclic antidepressants and their metabolites

Drug/metabolite	NA uptake	5-HT uptake
Imipramine	+++	++
Desmethylimipramine (DMI)	++++	+
Hydroxy-DMI	+++	–
Clomipramine (CMI)	++	+++
Desmethyl-CMI	+++	+
Amitriptyline (AMI)	++	++
Nortriptyline (desmethyl-AMI)	+++	++
Hydroxynortriptyline	++	++

Pharmacokinetic aspects

Tricyclic antidepressants are all rapidly absorbed when given orally and bind strongly to plasma albumin, most being 90–95% bound at therapeutic plasma concentrations. They also bind to extravascular tissues, which accounts for their generally very large distribution volumes (usually 10–50 l/kg; see Ch. 7) and low rates of elimination. Extravascular sequestration, together with strong binding to plasma albumin, means that haemodialysis is ineffective as a means of increasing drug elimination.

Tricyclic antidepressants are metabolised in the liver by two main routes (Fig. 39.2), namely N-*demethylation*, whereby tertiary amines are converted to secondary amines (e.g. **imipramine** to desmethylimipramine, **amitriptyline** to nortriptyline), and *ring hydroxylation*. Both the desmethyl and the hydroxylated metabolites commonly retain biological activity (see Table 39.2). During prolonged treatment with TCAs, the plasma concentration of these metabolites is usually comparable with that of the parent drug, although there is wide variation between individuals. Inactivation of the drugs occurs by glucuronide conjugation of the hydroxylated metabolites, the glucuronides being excreted in the urine.

The overall half-times for elimination of TCAs are generally long, ranging from 10 to 20 hours for **imipramine** and **desipramine** to about 80 hours for **protriptyline**. They are even longer in elderly patients. Therefore gradual accumulation is possible, leading to slowly developing side effects. The relationship between plasma concentrations and the therapeutic effect is not simple. Indeed, a study on nortriptyline (Fig. 39.5) showed that too high a plasma concentration actually *reduces* the antidepressant effect, and there is a narrow 'therapeutic window'.

Other non-selective uptake inhibitors

Other relatively non-selective amine uptake inhibitors (serotonin/noradrenaline reuptake inhibitors, or 'SNRIs'[4]) include **venlafaxine** and **duloxetine** (see Table 39.4).

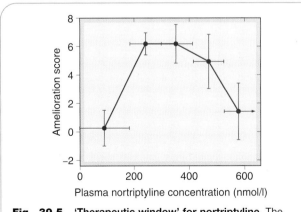

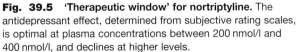

Fig. 39.5 'Therapeutic window' for nortriptyline. The antidepressant effect, determined from subjective rating scales, is optimal at plasma concentrations between 200 nmol/l and 400 nmol/l, and declines at higher levels.

---

[4]Don't be misled by a marketing term for a less selective drug than an SSRI.

> ### Tricyclic antidepressants
>
> - Tricyclic antidepressants are chemically related to phenothiazines, and some have similar non-selective receptor-blocking actions.
> - Important examples are imipramine, amitriptyline and clomipramine.
> - Most are long-acting, and they are often converted to active metabolites.
> - Important side effects: sedation (H_1 block); postural hypotension (α-adrenoceptor block); dry mouth, blurred vision, constipation (muscarinic block); occasionally mania and convulsions. Risk of ventricular dysrhythmias due to HERG channel block.
> - Dangerous in acute overdose: confusion and mania, cardiac dysrhythmias.
> - Liable to interact with other drugs (e.g. alcohol, anaesthetics, hypotensive drugs and non-steroidal anti-inflammatory drugs; should not be given with monoamine oxidase inhibitors).

> ### Clinical uses of tricyclic antidepressants and related drugs
>
> - Tricyclic antidepressants (e.g. **amitriptyline**, **imipramine**) and related drugs (e.g. **trazodone**) are used:
>   - for moderate to severe *endogenous depression*, especially with psychomotor features such as insomnia (a sedating drug such as **amitriptyline** is used) or poor appetite; **trazodone** has less marked antimuscarinic effects
>   - for *panic* and related disorders (e.g. **clomipramine** for obsessional and phobic states)
>   - for *neuropathic pain* (e.g. postherpetic and other forms of neuralgia; see Ch. 41)
>   - short-term treatment of nocturnal enuresis in older children (Ch. 24).
> - Points to note are as follow.
>   - Onset of action is slow: treatment should be for at least 4–6 weeks before concluding that an individual drug is ineffective. If there is a partial response, treatment should be continued for several more weeks before increasing the dose. Treatment should continue for at least 4 months following remission. Withdrawal is tapered over several weeks.
>   - Tricyclic antidepressants cause severe cardiotoxicity (dysrhythmia) in overdose; suicide risk should be assessed before prescribing.

SELECTIVE 5-HYDROXYTRYPTAMINE UPTAKE INHIBITORS

Drugs of this type (often termed *selective serotonin reuptake inhibitors* or *SSRIs*) include **fluoxetine**, **fluvoxamine**, **paroxetine**, **citalopram** and **sertraline** (see Table 39.4). They are the most commonly prescribed group of antidepressants. As well as showing selectivity with respect to 5-HT over noradrenaline uptake, they are less likely than TCAs to cause anticholinergic side effects and are less dangerous in overdose. In contrast to MAOIs (see below), they do not cause 'cheese reactions'. They are as effective as TCAs and MAOIs in treating depression of moderate degree, but probably less effective than TCAs in treating severe depression. They are also used to treat a particular type of anxiety disorder known as *obsessive compulsive disorder* (see Ch. 37).

Pharmacokinetic aspects

The SSRIs are well absorbed, and most have plasma half-lives of 15–24 hours (**fluoxetine** is longer acting: 24–96 hours). The delay of 2–4 weeks before the therapeutic effect develops is similar to that seen with other antidepressants. **Paroxetine** and **fluoxetine** are not used in combination with TCAs, whose hepatic metabolism they inhibit, for fear of increasing TCA toxicity.

Unwanted effects

Common side effects are nausea, anorexia, insomnia, loss of libido and failure of orgasm.

In combination with MAOIs, SSRIs can cause a 'serotonin syndrome' characterised by *tremor*, *hyperthermia* and *cardio-vascular collapse*, from which deaths have occurred.

There have been reports of increased aggression, and occasionally violence, in patients treated with fluoxetine, but these have not been confirmed by controlled studies. The use of SSRIs is not recommended for treating depression in children under 18, in whom efficacy is doubtful and adverse effects, including excitement, insomnia and aggression in the first few weeks of treatment, may occur. The possibility of increased suicidal ideation is a concern in this age group.

Despite the apparent advantages of 5-HT uptake inhibitors over TCAs in terms of side effects, the combined results of many trials show no overall difference in terms of patient acceptability (Song et al., 1993).

5-HT uptake inhibitors are used in a variety of psychiatric disorders, as well as in depression, including anxiety disorders, panic attacks and obsessive compulsive disorder.

MONOAMINE OXIDASE INHIBITORS

Monoamine oxidase inhibitors (MAOIs) were among the first drugs to be introduced clinically as antidepressants but were largely superseded by tricyclic and other types of antidepressants, whose clinical efficacies were considered better and whose side effects are generally less than those of MAOIs. The main examples are **phenelzine**, **tranylcypromine** and **iproniazid**. These drugs cause irreversible inhibition of the enzyme and do not distinguish between the two main isozymes (see below). Recently, the discovery of reversible inhibitors that show isozyme selectivity has rekindled

---

> ### Selective serotonin reuptake inhibitors (SSRIs) 🔑
>
> - Examples include fluoxetine, fluvoxamine, paroxetine, sertraline, citalopram. Venlafoxine is a less selective 5-HT uptake inhibitor.
> - Antidepressant actions are similar in efficacy and time course to those of TCA.
> - Acute toxicity (especially cardiotoxicity) is less than that of MAOI or TCA, so overdose risk is reduced.
> - Side effects include nausea, insomnia and sexual dysfunction. SSRI are less sedating and have less antimuscarinic side effects than the older TCAs.
> - No food reactions, but dangerous 'serotonin reaction' (hyperthermia, muscle rigidity, cardiovascular collapse) can occur if given with MAOI.
> - Currently the most commonly prescribed antidepressants; also used for some other psychiatric indications. Venlafaxine is licensed to treat generalized anxiety disorder as well as depressive illness.
> - There is concern about the use of SSRI in children and aolescents, due to reports of an increase in suicidal thoughts on starting treatment.

> ### Other monoamine uptake inhibitors 🔑
>
> - Group of noradrenaline-selective (e.g. reboxetine) or non-selective (e.g. venlafaxine, duloxetine) inhibitors.
> - Generally similar to tricyclic antidepressants but lack major receptor-blocking actions, so fewer side effects.
> - Less risk of cardiac effects, so safer in overdose than tricyclic antidepressants.

interest in this class of drug. Although several studies have shown a reduction in platelet MAO activity in certain groups of depressed patients, there is no clear evidence that abnormal MAO activity is involved in the pathogenesis of depression.

Monoamine oxidase (see Ch. 11) is found in nearly all tissues, and exists in two similar molecular forms coded by separate genes (see Table 39.3). MAO-A has a substrate preference for 5-HT and is the main target for the antidepressant MAOIs. MAO-B has a substrate preference for phenylethylamine, and both enzymes act on noradrenaline and dopamine. Type B is selectively inhibited by **selegiline**, which is used in the treatment of parkinsonism (see Ch. 35). Disruption of the MAO-A gene in mice causes increased brain accumulation of 5-HT and, to a lesser extent, noradrenaline, along with aggressive behaviour (Shih et al., 1999). A family has been reported with an inherited mutation leading to loss of MAO-A activity, whose members showed mental retardation and violent behaviour patterns. Most antidepressant MAOIs act on both forms of MAO, but clinical

Table 39.3 Substrates and inhibitors for type A and type B monoamine oxldase

	Type A	Type B
Preferred substrates	Noradrenaline 5-Hydroxytryptamine	Phenylethylamine Benzylamine
Non-specific substrates	Dopamine Tyramine	Dopamine Tyramine
Specific inhibitors	Clorgiline Moclobemide	Selegiline
Non-specific inhibitors	Pargyline Tranylcypromine Isocarboxazid	Pargyline Tranylcypromine Isocarboxazid

studies with subtype-specific inhibitors have shown clearly that antidepressant activity, as well as the main side effects of MAOIs, is associated with MAO-A inhibition. MAO is located intracellularly, mostly associated with mitochondria, and has two main functions.

- Within nerve terminals, MAO regulates the free intraneuronal concentration of noradrenaline or 5-HT, and hence the releasable stores of these transmitters. It is not involved in the inactivation of released transmitter. The biochemical role of MAO in noradrenergic nerves and the effect of MAOI on transmitter metabolism are discussed in Chapter 11.
- MAO is important in the inactivation of endogenous and ingested amines that would otherwise produce unwanted effects. An example is *tyramine*, an ingested amine that is a substrate for both MAO-A and MAO-B, and is important in producing some clinically important adverse interactions of MAOIs with foods and other drugs (see below).

Chemical aspects

Monoamine oxidase inhibitors are substrate analogues with a phenylethylamine-like structure, and most contain a reactive group (e.g. hydrazine, propargylamine, cyclopropylamine) that enables the inhibitor to bind covalently to the enzyme, resulting in a non-competitive and long-lasting inhibition. Recovery of MAO activity after inhibition takes several weeks with most drugs, but is quicker after **tranylcypromine**, which forms a less stable bond with the enzyme. **Moclobemide** acts as a reversible competitive inhibitor.

Monoamine oxidase inhibitors are not particularly specific in their actions, and inhibit a variety of other enzymes as well as MAO, including many enzymes involved in the metabolism of other drugs. This is responsible for some of the many clinically important drug interactions associated with MAOIs.

Pharmacological effects

Monoamine oxidase inhibitors cause a rapid and sustained increase in the 5-HT, noradrenaline and dopamine content of the brain, 5-HT being affected most and dopamine least. Similar changes occur in peripheral tissues such as heart, liver and intestine, and increases in the plasma concentrations of these amines are also detectable. Although these increases in tissue amine content are largely due to accumulation within neurons, transmitter release in response to nerve activity is not increased. In contrast to the effect of TCAs, MAOIs do not increase the response of peripheral organs, such as the heart and blood vessels, to sympathetic nerve stimulation. The main effect of MAOIs is to increase the cytoplasmic concentration of monoamines in nerve terminals, without greatly affecting the vesicular stores that form the pool that is releasable by nerve stimulation. The increased cytoplasmic pool results in an increased rate of spontaneous leakage of monoamines, and also an increased release by indirectly acting sympathomimetic amines such as **amphetamine** and **tyramine** (see Ch. 11). This occurs because these amines work by displacing noradrenaline from the vesicles into the nerve terminal cytoplasm, from which it may either leak out and produce a response, or be degraded by MAO (see Fig. 11.8). Inhibition of MAO increases the proportion that escapes and thus enhances the response. Tyramine thus causes a much greater rise in blood pressure in MAOI-treated animals than in controls. This mechanism is important in relation to the cheese reaction produced by MAOIs in humans (see later section).

In normal human subjects, MAOIs cause an immediate increase in motor activity, and euphoria and excitement develop over the course of a few days. This is in contrast to TCAs, which cause only sedation and confusion when given to non-depressed subjects. MAOIs (like TCAs) are also effective in reversing the behavioural effects of reserpine treatment. The effects of MAOIs on amine metabolism develop rapidly, and the effect of a single dose lasts for several days. There is a clear discrepancy, as with TCAs, between the rapid biochemical response and the delayed antidepressant effect.

The mechanisms underlying the antidepressant effects of MAOIs are not well understood, but MAOIs cause a delayed down-regulation of β-adrenoceptors and 5-HT$_2$-receptors similar to that produced by TCAs.

Unwanted effects and toxicity

Many of the unwanted effects of MAOIs result directly from MAO inhibition, but some are produced by other mechanisms.

Hypotension is a common side effect; indeed, **pargyline** was at one time used as an antihypertensive drug. One possible explanation for this effect—the opposite of what might have been expected—is that amines such as *dopamine* or *octopamine* accumulate within peripheral sympathetic nerve terminals and displace noradrenaline from the storage vesicles, thus reducing noradrenaline release associated with sympathetic activity.

Excessive central stimulation may cause tremors, excitement, insomnia and, in overdose, convulsions.

Increased appetite, leading to weight gain, can be so extreme as to require the drug to be discontinued.

Atropine-like side effects (dry mouth, blurred vision, urinary retention, etc.) are common with MAOIs, although they are less of a problem than with TCAs.

MAOIs of the hydrazine type (e.g. **phenelzine** and **iproniazid**) produce, very rarely (less than 1 in 10 000), severe hepatotoxicity,

---

Other antidepressant drugs

- Heterogeneous group including trazodone, mirtazapine and bupropion.
- No common mechanism of action. Act mainly as non-selective antagonists at presynaptic receptors, possibly enhancing amine release.
- Delay in therapeutic response is similar to that with tricyclic antidepressants and monoamine oxidase inhibitors. Mirtazapine may act more rapidly.
- Unwanted effects and acute toxicity vary but are generally less than with tricyclic antidepressants.

Monoamine oxidase inhibitors (MAOI)

- Main examples are phenelzine, tranylcypromine, isocarboxazid (irreversible, long-acting, non-selective between MAO-A and B) and moclobemide (reversible, short-acting, MAO-A-selective).
- Long acting MAOI:
  - Main side effects: postural hypotension (sympathetic block); atropine-like effects (as with TCA); weight gain; CNS stimulation, causing restlessness, insomniahepatotoxicity and neurotoxicity (rare).
  - Acute overdose causes CNS stimulation, sometimes convulsions.
  - 'Cheese reaction', ie. severe hypertensive response to tyramine-containing foods (e.g. cheese, beer, wine, well-hung game, yeast or soy extracts. Such reactions can occur up to 2 weeks after treatment is discontinued.
- Interaction with other amines (e.g. **ephedrine** in over the counter decongestants, **clomipramine** and other TCAs) and some other drugs (e.g. **pethidine**) are also potentially lethal.
- **Moclobemide** is used for major depression and social phobia. Cheese reaction and other drug interactions less severe and shorter-lasting than with long-lasting MAOIs.
- MAOI are used much less than other antidepressants because of their adverse effects and serious interactions.
- They are indicated for major depression in patients who have not responded to other drugs.

---

which seems to be due to the hydrazine moiety of the molecule. Their use in patients with liver disease is therefore unwise.

Interaction with other drugs and foods

Interaction with other drugs and foods is the most serious problem with MAOIs and is the main factor that caused their clinical use to decline. The special advantage claimed for the new reversible MAOIs, such as **moclobemide**, is that these interactions are reduced.

The *cheese reaction* is a direct consequence of MAO inhibition and occurs when normally innocuous amines (mainly tyramine) produced during fermentation are ingested. Tyramine is normally metabolised by MAO in the gut wall and liver, and little dietary tyramine reaches the systemic circulation. MAO inhibition allows tyramine to be absorbed, and also enhances its sympathomimetic effect, as discussed above. The result is acute hypertension, giving rise to a severe throbbing headache and occasionally even to intracranial haemorrhage. Although many foods contain some tyramine, it appears that at least 10 mg of tyramine needs to be ingested to produce such a response, and the main danger is from ripe cheeses and from concentrated yeast products such as Marmite. Administration of indirectly acting sympathomimetic amines (e.g. **ephedrine**, **amphetamine**) also causes severe hypertension in patients receiving MAOIs; directly acting agents such as noradrenaline (used for example in conjunction with local anaesthetics; see Ch. 44) are not hazardous. Moclobemide, a specific MAO-A inhibitor, does not cause the cheese reaction, probably because tyramine can still be metabolised by MAO-B.

Hypertensive episodes have been reported in patients given TCAs and MAOIs simultaneously. The probable explanation is that inhibition of noradrenaline reuptake further enhances the cardiovascular response to dietary tyramine, thus accentuating the cheese reaction. This combination of drugs can also produce excitement and hyperactivity.

Monoamine oxidase inhibitors can interact with **pethidine** (see Ch. 41) to cause severe hyperpyrexia, with restlessness, coma and hypotension. The mechanism is uncertain, but it is likely that an abnormal pethidine metabolite is produced because of inhibition of demethylation.

A comparison of the main characteristics of MAOIs and other antidepressant drugs is given in Table 39.4.

FUTURE ANTIDEPRESSANT DRUGS

Uncertainty about the biochemical pathogenesis of depression raises the possibility of finding new antidepressants acting on other (non–amine-related) targets. Many different approaches have been taken, and several compounds are in development (see Pacher & Kecsemeti, 2004). They include antagonists of neuropeptides—including CRH and substance P—as well as compounds active on NMDA, acetylcholine and histamine receptors, and compounds that act on the signal transduction pathways responsible for neurogenesis, neural plasticity and apoptosis. The aim is to satisfy the following criteria:

- fewer side effects (e.g. sedation and anticholinergic effects)
- lower toxicity in overdose
- rapid action
- greater efficacy (i.e. more complete relief of symptoms)
- efficacy in patients non-responsive to TCAs or MAOIs.

So far, although many compounds have shown some efficacy in clinical trials, none appear better than the existing drugs with respect to these criteria.

ELECTROCONVULSIVE THERAPY (ECT)

A faulty line of reasoning, namely that schizophrenia and epilepsy were believed to be mutually exclusive, led to the use of induced convulsions as therapy for psychological disorders in the 1930s; although useless in schizophrenia, its efficacy in treating severe depression has been repeatedly confirmed. ECT in humans involves stimulation through electrodes placed on either side of the head, with the patient lightly anaesthetised, paralysed with a short-acting neuromuscular-blocking drug (e.g. succinylcholine; Ch. 10) so as to avoid physical injury, and artificially ventilated. More recently, a technique involving transcranial magnetic stimulation, which does not require these precautions, has been introduced. Controlled trials have shown ECT to be at least as effective as antidepressant drugs, with response rates ranging between 60% and 80%; it appears to be the most effective treatment for severe suicidal depression. The main disadvantage of ECT is that it often causes confusion and memory loss lasting for days or weeks.

The effect of ECT on experimental animals has been carefully analysed to see if it provides clues as to the mode of action of antidepressant drugs, but the clues it gives are enigmatic. 5-HT synthesis and uptake are unaltered, and noradrenaline uptake is somewhat increased (in contrast to the effect of TCAs). Decreased β-adrenoceptor responsiveness, both biochemical and behavioural, occurs with both ECT and long-term administration of antidepressant drugs, but changes in 5-HT-mediated responses tend to go in opposite directions (see Maes & Meltzer, 1995).

CLINICAL EFFECTIVENESS OF ANTIDEPRESSANT TREATMENTS

The overall clinical efficacy of antidepressants has been established in many well-controlled clinical trials, although the degree of improvement is limited.[5] Moreover, it is clear that a substantial proportion of patients recover spontaneously, and that 30–40% of patients fail to improve with drug treatments. Although antidepressants produce significant benefit in patients with moderate or severe depression, their efficacy in mild cases has not been clearly demonstrated. Controlled trials show there is little to choose in terms of overall efficacy between any of the drugs currently in use, although clinical experience suggests that individual patients may, for unknown reasons, respond better to one drug than to another.

Pharmacogenetic factors

▼ The individual variation in response to antidepressants may be partly due to genetic factors, as well as to heterogeneity of the clinical condition. Two genetic factors have received particular attention, namely:

- polymorphism of the cytochrome P450 gene, especially *CYP2D6* (see Kirchheiner et al., 2004) which is responsible for hydroxylation of TCAs
- polymorphism of monoamine transporter genes (see Glatt & Reus, 2003).

Up to 10% of white people possess a dysfunctional *CYP2D6* gene, and consequently may be susceptible to side effects of TCAs and various other drugs (see Ch. 51) that are metabolised by this route. The opposite effect, caused by duplication of the gene, is common in Eastern European and East African populations, and may account for a lack of clinical efficacy in some individuals. There is some evidence to suggest that responsiveness to SSRIs is related to polymorphism of one of the serotonin transporter genes, but this remains controversial.

Although genotyping may prove to be a useful approach in the future to individualising antidepressant therapy, its practical realisation is some way off.

Suicide and antidepressants

▼ Various anecdotal reports, and some definitive studies, have suggested that antidepressants may increase the risk of 'suicidality' in depressed patients (see Licinio & Wong, 2005). The term *suicidality* encompasses suicidal thoughts and planning as well as unsuccessful attempts; actual suicide, although one of the major causes of death in young people, is much rarer than suicidality. Clinical trials to determine the relationship between antidepressants and suicidality are difficult, because of the clear association between depression and suicide, and have given variable results, with some studies suggesting that suicidality may be increased during the first few weeks of antidepressant treatment, although not thereafter, and some showing a small increase in the risk of actual suicide (see Cipriani et al., 2005). There is no evidence to suggest that SSRIs carry any greater risk than other antidepressants. Although inconclusive, these data have caused the regulatory authorities to issue warnings about the use of antidepressants. Their caution has been reinforced by detailed reappraisal of trials data, suggesting that the clinical efficacy of antidepressants is weaker than previously thought and significant only in cases of severe depression. This backlash of opinion regarding the use of antidepressants has sparked much controversy, with many clinicians arguing that, even if the suicide risk is real, for many patients the benefits greatly outweigh the risks.

MOOD-STABILISING DRUGS

These drugs are used to control the mood swings characteristic of manic-depressive (bipolar) illness. **Lithium** is most commonly used, but recently antiepileptic drugs such as **carbamazepine**, **valproate** and **gabapentin** (Ch. 40), which have fewer side effects than lithium, have also proved efficacious.

Used prophylactically in bipolar depression, mood-stabilising drugs prevent the swings of mood and thus reduce both the depressive and the manic phases of the illness. They are given over long periods, and their beneficial effects take 3–4 weeks to develop. Given in an acute attack, they are effective only in reducing mania, not during the depressive phase (although lithium is sometimes used as an adjunct to antidepressants in severe cases of unipolar depression).

LITHIUM

The psychotropic effect of lithium was discovered in 1949 by Cade, who had predicted that urate salts should prevent the induction by uraemia of a hyperexcitability state in guinea pigs. He found lithium urate to produce an effect, quickly discovered

---

[5]Placebo responses are particularly evident in antidepressant trials, patients being influenced by the attitude of the prescriber, who is in turn influenced by claims for the latest in a long line of drugs. A nightmare for hospital formulary committees!

Table 39.4   Types of antidepressant drugs and their characteristics

Type and examples	Action(s)	Unwanted effects	Risk of overdose	Pharmacokinetics	Notes
		MONOAMINE UPTAKE INHIBITORS			
TCA group	Inhibition of NA/5-HT reuptake	Sedation Anticholinergic effects (dry mouth, constipation, blurred vision, urinary retention, etc.) Postural hypotension Seizures Impotence Interaction with CNS depressants (especially alcohol, MAO inhibitors)	Ventricular dysrhythmias High risk in combination with CNS depressants	–	'First-generation' antidepressants, still very widely used, although newer compounds generally have fewer side effects and lower risk with overdose
Imipramine	Non-selective	As above	As above	$t_{1/2}$ 4–18 h; converted to desipramine	–
Desipramine	NA-selective	As above	As above	$t_{1/2}$ 12–24 h	–
Amitriptyline	Non-selective	As above	As above	$t_{1/2}$ 12–24 h; converted to nortriptyline	Widely used, also for neuropathic pain (Ch. 41)
Nortriptyline	NA-selective (slight)	As above	As above	Long $t_{1/2}$ (24–96 h)	Long duration, less sedative
Clomipramine	Non-selective	As above	As above	$t_{1/2}$ 18–24 h	Also used for anxiety disorders
Other non-selective uptake inhibitors Venlafaxine	Weak non-selective NA/5-HT uptake inhibitor Also non-selective receptor-blocking effects	As SSRIs (see below) Withdrawal effects common and troublesome if doses are missed	Safe in overdose	Short $t_{1/2}$ (~5 h)	Claimed to act more rapidly than other antidepressants, and to work better in 'treatment-resistant' patients Usually classed as non-selective NA/5-HT uptake blocker, although in vitro data show selectivity for 5-HT
St John's wort (active principle: hyperforin)	Weak non-selective NA/5-HT uptake inhibitor Also non-selective receptor-blocking effects	Few side effects reported	Risk of drug interactions due to enhanced drug metabolism (e.g. loss of efficacy of ciclosporin, antidiabetic drugs etc)	$t_{1/2}$ ~12 h	Freely available as crude herbal preparation Similar efficacy to other antidepressants, with fewer acute side effects but risk of serious drug interactions (see text)
Duloxetine	Potent non-selective NA/5-HT uptake inhibitor No action on monoamine receptors	Fewer side effects than venlafaxine Sedation, dizziness, nausea Sexual dysfunction	–	$t_{1/2}$ ~14 h	Also used to treat urinary incontinence (see Ch. 25) and for anxiety disorders

Table 39.4 (cont'd) Types of antidepressant drugs and their characteristics

Type and examples	Action(s)	Unwanted effects	Risk of overdose	Pharmacokinetics	Notes
Bupropion	Weak inhibitor of dopamine and NA uptake Mechanism poorly understood	Headache, dry mouth, agitation, insomnia	Seizures at high doses	$t_{1/2}$ ~12 h	Plasma half-life ~20 h Used mainly in depression associated with anxiety Slow-release formulation used to treat nicotine dependence (Ch. 43)
SSRIs	All highly selective for 5-HT	Nausea, diarrhoea, agitation, insomnia, anorgasmia Inhibit metabolism of other drugs, so risk of interactions	Low risk in overdose but must not be used in combination with MAO inhibitors	–	–
Fluoxetine	As above	As above	As above	Long $t_{1/2}$ (24–96 h)	–
Fluvoxamine	As above	As above	As above	$t_{1/2}$ 18–24 h	Less nausea than with other SSRIs
Paroxetine	As above	As above	As above	$t_{1/2}$ 18–24 h	Withdrawal reaction
Citalopram	As above	As above	As above	$t_{1/2}$ 24–36 h	Escitalopram is active S isomer of citalopram Fewer side effects reported
Sertraline	As above	As above	As above	$t_{1/2}$ 24–36 h	–
NA-selective uptake inhibitors Maprotiline	Selective NA uptake inhibitor	As TCAs; no significant advantages	As TCAs	Long $t_{1/2}$ ~40 h	No significant advantages over TCAs
Reboxetine	Selective NA uptake inhibitor	Dizziness Insomnia Anticholinergic effects	Safe in overdose (low risk of cardiac dysrhythmia)	$t_{1/2}$ ~12 h	Safer and fewer side effects than TCAs
MAO INHIBITORS					
	Inhibit MAO-A and/or MAO-B Earlier compounds have long duration of action due to covalent binding to enzyme				
Phenelzine	Non-selective	'Cheese reaction' to tyramine-containing foods (see text) Anticholinergic side effects Hypotension Insomnia Weight gain Liver damage (rare)	Many interactions (TCAs, opioids, sympathomimetic drugs)—risk of severe hypertension due to cheese reaction	$t_{1/2}$ 1–2 h Long duration of action due to irreversible binding	–

Table 39.4 (cont'd) Types of antidepressant drugs and their characteristics

Type and examples	Action(s)	Unwanted effects	Risk of overdose	Pharmacokinetics	Notes
Tranylcypromine	Non-selective	As phenelzine	As phenelzine	$t_{1/2}$ 1–2 h Long duration of action due to irreversible binding	–
Isocarboxazid	Non-selective	As phenelzine	As phenelzine	Long $t_{1/2}$ ~36 h	–
Moclobemide	MAO-A–selective Short acting	Nausea Insomnia, agitation	Interactions less severe than with other MAO inhibitors; no cheese reactions reported	$t_{1/2}$ 1–2 h	Safer alternative to earlier MAO inhibitors
MISCELLANEOUS ANTIDEPRESSANTS					
Trazodone	Weak 5-HT uptake inhibitor Also blocks 5-HT$_2$ and H$_1$ receptors (enhances NA/5-HT release)	Sedation Hypotension Cardiac dysrhythmias	Safe in overdose	$t_{1/2}$ 6–12 h	Nefazodone and mianserin are similar
Mirtazapine	Blocks α_2, 5-HT$_2$ and 5-HT$_3$ receptors	Dry mouth Sedation Weight gain	No serious drug interactions	$t_{1/2}$ 20–40 h	Claimed to have faster onset of action than other antidepressants

that it was due to lithium rather than urate, and went on to show that lithium produced a rapid improvement in a group of manic patients. Adoption of lithium for prophylaxis of mania was delayed in the USA by earlier American experience of lithium as an over-the-counter salt substitute for patients recommended a low salt diet because of heart failure, in whom it caused severe toxicity.

Other drugs (e.g. antipsychotics) are equally effective in treating acute mania; they act more quickly and are considerably safer, so the clinical use of lithium is mainly confined to prophylactic control of manic-depressive illness.

Pharmacological effects and mechanism of action

Lithium is clinically effective at a plasma concentration of 0.5–1 mmol/l, and above 1.5 mmol/l it produces a variety of toxic effects, so the therapeutic window is narrow. In normal subjects, 1 mmol/l lithium in plasma has no appreciable psychotropic effects. It does, however, produce many detectable biochemical changes, and it is still unclear how these may be related to its therapeutic effect.

Lithium is a monovalent cation that can mimic the role of Na^+ in excitable tissues, being able to permeate the voltage-gated Na^+ channels that are responsible for action potential generation (see Ch. 4). It is, however, not pumped out by the Na^+/K^+ ATPase, and therefore tends to accumulate inside excitable cells, leading to a partial loss of intracellular K^+, and depolarisation of the cell.

The biochemical effects of lithium are complex, and it inhibits many enzymes that participate in signal transduction pathways. Its therapeutic actions are generally ascribed to two mechanisms (see Phiel & Klein, 2001).

- Inhibition of inositol monophosphatase, which blocks the phosphatidyl inositol (PI) pathway (see Ch. 3) at the point where inositol phosphate is hydrolysed to free inositol, resulting in depletion of PI. This prevents agonist-stimulated inositol trisphosphate formation through various PI-linked receptors, and therefore blocks many receptor-mediated effects.
- Inhibition of glycogen synthase kinase, which phosphorylates a number of key enzymes involved in pathways leading to apoptosis and amyloid formation (see Phiel & Klein, 2001).

Lithium also inhibits hormone-induced cAMP production and blocks other cellular responses (e.g. the response of renal tubular cells to antidiuretic hormone, and of the thyroid to thyroid-stimulating hormone; see Chs 24 and 29, respectively). This is not, however, a pronounced effect in the brain.

The cellular selectivity of lithium appears to depend on its selective uptake, reflecting the activity of sodium channels in different cells. This could explain its relatively selective action in the brain and kidney, even though many other tissues use the same second messengers. Notwithstanding such insights, our ignorance of the nature of the disturbance underlying the mood swings in bipolar depression leaves us groping for links between the biochemical and prophylactic effects of lithium.

Pharmacokinetic aspects and toxicity

Lithium is given by mouth as the carbonate salt and is excreted by the kidney. About half of an oral dose is excreted within about 12 hours—the remainder, which presumably represents lithium taken up by cells, is excreted over the next 1–2 weeks. This very slow phase means that, with regular dosage, lithium accumulates slowly over 2 weeks or more before a steady state is reached. The narrow therapeutic window (approximately 0.5–1.5 mmol/l) means that monitoring of the plasma concentration is essential. Na^+ depletion reduces the rate of excretion by increasing the reabsorption of lithium by the proximal tubule, and thus increases the likelihood of toxicity. Diuretics that act distal to the proximal tubule (Ch. 24) also have this effect, and renal disease also predisposes to lithium toxicity.

The main toxic effects that may occur during treatment are as follows.

- Nausea, vomiting and diarrhoea.
- Tremor.
- Renal effects: polyuria (with resulting thirst) resulting from inhibition of the action of antidiuretic hormone. At the same time, there is some Na^+ retention associated with increased aldosterone secretion. With prolonged treatment, serious renal tubular damage may occur, making it essential to monitor renal function regularly in lithium-treated patients.

- Thyroid enlargement, sometimes associated with hypothyroidism.
- Weight gain.

Acute lithium toxicity results in various neurological effects, progressing from confusion and motor impairment to coma, convulsions and death if the plasma concentration reaches 3–5 mmol/l.

Mood-stabilising drugs

- Inorganic ion taken orally as lithium carbonate.
- Mechanism of action is not understood. The main biochemical possibilities are:
  — interference with inositol trisphosphate formation
  — inhibition of kinases.
- Alternative drugs (e.g. carbamazepine, valproate, gabapentin) are gaining favour for treatment of mania, because of better side effect and safety profile.

Clinical use of mood-stabilising drugs

- **Lithium** (as the carbonate) is the main drug. It is used:
  — in prophylaxis and treatment of *mania*, and in the prophylaxis of *bipolar* or *unipolar disorder* (manic depression or recurrent depression).
- Points to note include:
  — there is a narrow therapeutic window and long duration of action
  — acute toxic effects include cerebellar effects, nephrogenic diabetes insipidus (see Ch. 24) and renal failure
  — dose must be adjusted according to the plasma concentration
  — elimination is via the kidney and is reduced by proximal tubular reabsorption. Diuretics increase the activity of the reabsorptive mechanism and hence can precipitate lithium toxicity
  — thyroid disorders and mild cognitive impairment occur during chronic use.
- **Carbamazepine** and **valproic acid** (sodium channel blockers with antiepileptic, Ch. 40, and analgesic action, Ch. 41) are used, respectively, for the prophylaxis and treatment of manic episodes in patients with bipolar disorder unresponsive to lithium.

REFERENCES AND FURTHER READING

Pathogenesis of depressive illness

Baker G B, Dewhurst W G 1985 Biochemical theories of affective disorders. In: Dewhurst W G, Baker G B (eds) Pharmacotherapy of affective disorders. Croom Helm, Beckenham (*Useful review of earlier hypotheses relating monoamine disturbances to mood disorders*)

Charney D S, Manji M K 2004 Life stress, genes and depression: multiple pathways lead to increased risk and new opportunities for intervention. http://www.stke.org (*Detailed review of current understanding of the pathophysiology of depression, emphasising the role of neural plasticity, neurogenesis and apoptosis*)

Duman R S 2004 Depression: a case of neuronal life and death? Biol Psychiatry 56: 140–145 (*Reviews evidence suggesting that neuronal loss in the hippocampus and prefrontal cortex results in depressive symptoms, and*

that antidepressants act indirectly to promote neurogenesis)

Maes M, Meltzer H Y 1995 The serotonin hypothesis of major depression. In: Bloom F E, Kupfer D J (eds) Psychopharmacology: the fourth generation of progress. Raven Press, New York (*Review showing how emphasis has shifted towards the involvement of 5-HT, rather than noradrenaline, in the aetiology of depression*)

Manji H K, Drevets W C, Charney D S 2001 The cellular neurobiology of depression. Nat Med 7: 541–547 (*Speculative review of the possible mechanisms and role of neurodegeneration and neuroplasticity in depressive disorders, attempting to move beyond the monoamine theory*)

Porsolt R D 1985 Animal models of affective disorders. In: Dewhurst W G, Baker G B (eds) Pharmacotherapy of affective disorders. Croom Helm, Beckenham

(*Useful review of animal models, still mainly valid despite date*)

Santarelli L, Saxe M, Gross C et al. 2003 Requirement of hippocampal neurogenesis for the behavioural effects of antidepressants. Science 301: 805–809 (*Study in rats suggesting that growth of new hippocampal neurons is responsible for antidepressant effects; commentary in same issue of* Science, p. 757)

Shih J C, Chen K, Ridd M J 1999 Monoamine oxidase: from genes to behaviour. Annu Rev Neurosci 22: 197–217 (*Review of recent work on transgenic mice with MAO mutation or deletion*)

Wong M-L, Licinio J 2001 Research and treatment approaches to depression. Nat Rev Neurosci 2: 343–351 (*Excellent summary of the current—somewhat patchy—state of knowledge about the biochemical and genetic basis of depression, and the mechanism of action of antidepressant drugs)*

Antidepressant drugs

Bosker F J, Westerink B H, Cremers T I et al. 2004 Future antidepressants: what is in the pipeline and what is missing? CNS Drugs 18: 705–732 (*Focuses on new approaches to development of antidepressants*)

Cipriani A, Barbui C, Geddes J R 2005 Suicide, depression, and antidepressants. Br Med J 330: 373–374 (*Comment on detailed trials data in the same issue of the journal*)

Glatt C E, Reus V I 2003 Pharmacogenetics of monoamine transporters. Pharmacogenomics 4: 583–596 (*Discusses prospects for correlating transporter gene polymorphism to variation in response to psychoactive drugs*)

Holsboer F 1999 The rationale for corticotrophin-releasing hormone receptor (CRH-R) antagonists to treat depression and anxiety. J Psychiatr Res 33: 181–214 (*Reviews the evidence linking CRH with depressive illness*)

Kirchheiner J, Nickchen K, Bauer M et al. 2004 Pharmacogenetics of antidepressants and antipsychotics: the contribution of allelic variations to the phenotype of drug response. Mol Psychiatry 9: 442–473 (*Discusses effect of gene polymorphisms on antidepressant actions; principles are not yet incorporated into clinical practice*)

Licinio J, Wong M-L 2005 Depression, antidepressants and suicidality: a critical appraisal. Nat Rev Drug Discov 4: 165–171 (*Review of the equivocal evidence linking antidepressant use to suicide*)

Pacher P, Kecsemeti V 2004 Trends in the development of new antidepressants. Is there light at the end of the tunnel? Curr Med Chem 11: 925–943 (*Discusses new developments from the starting point of the monoamine theory*)

Song F, Freemantle N, Sheldon T A et al. 1993 Selective serotonin reuptake inhibitors: meta-analysis of efficacy and acceptability. Br Med J 306: 683–687 (*Summary of clinical trials data, showing limitations as well as advantages of SSRIs*)

Lithium

Phiel C J, Klein P S 2001 Molecular targets of lithium action. Annu Rev Pharmacol Toxicol 41: 789–813 (*Review of a topic that is still little understood*)

Antiepileptic drugs

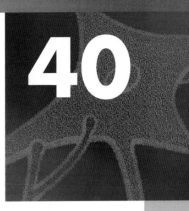

40

OVERVIEW

Epilepsy is a very common disorder, characterised by *seizures*, which take various forms and result from episodic neuronal discharges, the form of the seizure depending on the part of the brain affected. Epilepsy affects 0.5–1% of the population. Often, there is no recognisable cause, although it may develop after brain damage, such as trauma, infection or tumour growth, or other kinds of neurological disease, including various inherited neurological syndromes. Epilepsy is treated mainly with drugs, although brain surgery may be used for a very few suitable severe cases. Current antiepileptic drugs are effective in controlling seizures in about 70% of cases, but their use is often limited by side effects. In addition to their use in patients with epilepsy, antiepileptic drugs are used to treat or prevent convulsions caused by other brain diseases, for example trauma (including following neurosurgery), infection (as an adjunct to antibiotics), brain tumours and following cerebral infarction. For this reason, they are sometimes termed *anticonvulsants* rather than *antiepileptics*. A separate important use discussed in Chapter 41 is in

treating neuropathic pain. Many new antiepileptic drugs have been developed in the past 15–20 years —one of the most active areas of drug development— in attempts to improve their efficacy and side effect profile. Improvements have been steady rather than spectacular, and epilepsy remains a difficult problem, despite the fact that controlling reverberative neuronal discharges would seem, on the face of it, to be a much simpler problem than controlling those aspects of brain function that determine emotions, mood and cognitive function.

In this chapter, we describe the nature of epilepsy, the neurobiological mechanisms underlying it, and the animal models that can be used to study it. We then proceed to describe the various classes of drugs that are used to treat it, the mechanisms by which they work and their pharmacological characteristics. More information on the topics covered here is given by Eadie & Vajda (1999) and Levy et al. (2002).

Centrally acting muscle relaxants are discussed briefly at the end of the chapter.

THE NATURE OF EPILEPSY

The characteristic event in epilepsy is the *seizure*, which is associated with the episodic high-frequency discharge of impulses by a group of neurons in the brain. What starts as a local abnormal discharge may then spread to other areas of the brain. The site of the primary discharge and the extent of its spread determine the symptoms that are produced, which range from a brief lapse of attention to a full convulsive fit lasting for several minutes, as well as odd sensations or behaviours. The particular symptoms produced depend on the function of the region of the brain that is affected. Thus involvement of the motor cortex causes convulsions; involvement of the hypothalamus causes peripheral autonomic discharge, and involvement of the reticular formation in the upper brain stem leads to loss of consciousness.

Abnormal electrical activity during and following a seizure can be detected by electroencephalography (EEG) recording from electrodes distributed over the surface of the scalp. Various types of seizure can be recognised on the basis of the nature and distribution of the abnormal discharge (Fig. 40.1).

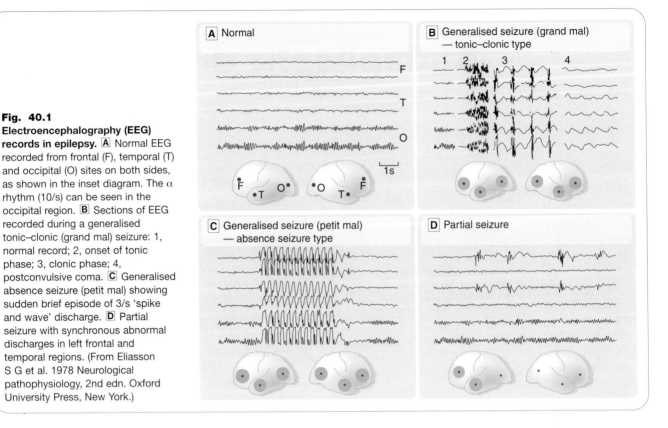

Fig. 40.1
Electroencephalography (EEG) records in epilepsy. [A] Normal EEG recorded from frontal (F), temporal (T) and occipital (O) sites on both sides, as shown in the inset diagram. The α rhythm (10/s) can be seen in the occipital region. [B] Sections of EEG recorded during a generalised tonic–clonic (grand mal) seizure: 1, normal record; 2, onset of tonic phase; 3, clonic phase; 4, postconvulsive coma. [C] Generalised absence seizure (petit mal) showing sudden brief episode of 3/s 'spike and wave' discharge. [D] Partial seizure with synchronous abnormal discharges in left frontal and temporal regions. (From Eliasson S G et al. 1978 Neurological pathophysiology, 2nd edn. Oxford University Press, New York.)

[A] Normal

[B] Generalised seizure (grand mal) — tonic–clonic type

[C] Generalised seizure (petit mal) — absence seizure type

[D] Partial seizure

TYPES OF EPILEPSY

The clinical classification of epilepsy defines two major categories, namely *partial* and *generalised* seizures, although there is some overlap and many varieties of each. Either form is classified as *simple* (if consciousness is not lost) or *complex* (if consciousness is lost).

PARTIAL SEIZURES

Partial seizures are those in which the discharge begins locally and often remains localised. The symptoms depend on the brain region or regions involved, and include involuntary muscle contractions, abnormal sensory experiences or autonomic discharge, or effects on mood and behaviour, often termed *psychomotor epilepsy*. The EEG discharge in this type of epilepsy is normally confined to one hemisphere (Fig. 40.1D). Partial seizures can often be attributed to local cerebral lesions, and their incidence increases with age. In complex partial seizures, loss of consciousness may occur at the outset of the attack, or somewhat later, when the discharge has spread from its site of origin to regions of the brain stem reticular formation.

An epileptic focus in the motor cortex results in attacks, sometimes called *jacksonian epilepsy*,[1] consisting of repetitive jerking of a particular muscle group, beginning on one side of the body, often in the thumb, big toe or angle of the mouth, which spreads and may involve much of the body within about 2 minutes before dying out. The patient loses voluntary control of the affected parts of the body but does not necessarily lose consciousness. In *psychomotor epilepsy*, which is often associated with a focus in the temporal lobe, the attack may consist of stereotyped purposive movements such as rubbing or patting movements, or much more complex behaviour such as dressing, walking or hair combing. The seizure usually lasts for a few minutes, after which the patient recovers with no recollection of the event. The behaviour during the seizure can be bizarre and accompanied by a strong emotional response.

GENERALISED SEIZURES

Generalised seizures involve the whole brain, including the reticular system, thus producing abnormal electrical activity throughout both hemispheres. Immediate loss of consciousness is characteristic of generalised seizures. Two important categories are *tonic–clonic seizures* (grand mal, Fig. 40.1B) and *absence seizures* (petit mal, Fig. 40.1C). A tonic–clonic seizure consists of an initial strong contraction of the whole musculature, causing a rigid extensor spasm and an involuntary cry. Respiration stops, and defecation, micturition and salivation often occur. This tonic phase lasts for about 1 minute, during which the face is suffused and becomes blue (an important clinical distinction from syncope, the main disorder from which fits must be distinguished, where the face is ashen pale), and is followed by a series of violent, synchronous jerks that gradually die out in 2–4 minutes. The patient stays unconscious for a few more minutes and then gradually recovers,

[1] After Hughlings Jackson, a distinguished 19th century Yorkshire neurologist who published his outstanding work in the *Annals of the West Riding Lunatic Asylum.*

feeling ill and confused. Injury may occur during the convulsive episode. The EEG shows generalised continuous high-frequency activity in the tonic phase and an intermittent discharge in the clonic phase.

Absence seizures occur in children; they are much less dramatic but may occur more frequently (many seizures each day) than tonic–clonic seizures. The patient abruptly ceases whatever he or she was doing, sometimes stopping speaking in mid-sentence, and stares vacantly for a few seconds, with little or no motor disturbance. Patients are unaware of their surroundings and recover abruptly with no after-effects. The EEG pattern shows a characteristic rhythmic discharge during the period of the seizure (Fig. 40.1C). The rhythmicity appears to be due to oscillatory feedback between the cortex and the thalamus, the special properties of the thalamic neurons being dependent on the calcium channels that they express (see Willoughby, 1999). The pattern differs from that of partial seizures, where a high-frequency asynchronous discharge spreads out from a local focus. Accordingly (see below), the drugs used specifically to treat absence seizures act mainly by blocking calcium channels, whereas drugs effective against other types of epilepsy act mainly by blocking sodium channels or enhancing GABA-mediated inhibition.

A particularly severe kind of epilepsy, *Lennox–Gastaut syndrome*, occurs in children and is associated with progressive mental retardation, possibly a reflection of excitotoxic neuro-degeneration (see Ch. 35). About one-third of cases of epilepsy are familial, and a few specific gene defects accounting for rare forms of the disorder have been identified (see Steinlein, 2004). Most of these encode neuronal ion channels closely involved in controlling action potential generation (see Ch. 4), such as voltage-gated sodium and potassium channels, $GABA_A$ receptors and nicotinic acetylcholine receptors. Other genes of unknown function may also be involved,[2] and it is clear that seizures can be the end result of many kinds of disorder at the cellular level. Therefore—a familiar theme in central nervous system drugs—antiepileptic drugs aim to inhibit the abnormal neuronal discharge rather than to correct the underlying cause.

With optimal drug therapy, epilepsy is controlled completely in about 75% of patients, but about 10% (50 000 in Britain) continue to have seizures at intervals of 1 month or less, which severely disrupts their life and work. There is therefore a need to improve the efficacy of therapy.

Status epilepticus refers to continuous uninterrupted seizures, requiring emergency medical treatment

NEURAL MECHANISMS AND ANIMAL MODELS OF EPILEPSY

▼ The underlying neuronal abnormality in epilepsy is poorly understood. In general, excitation will naturally tend to spread throughout a network of interconnected neurons but is normally prevented from doing so by inhibitory mechanisms. Thus *epileptogenesis* can arise if excitatory transmission is facilitated or inhibitory transmission is reduced. In certain respects, epileptogenesis resembles long-term potentiation (Ch. 33), and similar types of use-dependent synaptic plasticity may be involved (see Kulmann et al., 2000). Because detailed studies are difficult to carry out on epileptic patients, many different animal models of epilepsy have been investigated (see Sarkisian, 2001). These include a variety of genetic strains that show epilepsy-like characteristics (e.g. mice that convulse briefly in response to certain sounds, baboons that show photically induced seizures, and beagles with an inherited abnormality that closely resembles human epilepsy). Recently, several transgenic mouse strains have been reported that show spontaneous seizures. They include knockout mutations of various ion channels, receptors and other synaptic proteins. It is too early to say whether these will be useful as models of human epilepsy. Local cortical damage (e.g. by applying aluminium oxide paste or crystals of a cobalt salt) results in focal epilepsy. Local application of **penicillin** crystals has a similar effect, probably by interfering with inhibitory synaptic transmission. Convulsant drugs such as **pentylenetetrazol** (**PTZ**; see Ch. 42) are often used, particularly in the testing of antiepileptic agents, and seizures caused by electrical stimulation of the whole brain are used for the same purpose. It has been found empirically that drugs that inhibit PTZ-induced convulsions and

> **Nature of epilepsy**
>
> - Epilepsy affects about 0.5% of the population.
> - The characteristic event is the seizure, which may be associated with convulsions but often takes other forms.
> - The seizure is caused by an asynchronous high-frequency discharge of a group of neurons, starting locally and spreading to a varying extent to affect other parts of the brain. In absence seizures, the discharge is regular and oscillatory.
> - Partial seizures affect localised brain regions, and the attack may involve mainly motor, sensory or behavioural phenomena. Unconsciousness occurs when the reticular formation is involved. Generalised seizures affect the whole brain.
> - Two common forms of epilepsy are the tonic–clonic fit (grand mal) and the absence seizure (petit mal). Status epilepticus is a life-threatening condition in which seizure activity is uninterrupted.
> - Many animal models have been devised, including electrically and chemically induced generalised seizures, production of local chemical damage, and kindling. These provide good prediction of antiepileptic drug effects in humans.
> - The neurochemical basis of the abnormal discharge is not well understood. It may be associated with enhanced excitatory amino acid transmission, impaired inhibitory transmission, or abnormal electrical properties of the affected cells. Several susceptibility genes, mainly encoding neuronal ion channels, have been identified.
> - Repeated epileptic discharge can cause neuronal death (excitotoxicity).
> - Current drug therapy is effective in 70–80% of patients.

---

[2]In one type, the mutation turned out to be in a ubiquitous endogenous protease inhibitor, cystatin B, previously unsuspected of any connection with neuronal function. Comment of an expert in epilepsy genetics, quoted in *Science*: 'Boy, what a surprising thing!'

raise the threshold for production of electrically induced seizures are generally effective against absence seizures, whereas those that reduce the duration and spread of electrically induced convulsions are effective in focal types of epilepsy such as tonic–clonic seizures.

The *kindling model* may approximate the human condition more closely than directly evoked seizure models. Low-intensity electrical stimulation of certain regions of the limbic system, such as the amygdala, with implanted electrodes normally produces no seizure response. If a brief period of stimulation is repeated daily for several days, however, the response gradually increases until very low levels of stimulation will evoke a full seizure, and eventually seizures begin to occur spontaneously. Once produced, the kindled state persists indefinitely. This change is prevented by NMDA receptor antagonists, and may involve processes similar to those that cause long-term potentiation of synaptic transmission in the hippocampus (see Ch. 33). In human focal epilepsies, surgical removal of a damaged region of cortex often fails to cure the condition, as though the abnormal discharge from the region of primary damage had somehow produced a secondary hyperexcitability elsewhere in the brain. Furthermore, prophylactic treatment with antiepileptic drugs for 2 years following severe head injury reduces the subsequent incidence of post-traumatic epilepsy, which suggests that a phenomenon similar to kindling may underlie this form of epilepsy.

The *kainate model* entails a single injection of the glutamate receptor agonist kainic acid into the amygdaloid nucleus of a rat. After transient intense stimulation, spontaneous seizures begin to occur 2–4 weeks later, and then continue indefinitely. It is believed that excitotoxic damage to inhibitory neurons is responsible, associated with structural remodelling of excitatory synaptic connections, changes that may also be a factor in human epilepsies.

Neurons from which the epileptic discharge originates display an unusual type of electrical behaviour termed the *paroxysmal depolarising shift* (*PDS*), during which the membrane potential suddenly decreases by about 30 mV and remains depolarised for up to a few seconds before returning to normal. A burst of action potentials often accompanies this depolarisation (Fig. 40.2). This event probably results from the abnormally exaggerated and prolonged action of an excitatory transmitter. Activation of NMDA receptors (see Ch. 33) produces 'plateau-shaped' depolarising responses very similar to the PDS, as well as initiating seizure activity. This membrane response occurs because of the voltage-dependent blocking action of Mg^{2+} on channels operated by NMDA receptors (see Ch. 33). Glutamate must undoubtedly participate in the epileptic discharge, but efforts to develop glutamate antagonists as antiepileptic drugs have met with little success. It is known that repeated seizure activity can lead to neuronal degeneration, possibly due to excitotoxicity (Ch. 35).

Studies on experimental epilepsy in the kindling or kainate models have revealed a deficit in various biochemical markers of GABA-mediated inhibitory transmission, and an increase of markers associated with glutamate-mediated excitation (see Jarrott, 1999). Human studies have shown less consistent changes, although studies on brain samples removed at operation suggest that the epileptic focus contains more glutamate than normal; the GABA content is not affected. Potassium-stimulated glutamate release is also increased in the epileptic focus compared with in normal tissue.

Recent studies (see Binder et al., 2001) suggest that *neurotrophins*, particularly **brain-derived neurotrophic factor** (**BDNF**), may play a role in epileptogenesis. BDNF, which acts on a membrane receptor tyrosine kinase (Ch. 3), enhances membrane excitability and also stimulates synapse formation. Production and release of BDNF is increased in the kindling models, and there is also evidence for its involvement in human epilepsy. Specific blocking agents represent a possible future strategy for treating epilepsy but remain to be identified.

MECHANISM OF ACTION OF ANTIEPILEPTIC DRUGS

Three main mechanisms appear to be important in the action of antiepileptic drugs (see Meldrum, 1996; Rogawski & Löscher, 2004a):

- enhancement of GABA action
- inhibition of sodium channel function
- inhibition of calcium channel function.

Other mechanisms include inhibition of glutamate release and block of glutamate receptors. Many of the current antiepileptic drugs were developed empirically on the basis of activity in animal models. Their mechanism of action at the cellular level is not fully understood. As with drugs used to treat cardiac dysrhythmias (Ch. 18), the aim is to prevent the paroxysmal discharge without affecting normal transmission. It is clear that properties such as use-dependence and voltage-dependence of channel-blocking drugs (see Ch. 4) are important in achieving this selectivity, but our understanding remains fragmentary.

Enhancement of GABA action

Several antiepileptic drugs (e.g. **phenobarbital** and **benzodiazepines**) enhance the activation of $GABA_A$ receptors, thus facilitating the GABA-mediated opening of chloride channels (see Chs 3 and 37).[3] **Vigabatrin** (see below) acts by inhibiting the enzyme GABA transaminase, which is responsible

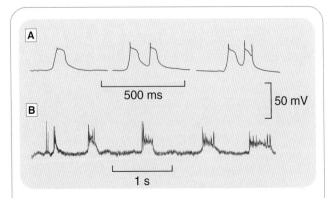

Fig. 40.2 **'Paroxysmal depolarising shift' (PDS) compared with experimental activation of glutamate receptors of the NMDA type.** **A** PDS recorded with an intracellular microelectrode from cortical neurons of anaesthetised cats. Seizure activity was induced by topical application of penicillin. **B** Intracellular recording from caudate nucleus of anaesthetised cat. The glutamate analogue NMDA was applied by ionophoresis from a nearby micropipette. Note the periodic waves of depolarisation, associated with a burst of action potentials, which closely resemble the PDS. (From: (A) Matsumoto H, Marsan C A 1964 Exp Neurol 9: 286; (B) Herrling P L et al. 1983 J Physiol 339: 207.)

---

[3]Absence seizures, paradoxically, are often exacerbated by drugs that enhance GABA activity (see Manning et al., 2003) and better treated by drugs acting by different mechanisms.

for inactivating GABA, and **tiagabine** inhibits GABA uptake; both thereby enhance the action of GABA as an inhibitory transmitter. **Gabapentin** (see below) was designed as an agonist at GABA$_A$ receptors, but ironically was found to be an effective antiepileptic drug despite having little or no effect on GABA receptors or on the transporter; it has high affinity for a particular subunit ($\alpha_2\delta$) of voltage-gated calcium channels (see Ch. 4), but its mechanism of action remains uncertain (see Macdonald, 1999).

Inhibition of sodium channel function

Several of the most important antiepileptic drugs (e.g. **phenytoin**, **carbamazepine**, **valproate**, **lamotrigine**) affect membrane excitability by an action on voltage-dependent sodium channels (see Ch. 4), which carry the inward membrane current necessary for the generation of an action potential. Their blocking action shows the property of use-dependence (see Ch. 4); in other words, they block preferentially the excitation of cells that are firing repetitively, and the higher the frequency of firing, the greater the block produced. This characteristic, which is relevant to the ability of drugs to block the high-frequency discharge that occurs in an epileptic fit without unduly interfering with the low-frequency firing of neurons in the normal state, arises from the ability of blocking drugs to discriminate between sodium channels in their resting, open and inactivated states. Depolarisation of a neuron (such as occurs in the PDS described above) increases the proportion of the sodium channels in the inactivated state. Antiepileptic drugs bind preferentially to channels in this state, preventing them from returning to the resting state, and thus reducing the number of functional channels available to generate action potentials.

Inhibition of calcium channels

Several antiepileptic drugs have minor effects on calcium channels (see Table 40.1), but only **ethosuximide** specifically blocks the T-type calcium channel, activation of which is believed to play a role in the rhythmic discharge associated with absence seizures (Khosravani et al., 2004). **Gabapentin** acts on L-type calcium channels by binding to the $\alpha_2\delta$ subunit (see below), but whether this is important for its antiepileptic properties is uncertain.

Other mechanisms

The action of many antiepileptic drugs remains poorly understood (see Meldrum, 1996; Macdonald, 1999; Levy et al., 2002). **Phenobarbital** is a barbiturate (see Ch. 37) that has a greater antiepileptic effect and relatively less sedative action than other barbiturates, although its GABA-potentiating action is similar. However, phenobarbital is as effective against electrically induced convulsions as it is against PTZ-induced convulsions in rats or mice, whereas benzodiazepines, which act similarly on GABA-mediated transmission, are without effect on electrically induced convulsions. Phenobarbital reduces the electrical activity of neurons within a chemically induced epileptic focus within the cortex, whereas diazepam (a benzodiazepine) does not suppress the focal activity but prevents it from spreading. The action of phenobarbital cannot therefore be due solely to its interaction with GABA, and it is likely that

> **Mechanism of action of antiepileptic drugs**
>
> - Current antiepileptic drugs are thought to act mainly by three main mechanisms:
>   — reducing electrical excitability of cell membranes, mainly through use-dependent block of sodium channels
>   — enhancing GABA-mediated synaptic inhibition; this may be achieved by an enhanced postsynaptic action of GABA, by inhibiting GABA transaminase, or by drugs with direct GABA agonist properties
>   — inhibiting T-type calcium channels (important in controlling absence seizures).
> - Newer drugs act by other mechanisms yet to be elucidated.
> - Drugs that block glutamate receptors are effective in animal models but are unsuitable for clinical use.

it also acts by inhibiting excitatory synaptic responses, although little is known about the mechanism.

Phenytoin has been studied in great detail. It not only causes use-dependent block of sodium channels (see above) but also affects other aspects of membrane function, including calcium channels and post-tetanic potentiation, as well as intracellular protein phosphorylation by calmodulin-activated kinases, which could also interfere with membrane excitability and synaptic function.

Newer antiepileptic drugs such as **levetiracetam** and **zonisamide** act by mechanisms that are as yet poorly understood, although they have weak effects on several of the targets discussed above.[4]

One theme, which has become familiar in earlier chapters in the central nervous system section of this book, is that antagonists at excitatory amino acid receptors have not, despite showing efficacy in animal models, proved useful in the clinic, because the margin between the desired anticonvulsant effect and unacceptable side effects, such as loss of motor coordination, is too narrow.

ANTIEPILEPTIC DRUGS

The term *antiepileptic* is used synonymously with *anticonvulsant* to describe drugs that are used to treat epilepsy (which does not necessarily cause convulsions) as well as non-epileptic convulsive disorders.

---

[4]The highly complex actions of current antiepileptic drugs are apt to make discouraging reading for those engaged in trying to develop new drugs on simple rational principles. Serendipity, not science, appears to be the path to therapeutic success.

Antiepileptic drugs are fully effective in controlling seizures in 50–80% of patients, although unwanted effects are common (see below). Patients with epilepsy usually need to take drugs continuously for many years, so avoidance of side effects is particularly important. This also explains why some drugs that are largely obsolete because of their adverse effects are still quite widely used even though they are not drugs of choice for newly diagnosed patients. There is clearly a need for more specific and effective drugs, and several new drugs have been recently introduced for clinical use. Long-established antiepileptic drugs (see Table 40.1) include **phenytoin, carbamazepine, valproate, ethosuximide** and **phenobarbital**, together with various benzodiazepines, such as **diazepam, clonazepam** and **clobazam**. Newer drugs include **vigabatrin, gabapentin, lamotrigine, felbamate, tiagabine, topiramate, levetiracetam** and **zonisamide**. The length of this list reflects the efforts being made to improve on the far from ideal properties of the earlier drugs. In general, the newer drugs are less likely to interact pharmacokinetically with other drugs (see Ch. 52) and have fewer adverse effects, although their efficacy in controlling seizures is no greater. The selection of drugs from this large available menu depends on many clinical factors and is covered in specialised textbooks.

PHENYTOIN

Phenytoin is the most important member of the hydantoin group of compounds, which are structurally related to the barbiturates. It is highly effective in reducing the intensity and duration of electrically induced convulsions in mice, although ineffective against PTZ-induced convulsions. Despite its many side effects and unpredictable pharmacokinetic behaviour, phenytoin is widely used, being effective against various forms of partial and generalised seizures, although not against absence seizures, which may even get worse.

Pharmacokinetic aspects

Phenytoin has certain pharmacokinetic peculiarities that need to be taken into account when it is used clinically. It is well absorbed when given orally, and about 80–90% of the plasma content is bound to albumin. Other drugs, such as salicylates, phenylbutazone and valproate, inhibit this binding competitively (see Ch. 52). This increases the free phenytoin concentration but also increases hepatic clearance of phenytoin, so may enhance or reduce the effect of the phenytoin in an unpredictable way. Phenytoin is metabolised by the hepatic mixed function oxidase system and excreted mainly as glucuronide. It causes enzyme induction, and thus increases the rate of metabolism of other drugs (e.g. oral anticoagulants). The metabolism of phenytoin itself can be either enhanced or competitively inhibited by various other drugs that share the same hepatic enzymes. Phenobarbital produces both effects, and because competitive inhibition is immediate whereas induction takes time, it initially enhances and later reduces the pharmacological activity of phenytoin. Ethanol has a similar dual effect.

The metabolism of phenytoin shows the characteristic of saturation (see Ch. 8), which means that over the therapeutic plasma concentration range the rate of inactivation does not increase in proportion to the plasma concentration. The consequences of this are as follow.

- The plasma half-life (approximately 20 hours) increases as the dose is increased.
- The steady-state mean plasma concentration, achieved when a patient is given a constant daily dose, varies disproportionately with the dose. Figure 40.3 shows that, in one patient, increasing the dose by 50% caused the steady-state plasma concentration to increase more than fourfold.

The range of plasma concentration over which phenytoin is effective without causing excessive unwanted effects is quite narrow (approximately 40–100 µmol/l). The very steep relationship between dose and plasma concentration, and the many interacting factors, mean that there is considerable individual variation in the plasma concentration achieved with a given dose. A radioimmunoassay for phenytoin in plasma is available, and its use has helped considerably in achieving an optimal therapeutic effect. The past tendency was to add further drugs in

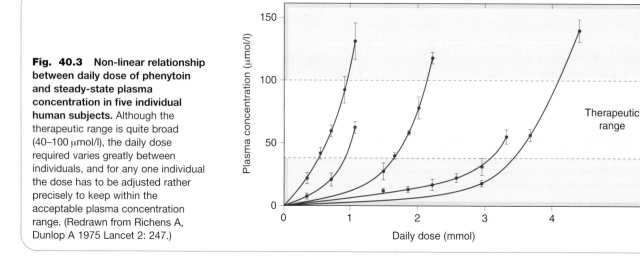

Fig. 40.3 Non-linear relationship between daily dose of phenytoin and steady-state plasma concentration in five individual human subjects. Although the therapeutic range is quite broad (40–100 µmol/l), the daily dose required varies greatly between individuals, and for any one individual the dose has to be adjusted rather precisely to keep within the acceptable plasma concentration range. (Redrawn from Richens A, Dunlop A 1975 Lancet 2: 247.)

cases where a single drug failed to give adequate control. It is now recognised that much of the unpredictability can be ascribed to pharmacokinetic variability, and regular monitoring of plasma concentration has reduced the use of polypharmacy.

Unwanted effects

Side effects of phenytoin begin to appear at plasma concentrations exceeding 100 µmol/l and may be severe above about 150 µmol/l. The milder side effects include vertigo, ataxia, headache and nystagmus, but not sedation. At higher plasma concentrations, marked confusion with intellectual deterioration occurs; a paradoxical increase in seizure frequency is a particular trap for the unwary prescriber. These effects occur acutely and are quickly reversible. Hyperplasia of the gums often develops gradually, as does hirsutism and coarsening of the features, which probably result from increased androgen secretion. Megaloblastic anaemia, associated with a disorder of folate metabolism, sometimes occurs, and can be corrected by giving folic acid (Ch. 22). Hypersensitivity reactions, mainly rashes, are quite common. Phenytoin has also been implicated as a cause of the increased incidence of fetal malformations in children born to epileptic mothers, particularly the occurrence of cleft palate, associated with the formation of an epoxide metabolite. Severe idiosyncratic reactions, including hepatitis, skin reactions and neoplastic lymphocyte disorders, occur in a small proportion of patients.

CARBAMAZEPINE

Carbamazepine, one of the most widely used antiepileptic drugs, is chemically derived from the tricyclic antidepressant drugs (see Ch. 39) and was found in a routine screening test to inhibit electrically-evoked seizures in mice. Pharmacologically and clinically, its actions resemble those of phenytoin, although it appears to be particularly effective in treating complex partial seizures (e.g. psychomotor epilepsy). It is also used to treat other conditions, such as neuropathic pain (Ch. 41) and manic-depressive illness (Ch. 39).

Pharmacokinetic aspects

Carbamazepine is well absorbed. Its plasma half-life is about 30 hours when it is given as a single dose, but it is a strong inducing agent, and the plasma half-life shortens to about 15 hours when it is given repeatedly. A slow-release preparation is used for patients who experience transient side effects coinciding with plasma concentration peaks following oral dosing (see below).

Unwanted effects

Carbamazepine produces a variety of unwanted effects ranging from drowsiness, dizziness and ataxia to more severe mental and motor disturbances. It can also cause water retention (and hence hyponatraemia; Ch. 28) and a variety of gastrointestinal and cardiovascular side effects. The incidence and severity of these effects is relatively low, however, compared with other drugs. Treatment is usually started with a low dose, which is built up gradually to avoid dose-related toxicity. Severe bone marrow depression, causing neutropenia, and other severe forms of hypersensitivity reaction can occur but are very rare.

Carbamazepine is a powerful inducer of hepatic microsomal enzymes, and thus accelerates the metabolism of many other drugs, such as **phenytoin**, oral contraceptives, **warfarin** and corticosteroids. In general, it is inadvisable to combine it with other antiepileptic drugs. **Ozcarbazepine**, introduced recently, is a prodrug that is metabolised to a compound closely resembling carbamazepine, with similar actions but less tendency to induce drug-metabolising enzymes.

VALPROATE

Valproate is a simple monocarboxylic acid, chemically unrelated to any other class of antiepileptic drug, and in 1963 it was discovered quite accidentally to have anticonvulsant properties in mice. It inhibits most kinds of experimentally induced convulsions and is effective in many kinds of epilepsy, being particularly useful in certain types of infantile epilepsy, where its low toxicity and lack of sedative action are important, and in adolescents in whom grand mal and petit mal coexist, because valproate (unlike most antiepileptic drugs) is effective against both. Like carbamazepine, valproate is also used in psychiatric conditions such as bipolar depressive illness (Ch. 39).

Mechanism of action

Valproate works by several mechanisms, of which the details remain uncertain (see Macdonald, 1999). It causes a significant increase in the GABA content of the brain and is a weak inhibitor of two enzyme systems that inactivate GABA, namely GABA transaminase and succinic semialdehyde dehydrogenase, but in vitro studies suggest that these effects would be very slight at clinical dosage. Other more potent inhibitors of these enzymes (e.g. **vigabatrin**; see below) also increase GABA content and have an anticonvulsant effect in experimental animals. There is some evidence that it enhances the action of GABA by a postsynaptic action, but no clear evidence that it affects inhibitory synaptic responses. It also inhibits sodium channels, but less so than phenytoin.

Valproate is well absorbed orally and excreted, mainly as the glucuronide, in the urine, the plasma half-life being about 15 hours.

Unwanted effects

Compared with most antiepileptic drugs, valproate is relatively free of unwanted effects. It causes thinning and curling of the hair in about 10% of patients. The most serious side effect is hepatotoxicity. An increase in serum glutamic oxaloacetic transaminase, which signals liver damage of some degree, commonly occurs, but proven cases of valproate-induced hepatitis are rare. The few cases of fatal hepatitis in valproate-treated patients may well have been caused by other factors. Valproate is teratogenic, causing spina bifida and other neural tube defects.

ETHOSUXIMIDE

Ethosuximide, which belongs to the succinimide class, is another drug developed empirically by modifying the barbituric acid ring structure. Pharmacologically and clinically, however, it is different from the drugs so far discussed, in that it is active against PTZ-induced convulsions in animals and against absence seizures in humans, with little or no effect on other types of epilepsy. It supplanted **trimethadione**, the first drug found to be effective in absence seizures, which had major side effects. Ethosuximide is used clinically for its selective effect on absence seizures.

The mechanism of action of ethosuximide and trimethadione appears to differ from that of other antiepileptic drugs. The main effect described is inhibition of T-type calcium channels, which may play a role in generating the 3/second firing rhythm in thalamic relay neurons that is characteristic of absence seizures.

Ethosuximide is well absorbed, and metabolised and excreted much like phenobarbital, with a plasma half-life of about 50 hours. Its main side effects are nausea and anorexia, sometimes lethargy and dizziness, and it is said to precipitate tonic–clonic seizures in susceptible patients. Very rarely, it can cause severe hypersensitivity reactions.

PHENOBARBITAL

▼ Phenobarbital was one of the first barbiturates to be developed, and its antiepileptic properties were recognised in 1912. In its action against experimentally induced convulsions and clinical forms of epilepsy, it closely resembles phenytoin; it affects the duration and intensity of artificially induced seizures, rather than the seizure threshold, and is (like phenytoin) ineffective in treating absence seizures. **Primidone**, now rarely used, acts by being metabolised to phenobarbital. It often causes hypersensitivity reactions. The clinical uses of phenobarbital are virtually the same as those of phenytoin, although phenytoin is preferred because of the absence of sedation.

Pharmacokinetic aspects

▼ Phenobarbital is well absorbed, and about 50% of the drug in the blood is bound to plasma albumin. It is eliminated slowly from the plasma (half-life, 50–140 hours). About 25% is excreted unchanged in the urine. Because phenobarbital is a weak acid, its ionisation and hence renal elimination are increased if the urine is made alkaline (see Ch. 8). The remaining 75% is metabolised, mainly by oxidation and conjugation, by the hepatic microsomal enzymes. Phenobarbital is a powerful inducer of liver P450 enzymes, and it lowers the plasma concentration of several other drugs (e.g. steroids, oral contraceptive, warfarin, tricyclic antidepressants) to an extent that is clinically important.

Unwanted effects

▼ The main unwanted effect of phenobarbital is sedation, which often occurs at plasma concentrations within the therapeutic range for seizure control. This is a serious drawback, because the drug may have to be used for years on end. Some degree of tolerance to the sedative effect seems to occur, but objective tests of cognition and motor performance show impairment even after long-term treatment. Other unwanted effects that may occur with clinical dosage include megaloblastic anaemia (similar to that caused by phenytoin), mild hypersensitivity reactions and osteomalacia. Like other barbiturates (see Ch. 52), it must not be given to patients with porphyria. In overdose, phenobarbital produces coma and respiratory and circulatory failure, as do all barbiturates.

Clinical use

▼ Phenobarbital is now seldom used in adults because of sedation. For some years, it was widely used in children, including as prophylaxis following febrile convulsions in infancy, but it can cause behavioural

---

The major antiepileptic drugs

The main drugs in current use are phenytoin, carbamazepine, valproate and ethosuximide.

- **Phenytoin:**
  - acts mainly by use-dependent block of sodium channels
  - effective in many forms of epilepsy, but not absence seizures
  - metabolism shows saturation kinetics, therefore plasma concentration can vary widely; monitoring is therefore needed
  - drug interactions are common
  - main unwanted effects are confusion, gum hyperplasia, skin rashes, anaemia, teratogenesis
  - widely used in treatment of epilepsy; also used as antidysrhythmic agent (Ch. 18).
- **Carbamazepine:**
  - derivative of tricyclic antidepressants
  - similar profile to that of phenytoin but with fewer unwanted effects
  - effective in most forms of epilepsy (except absence seizures); particularly effective in psychomotor epilepsy; also useful in trigeminal neuralgia
  - strong inducing agent, therefore many drug interactions
  - low incidence of unwanted effects, principally sedation, ataxia, mental disturbances, water retention.
- **Valproate:**
  - chemically unrelated to other antiepileptic drugs
  - mechanism of action not clear; weak inhibition of GABA transaminase, some effect on sodium channels
  - relatively few unwanted effects: baldness, teratogenicity, liver damage (rare, but serious).
- **Ethosuximide:**
  - the main drug used to treat absence seizures; may exacerbate other forms
  - acts by blocking T-type calcium channels
  - relatively few unwanted effects, mainly nausea and anorexia.
- **Secondary drugs include:**
  - phenobarbital: highly sedative
  - various benzodiazepines (e.g. clonazepam); diazepam used in treating status epilepticus.
- Newer agents that are becoming widely used because of their improved side effect profile include **vigabatrin, lamotrigine, felbamate, gabapentin, pregabalin, tiagabine, topiramate** and **zonisamide**.

disturbances and hyperkinesia, and is now seldom used at all in newly diagnosed patients.

BENZODIAZEPINES

Diazepam, given intravenously or rectally, is used to treat *status epilepticus*, a life-threatening condition in which epileptic seizures occur almost without a break. Its advantage in this situation is that it acts very rapidly compared with other antiepileptic drugs. With most benzodiazepines (see Ch. 37), the sedative effect is too pronounced for them to be used for maintenance therapy. **Clonazepam** and the related compound **clobazam** are claimed to be relatively selective as antiepileptic drugs. Sedation is the main side effect of these compounds, and an added problem may be the withdrawal syndrome, which results in an exacerbation of seizures if the drug is stopped abruptly.

NEWER ANTIEPILEPTIC DRUGS

For about 25 years, from the mid-1960s, the inventiveness of the pharmaceutical industry in producing improved antiepileptic drugs dried up. Around 1985, the muse returned, and a spate of new drugs was developed over the next 10–15 years (see Eadie & Vajda, 1999).

VIGABATRIN

Vigabatrin, the first 'designer drug' in the epilepsy field, is a vinyl-substituted analogue of GABA that was designed as an inhibitor of the GABA-metabolising enzyme GABA transaminase. Vigabatrin is extremely specific for this enzyme and works by forming an irreversible covalent bond. In animal studies, vigabatrin increases the GABA content of the brain and also increases the stimulation-evoked release of GABA, implying that GABA transaminase inhibition can increase the releasable pool of GABA and effectively enhance inhibitory transmission. In humans, vigabatrin increases the content of GABA in the cerebrospinal fluid. Although its plasma half-life is short, it produces a long-lasting effect because the enzyme is blocked irreversibly, and the drug can be given by mouth once daily. Evidence of neurotoxicity was found in animals but has not been found in humans, removing one of the main question marks hanging over this drug.

The main drawback of vigabatrin is the occurrence of depression, and occasionally psychotic disturbances, in a minority of patients; otherwise, it is relatively free from side effects.

Vigabatrin has been reported to be effective in a substantial proportion of patients resistant to the established drugs, and may represent an important therapeutic advance.

LAMOTRIGINE

Lamotrigine, although chemically unrelated, resembles phenytoin and carbamazepine in its pharmacological effects, acting on sodium channels and inhibiting the release of excitatory amino acids. It appears that, despite its similar mechanism of action, lamotrigine has a broader therapeutic profile than the earlier drugs, with significant efficacy against absence seizures (and is also used to treat unrelated psychiatric disorders). Its main side effects are nausea, dizziness and ataxia, and hypersensitivity reactions (mainly mild rashes, but occasionally more severe). Its plasma half-life is about 24 hours, with no particular pharmacokinetic anomalies, and it is taken orally.

FELBAMATE

Felbamate is an analogue of an obsolete anxiolytic drug, **meprobamate**. It is active in many animal seizure models and has a broader clinical spectrum than earlier antiepileptic drugs, but its mechanism of action at the cellular level is uncertain. It has only a weak effect on sodium channels and little effect on GABA, but causes some block of the NMDA receptor channel (Ch. 33). Its acute side effects are mild, mainly nausea, irritability and insomnia, but it occasionally causes severe reactions resulting in aplastic anaemia or hepatitis. For this reason, its recommended use is limited to a form of intractable epilepsy in children (Lennox–Gastaut syndrome) that is unresponsive to other drugs. Its plasma half-life is about 24 hours, and it can enhance the plasma concentration of other antiepileptic drugs given concomitantly.

GABAPENTIN

Gabapentin was designed as a simple analogue of GABA that would be sufficiently lipid-soluble to penetrate the blood–brain barrier. It turned out to be an effective anticonvulsant in several animal models but, surprisingly, not by acting on GABA receptors. Its main site of action appears to be on T-type calcium channel function, by binding to a particular channel subunit ($\alpha_2\delta$), and it inhibits the release of various neurotransmitters and modulators, but the details remain unclear. The side effects of gabapentin (mainly sedation and ataxia) are less severe than with many antiepileptic drugs. The absorption of gabapentin from the intestine depends on the amino acid carrier system and shows the property of saturability, which means that increasing the dose does not proportionately increase the amount absorbed. This makes gabapentin relatively safe and free of side effects associated with overdosing. Its plasma half-life is about 6 hours, requiring dosing two to three times daily. It is excreted unchanged in the urine and is free of interactions with other drugs. It has limited efficacy when used on its own, so is used mainly as add-on therapy. It is also used as an analgesic to treat neuropathic pain (Ch. 41). A recently introduced follow-up drug, **pregabalin**, is more potent than gabapentin but otherwise very similar. These drugs are excreted unchanged in the urine, and so must be used with care in patients whose renal function is impaired.

TIAGABINE

Tiagabine, an analogue of GABA that is able to penetrate the blood–brain barrier, acts by inhibiting the reuptake of GABA by neurons and glia, and was the product of rational drug design. It enhances the extracellular GABA concentration, as measured in microdialysis experiments, and also potentiates and prolongs GABA-mediated synaptic responses in the brain. It has a short plasma half-life, and its main side effects are drowsiness and confusion. The clinical usefulness of tiagabine has not yet been fully assessed.

TOPIRAMATE

Topiramate is a recently introduced drug that, mechanistically, appears to do a little of everything, blocking sodium channels, enhancing the action of GABA, blocking AMPA receptors and, for good measure, weakly inhibiting carbonic anhydrase. Its spectrum of action resembles that of phenytoin, and it is claimed to produce less severe side effects, as well as being devoid of the pharmacokinetic properties that cause trouble with phenytoin. Its main drawback is that (like many antiepileptic drugs) it is teratogenic in animals, so it should not be used in women of child-bearing age. Currently, it is recommended for use as add-on therapy in refractory cases of epilepsy.

LEVETIRACETAM

Levetiracetam was developed as an analogue of **piracetam**, a drug used to improve cognitive function (see Ch. 35), and discovered by accident to have antiepileptic activity in animal models. Unusually, it lacks activity in conventional models such as electroshock and PTZ tests, but is effective in the kindling model. It has little or no effect on known targets (ion channels and GABA-related mechanisms), and its mechanism of action is unknown. It is excreted unchanged in the urine.

ZONISAMIDE

Zonisamide is a sulfonamide compound originally intended as an antibacterial drug and found accidentally to have antiepileptic properties. It is believed to act by blocking sodium channels but may well have other effects. It is free of major unwanted effects, although it causes drowsiness, and of serious interaction with other drugs. It tends to suppress appetite and cause weight loss, and is sometimes used for this purpose. Zonisamide has a long plasma half-life of 60–80 hours, and is partly excreted unchanged and partly converted to a glucuronide metabolite.

OTHER USES OF ANTIEPILEPTIC DRUGS

Antiepileptic drugs have proved to have much wider clinical applications than was originally envisaged, and clinical trials have shown many of them to be effective in the following conditions:

- cardiac dysrhythmias (e.g. **phenytoin**—not used clinically, however; Ch. 18)
- bipolar disorder (**valproate, carbamazepine, oxcarbazepine, lamotrigine, topiramate**; Ch. 39)
- migraine prophylaxis (**valproate, gabapentin**)
- anxiety disorders (**gabapentin**; Ch. 37)
- neuropathic pain (**gabapentin, carbamazepine, lamotrigine**; Ch. 41).

This surprising multiplicity of clinical indications may reflect the fact that similar neurobiological mechanisms, involving synaptic

---

> **Clinical uses of antiepileptic drugs**
>
> - *Tonic–clonic* (grand mal) seizures:
>   - **carbamazepine** (preferred because of a relatively favourable effectiveness:risk ratio), **phenytoin**, **valproate**
>   - use of a single drug is preferred, when possible, to avoid pharmacokinetic interactions
>   - newer agents include **vigabatrin, lamotrigine, felbamate, gabapentin**.
> - *Partial (focal) seizures*: **carbamazepine, valproate**; alternatives are **clonazepam** or **phenytoin**.
> - *Absence seizures* (petit mal): **ethosuximide** or **valproate**
>   - valproate is used when absence seizures coexist with tonic–clonic seizures, because most other drugs used for tonic–clonic seizures can worsen absence seizures.
> - *Myoclonic seizures*: **diazepam** intravenously or (in absence of accessible veins) rectally.
> - *Neuropathic pain*: for example **carbamazepine, gabapentin** (see Ch. 41).
> - To stabilise mood in mono- or bipolar *affective disorder* (as an alternative to lithium): for example **carbamazepine, valproate** (see Ch. 39).

plasticity and increased excitability of interconnected populations of neurons, underlie each of these disorders (see Rogawski & Löscher, 2004b).

MUSCLE SPASM AND MUSCLE RELAXANTS

Many diseases of the brain and spinal cord produce an increase in muscle tone, which can be painful and disabling. Spasticity resulting from birth injury or cerebral vascular disease, and the paralysis produced by spinal cord lesions, are examples. Local injury or inflammation, as in arthritis, can have the same effect, and chronic back pain is also often associated with local muscle spasm.

Certain centrally acting drugs are available that have the effect of reducing the background tone of the muscle without seriously affecting its ability to contract transiently under voluntary control. The distinction between voluntary movements and 'background tone' is not clear-cut, and the selectivity of those drugs is not complete. Postural control, for example, is usually jeopardised by centrally acting muscle relaxants. Furthermore, drugs that affect motor control generally produce rather widespread effects on the central nervous system, and drowsiness and confusion turn out to be very common side effects of these agents. The main groups of drugs that have been used to control muscle tone are:

- **mephenesin** and related drugs
- **baclofen**
- **benzodiazepines** (see Ch. 37)

Table 40.1 Properties of the main antiepileptic drugs

Drug	Site of action				Main uses	Main unwanted effect(s)	Pharmacokinetics
	Sodium channel	*GABA$_A$ receptor*	*Calcium channel*	*Other*			
Phenytoin	++				All types *except* absence seizures	Ataxia, vertigo Gum hypertrophy Hirsutism Megaloblastic anaemia Fetal malformation Hypersensitivity reactions	Half-life ~24 h Saturation kinetics, therefore unpredictable plasma levels Plasma monitoring often required
Carbamazepine[a]	++				All types *except* absence seizures Especially temporal lobe epilepsy (Also used in trigeminal neuralgia) Most widely used antiepileptic drug	Sedation, ataxia Blurred vision Water retention Hypersensitivity reactions Leucopenia, liver failure (rare)	Half-life 12–18 h (longer initially) Strong induction of microsomal enzymes, therefore risk of drug interactions
Valproate	+	?+		GABA trans-aminase inhibition	Most types, including absence seizures	Generally less than with other drugs Nausea Hair loss Weight gain Fetal malformations	Half-life 12–15 h
Ethosuximide[b]			++		Absence seizures May exacerbate tonic–clonic seizures	Nausea, anorexia Mood changes Headache	Long plasma half-life (~60 h)
Phenobarbital[c]	?+	+			All types *except* absence seizures	Sedation, depression	Long plasma half-life (> 60 h) Strong induction of microsomal enzymes, therefore risk of drug interactions (e.g. with phenytoin)
Benzodiazepines (e.g. clonazepam, clobazam, diazepam)		++			All types Diazepam used intravenously to control *status epilepticus*	Sedation Withdrawal syndrome (see Ch. 37)	See Chapter 37
Vigabatrin				GABA trans-aminase inhibition	All types Appears to be effective in patients resistant to other drugs	Sedation Behavioural and mood changes (occasionally psychosis) Visual field defects	Short plasma half-life, but enzyme inhibition is long-lasting
Lamotrigine	++		?+	Inhibits gluta-mate release	All types	Dizziness Sedation Skin rashes	Plasma half-life 24–36 h
Gabapentin[a]			?+		Partial seizures	Few side effects, mainly sedation	Plasma half-life 6–9 h

Table 40.1 (cont'd)   Properties of the main antiepileptic drugs

Drug	Site of action				Main uses	Main unwanted effect(s)	Pharmacokinetics
	Sodium channel	GABA_A receptor	Calcium channel	Other			
Felbamate	?+			?NMDA receptor block	Used mainly for severe (Lennox–Gastaut syndrome) because of risk of idiosyncratic reaction	Few acute side effects but can cause aplastic anaemia and liver damage as rare idiosyncratic reaction	Plasma half-life ~20 h Excreted unchanged
Tiagabine				Inhibits GABA uptake	Partial seizures	Sedation	Plasma half-life ~7 h Hepatic metabolism
Topiramate	?+	?+	?+	Mechanism unknown	As phenytoin	Sedation Fewer pharmacokinetic interactions than phenytoin Fetal malformation	Plasma half-life ~20 h Excreted unchanged
Levetiracetam				Mechanism unknown	Partial seizures	Sedation (slight)	Plasma half-life ~7 h Excreted unchanged
Zonisamide	+				Partial seizures	Sedation (slight) Appetite suppression and weight loss	Plasma half-life ~70 h Excreted partly unchanged and partly as glucuronide

[a]**Oxcarbazepine**, recently introduced, is similar; claimed to have fewer side effects.
[b]**Trimethadione** is similar to ethosuximide in that it acts selectively against absence seizures. Its greater toxicity (especially the risk of severe hypersensitivity reactions) means that ethosuximide has largely replaced it in clinical use.
[c]**Primidone** is pharmacologically similar to phenobarbital and is converted to phenobarbital in the body. It has no clear advantages and is more liable to produce hypersensitivity reactions, so is now rarely used.

- **botulinum toxin** (see Ch. 10); injected into a muscle, this neurotoxin causes long-lasting paralysis confined to the site of injection, and its use to treat local muscle spasm is increasing
- **dantrolene** (see Ch. 4).

MEPHENESIN

Mephenesin is an aromatic ether that acts mainly on the spinal cord, causing a selective inhibition of polysynaptic excitation of motor neurons. Thus it strongly inhibits the polysynaptic flexor withdrawal reflex without affecting the tendon jerk reflex, which is monosynaptic, and it abolishes decerebrate rigidity. Its mechanism of action at the cellular level is unknown. Mephenesin is little used clinically, although it is sometimes given as an intravenous injection to reduce acute muscle spasm resulting from injury.

BACLOFEN

Baclofen (see Ch. 33) is a chlorophenyl derivative of GABA originally prepared as a lipophilic GABA-like agent in order to assist penetration of the blood–brain barrier, which is impermeable to GABA itself. Baclofen is a selective agonist at presynaptic GABA_B receptors (see Ch. 33). The antispastic action of baclofen is exerted mainly on the spinal cord, where it inhibits both monosynaptic and polysynaptic activation of motor neurons. It is effective when given by mouth, and is used in the treatment of spasticity associated with multiple sclerosis or spinal injury. However, it is ineffective in cerebral spasticity caused by birth injury.

Baclofen produces various unwanted effects, particularly drowsiness, motor incoordination and nausea, and it may also have behavioural effects. It is not useful in epilepsy.

CANNABIS

Anecdotal evidence suggests that smoking cannabis (Ch. 43) relieves the painful muscle spasms associated with multiple sclerosis. A full-scale controlled trial of **tetrahydrocannabinol** (see Ch. 15), however, showed no significant effect on muscle spasm, tremor, bladder control or disability, although the patients reported subjective improvements (Zajicek et al., 2003).

REFERENCES AND FURTHER READING

Pathogenesis and types of epilepsy

Binder D K, Croll S D, Gall C M, Scharfman H E 2001 BDNF and epilepsy: too much of a good thing? Trends Neurosci 24: 47–53 (*Recent ideas on possible role of BDNF in epileptogenesis*)

Jarrott B 1999 Epileptogenesis: biochemical aspects. Handb Exp Pharmacol 138: 87–121 (*Review article describing possible neurochemical mechanisms underlying epilepsy—mostly speculative*)

Khosravani H, Altier C, Simms B et al. 2004 Gating effects of mutations in the Cav3.2 T-type calcium channel associated with childhood absence epilepsy. J Biol Chem 279: 9681–9684 (*Study showing that calcium channel mutations seen in childhood absence seizures cause abnormal neuronal discharges in transgenic mice*)

Kulmann D M, Asztely F, Walker M C 2000 The role of mammalian ionotropic receptors in synaptic plasticity: LTP, LTD and epilepsy. Cell Mol Life Sci 57: 1551–1561 (*Draws parallels between epileptogenesis and other well-studied forms of synaptic plasticity*)

Manning J-P A, Richards D A, Bowery N G 2003 Pharmacology of absence epilepsy. Trends Pharmacol Sci 24: 542–549 (*Short review emphasising the differences between absence seizures and other types of epilepsy*)

Sarkisian M R 2001 Overview of the current animal models for human seizure and epileptic disorders. Epilepsy Behav 2: 201–216

Steinlein O K 2004 Genetic mechanisms that underlie epilepsy. Nat Rev Neurosci 5: 400–408 (*Describes the current, limited state of knowledge about genetic 'channelopathies' as a cause of epilepsy*)

Willoughby J O 1999 Epileptogenesis: electrophysiology. Handb Exp Pharmacol 138: 63–85 (*Review article*)

Antiepileptic drugs

Eadie M J, Vajda F J (eds) 1999 Antiepileptic drugs: pharmacology and therapeutics. Handb Exp Pharmacol 138 (*Useful collection of articles covering all aspects of antiepileptic drugs*)

Levy R H, Mattson R H, Meldrum B S, Perucca E (eds) 2002 Antiepileptic drugs, 5th edn. Lippincott, Williams & Wilkins, Philadelphia (*Comprehensive general textbook*)

Macdonald R L 1999 Cellular actions of antiepileptic drugs. Handb Exp Pharmacol 138: 123–150 (*Good review article including information on new drugs*)

Meldrum B S 1996 Update on the mechanism of action of antiepileptic drugs. Epilepsia 37(suppl 6): S4–S11 (*Excellent review article summarising knowledge on mechanisms*)

Rogawski M A, Löscher W 2004a The neurobiology of antiepileptic drugs. Nat Rev Neurosci 5: 553–564 (*Good general review article covering basic pharmacology and mechanisms of action of the major antiepileptic drugs*)

Rogawski M A, Löscher W 2004b The neurobiology of antiepileptic drugs for the treatment of nonepileptic conditions. Nat Med 10: 685–692

Zajicek J, Fox P, Sanders H et al. 2003 Cannabinoids for treatment of spasticity and other symptoms related to multiple sclerosis: multi-centre randomised placebo-controlled trial. Lancet 362: 1517–1526 (*Full-scale trial showing very limited efficacy of cannabinoids in multiple sclerosis*)

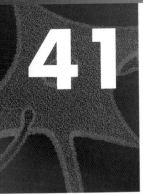

41 Analgesic drugs

OVERVIEW

Pain is a disabling accompaniment of many medical conditions, and pain control is one of the most important therapeutic priorities.

In this chapter, we discuss the neural mechanisms responsible for different types of pain, and the various drugs that are used to reduce it. The 'classic' analgesic drugs, notably opiates and non-steroidal anti-inflammatory drugs (NSAIDs; described in Ch. 14), have their origins in natural products that have been used for centuries. The original compounds, typified by morphine and aspirin, are still in widespread use, but many synthetic compounds that act by the same mechanisms have been developed. Opiate analgesics are described in this chapter. Next, we consider various other drug classes, such as antidepressants and antiepileptic drugs, which clinical experience has shown to be effective in certain types of pain. Finally, looking into the future, many potential new drug targets have emerged over the past decade or so as our knowledge of the neural mechanisms underlying pain has advanced. We describe briefly some of these new approaches at the end of the chapter.

NEURAL MECHANISMS OF PAIN

Pain is a subjective experience, hard to define exactly, even though we all know what we mean by it. Typically, it is a direct response to an untoward event associated with tissue damage, such as injury, inflammation or cancer, but severe pain can arise independently of any obvious predisposing cause (e.g. trigeminal neuralgia), or persist long after the precipitating injury has healed (e.g. phantom limb pain). It can also occur as a consequence of brain or nerve injury (e.g. following a stroke or herpes infection). Painful conditions of the latter kind, not directly linked to tissue injury, are very common and a major cause of disability and distress, and in general they respond less well to conventional analgesic drugs than do conditions where the immediate cause is clear. In these cases, we need to think of pain in terms of disordered neural function, comparable with schizophrenia or epilepsy, rather than simply as a 'normal' response to tissue injury. Therefore it is useful to distinguish two components, either or both of which may be involved in pathological pain states:

- the peripheral nociceptive afferent neuron, which is activated by noxious stimuli
- the central mechanisms by which the afferent input generates a pain sensation.

Good accounts of the neural basis of pain can be found in McMahon & Koltzenburg (2006).

NOCICEPTIVE AFFERENT NEURONS

Under normal conditions, pain is associated with impulse activity in small-diameter primary afferent fibres of peripheral nerves (see Raja et al., 1999). These nerves have sensory endings in peripheral tissues and are activated by stimuli of various kinds (mechanical, thermal, chemical; Julius & Basbaum, 2001; Julius & McCleskey, 2006). They are distinguished from other sorts of mechanical and thermal receptors by their higher threshold, because they are normally activated only by stimuli of noxious intensity—sufficient to cause some degree of tissue damage.

Recordings of activity in single afferent fibres in human subjects have shown that stimuli sufficient to excite these small afferent fibres also evoke a painful sensation. Many of these fibres are non-myelinated C fibres with low conduction velocities (< 1 m/s); this group is known as *C polymodal nociceptors*. Others are fine myelinated (Aδ) fibres, which conduct more rapidly but respond to similar peripheral stimuli. Although there are some species differences, the majority of the C fibres are associated with polymodal nociceptive endings. Afferents from muscle and viscera also convey nociceptive information. In the nerves from these tissues, the small myelinated Aδ fibres are connected to high-threshold mechanoreceptors, while the non-myelinated C fibres are connected to polymodal nociceptors, as in the skin.

Experiments on human subjects, in which recording or stimulating electrodes are applied to cutaneous sensory nerves, have shown that activity in the Aδ fibres causes a sensation of sharp, well-localised pain, whereas C fibre activity causes a dull, diffuse, burning pain.

With many pathological conditions, tissue injury is the immediate cause of the pain and results in the local release of a variety of chemicals that act on the nerve terminals, either activating them directly or enhancing their sensitivity to other forms of stimulation. The pharmacological properties of nociceptive nerve terminals are discussed in more detail below.

The cell bodies of spinal nociceptive afferent fibres lie in dorsal root ganglia; fibres enter the spinal cord via the dorsal roots, ending in the grey matter of the dorsal horn (Fig. 41.1). Most of the nociceptive afferents terminate in the superficial region of the dorsal horn, the C fibres and some Aδ fibres innervating cell bodies in laminae I and II, while other A fibres penetrate deeper into the dorsal horn (lamina V). Cells in laminae I and V give rise to the main projection pathways from the dorsal horn to the thalamus.

The non-myelinated afferent neurons contain several neuropeptides (see Ch. 16), particularly substance P and calcitonin gene–related peptide (CGRP). These are released as mediators at both the central and the peripheral terminals, and play an important role in the pathology of pain.

MODULATION IN THE NOCICEPTIVE PATHWAY

Acute pain is generally well accounted for in terms of *nociception*—an excessive noxious stimulus giving rise to an intense and unpleasant sensation. In contrast, most chronic pain states[1] are associated with aberrations of the normal physiological pathway, giving rise to *hyperalgesia* (an increased amount of pain associated with a mild noxious stimulus), *allodynia* (pain evoked by a non-noxious stimulus) or *spontaneous pain* without any precipitating stimulus. An analogy is with an old radio set that plays uncontrollably loudly (hyperalgesia), receives two stations at once (allodynia), or produces random shrieks and whistles (spontaneous pain spasms). These distortions in the transmission line are beginning to be understood in terms of various types of positive and negative modulation in the nociceptive pathway, discussed in more detail below. Some of the main mechanisms are summarised in Figure 41.2.

HYPERALGESIA AND ALLODYNIA

▼ Anyone who has suffered a burn or sprained ankle has experienced hyperalgesia and allodynia. Hyperalgesia involves both sensitisation of peripheral nociceptive nerve terminals and central facilitation of transmission at the level of the dorsal horn and thalamus—changes defined by the term *neuroplasticity*. The peripheral component is due to the action of mediators such as bradykinin and prostaglandins acting on the nerve terminals (see below). The central component reflects

---

[1]Defined as pain that outlasts the precipitating tissue injury. Many clinical pain states fall into this category. The dissociation of pain from noxious input is most evident in 'phantom limb' pain, which occurs after amputations and may be very severe. The pain is usually not relieved by local anaesthetic injections, implying that electrical activity in afferent fibres is not an essential component. At the other extreme, noxious input with no pain, there are many well-documented reports of mystics and showmen who subject themselves to horrifying ordeals with knives, burning embers, nails and hooks (undoubtedly causing massive afferent input) without apparently suffering pain.

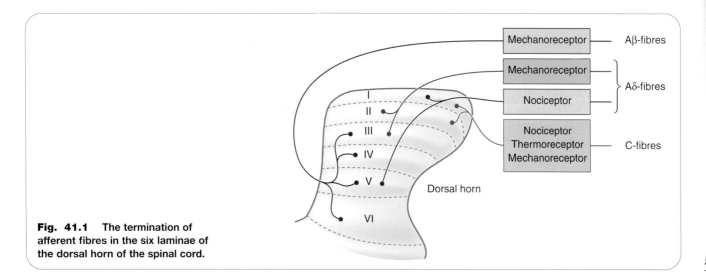

Fig. 41.1 The termination of afferent fibres in the six laminae of the dorsal horn of the spinal cord.

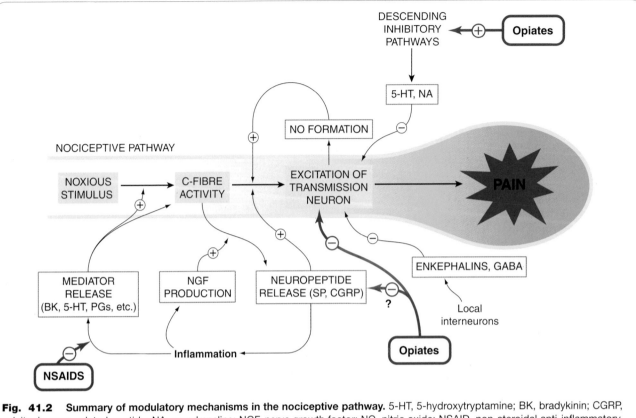

Fig. 41.2 **Summary of modulatory mechanisms in the nociceptive pathway.** 5-HT, 5-hydroxytryptamine; BK, bradykinin; CGRP, calcitonin gene–related peptide; NA, noradrenaline; NGF, nerve growth factor; NO, nitric oxide; NSAID, non-steroidal anti-inflammatory drug; PG, prostaglandin; SP, substance P.

facilitation of synaptic transmission. This has been well studied in the dorsal horn (see Yaksh, 1999). The synaptic responses of dorsal horn neurons to nociceptive inputs display the phenomenon of 'wind-up'—i.e. the synaptic potentials steadily increase in amplitude with each stimulus—when repeated stimuli are delivered at physiological frequencies (see Fig. 41.3). This activity-dependent facilitation of transmission has features in common with the phenomenon of long-term potentiation in the hippocampus, described in Chapter 33, and the chemical mechanisms underlying it may also be similar (see Ji et al., 2003). In the dorsal horn, the facilitation is blocked by NMDA receptor antagonists, also by antagonists of substance P, a slow excitatory transmitter released by nociceptive afferent neurons (see above), and by inhibitors of nitric oxide synthesis. Substance P produces a slow depolarising response in the postsynaptic cell, which builds up during repetitive stimulation, and is believed to enhance NMDA receptor–mediated transmission. This results in Ca^{2+} influx and activation of nitric oxide synthase (see Ch. 17), the released nitric oxide acting to facilitate transmission by mechanisms that have yet to be elucidated. Substance P and CGRP released from primary afferent neurons also act in the periphery, promoting inflammation by their effects on blood vessels and cells of the immune system (Ch. 13). This mechanism, known as *neurogenic inflammation*, amplifies and sustains the inflammatory reaction and the accompanying activation of nociceptive afferent fibres.

Central facilitation is an important component of pathological hyperalgesia (e.g. that associated with inflammatory responses; see Fig. 41.2). The mediators responsible for central facilitation include substance P and CGRP, as well as many others (see Ji et al., 2003). For example, *nerve growth factor (NGF)*, a cytokine-like mediator produced by peripheral tissues, particularly in inflammation, acts specifically on nociceptive afferent neurons, increasing their electrical excitability, chemosensitivity and peptide content, and also promoting the formation

of synaptic contacts. Increased NGF production may be an important mechanism by which nociceptive transmission becomes facilitated by tissue damage, leading to hyperalgesia (see McMahon, 1996). Increased gene expression in sensory neurons is induced by NGF and other inflammatory mediators; the up-regulated genes include those encoding various neuropeptide precursors, receptors and channels, and have the overall effect of facilitating transmission at the first synaptic relay in the dorsal horn. *Brain-derived neurotrophic factor* released from primary afferent nerve terminals activates pathways leading to sensitisation of glutamate receptors, and hence synaptic facilitation, in the dorsal horn.

Excitation of nociceptive sensory neurons depends, as in other neurons (see Ch. 4), on voltage-gated sodium channels. Certain sodium channel subtypes are found in these neurons but not elsewhere, and there is good evidence (see Lai et al., 2004; Chahine et al., 2005) that increased expression of these channels underlies the sensitisation to external stimuli that occurs in inflammatory pain and hyperalgesia. Consistent with this hypothesis is the fact that many antiepileptic and antidysrhythmic drugs, which act by blocking sodium channels (see Chs 18 and 40) also find clinical application as analgesics.

THE SUBSTANTIA GELATINOSA AND THE GATE CONTROL THEORY

Cells of lamina II of the dorsal horn (the *substantia gelatinosa, SG*) are mainly short inhibitory interneurons projecting to lamina I and lamina V, and they regulate transmission at the first synapse of the nociceptive pathway, between the primary afferent fibres and the spinothalamic tract transmission neurons. This gatekeeper function gave rise to the term *gate control theory*,

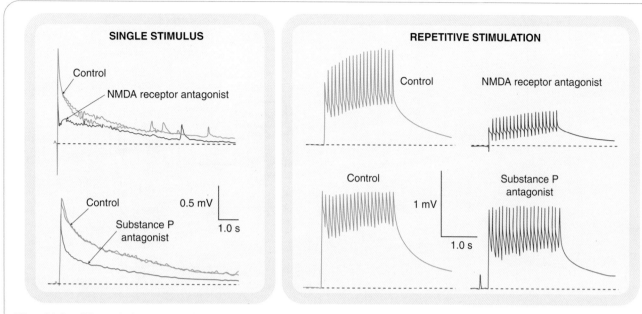

Fig. 41.3 Effect of glutamate and substance P antagonist on nociceptive transmission in the rat spinal cord. The rat paw was inflamed by ultraviolet irradiation 2 days before the experiment, a procedure that induces hyperalgesia and spinal cord facilitation. The synaptic response was recorded from the ventral root, in response to stimulation of C fibres in the dorsal root with single stimuli (left) or repetitive stimuli (right). The effects of the NMDA receptor antagonist D-AP-5 (see Ch. 33) and the substance P antagonist RP 67580 (selective for neurokinin type 2, NK$_2$, receptors) are shown. The slow component of the synaptic response is reduced by both antagonists (left-hand traces), as is the 'wind-up' in response to repetitive stimulation (right-hand traces). These effects are much less pronounced in the normal animal. Thus both glutamate, acting on NMDA receptors, and substance P, acting on NK$_2$ receptors, are involved in nociceptive transmission, and their contribution increases as a result of inflammatory hyperalgesia. (Records kindly provided by L Urban and S W Thompson.)

proposed by Wall and Melzack in 1965. According to this view (summarised in Fig. 41.4), the SG cells respond both to the activity of afferent fibres entering the cord (thus allowing the arrival of impulses via one group of afferent fibres to regulate the transmission of impulses via another pathway) and to the activity of descending pathways (see below). The SG is rich in both opioid peptides and opioid receptors, and may be an important site of action for morphine-like drugs (see later section). For a more detailed account of dorsal horn circuitry, see Fields et al. (2006). Similar 'gate' mechanisms also operate in the thalamus.

From the spinothalamic tracts, the projection fibres form synapses, mainly in the ventral and medial parts of the thalamus, with cells whose axons run to the somatosensory cortex. In the medial thalamus in particular, many cells respond specifically to noxious stimuli in the periphery, and lesions in this area cause analgesia. Functional imaging studies in conscious subjects (see Schnitzler & Ploner, 2000) suggest that the affective component of pain sensation (i.e. its unpleasantness) involves a specific region of the cingulate cortex, distinct from the somatosensory cortex.

DESCENDING INHIBITORY CONTROLS

As mentioned above, descending pathways (Fig. 41.5) constitute one of the gating mechanisms that control impulse transmission in the dorsal horn (see Millan, 2002). A key part of this descending system is the *periaqueductal grey (PAG) area* of the

midbrain, a small area of grey matter surrounding the central canal. In 1969, Reynolds found that electrical stimulation of this brain area in the rat caused analgesia sufficiently intense that abdominal surgery could be performed without anaesthesia and without eliciting any marked response. Non-painful sensations were unaffected. The PAG receives inputs from many other brain regions, including the hypothalamus, cortex and thalamus, and is the main pathway through which cortical and other inputs act to control the nociceptive gate in the dorsal horn.

The PAG projects first to an area of the medulla close to the midline, known as the nucleus raphe magnus (NRM), and thence via the dorsolateral funiculus of the spinal cord to the dorsal horn. Two important transmitters in this pathway are 5-hydroxytryptamine and enkephalin, which act directly or via interneurons to inhibit the discharge of spinothalamic neurons (Fig. 41.5).

The descending inhibitory pathway is probably an important site of action for opioid analgesics (see below). Both PAG and SG are particularly rich in enkephalin-containing neurons, and opioid antagonists such as **naloxone** (see later section) can prevent electrically induced analgesia, which would suggest that opioid peptides may function as transmitters in this system. The physiological role of opioid peptides in regulating pain transmission has been controversial, mainly because under normal conditions naloxone has relatively little effect on pain threshold. Under pathological conditions, however, when stress is present, naloxone causes hyperalgesia, implying that the opioid system is active.

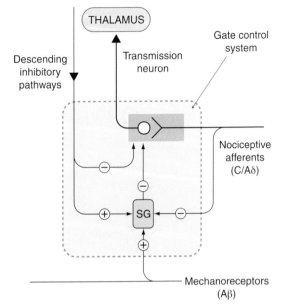

Fig. 41.4 Schematic diagram of the gate control system. This system regulates the passage of impulses from the peripheral afferent fibres to the thalamus via transmission neurons originating in the dorsal horn. Neurons in the *substantia gelatinosa* (*SG*) of the dorsal horn act to inhibit the transmission pathway. Inhibitory interneurons are activated by descending inhibitory neurons or by non-nociceptive afferent input. They are inhibited by nociceptive C-fibre input, so the persistent C-fibre activity facilitates excitation of the transmission cells by either nociceptive or non-nociceptive inputs. This autofacilitation causes successive bursts of activity in the nociceptive afferents to become increasingly effective in activating transmission neurons. Details of the interneuronal pathways are not shown. (From Melzack R, Wall P D 1982 The challenge of pain. Penguin, Harmondsworth.)

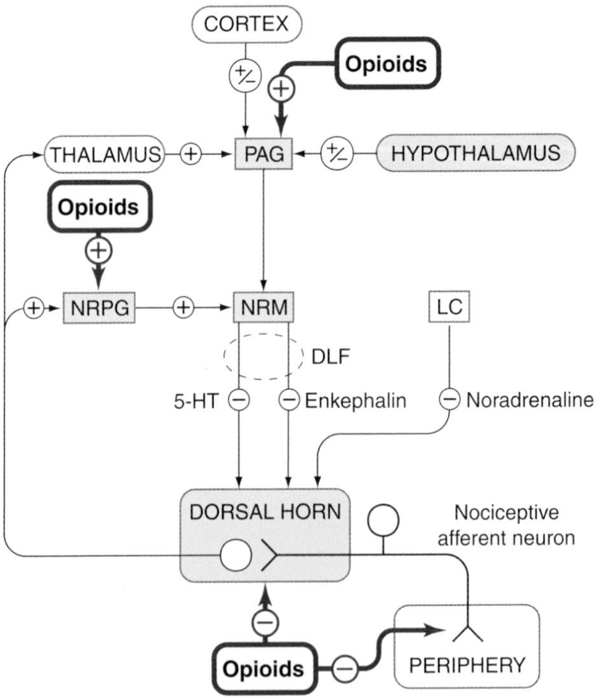

Fig. 41.5 The descending control system, showing the main sites of action of opioids on pain transmission. Opioids excite neurons in the periaqueductal grey matter (PAG) and in the *nucleus reticularis paragigantocellularis* (*NRPG*), which in turn project to the rostroventral medulla, which includes the *nucleus raphe magnus* (*NRM*). From the NRM, 5-hydroxytryptamine (5-HT)- and enkephalin-containing neurons run to the *substantia gelatinosa* of the dorsal horn, and exert an inhibitory influence on transmission. Opioids also act directly on the dorsal horn, as well as on the peripheral terminals of nociceptive afferent neurons. The *locus coeruleus* (*LC*) sends noradrenergic neurons to the dorsal horn, which also inhibit transmission. The pathways shown in this diagram represent a considerable oversimplification but depict the general organisation of the supraspinal control mechanisms. Shaded boxes represent areas rich in opioid peptides. (For more detailed information, see Fields & Basbaum, 1994.) DLF, dorsolateral funiculus.

There is also a noradrenergic pathway from the locus coeruleus (see Ch. 34), which has a similar inhibitory effect on transmission in the dorsal horn (Fig. 41.5). The use of tricyclic antidepressants to control pain (see below) probably depends on this pathway.

NEUROPATHIC PAIN

Neurological disease affecting the sensory pathway can produce severe chronic pain—termed *neuropathic pain*—unrelated to any peripheral tissue injury. This occurs with central nervous system (CNS) disorders such as stroke and multiple sclerosis, or with conditions associated with peripheral nerve damage, such as mechanical injury, diabetic neuropathy or herpes zoster infection (shingles). The pathophysiological mechanisms underlying this kind of pain are poorly understood, although spontaneous activity in damaged sensory neurons, due to overexpression or redistribution of voltage-gated sodium channels (see above), is thought to be a factor (see Chahine et al., 2005). The sympathetic nervous system also plays a part, because damaged sensory neurons can express α adrenoceptors and develop a sensitivity to noradrenaline (norepinephrine) that they do not possess

under normal conditions. Thus physiological stimuli that evoke sympathetic responses can produce severe pain, a phenomenon described clinically as *sympathetically mediated pain*. Neuropathic pain, which appears to be a component of many types of clinical pain (including common conditions such as back pain and cancer pain, as well as amputation pain), is generally difficult to control with conventional analgesic drugs. Potential new drug targets are discussed below.

PAIN AND NOCICEPTION

▼ As emphasised above, the perception of noxious stimuli (termed *nociception* by Sherrington) is not the same thing as pain, which is a subjective experience and includes a strong emotional (affective) component. The amount of pain that a particular stimulus produces depends on many factors other than the stimulus itself. A stabbing sensation in the chest will cause much more pain if it occurs

Modulation of pain transmission

- Transmission in the dorsal horn is subject to various modulatory influences, constituting the 'gate control' mechanism.
- Descending pathways from the midbrain and brain stem exert a strong inhibitory effect on dorsal horn transmission. Electrical stimulation of the midbrain periaqueductal grey area causes analgesia through this mechanism.
- The descending inhibition is mediated mainly by enkephalins, 5-hydroxytryptamine, noradrenaline and adenosine. Opioids cause analgesia partly by activating these descending pathways, partly by inhibiting transmission in the dorsal horn, and partly by inhibiting excitation of sensory nerve terminals in the periphery.
- Repetitive C-fibre activity facilitates transmission through the dorsal horn ('wind-up') by mechanisms involving activation of NMDA and substance P receptors.

spontaneously in a middle-aged man than if it is due to a 2-year-old poking him in the ribs with a sharp stick. The nociceptive component may be much the same, but the affective component is quite different. Animal tests of analgesic drugs commonly measure nociception and involve testing the reaction of an animal to a mildly painful stimulus, often mechanical or thermal. Such measures include the tail flick test (measuring the time taken for a rat to withdraw its tail when a standard radiant heat stimulus is applied) or the paw pressure test (measuring the withdrawal threshold when a normal or inflamed paw is pinched with increasing force). Similar tests can be used on human subjects, who simply indicate when a stimulus begins to feel painful, but the pain in these circumstances lacks the affective component. Clinically, spontaneous pain and allodynia of neuropathic origin is coming to be recognised as particularly important, but this is more difficult to model in animal studies. It is recognised clinically that many analgesics, particularly those of the morphine type, can greatly reduce the distress associated with pain even though the patient reports no great change in the intensity of the actual sensation. It is much more difficult to devise tests that measure this affective component, and important to realise that it may be at least as significant as the antinociceptive component in the action of these drugs. There is often a poor correlation between the activity of analgesic drugs in animal tests (which mainly assess antinociceptive activity) and their clinical effectiveness.

CHEMICAL SIGNALLING IN THE NOCICEPTIVE PATHWAY

CHEMOSENSITIVITY OF NOCICEPTIVE NERVE ENDINGS

In most cases, stimulation of nociceptive endings in the periphery is chemical in origin. Excessive mechanical or thermal stimuli can obviously cause acute pain, but the persistence of such pain after the stimulus has been removed, or the pain resulting from inflammatory or ischaemic changes in tissues, generally reflects an altered chemical environment of the pain afferents. The field was opened up in the 1960s by Keele and Armstrong, who developed a simple method for measuring the pain-producing effect of

various substances that act on cutaneous nerve endings. They produced small blisters on the forearm of human subjects, and applied chemicals to the blister base, recording the degree of pain that the subjects reported. Since then, electrical recording from sensory nerves and studies of the membrane responses of neurons in culture, coupled with molecular biology techniques to identify receptors and signal transduction pathways in nociceptive neurons, have produced a wealth of new information, and the humble nociceptive neuron has bathed in a limelight that more aristocratic neurons might envy. The current state of knowledge is reviewed by McMahon et al. (2006) and summarised in Figure 41.6.

The main groups of substances that stimulate pain endings in the skin are discussed below.

The vanilloid receptor (TRPV1)

▼ Capsaicin, the substance in chilli peppers that gives them their pungency, selectively excites nociceptive nerve terminals, causing intense pain if injected into the skin or applied to sensitive structures such as the cornea.[2] It produces this effect by binding to a receptor expressed by nociceptive afferent neurons. The receptor, originally known as the vanilloid receptor because many capsaicin-like compounds are based on the structure of vanillic acid, is a typical ligand-gated cation channel known as the *transient receptor potential vanilloid receptor 1* (TRPV1) (see Ch. 3). Agonists such as capsaicin open the channel, which is permeable to Na^+, Ca^{2+} and other cations, causing depolarisation and initiation of action potentials. TRPV1 responds not only to capsaicin-like agonists but also to other stimuli, including temperatures in excess of about 45°C (the threshold for pain) and proton concentrations in the micromolar range (pH 5.5 and below), which also cause pain. The receptor thus has unusual 'polymodal' characteristics that closely match those of nociceptive neurons, and it is believed to play a central role in nociception (see Wang & Woolf, 2005). TRPV1 is, like many other ionotropic receptors, modulated by phosphorylation, and several of the pain-producing substances that act through G-protein–coupled receptors (e.g. **bradykinin**; see below) work by sensitising TRPV1. A search for endogenous ligands for TRPV1 revealed, surprisingly, that **anandamide** (a lipid mediator previously identified as an agonist at cannabinoid receptors; see Ch. 43) is also a TRPV1 agonist, although less potent than capsaicin. Other endogenous lipid mediators, collectively known as *endovanilloids* (van der Stelt & Di Marzo, 2004) have since been identified, but their role in nociception is not currently known. Confirming the role of TRPV1 in nociception, it has been found that TRPV1 knockout mice show reduced responsiveness to noxious heat and also fail to show thermal hyperalgesia in response to inflammation. The latter observation is interesting, because TRPV1 expression is known to be increased by inflammation (see Wang & Woolf, 2005), and this may be a key mechanism by which primary hyperalgesia is produced.

The TRPV1 channels may represent the common pathway through which many pain-producing mediators exert their excitatory effects on nociceptors, and are considered to be a possible target for future analgesic drugs (see Krause et al., 2005).

Capsaicin and related irritant substances

▼ Capsaicin is a potent TRPV1 agonist that selectively stimulates nociceptive nerve endings, as described above. Similar substances exist in other pungent plants (ginger, black pepper, etc.), but none are as potent as capsaicin. **Resiniferatoxin**, a compound produced by some plants

---
[2]Anyone who has rubbed their eyes after cutting up chilli peppers will know this.

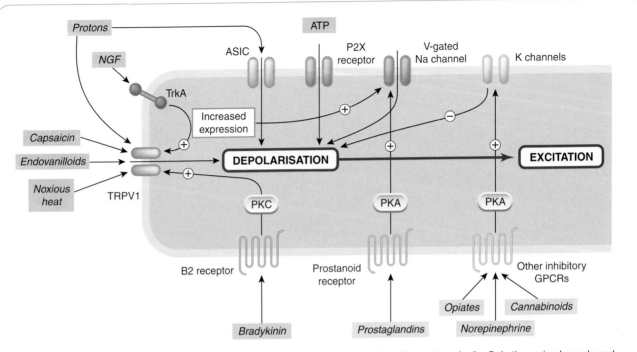

Fig. 41.6   Channels, receptors and transduction mechanisms of nociceptive afferent terminals. Only the main channels and receptors are shown. Ligand-gated channels include acid-sensitive ion channels (ASICs), ATP-sensitive channels (P_{2X} receptors) and the capsaicin-sensitive channel (TRPV1), which is also sensitive to protons and to temperature. Various facilitatory and inhibitory G-protein–coupled receptors (GPCRs) are shown, which regulate channel function through various second messenger systems. Growth factors such as nerve growth factor (NGF) act via kinase-linked receptors (TrkA) to control ion channel function and gene expression. B_2 receptor, bradykinin type 2 receptor; PKA, protein kinase A; PKC, protein kinase C.

of the *Euphorbia* family, whose sap causes painful skin irritation, is so far the most potent agonist known.

There are several interesting features of the action of capsaicin.

- The large influx of Ca^{2+} into nerve terminals that it produces results in peptide release (mainly substance P and CGRP), causing intense vascular and other physiological responses. The Ca^{2+} influx may be enough to cause nerve terminal degeneration, which takes days or weeks to recover. Attempts to use topically applied capsaicin to relieve painful skin conditions have had some success, but the initial strong irritant effect is a major disadvantage.
- Capsaicin applied to the bladder causes degeneration of primary afferent nerve terminals, and has been used to treat incontinence associated with bladder hyperreactivity in stroke or spinal injury patients. C-fibre afferents in the bladder serve a local reflex function, which promotes emptying when the bladder is distended, the reflex being exaggerated when central control is lost.
- Given to neonatal animals, capsaicin causes an irreversible loss of polymodal nociceptors, because the cell bodies (not just the terminals) are killed. The animals grow up with greatly reduced responses to painful stimuli. This has been used as an experimental procedure for investigating the role of these neurons.
- Unlike mammals, birds do not respond to capsaicin, because avian TRPV1 differs from mammalian TRPV1. Consequently, birds eat chilli peppers and distribute their seeds, while mammals (other than humans—the only masochistic mammal) avoid them.

Kinins

The most active substances are **bradykinin** and **kallidin** (see Ch. 13), two closely related peptides produced under conditions of tissue injury by the proteolytic cleavage of the active kinins

from a precursor protein contained in the plasma (reviewed by Dray & Perkins, 1993). Bradykinin is a potent pain-producing substance, acting partly by release of prostaglandins, which strongly enhance the direct action of bradykinin on the nerve terminals (Fig. 41.7). Bradykinin acts by combining with specific G-protein–coupled receptors, of which there are two subtypes, B_1 and B_2. In nociceptive neurons, B_2-receptors are coupled to activation of a specific isoform of protein kinase C (PKCε), which phosphorylates TRPV1 and facilitates opening of the TRPV1 channel.

Bradykinin acts on B_2-receptors but is converted in tissues by removal of a terminal arginine residue to **des-Arg^9 bradykinin**, which acts selectively on B_1-receptors. B_2 and B_1-receptors are both involved in the pathogenesis of pain and inflammation. B_1 receptors are unusual in that they are normally expressed at very low levels, but their expression is strongly up-regulated in inflamed tissues (see Calixto et al., 2004). Transgenic knockout animals lacking either type of receptor show reduced inflammatory hyperalgesia. Specific competitive antagonists for both B_1 and B_2-receptors are known, including peptides such as the B_2 antagonist **icatibant** (Ch. 13), as well as non-peptides. These show analgesic and anti-inflammatory properties, and may prove suitable for clinical use as analgesics (see Marceau & Regoli, 2004).

Prostaglandins

Prostaglandins do not themselves cause pain, but they strongly enhance the pain-producing effect of other agents such as 5-

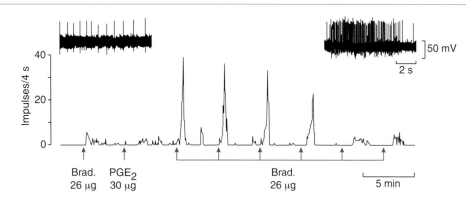

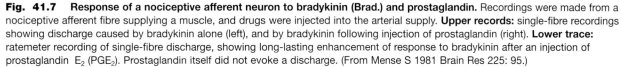

Fig. 41.7 **Response of a nociceptive afferent neuron to bradykinin (Brad.) and prostaglandin.** Recordings were made from a nociceptive afferent fibre supplying a muscle, and drugs were injected into the arterial supply. **Upper records:** single-fibre recordings showing discharge caused by bradykinin alone (left), and by bradykinin following injection of prostaglandin (right). **Lower trace:** ratemeter recording of single-fibre discharge, showing long-lasting enhancement of response to bradykinin after an injection of prostaglandin E_2 (PGE$_2$). Prostaglandin itself did not evoke a discharge. (From Mense S 1981 Brain Res 225: 95.)

hydroxytryptamine or bradykinin (Fig. 41.7). Prostaglandins of the E and F series are released in inflammation (Ch. 13) and also during tissue ischaemia. They sensitise nerve terminals to other agents partly by inhibiting potassium channels and partly by facilitating—through second messenger–mediated phosphorylation reactions (see Ch. 3)—the cation channels opened by noxious agents. It is of interest that bradykinin itself causes prostaglandin release, and thus has a powerful 'self-sensitising' effect on nociceptive afferents. Other eicosanoids, including prostacyclin, leukotrienes and the unstable hydroxyeicosatetraenoic acid (HETE) derivatives (Ch. 13), may also be important (see Samad et al., 2002). The analgesic effects of NSAIDs (Ch. 14) result from inhibition of prostaglandin synthesis.

Other peripheral mediators

Various metabolites and substances are released from damaged or ischaemic cells, or inflamed tissues, including ATP, protons (produced by lactic acid), 5-hydroxytryptamine, histamine and K^+, many of which affect nociceptive nerve terminals.

ATP excites nociceptive nerve terminals by acting on P_{2X3} receptors, a form of ligand-gated ion channel that is selectively expressed by these neurons. Down-regulation of P_{2X3} receptors, by antisense DNA technology, reduces inflammatory pain.[3] Antagonists at this receptor may be developed for clinical use. ATP and other purine mediators, such as adenosine, also play a role in the dorsal horn, and other types of purinoceptor may also be targeted by analgesic drugs in the future (see Liu & Salter, 2005).

Low pH excites nociceptive afferent neurons partly by opening proton-activated cation channels (acid-sensitive ion channels) and partly by facilitation of TRPV1 (see above).

5-Hydroxytryptamine causes excitation, but studies with antagonists suggest that it plays at most a minor role. Histamine is also

Mechanisms of pain and nociception

- *Nociception* is the mechanism whereby noxious peripheral stimuli are transmitted to the central nervous system. *Pain* is a subjective experience not always associated with nociception.
- Polymodal nociceptors (PMNs) are the main type of peripheral sensory neuron that responds to noxious stimuli. The majority are non-myelinated C fibres whose endings respond to thermal, mechanical and chemical stimuli.
- Chemical stimuli acting on PMNs to cause pain include bradykinin, protons, ATP and vanilloids (e.g. capsaicin). PMNs are sensitised by prostaglandins, which explains the analgesic effect of aspirin-like drugs, particularly in the presence of inflammation.
- The vanilloid receptor TRPV1 (transient receptor potential vanilloid receptor 1) responds to noxious heat as well as capsaicin-like agonists. The lipid mediator anandamide is an agonist at vanilloid receptors, as well as being an endogenous cannabinoid receptor agonist.
- Nociceptive fibres terminate in the superficial layers of the dorsal horn, forming synaptic connections with transmission neurons running to the thalamus.
- PMN neurons release glutamate (fast transmitter) and various peptides (especially substance P) that act as slow transmitters. Peptides are also released peripherally and contribute to neurogenic inflammation.
- Neuropathic pain, associated with damage to neurons of the nociceptive pathway rather than an excessive peripheral stimulus, is frequently a component of chronic pain states and may respond poorly to opioid analgesics.

---

[3]P_{2X3} knockout mice are, in contrast, fairly normal in this respect, presumably because other mechanisms take over.

active but causes itching rather than actual pain. Both these substances are released locally in inflammation (see Ch. 13).

Opioid peptides released peripherally inhibit nociceptor excitability, as do cannabinoids. These agents act through G-protein–coupled receptors that are negatively coupled to adenylate cyclase, and hence their effects oppose those of prostaglandins. The physiological significance of these mediators in the periphery is uncertain.

In summary, pain endings can be activated or sensitised by a wide variety of endogenous mediators, the receptors for which are often up- or down-regulated under pathophysiological conditions. Neuroplasticity plays an important role in persistent pain states, irrespective of their primary cause; not surprisingly, the signalling pathways have much in common with, and are at least as complex as, those involved in other neuroplasticity-based CNS pathologies discussed in earlier chapters. The strategies for developing the next wave of analgesic drugs therefore follow similar lines.[4]

TRANSMITTERS AND MODULATORS IN THE NOCICEPTIVE PATHWAY

The family of opioid peptides (see Ch. 16) plays a key role in nociceptive transmission; its role in descending inhibitory controls is summarised in Figure 41.5. Opiate analgesics (see below) act on the various receptors for these peptides.

Another peptide family thought to play a key role is the tachykinin family (see Ch. 16), of which substance P is the best-known member. Substance P is expressed by nociceptive afferent neurons and released at their peripheral and central terminals. In the periphery, it produces some of the features of neurogenic inflammation (see above), and in the dorsal horn it may be involved in wind-up and central sensitisation. In animal models, substance P antagonists are effective analgesic drugs, but clinical trials have failed to confirm this in humans, so the high hopes for developing a new type of analgesic for clinical use have been dashed. The reason for this failure is not clear, but it may imply that substance P is less important as a pain mediator in humans than in rats.

Other mediators include the following.

- Glutamate (see Ch. 33) is released from primary afferent neurons and, acting on AMPA receptors, is responsible for fast synaptic transmission at the first synapse in the dorsal horn. There is also a slower NMDA receptor–mediated response, which is important in relation to the wind-up phenomenon (see Fig. 41.3).
- GABA (see Ch. 33) is released by spinal cord interneurons and inhibits transmitter release by primary afferent terminals in the dorsal horn.
- 5-Hydroxytryptamine is the transmitter of inhibitory neurons running from NRM to the dorsal horn.

- Noradrenaline is the transmitter of the inhibitory pathway from the locus coeruleus to the dorsal horn, and possibly also in other antinociceptive pathways.
- Adenosine plays a dual role in regulating nociceptive transmission, activation of A_1 receptors causing analgesia, by acting on both peripheral nerve terminals and dorsal horn neurons, while activation of A_2 receptors in the periphery does the reverse (see Liu & Salter, 2005). There is evidence for descending inhibitory purinergic pathways acting on pain transmission through A_1 receptors.

ANALGESIC DRUGS

MORPHINE-LIKE DRUGS

The term *opioid* applies to any substance, whether endogenous or synthetic, that produces morphine-like effects that are blocked by antagonists such as naloxone. The older term, *opiate*, is restricted to synthetic morphine-like drugs with non-peptidic structures. The field is reviewed thoroughly by Herz (1993).

Opium is an extract of the juice of the poppy *Papaver somniferum*, which has been used for social and medicinal purposes for thousands of years as an agent to produce euphoria, analgesia and sleep, and to prevent diarrhoea. It was introduced in Britain at the end of the 17th century, usually taken orally as 'tincture of laudanum', addiction to which acquired a certain social cachet during the next 200 years. The situation changed when the hypodermic syringe and needle were invented in the mid-19th century, and opiate dependence began to take on a more sinister significance.

CHEMICAL ASPECTS

Opium contains many alkaloids related to morphine. The structure of morphine (Fig. 41.8) was determined in 1902, and since then many semisynthetic compounds (produced by chemical modification of morphine) and fully synthetic opiates have been studied. In addition to morphine-like compounds, opium also contains papaverine, a smooth muscle relaxant (see Ch. 19).

The main groups of drugs that are discussed in this section are as follow.

- Morphine analogues. These are compounds closely related in structure to morphine and often synthesised from it. They may be agonists (e.g. **morphine**, **diamorphine** [heroin] and **codeine**), partial agonists (e.g. **nalorphine** and **levallorphan**) or antagonists (e.g. **naloxone**).
- Synthetic derivatives with structures unrelated to morphine:
  —phenylpiperidine series (e.g. **pethidine** and **fentanyl**)
  —methadone series (e.g. **methadone** and **dextropropoxyphene**)
  —benzomorphan series (e.g. **pentazocine** and **cyclazocine**)
  —semisynthetic thebaine derivatives (e.g. **etorphine** and **buprenorphine**).

Mention should also be made of **loperamide**, an opiate that does not enter the brain and therefore lacks analgesic activity. Like other opiates (see below), it inhibits peristalsis, and it is used to control diarrhoea (see Ch. 25).

---

[4]And, sceptics may argue, face similar obstacles in relation to specificity and unwanted effects.

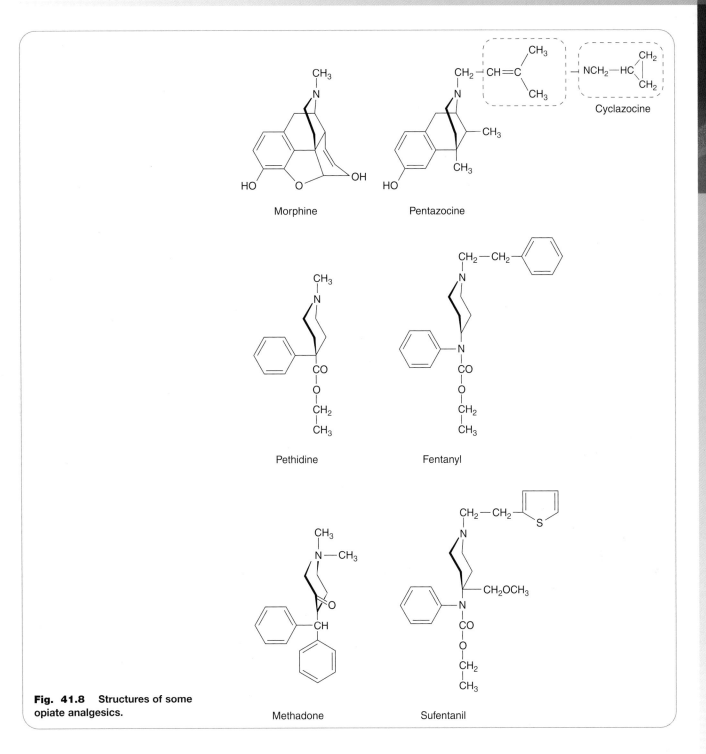

Fig. 41.8 Structures of some opiate analgesics.

Morphine analogues

Morphine is a phenanthrene derivative with two planar rings and two aliphatic ring structures, which occupy a plane roughly at right angles to the rest of the molecule (Fig. 41.8). Variants of the morphine molecule have been produced by substitution at one or both of the hydroxyl groups or at the nitrogen atom.

Synthetic derivatives

Phenylpiperidine series. Pethidine (known as meperidine in the USA), the first fully synthetic morphine-like drug, was discovered accidentally when new atropine-like drugs were being

sought. It is chemically unlike morphine, although its pharmacological actions are very similar. Fentanyl and sufentanil (the latter not used in the UK) are more potent and shorter-acting derivatives that are used intravenously, or for chronic pain via patches applied to the skin, to treat severe pain or as an adjunct to anaesthesia.

Methadone series. Methadone, although its structural formula bears no obvious chemical relationship to that of morphine, assumes a similar conformation in solution and was designed by reference to the common three-dimensional structural features of morphine and pethidine (Fig. 41.8). It is longer acting than morphine but otherwise very similar to it. Dextropropoxyphene is very similar and was used clinically for treating mild or moderate pain (no longer recommended on account of cardiotoxicity).

Benzomorphan series. The most important members of this class are pentazocine and cyclazocine (Fig. 41.8). These drugs differ from morphine in their receptor-binding profile (see below), and so have somewhat different actions and side effects. Cyclazocine is not used in the UK, and the use of pentazocine is declining.

Thebaine derivatives. Etorphine is a highly potent morphine-like drug used mainly in veterinary practice. Buprenorphine resembles morphine but is a partial agonist (see below); therefore, although very potent, its maximal effect is less than that of morphine, and it antagonises the effect of other opiates.

OPIOID RECEPTORS

The discovery of endogenous opiod peptides (enkephalins, see Ch. 16) by Hughes and Kosterlitz in 1972 was quickly followed by the discovery by Snyder and his collegues of specific binding sites in the brain, and the identification of these as specific opioid receptors, the existence of which had been proposed much earlier to account for the actions of drugs that antagonised the effects of morphine. Various pharmacological observations implied that more than one type of receptor was involved, the original suggestion of multiple receptor types arising from in vivo studies of the spectrum of actions (analgesia, sedation, pupillary constriction, bradycardia, etc.) produced by different drugs. It was also found that some opiates, but not all, were able to relieve withdrawal symptoms in morphine-dependent animals, and this was interpreted in terms of distinct receptor subtypes. The conclusion (see Dhawan et al., 1996) from these and many

subsequent pharmacological studies, later confirmed by receptor cloning, is that three types of opioid receptor, termed μ, δ and κ[5] (all of them typical G-protein–coupled receptors; see Ch. 3), mediate the main pharmacological effects of opiates, as summarised in Table 41.1.[6] There is pharmacological evidence for further subdivisions of each of these three subtypes; it is possible that splice variants and receptor dimerisation (see Ch. 3) can account for this pharmacological diversity. Studies on the characteristics of transgenic mouse strains lacking each of the three main subtypes (see Law et al., 2000) show that the major pharmacological effects of morphine, including analgesia, are mediated by the μ-receptor.

The interaction of various opioid drugs and peptides with the various receptor types is summarised in Table 41.2. In addition to endogenous peptides and drugs in clinical use, some agents that are used as experimental tools for distinguishing the different receptor subtypes are also shown.

Table 41.1 Functional effects associated with the main types of opioid receptor

	μ	δ	κ
Analgesia			
Supraspinal	+++	−	−
Spinal	++	++	+
Peripheral	++	−	++
Respiratory depression	+++	++	−
Pupil constriction	++	−	+
Reduced gastrointestinal motility	++	++	+
Euphoria	+++	−	−
Dysphoria	−	−	+++
Sedation	++	−	++
Physical dependence	+++	−	+

Opioid analgesics

- Opioid drugs include:
  - phenanthrene derivatives structurally related to morphine
  - synthetic compounds with a variety of dissimilar structures but similar pharmacological effects.
- Important morphine-like agonists include diamorphine and codeine; other structurally related compounds are partial agonists (e.g. nalorphine and levallorphan) or antagonists (e.g. naloxone).
- The main groups of synthetic analogues are the piperidines (e.g. pethidine and fentanyl), the methadone-like drugs, the benzomorphans (e.g. pentazocine) and the thebaine derivatives (e.g. buprenorphine).
- Opioid analgesics may be given orally, by injection, or intrathecally to produce analgesia.

[5]A fourth subtype, σ, was also postulated in order to account for the 'dysphoric' effects (anxiety, hallucinations, bad dreams, etc.) produced by some opiates. These are, however, not true opioid receptors, because many other types of psychotropic drug also interact with them, and their biological role remains unclear (see Walker et al., 1990). Of the opiate drugs, only benzomorphans, such as pentazocine and cyclazocine, bind appreciably to σ receptors, which is consistent with their known psychotomimetic properties.

[6]The opiod system is unusual among mediator system directed by G-protein-coupled receptors, in that there are many (20 or more) opioid peptides but only three receptors. In contrast, 5-hydroxytryptamine, for example, is a single mediator interacting with many (about 14) receptors, which is the more common pattern.

Opioid receptors

- μ-Receptors are thought to be responsible for most of the analgesic effects of opioids, and for some major unwanted effects (e.g. respiratory depression, euphoria, sedation and dependence). Most of the analgesic opioids are μ-receptor agonists.
- δ-Receptors are probably more important in the periphery but may also contribute to analgesia.
- κ-Receptors contribute to analgesia at the spinal level and may elicit sedation and dysphoria, but produce relatively few unwanted effects and do not contribute to dependence. Some analgesics are relatively κ-selective.
- σ-Receptors are not true opioid receptors but are the site of action of certain psychotomimetic drugs, with which some opioids interact.
- All opioid receptors are linked through G-proteins to inhibition of adenylate cyclase. They also facilitate opening of potassium channels (causing hyperpolarisation) and inhibit opening of calcium channels (inhibiting transmitter release). These membrane effects are not linked to the decrease in cAMP formation.
- Functional heterodimers, formed by combination of different types of opioid receptor, may occur and give rise to further pharmacological diversity.

AGONISTS AND ANTAGONISTS

Opiates vary not only in their receptor specificity but also in their efficacy at the different types of receptor. Thus some agents act as agonists on one type of receptor, and antagonists or partial agonists at another, producing a very complicated pharmacological picture. Some of this complexity may reflect the existence of receptor heterodimers whose functional properties differ from those of the well-studied monomeric opiate receptors. 'Agonist-directed trafficking' (see Ch. 3), whereby different ligands acting on the same receptor can elicit different cellular responses, may also account for some of the complexity. Current understanding of why different opiates have different actions is far from complete.

Three main pharmacological categories are recognised (Table 41.2).

- *Pure agonists.* This group includes most of the typical morphine-like drugs. They all have high affinity for μ receptors and generally lower affinity for δ and κ sites. Some drugs of this type, notably codeine, methadone and dextropropoxyphene, are sometimes referred to as weak agonists because their maximal effects, both analgesic and unwanted, are less than those of morphine, and they do not cause dependence. Whether they are truly partial agonists is not established.

Table 41.2 Selectivity of opioid drugs and peptides for receptor subtypes

	μ	δ	κ
Endogenous peptides			
β-Endorphin	+++	+++	+++
Leu-enkephalin	+	+++	−
Met-enkephalin	++	+++	−
Dynorphin	++	+	+++
Opiate drugs			
Pure agonists			
Morphine, codeine, oxymorphone, dextropropoxyphene	+++	+	+
Methadone	+++	−	−
Meperidine	++	+	+
Etorphine, bremazocine	+++	+++	+++
Fentanyl, sufentanil	+++	+	−
Partial/mixed agonists			
Pentazocine, ketocyclazocine	+	+	++
Nalbuphine	+	+	(++)
Nalorphine	++	−	(++)
Buprenorphine	(+++)	−	++
Antagonists			
Naloxone	+++	+	++
Naltrexone	+++	+	+++
Research tools (receptor-selective)			
DAMGO[a]	+++	−	−
DPDPE[a]	−	++	−
U50488[b]	−	−	+++
CTOP[a]	+++	−	−
Naltrindole, diprenorphine	−	+++	−
Nor-binaltorphimine	+	+	+++

Note: Blue + symbols represent **agonists** activity; partial agonists in parentheses
Black + symbols denote **antagonist** activity.
− symbols represent weak or no activity.
[a]DAMGO, DPDPE and CTOP are synthetic opioid-like peptides, more receptor-selective than endogenous opioids.
[b]U50488 is a synthetic opiate.

- *Partial agonists and mixed agonist–antagonists.* These drugs, typified by nalorphine and pentazocine, combine a degree of agonist and antagonist activity on different receptors. Nalorphine, for example, is an agonist when tested on guinea pig ileum, but it also inhibits competitively the effect of morphine on this tissue (consistent with a partial agonist profile; see Ch. 2). In vivo, it shows a similar mixture of agonist and antagonist actions. Pentazocine and cyclazocine, on the other hand, are antagonists at μ-receptors but partial agonists on δ and κ-receptors. Most of the drugs in this group tend to cause dysphoria rather than euphoria, probably by acting on the κ-receptor.

- *Antagonists*. These drugs produce very little effect when given on their own but block the effects of opiates. The most important examples are naloxone and naltrexone.

MECHANISM OF ACTION OF OPIATES

The opiates have probably been studied more intensively than any other group of drugs in the effort to understand their powerful effects in molecular, biochemical and physiological terms, and to use this understanding to develop opiate drugs as analgesics with significant advantages over morphine. While the receptor biology is well worked out (see Waldhoer et al., 2004), the physiological pathways that are regulated by opiates, which underlie their analgesic and other actions, are only partly understood. Even so, morphine—described by Osler as 'God's own medicine'—remains the standard against which any new analgesic is assessed. For a review on the neuropharmacology of opiates, see Yaksh (1997).

Cellular actions

Opioid receptors belong to the family of G-protein–coupled receptors, and all three receptor subtypes inhibit adenylyl cyclase, so reducing the intracellular cAMP content (see Dhawan et al., 1996), secondarily affecting protein phosphorylation pathways and hence cell function. They also exert effects on ion channels through a direct G-protein coupling to the channel. By these means, opiates promote the opening of potassium channels and inhibit the opening of voltage-gated calcium channels, which are the main effects seen at the membrane level. These membrane effects reduce both neuronal excitability (because the increased K^+ conductance causes hyperpolarisation of the membrane) and transmitter release (due to inhibition of Ca^{2+} entry). The overall effect is therefore inhibitory at the cellular level. Nonetheless, opiates increase activity in some neuronal pathways (see below) by suppressing the firing of inhibitory interneurons. At the cellular level, all three receptor subtypes mediate very similar effects, although the heterogeneous distribution of the receptors means that particular neurons and pathways are affected selectively by different agonists.

Effects on the nociceptive pathway

Opioid receptors are widely distributed in the brain, and their relationship to the nociceptive pathway is summarised in Figure 41.5. Opiates are effective as analgesics when given intrathecally in minute doses, implying that a central action can account for their analgesic effect. Injection of morphine into the PAG region causes marked analgesia, which can be prevented by surgical interruption of the descending pathway to NRM or by blocking 5-hydroxytryptamine synthesis pharmacologically with *p*-chlorophenylalanine. This latter procedure blocks the 5-hydroxytryptamine pathway running from NRM to the dorsal horn. Moreover, systemic morphine is rendered less effective in suppressing nociceptive spinal reflexes by transection of the spinal cord in the neck, and the firing of neurons associated with the descending inhibitory pathways is increased by morphine, confirming that there is a significant supraspinal component of the overall effect.

At the spinal level, morphine inhibits transmission of nociceptive impulses through the dorsal horn and suppresses nociceptive spinal reflexes, even in patients with spinal cord transection. It can inhibit release of substance P from primary afferent terminals in the dorsal horn neurons, but does not appear to do so in rats when given systemically in analgesic doses, implying that an action on primary afferent terminals may not be important in producing its therapeutic effect.

There is also evidence (see Sawynok, 2003) that opiates inhibit the discharge of nociceptive afferent terminals in the periphery, particularly under conditions of inflammation, in which the expression of opioid receptors by sensory neurons is increased. Injection of morphine into the knee joint following surgery to the joint provides effective analgesia, undermining the age-old belief that opiate analgesia is exclusively a central phenomenon.

PHARMACOLOGICAL ACTIONS

Morphine is typical of many opiate analgesics and will be taken as the reference compound.

The most important effects of morphine are on the CNS and the gastrointestinal tract, although numerous effects of lesser significance on many other systems have been described.

Effects on the central nervous system

Analgesia

Morphine is effective in most kinds of acute and chronic pain, although opiates in general are less useful in neuropathic pain syndromes (such as phantom limb and other types of deafferentation pain, and trigeminal neuralgia) than in pain associated with tissue injury, inflammation or tumour growth.

As well as being antinociceptive, morphine also reduces the affective component of pain. This reflects its supraspinal action, possibly at the level of the limbic system, which is probably involved in the euphoria-producing effect. Drugs such as nalorphine and pentazocine share the antinociceptive actions of morphine but have much less effect on the psychological response to pain.

Euphoria

Morphine causes a powerful sense of contentment and well-being. This is an important component of its analgesic effect, because the agitation and anxiety associated with a painful illness or injury are thereby reduced. If morphine or diamorphine (heroin) is given intravenously, the result is a sudden 'rush' likened to an 'abdominal orgasm'. The euphoria produced by morphine depends considerably on the circumstances. In patients who are distressed it is pronounced, but in patients who become accustomed to chronic pain, morphine causes analgesia with little or no euphoria. Some patients report restlessness rather than euphoria under these circumstances.

Euphoria appears to be mediated through μ receptors, and to be balanced by the dysphoria associated with κ-receptor activation (see Table 41.1). Thus, different opiate drugs vary greatly in the amount of euphoria that they produce. It does not occur with codeine or with pentazocine to any marked extent, and nalorphine, in doses sufficient to cause analgesia, produces dysphoria.

Respiratory depression

Respiratory depression, resulting in increased arterial P_{CO_2}, occurs with a normal analgesic dose of morphine or related compounds. Analgesia and respiratory depression are both mediated by μ-receptors, and the balance between them is therefore the same for most opiates. The depressant effect is associated with a decrease in the sensitivity of the respiratory centre to P_{CO_2}. Neurons in the medullary respiratory centre itself do not appear to be directly depressed, but opiates applied to the ventral surface of the medulla in the region where CO_2 chemosensitivity is maximal have a powerful depressant effect on respiration.

Respiratory depression by opiates is not accompanied by depression of the medullary centres controlling cardiovascular function (in contrast to the action of anaesthetics and other general depressants). This means that respiratory depression produced by opiates is much better tolerated than a similar degree of depression caused by, say, a barbiturate. Nonetheless, respiratory depression is the most troublesome unwanted effect of these drugs and, unlike that due to general CNS depressant drugs, it occurs at therapeutic doses. It is the commonest cause of death in acute opiate poisoning.

Depression of cough reflex

Cough suppression, surprisingly, does not correlate closely with the analgesic and respiratory depressant actions of opiates, and its mechanism at the receptor level is unclear. In general, increasing substitution on the phenolic hydroxyl group of morphine increases antitussive relative to analgesic activity. Thus codeine suppresses cough in subanalgesic doses and is often used in cough medicines (see Ch. 23). **Pholcodine** is even more selective, although these agents cause constipation as an unwanted effect.

Nausea and vomiting

Nausea and vomiting occur in up to 40% of patients to whom morphine is given, and do not seem to be separable from the analgesic effect among a range of opiate analgesics. The site of action is the area postrema (chemoreceptor trigger zone), a region of the medulla where chemical stimuli of many kinds may initiate vomiting (see Ch. 25).[7] Nausea and vomiting following morphine injection are usually transient and disappear with repeated administration.

Pupillary constriction

Pupillary constriction is caused by μ and κ receptor–mediated stimulation of the oculomotor nucleus. Pinpoint pupils are an important diagnostic feature in opiate poisoning,[8] because most other causes of coma and respiratory depression produce pupillary dilatation.

Effects on the gastrointestinal tract

Morphine increases tone and reduces motility in many parts of the gastrointestinal system, resulting in constipation, which may be severe and very troublesome to the patient. The resulting delay in gastric emptying can considerably retard the absorption of other drugs. Pressure in the biliary tract increases because of contraction of the gall bladder and constriction of the biliary sphincter. Opiates should be avoided in patients suffering from biliary colic due to gallstones, in whom pain may be increased rather than relieved. The rise in intrabiliary pressure can cause a transient increase in the concentration of amylase and lipase in the plasma.

The action of morphine on visceral smooth muscle is probably mediated mainly through the intramural nerve plexuses, because the increase in tone is reduced or abolished by atropine. It is partly mediated by a central action of morphine, because intraventricular injection of morphine inhibits propulsive gastrointestinal movements. The local effect of morphine and other opiates on neurons of the myenteric plexus is inhibitory, associated with hyperpolarisation resulting from an increased K^+ conductance. The receptors involved in these effects are of the μ, κ and δ type, with much variation between different preparations and different species.

Other actions of opiates

Morphine releases histamine from mast cells by an action unrelated to opioid receptors. This release of histamine can cause local effects, such as urticaria and itching at the site of the injection, or systemic effects, namely bronchoconstriction and hypotension. The bronchoconstrictor effect can have serious consequences for

---

> **Actions of morphine**
>
> - The main pharmacological effects are:
>   - analgesia
>   - euphoria and sedation
>   - respiratory depression and suppression of cough
>   - nausea and vomiting
>   - pupillary constriction
>   - reduced gastrointestinal motility, causing constipation
>   - histamine release, causing bronchoconstriction and hypotension.
> - The most troublesome unwanted effects are constipation and respiratory depression.
> - Morphine may be given by injection (intravenous or intramuscular) or by mouth, often as slow-release tablets.
> - Acute overdosage with morphine produces coma and respiratory depression.
> - Morphine is metabolised to morphine-6-glucuronide, which is more potent as an analgesic.
> - Morphine and morphine-6-glucuronide are the active metabolites of diamorphine and codeine.

---

[7]The chemically related compound apomorphine is more strongly emetic than morphine, through its action as a dopamine agonist; despite its name, it is inactive on opioid receptors. It was at one time used as a conditioned 'aversion therapy' for treating various kinds of unwanted behaviour.

[8]The exception is pethidine, which causes pupillary dilatation because it blocks muscarinic receptors.

asthmatic patients, to whom morphine should not be given. Pethidine does not produce this effect.

Hypotension and bradycardia occur with large doses of most opiates, due to an action on the medulla. With morphine and similar drugs, histamine release may contribute to the hypotension.

Effects on smooth muscle other than that of the gastrointestinal tract and bronchi are slight, although spasms of the ureters, bladder and uterus sometimes occur. The Straub tail reaction, an improbable phenomenon beloved of pharmacologists, consists of a raising and stiffening of the tail of rats or mice given opiate drugs, and is due to spasm of a muscle at the base of the tail. It was through this effect that the analgesic action of pethidine was discovered.

Opiates also exert complex immunosuppressant effects, which may be important as a link between the nervous system and immune function (see Vallejo et al., 2004). The pharmacological significance of this is not yet clear, but there is evidence in humans that the immune system is depressed by long-term opiate abuse, leading to increased susceptibility to infections.

TOLERANCE AND DEPENDENCE

Tolerance to opiates (i.e. an increase in the dose needed to produce a given pharmacological effect) develops within a few days and is readily demonstrated. *Physical dependence* refers to a state in which withdrawal of the drug causes adverse physiological effects, i.e. the *abstinence syndrome*. These phenomena occur to some degree whenever opiates are administered for more than a few days. They must not be confused with addiction (see Ch. 43), in which physical dependence is much more pronounced and psychological dependence (or 'craving') is the main driving force. Addiction is rare in patients receiving opiates to control pain. The opiate withdrawal syndrome can be reproduced in experimental animals and appears to be closely related to tolerance.

Tolerance

Tolerance can be detected within 12–24 hours of morphine administration. Figure 41.9 shows the increase in the equianalgesic dose of morphine (measured by the hotplate test) that occurred when a slow-release pellet of morphine was implanted subcutaneously in mice. The pellet was removed 8 hours before the test, to allow morphine absorbed from it to be eliminated before the test was carried out. Within 3 days, the equianalgesic dose increased about fivefold. Sensitivity returned to normal within about 3 days of removing the pellet. Tolerance extends to most of the pharmacological effects of morphine, including analgesia, emesis, euphoria and respiratory depression, but affects the constipating and pupil-constricting actions much less. Therefore addicts may take 50 times the normal analgesic dose of morphine with relatively little respiratory depression but marked constipation and pupillary constriction.

The cellular mechanisms responsible for tolerance are discussed in Chapter 43. Certain possibilities can be excluded, such as increased metabolic degradation, reduced affinity of opiates for their receptors, down-regulation of opioid receptors and inhibition of the release of endogenous opioids. Tolerance is a general

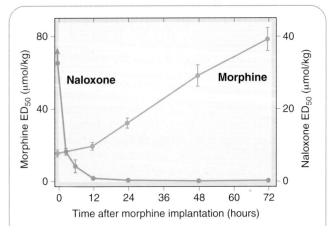

Fig. 41.9 Development of morphine tolerance in mice. The median effective dose (ED_{50}) for analgesia (hotplate test) produced by subcutaneous injection of a test dose of morphine (orange line) was measured at intervals after implantation of a slow-release pellet of morphine, the pellet being removed 8 hours before the assay in order to allow the circulating morphine concentration to fall to zero before the test dose was given. The ED_{50} increases about fivefold after 72 hours. Simultaneously, the dose of naloxone needed to precipitate withdrawal symptoms (green line) decreases very markedly. (From Way E L et al. 1969 J Pharmacol Exp Ther 167: 1.)

phenomenon of opioid receptor ligands, irrespective of which type of receptor they act on. Cross-tolerance occurs between drugs acting at the same receptor, but not between opiates that act on different receptors. In clinical settings, the opiate dose required for effective pain relief may increase as a result of developing tolerance, but it does not constitute a major problem.

Physical dependence

Physical dependence is characterised by a clear-cut abstinence syndrome. In experimental animals (e.g. rats), abrupt withdrawal of morphine after chronic administration for a few days causes an increased irritability, loss of weight and a variety of abnormal behaviour patterns, such as body shakes, writhing, jumping and signs of aggression. These reactions decrease after a few days, but abnormal irritability and aggression persist for many weeks. The signs of physical dependence are much less intense if the opiate is withdrawn gradually. Humans often experience an abstinence syndrome when opiates are withdrawn after being used for pain relief over days or weeks, with symptoms of restlessness, runny nose, diarrhoea, shivering and piloerection.[9] The intensity of the abstinence syndrome varies greatly, and dependence rarely progresses to addiction, in which psychological dependence (i.e. craving for the drug) is the predominant feature.

Many physiological changes have been described in relation to the abstinence syndrome. For example, spinal reflex hyperexcitability occurs in morphine-dependent animals and can be produced by chronic intrathecal as well as systemic administration

---

[9]Causing goose pimples. This is the origin of the phrase 'cold turkey' used to describe the effect of morphine withdrawal.

of morphine. The noradrenergic pathways emanating from the locus coeruleus (see above) may also play an important role in causing the abstinence syndrome, and the α_2-adrenoceptor agonist **clonidine** (Ch. 11, p. 170) is sometimes used to alleviate it. In animal models, and also in humans, the abstinence syndrome is reduced by giving NMDA receptor antagonists (e.g. **ketamine**; see Ch. 33).[10] The rate of firing of locus coeruleus neurons is reduced by opiates and increased during the abstinence syndrome. Similar changes affect dopaminergic neurons in the ventral tegmental area that project to the nucleus accumbens. These cells receive input from opioid-containing neurons and constitute the 'reward pathway' responsible for the strong reinforcing effect of opiates (see Ch. 43).

PHARMACOKINETIC ASPECTS

Table 41.3 summarises the pharmacokinetic properties of the main opiate analgesics. The absorption of morphine congeners by mouth is variable. Morphine itself is slowly and erratically absorbed, and is commonly given by intravenous or intramuscular injection to treat acute severe pain; oral morphine is, however, often used in treating chronic pain, and slow-release preparations are available to increase its duration of action.

Tolerance and dependence

- Tolerance develops rapidly, accompanied by physical withdrawal syndrome.
- The mechanism of tolerance may involve adaptive up-regulation of adenylyl cyclase. It is not pharmacokinetic in origin, and receptor down-regulation is not a major factor.
- Dependence is satisfied by μ-receptor agonists, and the withdrawal syndrome is precipitated by μ-receptor antagonists.
- Dependence comprises two components: (i) physical dependence, associated with the withdrawal syndrome and lasting for a few days; and (ii) psychological dependence, associated with craving and lasting for months or years. Psychological dependence rarely occurs in patients being given opioids as analgesics.
- Weak, long-acting μ-receptor agonists such as methadone may be used to relieve withdrawal symptoms.
- Certain opioid analgesics, such as codeine, pentazocine, buprenorphine and tramadol, are much less likely to cause physical or psychological dependence.

Codeine is well absorbed and normally given by mouth. Most morphine-like drugs undergo considerable first-pass metabolism, and are therefore markedly less potent when taken orally than when injected.

The plasma half-life of most morphine analogues is 3–6 hours. Hepatic metabolism is the main mode of inactivation, usually by conjugation with glucuronide. This occurs at the 3- and 6-OH groups, and these glucuronides constitute a considerable fraction of the drug in the bloodstream. Morphine-6-glucuronide is, surprisingly, more active as an analgesic than morphine itself, and contributes substantially to the pharmacological effect. Morphine-3-glucuronide has been claimed to antagonise the analgesic effect of morphine, but the significance of this experimental finding is uncertain. Morphine glucuronides are excreted in the urine, so the dose needs to be reduced in cases of renal failure. Glucuronides also reach the gut via biliary excretion, where they are hydrolysed, most of the morphine being reabsorbed (enterohepatic circulation). Because of low conjugating capacity in neonates, morphine-like drugs have a much longer duration of action; because even a small degree of respiratory depression can be hazardous, morphine congeners should not be used in the neonatal period, nor used as analgesics during childbirth. Pethidine (see below) is a safer alternative for this purpose.

Analogues that have no free hydroxyl group in the 3-position (i.e. diamorphine, codeine) are metabolised to morphine, which accounts for all or part of their pharmacological activity. Morphine produces very effective analgesia when administered intrathecally, and is often used in this way by anaesthetists, the advantage being that the sedative and respiratory depressant effects are reduced, although not completely avoided.

For the treatment of chronic or postoperative pain, opiates are being increasingly used 'on demand' (patient-controlled analgesia). The patients are provided with an infusion pump that they control, the maximum possible rate of administration being limited to avoid acute toxicity. Contrary to fears, patients show little tendency to use excessively large doses and become dependent; instead, the dose is adjusted to achieve analgesia without excessive sedation, and is reduced as the pain subsides. Being in control of their own analgesia, the patients' anxiety and distress is reduced, and analgesic consumption actually tends to decrease.

UNWANTED EFFECTS

The main unwanted effects of morphine and related drugs are listed in Table 41.3.

Acute overdosage with morphine results in coma and respiratory depression, with characteristically constricted pupils. It is treated by giving naloxone intravenously. This also serves as a diagnostic test, for failure to respond to naloxone suggests a cause other than opiate poisoning for the comatose state.[11] There is a danger of precipitating a severe withdrawal syndrome with naloxone, because opiate poisoning occurs mainly in addicts.

---

[10]The opiate drug dextromethorphan has NMDA receptor blocking activity as well as being a μ-opioid receptor agonist, and appears to be less liable than other opiates to induce physical dependence.

[11]For unknown reasons, naloxone may be ineffective in reversing the effects of 'weak' opiates such as buprenorphine or dextropropoxyphene.

Individual variability

▼ Individuals vary by as much as 10-fold in their sensitivity to opioid analgesics. This is due to differences in the plasma concentration needed to produce a given effect, and therefore reflects pharmacodynamic rather than pharmacokinetic variability. It may be related to polymorphism of the μ-opioid receptor gene (see Ikeda et al., 2005). Genotyping could in principle be used to identify opioid-resistant individuals, but this approach has not yet been tested in practice.

OTHER OPIATE ANALGESICS

Diamorphine (heroin) is the diacetyl derivative of morphine. A strong smell of vinegar commonly provides the lead to illicit heroin producers, at least in fiction. In the body, it is rapidly deacetylated to morphine, and its effects are indistinguishable following oral administration. However, because of its greater lipid solubility, it crosses the blood–brain barrier more rapidly than morphine and gives a greater rush when injected intravenously. It is said to be less emetic than morphine, but the evidence for this is slight. It is still available in Britain for use as an analgesic, although it is banned in many countries. Its only advantage over morphine is its greater solubility, which allows smaller volumes to be given orally, subcutaneously or intrathecally. It exerts the same respiratory depressant effect as morphine, and if given intravenously is more likely to cause dependence.

Codeine (3-methylmorphine) is more reliably absorbed by mouth than morphine, but has only 20% or less of the analgesic potency. Furthermore, its analgesic effect does not increase appreciably at higher dose levels. It is therefore used mainly as an oral analgesic for mild types of pain (headache, backache, etc.). Unlike morphine, it causes little or no euphoria and is rarely addictive, so is available freely without prescription. It is often combined with paracetamol in proprietary analgesic preparations. In relation to its analgesic effect, codeine produces the same degree of respiratory depression as morphine, but the limited response even at high doses means that it is seldom a problem in practice. It does, however, cause constipation. Codeine has marked antitussive activity and is often used in cough mixtures (see Ch. 23). **Dihydrocodeine** is pharmacologically very similar, having no substantial advantages or disadvantages over codeine. About 10% of the population is resistant to the analgesic effect of codeine, because they lack the demethylating enzyme that converts it to morphine.

Pethidine (meperidine) is very similar to morphine in its pharmacological effects, except that it tends to cause restlessness rather than sedation, and it has an additional antimuscarinic action that may cause dry mouth and blurring of vision as side effects. It produces a very similar euphoric effect and is equally liable to cause dependence. Its duration of action is similar to that of morphine, but the route of metabolic degradation is different. Pethidine is partly *N*-demethylated in the liver to norpethidine, which has a hallucinogenic and convulsant effect. This becomes significant with large oral doses of pethidine, producing an overdose syndrome rather different from that of morphine. Pethidine is preferred to morphine for analgesia during labour, because it does not reduce the force of uterine contraction. Pethidine is only slowly eliminated in the neonate,

and naloxone may be needed to reverse respiratory depression in the baby. (Morphine is even more problematic in this regard, because the conjugation reactions on which the excretion of morphine, but not of pethidine, depends are deficient in the newborn). Severe reactions, consisting of excitement, hyperthermia and convulsions, have been reported when pethidine is given to patients receiving monoamine oxidase inhibitors. This seems to be due to inhibition of an alternative metabolic pathway, leading to increased norpethidine formation, but the details are not known.

Fentanyl and **sufentanil** are highly potent phenylpiperidine derivatives, with actions similar to those of morphine but with a more rapid onset and shorter duration of action, particularly sufentanil. Their main use is in anaesthesia, and they may be given intrathecally. They are also used in patient-controlled infusion systems, where a short duration of action is advantageous, and in severe chronic pain, when they are administered via patches applied to the skin.

Etorphine is a morphine analogue of remarkable potency, more than 1000 times that of morphine, but otherwise very similar in its actions. Its high potency confers no particular clinical advantage, but it is used to immobilise wild animals for trapping and research purposes, because the required dose, even for an elephant, is small enough to be incorporated into a dart or pellet.

Methadone is also pharmacologically similar to morphine, the main difference being that its duration of action is considerably longer (plasma half-life > 24 hours), and it is claimed to have less sedative action. The increased duration seems to occur because the drug is bound in the extravascular compartment and slowly released. One consequence is that the physical abstinence syndrome is less acute than with morphine or other short-acting drugs, although the psychological dependence is no less pronounced. Methadone is widely used as a means of treating morphine and diamorphine addiction. In the presence of methadone, an injection of morphine does not cause the normal euphoria, and the lack of a physical abstinence syndrome makes it possible to wean addicts from morphine or diamorphine by giving regular oral doses of methadone—an improvement if not a cure.[12]

Pentazocine is a mixed agonist–antagonist (see earlier section) with analgesic properties similar to those of morphine. However, it causes marked dysphoria, with nightmares and hallucinations, rather than euphoria, and is now rarely used.

Buprenorphine is a partial agonist on μ receptors. It is less liable to cause dysphoria than pentazocine but more liable to cause respiratory depression. It has a long duration of action. Its abuse liability is probably less than that of morphine.

Meptazinol is a recently introduced opiate of unusual chemical structure. It can be given orally or by injection and has a duration of action shorter than that of morphine. It seems to be relatively free of morphine-like side effects, causing neither euphoria nor dysphoria, nor severe respiratory depression. It does, however, produce nausea, sedation and dizziness, and has

---

[12]The benefits come mainly from removing the risks of self-injection and the need to finance the drug habit through crime.

atropine-like side effects. Because of its short duration of action and lack of respiratory depression, it may have advantages for obstetric analgesia.

Tramadol is widely used as an analgesic for postoperative pain. It is a weak agonist at µ-opioid receptors, and also a weak inhibitor of noradrenaline reuptake. It is effective as an analgesic and appears to have a better side effect profile than most opiates, although psychiatric reactions have been reported. It is given by mouth or by intramuscular or intravenous injection for moderate to severe pain.

OPIOID ANTAGONISTS

Nalorphine is closely related in structure to morphine, was the first specific antagonist to be discovered, and provided the first clear evidence in favour of a specific receptor for morphine, recognition of which led to the successful search for endogenous mediators. Nalorphine has, in fact, a more complicated action than that of a simple competitive antagonist (Table 41.2). In low doses, it is a competitive antagonist and blocks most actions of morphine in whole animals or isolated tissues. Higher doses, however, are analgesic and mimic the effects of morphine. These effects probably reflect an antagonist action on µ-receptors, coupled with a partial agonist action on δ and κ-receptors, the latter causing dysphoria, which makes it unsuitable for use as an analgesic. Nalorphine can itself produce physical dependence, but can also precipitate a withdrawal syndrome in morphine or diamorphine addicts. Nalorphine now has few clinical uses.

Naloxone was the first pure opioid antagonist, with affinity for all three opioid receptors. It blocks the actions of endogenous opioid peptides as well as those of morphine-like drugs, and has been extensively used as an experimental tool to determine the physiological role of these peptides, particularly in pain transmission.

Given on its own, naloxone produces very little effect in normal subjects but produces a rapid reversal of the effects of morphine and other opiates, including partial agonists such as pentazocine and nalorphine. It has little effect on pain threshold under normal conditions but causes hyperalgesia under conditions of stress or inflammation, when endogenous opioids are produced. This occurs, for example, in patients undergoing dental surgery, or in animals subjected to physical stress. Naloxone also inhibits acupuncture analgesia, which is known to be associated with the release of opioid peptides. Analgesia produced by PAG stimulation is also prevented.

The main clinical uses of naloxone are to treat respiratory depression caused by opiate overdosage, and occasionally to reverse the effect of opiate analgesics, used during labour, on the respiration of the newborn baby. It is usually given intravenously, and its effects are produced immediately. It is rapidly metabolised by the liver, and its effect lasts only 2–4 hours, which is considerably shorter than that of most morphine-like drugs. Therefore it may have to be given repeatedly.

Naloxone has no important unwanted effects of its own but precipitates withdrawal symptoms in addicts. It can be used to detect opiate addiction.

Naltrexone is very similar to naloxone but with the advantage of a much longer duration of action (half-life about 10 hours). It may be of value in addicts who have been 'detoxified', because it nullifies the effect of a dose of opiate should the patient's resolve fail. Its use in other conditions, such as alcoholism and septic shock, is being investigated, although the role of opioid peptides in these conditions is controversial.

Specific antagonists at µ, δ and κ-receptors are available for experimental use (Table 41.2) but not yet for clinical purposes.

PARACETAMOL

The NSAIDs (covered in detail in Ch. 14) are widely used to treat painful inflammatory conditions. **Paracetamol** (known as **acetaminophen** in the USA) deserves special mention. It was first synthesised more than a century ago, and since the 1950s has (alongside aspirin) been the most widely used over-the-counter remedy for minor aches and pains. Paracetamol differs from other NSAIDs in producing analgesic and antipyretic effects while lacking anti-inflammatory effects. It also lacks the tendency of other NSAIDs to cause gastric ulceration and bleeding. The reason for the difference between paracetamol and other NSAIDs is unclear. Biochemical tests showed it to be only a weak cyclo-oxygenase (COX) inhibitor, with some selectivity for brain COX. More recently, it was claimed to act on a novel COX variant (COX-3), which turned out to be a splice variant of the main COX isoform COX-1 (see Ch. 14). There is still uncertainty about the role of COX-3 in humans, and disagreement about its significance as a target for paracetamol (see Graham & Scott, 2003; Davies et al, 2004).

Paracetamol is well absorbed by mouth, and its plasma half-life is about 3 hours. It is metabolised by hydroxylation, conjugated mainly as glucuronide, and excreted in the urine. In therapeutic

---

Opioid antagonists

- Pure antagonists include naloxone (short acting) and naltrexone (long acting). They block µ, δ and κ-receptors more or less equally. Selective antagonists are available as experimental tools.
- Other drugs, such as nalorphine and pentazocine, produce a mixture of agonist and antagonist effects.
- Naloxone does not affect pain threshold normally but blocks stress-induced analgesia and can exacerbate clinical pain.
- Naloxone rapidly reverses opioid-induced analgesia and respiratory depression, and is used mainly to treat opioid overdose or to improve breathing in newborn babies affected by opioids given to the mother.
- Naloxone precipitates withdrawal symptoms in morphine-dependent patients or animals. Pentazocine may also do this.

Table 41.3   Characteristics of the main opioid analgesic drugs

Drug	Use(s)	Route(s) of administration	Pharmacokinetic aspects	Main adverse effects	Notes
Morphine	Widely used for acute and chronic pain	Oral, including sustained-release form Injection[a] Intrathecal	Half-life 3–4 h Converted to active metabolite (morphine 6-glucuronide)	Sedation Respiratory depression Constipation Nausea and vomiting Itching (histamine release) Tolerance and dependence Euphoria	Tolerance and withdrawal effects not common when used for analgesia
Diamorphine	Acute and chronic pain	Oral Injection	Acts more rapidly than morphine because of rapid brain penetration Metabolised to morphine	As morphine	Not available in all countries Considered (irrationally) to be analgesic of last resort. Also known as heroin
Hydromorphone	Acute and chronic pain	Oral Injection	Half-life 2–4 h No active metabolites	As morphine but allegedly less sedative	Levorphanol is similar, with longer duration of action
Methadone	Chronic pain Maintenance of addicts	Oral Injection	Long half-life (> 24 h) Slow onset	As morphine but little euphoric effect Accumulation may occur because of long half-life	Slow recovery results in attenuated withdrawal syndrome
Pethidine	Acute pain	Oral Intramuscular injection	Half-life 2–4 h Active metabolite (norpethidine) may account for stimulant effects	As morphine, anticholinergic effects Risk of excitement and convulsions	Known as meperidine in USA Interacts with monoamine oxidase inhibitors (Ch. 39)
Buprenorphine	Acute and chronic pain	Sublingual Injection Intrathecal	Half-life about 12 h Slow onset Inactive orally because of first-pass metabolism	As morphine but less pronounced Respiratory depression not reversed by naloxone (therefore not suitable for obstetric use)	Useful in chronic pain with patient-controlled injection systems
Pentazocine	Mainly acute pain	Oral Injection	Half-life 2–4 h	Psychotomimetic effects (dysphoria) Irritation at injection site. May precipitate morphine withdrawal syndrome (μ-antagonist effect)	Nalbuphine is similar
Fentanyl	Acute pain Anaesthesia	Intravenous Epidermal Transdermal patch	Half-life 1–2 h	As morphine	High potency allows transdermal administration Sufentanil is similar Remifentanil is similar with more rapid onset and recovery

Table 41.3 (cont'd)   Characteristics of the main opioid analgesic drugs

Drug	Use(s)	Route(s) of administration	Pharmacokinetic aspects	Main adverse effects	Notes
Codeine	Mild pain	Oral	Acts as prodrug Metabolised to morphine and other active opioids	Mainly constipation No dependence liability	Effective only in mild pain Also used to suppress cough Dihydrocodeine is similar
Dextropropoxyphene	Mild pain	Mainly oral	Half-life ~4 h Active metabolite (norpropoxyphene) with half-life ~24 h	Respiratory depression May cause convulsions (possibly by action of norpropoxyphene)	Similar to codeine No longer recommended
Tramadol	Acute (mainly postoperative) and chronic pain	Oral Intravenous	Well absorbed Half-life 4–6 h	Dizziness May cause convulsions No respiratory depression	Metabolite of trazodone (Ch. 39) Mechanism of action uncertain Weak agonist at opioid receptors Also inhibits noradrenaline uptake

[a]Injections may by given intravenously, intramuscularly or subcutaneously for most drugs.

doses, it has few adverse effects. However, in overdose paracetamol causes severe liver damage, which is commonly fatal (see Chs 14 and 53), and the drug is often used in attempted suicide.

OTHER ANALGESIC DRUGS

▼ Several other drugs are used as analgesics, particularly to treat neuropathic pain states, which respond poorly to conventional analgesic drugs and pose a major clinical problem.

This group includes the following.

- *Tricyclic antidepressants*, particularly **imipramine** and **amitriptyline** (Ch. 39). These drugs act centrally by inhibiting noradrenaline reuptake and are highly effective in relieving neuropathic pain in some, but not all, cases. Their action is independent of their antidepressant effects, and selective serotonin reuptake inhibitors are not effective.
- *Antiepileptic drugs* (Ch. 40). **Carbamazepine**, **gabapentin** and occasionally **phenytoin** are sometimes effective in neuropathic pain. Carbamazepine and phenytoin act on voltage-gated sodium channels. The target for gabapentin is the $\alpha_2\delta$ subunit of the L-type calcium channel (see Ch. 3).
- **Ketamine**, a dissociative anaesthetic (Ch. 36) that works by blocking NMDA receptor channels, has analgesic properties probably directed at the wind-up phenomenon in the dorsal horn (Fig. 41.3). Given intrathecally, its effects on memory and cognitive function are largely avoided.
- Intravenous **lignocaine (lidocaine)**, a local anaesthetic drug (Ch. 44) with a short plasma half-life, can give long-lasting relief in neuropathic pain states. It probably acts by blocking spontaneous discharges from damaged sensory nerve terminals, but the reason for its persistent analgesic effect is not clear.

Other analgesic drugs

- Paracetamol resembles non-steroidal anti-inflammatory drugs and is effective as an analgesic, but it lacks anti-inflammatory activity. It may act by inhibiting cyclo-oxygenase (COX)-3, a splice variant of COX-1, but probably has other effects as well. In overdose, it causes hepatotoxicity.
- Various antidepressants (e.g. amitriptyline), as well as antiepileptic drugs (e.g. carbamazepine, gabapentin), are used mainly to treat neuropathic pain.
- Other drugs occasionally used include the NMDA receptor antagonist ketamine and the local anaesthetic drug lignocaine (lidocaine).

NEW APPROACHES

▼ As in other fields of neuropharmacology, increasing knowledge of the various chemical mediators and signalling pathways responsible for pain sensation suggests many new approaches to the control of pain. Currently, opiates and NSAIDs are the mainline treatments, with various other drugs listed above—all discovered by accident rather than by design—being used for special purposes. Nevertheless, pain treatment is currently far from perfect, and several new approaches are being explored.

- Enkephalinase inhibitors such as **thiorphan** act by inhibiting the metabolic degradation of endogenous opioid peptides, and have been

Clinical uses of analgesic drugs (1)

- Analgesics are used to treat and prevent pain, for example:
  - pre- and postoperatively
  - common painful conditions including headache, dysmenorrhoea, labour, trauma, burns
  - many medical and surgical emergencies (e.g. myocardial infarction and renal colic)
  - terminal disease (especially metatastic cancer).
- Opioid analgesics are used in some non-painful conditions, for example acute heart failure (because of their haemodynamic effects) and terminal chronic heart failure (to relieve distress).
- The choice and route of administration of analgesic drugs depends on the nature and duration of the pain.
- A progressive approach is often used, starting with non-steroidal anti-inflammatory drugs (NSAIDs), supplemented first by weak opioid analgesics and then by strong opioids.
- In general, severe acute pain is treated with strong opioids (e.g. morphine, fentanyl) given by injection. Mild inflammatory pain (e.g. sprains, mild arthralgia) is treated with NSAIDs (e.g. ibuprofen) or by paracetamol supplemented by weak opioids (e.g. codeine, dextropropoxyphene). Severe pain (e.g. cancer pain) is treated with strong opioid given orally, intrathecally, epidurally or by subcutaneous injection. Patient-controlled infusion systems are useful postoperatively.
- Chronic neuropathic pain is often unresponsive to opioids and is treated with tricyclic antidepressants (e.g. amitriptyline) or anticonvulsants (e.g. carbamazepine, gabapentin).

Clinical use of analgesic drugs (2)

- **Non-steroidal anti-inflammatory drugs** (see clinical box on p. 234) including **paracetamol** are useful for musculoskeletal and dental pain and for dysmenorrhoea. They reduce opioid requirements in acute (e.g. postoperative) and chronic (e.g. bone metastasis) pain.
- Weak opioids (e.g. **codeine**) combined with paracetamol are useful in moderately severe pain if non-opioids are not sufficient. **Tramadol** (a weak opioid with additional action on 5-hydroxytryptamine and noradrenaline uptake; p. 606) is an alternative.
- Strong opioids (e.g. **morphine**) are used for severe pain, particularly of visceral origin.
- Note that:
  - the intravenous route provides rapid relief from pain and distress
  - the intravenous dose is much lower than the oral dose because of presystemic metabolism
  - morphine is given orally as a solution or as 'immediate-release' tablets every 4 hours
  - dose is titrated; when the daily requirement is apparent, the preparation is changed to a modified-release formulation to allow once- or twice-daily dosing
  - transdermal administration (e.g. patches of **fentanyl**) is an alternative
  - adverse effects (nausea, constipation) are anticipated and treated preemptively
  - addiction is *not* an issue in the setting of terminal care
  - intravenous morphine has a distinct use for acute left ventricular failure (Chs 18 and 19).
- *Neuropathic pain* responds to drugs that interfere with amine uptake (e.g. **amitriptyline**; p. 562) or block sodium channels (e.g. **gabapentin** or **carbamazepine**; p. 583).
- Subanaesthetic doses of **nitrous oxide** (Ch. 36, p. 531) are analgesic, and self-administration of a mixture of nitrous oxide with oxygen is widely used during labour, for painful dressing changes and in ambulances.

shown to produce analgesia, together with other morphine-like effects, without causing dependence.

- The various ion channels that play a role in nociceptive nerves (Fig. 41.6) may represent useful drug targets. They include the TRPV1 receptor, for which antagonists have been identified (see Krause et al., 2005), and certain sodium channel subtypes that are specific for these nerve terminals (see Lai et al., 2004).
- Various neuropeptides, such as somatostatin (see Ch. 28) and calcitonin (see Ch. 29), produce powerful analgesia when applied intrathecally, and there are clinical reports suggesting that they may have similar effects when used systemically to treat endocrine disorders.
- Glutamate antagonists acting on NMDA or AMPA receptors show analgesic activity in animal models, but it has not yet been possible to obtain this effect in humans without unacceptable side effects. Antagonists at the metabotropic glutamate receptor mGluR$_5$ are currently in development and have fewer side effects.
- Adenosine analogues and adenosine kinase inhibitors could mimic or enhance the inhibitory effect of adenosine on nociceptive pathways.

- Agonists at nicotinic acetylcholine receptors, based on **epibatidine** (an alkaloid from frog skin, which is a potent nicotinic agonist and—unexpectedly—a potent analgesic as well), may be analgesic. Derivatives with fewer side effects are under investigation.
- Agonists at cannabinoid receptors, including **tetrahydrocannabinol** (Ch. 15) have strong analgesic effects in animal models, supported by anecdotal reports from dope smokers. Cannabinoid receptors have an inhibitory effect on nociceptive afferent terminals, and also on dorsal horn transmission. Formal trials are in progress to assess the clinical value of such compounds.

For more information on new approaches, see Sawynok (2003) and Ahmad & Dray (2004).

We should recall that analgesia was, for the best part of a century, a therapeutic need addressed only by opiates and NSAIDs, and the only new drugs to be developed as analgesics in recent years have been lookalikes in these two families. As often happens, clinical observation rather than pharmacological inventiveness has expanded the range by discovering, for example, the efficacy of tricyclic antidepressants in pain treatment. The long list of new possibilities under investigation suggests that the tide of inventiveness may have resumed after a long gap, but it is too early to say whether it will lead to better therapies (see Hill, 2006). Morphine is, as expected of 'God's own medicine', very hard to beat!

REFERENCES AND FURTHER READING

General

Fields H L, Basbaum A I 1994 Central nervous system mechanisms of pain modulation. In: Wall P D, Melzack R (eds) Textbook of pain. Churchill Livingstone, Edinburgh

Fields H L, Basbaum A I, Heinricher M M 2006 Central nervous system mechanisms of pain mudulation. In: McMahon S B, Koltzenburg M (eds) Wall & Melzack's textbook of pain, 5th edn. Elsevier, Edinburgh, pp. 125–142 (*Detailed account of central pathways that inhibit or enhance transmission in the dorsal horn*)

Hill R G 2006 Analgesic drugs in development. In: McMahon S B, Koltzenburg M (eds) Wall & Melzack's textbook of pain, 5th edn. Elsevier, Edinburgh, pp. 541–552 (*Balanced account of current approaches to develop novel analgesic drugs*)

Julius D, McCleskey E W 2006 Cellular and molecular properties of primary afferent neurons. In: McMahon S B, Koltzenburg M (eds) Wall & Melzack's textbook of pain, 5th edn. Elsevier, Edinburgh, pp. 35–48 (*Describes receptors, ion channels and signalling mechanisms of nociceptive neurons*)

McMahon S B, Koltzenburg M (eds) 2006 Wall & Melzack's textbook of pain, 5th edn. Elsevier, Edinburgh (*Large multiauthor reference book*)

Millan M J 2002 Descending control of pain. Prog Neurobiol 66: 355–474 (*Comprehensive review article covering inhibitory and facilitatory mechanisms in great detail*)

Raja S N, Meyer R A, Ringkamp M, Campbell J N 1999 Chapter 1. In: Wall P D, Melzack R (eds) 1999 Textbook of pain, 4th edn. Churchill Livingstone, Edinburgh, pp. 11–57 (*Good general account of peripheral nociceptor functions*)

Sawynok J 2003 Topical and peripherally acting analgesics. Pharmacol Rev 55: 1–20 (*Review of the numerous mechanisms by which drugs interfere with nociceptive mechanisms in the periphery*)

Schnitzler A, Ploner M 2000 Neurophysiology and functional neuroanatomy of pain perception. J Clin Neurophysiol 17: 592–603 (*Reviews findings of neuroimaging studies of pain in humans, showing that the affective component of pain involves brain regions distinct from the major somatosensory pathways*)

Yaksh T L 1999 Spinal systems and pain processing: development of novel analgesic drugs with mechanistically defined models. Trends Pharmacol Sci 20: 329–337 (*Good general review article on spinal cord mechanisms—more general than its title suggests*)

Ion channels

Chahine M, Ziane R, Vijayaragavan K, Okamura Y 2005 Regulation of Na_v channels in sensory neurons. Trends Pharmacol Sci 26: 496–502 (*Discusses role of regulation of expression and gating characteristics of voltage-gated sodium channels in pathogenesis of pain*)

Clapham D E 2003 TRP channels as cellular sensors. Nature 426: 517–524

Julius D, Basbaum A I 2001 Molecular mechanisms of nociception. Nature 413: 203–210 (*Review article focusing mainly on receptors and channels involved in activation of sensory nerves by noxious stimuli*)

Krause J E, Chenard B L, Cortright D N 2005 Transient receptor potential ion channels as targets for the discovery of pain therapeutics. Curr Opin Investig Drugs 6: 48–57 (*A look ahead to the possibilities of developing transient receptor potential channel ligands as analgesic drugs*)

Lai J, Porreca F, Hunter J C, Gold M S 2004 Voltage-gated sodium channels and hyperalgesia. Annu Rev Pharmacol Toxicol 44: 371–197 (*Useful review article on biology of sodium channels in relation to pain mechanisms*)

van der Stelt M, Di Marzo V 2004 Endovanilloids. Putative endogenous ligands of transient receptor potential vanilloid 1 channels. Eur J Biochem 271: 1827–1834

Wang H, Woolf C J 2005 Pain TRPs. Neuron 46: 9–12 (*Useful review of current knowledge about the role of transient receptor potential channels in pain*)

Chemical mediators and receptors

Ahmad S, Dray A 2004 Novel G-protein–coupled receptors as pain targets. Curr Opin Investig Drugs 5: 67–70 (*A look at future possibilities for analgesic drugs*)

Calixto J B, Medeiros R, Fernandes E S 2004 Kinin B_1 receptors: key G-protein–coupled receptors and their role in inflammatory and painful processes Br J Pharmacol 143: 803–818 (*Review emphasising the role of inducible B_1 receptors in various conditions, including inflammatory pain*)

Dray A, Perkins M 1993 Bradykinin and inflammatory pain. Trends Neurosci 16: 99–104

Ji R-R, Kohno T, Moore K A, Woolf C J 2003 Central sensitisation and LTP: do pain and memory share similar mechanisms? Trends Neurosci 25: 696–705 (*Review that emphasises the mechanistic parallels between pain and memory*)

Liu X J, Salter M W 2005 Purines and pain mechanisms: recent developments. Curr Opin Investig Drugs 6: 65–75

Marceau F, Regoli D 2004 Bradykinin receptor ligands: therapeutic perspectives. Nat Rev Drug Discov 3: 845–852

McMahon S B 1996 NGF as a mediator of inflammatory pain. Philos Trans R Soc Lond 351: 431–440 (*Review of evidence implicating NGF as a mediator of inflammatory pain and hyperalgesia, including studies of a novel type of NGF inhibitor*)

McMahon S B, Bennett D H L, Bevan S J 2006 Inflammatory mediators and modulators of pain. In: McMahon S B, Koltzenburg M (eds) Wall & Melzack's textbook of pain, 5th edn. Elsevier, Edinburgh, pp. 49–72 (*Review of the actions of many peripheral mediators on nociceptive nerve terminals*)

Samad T A, Sapirstein A, Woolf C J 2002 Prostanoids and pain: unravelling mechanisms and revealing therapeutic targets. Trends Mol Med 8: 390–396 (*Useful review article*)

Opiates

Dhawan B N, Cesselin F, Raghubir R et al. 1996 Classification of opioid receptors. Pharmacol Rev 48: 567–592 (*The last word on opioid receptor classification, from the International Union of Pharmacology subcommittee entrusted with the task*)

Henderson G, McKnight A T 1997 The orphan opioid receptor and its endogenous ligand-nociceptin/orphanin FQ. Trends Pharmacol Sci 18: 293–300 (*Review article summarising what we know about the newly discovered opioid peptide and its receptor*)

Herz A (ed) 1993 Opioids. Handb Exp Pharmacol 104 (*Definitive compendium of reviews on all aspects of opioid pharmacology*)

Ikeda K, Ide S, Han W et al. 2005 How individual sensitivity to opiates can be predicted by gene analysis. Trends Pharmacol Sci 26: 311–317 (*Focuses on polymorphism of μ-opioid receptor gene as a cause of individual variation*)

Law P Y, Wong Y H, Loh H H 2000 Molecular mechanisms and regulation of opioid receptor signaling. Annu Rev Pharmacol Toxicol 40: 389–430

Vallejo R, de Leon-Casasola O, Benyamin R 2004 Opioid therapy and immunosuppression: a review. Am J Ther 11: 354–365

Waldhoer M, Bartlett S E, Whistler J I 2004 Opioid receptors. Annu Rev Biochem 73: 953–990 (*Comprehensive review article with discussion of mechanisms underlying tolerance and dependence*)

Walker J M, Bowen W D, Walker F O et al. 1990 Sigma receptors: biology and function. Pharmacol Rev 42: 355–402

Yaksh T L 1997 Pharmacology and mechanisms of opioid analgesic activity. Acta Anaesthesiol Scand 41: 94–111 (*Review of evidence relating to sites of action and receptor specificity of analgesic effect of opioids*)

Paracetamol

Davies N M, Good R L, Roupe K A et al. 2004 Cyclooxygenase-3: axiom, dogma, anomaly or splice error?—not as easy as 1, 2, 3. J Pharm Pharm Sci 7: 217–226 (*Update on the confusing role of COX-3 as a target for paracetamol*)

Graham G G, Scott K F 2003 Mechanisms of action of paracetamol and related analgesics. Inflammopharmacology 11: 401–413

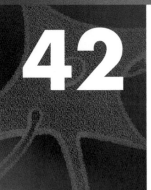

42

CNS stimulants and psychotomimetic drugs

OVERVIEW

In this chapter, we describe drugs that have a predominantly stimulant effect on the central nervous system (CNS); these fall into three broad categories:

- convulsants and respiratory stimulants
- psychomotor stimulants
- psychotomimetic drugs, also known as hallucinogens.

Drugs in the first category have relatively little effect on mental function and appear to act mainly on the brain stem and spinal cord, producing exaggerated reflex excitability, an increase in activity of the respiratory and vasomotor centres and, with higher dosage, convulsions.

Drugs in the second category have a marked effect on mental function and behaviour, producing excitement and euphoria, reduced sensation of fatigue, and an increase in motor activity.

Drugs in the third category mainly affect thought patterns and perception, distorting cognition in a complex way and producing effects that superficially resemble psychotic illness.

Table 42.1 summarises the classification of the drugs that are discussed in this chapter.

Several of these drugs have no clinical uses but are recognised as drugs of abuse on the strength of their tendency to produce dependence. This aspect is discussed in Chapter 43.

CONVULSANTS AND RESPIRATORY STIMULANTS

Convulsants and respiratory stimulants (sometimes called *analeptics*) are a chemically diverse group of substances whose mechanisms of action are, with some exceptions, not well understood. Such drugs were once used to treat patients in terminal coma or with severe respiratory failure, but their use has largely been replaced by mechanical means of assisting ventilation. Although temporary restoration of function could sometimes be achieved, mortality was not reduced, and the treatment carried a considerable risk of causing convulsions, which left the patient more deeply comatose than before. There remains a very limited clinical use for respiratory stimulants in treating acute ventilatory failure (see Ch. 23), **doxapram** (Table 42.1) being most commonly used, because it carries less risk of causing convulsions than earlier compounds.

Also included in this group are various compounds, such as **strychnine**, **picrotoxin** and **pentylenetetrazol** (**PTZ**), which are of interest as experimental tools but have no clinical uses.

Strychnine is an alkaloid found in the seeds of an Indian tree, which has been used for centuries as a poison (mainly vermin, but also human; it is much favoured in detective stories of a certain genre). It is a powerful convulsant and acts throughout the CNS but particularly on the spinal cord, causing violent extensor spasms that are triggered by minor sensory stimuli, the head being thrown back and the face fixed, we are told, in a hideous grin. These effects result from blocking receptors for glycine, which is the main inhibitory transmitter acting on motor neurons. The action of strychnine superficially resembles that of **tetanus toxin**, a protein neurotoxin produced by the anaerobic bacterium *Clostridium tetani*, which blocks the release of glycine from inhibitory interneurons. This is very similar to the action of botulinum toxin (see Ch. 10), which is produced by another bacterium of the *Clostridium* genus and causes paralysis by blocking acetylcholine release. In small doses, strychnine causes a measurable improvement in visual and auditory acuity; it was until quite recently included in various 'tonics' on the basis that CNS stimulation should restore both the weary brain and the debilitated body.

Bicuculline, also a plant alkaloid, resembles strychnine in its effects but acts by blocking receptors for GABA rather than glycine. Its action is confined to GABA$_A$ receptors, which control Cl$^-$ permeability, and it does not affect GABA$_B$ receptors (see Ch. 33). Its main effects are on the brain rather than the spinal cord, and it is a useful experimental tool for studying GABA-mediated transmission; it has no clinical uses.

Picrotoxin (obtained from the fishberry) also blocks the action of GABA on chloride channels, although not competitively. The plant's name reflects the native practice of incapacitating fish by throwing berries into the water. Picrotoxin, like bicuculline, causes convulsions and has no clinical uses.

Pentylenetetrazol acts similarly, although its precise mechanism is unknown. Inhibition of PTZ-induced convulsions by antiepileptic drugs (see Ch. 40) correlates quite well with their effectiveness against absence seizures, and PTZ has occasionally been used diagnostically in humans, because it can precipitate the typical EEG pattern of absence seizures in susceptible patients.

Doxapram is similar to the above drugs but has a bigger margin of safety between respiratory stimulation and convulsions. It also causes nausea, coughing and restlessness, which limit its usefulness. It is rapidly eliminated, and it is occasionally used as an intravenous infusion in patients with acute respiratory failure.

PSYCHOMOTOR STIMULANTS

AMPHETAMINES AND RELATED DRUGS

Amphetamine and its active dextroisomer **dextroamphetamine**, together with **methamphetamine** and **methylphenidate**, comprise a group of drugs with very similar pharmacological properties (see Fig. 42.1), which includes 'street drugs' such as

methylenedioxymethamphetamine (**MDMA** or 'ecstasy'; see below). **Fenfluramine**, although chemically similar, has slightly different pharmacological effects. All these drugs act by releasing monoamines from nerve terminals in the brain (see Seiden et al., 1993; Green et al., 2003). They are substrates for the neuronal uptake transporters for noradrenaline (norepinephrine), serotonin and dopamine, and cause release of these mediators, as described in Chapter 34, producing the acute effects described below. With prolonged use, they are neurotoxic, causing degeneration of

---

Convulsants and respiratory stimulants

- This is a diverse group of drugs that have little clinical use, although several are useful as experimental tools.
- Certain short-acting respiratory stimulants (e.g. **doxapram**) can be used in acute respiratory failure.
- **Strychnine** is a convulsant poison that acts mainly on the spinal cord by blocking receptors for the inhibitory transmitter glycine.
- **Picrotoxin** and **bicuculline** act as GABA$_A$ antagonists; bicuculline blocks the GABA$_A$ receptor site, whereas picrotoxin appears to block the ion channel.
- **Pentylenetetrazol** (**PTZ**) works by an unknown mechanism. PTZ-induced convulsions provide an animal model for testing antiepileptic drugs, giving good correlation with effectiveness in preventing absence seizures.

Table 42.1 Central nervous system stimulants and psychotomimetic drugs

Category	Example(s)	Mode(s) of action	Clinical significance
Convulsants and respiratory stimulants (analeptics) Respiratory stimulant	Doxapram	Not known	Short-acting respiratory stimulant sometimes given by intravenous infusion to treat acute respiratory failure
Miscellaneous convulsants	Strychnine	Antagonist of glycine Main action is to increase reflex excitability of spinal cord	No clinical uses
	Bicuculline	Competitive antagonist of GABA	No clinical uses
	Picrotoxin	Non-competitive antagonist of GABA	Clinical use as respiratory stimulant (now obsolete) Risk of convulsions
	Pentylenetetrazol	Not known	No clinical use Convulsant activity in experimental animals provides a useful model for testing antiepileptic drugs (see Ch. 40)

Table 42.1 (cont'd)   Central nervous system stimulants and psychotomimetic drugs

Category	Example(s)	Mode(s) of action	Clinical significance
Psychomotor stimulants	Amphetamine and related compounds (e.g. dexamphetamine, methylamphetamine, methylphenidate, fenfluramine)	Release of catecholamines Inhibition of catecholamine uptake	Methylphenidate and dexamphetamine used to treat ADHD in children; otherwise very limited clinical use Some agents used occasionally as appetite suppressants Risk of dependence, sympathomimetic side effects and pulmonary hypertension Mainly important as drugs of abuse
	Cocaine	Inhibition of catecholamine uptake Local anaesthetic	Important as drug of abuse Risk of fetal damage Occasionally used for nasopharyngeal and ophthalmic anaesthesia (see Ch. 44)
	Methylxanthines (e.g. caffeine, theophylline)	Inhibition of phosphodiesterase Antagonism of adenosine A_2 receptors (relevance of these actions to central effects is not clear)	Clinical uses unrelated to stimulant activity, although caffeine is included in various 'tonics' Theophylline used for action on cardiac and bronchial muscle (Chs 18, 23) Constituents of beverages
Psychotomimetic drugs (hallucinogens)	LSD	Agonist at 5-HT_{2A} receptors (see Ch. 11)	No clinical use Important as drug of abuse
	MDMA	Releases 5-HT and blocks reuptake	No clinical use Important as drug of abuse
	Mescaline	Not known Chemically similar to amphetamine	–
	Psilocybin	Chemically related to 5-HT; probably acts on 5-HT receptors	–
	Phencyclidine	Chemically similar to ketamine (see Ch. 36) Blocks NMDA receptor–operated ion channels (see Ch. 33) Also blocks σ receptors (Ch. 41)	Originally proposed as an anaesthetic, now important as drug of abuse and as a model for schizophrenia

5-HT, 5-hydroxytryptamine; ADHD, attention deficit hyperactivity disorder; LSD, lysergic acid diethylamide; MDMA, methylenedioxymethamphetamine.

amine-containing nerve terminals and eventually cell death. This effect is probably due to the accumulation of reactive metabolites of the parent compounds within the nerve terminals. It has been well documented in experimental animals, and is believed to occur also in humans, possibly accounting for long-term adverse psychological effects in habitual users of amphetamine derivatives.

Further information on the pharmacology, uses and dangers of amphetamines can be found in the monograph by Iversen (2006).

Pharmacological effects

The main central effects of amphetamine-like drugs are:

- locomotor stimulation
- euphoria and excitement
- stereotyped behaviour
- anorexia.

In addition, amphetamines have peripheral sympathomimetic actions, producing a rise in blood pressure and inhibition of gastrointestinal motility.

In experimental animals, amphetamines cause increased alertness and locomotor activity, and increased grooming; they also increase aggressive behaviour. On the other hand, systematic exploration of novel objects by unrestrained rats is reduced by amphetamine. The animals run around more but appear less

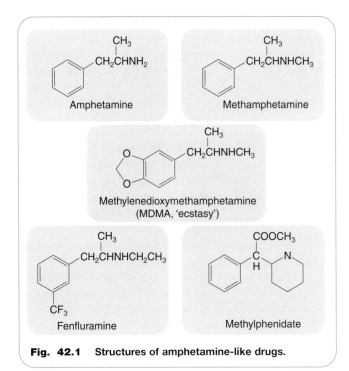

Fig. 42.1 Structures of amphetamine-like drugs.

attentive to their surroundings. Studies of conditioned responses suggest that amphetamines increase the overall rate of responding without affecting the training process markedly. Thus, in a fixed interval schedule where a reward for lever pressing is forthcoming only after a fixed interval (say 10 minutes) following the last reward, trained animals normally press the lever very infrequently in the first few minutes after the reward, and increase the rate towards the end of the 10-minute interval when another reward is due. The effect of amphetamine is to increase the rate of unrewarded responses at the beginning of the 10-minute interval without affecting (or even reducing) the rate towards the end of the period. The effects of amphetamine on more sophisticated types of conditioned response, for example those involving discriminative tasks, are not clear-cut, and there is no clear evidence that either the rate of learning of such tasks or the final level of performance that can be achieved is affected by the drug. Put crudely, amphetamine makes the animals busier rather than brighter.

With large doses of amphetamines, stereotyped behaviour occurs. This consists of repeated actions, such as licking, gnawing, rearing or repeated movements of the head and limbs. These activities are generally inappropriate to the environment, and with increasing doses of amphetamine they take over more and more of the behaviour of the animal. These behavioural effects are evidently produced by the release of catecholamines in the brain, because pretreatment with 6-hydroxydopamine, which depletes the brain of both noradrenaline and dopamine, abolishes the effect of amphetamine, as does pretreatment with α-methyltyrosine, an inhibitor of catecholamine biosynthesis (see Ch. 11). Similarly, tricyclic antidepressants and monoamine oxidase inhibitors (see Ch. 39) potentiate the effects of amphetamine, presumably by blocking amine reuptake or metabolism. Interestingly, reserpine, which inhibits vesicular storage

of catecholamines (see Ch. 11), does not block the behavioural effects of amphetamine. This is probably because amphetamine releases cytosolic rather than vesicular catecholamines (see Ch. 11). The behavioural effects of amphetamine are probably due mainly to release of dopamine rather than noradrenaline. The evidence for this is that destruction of the central noradrenergic bundle does not affect locomotor stimulation produced by amphetamine, whereas destruction of the dopamine-containing nucleus accumbens (see Ch. 34) or administration of antipsychotic drugs that antagonise dopamine (see Ch. 38) inhibits this response.

Amphetamine-like drugs cause marked anorexia, but with continued administration this effect wears off in a few days and food intake returns to normal. The effect is most marked with **fenfluramine** and its D isomer **dexfenfluramine**, which preferentially affect 5-hydroxytryptamine (5-HT) release.

In humans, amphetamine causes euphoria; with intravenous injection, this can be so intense as to be described as 'orgasmic'. Subjects become confident, hyperactive and talkative, and sex drive is said to be enhanced. Fatigue, both physical and mental, is reduced by amphetamine, and many studies have shown improvement of both mental and physical performance in fatigued, although not in well-rested, subjects. Mental performance is improved for simple tedious tasks much more than for difficult tasks, and amphetamines have been used to improve the performance of soldiers, military pilots and others who need to remain alert under extremely fatiguing conditions. It has also been in vogue as a means of helping students to concentrate before and during examinations, but the improvement caused by reduction of fatigue can be offset by the mistakes of overconfidence.[1] The use of amphetamines in sport is described in Chapter 54.

Tolerance and dependence

If amphetamine is taken repeatedly over the course of a few days, which occurs when users seek to maintain the euphoric 'high' that a single dose produces, a state of 'amphetamine psychosis' can develop, which closely resembles an acute schizophrenic attack (see Ch. 38), with hallucinations accompanied by paranoid symptoms and aggressive behaviour. At the same time, repetitive stereotyped behaviour may develop (e.g. polishing shoes or stringing beads). The close similarity of this condition to schizophrenia, and the effectiveness of antipsychotic drugs in controlling it, is consistent with the dopamine theory of schizophrenia discussed in Chapter 38. When the drug is stopped after a few days, there is usually a period of deep sleep, and on awakening the subject feels lethargic, depressed, anxious (sometimes even suicidal) and hungry. Even a single dose of amphetamine, insufficient to cause psychotic symptoms, usually leaves the subject later feeling tired and depressed. These after-effects may be the result of depletion of the normal stores of

---

[1]Pay heed to the awful warning of the medical student who, it is said, having taken copious amounts of dextroamphetamine, left the examination hall in confident mood, having spent 3 hours writing his name over and over again.

noradrenaline and dopamine, but the evidence for this is not clear-cut. A state of amphetamine dependence can be produced in experimental animals—thus rats quickly learn to press a lever in order to obtain a dose of amphetamine, and also become inactive and irritable in the withdrawal phase. These effects do not occur with **fenfluramine**.

Tolerance develops rapidly to the peripheral sympathomimetic and anorexic effects of amphetamine, but more slowly to the other effects (locomotor stimulation and stereotyped behaviour). Dependence on amphetamine appears to be a consequence of the unpleasant after-effect that it produces and to the insistent memory of euphoria, which leads to a desire for a repeat dose. There is no clear-cut physical withdrawal syndrome such as occurs with opiates. It is estimated that only about 5% of users progress to full dependence, the usual pattern being that the dose is increased as tolerance develops, and then uncontrolled 'binges' occur in which the user takes the drug repeatedly over a period of a day or more, remaining continuously intoxicated. Large doses may be consumed in such binges, with a high risk of acute toxicity, and the demand for the drug displaces all other considerations.

Experimental animals, given unlimited access to amphetamine, take it in such large amounts that they die from the cardiovascular effects within a few days. Given limited amounts, they too develop a binge pattern of dependence.

Pharmacokinetic aspects

Amphetamine is readily absorbed from the gastrointestinal tract and freely penetrates the blood–brain barrier. It does this more readily than other indirectly acting sympathomimetic amines such as **ephedrine** or **tyramine** (Ch. 11), which probably explains why it produces more marked central effects than those drugs. Amphetamine is mainly excreted unchanged in the urine, and the rate of excretion is increased when the urine is made more acidic (see Ch. 8). The plasma half-life of amphetamine varies from about 5 hours to 20–30 hours, depending on urine flow and urinary pH.

Clinical use and unwanted effects

The main use of amphetamines is in the treatment of *attention deficit–hyperactivity disorder (ADHD)*, particularly in children, **methylphenidate** being the drug most commonly used, at doses lower than those causing euphoria and other side effects. ADHD is a common condition in children whose incessant overactivity and very limited attention span disrupt their education and social development. The efficacy of amphetamines has been confirmed in many controlled trials. Disorders of dopamine pathways are suspected to underlie ADHD symptomatology, but the mechanism of action of amphetamines is unclear.

Narcolepsy is a disabling condition, probably a form of epilepsy, in which the patient suddenly and unpredictably falls asleep at frequent intervals during the day. Amphetamine is helpful but not completely effective.

As appetite suppressants in humans, for use in treating obesity, amphetamine derivatives proved relatively ineffective and have been largely abandoned because of their tendency to cause pulmonary hypertension, which can be so severe as to necessitate heart–lung transplantation.

The limited clinical usefulness of amphetamine is offset by its many unwanted effects, including hypertension, insomnia, anorexia, tremors, risk of exacerbating schizophrenia, and risk of dependence.

Sudden deaths have occurred in ecstasy users, even after a single, moderate dose. The drug can induce a condition resembling heatstroke, associated with muscle damage and renal failure, and also causes inappropriate secretion of antidiuretic hormone, leading to thirst, over-hydration and hyponatraemia ('water intoxication'). Cerebral haemorrhage has also been reported after amphetamine use, possibly the result of acutely raised blood pressure. There is evidence that habitual use of amphetamines is associated with long-term psychological effects of many kinds, including psychotic symptoms, anxiety, depression and cognitive impairment, although interpretation is made difficult by the fact that drug users generally take many different substances, and the association may reflect increased drug use by psychologically disturbed individuals rather than the psychological after-effects of the drug. Taken in conjunction with animal data, however, the human data suggest that amphetamines can cause long-term damage.

COCAINE

Cocaine (see reviews by Gawin & Ellinwood, 1988; Johanson & Fischman, 1989) is found in the leaves of a South American shrub, coca. These leaves are used for their stimulant properties by natives of South America, particularly those in mountainous areas, who use it to reduce fatigue during work at high altitude. Considerable mystical significance was attached to the powers of cocaine to boost the flagging human spirit, and Freud tested it extensively on his patients and his family, publishing an influential

---

Amphetamines

- The main effects are:
  - increased motor activity
  - euphoria and excitement
  - anorexia
  - with prolonged administration, stereotyped and psychotic behaviour.
- Effects are due mainly to release of catecholamines, especially noradrenaline and dopamine.
- Stimulant effect lasts for a few hours and is followed by depression and anxiety.
- Tolerance to the stimulant effects develops rapidly, although peripheral sympathomimetic effects may persist.
- Amphetamines may be useful in treating narcolepsy, and also (paradoxically) to control hyperkinetic children. They are no longer used as appetite suppressants because of the risk of pulmonary hypertension.
- Amphetamine psychosis, which closely resembles schizophrenia, can develop after prolonged use.
- Their main importance is in drug abuse.

monograph in 1884 advocating its use as a psychostimulant.[2] Freud's ophthalmologist colleague, Köller, obtained supplies of the drug and discovered its local anaesthetic action (Ch. 44), but the psychostimulant effects of cocaine have not proved to be clinically useful. On the other hand, they led to it becoming a widespread drug of abuse in western countries. The mechanisms and treatment of cocaine abuse are discussed in Chapter 43.

Pharmacological effects

Cocaine inhibits catecholamine uptake by the noradrenaline and dopamine transporters (see Ch. 11), thereby enhancing the peripheral effects of sympathetic nerve activity and producing a marked psychomotor stimulant effect. The latter produces euphoria, garrulousness, increased motor activity and a magnification of pleasure, similar to the effects of amphetamine. Its effects resemble those of amphetamines, although it has less tendency to produce stereotyped behaviour, delusions, hallucinations and paranoia. With excessive dosage, tremors and convulsions, followed by respiratory and vasomotor depression, may occur. The peripheral sympathomimetic actions lead to tachycardia, vasoconstriction and an increase in blood pressure. Body temperature may increase, owing to the increased motor activity coupled with reduced heat loss. Like amphetamine, cocaine produces no clear-cut physical dependence syndrome but tends to cause depression and dysphoria, coupled with craving for the drug (see Ch. 43), following the initial stimulant effect. Withdrawal of cocaine after administration for a few days causes a marked deterioration of motor performance and learned behaviour, which are restored by resuming dosage with the drug. There is thus a considerable degree of psychological dependence. The pattern of dependence, evolving from occasional use through escalating dosage to compulsive binges, is identical to that seen with amphetamines.

The duration of action of cocaine (about 30 minutes when given intravenously) is much shorter than that of amphetamine.

Pharmacokinetic aspects

Cocaine is readily absorbed by many routes. For many years, illicit supplies consisted of the hydrochloride salt, which could be given by nasal inhalation or intravenously. The latter route produces an intense and immediate euphoria, whereas nasal inhalation produces a less dramatic sensation and also tends to cause atrophy and necrosis of the nasal mucosa and septum. Cocaine use increased dramatically when the freebase form ('crack') became available as a street drug. Unlike the salt, this can be smoked, giving an effect nearly as rapid as that of intravenous administration, with less inconvenience and social stigma. The social, economic and even political consequences of this small change in formulation have been far-reaching.

---

[2]In the 1860s, a Corsican pharmacist, Mariani, devised cocaine-containing beverages, Vin Mariani and Thé Mariani, which were sold very successfully as tonics. Imitators soon moved in, and Thé Mariani became the forerunner of Coca Cola. In 1903, cocaine was removed from Coca Cola because of its growing association with addiction and criminality (see Courtwright, 2001, for a lively account).

A cocaine metabolite is deposited in hair, and analysis of its content along the hair shaft allows the pattern of cocaine consumption to be monitored, a technique that has revealed a much higher incidence of cocaine use than was voluntarily reported. Cocaine exposure in utero can be estimated from analysis of the hair of neonates.

Cocaine is still occasionally used topically as a local anaesthetic, mainly in ophthalmology and minor nose and throat surgery, but has no other clinical uses. It is a valuable pharmacological tool for the study of catecholamine release and reuptake, because of its relatively specific action in blocking noradrenaline and dopamine uptake.

Adverse effects

Toxic effects occur commonly in cocaine abusers. The main acute dangers are serious cardiovascular events (cardiac dysrhythmias, aortic dissection, and myocardial or cerebral infarction or haemorrhage). Progressive myocardial damage can lead to heart failure, even in the absence of a history of acute cardiac effects.

Cocaine can severely impair brain development in utero (see Volpe, 1992). The brain size is significantly reduced in babies exposed to cocaine in pregnancy, and neurological and limb malformations are increased. The incidence of ischaemic and haemorrhagic brain lesions, and of sudden infant death, is also higher in cocaine-exposed babies. Interpretation of the data is difficult because many cocaine abusers also take other illicit drugs that may affect fetal development, but the probability is that cocaine is highly detrimental.

Dependence, the main psychological adverse effect of amphetamines and cocaine, has potentially severe effects on quality of life (Ch. 43).

METHYLXANTHINES

Various beverages, particularly tea, coffee and cocoa, contain methylxanthines, to which they owe their mild central stimulant effects. The main compounds responsible are **caffeine** and **theophylline**. The nuts of the cola plant also contain caffeine, which is present in cola-flavoured soft drinks. However, the most important sources, by far, are coffee and tea, which account

---

Cocaine

- Cocaine acts by inhibiting catecholamine uptake (especially dopamine) by nerve terminals.
- Behavioural effects of cocaine are very similar to those of amphetamines, although psychotomimetic effects are rarer. Duration of action is shorter.
- Cocaine used in pregnancy impairs fetal development and may produce fetal malformations.
- As drugs of abuse, amphetamines and cocaine produce strong psychological dependence and carry a high risk of severe adverse reactions.

for more than 90% of caffeine consumption. A cup of instant coffee or strong tea contains 50–70 mg of caffeine, while filter coffee contains about twice as much. Among adults in tea- and coffee-drinking countries, the average daily caffeine consumption is about 200 mg. Further information on the pharmacology and toxicology of caffeine is presented by Fredholm et al. (1999).

Pharmacological effects

Methylxanthines have the following major pharmacological actions:

- CNS stimulation
- diuresis (see Ch. 24)
- stimulation of cardiac muscle (see Ch. 18)
- relaxation of smooth muscle, especially bronchial muscle (see Ch. 23).

The latter two effects resemble those of β-adrenoceptor stimulation (see Ch. 11). This is thought to be because methylxanthines (especially **theophylline**) inhibit phosphodiesterase, which is responsible for the intracellular metabolism of cAMP (Ch. 3). They thus increase intracellular cAMP and produce effects that mimic those of mediators that stimulate adenylyl cyclase. Methylxanthines also antagonise many of the effects of adenosine, acting on both A_1 and A_2 receptors (see Ch. 12). Transgenic mice lacking functional A_2 receptors are abnormally active and aggressive, and fail to show increased motor activity in response to caffeine (Ledent et al., 1997), suggesting that antagonism at A_2 receptors accounts for part, at least, of its CNS stimulant action. The concentration of caffeine reached in plasma and brain after two or three cups of strong coffee—about 100 μM—is sufficient to produce appreciable adenosine receptor block and a small degree of phosphodiesterase inhibition. The diuretic effect probably results from vasodilatation of the afferent glomerular arteriole, causing an increased glomerular filtration rate.

Caffeine and theophylline have very similar stimulant effects on the CNS. Human subjects experience a reduction of fatigue, with improved concentration and a clearer flow of thought. This is confirmed by objective studies, which have shown that caffeine reduces reaction time and produces an increase in the speed at which simple calculations can be performed (although without much improvement in accuracy). Performance at motor tasks, such as typing and simulated driving, is also improved, particularly in fatigued subjects. Mental tasks, such as syllable learning, association tests and so on, are also facilitated by moderate doses (up to about 200 mg of caffeine, or about three cups of coffee) but impaired by larger doses. Insomnia is common. By comparison with amphetamines, methylxanthines produce less locomotor stimulation and do not induce euphoria, stereotyped behaviour patterns or a psychotic state, but their effects on fatigue and mental function are similar.

Tolerance and habituation develop to a small extent, but much less than with amphetamines, and withdrawal effects are slight. Caffeine does not lead to self-administration in animals, and it cannot be classified as a dependence-producing drug.

Clinical use and unwanted effects

There are few clinical uses for caffeine. It is included with aspirin in some preparations for treating headaches and other aches and pains, and with ergotamine in some antimigraine preparations, the object being to produce a mildly agreeable sense of alertness. Theophylline is used mainly as a bronchodilator in treating severe asthmatic attacks (see Ch. 23). Caffeine has few unwanted side effects and is safe even in very large doses. In vitro tests show that it has mutagenic activity, and large doses are teratogenic in animals. However, epidemiological studies have shown no evidence of carcinogenic or teratogenic effects of tea or coffee drinking in humans.

PSYCHOTOMIMETIC DRUGS

Psychotomimetic drugs (also referred to as *psychedelic* or *hallucinogenic* drugs) affect thought, perception and mood, without causing marked psychomotor stimulation or depression (see review by Nichols, 2004). Thoughts and perceptions tend to become distorted and dreamlike, rather than being merely sharpened or dulled, and the change in mood is likewise more complex than a simple shift in the direction of euphoria or depression. Importantly, psychotomimetic drugs do not cause dependence or addiction, even though their psychological effects overlap those of highly addictive major psychostimulants such as cocaine and amphetamines.

Psychotomimetic drugs fall broadly into two groups.

- Drugs that act on 5-HT transporters or receptors. These include **lysergic acid diethylamide** (**LSD**), **psilocybin** and **mescaline**, which are agonists at $5\text{-}HT_2$ receptors (see Ch. 12), and **MDMA** (ecstasy; see above), which acts mainly by inhibiting 5-HT uptake. MDMA also acts on many other receptors and transporters (see Green et al., 2003), and has powerful psychostimulant effects typical of amphetamines, as well as psychotomimetic effects.
- Antagonists at NMDA-type glutamate receptors (e.g. **phencyclidine**).

Methylxanthines

- Caffeine and theophylline produce psychomotor stimulant effects.
- Average caffeine consumption from beverages is about 200 mg/day.
- Main psychological effects are reduced fatigue and improved mental performance, without euphoria. Even large doses do not cause stereotyped behaviour or psychotomimetic effects.
- Methylxanthines act mainly by antagonism at A_2 purine receptors, and partly by inhibiting phosphodiesterase, thus producing effects similar to those of β-adrenoceptor agonists.
- Peripheral actions are exerted mainly on heart, smooth muscle and kidney.
- Theophylline is used clinically as a bronchodilator; caffeine is not used clinically.

LSD, PSILOCYBIN AND MESCALINE

LSD is an exceptionally potent psychotomimetic drug capable of producing strong effects in humans in doses less than $1 \mu g/kg$. It is a chemical derivative of lysergic acid, which occurs in the cereal fungus ergot (see Ch. 12), and was first synthesised by Hoffman in 1943. Hoffman deliberately swallowed about $250 \mu g$ of LSD and wrote 30 years later of the experience: 'the faces of those around me appeared as grotesque coloured masks ... marked motoric unrest, alternating with paralysis ... heavy feeling in the head, limbs and entire body, as if they were filled with lead ... clear recognition of my condition, in which state I sometimes observed, in the manner of an independent observer, that I shouted half insanely'. These effects lasted for a few hours, after which Hoffman fell asleep, 'and awoke next morning feeling perfectly well'. Apart from these dramatic psychological effects, LSD has few physiological effects. **Mescaline**, which is derived from a Mexican cactus and has been known as a hallucinogenic agent for many centuries, was made famous by Aldous Huxley in *The Doors of Perception*. It is chemically related to amphetamine and acts as an inhibitor of monoamine transport, in addition to its agonist action on $5HT_2$ receptors. **Psilocybin** is obtained from a fungus and has very similar properties to LSD. The psychotomimetic effects of all three drugs are the same.

Pharmacological effects

The main effects of these drugs are on mental function, most notably an alteration of perception in such a way that sights and sounds appear distorted and fantastic. Hallucinations visual, auditory, tactile or olfactory also occur, and sensory modalities may become confused, so that sounds are perceived as visions. Thought processes tend to become illogical and disconnected, but subjects retain insight into the fact that their disturbance is drug-induced, and generally find the experience exhilarating. Occasionally, LSD produces a syndrome that is extremely disturbing to the subject (the 'bad trip'), in which the hallucinatory experience takes on a menacing quality and may be accompanied by paranoid delusions. This sometimes goes so far as to produce homicide or suicide attempts, and in many respects the state has features in common with acute schizophrenic illness. Furthermore, 'flashbacks' of the hallucinatory experience have been reported weeks or months later.

LSD acts on various 5-HT-receptor subtypes (see Ch. 12), and in the CNS it is believed to work mainly as a 5-HT_{2A}-receptor agonist (see Nichols, 2004). It inhibits the firing of 5-HT-containing neurons in the raphe nuclei (see Ch. 34), apparently by acting as an agonist on the inhibitory autoreceptors of these cells. The action of mescaline is apparently different, however, and exerted mainly on noradrenergic neurons. It is still quite unclear how changes in cell firing rates might be related to the psychotomimetic action of these drugs.

The main effects of psychotomimetic drugs are subjective, so it is not surprising that animal tests that reliably predict psychotomimetic activity in humans have not been devised. Attempts to measure changes in perception by behavioural conditioning studies have given variable results, but some authors have claimed that effects consistent with increased sensory 'generalisation' (i.e. a tendency to respond similarly to any sensory stimulus) can be detected in this way. One of the more bizarre tests involves spiders, whose normal elegantly symmetrical webs become jumbled and erratic if the animals are treated with LSD.

Dependence and adverse effects

Psychotomimetic agents (except for phencyclidine; see below) are not self-administered by experimental animals. Indeed, in contrast to most of the drugs that are widely abused by humans, they have aversive rather than reinforcing properties in behavioural tests. Tolerance to their effects develops quite quickly.

There is no physical withdrawal syndrome in animals or humans.

There has been much concern over reports that LSD and other psychotomimetic drugs, as well as causing potentially dangerous bad trips, can lead to more persistent mental disorder (see Abraham & Aldridge, 1993). There are recorded instances in which altered perception and hallucinations have lasted for up to 3 weeks following a single dose of LSD, and of precipitation of attacks in schizophrenic patients. Furthermore, it is possible that LSD may occasionally initiate long-lasting schizophrenia, although conclusive evidence is lacking. This possibility, coupled with the fact that the occasional bad trip can result in severe injury through violent behaviour, means that LSD and other psychotomimetics must be regarded as highly dangerous drugs, far removed from the image of peaceful 'experience enhancers' that the hippy subculture[3] of the 1960s so enthusiastically espoused.

MDMA

MDMA is an amphetamine derivative with complex effects on monoamine function (see Green et al., 2003; Morton, 2005; Iversen 2006). It inhibits monoamine transporters, principally the 5-HT transporter, and also releases 5-HT, the net effect being a large increase in free 5-HT in certain brain regions, followed by depletion. Similar but smaller changes occur in relation to dopamine and noradrenaline. Simplistically, the effects on 5-HT function determine the psychotomimetic effects, while dopamine and noradrenaline changes account for the initial euphoria and later rebound dysphoria. MDMA is widely used as a 'party drug' because of the euphoria, loss of inhibitions and energy surge that it induces. Although not addictive, MDMA carries serious risks, both acute and long term.

Sudden illness and death can occur even after small doses of MDMA. The syndrome appears to result from acute hyperthermia, resulting in damage to skeletal muscle and renal failure. This may reflect an action of MDMA on mitochondrial function, exacerbated by energetic dancing and high ambient temperature. It appears that certain individuals may be particularly susceptible to this danger.

---

[3]You may recall the Beatles' lyric *Lucy in the Sky with Diamonds*, also the phrase 'Drop out; tune in; turn on' coined by Timothy Leary, whose ashes were sent into orbit in 1997.

The after-effects of MDMA persist for a few days and comprise depression, anxiety, irritability and increased aggression—the 'midweek blues'. There is also evidence of long-term deleterious effects on memory and cognitive function in heavy MDMA users. In animal studies, MDMA can cause degeneration of 5-HT and dopamine neurons, but whether this occurs in humans is uncertain. In summary, recreational use of MDMA cannot be considered safe.

PHENCYCLIDINE

Phencyclidine was originally intended as an intravenous anaesthetic agent, but was found to produce in many patients a period of disorientation and hallucinations following recovery of consciousness. **Ketamine** (see Ch. 36), a close analogue of phencyclidine, is better as an anaesthetic, although it too can cause symptoms of disorientation. Phencyclidine is now of interest mainly as a drug of abuse ('Angel dust', now declining in popularity).

Pharmacological effects

The effects of phencyclidine resemble those of other psychotomimetic drugs (see Johnson & Jones, 1990) but also include analgesia, which was one of the reasons for its introduction as an anaesthetic agent. It can also cause stereotyped motor behaviour, like amphetamine. It has the same reported tendency as LSD to cause occasional bad trips and to lead to recurrent psychotic episodes. Its main pharmacological effect is to block the NMDA receptor channel (see Ch. 33), but it is also an antagonist at σ-receptors, which are activated by various opioids of the benzomorphan type (Ch. 41). It is believed that the NMDA channel–blocking action is primarily responsible for the psychotomimetic effects, which mimic, both behaviourally and biochemically, the manifestations of human schizophrenia (Morris et al., 2005). Phencyclidine is known to exacerbate symptoms in stabilised schizophrenic patients, but it is not known whether habitual use can cause the disorder to develop.

> ### Psychotomimetic drugs
>
> - The main types are:
>   - lysergic acid diethylamide (LSD), psilocybin and mescaline (actions related to 5-hydroxytryptamine (5-HT) and catecholamines)
>   - methylenedioxymethamphetamine (MDMA, 'ecstasy')
>   - phencyclidine.
> - Their main effect is to cause sensory distortion of a fantastic and hallucinatory nature.
> - LSD is exceptionally potent, producing a long-lasting sense of dissociation and disordered thought, sometimes with frightening hallucinations and delusions, which can lead to violence. Hallucinatory episodes can recur after a long interval.
> - LSD and phencyclidine precipitate schizophrenic attacks in susceptible patients, and LSD may cause long-lasting psychopathological changes.
> - LSD appears to act as an agonist at 5-HT$_2$-receptors, and suppresses electrical activity in 5-HT raphe neurons, an action that appears to correlate with psychotomimetic activity.
> - MDMA is an amphetamine analogue that has powerful psychostimulant as well as psychotomimetic effects.
> - MDMA can cause an acute hyperthermic reaction, sometimes fatal. It also has severe long-term psychological effects, similar to LSD.
> - Psychotomimetic drugs do not cause physical dependence and tend to be aversive, rather than reinforcing, in animal models.
> - Phencyclidine acts by blocking the glutamate-activated NMDA receptor channel, and also blocks σ-receptors.

REFERENCES AND FURTHER READING

General reference

Courtwright D T 2001 Forces of habit: drugs and the making of the modern world. Harvard University Press, Cambridge (*A lively historical account of habit-forming drugs*)

Psychostimulants

Fredholm B B, Battig K, Holmes J et al. 1999 Actions of caffeine in the brain with special reference to factors that contribute to its widespread use. Pharmacol Rev 51: 83–133 (*Comprehensive review covering pharmacological, behavioural and social aspects*)

Gawin F H, Ellinwood E H 1988 Cocaine and other stimulants. N Engl J Med 318: 1173–1182

Iversen LL 2006 Speed, Ecstasy, ritalin. The science of amphetamines. Oxford University Press. (*Authoritative book on all aspects of the properties, use and abuse of amphetamines.*)

Johanson C-E, Fischman M W 1989 The pharmacology of cocaine related to its abuse. Pharmacol Rev 41: 3–47

Ledent C et al. 1997 Aggressiveness, hypoalgesia and high blood pressure in mice lacking the adenosine A$_{2a}$ receptor. Nature 388: 674–678 (*Study of transgenic mice, showing loss of stimulant effects of caffeine in mice lacking A$_2$ receptors*)

Nehlig A, Daval J-L, Debry G 1992 Caffeine and the central nervous system: mechanisms of action, biochemical, metabolic and psychostimulant effects. Brain Res Rev 17: 139–170

Seiden L S, Sabol K E, Ricaurte G A 1993 Amphetamine: effects on catecholamine systems and behavior. Annu Rev Pharmacol Toxicol 33: 639–677

Volpe J J 1992 Effect of cocaine on the fetus. N Engl J Med 327: 399–407

Psychotomimetics

Abraham H D, Aldridge A M 1993 Adverse consequences of lysergic acid diethylamide. Addiction 88: 1327–1334

Green A R, Mechan A O, Elliott J M et al. 2003 The pharmacology and clinical pharmacology of 3,4-methylenedioxymethamphetamine (MDMA, 'Ecstasy'). Pharm Rev 55: 463–508

Johnson K M, Jones S M 1990 Neuropharmacology of phencyclidine: basic mechanisms and therapeutic potential. Annu Rev Pharmacol Toxicol 30: 707–750

Morris B J, Cochran S M, Pratt J A 2005 PCP: from pharmacology to modelling schizophrenia. Curr Opin Pharmacol 5: 101–106 (*Review arguing that NMDA channel block by phencyclidine closely models human schizophrenia*)

Morton J 2005 Ecstasy: pharmacology and neurotoxicity. Curr Opin Pharmacol 5: 79–86 (*Useful short review focusing on adverse effects of MDMA*)

Nichols D E 2004 Hallucinogens. Pharmacol Ther 101: 131–181 (*Comprehensive review article focusing on 5HT$_{2A}$ receptors as the target of psychotomimetic drugs*)

Drug addiction, dependence and abuse

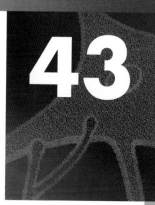

43

OVERVIEW

In earlier chapters, we have discussed several drugs (e.g. benzodiazepines, opiates, psychostimulants) that can cause dependence. There are also many drugs that human beings consume because they choose to, and not because they are advised to by doctors. Society in general disapproves, because in most cases there is a social cost; for certain drugs, this is judged to outweigh the individual benefit, and their use is banned in many countries. In western societies, the three most commonly used non-therapeutic drugs are caffeine, nicotine and ethanol, all of which are legally and freely available. Many other drugs are widely used although their manufacture, sale and consumption has been declared illegal in most

western countries—but very big business, nevertheless[1]—except when it is under the direction of the medical profession. A list of the more important ones is given in Table 43.1. Other 'lifestyle' and 'sport' drugs are discussed in Chapter 54.

The reasons why particular drugs should come to be used in a way that constitutes a problem to society are complex and largely outside the scope of this book. The drug and its pharmacological activity are only the starting point, although drug taking is clearly seen by society in a quite different light from other forms of addictive self-gratification, such as opera going, football or sex. At first sight, the 'drugs of abuse' form an extremely heterogeneous pharmacological group; we can find little in common at the molecular and cellular level between say, morphine, cocaine and barbiturates. What links them is that people find their effect pleasurable (hedonic) and tend to want to repeat it, an action that reflects the effect—common to all dependence-producing drugs—of activating mesolimbic dopaminergic neurons (see below). This hedonic effect becomes a problem when:

* the want becomes so insistent that it dominates the lifestyle of the individual and damages his or her quality of life
* the habit itself causes actual harm to the individual or the community.

Examples of the latter are the mental incapacity and liver damage caused by ethanol, the many diseases associated with smoking, the high risk of infection (especially with HIV), the serious risk of overdosage with most narcotics, and the criminal behaviour resorted to when addicts need to finance their habit.

In this chapter, we discuss some general aspects of drug dependence and drug abuse, and describe the pharmacology of three important drugs that

---

[1]Globally, according to UN estimates, annual sales of illegal drugs were about $800 billion in the late 1990s, accounting for 8% of all international trade, similar to oil sales and roughly three times that of prescription drugs.

have no place in therapy but are consumed in large amounts, namely nicotine, ethanol and cannabis. Other drugs with abuse potential are described elsewhere in this book (see Table 43.1). For further information on various aspects of drug abuse, see Friedman et al. (1996), Karch (1997), Hyman & Malenka (2001) and Winger et al. (2004).

THE NATURE OF DRUG ADDICTION

Several related terms are used, sometimes interchangeably, to describe the consequences of continued administration of hedonic drugs. *Drug dependence* and the older term *drug addiction* describe the human condition in which drug taking becomes compulsive, taking precedence over other needs, often with serious adverse consequences. This generally implies a state of physical, as well as psychological, dependence (see below). Drug dependence can be viewed as a reversible pharmacological phenomenon, readily induced in animals, whereas addiction is a chronic, relapsing human condition, as distinct from an acute illness that can be cured by abstinence. *Drug abuse* and *substance abuse* are more general terms, meaning any recurrent use of substances that are illegal or that cause harm to the individual, including drugs in sport. *Tolerance*—the decrease in pharmacological effect on repeated administration of the drug—often accompanies the state of dependence, and it is possible that related mechanisms account for both phenomena (see below). *Withdrawal syndrome* or *abstinence syndrome* describes the adverse effects, both physical and psychological and lasting for a few days or weeks, of stopping taking a drug. Several psychotropic drugs, including antidepressant and antipsychotic agents, produce withdrawal symptoms but are not addictive, so it is important to distinguish this type of commonly observed 'rebound' phenomenon from true dependence.

The common feature of the various types of psychoactive drugs that are addictive is that all produce a *rewarding* effect. In animal studies, where this cannot be inferred directly, it is manifest as positive reinforcement (i.e. an increase in the probability of occurrence of any behaviour that results in the drug being administered). Thus, with all dependence-producing drugs, spontaneous self-administration can be induced in animal studies. Coupled with the direct rewarding effect of the drug, there is usually also a process of *habituation,* or *adaptation,* when the drug is given repeatedly or continuously, such that cessation of the drug has an *aversive* effect, negative reinforcement, from which the subject will attempt to escape by self-administration of the drug. The physical withdrawal syndrome, associated with the state of physical dependence, is one manifestation of this type of habituation; the intensity and nature of physical withdrawal symptoms varies from one class of drug to another, being particularly marked with opioids. It is less important in sustaining drug-seeking behaviour than psychological habituation, which is associated with a craving that is not related to physical symptoms. A degree of physical dependence is common when patients receive opioid analgesics in hospital for several days, but this rarely leads to addiction. On the other hand, addicts who are nursed through and recover fully from the physical abstinence syndrome are still extremely likely to revert to drug taking later. Therefore physical dependence is not the major factor in long-term drug dependence. In addition to the positive and negative reinforcement associated with drug administration and withdrawal, *conditioning* plays a significant part in sustaining drug dependence (see Weiss, 2005). When a particular environment or location, or the sight of a syringe or cigarette, becomes associated with the pleasurable experience of drug taking, the antecedent

Table 43.1 The main drugs of abuse

Type	Examples	Dependence liability	Chapter in which discussed
Narcotic analgesics	Morphine	Very strong	41
	Diamorphine	Very strong	41
General central nervous system depressants	Ethanol	Strong	This chapter
	Barbiturates	Strong	37
	Methaqualone	Moderate	37
	Glutethimide	Moderate	37
	Anaesthetics	Moderate	36
	Solvents	Strong	–
Anxiolytic drugs	Benzodiazepines	Moderate	37
Psychomotor stimulants	Amphetamines	Strong	42
	Cocaine	Very strong	42
	Caffeine	Weak	42
	Nicotine	Very strong	This chapter
Psychotomimetic agents	Lysergic acid diethylamide	Weak or absent	42
	Mescaline	Weak or absent	42
	Phencyclidine	Moderate	42
	Cannabis	Weak	This chapter

stimulus itself evokes the response, as with Pavlov's dogs. The same happens in reverse, so that the antecedents of not taking the drug become aversive. This kind of conditioning is generally more persistent and less easily extinguished than unconditioned reinforcement, and probably accounts for the high relapse rate of 'weaned' addicts. The psychological factors in drug dependence are discussed by Koob (1996) and summarised in Figure 43.1.

▼ Animal models of drug dependence rely mainly on *self-administration* protocols, in which a dose of the drug is given in response to a behaviour such as bar pressing. Some drugs, for example ethanol, are spontaneously self-administered by laboratory animals; others, for example cocaine, are self-administered only after dependence has been induced by previous administration of the drug. Humans, of course, self-administer drugs such as ethanol without necessarily becoming addicted. To model the compulsive nature of addiction more accurately, extensions to the self-administration paradigm may be employed (see Deroche-Gamonet et al., 2004). Rats treated for a short time with 'non-addictive' doses of cocaine will self-administer the drug by bar pressing but stop bar pressing when a signal is shown to indicate that the drug injector is disconnected, or if the drug injection is accompanied by punishment in the form of a foot shock. With more intense 'addictive' pretreatment, bar pressing persists at a high rate under these conditions. Models of this sort are considered more likely to replicate the situation of addiction in humans, as a basis for testing therapeutic approaches, but in humans drug dependence represents a *stable* change in brain function sustained by processes that are more complex and long lasting than the neurobiological changes so far studied in experimental animals.

REWARD PATHWAYS

▼ Virtually all dependence-producing drugs so far tested, including opioids, nicotine, amphetamines, ethanol and cocaine, activate the *reward pathway*—the mesolimbic dopaminergic pathway (see Ch. 34), which runs, via the medial forebrain bundle, from the ventral tegmental area of the midbrain (A10 cell group in rats) to the nucleus accumbens and limbic region (see Nestler, 2001). Even though their primary sites of action are generally elsewhere in the brain, all these drugs increase the release of dopamine in the nucleus accumbens, as shown by microdialysis

and other techniques (see Spanagel & Weiss, 1999). Some stimulate firing of A10 cells, whereas others, such as amphetamine and cocaine, release dopamine or prevent its reuptake (see Ch. 11). Their *hedonic* effect results from activation of this pathway, rather than from a subjective appreciation of the diverse other effects (such as alertness or disinhibition) that the drugs produce. Chemical or surgical interruption of this dopaminergic pathway impairs drug-seeking behaviours in many experimental situations. Deletion of D_2 receptors in a transgenic mouse strain eliminated the reward properties of morphine administration without eliminating other opiate effects, and it did not prevent the occurrence of physical withdrawal symptoms in morphine-dependent animals (Maldonado et al., 1997), suggesting that the dopaminergic pathway is responsible for the positive reward but not for the negative withdrawal effects. However, D_2-receptor antagonists (antipsychotic drugs; see Ch. 38) have not been successful in treating addiction, and more recent evidence (see Heidbreder & Hagan, 2005) suggests that D_3-receptors play an important role. Other mediators, particularly 5-hydroxytryptamine, glutamate and GABA, have also been implicated in the conditioning mechanisms that reinforce drug-seeking behaviour, and a variety of pharmacological strategies based on blocking these pathways are being explored (see Heidbreder & Hagan, 2005). In this regard, the field of drug addiction resembles many of the topics discussed in other chapters dealing with central nervous system (CNS) drugs, where many of the same mediators appear to be involved, and many of the same pharmacological strategies have been proposed to treat addiction, so far with limited success (see below).

BIOCHEMICAL MECHANISMS

▼ The cellular mechanisms involved in habituation to the effects of drugs such as opioids and cocaine have been studied in some detail (see Nestler, 2004). Both classes of drug produce, on chronic administration, an increase in the activity of adenylyl cyclase in brain regions such as the nucleus accumbens, which compensates for their acute inhibitory effect on cAMP formation and produces a rebound increase in cAMP when the drug is terminated (Fig. 43.2). Chronic opioid treatment increases the amount not only of adenylyl cyclase itself, but also of other components of the signalling pathway, including the G-proteins and various protein kinases. This increase in cAMP affects many cellular functions through the increased activity of various cAMP-dependent protein kinases, which

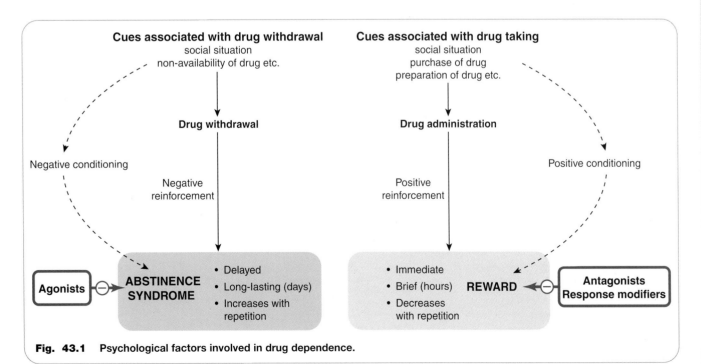

Fig. 43.1 **Psychological factors involved in drug dependence.**

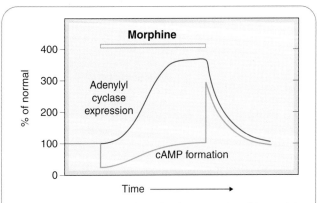

Fig. 43.2 Biochemical mechanism postulated to explain morphine tolerance and dependence. Morphine inhibits adenylyl cyclase, thus reducing cAMP formation (green line). A secondary rise in adenylyl cyclase expression occurs (red line), so that cAMP production recovers in the presence of morphine (i.e. tolerance develops). On cessation of morphine treatment, excessive cAMP production occurs, causing withdrawal symptoms, until the high level of adenylyl cyclase expression returns to normal. Later work has shown that other elements in the cAMP signalling pathway, in addition to adenylyl cyclase itself, are similarly affected by chronic drug exposure, in vivo as well as in vitro. (From Sharma S K et al. 1975 Proc Natl Acad Sci USA 72: 3092.)

control the activity of ion channels (making the cells more excitable), as well as various enzymes and transcription factors. One particular transcription factor, cAMP response element–binding protein (CREB), which is up-regulated in the nucleus accumbens by prolonged administration of opiates or cocaine, plays a key role in regulating various components of cAMP signalling pathways, and transgenic animals lacking CREB show reduced withdrawal symptoms (see Chao & Nestler, 2004). These changes (see Fig. 43.3) probably account for the relatively short-term (days to weeks) phenomena of tolerance and dependence, but the long-term processes responsible for craving and relapse—the major issues in human addiction—are very poorly understood at the neurochemical level.

Adenosine, which is an important CNS mediator (see Ch. 12), has also been implicated in drug dependence. Withdrawal of opiates, cocaine or alcohol results in increased adenosine production, due partly to the conversion of high levels of cAMP to adenosine (see Hack & Christie, 2003). Adenosine, acting on presynaptic A_1-receptors, acts to inhibit glutamate release at excitatory synapses, and thus counteracts the neuronal hyperexcitability that occurs during drug withdrawal, suggesting the possibility—not yet clinically proven—that adenosine agonists might prove useful in treating drug dependence.

Family studies show clearly that susceptibility to addiction is an inherited characteristic, and many candidate genes have been reported, with a particular focus on genes involved in transmitter metabolism, receptors, etc. (see Mayer & Höllt, 2005). The general conclusion is that variants of many different genes each make a small contribution to the overall susceptibility of an individual to addiction—a familiar scenario that provides few pointers for therapeutic intervention. Polymorphisms in ethanol-metabolising genes (see below) are the best example of genes that directly affect the tendency to abuse a drug.

PHARMACOLOGICAL APPROACHES TO TREATING DRUG ADDICTION

From the discussion above, it will be clear that drug addiction involves many psychosocial and some genetic factors, as well as neuropharmacological mechanisms, so drug treatment is only one component of the therapeutic approaches that are used.

The main pharmacological approaches (see O'Brien, 1997; Heidbreder & Hagan, 2005) are summarised in Table 43.2.

NICOTINE AND TOBACCO

Tobacco growing, chewing and smoking was indigenous throughout the American subcontinent and Australia at the time that European explorers first visited these places. Smoking spread through Europe during the 16th century, coming to England mainly as a result of its enthusiastic espousal by Raleigh at the court of Elizabeth I. James I strongly disapproved of both Raleigh and tobacco, and initiated the first antismoking campaign in the early 17th century with the support of the Royal College of Physicians. Parliament responded by imposing a substantial duty on tobacco, thereby setting up the dilemma (from which we show no sign of being able to escape) of giving the State an economic interest in the continuation of smoking at the same time that its official expert advisers were issuing emphatic warnings about its dangers.

	Drug-taking		**Drug withdrawal**	
State produced:	Acute drugged state	*Days–weeks* → Chronic drugged state	Acute abstinence	*Months–years* → Chronic abstinence
Effect:	Reward	Tolerance, dependence	Withdrawal syndrome	Craving
Mechanism:	Activation of mesolimbic DA pathway. ? Other reward pathways	Adaptive changes in receptors, transporters, 2nd messengers, etc. (e.g. ↑adenylyl cyclase, DA ↑transporter)	Uncompensated adaptive changes (e.g. ↓DA, ↑glutamate)	Not known

Fig. 43.3 Cellular and physiological mechanisms involved in drug dependence showing the relationship between the immediate and delayed effects of drug-taking and drug withdrawal. DA, dopamine.

Table 43.2 Pharmacological approaches to treating drug dependence

Mechanism	Example(s)
Substitution to alleviate withdrawal symptoms	Methadone used short term to blunt opiate withdrawal Benzodiazepines to blunt alcohol withdrawal α_2-Adrenoceptor agonists (e.g. clonidine, lofexidine) to diminish withdrawal symptoms
Long-term substitution	Methadone substitution for opiate addiction Nicotine patches or chewing gum
Blocking response	Naltrexone to block opiate effects Mecamylamine to block nicotine effects Immunisation against cocaine and nicotine to produce circulating antibody (not yet proven)
Aversive therapies	Disulfiram to induce unpleasant response to ethanol
Modification of craving	Bupropion (antidepressant) Naltrexone (blocks opiate receptors—also of value in treating other addictions) Clonidine (α_2-adrenoceptor agonist) Acamprosate (NMDA receptor antagonist) used to treat alcoholism

Until the latter half of the 19th century, tobacco was smoked in pipes, and by men. Cigarette manufacture began at the end of the 19th century, and now cigarettes account for 98% of tobacco consumption. The trend in cigarette consumption in the 20th century is shown in Figure 43.4. From a peak in the early 1970s, cigarette consumption in the UK dropped by about 50%, the main factors being increased price, adverse publicity, restrictions on advertising, and the compulsory publication of health warnings. Filter cigarettes (which give a somewhat lower delivery of tar and nicotine than standard cigarettes) and 'low-tar' cigarettes (which are also low in nicotine) constitute an increasing proportion of the total.[2] The proportion of cigarette smokers in the UK is currently about 27%, with little difference between men and women, and has remained at this level since the early 1990s. About 10% of children aged 10–15 are regular smokers. Currently, there are about 1.1 billion smokers in the world (18% of the population), and the number in developing countries is increasing rapidly. Five trillion (5×10^{12}) cigarettes are sold each year, about 5000 per smoker.

For reviews on nicotine and smoking, see Balfour & Fagerstrom (1996) and Benowitz (1996).

PHARMACOLOGICAL EFFECTS OF SMOKING

Nicotine[3] is the only pharmacologically active substance in tobacco smoke, apart from carcinogenic tars and carbon monoxide (see

Drug dependence

- Dependence is defined as a compulsive craving that develops as a result of repeated administration of the drug.
- Dependence occurs with a wide range of psychotropic drugs, acting by many different mechanisms.
- The common feature of dependence-producing drugs is that they have a positive reinforcing action ('reward') associated with activation of the mesolimbic dopaminergic pathway.
- Dependence is often associated with (i) tolerance to the drug, which can arise by various biochemical mechanisms; (ii) a physical abstinence syndrome, which varies in type and intensity for different classes of drug; (iii) psychological dependence (craving), which may be associated with the tolerance-producing biochemical changes.
- Psychological dependence, which usually outlasts the physical withdrawal syndrome, is the major factor leading to relapse among treated addicts.
- Although genetic factors contribute to drug-seeking behaviour, no specific genes have yet been identified.

---

[2]Smokers adapt by smoking more low-tar cigarettes so as to maintain their nicotine consumption.

[3]From the plant *Nicotiana*, named after Jean Nicot, French ambassador to Portugal, who presented seeds to the French king in 1560, having been persuaded of the medical value of smoking tobacco leaves by natives of South America. Smoking was believed to protect against illness, particularly the plague.

below). The acute effects of smoking can be mimicked by injection of nicotine and are blocked by **mecamylamine**, an antagonist at neuronal nicotinic acetylcholine receptors (nAChRs) (see Ch. 10).

Effects on the central nervous system

The central effects of nicotine are complex and cannot be summed up overall simply in terms of stimulation or inhibition. At the

Clinical use of drugs in substance dependence

- *Tobacco dependence*:
  - short-term **nicotine** is the drug of choice as adjunct to behavioural therapy in smokers committed to giving up
  - **bupropion** is also effective but lowers seizure threshold, so is contraindicated in people with risk factors for seizures.
- *Alcohol dependence*:
  - long-acting benzodiazepines (e.g. **chlordiazepoxide**) can be used to reduce withdrawal symptoms and the risk of seizures; they should be tapered over 1–2 weeks and then discontinued because of their abuse potential
  - **disulfiram** is used as an adjunct to behavioural therapy in suitably motivated alcoholics after detoxification; it is contraindicated for patients in whom a hypotensive acetaldehyde-induced reaction (p. 632) would be dangerous (e.g. those with coronary or cerebral vascular disease)
  - **acamprosate** can help to maintain abstinence; it is started as soon as abstinence has been achieved and maintained if relapse occurs, and it is continued for 1 year.
- *Opioid dependence*:
  - opioid agonists or partial agonists (e.g., respectively, **methadone** and **buprenorphine**) administered orally or sublingually may be substituted for injectable narcotics, many of whose harmful effects are attributable to the route of administration
  - **naltrexone**, a long-acting opioid antagonist, is used as an adjunct to help prevent relapse in detoxified addicts (opioid-free for at least 1 week)
  - **lofexidine**, an α_2 agonist (cf. **clonidine**; Ch. 11) is used short term (usually up to 10 days) to ameliorate symptoms of opioid withdrawal, and is then tapered over a further 2–4 days.

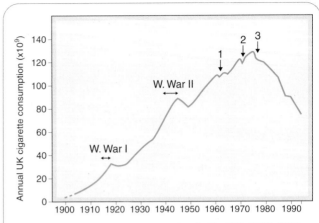

Fig. 43.4 Cigarette consumption in the UK, 1900–1994. Numbers 1, 2 and 3 refer to publication of Royal College of Physicians reports on smoking and health. Since 1980, the drop in consumption has closely followed price increases. Since 1994, cigarette consumption has levelled off. (Data from Ashton H, Stepney R 1982 Smoking psychology and pharmacology. Tavistock Publications, London; Townsend 1996 Price and consumption of tobacco. Br Med Bull 52: 132–142.)

Tobacco smoking

- Cigarette consumption in the UK is now declining after reaching a peak in the mid-1970s.
- The worldwide prevalence of smoking is now about 18% of the adult population, each smoker using on average 5000 cigarettes per year.
- Nicotine is the only pharmacologically active agent in tobacco, apart from carcinogenic tars and carbon monoxide.
- The amount of nicotine absorbed from an average cigarette is about 1–1.5 mg, which causes the plasma nicotine concentration to reach 130–200 nmol/l. These values depend greatly on the type of cigarette and on the extent of inhalation of the smoke.

cellular level, nicotine acts on nAChRs of the $\alpha_4\beta_2$ subtype (see Ch. 34), which are widely expressed in the brain, particularly in the cortex and hippocampus, and are believed to play a role in cognitive function, as well as in the ventral tegmental area, from which dopaminergic neurons project to the nucleus accumbens (the reward pathway, see above). These receptors are ligand-gated cation channels located both pre- and postsynaptically, causing, respectively, enhanced transmitter release and neuronal excitation (see Wonnacott et al., 2005). As well as activating the receptors, nicotine also causes desensitisation, which may be an important component of its effects, because the effects of a dose of nicotine are diminished in animals after sustained exposure to the drug. Chronic nicotine administration leads to a substantial increase in the number of nAChRs (an effect opposite to that produced by sustained administration of most receptor agonists), which may represent an adaptive response to prolonged receptor desensitisation. It is likely that the overall effect of nicotine reflects a balance between activation of nAChRs, causing neuronal excitation, and desensitisation, causing synaptic block.

At the spinal level, nicotine inhibits spinal reflexes, causing skeletal muscle relaxation that can be measured by electromyography. This may be due to stimulation of the inhibitory Renshaw cells in the ventral horn of the spinal cord. The higher level functioning of the brain, as reflected in the subjective sense of alertness or by the electroencephalography (EEG) pattern, can be affected in either direction by nicotine, according to dose and circumstances. Smokers report that smoking wakes them up when they are drowsy and calms them down when they are tense, and EEG recordings broadly bear this out. It also seems that small doses of nicotine tend to cause arousal, whereas large doses do the reverse. Tests of motor and sensory performance (e.g. reaction time measurements or vigilance tests) in humans generally show improvement after smoking, and nicotine enhances learning in rats. Some elaborate tests have been conducted to see, for example, whether the effect of nicotine on performance and aggression varies according to the amount of stress. In one such test, the subject first has to name the colours of a series of squares (low stress), and then has to name the colours in which the names of other colours are written (high stress). The difference between the scores, reflecting the extent by which performance is affected by stress, was diminished by smoking. Some tests border on nasty-mindedness, such as one in which subjects played a complicated logical game with a computer that initially played fair and then began to cheat randomly, causing stress and aggression in the subjects and a decline in their performance. Smoking, it was reported, did not reduce the anger but did reduce the decline in performance.

Nicotine and other agonists such as **epibatidine** (Ch. 41) have significant analgesic activity.

Peripheral effects

The peripheral effects of small doses of nicotine result from stimulation of autonomic ganglia (see Ch. 10) and of peripheral sensory receptors, mainly in the heart and lungs. Stimulation of these receptors elicits various autonomic reflex responses, causing tachycardia, increased cardiac output and increased arterial pressure, reduction of gastrointestinal motility, and sweating. When people smoke for the first time, they usually experience nausea and sometimes vomit, probably because of stimulation of sensory receptors in the stomach. All these effects decline with repeated dosage, although the central effects remain. Secretion of adrenaline and noradrenaline from the adrenal medulla contributes to the cardiovascular effects, and release of antidiuretic hormone from the posterior pituitary causes a decrease in urine flow. The plasma concentration of free fatty acids is increased, probably owing to sympathetic stimulation and adrenaline secretion.

Smokers weigh, on average, about 4 kg less than non-smokers, mainly because of reduced food intake; giving up smoking usually causes weight gain associated with increased food intake.

PHARMACOKINETIC ASPECTS

An average cigarette contains about 0.8 g of tobacco and 9–17 mg of nicotine, of which about 10% is normally absorbed by the smoker. This fraction varies greatly with the habits of the smoker and the type of cigarette.

Nicotine in cigarette smoke is rapidly absorbed from the lungs but poorly from the mouth and nasopharynx. Therefore inhalation is required to give appreciable absorption of nicotine, each puff delivering a distinct bolus of drug to the CNS. Pipe or cigar smoke is less acidic than cigarette smoke, and the nicotine tends to be absorbed from the mouth and nasopharynx rather than the lungs. Absorption is considerably slower than from inhaled cigarette smoke, resulting in a later and longer lasting peak in the plasma nicotine concentration (Fig. 43.5). An average cigarette, smoked over 10 minutes, causes the plasma nicotine concentration to rise to 15–30 ng/ml (100–200 nmol/l), falling to about half within 10 minutes and then more slowly over the next 1–2 hours. The rapid decline results mainly from redistribution between the blood and other tissues; the slower decline is due to hepatic metabolism, mainly by oxidation to an inactive ketone metabolite, *cotinine*. This has a long plasma half-life, and measurement of plasma cotinine concentration provides a useful measure of smoking behaviour. A nicotine patch applied for 24 hours causes the plasma concentration to rise to 75–150 nmol/l over 6 hours and to remain fairly constant for about 20 hours. Administration by nasal spray or chewing gum results in a time course intermediate between that of smoking and the nicotine patch.

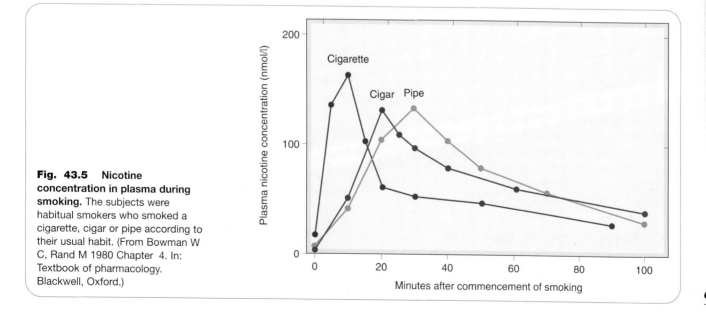

Fig. 43.5 Nicotine concentration in plasma during smoking. The subjects were habitual smokers who smoked a cigarette, cigar or pipe according to their usual habit. (From Bowman W C, Rand M 1980 Chapter 4. In: Textbook of pharmacology. Blackwell, Oxford.)

TOLERANCE AND DEPENDENCE

As with other dependence-producing drugs, three separate but related processes—tolerance, physical dependence and psychological dependence—contribute to the overall state of dependence, in which taking the drug becomes compulsive.

The effects of nicotine associated with peripheral ganglionic stimulation show rapid tolerance, perhaps as a result of desensitisation of nAChRs by nicotine. With large doses of nicotine, this desensitisation produces a block of ganglionic transmission rather than stimulation (see Ch. 10). Tolerance to the central effects of nicotine (e.g. in the arousal response) is much less than in the periphery. The increase in the number of nicotinic receptors in the brain produced by chronic nicotine administration in animals (see above) also occurs in heavy smokers. Because the cellular effects of nicotine are diminished, it is possible that the additional binding sites represent desensitised rather than functional receptors.

The addictiveness of smoking is due solely to nicotine. Rats choose to drink dilute nicotine solution in preference to water if given a choice, and in a situation in which lever pressing causes an injection of nicotine to be delivered, they quickly learn to self-administer it. Similarly, monkeys who have been trained to smoke, by providing a reward in response to smoking behaviour, will continue to do so spontaneously (i.e. unrewarded) if the smoking medium contains nicotine, but not if nicotine-free tobacco is offered instead. Like other addictive drugs (see above), nicotine causes excitation of the mesolimbic reward pathway and increased dopamine release in the nucleus accumbens. Transgenic mice lacking the β_2 subunit of the acetylcholine receptor lose the rewarding effect of nicotine and its dopamine-releasing effect, confirming the role of this nAChR subtype and mesolimbic dopamine release in the response to nicotine. In contrast to normal mice, the mutant mice could not be induced to self-administer nicotine, even though they did so with cocaine. Further evidence implicating brain nAChRs in the addictive property of nicotine comes from experiments with **mecamylamine**, an antagonist at nAChRs. If monkeys are habituated to tobacco smoking so that they choose to puff smoke in preference to air, administration of mecamylamine causes them to switch to puffing air instead of smoke.

A physical withdrawal syndrome occurs in both humans and experimental animals accustomed to regular nicotine administration. Its main features are increased irritability, impaired performance of psychomotor tasks, aggressiveness and sleep disturbance. The withdrawal syndrome is much less severe than that produced by opiates, and it can be alleviated not only by nicotine but also by amphetamine, a finding consistent with the postulated role of dopamine in the reward pathway. The nicotine withdrawal syndrome lasts for 2–3 weeks, although the craving for cigarettes persists for much longer than this; relapses during attempts to give up cigarette smoking occur most commonly at a time when the physical withdrawal syndrome has long since subsided.

HARMFUL EFFECTS OF SMOKING

The life expectancy of smokers is shorter than that of non-smokers. For example, in a 1971 study of British doctors, the proportion of heavy smokers dying between the ages of 35 and 65 was estimated

---

> **Pharmacology of nicotine**
>
> - At a cellular level, nicotine acts on nicotinic acetylcholine receptors (nAChRs), mainly of the $\alpha_4\beta_2$ subtype, to cause neuronal excitation. Its central effects are blocked by receptor antagonists such as mecamylamine.
> - At the behavioural level, nicotine produces a mixture of inhibitory and excitatory effects.
> - Nicotine shows reinforcing properties, associated with increased activity in the mesolimbic dopaminergic pathway, and self-administration can be elicited in animal studies.
> - Electroencephalography changes show an arousal response, and subjects report increased alertness accompanied by a reduction of anxiety and tension.
> - Learning, particularly under stress, is facilitated by nicotine.
> - Peripheral effects of nicotine are due mainly to ganglionic stimulation: tachycardia, increased blood pressure and reduced gastrointestinal motility. Tolerance develops rapidly to these effects.
> - Nicotine is metabolised, mainly in the liver, within 1–2 hours. The inactive metabolite, cotinine, has a long plasma half-life and can be used as a measure of smoking habits.
> - Nicotine gives rise to tolerance, physical dependence and psychological dependence (craving), and is highly addictive. Attempts at long-term cessation succeed in only about 20% of cases.
> - Nicotine replacement therapy (chewing gum or skin patch preparations) improves the chances of giving up smoking but only when combined with active counselling.

---

to be 40%, compared with 15% for non-smokers. For a recent analysis, see Peto et al. (1996). Smoking is, by a large margin, the biggest preventable cause of death, responsible for about 1 in 10 adult deaths worldwide. Apart from AIDS, smoking is the only major cause of death that is increasing rapidly. In 1990, smoking was responsible for 10% (3 million out of 30 million) of deaths worldwide; by 2030, this is expected to increase to 17% (10 million out of 60 million), mainly due to the growth of smoking in Asia, Africa and Latin America (Peto et al., 1999).

The main health risks are as follow.

- *Cancer, particularly of the lung and upper respiratory tract but also of the oesophagus, pancreas and bladder.* Smoking 20 cigarettes per day is estimated to increase the risk of lung cancer about 10-fold. About 90% of lung cancers are caused by smoking. Pipe and cigar smoking carry much less risk than cigarette smoking, although the risk is still appreciable. Tar, rather than nicotine, is responsible for the cancer risk.

- *Coronary heart disease and other forms of peripheral vascular disease.* The mortality among men aged 55–64 from coronary thrombosis is about 60% greater in men who smoke 20 cigarettes per day than in non-smokers. Although the increase in risk is less than it is for lung cancer, the actual number of excess deaths associated with smoking is larger, because coronary heart disease is so common. Other kinds of vascular disease (e.g. stroke, intermittent claudication and diabetic gangrene) are also strongly smoking-related. Many studies have suggested that nicotine is mainly responsible for the adverse effect of smoking on the incidence of cardiovascular disease. Another factor may be *carbon monoxide* (see below). Surprisingly, there is no clear increase in ischaemic heart disease in pipe and cigar smokers, even though similar blood nicotine and carboxyhaemoglobin concentrations are reached, suggesting that nicotine and carbon monoxide may not be the only causative factors.

- *Chronic bronchitis.* Chronic bronchitis is much more common in smokers than in non-smokers. Nonetheless, in contrast to lung cancer, chronic bronchitis has declined in prevalence over the past 50 years. This is generally attributed to cleaner air and other social changes, and smoking now appears to be the most important remaining cause. Its effect is probably due to tar and other irritants rather than nicotine.

- *Harmful effects in pregnancy.* Smoking, particularly during the latter half of pregnancy, significantly reduces birth weight (by about 8% in women who smoke 25 or more cigarettes per day during pregnancy) and increases perinatal mortality (by an estimated 28% in babies born to mothers who smoke in the last half of pregnancy). There is evidence that children born to smoking mothers remain behind, in both physical and mental development, for at least 7 years. By 11 years of age, the difference is no longer significant. These effects of smoking, although measurable, are much smaller than the effects of other factors, such as social class and birth order. Various other complications of pregnancy are also more common in women who smoke, including spontaneous abortion (increased 30–70% by smoking), premature delivery (increased about 40%) and placenta praevia (increased 25–90%). Nicotine is excreted in breast milk in sufficient amounts to cause tachycardia in the infant.

Parkinson's disease is approximately twice as common in non-smokers as in smokers. It is possible that this reflects a protective effect of nicotine, but it could be that common genetic or environmental factors underlie smoking behaviour and susceptibility to Parkinson's disease. Symptoms from *inflammatory bowel disease* may be reduced by cigarette smoking. Earlier reports that Alzheimer's disease is less common in smokers have not been confirmed.

The agents probably responsible for the harmful effects are as follow.

- *Tar and irritants*, such as nitrogen dioxide and formaldehyde. Cigarette smoke tar contains many known carcinogenic hydrocarbons, as well as tumour promoters, which account

for the high cancer risk. It is likely that the various irritant substances are also responsible for the increase in bronchitis and emphysema.

- *Nicotine* probably accounts for retarded fetal development because of its vasoconstrictor properties.

- *Carbon monoxide.* The average carbon monoxide content of cigarette smoke is about 3%. Carbon monoxide has a high affinity for haemoglobin, and the average carboxyhaemoglobin content in the blood of cigarette smokers is about 2.5% (compared with 0.4% for non-smoking urban dwellers). In very heavy smokers, up to 15% of haemoglobin may be carboxylated, a level that affects fetal development in rats. This factor may also contribute to the increased incidence of heart and vascular disease. Fetal haemoglobin has a higher affinity for carbon monoxide than adult haemoglobin, and the proportion of carboxyhaemoglobin is higher in fetal than in maternal blood.

- Increased *oxidative stress* may be responsible for *atherogenesis* (Ch. 20) and *chronic obstructive lung disease* (Ch. 23).

Low-tar cigarettes give a lower yield of both tar and nicotine than standard cigarettes. However, it has been shown that smokers puff harder, inhale more, and smoke more cigarettes when low-tar brands are substituted for standard brands. The end result may be a slightly reduced intake of tar and nicotine but an increase in carbon monoxide intake, with no net gain in terms of safety.

PHARMACOLOGICAL APPROACHES TO TREATMENT OF NICOTINE DEPENDENCE

Most smokers would like to quit, but few succeed.[4] The most successful smoking cure clinics, using a combination of psychological and pharmacological treatments, achieve a success rate of

---

Harmful effects of smoking

- Smoking accounts for about 10% of deaths worldwide, mainly due to:
  - cancer, especially lung cancer, of which about 90% of cases are smoking-related; carcinogenic tars are responsible
  - ischaemic heart disease; both nicotine and carbon monoxide may be responsible
  - chronic bronchitis; tars are mainly responsible.
- Smoking in pregnancy reduces birth weight and retards childhood development. It also increases abortion rate and perinatal mortality. Nicotine and possibly carbon monoxide are responsible.
- The incidence of Parkinson's disease is lower in smokers than in non-smokers.

---

[4]Freud tried unsuccessfully to give up cigars for 45 years before dying of cancer of the mouth at the age of 83.

about 25%, measured as the percentage of patients still abstinent after 1 year. The two main pharmacological treatments (see George & O'Malley, 2004) are **nicotine replacement therapy** and **bupropion** (also used to treat depression; see Table 39.2).

Nicotine replacement therapy is used mainly to assist smokers to quit by relieving the psychological and physical withdrawal syndrome. Because nicotine is relatively short-acting and not well absorbed from the gastrointestinal tract, it is given either in the form of chewing gum, used several times daily, or as a transdermal patch that is replaced daily. These preparations cause various side effects, particularly nausea and gastrointestinal cramps, cough, insomnia and muscle pains. There is a risk that nicotine may cause coronary spasm in patients with heart disease. Transdermal patches often cause local irritation and itching. The conclusion of many double-blind trials of nicotine against placebo is that these preparations, combined with professional counselling and supportive therapy, roughly double the chances of successfully breaking the smoking habit, but the success rate measured as abstinence 1 year after ceasing treatment is still only about 25%. Nicotine on its own, without counselling and support, is no more effective than placebo, so its use as an over-the-counter smoking remedy has little justification. Although of limited value as an aid to abstinence, the long-term use of nicotine can significantly reduce cigarette consumption by smokers. In Sweden, the use of 'smokeless tobacco' is encouraged and smoking-related death rate is much lower than elsewhere in Europe or North America.

The identification of the $\alpha_4\beta_2$ nAChR subtype as the putative 'nicotine receptor' in the brain may allow selective agonists to be developed as nicotine substitutes with fewer side effects, but this remains theoretical at present.

Bupropion (Ch. 39), in recent trials, appears to be as effective as nicotine replacement therapy, even in non-depressed patients, and has fewer side effects. However, bupropion lowers the seizure threshold so should not be prescribed if there are other risk factors for seizures (including other drugs that lower seizure threshold). It is also contraindicated if there is a history of eating disorders or of bipolar mood disorder, and is used only with caution in patients with liver or renal disease. Because of these problems, nicotine remains the pharmacological treatment of choice in most cases.

Bupropion may act by increasing dopamine activity in the nucleus accumbens. It is a weak blocker of dopamine and noradrenaline uptake, but it is not clear that this accounts for its efficacy in treating nicotine dependence. It is usually given as a slow-release formulation.

Many other drugs have been tested clinically and shown to be useful in some cases. They include the following.

- **Clonidine**, an α_2-adrenoceptor agonist (see Ch. 11), which reduces the withdrawal effects of several dependence-producing drugs, including opioids and **cocaine**, as well as nicotine.[5] Clonidine may be given orally or as a transdermal patch, and is about as effective as nicotine substitution in assisting abstinence. The side effects of clonidine (hypotension, dry mouth, drowsiness) are troublesome, however, and it is not widely used.

- **Tricyclic antidepressants, selective serotonin reuptake inhibitors** and **monoamine oxidase inhibitors,** used mainly as antidepressants (Ch. 39). The rationale may be that depressive episodes, which often lead to resumption of smoking, are prevented.

- **Mecamylamine**, which antagonises the effects of nicotine, is not promising. Small doses actually increase smoking, presumably because the antagonism can be overcome by increasing the amount of nicotine. Larger doses of mecamylamine, which abolish the effects of nicotine more effectively, have many autonomic side effects (see Ch. 10), and compliance is poor. The rationale is questionable because, although mecamylamine reduces the reward effect of nicotine, it does not affect the craving associated with abstinence.

A new approach to the treatment of drug dependence, so far applied mainly to nicotine and cocaine, is the development of vaccines (see Bunce et al., 2003) consisting of the drug molecule complexed to a protein. Antibodies produced in response to injection of the complex also bind the free drug, thereby preventing it from reaching the brain. This strategy is effective in animal models involving self-administration, and clinical trials in humans are in progress.

ETHANOL

Judged on a molar basis, the consumption of ethanol far exceeds that of any other drug. The ethanol content of various drinks ranges from about 2.5% (weak beer) to about 55% (strong spirits), and the size of the normal measure is such that a single drink usually contains about 8–12 g (0.17–0.26 moles) of ethanol. It is by no means unusual to consume 1–2 moles at a sitting, equivalent to about 0.5 kg of most other drugs. Its low pharmacological potency is reflected in the range of plasma concentrations needed to produce pharmacological effects: minimal effects occur at about 10 mmol/l (46 mg/100 ml), and 10 times this concentration may be lethal. The average per capita ethanol consumption in European countries is about 10 litres/year (expressed as pure ethanol), a figure that has changed little over the past 20 years, the main change having been a growing consumption of wine in preference to beer.

For practical purposes, ethanol intake is often expressed in terms of units. One unit is equal to 8 g (10 ml) of ethanol, and is the amount contained in half a pint of normal strength beer, one measure of spirits or one small glass of wine. Based on the health risks described below, the current official recommendation is a maximum of 21 units/week for men and 14 units/week for women. It is estimated that in the UK, about 33% of men and 13% of women exceed these levels. The annual tax revenue from drink amounts to about £7 billion, whereas the health cost is estimated at £3 billion, and the social cost undoubtedly greater. Governments in most developed countries are attempting to curb alcohol consumption.

---

[5]It also reduces postmenopausal flushing, which may represent a physiological oestrogen withdrawal response.

PHARMACOLOGICAL EFFECTS OF ETHANOL

Effects on the central nervous system

The main effects of ethanol are on the CNS (see review by Charness et al., 1989), where its depressant actions resemble those of volatile anaesthetics (Ch. 36). At a cellular level, the effect of ethanol is purely depressant, although it increases neuronal activity—presumably by disinhibition—in some parts of the CNS, notably in the mesolimbic dopaminergic neurons that are involved in the reward pathway described above. The main theories of ethanol action (see reviews by Little, 1991; Lovinger, 1997; Tabakoff & Hoffman, 1996) are:

- enhancement of GABA-mediated inhibition, similar to the action of benzodiazepines (see Ch. 37)
- inhibition of Ca^{2+} entry through voltage-gated calcium channels
- inhibition of NMDA receptor function
- inhibition of adenosine transport.

Ethanol enhances the action of GABA acting on $GABA_A$ receptors in a similar way to benzodiazepines (see Ch. 37). Its effect is, however, smaller and less consistent than that of benzodiazepines, and no clear effect on inhibitory synaptic transmission in the CNS has been demonstrated for ethanol. The benzodiazepine antagonist **flumazenil** (see Ch. 37) reverses the central depressant actions of ethanol, but this appears to result from physiological antagonism rather than from a direct pharmacological interaction. The use of flumazenil to reverse ethanol intoxication and treat dependence has not found favour for several reasons. Because flumazenil is an inverse agonist (see Ch. 2) at benzodiazepine receptors, it carries a risk of causing seizures, and it could cause an increase in ethanol consumption and thus increase long-term toxic manifestations.

Ethanol inhibits transmitter release in response to nerve terminal depolarisation by inhibiting the opening of voltage-sensitive calcium channels in neurons.

The excitatory effects of glutamate are inhibited by ethanol at concentrations that produce CNS depressant effects in vivo. NMDA receptor activation is inhibited at lower ethanol concentrations than are required to affect AMPA receptors (see Ch. 34). Other effects produced by ethanol include an enhancement of the excitatory effects produced by activation of nAChRs and $5-HT_3$ receptors. The relative importance of these various effects in the overall effects of ethanol on CNS function is not clear at present.

The depressant effects of ethanol on neuronal function resemble those of adenosine acting on A_1-receptors (see Ch. 12). Ethanol in cell culture systems increases extracellular adenosine by inhibiting adenosine uptake, and there is some evidence that inhibition of the adenosine transporter may account for some of its CNS effects (Melendez & Kalivas, 2004).

Endogenous opioids also play a role in the CNS effects of ethanol, because both human and animal studies show that the opioid receptor antagonist **naltrexone** reduces the reward associated with ethanol.

The effects of acute ethanol intoxication in humans are well known and include slurred speech, motor incoordination, increased self-confidence and euphoria. The effect on mood varies among individuals, most becoming louder and more outgoing, but some becoming morose and withdrawn. At higher levels of intoxication, the mood tends to become highly labile, with euphoria and melancholy, aggression and submission, often occurring successively. The association between alcohol and violence is well documented.

Intellectual and motor performance and sensory discrimination show uniform impairment by ethanol, but subjects are generally unable to judge this for themselves. For example, bus drivers were asked to drive through a gap that they selected as the minimum for their bus to pass through; ethanol caused them not only to hit the barriers more often at any given gap setting, but also to set the gap to a narrower dimension, often narrower than the bus.

Much effort has gone into measuring the effect of ethanol on driving performance in real life, as opposed to artificial tests under experimental conditions. In an American study of city drivers, it was found that the probability of being involved in an accident was unaffected at blood ethanol concentrations up to 50 mg/100 ml (10.9 mmol/l); by 80 mg/100 ml (17.4 mmol/l), the probability was increased about fourfold, and by 150 mg/100 ml (32.6 mmol/l) about 25-fold. In the UK, driving with a blood ethanol concentration greater than 80 mg/100 ml constitutes a legal offence.

The relationship between plasma ethanol concentration and effect is highly variable. A given concentration produces a larger effect when the concentration is rising than when it is steady or falling. A substantial degree of tissue tolerance develops in habitual drinkers, with the result that a higher plasma ethanol concentration is needed to produce a given effect (see below). In one study, 'gross intoxication' (assessed by a battery of tests that measured speech, gait and so on) occurred in 30% of subjects between 50 and 100 mg/100 ml and in 90% of subjects with more than 150 mg/100 ml. Coma generally occurs at about 400 mg/100 ml, and death from respiratory failure is likely at levels exceeding 500 mg/100 ml.

In addition to the acute effects of ethanol on the nervous system, chronic administration also causes irreversible neurological effects (see Harper & Matsumoto, 2005). These may be due to ethanol itself, or to metabolites such as acetaldehyde or fatty acid esters. The majority of heavy drinkers develop irreversible dementia and motor impairment associated with thinning of the cerebral cortex (apparent as ventricular enlargement) detectable by brain-imaging techniques. Degeneration in the cerebellum and other specific brain regions can also occur, as well as peripheral neuropathy. Some of these changes are not due to ethanol itself but to accompanying thiamine deficiency, which is common in alcoholics.

Ethanol significantly enhances—sometimes to a dangerous extent—the CNS depressant effects of many other drugs, including benzodiazepines, antidepressants, antipsychotic drugs and opiates.

Effects on other systems

The main acute cardiovascular effect of ethanol is to produce cutaneous vasodilatation, central in origin, which causes a warm feeling but actually increases heat loss. Paradoxically, there is a positive correlation between ethanol consumption and hypertension, possibly because ethanol withdrawal causes increased sympathetic activity. The beneficial effect of moderate drinking on cardiovascular function is discussed below.

Ethanol increases salivary and gastric secretion. This is partly a reflex effect produced by the taste and irritant action of ethanol.

However, heavy consumption of spirits causes damage directly to the gastric mucosa, causing chronic gastritis. Both this and the increased acid secretion are factors in the high incidence of gastric bleeding in alcoholics.

Ethanol produces a variety of endocrine effects. In particular, it increases the output of adrenal steroid hormones by stimulating the anterior pituitary gland to secrete adrenocorticotrophic hormone. However, the increase in plasma hydrocortisone usually seen in alcoholics (producing a 'pseudo-Cushing's syndrome'; Ch. 28) is due partly to inhibition by ethanol of hydrocortisone metabolism in the liver.

Diuresis is a familiar effect of ethanol. It is caused by inhibition of antidiuretic hormone secretion, and tolerance develops rapidly, so that the diuresis is not sustained. There is a similar inhibition of oxytocin secretion, which can delay parturition. Attempts have been made to use this effect in premature labour, but the dose needed is large enough to cause obvious drunkenness in the mother. If the baby is born prematurely despite the ethanol, it too may be intoxicated at birth, sufficiently for respiration to be depressed. The procedure evidently has serious disadvantages.

Chronic male alcoholics are often impotent and show signs of feminisation. This is associated with impaired testicular steroid synthesis, but induction of hepatic microsomal enzymes by ethanol, and hence an increased rate of testosterone inactivation, also contributes.

Effects of ethanol on the liver

Together with brain damage, liver damage is the most serious long-term consequence of excessive ethanol consumption (see Lieber, 1995). In the sequence of effects, increased fat accumulation (fatty liver) progresses to hepatitis (i.e. inflammation of the liver) and eventually to irreversible hepatic necrosis and fibrosis. Diversion of portal blood flow around the fibrotic liver often causes oesophageal varices to develop, which can bleed suddenly and catastrophically. Increased fat accumulation in the liver occurs, in rats or in humans, after a single large dose of ethanol. The mechanism is complex, the main factors being:

- increased release of fatty acids from adipose tissue, which is the result of increased stress, causing sympathetic discharge
- impaired fatty acid oxidation, because of the metabolic load imposed by the ethanol itself.

With chronic ethanol consumption, many other factors contribute to the liver damage. One is malnutrition, for alcoholic individuals may satisfy much of their calorie requirement from ethanol itself. Three hundred grams of ethanol (equivalent to one bottle of whisky) provides about 2000 kcal but, unlike a normal diet, it provides no vitamins, amino acids or fatty acids. Thiamine deficiency is an important factor in causing chronic neurological damage (see above). The hepatic changes occurring in alcoholics are partly due to chronic malnutrition but mainly to the cellular toxicity of ethanol, which promotes inflammatory changes in the liver.

The overall incidence of chronic liver disease is a function of cumulative ethanol consumption over many years. Therefore overall consumption, expressed as g/kg of body weight per day multiplied by years of drinking, provides an accurate predictor of the incidence of cirrhosis. An increase in the plasma concentration of the liver enzyme γ-glutamyl transpeptidase provides an index of liver damage, although not specific to ethanol.

Effects on lipid metabolism, platelet function and atherosclerosis

Moderate drinking reduces mortality associated with coronary heart disease, the maximum effect—about 30% reduction of mortality overall—being achieved at a level of 2–3 units/day (see Groenbaek et al., 1994). The effect is much more pronounced (> 50% reduction) in men with high plasma concentrations of low-density lipoprotein cholesterol (see Ch. 20).[6] Most evidence suggests that ethanol, rather than any specific beverage, such as red wine, is the essential factor.

Two mechanisms have been proposed. The first involves the effect of ethanol on the plasma lipoproteins that are the carrier molecules for cholesterol and other lipids in the bloodstream (see Ch. 20). Epidemiological studies, as well as studies on volunteers, have shown that ethanol, in daily doses too small to produce obvious CNS effects, can over the course of a few weeks increase plasma high-density lipoprotein concentration, thus exerting a protective effect against atheroma formation.

Ethanol may also protect against ischaemic heart disease by inhibiting platelet aggregation. This effect occurs at ethanol concentrations in the range achieved by normal drinking in humans (10–20 mmol/l) and probably results from inhibition of arachidonic acid formation from phospholipid. In humans, the magnitude of the effect depends critically on dietary fat intake, and it is not yet clear how important it is clinically.

The effect of ethanol on fetal development

The adverse effect of ethanol consumption during pregnancy on fetal development was demonstrated in the early 1970s, when the term *fetal alcohol syndrome* (*FAS*) was coined.

The features of full FAS include:

- abnormal facial development, with wide-set eyes, short palpebral fissures and small cheekbones
- reduced cranial circumference
- retarded growth
- mental retardation and behavioural abnormalities, often taking the form of hyperactivity and difficulty with social integration
- other anatomical abnormalities, which may be major or minor (e.g. congenital cardiac abnormalities, malformation of the eyes and ears).

A lesser degree of impairment, termed *alcohol-related neurodevelopmental disorder* (*ARND*), results in behavioural problems, and cognitive and motor deficits, often associated with reduced brain size. Full FAS occurs in about 3 per 1000 live births and affects about 30% of children born to alcoholic mothers. It is rare with mothers who drink less than about 5 units/day, and most common in 'binge drinkers' who sporadically consume much larger amounts, resulting in high peak levels of ethanol. ARND

---

[6]This beneficial effect of moderate drinking outweighs the risk of adverse effects (e.g. accidents, cancers, liver damage) only in men over 45 and women over 55.

is about three times as common. Although there is no clearly defined safe threshold, there is no evidence that amounts less than about 2 units/day are harmful. There is no critical period during pregnancy when ethanol consumption is likely to lead to FAS, although one study suggests that FAS incidence correlates most strongly with ethanol consumption very early in pregnancy, even before pregnancy is recognised, implying that not only pregnant women, but also women who are likely to become pregnant, must be advised not to drink heavily. Experiments on rats and mice suggest that the effect on facial development may be produced very early in pregnancy (up to 4 weeks in humans), while the effect on brain development is produced rather later (up to 10 weeks).

Other adverse effects of chronic ethanol consumption include gastritis, associated with increased acid secretion and the direct irritant effect of ethanol; immunosuppression, leading to increased incidence of infections such as pneumonia; and increased cancer risk, particularly of the mouth, larynx and oesophagus.

Effects of ethanol

- Ethanol consumption is generally expressed in units of 10 ml (8 g) of pure ethanol. Per capita consumption in Europe is about 10 l/year.
- Ethanol acts as a general central nervous system depressant, similar to volatile anaesthetic agents, producing the familiar effects of acute intoxication.
- Several cellular mechanisms are postulated: inhibition of calcium channel opening, enhancement of GABA action, and inhibitory action at NMDA-type glutamate receptors.
- Effective plasma concentrations:
  — threshold effects: about 40 mg/100 ml (5 mmol/l)
  — severe intoxication: about 150 mg/100 ml
  — death from respiratory failure: about 500 mg/100 ml.
- Main peripheral effects are self-limiting diuresis (reduced antidiuretic hormone secretion), cutaneous vasodilatation, and delayed labour (reduced oxytocin secretion).
- Neurological degeneration occurs in heavy drinkers, causing dementia and peripheral neuropathies.
- Long-term ethanol consumption causes liver disease, progressing to cirrhosis and liver failure.
- Moderate ethanol consumption has a protective effect against ischaemic heart disease.
- Excessive consumption in pregnancy causes impaired fetal development, associated with small size, abnormal facial development and other physical abnormalities, and mental retardation.
- Tolerance, physical dependence and psychological dependence all occur with ethanol.
- Drugs used to treat alcohol dependence include disulfiram (aldehyde dehydrogenase inhibitor), naltrexone (opiate antagonist) and acamprosate (NMDA receptor antagonist).

PHARMACOKINETIC ASPECTS

Metabolism of ethanol

Ethanol is rapidly absorbed, an appreciable amount being absorbed from the stomach. A substantial fraction is cleared by first-pass hepatic metabolism. Hepatic metabolism of ethanol shows saturation kinetics (see Ch. 8) at quite low ethanol concentrations, so the fraction of ethanol removed decreases as the concentration reaching the liver increases. Thus, if ethanol absorption is rapid and portal vein concentration is high, most of the ethanol escapes into the systemic circulation, whereas with slow absorption more is removed by first-pass metabolism. This is one reason why drinking ethanol on an empty stomach produces a much greater pharmacological effect. Ethanol is quickly distributed throughout the body water, the rate of its redistribution depending mainly on the blood flow to individual tissues, as with volatile anaesthetics (see Ch. 36).

Ethanol is about 90% metabolised, 5–10% being excreted unchanged in expired air and in urine. This fraction is not pharmacokinetically significant but provides the basis for estimating blood ethanol concentration from measurements on breath or urine. The ratio of ethanol concentrations in blood and alveolar air, measured at the end of deep expiration, is relatively constant, 80 mg/100 ml of ethanol in blood producing 35 µg/100 ml in expired air, this being the basis of the breathalyser test. The concentration in urine is more variable and provides a less accurate measure of blood concentration.

Ethanol metabolism occurs almost entirely in the liver, and mainly by a pathway involving successive oxidations, first to acetaldehyde and then to acetic acid (Fig. 43.6). Since ethanol is often consumed in large quantities (compared with most drugs), 1–2 moles daily being by no means unusual, it constitutes a substantial load on the hepatic oxidative systems. The oxidation of 2 moles of ethanol consumes about 1.5 kg of the cofactor nicotinamide adenine dinucleotide (NAD⁺). Availability of NAD⁺ limits the rate of ethanol oxidation to about 8 g/hour in a normal adult, independently of ethanol concentration (Fig. 43.7), causing the process to show saturating kinetics (Ch. 8). It also leads to competition between the ethanol and other metabolic substrates for the available NAD⁺ supplies, which may be a factor in ethanol-induced liver damage (see Ch. 53). The intermediate metabolite, acetaldehyde, is a reactive and toxic compound, and this may also contribute to the hepatotoxicity. A small degree of esterification of ethanol with various fatty acids also occurs in the tissues, and these esters may also contribute to long-term toxicity.

Alcohol dehydrogenase is a soluble cytoplasmic enzyme, confined mainly to liver cells, which oxidises ethanol at the same time as reducing NAD⁺ to NADH (Fig. 43.6). Ethanol metabolism causes the ratio of NAD⁺ to NADH to fall, and this has other metabolic consequences (e.g. increased lactate and slowing down of the Krebs cycle). The limitation on ethanol metabolism imposed by the limited rate of NAD⁺ regeneration has led to attempts to find a 'sobering up' agent that works by regenerating NAD⁺ from NADH. One such agent is **fructose**, which is reduced by an NADH-requiring enzyme. In large doses, it causes a measurable increase in the rate of ethanol metabolism, but not enough to have a useful effect on the rate of return to sobriety.

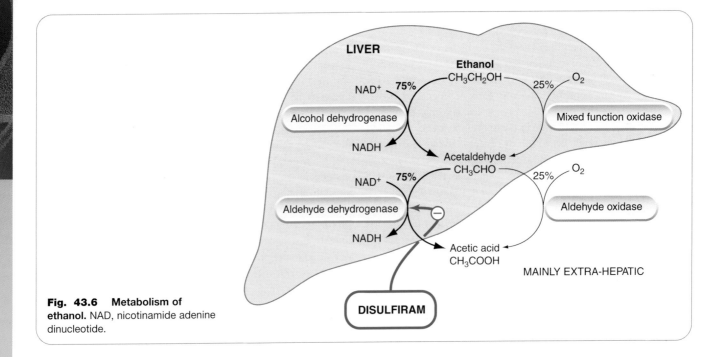

Fig. 43.6 **Metabolism of ethanol.** NAD, nicotinamide adenine dinucleotide.

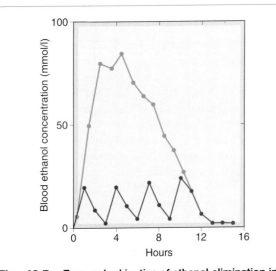

Fig. 43.7 **Zero-order kinetics of ethanol elimination in rats.** Rats were given ethanol orally (104 mmol/kg) either as a single dose or as four divided doses. The single dose results in a much higher and more sustained blood ethanol concentration than the same quantity given as divided doses. Note that, after the single dose, ethanol concentration declines linearly, the rate of decline being similar after a small or large dose, because of the saturation phenomenon. (From Kalant H et al. 1975 Biochem Pharmacol 24: 431.)

Normally, only a small amount of ethanol is metabolised by the microsomal mixed function oxidase system (see Ch. 8), but induction of this system occurs in alcoholics. Ethanol can affect the metabolism of other drugs that are metabolised by the mixed function oxidase system (e.g. **phenobarbitone, warfarin** and **steroids**), with an initial inhibitory effect produced by competition, followed by enhancement due to enzyme induction.

Nearly all the acetaldehyde produced is converted to acetate in the liver by aldehyde dehydrogenase (Fig. 43.6). Normally, only a little acetaldehyde escapes from the liver, giving a blood acetaldehyde concentration of 20–50 μmol/l after an intoxicating dose of ethanol in humans. The circulating acetaldehyde usually has little or no effect, but the concentration may become much larger under certain circumstances and produce toxic effects. This occurs if aldehyde dehydrogenase is inhibited by drugs such as **disulfiram.** In the presence of disulfiram, which produces no marked effect when given alone, ethanol consumption is followed by a severe reaction comprising flushing, tachycardia, hyperventilation, and considerable panic and distress, which is due to excessive acetaldehyde accumulation in the bloodstream. This reaction is extremely unpleasant but not harmful, and disulfiram can be used as aversion therapy to discourage people from taking ethanol. Some other drugs (e.g. **metronidazole**; see Ch. 46) produce similar reactions to ethanol. Interestingly, a Chinese herbal medicine, used traditionally to cure alcoholics, contains **daidzin**, a specific inhibitor of aldehyde dehydrogenase. In hamsters (which spontaneously consume alcohol in amounts that would defeat even the hardest two-legged drinker, while remaining, as far as one can tell in a hamster, completely sober), daidzin markedly inhibits alcohol consumption.

Genetic factors

In 50% of Asian people, an inactive genetic variant of one of the aldehyde dehydrogenase isoforms (ALDH-2) is expressed; these individuals experience a disulfiram-like reaction after alcohol, and the incidence of alcoholism in this group is extremely low (see Tanaka et al., 1997; Tyndale, 2003).

Metabolism and toxicity of methanol

▼ Methanol is metabolised in the same way as ethanol but produces formaldehyde instead of acetaldehyde from the first oxidation step.

Metabolism of ethanol

- Ethanol is metabolised mainly by the liver, first by alcohol dehydrogenase to acetaldehyde, then by aldehyde dehydrogenase to acetate. About 25% of the acetaldehyde is metabolised extrahepatically.
- Small amounts of ethanol are excreted in urine and expired air. Hepatic metabolism shows saturation kinetics, mainly because of limited availability of nicotinamide adenine dinucleotide (NAD^+). Maximal rate of ethanol metabolism is about 10 ml/hour. Thus plasma concentration falls linearly rather than exponentially.
- Acetaldehyde may produce toxic effects. Inhibition of aldehyde dehydrogenase by disulfiram accentuates nausea, etc., caused by acetaldehyde, and can be used in aversion therapy.
- Methanol is similarly metabolised to formic acid, which is toxic, especially to retina.
- Asian people show a high rate of genetic polymorphism of alcohol and aldehyde dehydrogenase, associated with alcoholism and alcohol intolerance, respectively.

Formaldehyde is more reactive than acetaldehyde and reacts rapidly with proteins, causing the inactivation of enzymes involved in the tricarboxylic acid cycle. It is converted to another toxic metabolite, formic acid. This, unlike acetic acid, cannot be utilised in the tricarboxylic acid cycle and is liable to cause tissue damage. Conversion of alcohols to aldehydes occurs not only in the liver but also in the retina, catalysed by the dehydrogenase responsible for retinol–retinal conversion. Formation of formaldehyde in the retina accounts for one of the main toxic effects of methanol, namely blindness, which can occur after ingestion of as little as 10 g. Formic acid production and derangement of the tricarboxylic acid cycle also produce severe acidosis. Methanol is used as an industrial solvent and also to adulterate industrial ethanol in order to make it unfit to drink. Methanol poisoning is quite common, and it is treated by administration of large doses of ethanol, which acts to retard methanol metabolism by competition for alcohol dehydrogenase. This is often done in conjunction with haemodialysis to remove unchanged methanol, which has a small volume of distribution.

TOLERANCE AND DEPENDENCE

Tolerance to the effects of ethanol can be demonstrated in both humans and experimental animals, to the extent of a two- to threefold reduction in potency occurring over 1–3 weeks of continuing ethanol administration. A small component of this is due to the more rapid elimination of ethanol. The major component is tissue tolerance, which accounts for a roughly twofold decrease in potency and which can be observed in vitro (e.g. by measuring the inhibitory effect of ethanol on transmitter release from synaptosomes) as well as in vivo. The mechanism of this tolerance is not known for certain (see Little, 1991). Ethanol tolerance is associated with tolerance to many anaesthetic agents, and alcoholics are often difficult to anaesthetise with drugs such as halothane.

Chronic ethanol administration produces various changes in CNS neurons, which tend to oppose the acute cellular effects that it produces (see above). There is a small reduction in the density of $GABA_A$ receptors, and a proliferation of voltage-gated calcium channels and NMDA receptors. The effect on calcium channels has received particular attention (see Charness et al., 1989). The acute effect of ethanol (see above) is to reduce Ca^{2+} entry through voltage-gated calcium channels, and thus to reduce transmitter release. During chronic exposure to ethanol, Ca^{2+} entry recovers owing to a proliferation of calcium channels, and when ethanol is withdrawn depolarisation-evoked Ca^{2+} entry and transmitter release are increased above normal, which is possibly associated with the physical withdrawal symptoms. Consistent with this explanation, calcium channel–blocking drugs of the dihydropyridine type (see Ch. 19) reduce the effects of ethanol withdrawal in experimental animals (see Little, 1991).

A well-defined physical abstinence syndrome develops in response to ethanol withdrawal. As with most other dependence-producing drugs, this is probably important as a short-term factor in sustaining the drug habit, but other (mainly psychological) factors are more important in the longer term. The physical abstinence syndrome usually subsides in a few days, but the craving for ethanol and the tendency to relapse last for very much longer.

The physical abstinence syndrome in humans, in severe form, develops after about 8 hours. In the first stage, the main symptoms are tremor, nausea, sweating, fever, and sometimes hallucinations. These last for about 24 hours. This phase may be followed by seizures ('rum fits'). Over the next few days, the condition of 'delirium tremens' develops, in which the patient becomes confused, agitated and often aggressive, and may suffer much more severe hallucinations. A similar syndrome of central and autonomic hyperactivity can be produced in experimental animals by ethanol withdrawal.

Alcohol dependence ('alcoholism') is common (4–5% of the population) and, as with smoking, difficult to treat effectively. The main pharmacological approaches (see Zernig et al., 1997; Table 43.2) are the following.

- To alleviate the acute abstinence syndrome during 'drying out', **benzodiazepines** (see Ch. 37) are effective; **clonidine** and **propranolol** are also useful. Clonidine (α_2-adrenoceptor agonist) is believed to act by inhibiting the exaggerated transmitter release that occurs during withdrawal, while propranolol (β-adrenoceptor antagonist) blocks some of the effects of excessive sympathetic activity.
- To render alcohol consumption unpleasant, **disulfiram** (see above).
- To reduce alcohol-induced reward, **naltrexone** (see above) is effective.
- To reduce craving, **acamprosate** is used. This taurine analogue is a weak antagonist at NMDA receptors, and may work by interfering in some way with synaptic plasticity. Several clinical trials have shown it to improve the success rate in achieving alcohol abstinence, with few unwanted effects.

CANNABIS

Extracts of the hemp plant, *Cannabis sativa*, which grows freely in temperate and tropical regions, contain the active substance Δ^9-tetrahydrocannabinol (THC; Fig. 43.8). Marijuana is the name given to the dried leaves and flower heads, prepared as a smoking mixture; hashish is the extracted resin. For centuries, these substances have been used for various medicinal purposes and as intoxicant preparations. Marijuana was brought to North America by immigrants, mainly in the 19th century, and began to be regarded as a social problem in the early years of the 20th century; it was banned during the 1930s. Its use increased dramatically in the 1960s, and recent figures suggest that about 15% of the adult population in America and Western Europe have taken cannabis at some time, with a much higher proportion (close to 50%) among teenagers and young adults. A good scientific account is given by Iversen & Snyder (2000).

CHEMICAL ASPECTS

Cannabis extracts contain numerous related compounds, called cannabinoids, most of which are insoluble in water. The most abundant cannabinoids are THC, its precursor **cannabidiol** and **cannabinol**, which is formed spontaneously from THC. THC is the most active pharmacologically and also the most abundant, constituting roughly 1–10% by weight of marijuana and hashish preparations. A metabolite, 11-hydroxy-THC, is more active than THC itself and probably contributes to the pharmacological effect. Radioimmunoassays have been developed for cannabinoids, but they lack sufficient chemical specificity to be able to distinguish THC from numerous other cannabinoids found in crude extracts, and from the various metabolites that are formed in vivo. Therefore the assay of pharmacologically active THC in biological fluids still presents a problem.

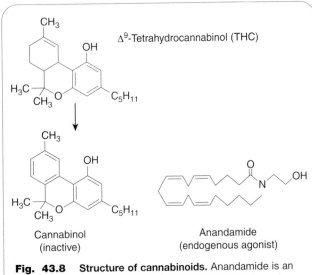

Fig. 43.8 **Structure of cannabinoids.** Anandamide is an arachidonic acid derivative that is present in the brain and believed to be an endogenous agonist for cannabinoid receptors.

PHARMACOLOGICAL EFFECTS

Δ^9-Tetrahydrocannabinol acts on cannabinoid CB_1-receptors (Ch. 15), which are widely distributed in the brain, producing a mixture of psychotomimetic and depressant effects (see Iversen, 2003), together with various centrally mediated peripheral autonomic effects. CB_1-receptors are typical G-protein–coupled receptors (see Ch.3), linked to inhibition of adenylyl cyclase. The receptors are also coupled to potassium channel activation and calcium channel inhibition, and thereby exert an inhibitory effect on transmitter release. These cellular effects closely resemble those of opioids. CB_1-receptors are abundant in the hippocampus (memory impairment), cerebellum and substantia nigra (motor disturbance), and mesolimbic dopamine pathways (reward), as well as in the cortex.

The main subjective effects in humans consist of:

- a feeling of relaxation and well-being, similar to the effect of ethanol but without the accompanying aggression
- a feeling of sharpened sensory awareness, with sounds and sights seeming more intense and fantastic.

These effects are similar to but usually less pronounced than those produced by psychotomimetic drugs such as LSD (see Ch. 42). Subjects report that time passes extremely slowly. The frightening sensations and paranoid delusions that often occur with LSD occur rarely and only after high doses of cannabis.

Central effects that can be directly measured in human and animal studies include:

- impairment of short-term memory and simple learning tasks—subjective feelings of confidence and heightened creativity are not reflected in actual performance
- impairment of motor coordination (e.g. driving performance)
- catalepsy—the retention of fixed unnatural postures, seen with large doses of cannabis in animals
- analgesia
- antiemetic action
- increased appetite.

The main peripheral effects of cannabis are:

- tachycardia, which can be prevented by drugs that block sympathetic transmission
- vasodilatation, which is particularly marked on the scleral and conjunctival vessels, producing a bloodshot appearance characteristic of cannabis smokers
- reduction of intraocular pressure
- bronchodilatation.

A potent CB_1-receptor antagonist, SR141716A, produces effects opposite to those of cannabinoid agonists, namely increased locomotor activity and improved short-term memory, as well as enhanced transmitter release in peripheral tissues, implying a degree of tonic activation of CB_1-receptors under physiological conditions.

The effects of cannabis on intraocular pressure, bronchial smooth muscle, pain perception and the vomiting reflex are of potential therapeutic value, and certain cannabinoid derivatives, for example **nabilone**, have been developed as therapeutic agents. The pronounced central effects produced by these compounds, including their possible addictive properties (see below), limit their usefulness.

As there is little evidence for subtypes of the CB_1-receptor—which might offer the possibility of developing ligands with more selective central effects—therapeutic developments on this front are currently stalled.

A second cannabinoid receptor subtype, CB2, occurs mainly in cells of the immune system, controlling cell migration and cytokine release. Its importance as a factor in the effects of THC and other cannabinoids is not clear.

TOLERANCE AND DEPENDENCE

Tolerance to cannabis, and physical dependence, occur to only a minor degree and mainly in heavy users. The abstinence symptoms are similar to those of ethanol or opiate withdrawal, namely nausea, agitation, irritability, confusion, tachycardia, sweating, etc., but are relatively mild and do not result in a compulsive urge to take the drug. Psychological dependence, accompanied by craving, does, however, occur to some extent with cannabis, although it is insufficient to classify cannabis as truly addictive. Self-administration does not occur in animal models, although the CB_1-receptor antagonist **rimonabant** given after treatment with cannabis for a few days induces a withdrawal syndrome in rats similar to opiate withdrawal.

PHARMACOKINETIC ASPECTS

The effect of cannabis, taken by smoking or by intravenous injection, takes about 1 hour to develop fully and lasts for 2–3 hours. A small fraction is converted to 11-hydroxy-THC, which is more active than THC itself, but most is converted to inactive metabolites. It is partly conjugated and undergoes enterohepatic recirculation. Being highly lipophilic, THC and its metabolites are sequestered in body fat, and excretion continues for several days after a single dose.

ADVERSE EFFECTS

In overdose, THC is relatively safe, producing drowsiness and confusion but not respiratory or cardiovascular effects that threaten life. In this respect, it is safer than most abused substances, particularly opiates and ethanol. Even in low doses, THC and synthetic derivatives such as **nabilone** produce euphoria and drowsiness, sometimes accompanied by sensory distortion and hallucinations. The risk of road accidents is significantly increased by recent use of cannabis.

In rodents, THC produces teratogenic and mutagenic effects, and an increased incidence of chromosome breaks in circulating white cells has been reported in humans. Such breaks are, however, by no means unique to cannabis, and epidemiological studies have not shown any increased risk of fetal malformation or cancer among cannabis users.

Certain endocrine effects occur in humans, notably a decrease in plasma testosterone and a reduction of sperm count. One study showed a reduction of more than 50% in both plasma testosterone and sperm count in subjects smoking 10 or more marijuana cigarettes per week.

Recently, major concern has arisen about the risk of long-term neurological and psychological disturbances resulting from

Cannabis

- Main active constituent is Δ^9-tetrahydrocannabinol (THC), although pharmacologically active metabolites may be important.
- Actions on central nervous system (CNS) include both depressant and psychotomimetic effects.
- Subjectively, subjects experience euphoria and a feeling of relaxation, with sharpened sensory awareness.
- Objective tests show impairment of learning, memory and motor performance.
- THC also shows analgesic and antiemetic activity, as well as causing catalepsy and hypothermia in animal tests.
- Peripheral actions include vasodilatation, reduction of intraocular pressure, and bronchodilatation.
- Cannabinoid receptors belong to the G-protein–coupled receptor family, linked to inhibition of adenylyl cyclase and effects on calcium and potassium channel function, causing inhibition of synaptic transmission. The brain receptor (CB_1) differs from the peripheral receptor (CB_2), which is expressed mainly in cells of the immune system. Selective agonists and antagonists have been developed.
- Anandamide, an arachidonic acid derivative, is an endogenous ligand for the CNS cannabinoid receptor; its function has not yet been ascertained.
- Cannabinoids are less liable than opiates, nicotine or alcohol to cause dependence but may have long-term psychological effects.
- Nabilone, a THC analogue, has been developed for its antiemetic property.
- Although cannabinoids are not available for clinical use, trials are in progress for symptomatic treatment of multiple sclerosis and AIDS.

cannabis use. Epidemiological studies have suggested an association between heavy cannabis use and poor cognitive function (see Kalant, 2004), but this does not necessarily imply causation, and there is little direct evidence that cannabis can cause neurodegeneration or irreversible cognitive impairment (see Iversen, 2005). The possibility that cannabis can cause psychotic illness has received much attention following reports that cannabis smoking during adolescence increased the likelihood of schizophrenia more than sixfold (see Arsenault et al., 2004). The issue is highly controversial, but it is generally believed that cannabis use during adolescence can cause psychosis to become manifest in 'prepsychotic' individuals earlier than it otherwise would, and that it can make the symptoms worse. It has been estimated that elimination of cannabis use in under-15s would reduce the incidence of schizophrenia by 8% (see Arsenault et al., 2004). Whether cannabis can induce psychosis in individuals who would not otherwise have become ill remains unclear.

The long-running argument over the legalisation of cannabis centres mainly on the seriousness of these adverse effects. Opponents of legalisation argue that it would be folly to change the law in favour of the use by the public at large of a substance that could turn out to have serious toxic effects. Proponents of a change argue that the present law is clearly ineffective and encourages crime, and that cannabis undoubtedly carries less health risk than either ethanol or tobacco.

CLINICAL USE OF CANNABIS: A CONTROVERSIAL TOPIC

Anecdotal evidence suggests that smoking cannabis may be efficacious in a number of conditions, particularly the following: relief of pain and muscle spasms associated with multiple sclerosis; relief of other types of chronic neuropathic pain, including AIDS-related pain; improvement of appetite and prevention of wasting in AIDS; and relief of chemotherapy-induced nausea. Currently, cannabis products cannot be prescribed for medical use in most countries.[7] There is strong pressure from patient groups to press ahead with licensing THC for clinical use, and clinical trials are in progress in a number of indications. The results so far have been equivocal, and neither THC nor synthetic cannabinoids have been approved for clinical use in Europe or the USA. Cannabis appears to have a significant but limited effect in reducing spasticity and pain associated with multiple sclerosis, without producing major adverse effects, and similar results have been reported in other neuropathic pain states (see Iversen, 2005). Trials are also underway in other conditions, including head injury, Tourette's syndrome and anorexia. Whether cannabinoids will prove to be a therapeutic panacea or a flop remains unclear, and passions are high on both sides of the argument.

---

[7]Dronabinol (purified THC, as distinct from the plant extract, which contains other active substances) is approved in the USA for treating chemotherapy-induced vomiting and to stimulate appetite in AIDS patients.

REFERENCES AND FURTHER READING

General

Bunce C J, Loudon P T, Akers C et al. 2003 Development of vaccines to help treat drug dependence. Curr Opin Mol Ther 5: 58–63

Chao J, Nestler E J 2004 Molecular neurobiology of addiction. Annu Rev Med 55: 113–132 (*Useful review article by leading scientists in addiction research*)

Deroche-Gamonet V, Belin D, Piazza P V 2004 Evidence for addiction-like behaviour in the rat. Science 305: 1014–1017 (*See also commentary by Robinson, ibid. 951–953,* Experimental strategy for distinguishing between self-administration and addiction-like behaviour in rats)

Friedman L, Fleming N F, Roberts D H, Hyman S E 1996 Source book of substance abuse and addiction. Williams & Wilkins, Baltimore (*Useful source of factual information*)

Hack S P, Christie M J 2003 Adaptations in adenosine signalling in drug dependence: therapeutic implications. Crit Rev Neurobiol 15: 235–274

Heidbreder C A, Hagan J J 2005 Novel pharmacological approaches for the treatment of drug addiction and craving. Curr Opin Pharmacol 5: 107–118 (*Describes the numerous theoretical strategies, based mainly on monoamine pharmacology, for treating addiction*)

Hyman S E, Malenka R C 2001 Addiction and the brain: the neurobiology of compulsion and its persistence. Nat Rev Neurosci 2: 695–705 (*Reviews long-term changes in the brain associated with addiction, emphasising semipermanent alterations in gene expression*)

Karch S B (ed) 1997 Drug abuse handbook. CRC Press, Boca Raton

Koob G F 1996 Drug addiction: the yin and yang of hedonic homeostasis. Neuron 16: 893–896

Maldonado R, Saiardi A, Valverde O et al. 1997 Absence of opiate rewarding effects in mice lacking dopamine D$_2$ receptors. Nature 388: 586–589 (*Use of transgenic animals to demonstrate role of dopamine receptors in reward properties of opiates*)

Mayer P, Höllt V 2005 Genetic disposition to addictive disorders—current knowledge and future perspectives. Curr Opin Pharmacol 5: 4–8 (*Describes the current inconclusive understanding of the genetic basis of addiction*)

Nestler E J 2001 Molecular basis of long-term plasticity underlying addiction. Nat Rev Neurosci 2: 119–128 (*Good review article focusing on long-term changes in gene expression associated with drug dependence*)

Nestler E J 2004 Molecular mechanisms of drug addiction. Neuropharmacology 47(suppl 1): 24–32

O'Brien C P 1997 A range of research-based pharmacotherapies for addiction. Science 278: 66–70 (*Useful overview of pharmacological approaches to treatment*)

Spanagel R, Weiss F 1999 The dopamine hypothesis of reward: past and current research. Trends Neurosci 22: 521–527 (*Summarises evidence for activation of mesolimbic dopamine pathways as a factor in drug dependence*)

Weiss F 2005 Neurobiology of craving, conditioned reward and relapse. Curr Opin Pharmacol 5: 9–19 (*Review of recent studies on the neurobiology of addiction, focusing mainly on animal models*)

Winger G, Woods J H, Hofmann F G 2004 A handbook on drug and alcohol abuse, 4th edn. Oxford University Press, New York (*Short and informative textbook on biomedical aspects*)

Nicotine

Balfour D J K, Fagerstrom K O 1996 Pharmacology of nicotine and its therapeutic use in smoking cessation and neurodegenerative disorders. Pharmacol Ther 72: 51–81 (*Review of the pharmacology of nicotine and its usefulness as replacement therapy*)

Benowitz N L 1993 Nicotine replacement therapy. Drugs 45: 157–170

Benowitz N L 1996 Pharmacology of nicotine: addiction and therapeutics. Annu Rev Pharmacol 36: 597–613 (*General review article including information on potential therapeutic uses of nicotine other than reduction of smoking*)

George T P, O'Malley S S 2004 Current pharmacological treatments for nicotine dependence. Trends Pharmacol Sci 25: 42–48

Peto R, Chen Z-M, Boreham J 1999 Tobacco—the growing epidemic. Nat Med 3: 15–17

Peto R, Lopez A D, Boreham J et al. 1996 Mortality from smoking worldwide. Br Med Bull 52: 12–21

Wonnacott S, Sidhpura N, Balfour D J K 2005 Nicotine: from molecular mechanisms to behaviour. Curr Opin Pharmacol 5: 53–59 (*Useful review on the acute and long-term CNS effects of nicotine*)

Ethanol

Charness M E, Simon R P, Greenberg D A 1989 Ethanol and the nervous system. N Engl J Med 321: 442–454

Groenbaek M et al. 1994 Influence of sex, age, body mass index and smoking on alcohol intake and mortality. Br Med J 308: 302–306 (*Large-scale Danish study showing reduced coronary mortality at moderate levels of drinking, with increase at high levels*)

Harper C, Matsumoto I 2005 Ethanol and brain damage. Curr Opin Pharmacol 5: 73–78 (*Describes deleterious effects of long-term alcohol abuse on brain function*)

Keung W-M, Vallee B L 1993 Daidzin and daidzein suppress free-choice ethanol intake by Syrian golden hamsters. Proc Natl Acad Sci USA 90: 10008–10012

Lieber C S 1995 Medical disorders of alcoholism. N Engl J Med 333: 1058–1065 (*Review focusing on ethanol-induced liver damage in relation to ethanol metabolism*)

Little H J 1991 Mechanisms that may underlie the behavioural effects of ethanol. Prog Neurobiol 36: 171–194

Lovinger D M 1997 Alcohols and neurotransmitters-gated ion channels: past present and future. Naunyn-Schmiedebergs Arch Pharmacol 356: 267–282 (*Review article arguing that alcohol effects depend on interaction with synaptic ion channels*)

Melendez R I, Kalivas P W 2004 Last call for adenosine transporters. Nat Neurosci 7: 795–796 (*Commentary on a study supporting a role for adenosine in the CNS effects of ethanol*)

Tabakoff B, Hoffman P L 1996 Alcohol addiction: an enigma among us. Neuron 16: 909–912 (*Review of alcohol actions at the cellular and molecular level—ignore the silly title*)

Tanaka F, Shiratori Y, Yokusuka O et al. 1997 Polymorphism of alcohol-metabolizing genes affects drinking behaviour and alcoholic liver disease in Japanese men. Alcohol Clin Exp Res 21: 596–601 (*Describes polymorphism of aldehyde and alcohol dehydrogenases, and their effect on drinking behaviour*)

Tyndale R F 2003 Genetics of alcohol and tobacco use in humans. Ann Med 35: 94–121 (*Detailed review of the many genetic factors implicated in alcohol and nicotine consumption habits*)

Zernig G, Fabisch K, Fabisch H 1997 Pharmacotherapy of alcohol dependence. Trends Pharmacol Sci 18: 229–231 (*Short review of drug therapies used in alcoholism*)

Cannabis

Arsenault L, Cannon M, Whitton J, Murray R M 2004 Causal association between cannabis and psychosis: examination of the evidence. Br J Psychiatry 184: 110–117 (*Summarises evidence relating to cannabis as a possible cause of schizophrenia*)

Dewey W L 1986 Cannabinoid pharmacology. Pharmacol Rev 38: 151–178

Iversen L L 2003 Cannabis and the brain. Brain 126: 1252–1270 (*Useful review on neuropharmacology of cannabis and assessment of risk to humans*)

Iversen L L 2005 Long-term effects of exposure to cannabis. Curr Opin Pharmacol 5: 69–72 (*Review suggesting that the dangers of cannabis have been overstated*)

Iversen L L, Snyder S H 2000 The science of marijuana. Oxford University Press, New York (*Short textbook presenting all aspects of cannabis*)

Kalant H 2004 Adverse effects of cannabis on health: an update of the literature since 1996. Prog Neuropsychopharmacol Biol Psychiatry 28: 849–863

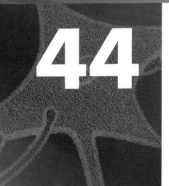

44

Local anaesthetics and other drugs affecting sodium channels

OVERVIEW

As described in Chapter 4, the property of electrical excitability is what enables the membranes of nerve and muscle cells to generate propagated action potentials, which are essential for communication in the nervous system and for the initiation of mechanical activity in striated and cardiac muscle. Electrical excitability depends mainly on voltage-gated sodium channels, which open transiently when the membrane is depolarised. Also important are the voltage-dependent potassium channels and calcium channels, which function similarly, although they serve quite different physiological functions and are affected by different classes of drugs (Chs 4, 18 and 19). Here we discuss local anaesthetics, which act mainly by blocking sodium channels, and mention briefly other drugs that affect sodium channel function.

There are, broadly speaking, two ways in which channel function may be modified, namely block of the channels and modification of gating behaviour. Either mechanism can cause an increase or a decrease of electrical excitability. Thus blocking sodium channels reduces excitability, whereas block of potassium channels tends to increase it. Similarly, an agent that affects sodium channel gating so as to increase channel opening will tend to increase excitability, and vice versa.

LOCAL ANAESTHETICS

Although many drugs block voltage-sensitive sodium channels and inhibit the generation of the action potential, the only drugs in this category that are clinically useful are the local anaesthetics, various antiepileptic drugs (see Ch. 40) and class I antidysrhythmic drugs (see Ch. 18).

History

Coca leaves have been chewed for their psychotropic effects for thousands of years (see Ch. 42) by South American Indians, who knew about the numbing effect they produced on the mouth and tongue. Cocaine was isolated in 1860 and proposed as a local anaesthetic for surgical procedures. Sigmund Freud, who tried unsuccessfully to make use of its 'psychic energising' power, gave some cocaine to his ophthalmologist friend in Vienna, Carl Köller, who reported in 1884 that reversible corneal anaesthesia could be produced by dropping cocaine into the eye. The idea was rapidly taken up, and within a few years cocaine anaesthesia was introduced into dentistry and general surgery. A synthetic substitute, **procaine**, was discovered in 1905, and many other useful compounds were later developed.

Chemical aspects

Local anaesthetic molecules consist of an aromatic part linked by an ester or amide bond to a basic side-chain (Fig. 44.1). They are weak bases, with pK_a values mainly in the range 8–9, so that they are mainly, but not completely, ionised at physiological pH. This is important in relation to their ability to penetrate the nerve sheath and axon membrane; quaternary derivatives, which are fully ionised irrespective of pH, are ineffective as local anaesthetics. **Benzocaine,** an atypical local anaesthetic, has no basic group.

The presence of the ester or amide bond in local anaesthetic molecules is important because of its susceptibility to metabolic hydrolysis. The ester-containing compounds are usually inactivated in the plasma and tissues (mainly liver) by non-specific esterases. Amides are more stable, and these anaesthetics generally have longer plasma half-lives.

Mechanism of action

Local anaesthetics block the initiation and propagation of action potentials by preventing the voltage-dependent increase in Na^+ conductance (see Fig. 4.5). Although they exert a variety of non-specific effects on membrane function, their main action is to block sodium channels, which they do by physically plugging the transmembrane pore, interacting with residues of the S6 transmembrane helical domain of the channel protein (see Strichartz & Ritchie, 1987; Ragsdale et al., 1994; Hille, 2001).

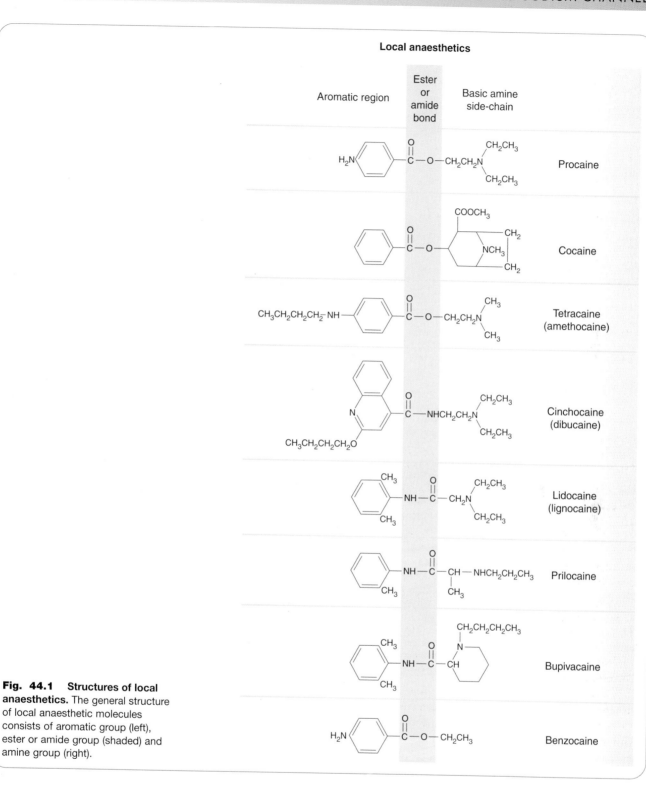

Fig. 44.1 Structures of local anaesthetics. The general structure of local anaesthetic molecules consists of aromatic group (left), ester or amide group (shaded) and amine group (right).

▼ Local anaesthetic activity is strongly pH-dependent, being increased at alkaline pH (i.e. when the proportion of ionised molecules is low) and reduced at acid pH. This is because the compound needs to penetrate the nerve sheath and the axon membrane to reach the inner end of the sodium channel (where the local anaesthetic–binding site resides). Because the ionised form is not membrane-permeant, penetration is very poor at acid pH. Once inside the axon, it is the ionised form of the local anaesthetic molecule that binds to the channel (Fig. 44.2). This pH dependence can be clinically important, because inflamed tissues are often acidic and thus somewhat resistant to local anaesthetic agents.

Further analysis of local anaesthetic action (see Strichartz & Ritchie, 1987) has shown that many drugs exhibit the property of 'use-dependent' block of sodium channels, as well as affecting, to some extent, the gating of the channels. Use-dependence means that the more the channels are opened, the greater the block becomes. It is a prominent feature of the action of many class I antidysrhythmic drugs (Ch. 18) and antiepileptic drugs (Ch. 40), and occurs because the blocking molecule enters the channel much more readily when the channel is open than when it is closed. With quaternary local anaesthetics working from the inside of the membrane, the channels must be cycled through their open state a few

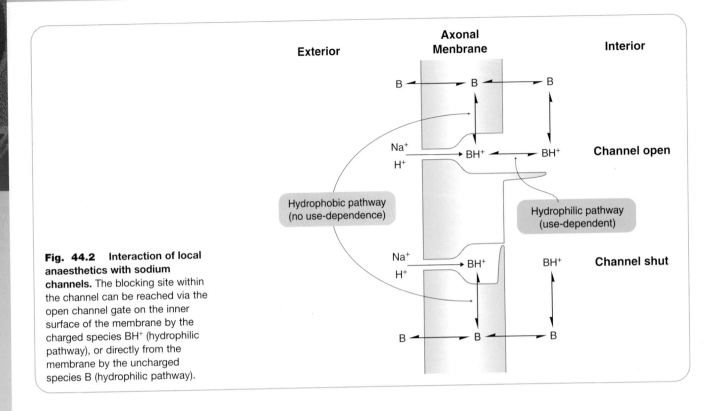

Fig. 44.2 **Interaction of local anaesthetics with sodium channels.** The blocking site within the channel can be reached via the open channel gate on the inner surface of the membrane by the charged species BH⁺ (hydrophilic pathway), or directly from the membrane by the uncharged species B (hydrophilic pathway).

times before the blocking effect appears. With tertiary local anaesthetics, on the other hand, block can develop even if the channels are not open, and it is likely that the blocking molecule (uncharged) can reach the channel either directly from the membrane phase or via the open gate (Fig. 44.2). The relative importance of these two blocking pathways—the hydrophobic pathway via the membrane, and the hydrophilic pathway via the inner mouth of the channel—varies according to the lipid solubility of the drug, and the degree of use-dependence varies correspondingly.

As discussed in Chapter 4, the channel can exist in three functional states: resting, open and inactivated. Many local anaesthetics bind most strongly to the inactivated state of the channel. Therefore, at any given membrane potential, the equilibrium between resting and inactivated channels will, in the presence of a local anaesthetic, be shifted in favour of the inactivated state, and this factor contributes to the overall blocking effect. The passage of a train of action potentials causes the channels to cycle through the open and inactivated states, both of which are more likely to bind local anaesthetic molecules than the resting state; thus both mechanisms contribute to use-dependence.

In general, local anaesthetics block conduction in small-diameter nerve fibres more readily than in large fibres. Because nociceptive impulses are carried by Aδ and C fibres (Ch. 41), pain sensation is blocked more readily than other sensory modalities (touch, proprioception, etc.). Motor axons, being large in diameter, are also relatively resistant. The differences in sensitivity among different nerve fibres, although easily measured experimentally, are not of much practical importance, and it is not possible to produce a block of pain sensation without affecting other sensory modalities.

Local anaesthetics, as their name implies, are mainly used to produce local nerve block. In concentrations too low to cause nerve block, however, they are able to suppress the spontaneous discharge in sensory neurons that is believed to be responsible for neuropathic pain (see Ch. 41). **Lidocaine (lignocaine; see below)**

can be used intravenously to control neuropathic pain, and some antidysrhythmic drugs (e.g. **mexiletine, tocainide, flecainide;** see Ch. 18) can be used orally (see Lai et al., 2004), although not licensed for this indication.

Action of local anaesthetics

- Local anaesthetics block action potential generation by blocking sodium channels.
- Local anaesthetics are amphiphilic molecules with a hydrophobic aromatic group and a basic amine group.
- Local anaesthetics probably act in their cationic form but must reach their site of action by penetrating the nerve sheath and axonal membrane as unionised species; they therefore have to be weak bases.
- Many local anaesthetics show use-dependence (depth of block increases with action potential frequency). This arises:
  - because anaesthetic molecules gain access to the channel more readily when the channel is open
  - because anaesthetic molecules have higher affinity for inactivated than for resting channels.
- Use-dependence is mainly of importance in relation to antidysrhythmic and antiepileptic effects of sodium channel blockers.
- Local anaesthetics block conduction in the following order: small myelinated axons, non-myelinated axons, large myelinated axons. Nociceptive and sympathetic transmission is thus blocked first.

The properties of individual local anaesthetic drugs are summarised in Table 44.1.

Unwanted effects

The main unwanted effects of local anaesthetics involve the central nervous system (CNS) and the cardiovascular system, and they constitute the main source of hazard when local anaesthetics are used clinically. Most local anaesthetics produce a mixture of depressant and stimulant effects on the CNS. Depressant effects predominate at low plasma concentrations, giving way to stimulation at higher concentrations, resulting in restlessness, tremor and sometimes convulsions, accompanied by subjective effects ranging from confusion to extreme agitation. Further increasing the dose produces profound CNS depression. The main threat to life comes from respiratory depression in this phase. The only local anaesthetic with markedly different CNS effects is **cocaine** (see Ch. 42), which produces euphoria at doses well below those that cause other CNS effects. This relates to its specific effect on monoamine uptake (see Ch. 42), an effect not shared by other local anaesthetics. **Procaine** is particularly liable to produce unwanted central effects, and has been superseded in clinical use by agents such as **lidocaine (lignocaine)** and **prilocaine,** whose central effects are much less pronounced. Studies with **bupivacaine** (Table 44.1), a widely used long-acting local anaesthetic prepared as a racemic mixture of two optical isomers, suggested that its CNS and cardiac effects were mainly due to the $S(+)$ isomer. The $R(-)$ isomer (**levobupivacaine**) proved to have a better margin of safety and has now been introduced.

The adverse cardiovascular effects of local anaesthetics are due mainly to myocardial depression, conduction block and vasodilatation. Reduction of myocardial contractility probably results indirectly from an inhibition of the Na^+ current in cardiac muscle (see Ch. 18). The resulting decrease of $[Na^+]_i$ in turn reduces intracellular Ca^{2+} stores (see Ch. 4), and this reduces the force

---

Table 44.1   **Properties of local anaesthetics**

Drug	Onset	Duration	Tissue penetration	Plasma half-life (h)	Main unwanted effects	Notes
Cocaine	Medium	Medium	Good	~1	Cardiovascular and CNS effects owing to block of amine uptake	Rarely used, only as spray for upper respiratory tract
Procaine	Medium	Short	Poor	< 1	CNS: restlessness, shivering, anxiety, occasionally convulsions followed by respiratory depression. Cardiovascular system: bradycardia and decreased cardiac output; vasodilatation, which can cause cardiovascular collapse	The first synthetic agent. No longer used
Lidocaine (lignocaine)	Rapid	Medium	Good	~2	As procaine but less tendency to cause CNS effects	Widely used for local anaesthesia. Also used intravenously for treating ventricular dysrhythmias (Ch. 18). Mepivacaine is similar
Tetracaine (amethocaine)	Rapid	Medium	Moderate	~1	As lidocaine	Used mainly for spinal and corneal anaesthesia
Bupivacaine	Slow	Long	Moderate	~2	As lidocaine but greater cardiotoxicity	Widely used because of long duration of action. Ropivacaine is similar, with less cardiotoxicity. Levobupivacaine, recently introduced, causes less cardiotoxicity and CNS depression than the racemate, bupivacaine
Prilocaine	Medium	Medium	Moderate	~2	No vasodilator activity. Can cause methaemoglobinaemia	Widely used; not for obstetric analgesia because of risk of neonatal methaemoglobinaemia

CNS, central nervous system.

of contraction. Interference with atrioventricular conduction can result in partial or complete heart block, as well as other types of dysrhythmia.

Vasodilatation, mainly affecting arterioles, is due partly to a direct effect on vascular smooth muscle, and partly to inhibition of the sympathetic nervous system. The combined myocardial depression and vasodilatation leads to a fall in blood pressure, which may be sudden and life-threatening. Cocaine is an exception in respect of its cardiovascular effects, because of its ability to inhibit noradrenaline reuptake (see Ch. 11). This enhances sympathetic activity, leading to tachycardia, increased cardiac output, vasoconstriction and increased arterial pressure.

Although local anaesthetics are usually administered in such a way as to minimise their spread to other parts of the body, they are ultimately absorbed into the systemic circulation. They may also be injected into veins or arteries by accident. The most dangerous unwanted effects result from actions on the central nervous and cardiovascular systems discussed above, namely restlessness and convulsions followed by respiratory depression, and hypotension, or even cardiac arrest. Hypersensitivity reactions sometimes occur with local anaesthetics, usually in the form of allergic dermatitis but rarely as an acute anaphylactic reaction. Other unwanted effects that are specific to particular drugs include mucosal irritation (cocaine) and methaemoglobinaemia (which occurs after large doses of **prilocaine,** because of the production of a toxic metabolite).

Pharmacokinetic aspects

Local anaesthetics vary a good deal in the rapidity with which they penetrate tissues, and this affects the rate at which they cause nerve block when injected into tissues, and the rate of onset of, and recovery from, anaesthesia (Table 44.1). It also affects their usefulness as surface anaesthetics for application to mucous membranes.

Most of the ester-linked local anaesthetics (e.g. **tetracaine**) are hydrolysed by plasma cholinesterase, so their plasma half-life is relatively short. **Procaine**—now rarely used—is hydrolysed to *p*-aminobenzoic acid, a folate precursor that interferes with the antibacterial effect of sulfonamides (see Ch. 46). The amide-linked drugs (e.g. **lidocaine [lignocaine]** and **prilocaine**) are metabolised mainly in the liver, usually by *N*-dealkylation rather than cleavage of the amide bond, and the metabolites are often pharmacologically active.

Benzocaine is an unusual local anaesthetic of very low solubility, which is used as a dry powder to dress painful skin ulcers, or as throat lozenges. The drug is slowly released and produces long-lasting surface anaesthesia.

The routes of administration, uses and main adverse effects of local anaesthetics are summarised in Table 44.2.

Most local anaesthetics have a direct vasodilator action, which increases the rate at which they are absorbed into the systemic circulation, thus increasing their potential toxicity and reducing their local anaesthetic action. Adrenaline (epinephrine) is often added to local anaesthetic solutions injected locally in order to cause vasoconstriction, although care is needed to avoid adrenaline-induced cardiovascular changes.

Future directions

Blocking specific sodium channel subtypes is seen as a promising therapeutic strategy for a variety of clinical conditions, including epilepsy, neurodegenerative diseases, stroke, neuropathic pain and myopathies.

Currently available local anaesthetic agents do not distinguish between different sodium channel subtypes (see Lai et al., 2004), and consequently produce a variety of unwanted effects when given systemically. It is expected that, with a better understanding of the role of specific sodium channel subtypes in different pathophysiological situations, it may be possible to develop selective blocking agents for use in different clinical situations. There is much activity in this area, but progress is slow, as it is proving difficult to identify blocking agents that are highly selective for different sodium channel subtypes.

Most local anaesthetics act for 2–3 hours when injected locally, which is often insufficient for pain relief. To increase the duration of action, special formulations consisting of local anaesthetics encapsulated in lipid vesicles (liposomes) are being developed as slow-release preparations.

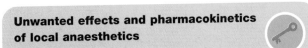

Unwanted effects and pharmacokinetics of local anaesthetics

- Local anaesthetics are either esters or amides. Esters are rapidly hydrolysed by plasma cholinesterase, and amides are metabolised in the liver. Plasma half-lives are generally short, about 1–2 hours.
- Unwanted effects are due mainly to escape of local anaesthetics into systemic circulation.
- Main unwanted effects are:
  — central nervous system effects, agitation, confusion, tremors progressing to convulsions and respiratory depression
  — cardiovascular effects, namely myocardial depression and vasodilatation, leading to fall in blood pressure
  — occasional hypersensitivity reactions.
- Local anaesthetics vary in the rapidity with which they penetrate tissues, and in their duration of action. Lidocaine (lignocaine) penetrates tissues readily and is suitable for surface application; bupivacaine has a particularly long duration of action.

OTHER DRUGS THAT AFFECT SODIUM CHANNELS

TETRODOTOXIN AND SAXITOXIN

▼ We should not be surprised that nature, rather than medicinal chemistry, has provided the most potent and selective agents that block sodium channels of excitable tissues. Tetrodotoxin (TTX) is produced by a marine bacterium and accumulates in the tissues of a poisonous Pacific fish, the puffer fish, so called because when alarmed it inflates itself to an almost spherical spiny ball. It is evidently a species highly preoccupied with defence, but the Japanese are not easily put off and the puffer fish is

Table 44.2 Methods of administration, uses and adverse effects of local anesthetics

Method	Uses	Drug(s)	Notes and adverse effects
Surface anaesthesia	Nose, mouth, bronchial tree (usually in spray form), cornea, urinary tract Not effective for skin[a]	Lidocaine, tetracaine, (amethocaine), dibucaine, benzocaine	Risk of systemic toxicity when high concentrations and large areas are involved
Infiltration anaesthesia	Direct injection into tissues to reach nerve branches and terminals Used in minor surgery	Most	Adrenaline or felypressin often added as vasoconstrictors (not with fingers or toes, for fear of causing ischaemic tissue damage) Suitable for only small areas, otherwise serious risk of systemic toxicity
Intravenous regional anaesthesia	LA injected intravenously distal to a pressure cuff to arrest blood flow; remains effective until the circulation is restored Used for limb surgery	Mainly lidocaine, prilocaine	Risk of systemic toxicity when cuff is released prematurely; risk is small if cuff remains inflated for at least 20 minutes
Nerve block anaesthesia	LA is injected close to nerve trunks (e.g. brachial plexus, intercostal or dental nerves) to produce a loss of sensation peripherally Used for surgery, dentistry, analgesia	Most	Less LA needed than for infiltration anaesthesia Accurate placement of the needle is important Onset of anaesthesia may be slow Duration of anaesthesia may be increased by addition of vasoconstrictor
Spinal anaesthesia	LA injected into the subarachnoid space (containing cerebrospinal fluid) to act on spinal roots and spinal cord Glucose sometimes added so that spread of LA can be limited by tilting patient Used for surgery to abdomen, pelvis or leg, mainly when general anesthesia cannot be used	Mainly lidocaine	Main risks are bradycardia and hypotension (owing to sympathetic block), respiratory depression (owing to effects on phrenic nerve or respiratory center); avoided by minimising cranial spread Postoperative urinary retention (block of pelvic autonomic outflow) is common
Epidural anaesthesia[b]	LA injected into epidural space, blocking spinal roots Uses as for spinal anesthesia; also for painless childbirth	Mainly lidocaine, bupivacaine	Unwanted effects similar to those of spinal anaesthesia but less probable, because longitudinal spread of LA is reduced Postoperative urinary retention common

LA, local anaesthetic.
[a]Surface anaesthesia does not work well on the skin, although a non-crystalline mixture of lidocaine and prilocaine (eutectic mixture of local anaesthetics or EMLA) has been developed for application to the skin, producing complete anaesthesia in about 1 hour.
[b]Intrathecal or epidural administration of LA in combination with an opiate (see Ch. 41) produces more effective analgesia than can be achieved with the opiate alone. Only a small concentration of LA is needed, insufficient to produce appreciable loss of sensation or other side effects. The mechanism of this synergism is unknown, but the procedure is proving useful in pain treatment.

regarded by them as a special delicacy partly because of the mild tingling sensation that follows eating its flesh. To serve it in public restaurants, however, the chef must be registered as sufficiently skilled in removing the toxic organs (especially liver and ovaries) so as to make the flesh safe to eat. (The alternative strategy, of farming puffer fish so that they do not accumulate the toxin and then adding a safe dose of TTX—obtained, say, from Sigma—sufficient to provide the tingling sensation, has never caught on, whether for cultural or gastronomic reasons one can only guess.)

Accidental TTX poisoning is quite common, nonetheless. Historical records of long sea voyages often contained reference to attacks of severe weakness, progressing to complete paralysis and death, caused by eating puffer fish.

Saxitoxin (STX) is produced by a marine micro-organism that sometimes proliferates in very large numbers and even colours the sea, giving the 'red tide' phenomenon. At such times, marine shellfish can accumulate the toxin and become poisonous to humans.

These toxins, unlike conventional local anaesthetics, act exclusively from the outside of the membrane. Both are complex molecules, bearing a positively charged guanidinium moiety. The guanidinium ion is able to permeate voltage-sensitive sodium channels, and this part of the TTX or STX molecule lodges in the channel, while the rest of the molecule blocks its outer mouth. In contrast to the local anaesthetics, there is no interaction between the gating and blocking reactions with TTX or STX—their association and dissociation are independent of whether the channel is open or closed. Some voltage-sensitive sodium channels are insensitive to TTX, notably those of cardiac muscle and nociceptive peripheral sensory neurons, the latter being of interest as a possible target for novel analgesic agents (see Ch. 41).

Both TTX and STX are unsuitable for clinical use as local anaesthetics, being expensive to obtain from their exotic sources and poor at penetrating tissues because of their very low lipid solubility. They have, however, been important as experimental tools for the isolation and cloning of sodium channels (see Ch. 4).

AGENTS THAT AFFECT SODIUM CHANNEL GATING

▼ Various substances, mostly complex and ornate molecules, are known that modify sodium channel gating in such a way as to increase the probability of opening of the channels (see Hille, 2001). They include various toxins, mainly from frog skin (e.g. **batrachotoxin**), scorpion or sea anemone venoms; plant alkaloids such as **veratridine**; and insecticides such as **DDT** and the **pyrethrins**. They facilitate sodium channel activation so that sodium channels open at the normal resting potential; they also inhibit inactivation, so that the channels fail to close if the membrane remains depolarised. The membrane thus becomes hyperexcitable, and the action potential is prolonged. Spontaneous discharges occur at first, but the cells eventually become permanently depolarised and inexcitable. All these substances affect the heart, producing extrasystoles and other dysrhythmias, culminating in fibrillation; they also cause spontaneous discharges in nerve and muscle, leading to twitching and convulsions. The very high lipid solubility of substances like DDT makes them effective as insecticides, for they are readily absorbed through the integument. Drugs in this class are useful as experimental tools for studying sodium channels but have no clinical uses.

Clinical use of local anaesthetics

- Local anaesthetics may be infiltrated into soft tissue (e.g. of gums) or to block a nerve or nerve plexus.
- Coadministration of a vasoconstrictor (e.g. **adrenaline**) prolongs the local effect.
- Lipid-soluble drugs (e.g. **lidocaine [lignocaine]**) are absorbed from mucous membranes and are used as surface anaesthetics.
- **Bupivacaine** has a slow onset but long duration. It is often used for epidural blockade (e.g. to provide continuous epidural blockade during labour) and spinal anaesthesia. Its isomer **levobupivacaine** is less cardiotoxic if it is inadvertently administered into a blood vessel.

REFERENCES AND FURTHER READING

Hille B 2001 Ionic channels of excitable membranes. Sinauer, Sunderland (*Excellent, clearly written textbook for those wanting more than the basic minimum*)

Lai J, Porreca F, Hunter J C, Gold M S 2004 Voltage-gated sodium channels and hyperalgesia. Annu Rev Pharmacol 44: 371–397 (*Review summarising the role of particular sodium channel subtypes in the pathogenesis of pain, and the use of local anaesthetic and antidysrhythmic drugs in controlling neuropathic pain*)

Ragsdale D R, McPhee J C, Scheuer T, Catterall W A 1994 Molecular determinants of state-dependent block of Na⁺ channels by local anesthetics. Science 265: 1724–1728 (*Use of site-directed mutations of the sodium channel to show that local anaesthetics bind to residues in the S6 transmembrane domain*)

Strichartz G R, Ritchie J M 1987 The action of local anaesthetics on ion channels of excitable tissues. Handb Exp Pharmacol 81: 21–52 (*Excellent review of actions of local anaesthetics—other articles in the same volume cover more clinical aspects*)

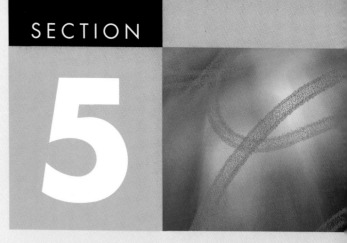

DRUGS USED IN THE TREATMENT OF INFECTIONS AND CANCER

Drugs used in the treatment of infections and cancer

45

OVERVIEW

Chemotherapy is the term originally used to describe the use of drugs that are 'selectively toxic' to invading micro-organisms while having minimal effects on the host. The term also embraces the use of drugs that target tumours and in fact has now come to be associated specifically with that branch of pharmacology. In this chapter, we use the term to cover both usages, although, in the public mind at least, chemotherapy is specifically associated with those types of anticancer drugs that cause side effects such as loss of hair, nausea and vomiting.

All living organisms are prey to infection. Humans, being no exception to this rule, are susceptible to diseases caused by viruses, bacteria, protozoa, fungi and helminths. The use of chemotherapeutic agents dates back to the work of Ehrlich and others and to the development of arsenical drugs such as *salvarsan* for the treatment of syphilis.[1] The successful development of such agents during the past 80 years, particularly the 'antibiotic revolution', constitutes one of the most important therapeutic advances in the entire history of medicine.

Clearly, the feasibility of selective toxicity depends on the ability to exploit such biochemical differences as may exist between the infecting organism (or indeed cancer cells, our internal 'invaders') and the host. The bulk of the chapters in this section of the book describe the drugs used to combat infections, but in this introductory chapter we consider, very broadly, the nature of these biochemical differences and outline the molecular targets of drug action.

Unhappily, our success in developing drugs to attack these invaders has been paralleled by their own success in counteracting the effects of the drugs, resulting in the emergence of drug resistance. And at present, the invaders—particularly some bacteria—seem close to getting the upper hand. This is a very important problem, and we will devote some space to the mechanisms of resistance and the means by which it is spread.

BACKGROUND

The term chemotherapy was coined by Ehrlich himself at the beginning of the 20th century to describe the use of synthetic chemicals to destroy infective agents. In recent years, the definition of the term has been broadened to include *antibiotics*—substances produced by some micro-organisms (or by pharmaceutical chemists) that kill or inhibit the growth of other micro-organisms. Here, we broaden it still further to include agents that kill or inhibit the growth of cancer cells.

THE MOLECULAR BASIS OF CHEMOTHERAPY

Chemotherapeutic agents then, are chemicals that are intended to be toxic for the pathogenic organism (or cancer cells) but innocuous to the host. Before discussing the molecular basis of such selective toxicity, we need to define what we mean by infectious organism. The word 'microbe' is generally used to describe bacteria, viruses and fungi, and the word 'parasite' to describe protozoa and helminths. However, we are concerned only with those organisms that cause disease, and the immune response of the human host

---

[1]Mercury-containing compounds were also once used for treating syphilis. 'One night with Venus, a lifetime with Mercury' was a saying of that time.

makes no distinction between the above categories, which are of purely semantic convenience. We will use the term *pathogens* to describe these invaders. It is important to remember that many micro-organisms share our body spaces (e.g. the gut) without causing disease (these are called *commensals*), although these may become pathogenic under adverse circumstances (i.e if the host is immunocompromised).

Living organisms are classified as either prokaryotes, cells without nuclei (the bacteria), or eukaryotes, cells with nuclei (e.g. protozoa, fungi, helminths). In a separate category are the viruses, which are not really cells at all because they do not have their own biochemical machinery for generating energy or for any sort of synthesis. Viruses need to utilise the metabolic machinery of the host cell, and they thus present a particular kind of problem for chemotherapeutic attack. There remain those mysterious protein-aceous agents, the prions (see Ch. 35), which cause disease but resist all attempts at classification, and for which there is no known antidote at present.

In yet another category still are cancer cells—host cells that have somehow escaped from the normal regulatory mechanisms that limit cell division. Cancer cells are clearly more similar to normal host cells than are any of the pathogenic invaders, and this makes the problem of implementing selective toxicity especially difficult. Nevertheless, major advances have been made, mainly following in the wake of the pioneering work of George Hitchings and Gertrude Elion, whose 'rational drug design' approach led to the development of many important 'antimetabolite' drugs, including antileukaemia agents.

Virtually all creatures, host and parasite alike, have the same basic blueprint—DNA (an exception being the RNA viruses)—so some biochemical processes are common to most, if not all,

organisms. Finding agents that affect pathogens or cancers but not other human cells necessitates finding either qualitative or quan-titative biochemical differences between them.

Bacteria cause most infectious diseases, and Figure 45.1 shows in simplified diagrammatic form the main structures and functions of a 'generalised' bacterial cell. Surrounding the cell is the *cell wall*, which characteristically contains peptidoglycan in all forms of bacteria except *mycoplasma*. Peptidoglycan is unique to prokaryotic cells and has no counterpart in eukaryotes. Within the cell wall is the *plasma membrane*, which, similar to that of eukaryotic cells, consists of a phospholipid bilayer and proteins. It functions as a selectively permeable membrane with specific transport mechanisms for various nutrients. However, in bacteria the plasma membrane does not contain any *sterols*, and this may alter the penetration of some chemicals.

The function of the cell wall is to support the underlying plasma membrane, which is subject to an internal osmotic pressure of about 5 atmospheres in *Gram-negative* organisms, and about 20 atmospheres in *Gram-positive* organisms (see below). The plasma membrane and cell wall together comprise the bacterial *envelope*.

Within the plasma membrane is the *cytoplasm*. As in eukaryotic cells, this contains soluble enzymes and other proteins, the *ribosomes* involved in protein synthesis, and the small-molecule intermediates involved in metabolism, as well as inorganic ions. However, unlike the eukaryotic cell, the bacterial cell has no nucleus; instead, the genetic material, in the form of a single *chromosome* containing all the genetic information, lies in the cytoplasm with no surrounding nuclear membrane. In further contrast to eukaryotic cells, there are no mitochondria—cellular energy is generated by enzyme systems located in the plasma membrane.

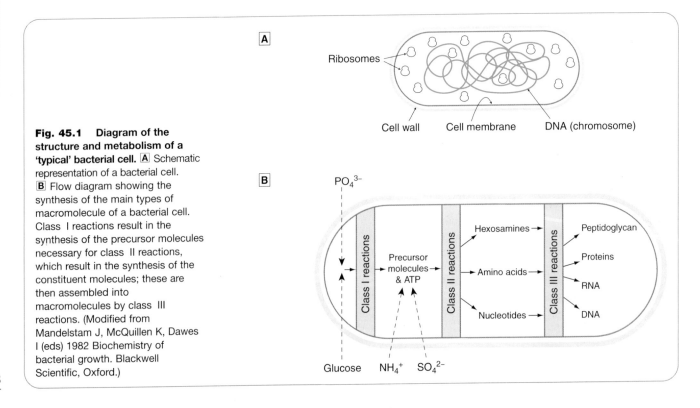

Fig. 45.1 Diagram of the structure and metabolism of a 'typical' bacterial cell. [A] Schematic representation of a bacterial cell. [B] Flow diagram showing the synthesis of the main types of macromolecule of a bacterial cell. Class I reactions result in the synthesis of the precursor molecules necessary for class II reactions, which result in the synthesis of the constituent molecules; these are then assembled into macromolecules by class III reactions. (Modified from Mandelstam J, McQuillen K, Dawes I (eds) 1982 Biochemistry of bacterial growth. Blackwell Scientific, Oxford.)

Some bacteria have additional components such as a *capsule* and/or one or more *flagella*, but the only additional structure with relevance for chemotherapy is the *outer membrane* outside the cell wall. The nature of this structure is important for taxonomic reasons, as it enables bacteria to be classified according to whether they take up Gram's stain ('Gram-positive') or not ('Gram-negative'; for more details, see Ch. 46). In Gram-negative bacteria, this membrane may prevent penetration of antibacterial agents, and it also prevents easy access of *lysozyme* (a microbiocidal enzyme found in white blood cells, tears and other tissue fluids that breaks down peptidoglycan).

The biochemical reactions that are potential targets for antibacterial drugs are shown in Figure 45.1. There are three groups.

- *Class I*: the utilisation of glucose or some alternative carbon source for the generation of energy (ATP) and synthesis of simple carbon compounds used as precursors in the next class of reactions.
- *Class II*: the utilisation of these precursors in an energy-dependent synthesis of all the amino acids, nucleotides, phospholipids, amino sugars, carbohydrates and growth factors required by the cell for survival and growth.
- *Class III*: assembly of small molecules into macromolecules—proteins, RNA, DNA, polysaccharides and peptidoglycan.

Other potential targets are the *formed structures*, for example the cell membrane, or in higher organisms (e.g. fungi and cancer cells) the *microtubules* or other specific tissues (e.g. muscle tissue in helminths). In considering these targets, emphasis will be placed on bacteria, but reference will also be made to protozoa, helminths, fungi, cancer cells and, where possible, viruses as well. The classification that follows is clearly not rigid; a drug may affect more than one class of reactions or more than one subgroup of reactions within a class.

The molecular basis of chemotherapy

- Chemotherapeutic drugs should be toxic to invading organisms and innocuous to the host. Such selective toxicity depends on the discovery of biochemical differences between the pathogen and the host that can be appropriately exploited.
- Three general classes of biochemical reaction are potential targets for chemotherapy of bacteria.
  - *Class I:* reactions that utilise glucose and other carbon sources are used to produce ATP and simple carbon compounds.
  - *Class II:* pathways utilising energy and class I compounds to make small molecules (e.g. amino acids and nucleotides).
  - *Class III:* pathways that convert small molecules into macromolecules such as proteins, nucleic acids and peptidoglycan.

BIOCHEMICAL REACTIONS AS POTENTIAL TARGETS

CLASS I REACTIONS

Class I reactions are not promising targets for two reasons. First, bacterial and human cells use similar mechanisms (the *Embden–Meyerhof pathway* and the *tricarboxylic acid cycle*) to obtain energy from glucose. Second, even if glucose oxidation was blocked, many other compounds (amino acids, lactate, etc.) could be utilised by bacteria as an alternative energy source.

CLASS II REACTIONS

Class II reactions are better targets because some pathways exist in parasitic but not in human cells. For instance, human cells lack the ability, possessed by bacteria, to synthesise the so-called 'essential' amino acids as well as certain growth factors (termed *vitamins* in human physiology). Differences such as these represent a potential target. Another opportunity occurs when a pathway is identical in both bacteria and humans but exhibits a differential sensitivity to drugs.

Folate

Folate biosynthesis is an example of a metabolic pathway found in bacteria but not in humans. Folate is required for DNA synthesis in both bacteria and in humans (see Chs 22 and 46). Humans cannot synthesise folate and must obtain it from the diet, and specific uptake mechanisms have evolved to transport it into cells. By contrast, most species of bacteria, as well as the asexual forms of malarial protozoa, lack the necessary transport mechanisms and cannot make use of preformed folate but must synthesise their own *de novo*. This is a prime example of a difference that has proved to be extremely useful for chemotherapy. **Sulfonamides** contain the sulfanilamide moiety—a structural analogue of *p*-aminobenzoic acid (PABA), which is essential in the synthesis of folate (see Figs 22.2 and 46.1). Sulfonamides compete with PABA for the enzyme involved in folate synthesis, and thus inhibit the metabolism of the bacteria. They are consequently *bacteriostatic* not *bactericidal*[2] (i.e. they suppress division of the cells but do not kill them), and are therefore only really effective in the presence of adequate host defences (which are discussed in Ch. 13).

The utilisation of folate, in the form of tetrahydrofolate, as a cofactor in thymidylate synthesis (see Figs 22.3 and 46.2) is a good example of a pathway where human and bacterial enzymes exhibit a differential sensitivity to chemicals (Table 45.1). Although the pathway is virtually identical in micro-organisms and humans, one of the key enzymes, *dihydrofolate reductase*, which reduces dihydrofolate to tetrahydrofolate (Fig. 22.2), is many times more sensitive to the folate antagonist **trimethoprim** in bacteria than in humans. In some malarial protozoa, this enzyme is somewhat less sensitive than the bacterial enzyme to trimethoprim but more

---

[2]Whether a drug is bactericidal rather than bacteriostatic is determined on a strict technical criterion, but in practice it can be difficult to differentiate the two actions during therapy.

Table 45.1   Specificity of inhibitors of dihydrofolate reductase

Inhibitor	IC$_{50}$ (μmol/l) for dihydrofolate reductase		
	Human	*Protozoal*	*Bacterial*
Trimethoprim	260	0.07	0.005
Pyrimethamine	0.7	0.0005	2.5
Methotrexate	0.001	~0.1[a]	Inactive

[a]Tested on *Plasmodium berghei*, a rodent malaria.

sensitive to **pyrimethamine** and **proguanil**, which are used as antimalarial agents (Ch. 49). The relative IC$_{50}$ values (the concentration causing 50% inhibition) for bacterial, malarial, protozoal and mammalian enzymes are given in Table 45.1. The human enzyme, by comparison, is very sensitive to the effect of the folate analogue **methotrexate** (Table 45.1), which is used in cancer chemotherapy (see Ch. 51). Methotrexate is inactive in bacteria because, being very similar in structure to folate, it requires active uptake by cells. Trimethoprim and pyrimethamine enter the cells by diffusion.

The use of sequential blockade with a combination of two drugs that affect the same pathway at different points, for example sulfonamides and the folate antagonists (Fig. 46.2), may be more successful than the use of either alone (e.g. in the treatment of *Pneumocystis carinii* pneumonia), and lower concentrations are effective when the two are used together. Thus pyrimethamine and a sulfonamide (**sulfadoxine**) are used to treat *falciparum* malaria (p. 702). An antibacterial formulation that contains both a sulfonamide and trimethoprim is **co-trimoxazole** (p. 664); once widely used, this combination has become progressively less effective because of the development of sulfonamide resistance.

Pyrimidine and purine analogues

The pyrimidine analogue **fluorouracil**, which is used in cancer chemotherapy (Ch. 51), is converted to a fraudulent nucleotide that interferes with thymidylate synthesis. Other cancer chemotherapy agents that give rise to fraudulent nucleotides are the purine analogues **mercaptopurine** and **thioguanine. Flucytosine,** an antifungal drug (Ch. 48), is deaminated to fluorouracil within fungal cells but to a much lesser extent in human cells, conferring a degree of selectivity.

CLASS III REACTIONS

As cells cannot take up their own unique macromolecules from the environment, class III reactions are particularly good targets for selective toxicity, and there are distinct differences between mammalian cells and parasitic cells in the class III pathways.

The synthesis of peptidoglycan

The cell wall of bacteria contains peptidoglycan, a substance that does not occur in eukaryotes. It is the equivalent of a non-stretchable

string bag enclosing the whole bacterium. In some bacteria (the Gram-negative organisms), this bag consists of a single thickness, but for others (Gram-positive organisms) there may be as many as 40 layers of peptidoglycan. Each layer consists of multiple backbones of amino sugars—alternating *N*-acetylglucosamine and *N*-acetylmuramic acid residues (Fig. 45.2)—the latter having short peptide side-chains that are cross-linked to form a polymeric lattice, which is strong enough to resist the high internal osmotic pressure and may constitute up to 10–15% of the dry weight of the cell. The cross-links differ in different species. In staphylococci, they consist of five glycine residues.

To build up this very large insoluble peptidoglycan layer on the outside of the cell membrane, the bacterial cell has the problem of how to transport the hydrophilic cytoplasmic 'building blocks' through the hydrophobic cell membrane structure. This is accomplished by linking them to a very large lipid carrier, containing 55 carbon atoms, which 'tows' them across the membrane. The process of peptidoglycan synthesis is outlined in Figure 45.3. First, *N*-acetylmuramic acid, attached to uridine diphosphate (UDP) and a pentapeptide, is transferred to the C55 lipid carrier in the membrane, with the release of uridine monophosphate. This is followed by a reaction with UDP–*N*-acetylglucosamine, resulting in the formation of a disaccharide pentapeptide complex attached to the carrier. This complex is the basic building block of the peptidoglycan. In *Staphylococcus aureus*, the five glycine residues are attached to the peptide chain at this stage. The building block is now transported to the outside of the cell and added to the growing end of the peptidoglycan, the

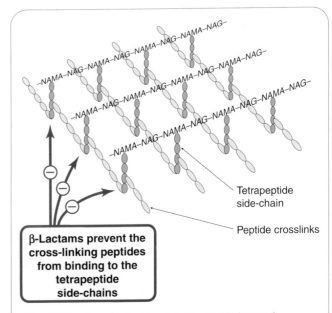

β-Lactams prevent the cross-linking peptides from binding to the tetrapeptide side-chains

Fig. 45.2 Schematic diagram of a single layer of peptidoglycan from a bacterial cell (e.g. *Staphylococcus aureus*), showing the site of action of the β-lactam antibiotics. In *S. aureus*, the peptide cross-links consist of five glycine residues. Gram-positive bacteria have several layers of peptidoglycan. (NAMA, N-acetylmuramic acid; NAG, N-acetylglucosamine: more detail in Figure 45.3).

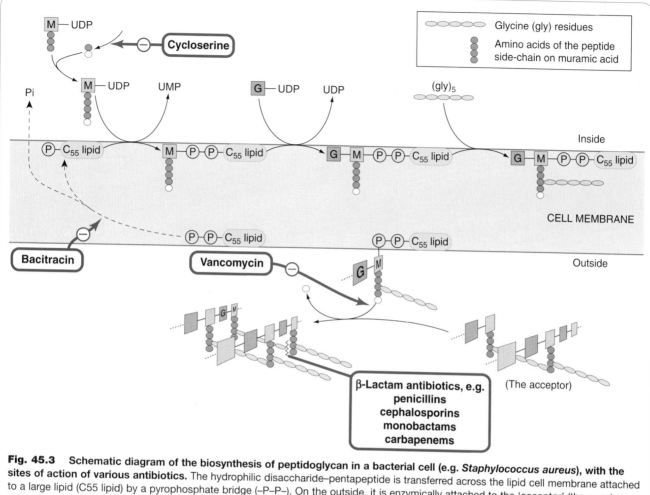

Fig. 45.3 **Schematic diagram of the biosynthesis of peptidoglycan in a bacterial cell (e.g. *Staphylococcus aureus*), with the sites of action of various antibiotics.** The hydrophilic disaccharide–pentapeptide is transferred across the lipid cell membrane attached to a large lipid (C55 lipid) by a pyrophosphate bridge (–P–P–). On the outside, it is enzymically attached to the 'acceptor' (the growing peptidoglycan layer). The final reaction is a transpeptidation, in which the loose end of the (gly)₅ chain is attached to a peptide side-chain of an M in the acceptor and during which the terminal amino acid (alanine) is lost. The lipid is regenerated by loss of a phosphate group (Pi) before functioning again as a carrier. G, *N*-acetylglucosamine; M, *N*-acetylmuramic acid; UDP, uridine diphosphate; UMP, uridine monophosphate.

'acceptor', with the release of the C55 lipid, which still has two phosphates attached. The lipid carrier then loses one phosphate group and thus becomes available for another cycle. Cross-linking between the peptide side-chains of the sugar residues in the peptidoglycan layer then occurs, the hydrolytic removal of the terminal alanine supplying the requisite energy.

This synthesis of peptidoglycan is a vulnerable step and can be blocked at several points by antibiotics (Fig. 45.3 and Ch. 46). **Cycloserine**, which is a structural analogue of D-alanine, prevents the addition of the two terminal alanine residues to the initial tripeptide side-chain on *N*-acetylmuramic acid by competitive inhibition. **Vancomycin** inhibits the release of the building block unit from the carrier, thus preventing its addition to the growing end of the peptidoglycan. **Bacitracin** interferes with the regeneration of the lipid carrier by blocking its dephosphorylation. **Penicillins, cephalosporins** and other β-**lactams** inhibit the final transpeptidation by forming covalent bonds with penicillin-binding

proteins that have transpeptidase and carboxypeptidase activities, thus preventing formation of the cross-links.

Protein synthesis

Protein synthesis takes place in the ribosomes. Eukaryotic and prokaryotic ribosomes are different, and this provides the basis for the selective antimicrobial action of some antibiotics. The bacterial ribosome consists of a 50S subunit and a 30S subunit (Fig. 45.4), whereas in the mammalian ribosome the subunits are 60S and 40S. The other elements involved in peptide synthesis are messenger RNA (mRNA), which forms the template for protein synthesis, and transfer RNA (tRNA), which specifically transfers the individual amino acids to the ribosome. The ribosome has three binding sites for tRNA, termed the *A, P* and *E* sites.

A simplified version of protein synthesis in bacteria is shown in Figure 45.4. To initiate translation, mRNA, transcribed from

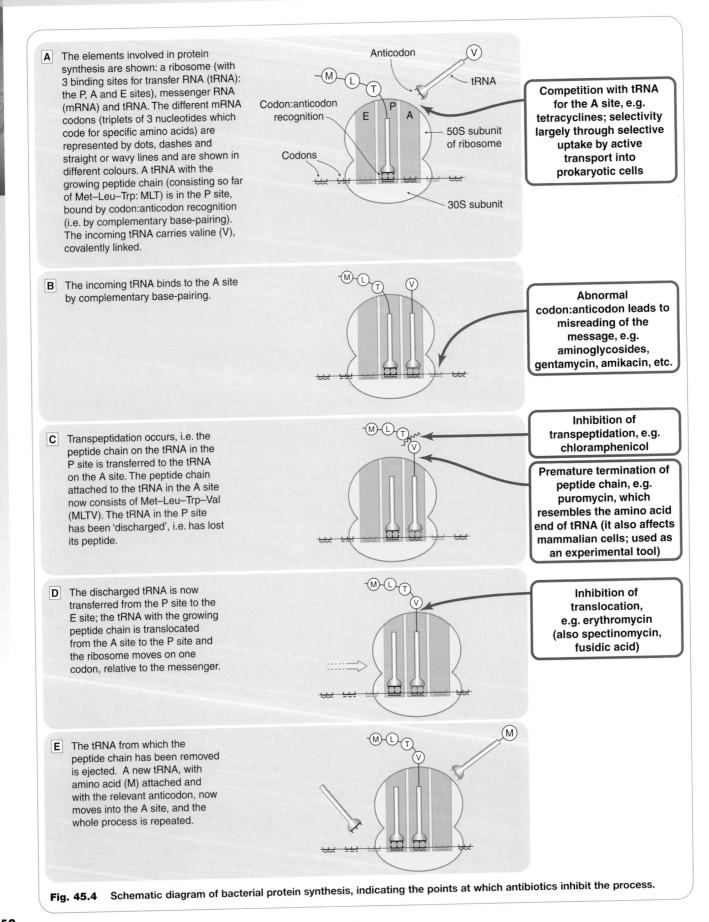

A The elements involved in protein synthesis are shown: a ribosome (with 3 binding sites for transfer RNA (tRNA): the P, A and E sites), messenger RNA (mRNA) and tRNA. The different mRNA codons (triplets of 3 nucleotides which code for specific amino acids) are represented by dots, dashes and straight or wavy lines and are shown in different colours. A tRNA with the growing peptide chain (consisting so far of Met–Leu–Trp: MLT) is in the P site, bound by codon:anticodon recognition (i.e. by complementary base-pairing). The incoming tRNA carries valine (V), covalently linked.

Anticodon

tRNA

Codon:anticodon recognition

E   P   A

Codons

50S subunit of ribosome

30S subunit

Competition with tRNA for the A site, e.g. tetracyclines; selectivity largely through selective uptake by active transport into prokaryotic cells

B The incoming tRNA binds to the A site by complementary base-pairing.

Abnormal codon:anticodon leads to misreading of the message, e.g. aminoglycosides, gentamycin, amikacin, etc.

C Transpeptidation occurs, i.e. the peptide chain on the tRNA in the P site is transferred to the tRNA on the A site. The peptide chain attached to the tRNA in the A site now consists of Met–Leu–Trp–Val (MLTV). The tRNA in the P site has been 'discharged', i.e. has lost its peptide.

Inhibition of transpeptidation, e.g. chloramphenicol

Premature termination of peptide chain, e.g. puromycin, which resembles the amino acid end of tRNA (it also affects mammalian cells; used as an experimental tool)

D The discharged tRNA is now transferred from the P site to the E site; the tRNA with the growing peptide chain is translocated from the A site to the P site and the ribosome moves on one codon, relative to the messenger.

Inhibition of translocation, e.g. erythromycin (also spectinomycin, fusidic acid)

E The tRNA from which the peptide chain has been removed is ejected. A new tRNA, with amino acid (M) attached and with the relevant anticodon, now moves into the A site, and the whole process is repeated.

Fig. 45.4 Schematic diagram of bacterial protein synthesis, indicating the points at which antibiotics inhibit the process.

the DNA template (see below), is attached to the 30S subunit of the ribosome. The 50S subunit then binds to the 30S subunit to form a 70S[3] subunit, which moves along the mRNA such that successive codons of the messenger pass along the ribosome from the A position to the P position. Antibiotics may affect protein synthesis at any one of these stages (Fig. 45.4 and Ch. 46).

Nucleic acid synthesis

The nucleic acids of the cell are DNA and RNA. There are three types of RNA: mRNA, tRNA and ribosomal RNA (rRNA). The last of these is an integral part of the ribosome and is necessary for its assembly as well as for facilitating mRNA binding. The assembled ribosome also exhibits peptidyl transferase activity.

DNA is the template for the synthesis of both DNA and RNA. It exists in the cell as a double helix, each strand of which is a linear polymer of nucleotides. Each nucleotide consists of a base linked to a sugar (deoxyribose) and a phosphate. There are two purine bases, adenine (A) and guanine (G), and two pyrimidine bases, cytosine (C) and thymine (T). Single-strand DNA comprises alternating sugar and phosphate groups with the bases attached (Fig. 45.5). Specific hydrogen bonding between G and C and between A and T on each strand (i.e. complementary base pairing) is the basis of the double-stranded helical structure of DNA. The DNA helix is itself further coiled. In the test tube, the coil has 10 base pairs per turn. In vivo, the coil is unwound by about 1 turn in 20, forming a *negative supercoil*.

Initiation of DNA synthesis requires first the activity of a protein that causes separation of the strands. The replication process inserts a positive supercoil, which is relaxed by *DNA gyrase* (also called *topoisomerase II*; Fig. 45.6). During the synthesis of DNA, nucleotide units—each consisting of a base linked to a sugar and three phosphate groups—are added by base pairing with the complementary residues on the template. Condensation occurs by elimination of two phosphate groups, catalysed by *DNA polymerase*.

RNA exists only in single-stranded form. The sugar moiety here is ribose, and the ribonucleotides contain the bases adenine, guanine, cytosine and uracil (U).

It is possible to interfere with nucleic acid synthesis in five different ways:

- by inhibiting the synthesis of the nucleotides
- by altering the base-pairing properties of the template
- by inhibiting either DNA or RNA polymerase
- by inhibiting DNA gyrase
- by a direct effect on DNA itself.

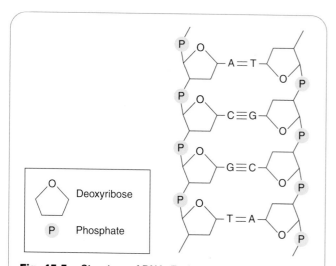

Fig. 45.5   Structure of DNA. Each strand of DNA consists of a sugar–phosphate backbone with purine or pyrimidine bases attached. The purines are adenine (A) or guanine (G) and the pyrimidines are cytosine (C) or thymine (T). The sugar is deoxyribose. Complementarity between the two strands of DNA is maintained by hydrogen bonds (either two or three) between bases.

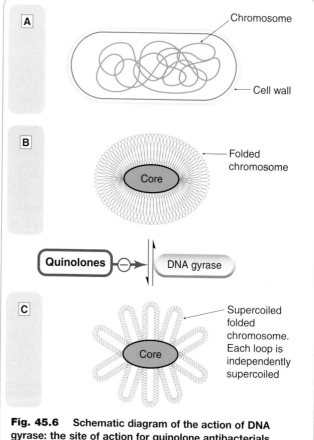

Fig. 45.6   Schematic diagram of the action of DNA gyrase: the site of action for quinolone antibacterials.
[A] Conventional diagram used to depict a bacterial cell and chromosome (e.g. *Escherichia coli*). Note that the *E. coli* chromosome is 1300 mm long and is contained in a cell envelope of 2 μm × 1 μm; this is approximately equivalent to a 50-m length of cotton folded into a matchbox.
[B] Chromosome folded around RNA core, and then
[C] supercoiled by DNA gyrase (topoisomerase II). Quinolone and antibacterials interfere with the action of this enzyme. (Modified from Smith J T 1985 In: Greenwood D, O'Grady F (eds) Scientific basis of antimicrobial therapy. Cambridge University Press, Cambridge, p. 69.)

---

[3]You query whether 30S + 50S = 70S? Yes it does, because we are talking about *Svedberg units*, which measure sedimentation rate not mass.

Inhibition of the synthesis of the nucleotides

This can be accomplished by an effect on the metabolic pathways that generate nucleotide precursors. Examples of agents that have such an effect have been described under class II reactions.

Alteration of the base-pairing properties of the template

Agents that intercalate in the DNA have this effect. Examples include acridines (**proflavine** and **acriflavine**), which are used topically as antiseptics. The acridines double the distance between adjacent base pairs and cause a frameshift mutation (Fig. 45.7), whereas some purine and pyrimidine analogues cause base *mispairing*.

mRNA (normal)	UCU Ser	UUU Phe	CUU Leu	AUU Ile	GUU Val	UCU... Ser
mRNA (mutant)	UCU Ser	UUG Leu	UCU Ser	UAU Tyr	UGU Cys	UUC... Phe

Fig. 45.7 An example of the effect on RNA and protein synthesis of a frameshift mutation in DNA. A frameshift mutation is one that involves a deletion of a base or an insertion of an extra base. In the above example, an extra cytosine has been inserted in the DNA template, with the result that when mRNA is formed it has an additional guanine (G), as indicated in orange. The effect is to alter that codon and all the succeeding ones (shown in blue), so that a completely different protein is synthesised, as indicated by the different amino acids (Leu instead of Phe, Ser instead of Leu, etc.). A, adenine; C, cytosine; U, uracil.

Inhibition of either DNA or RNA polymerase

Dactinomycin (**actinomycin D**) binds to the guanine residues in DNA and blocks the movement of RNA polymerase, thus preventing transcription and inhibiting protein synthesis. The drug is used in cancer chemotherapy in humans (Ch. 51) and also as an experimental tool, but it is not useful as an antibacterial agent. Specific inhibitors of bacterial RNA polymerase that act by binding to this enzyme in prokaryotic but not in eukaryotic cells include **rifamycin** and **rifampicin**, which are particularly useful for treating *Mycobacterium tuberculosis* (which causes tuberculosis; see Ch. 46). **Aciclovir** (an analogue of guanine) is phosphorylated in cells infected with herpes virus, the initial phosphorylation being by a virus-specific kinase to give the aciclovir trisphosphate, which has an inhibitory action on the DNA polymerase of the herpes virus (Ch. 47 and Fig. 45.8).

RNA retroviruses have a reverse transcriptase (viral RNA–dependent DNA polymerase) that copies the viral RNA into DNA that integrates into the host cell genome as a *provirus*. Various agents (**zidovudine, didanosine**) are phosphorylated by cellular enzymes to the trisphosphate forms, which compete with the host cell precursors essential for the formation by the viral reverse transcriptase of proviral DNA.

Cytarabine (cytosine arabinoside) is used in cancer chemotherapy (Ch. 51). Its trisphosphate derivative is a potent inhibitor of DNA polymerase in mammalian cells. **Foscarnet** inhibits viral RNA polymerase by attaching to the pyrophosphate-binding site.

Inhibition of DNA gyrase

Figure 45.6 is a simplified scheme showing the action of DNA gyrase. The **fluoroquinolones** (**cinoxacin, ciprofloxacin, nalidixic acid** and **norfloxacin**) act by inhibiting DNA gyrase, and these

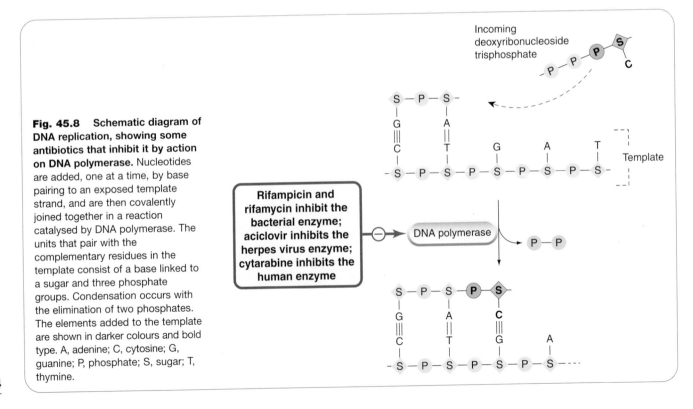

Fig. 45.8 Schematic diagram of DNA replication, showing some antibiotics that inhibit it by action on DNA polymerase. Nucleotides are added, one at a time, by base pairing to an exposed template strand, and are then covalently joined together in a reaction catalysed by DNA polymerase. The units that pair with the complementary residues in the template consist of a base linked to a sugar and three phosphate groups. Condensation occurs with the elimination of two phosphates. The elements added to the template are shown in darker colours and bold type. A, adenine; C, cytosine; G, guanine; P, phosphate; S, sugar; T, thymine.

Rifampicin and rifamycin inhibit the bacterial enzyme; aciclovir inhibits the herpes virus enzyme; cytarabine inhibits the human enzyme chemotherapeutic agents are used particularly in infections with Gram-negative organisms (Ch. 46). These drugs are selective for the bacterial enzyme because it is structurally different from the mammalian enzyme. Some anticancer agents, for example doxorubicin, act on the mammalian topoisomerase II.

Direct effects on DNA itself

Alkylating agents form covalent bonds with bases in the DNA and prevent replication. Compounds with this action are used only in cancer chemotherapy and include nitrogen mustard derivatives and nitrosoureas (Ch. 51). **Mitomycin** also binds covalently to DNA. No antibacterial agents work by these mechanisms. **Bleomycin,** an anticancer drug, causes fragmentation of the DNA strands following free radical formation (Ch. 51).

THE FORMED STRUCTURES OF THE CELL AS POTENTIAL TARGETS

THE MEMBRANE

The plasma membrane of bacterial cells is similar to that in mammalian cells in that it consists of a phospholipid bilayer in which proteins are embedded, but it can be more easily disrupted in certain bacteria and fungi.

Polymixins are cationic peptide antibiotics, containing both hydrophilic and lipophilic groups, which have a selective effect on bacterial cell membranes. They act as detergents, disrupting

the phospholipid components of the membrane structure, thus killing the cell.

Unlike mammalian and bacterial cells, fungal cell membranes have large amounts of *ergosterol*. This facilitates the attachment of polyene antibiotics (e.g. **nystatin** and **amphotericin;** Ch. 48), which act as ionophores and cause leakage of cations.

Azoles such as **itraconazole** kill fungal cells by inhibiting ergosterol synthesis, thereby disrupting the function of membrane-associated enzymes. The azoles also affect Gram-positive bacteria, their selectivity being associated with the presence of high levels of free fatty acids in the membrane of susceptible organisms (Ch. 48).

INTRACELLULAR ORGANELLES

Microtubules and/or microfilaments

The benzimidazoles (e.g. **albendazole**) exert their antihelminthic action by binding selectively to parasite tubulin and preventing microtubule formation (Ch. 50). The vinca alkaloids **vinblastine** and **vincristine** are anticancer agents that disrupt the functioning of microtubules during cell division (Ch. 51).

Food vacuoles

The erythrocytic form of the malaria plasmodium feeds on host haemoglobin, which is digested by proteases in the parasite food vacuole, the final product, haem, being detoxified by polymerisation. **Chloroquine** exerts its antimalarial action by inhibiting plasmodial haem polymerase (Ch. 49).

MUSCLE FIBRES

Some antihelminthic drugs have a selective action on helminth muscle cells (Ch. 50). **Piperazine** acts as an agonist on parasite-specific chloride channels gated by GABA in nematode muscle, hyperpolarising the muscle fibre membrane and paralysing the worm; **avermectins** increase Cl$^-$ permeability in helminth muscle—possibly by a similar mechanism. **Pyrantel** (now seldom used) and **levamisole** act as agonists at nematode acetylcholine nicotinic receptors on muscle, causing contraction followed by paralysis (Ch. 50).

> **Biochemical reactions as potential targets for chemotherapy**
>
> - Class I reactions are poor targets.
> - Class II reactions are better targets:
>   - folate synthesis in bacteria is inhibited by sulfonamides
>   - folate utilisation is inhibited by folate antagonists, for example trimethoprim (bacteria), pyrimethamine (malarial parasite), methotrexate (cancer cells)
>   - pyrimidine analogues (e.g. fluorouracil) and purine analogues (e.g. mercaptopurine) give rise to fraudulent nucleotides and are used to treat cancer.
> - Class III reactions are important targets:
>   - peptidoglycan synthesis in bacteria can be selectively inhibited by β-lactam antibiotics (e.g. penicillin)
>   - bacterial protein synthesis can be selectively inhibited by antibiotics that prevent binding of tRNA (e.g. tetracyclines), promote misreading of mRNA (e.g. aminoglycosides), inhibit transpeptidation (e.g. chloramphenicol) or inhibit translocation of tRNA from A site to P site (e.g. erythromycin).
>   - nucleic acid synthesis can be inhibited by altering base pairing of DNA template (e.g. the antiviral vidarabine), by inhibiting DNA polymerase (e.g. the antivirals aciclovir and foscarnet) or by inhibiting DNA gyrase (e.g. the antibacterial ciprofloxacin).

RESISTANCE TO ANTIBACTERIAL DRUGS

Since the 1940s, the development of effective and safe drugs to deal with bacterial and other infections has revolutionised medical treatment, and the morbidity and mortality associated with these diseases has been dramatically reduced. Unfortunately, the development of effective antibacterial drugs has been accompanied by the emergence of drug-resistant organisms. This is not unexpected, because the short generation time of many bacterial species affords ample opportunity for evolutionary adaptation. The phenomenon of resistance imposes serious constraints on the options available for the medical treatment of many bacterial infections. Resistance to chemotherapeutic agents can also develop in protozoa, in multicellular parasites (see Foley & Tilley, 1997; Martin & Robertson, 2000; St Georgiev, 2000) and in populations of malignant cells

> **Formed structures of the cell that are targets for chemotherapy** 🔑
>
> - The plasma membrane is affected by:
>   - amphotericin, which acts as an ionophore in fungal cells
>   - azoles, which inhibit fungal membrane ergosterol synthesis.
> - Microtubule function is disrupted by:
>   - vinca alkaloids (anticancer drugs)
>   - benzimidazoles (antihelminthics).
> - Muscle fibres are affected by:
>   - avermectins (antihelminthics), which increase Cl⁻ permeability
>   - pyrantel (antihelminthic), which stimulates nematode nicotinic receptors, eventually causing muscle paralysis.

(discussed in Ch. 51). Here, however, we will confine discussion mainly to the mechanisms of resistance in bacteria.

Antibiotic resistance in bacteria spreads in three ways:

- by transfer of bacteria between people
- by transfer of resistance genes between bacteria (usually on *plasmids*)
- by transfer of resistance genes between genetic elements within bacteria, on *transposons*.

Understanding the mechanisms involved in antibiotic resistance is crucial for the sensible clinical use of existing medicines and in the design of new antibacterial drugs. One by-product of the studies of resistance in bacteria was the development of plasmid-based techniques for DNA cloning, leading to the use of bacteria to produce recombinant proteins for therapeutic use (see Ch. 55).

GENETIC DETERMINANTS OF ANTIBIOTIC RESISTANCE

CHROMOSOMAL DETERMINANTS: MUTATIONS

The spontaneous mutation rate in bacterial populations for any particular gene is very low, and the probability is that approximately only 1 cell in 10 million will, on division, give rise to a daughter cell containing a mutation in that gene. However, as there are likely to be very many more cells than this over the course of an infection, the probability of a mutation causing a change from drug sensitivity to drug resistance can be quite high with some species of bacteria and with some drugs. Fortunately, in most cases, a few mutants are not sufficient to produce resistance as, despite the selective advantage that the resistant mutants possess, the drastic reduction of the population by the antibiotic usually enables the host's natural defences (see Ch. 13) to prevail. However, this may not occur if the primary infection is caused by a drug-resistant strain.

Resistance resulting from chromosomal mutation is important in some instances, notably infections with **methicillin**-resistant *S. aureus* (MRSA; see below) and in tuberculosis, but this type of resistance is of limited clinical relevance, possibly because the mutants often have reduced pathogenicity.

EXTRACHROMOSOMAL DETERMINANTS: PLASMIDS

In addition to the chromosome itself, many species of bacteria contain extrachromosomal genetic elements called *plasmids* that exist free in the cytoplasm. These are also genetic elements that can replicate independently. Structurally, they are closed loops of DNA that may comprise a single gene or as many as 500 or even more. Only a few plasmid copies may exist in the cell but often multiple copies are present, and there may also be more than one type of plasmid in each bacterial cell. Plasmids that carry genes for resistance to antibiotics (*r genes*) are referred to as *R plasmids*. Much of the drug resistance encountered in clinical medicine is plasmid-determined. It is not known how these genes arose.

THE TRANSFER OF RESISTANCE GENES BETWEEN GENETIC ELEMENTS WITHIN THE BACTERIUM

Transposons

Some stretches of DNA are readily transferred (transposed) from one plasmid to another and also from plasmid to chromosome or vice versa. This is because integration of these segments of DNA, which are called *transposons*, into the acceptor DNA can occur independently of the normal mechanism of homologous genetic recombination. Unlike plasmids, transposons are not able to replicate independently, although some may replicate during the process of integration (Fig. 45.9), resulting in a copy in both the donor and the acceptor DNA molecules. Transposons may carry one or more resistance genes (see below) and can 'hitch-hike' on a plasmid to a new species of bacterium. Even if the plasmid is unable to replicate in the new host, the transposon may integrate

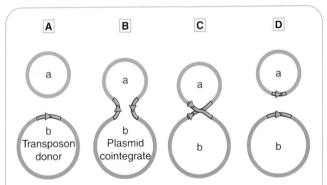

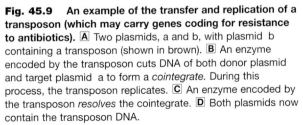

Fig. 45.9 **An example of the transfer and replication of a transposon (which may carry genes coding for resistance to antibiotics).** **A** Two plasmids, a and b, with plasmid b containing a transposon (shown in brown). **B** An enzyme encoded by the transposon cuts DNA of both donor plasmid and target plasmid a to form a *cointegrate*. During this process, the transposon replicates. **C** An enzyme encoded by the transposon *resolves* the cointegrate. **D** Both plasmids now contain the transposon DNA.

into the new host's chromosome or into its indigenous plasmids. This probably accounts for the widespread distribution of certain of the resistance genes on different R plasmids and among unrelated bacteria.

Gene cassettes and integrons

Plasmids and transposons do not complete the tally of mechanisms that natural selection has provided to confound the hopes of the microbiologist/chemotherapist. Resistance—in fact, *multidrug resistance*—can also be spread by another mobile element, the *gene cassette*, which consists of a resistance gene attached to a small recognition site. Several cassettes may be packaged together in a *multicassette array*, which can, in turn, be integrated into a larger mobile DNA unit termed an *integron*. The integron (which may be located on a transposon) contains a gene for an enzyme, *integrase* (recombinase), which inserts the cassette(s) at unique sites on the integron. This system—transposon/integron/multiresistance cassette array—allows particularly rapid and efficient transfer of multidrug resistance between genetic elements both within and between bacteria.

THE TRANSFER OF RESISTANCE GENES BETWEEN BACTERIA

The transfer of resistance genes between bacteria of the same and indeed of different species is of fundamental importance in the spread of antibiotic resistance. The most important mechanism in this context is *conjugation*. Other gene transfer mechanisms, *transduction* and *transformation*, are of little importance in spreading resistance genes.

Conjugation

Conjugation involves cell-to-cell contact during which chromosomal or extrachromosomal DNA is transferred from one bacterium to another, and is the main mechanism for the spread of resistance. The ability to conjugate is encoded in *conjugative plasmids*; these are plasmids that contain transfer genes, which, in *coliform* bacteria, code for the production by the host bacterium of proteinaceous surface tubules, termed *sex pili*, that connect the two cells. The conjugative plasmid then passes across from one bacterial cell to another (generally of the same species). Many Gram-negative and some Gram-positive bacteria can conjugate. Some *promiscuous plasmids* can cross the species barrier, accepting one host as readily as another. Many R plasmids are conjugative. Non-conjugative plasmids, if they coexist in a 'donor' cell with conjugative plasmids, can hitch-hike from one bacterium to the other with the conjugative plasmids. The transfer of resistance by conjugation is significant in populations of bacteria that are normally found at high densities, as in the gut.

Transduction

Transduction is a process by which plasmid DNA is enclosed in a bacterial virus (or *phage*) and transferred to another bacterium of the same species. It is a relatively ineffective means of transfer of genetic material but is clinically important in the transmission of resistance genes between strains of staphylococci and of streptococci.

Transformation

A few species of bacteria can, under natural conditions, undergo *transformation* by taking up DNA from the environment and incorporating it into the genome by normal homologous recombination. Transformation is probably not of importance clinically.

BIOCHEMICAL MECHANISMS OF RESISTANCE TO ANTIBIOTICS

THE PRODUCTION OF AN ENZYME THAT INACTIVATES THE DRUG

Inactivation of β-lactam antibiotics

The most important example of resistance caused by inactivation is that of the *β-lactam antibiotics*. The enzymes concerned are *β-lactamases*, which cleave the β-lactam ring of penicillins and **cephalosporins** (see Ch. 46). Cross-resistance between the two classes of antibiotic is not complete, because some β-lactamases have a preference for penicillins and some for cephalosporins.

▼ *Staphylococci* are the principal bacteria producing β-lactamase, and the genes coding for the enzymes are on plasmids that can be transferred by transduction. In staphylococci, the enzyme is inducible (i.e. its synthesis is not expressed in the absence of the drug), and minute, subinhibitory concentrations of antibiotics derepress the gene and result in a 50- to 80-fold increase in expression. The enzyme passes through the bacterial envelope and inactivates antibiotic molecules in the surrounding medium. The grave clinical problem posed by resistant staphylococci secreting β-lactamase was tackled by developing semisynthetic penicillins (such as methicillin) and new β-lactam antibiotics (the

---

Resistance to antibiotics

- Resistance in bacterial populations can be spread from person to person by bacteria, from bacterium to bacterium by plasmids, from plasmid to plasmid (or chromosome) by transposons.
- Plasmids are extrachromosomal genetic elements that can replicate independently and can carry genes coding for resistance to antibiotics (r genes).
- The main method of transfer of r genes from one bacterium to another is by conjugative plasmids. The bacterium forms a connecting tube with other bacteria through which the plasmids pass.
- A less common method of transfer is by transduction, i.e. the transmission by a bacterial virus (phage) of a plasmid bearing an r gene into another bacterium.
- Transposons are stretches of DNA that can be transposed from one plasmid to another, from a plasmid to a chromosome or vice versa. A plasmid containing an r gene–bearing transposon may code for enzymes that cause the plasmid to be integrated with another. Following their separation, this transposon replicates so that both plasmids then contain the r gene.

monobactams and **carbapenems**), and cephalosporins (such as **cephamandole**), that are less susceptible to inactivation. The growing problem of MRSA is discussed below.

Gram-negative organisms can also produce β-lactamases, and this is a significant factor in their resistance to the semisynthetic broad-spectrum β-lactam antibiotics. In these organisms, the enzymes may be coded by either chromosomal or plasmid genes. In the former case, the enzymes may be inducible, but in the latter they are produced constitutively. When this occurs, the enzyme does not inactivate the drug in the surrounding medium but instead remains attached to the cell wall, preventing access of the drug to membrane-associated target sites. Many of these β-lactamases are encoded by transposons, some of which may also carry resistance determinants to several other antibiotics.

Inactivation of chloramphenicol

Chloramphenicol is inactivated by *chloramphenicol acetyltransferase*, an enzyme produced by resistant strains of both Gram-positive and Gram-negative organisms, the resistance gene being plasmid-borne. In Gram-negative bacteria, the enzyme is produced constitutively, resulting in levels of resistance fivefold higher than in Gram-positive bacteria, in which the enzyme is inducible.

Inactivation of aminoglycosides

Aminoglycosides are inactivated by phosphorylation, adenylation or acetylation, and the requisite enzymes are found in both Gram-negative and Gram-positive organisms. The resistance genes are carried on plasmids, and several are found on transposons.

ALTERATION OF DRUG-SENSITIVE OR DRUG-BINDING SITE

The aminoglycoside-binding site on the 30S subunit of the ribosome may be altered by chromosomal mutation. A plasmid-mediated alteration of the binding site protein on the 50S subunit also underlies resistance to **erythromycin**, and decreased binding of fluoroquinolones because of a point mutation in DNA gyrase A has recently been described. An altered DNA-dependent RNA polymerase determined by a chromosomal mutation is reported to be the basis for rifampicin resistance.

In addition to acquiring resistance to β-lactams susceptible to β-lactamase, some strains of *S. aureus* have even become resistant to some antibiotics that are not significantly inactivated by β-lactamase (e.g. methicillin), because they express an additional β-lactam–binding protein coded for by a mutated chromosomal gene.

DECREASED DRUG ACCUMULATION IN THE BACTERIUM

An important example of decreased drug accumulation is the plasmid-mediated resistance to **tetracyclines** encountered in both Gram-positive and Gram-negative bacteria. In this case, resistance genes in the plasmid code for inducible proteins in the bacterial membrane, which promote energy-dependent efflux of the tetracyclines, and hence resistance. This type of resistance is common

and has greatly reduced the therapeutic value of the tetracyclines in human and veterinary medicine. Resistance of *S. aureus* to erythromycin and the other macrolides, and to fluoroquinolones, is also brought about by energy-dependent efflux.

There is also recent evidence of plasmid-determined inhibition of *porin* synthesis, which could affect those hydrophilic antibiotics that enter the bacterium through these water-filled channels in the outer membrane. Altered permeability as a result of chromosomal mutations involving the polysaccharide components of the outer membrane of Gram-negative organisms may confer enhanced resistance to **ampicillin**. Mutations affecting envelope components have been reported to affect the accumulation of aminoglycosides, β-lactams, chloramphenicol, peptide antibiotics and tetracycline.

THE DEVELOPMENT OF A PATHWAY THAT BYPASSES THE REACTION INHIBITED BY THE ANTIBIOTIC

Resistance to trimethoprim is the result of plasmid-directed synthesis of a *dihydrofolate reductase* with low or zero affinity for trimethoprim. It is transferred by transduction and may be spread by transposons.

Sulfonamide resistance in many bacteria is plasmid-mediated and results from the production of a form of *dihydropteroate synthetase* with a low affinity for sulfonamides but no change in affinity for PABA. Bacteria causing serious infections have been found to carry plasmids with resistance genes to both sulfonamides and trimethoprim.

CURRENT STATUS OF ANTIBIOTIC RESISTANCE IN BACTERIA

The most disturbing development of resistance has been in staphylococci, one of the commonest causes of hospital bloodstream infections, many strains of which are now resistant to almost all currently available antibiotics. In addition to resistance to some

---

Biochemical mechanisms of resistance to antibiotics

- The principal mechanisms are as follow.
  - *Production of enzymes that inactivate the drug:* for example β-lactamases, which inactivate penicillin; acetyltransferases, which inactivate chloramphenicol; kinases and other enzymes, which inactivate aminoglycosides.
  - *Alteration of the drug-binding sites:* this occurs with aminoglycosides, erythromycin, penicillin.
  - *Reduction of drug uptake by the bacterium:* for example tetracyclines.
  - *Alteration of enzyme pathways:* for example dihydrofolate reductase becomes insensitive to trimethoprim.

β-lactams through production of β-lactamase and the production of an additional β-lactam–binding protein that also renders them resistant to methicillin, *S. aureus* may also manifest resistance to other antibiotics as follows:

- to **streptomycin** (because of chromosomally determined alterations of target site)
- to aminoglycosides in general (because of altered target site and plasmid-determined inactivating enzymes)
- to chloramphenicol and the macrolides (because of plasmid-determined enzymes)
- to trimethoprim (because of transposon-encoded drug-resistant dihydrofolate reductase)
- to sulfonamides (because of chromosomally determined increased production of PABA)
- to rifampicin (because of chromosomally and plasmid-determined increases in efflux of the drug)
- to **fusidic acid** (because of chromosomally determined decreased affinity of the target site or a plasmid-encoded decreased permeability to the drug)
- to quinolones, for example ciprofloxacin and norfloxacin (because of chromosomally determined reduced uptake).

Infections with MRSA have become a major problem, particularly in hospitals, where they can spread rapidly among elderly and/or seriously ill patients, and patients with burns or wounds. In a number of hospitals, surgical wards have been closed because of the high rates of infection among patients. Until recently, the glycopeptide vancomycin was the antibiotic of last resort against MRSA but, ominously, strains of MRSA showing decreased susceptibility to this drug were isolated from hospitalised patients in the USA and Japan in 1997.[4] MRSA infections are rising; Bax et al. (2000) report prevalence in US hospitals as rising from 11–13% in 1985/6 to 26% in 1998.

The fact that vancomycin resistance seems to have developed spontaneously could have major clinical implications—and not only for nosocomial (those contracted in hospital) MRSA infections. It had been thought that antibiotic-resistant bacteria were dangerous only to seriously ill, hospitalised patients, in that the genetic burden of multiple resistance genes would lead to reduced virulence. Distressingly, however, there is now evidence that the spectrum and frequency of disease produced by methicillin-susceptible and methicillin-resistant staphylococci are similar.

In the past few years, *enterococci* have been rapidly developing resistance to many chemotherapeutic agents and have emerged as the second most common nosocomial pathogen. Non-pathogenic enterococci are ubiquitous in the intestine, have intrinsic resistance to many antibacterial drugs, and can readily become resistant to other agents by taking up plasmids and transposons carrying the relevant resistance genes. Such resistance is easily transferred to invading pathogenic enterococci.

Enterococci, already multiresistant, have recently developed resistance to vancomycin. This is apparently achieved by substitution of D-Ala-D-Ala with D-Ala-D-lactate in the peptide chain attached to *N*-acetylglucosamine-*N*-acetylmuramic acid (G-M) during the first steps of peptidoglycan synthesis (see Fig. 45.3 and Ch. 46). This is becoming a major problem in hospitalised patients, and in the USA vancomycin resistance has increased from 0.5% to 18% in less than a decade (Bax et al., 2000). A particular concern is the possibility of transfer of vancomycin resistance from enterococci to staphylococci, because they can coexist in the same patient.

Many other pathogens are developing or have developed resistance to commonly used drugs. This list includes *Pseudomonas aeruginosa, Streptococcus pyogenes, Streptococcus pneumoniae, Neisseria meningitidis, N. gonorrhoeae, Haemophilius influenzae* and *H. ducreyi*, as well as *Mycobacterium, Campylobacter* and *Bacteroides* species. Some strains of *M. tuberculosis* are now able to evade every antibiotic in the clinician's armamentarium, and tuberculosis, once easily treatable, is now reported to be causing more deaths worldwide than malaria and AIDS together. The only antibiotic that seems to defy resistance (at least at the time of writing) is **linezolid**, a relatively new oxazolidinone drug with a novel mechanism of action (see Zurenko et al., 2001, and Ch. 46).

Prescribers and consumers must also bear a responsibility for the burgeoning problem of resistance. Indiscriminate use of antibiotics in human and veterinary medicine, and their use in animal foodstuffs, has undoubtedly encouraged the growth of resistant strains. Some governmental and regulatory bodies (e.g. the European Union) have devised political and social measures to curb such excesses, and these have been at least partly successful (reviewed by Bax et al., 2000).

The issue around declining antibiotic efficacy is, however, not solely to do with bacterial countermeasures. The fact is that there has been a declining interest in the pharmaceutical industry in researching novel antibiotics. Historically, the area has been one of the mainstays of the industry, but most of the drugs available today are the result of incremental changes in the structures of a relatively small number of basic molecular structures, such as the β-lactam nucleus. By common consent, the days when it was possible to discover new and effective drugs in this way are long gone.

Hubris has also played a part. In 1967, the US Surgeon General effectively announced that infectious diseases had been vanquished, and that the researchers should turn their attention to chronic diseases instead. As a result, many pharmaceutical companies scaled down their efforts in the area, and only in the past few years has activity been resumed as the pressing need for novel compounds has been recognised (see Bax et al., 2000; Barrett & Barrett, 2003).

However, nature has endowed micro-organisms with fiendishly effective adaptive mechanisms for outwitting our best therapeutic strategies, and so far several have been effortlessly keeping pace with our attempts to eradicate them. This challenging situation has been reviewed in depth by Shlaes (2003) and Barrett & Barrett (2003).

---

[4]Noble et al. have transferred vancomycin resistance from enterococci to staphylococci. If this occured in a clinical environment, it would be disastrous. Some microbiologists have suggested that Noble and his team should be autoclaved.

Multidrug resistance

- Many pathogenic bacteria have developed resistance to the commonly used antibiotics. Examples include:
  - some strains of staphylococci and enterococci that are resistant to virtually all current antibiotics, the resistance being transferred by transposons and/or plasmids; such organisms can cause serious and virtually untreatable nosocomial infections
  - some strains of Mycobacterium tuberculosis that have become resistant to most antituberculosis agents.

REFERENCES AND FURTHER READING

General reading

Amyes S G B 2001 Magic bullets, lost horizons: the rise and fall of antibiotics. Taylor & Francis, London (*Thought-provoking book by a bacteriologist with wide experience in bacterial resistance and genetics; he opines that unless the problem of antibiotic resistance is solved in the next 5 years, 'we are going to slip further into the abyss of uncontrollable infection'*)

Bush K, Macielag M 2000 New approaches in the treatment of bacterial infections. Curr Opin Chem Biol 4: 433–439 (*Concise discussion of new antibacterial agents in phase II or phase III trial or already approved*)

Croft S L 1997 The current status of antiparasite chemotherapy. Parasitology 114: S3–S15 (*Comprehensive coverage of current drugs for protozoal, coccidial and helminth infections, with outline of approaches to possible future agents*)

Knodler L A, Celli J, Finlay B B 2001 Pathogenic trickery: deception of host cell processes. Mol Cell Biol 2: 578–588 (*Discusses bacterial ploys to subvert or block normal host cellular processes: mimicking the ligands for host cell receptors or signalling pathways. Useful list of examples.*)

Martin R J, Robertson A P 2000 Electrophysiological investigation of anthelmintic resistance. Parasitology 120(suppl): S87–S94 (*Uses patch clamp technique to study ion channels in resistant and non-resistant nematode tissue*)

Recchia G D, Hall R M 1995 Gene cassettes: a new class of mobile element. Microbiology 141: 3015–3027 (*Detailed coverage of this unusual mechanism*)

Shlaes D M 2003 The abandonment of antibacterials: why and wherefore? Curr Opin Pharmacol 3: 470–473 (*A good review that explains the reasons underlying the resistance problem and the regulatory and other hurdles that must be overcome before new antibacterials appear on to the market; almost apocalyptic in tone*)

Tan Y T, Tillett D J, McKay I A 2000 Molecular strategies for overcoming antibiotic resistance in bacteria. Mol Med Today 6: 309–314 (*Succinct article reviewing strategies to exploit advances in molecular biology to develop new antibiotics that overcome resistance; useful glossary of relevant terms*)

Zasloff M 2002 Antimicrobial peptides of multicellular organisms. Nature 415: 389–395 (*Thought-provoking article about the potent broad-spectrum antimicrobial peptides possessed by both animals and plants, which are used to fend off a wide range of microbes; it is suggested that exploiting these might be one answer to the problem of antibiotic resistance*)

Zurenko G E, Gibson J K, Shinabarger D L et al. 2001. Oxazolidinones: a new class of antibacterials. Curr Opin Pharmacol 1: 470–476 (*A ray of hope!*)

Drug resistance

Barrett C T, Barrett J F 2003 Antibacterials: are the new entries enough to deal with the emerging resistance problem? Curr Opin Biotechnol 14: 621–626 (*Good general review with some compelling examples and a round-up of new drug candidates*)

Bax R, Mullan N, Verhoef J 2000 The millennium bugs—the need for and development of new antibacterials. Int J Antimicrob Agents 16: 51–59 (*Excellent review of the problem of resistance and some of the new agents in the pipeline*)

Courvalin P, Trieu-Cout 2001 Minimizing potential resistance: the molecular view. Clin Infect Dis 33: S138–S146 (*Reviews the potential contribution of molecular biology to preventing the spread of resistant bacteria*)

Foley M, Tilley L 1997 Quinoline antimalarials: mechanisms of action and resistance. Int J Parasitol 27: 231–240 (*Good, short review; useful diagrams*)

Hawkey P M 1998 The origins and molecular basis of antibiotic resistance. Br Med J 7159: 657–659 (*Succinct overview of resistance; useful, simple diagrams; this is one of 12 papers on resistance in this issue of the journal*)

Jones M E, Peters E et al. 1997 Widespread occurrence of integrons causing multiple antibiotic resistance in bacteria. Lancet 349: 1742–1743

Levy S B 1998a Antibacterial resistance: bacteria on the defence. Br Med J 7159: 612–613 (*Resistance seen from the point of view of the bacterium; this is one of seven editorial articles on the subject of resistance in this issue of the journal*)

Levy S B 1998b The challenge of antibiotic resistance. Sci Am March: 32–39 (*Simple, clear review by an expert in the field; excellent diagrams*)

Michel M, Gutman L 1997 Methicillin-resistant *Staphylococcus aureus* and vancomycin-resistant enterococci: therapeutic realities and possibilities. Lancet 349: 1901–1906 (*Good review article; useful diagram; suggests schemes for medical management of infections caused by resistant organisms*)

Noble W C 1992 FEMS Microbiol Lett 72: 195–198.

St Georgiev V 2000 Membrane transporters and antifungal drug resistance. Curr Drug Targets 1: 184–261 (*Discusses various aspects of multidrug resistance in disease-causing fungi in the context of targeted drug development*)

van Belkum A 2000 Molecular epidemiology of methicillin-resistant *Staphylococcus aureus* strains: state of affairs and tomorrow's possibilities. Microb Drug Resist 6: 173–187

Walsh C 2000 Molecular mechanisms that confer antibacterial drug resistance. Nature 406: 775–781 (*Excellent review outlining the mechanisms of action of antibiotics and the resistance ploys of bacteria; very good diagrams*)

Woodford N 2005 Biological counterstrike: antibiotic resistance mechanisms of Gram-positive cocci. Clin Microbiol Infect 3: 2–21 (*A useful reference that classifies antibiotic resistance as one of the major public health concerns of the 21st century and discusses drug treatment for resistant strains*)

Antibacterial drugs

46

OVERVIEW

A detailed classification of the bacteria of medical importance is beyond the scope of this book, but a short list of common clinically important micro-organisms is given in Table 46.1, together with the principal chemotherapeutic agents in use and a general indication of their antibacterial actions. Characteristic diseases caused by these organisms are also highlighted, but it must be understood that most of these pathogens can produce a spectrum of illness.

INTRODUCTION

Many organisms (see Table 46.1) can be classified as being either *Gram-positive* or *Gram-negative* depending on whether or not they stain with Gram's stain.[1] This is not merely a taxonomic device, as it reflects several fundamental differences in (for example) the structure of their cell walls, and this in turn has implications for the action of antibiotics.

The cell wall of Gram-positive organisms is a relatively simple structure, 15–50 nm thick. It comprises about 50% peptidoglycan (see Ch. 45), 40–45% acidic polymer (which results in the cell surface being highly polar and carrying a negative charge) and 5–10% proteins and polysaccharides. The strongly polar polymer layer influences the penetration of ionised molecules and favours the penetration into the cell of positively charged compounds such as **streptomycin**.

The cell wall of Gram-negative organisms is much more complex. From the plasma membrane outwards, it consists of the following:

- a *periplasmic space* containing enzymes and other components
- a *peptidoglycan layer* 2 nm in thickness, forming 5% of the cell wall mass, that is often linked to outwardly projecting lipoprotein molecules
- an *outer membrane* consisting of a lipid bilayer, similar in some respects to the plasma membrane, that contains protein molecules and (on its inner aspect) lipoproteins linked to the peptidoglycan. Other proteins form transmembrane water-filled channels, termed *porins*, through which hydrophilic antibiotics can move freely.
- *complex polysaccharides* forming important components of the outer surface. These differ between strains of bacteria and are the main determinants of the antigenicity. The complex polysaccharides constitute the source of *endotoxin*, which, in vivo, trigger various aspects of the inflammatory reaction by activating complement, causing fever, etc. (see Ch. 13).

Difficulty in penetrating this complex outer layer is probably the reason why some antibiotics are less active against Gram-negative

---

[1]Named after the eponymous Danish physician who devised the technique.

e 46.1 General choice of antibiotics against common or important micro-organisms[a]

Micro-organism(s)[b]	First-choice antibiotic(s)[c]	Second-choice antibiotic(s)[c]
Gram-positive cocci		
Staphylococcus (boils, infection of wounds, etc.)		
Non–β-lactamase-producing	Benzylpenicillin (penicillin G) or phenoxymethylpenicillin (penicillin V)	A cephalosporin or vancomycin
β-lactamase-producing	A β-lactamase–resistant penicillin (e.g. flucloxacillin)	A cephalosporin or vancomycin, or a macrolide, or a quinolone
Methicillin-resistant	Vancomycin ± gentamicin ± rifampicin (rifampin)	Co-trimoxazole, or ciprofloxacin, or a macrolide ± fusidic acid, or rifampicin
Methicillin/vancomycin-resistant	Quinupristin/dalfopristin or linezolid	–
Streptococcus, haemolytic types (septic infections, e.g. bacteraemia, scarlet fever, toxic shock syndrome)	Benzylpenicillin or phenoxymethylpenicillin ± an aminoglycoside	A cephalosporin, or a macrolide, or vancomycin.
Enterococcus (endocarditis)	Benzylpenicillin + gentamicin	Vancomycin
Pneumococcus (pneumonia)	Benzylpenicillin or phenoxymethylpenicillin or ampicillin, or a macrolide	A cephalosporin
Gram-negative cocci		
Morasella catarrhalis (sinusitis)	Amoxicillin + clavulanic acid	Ciproxafloxacin
Neisseria gonorrhoeae (gonorrhoea)	Amoxicillin + clavulanic acid, or ceftriaxone	Cefotaxime, or a quinolone
Neisseria meningitidis (meningitis)	Benzylpenicillin	Chloramphenicol, or cefotaxime, or minocycline
Gram-positive rods		
Corynebacterium (diphtheria)	A macrolide	Benzylpenicillin
Clostridium (tetanus, gangrene)	Benzylpenicillin	A tetracycline, or a cephalosporin
Listeria monocytogenes (rare cause of meningitis and generalised infection in neonates)	Amoxicillin ± an aminoglycoside	Erythromycin ± an aminoglycoside
Gram-negative rods		
Enterobacteriaceae (coliform organisms) *Escherichia coli, Enterobacter, Klebsiella*		
Infections of urinary tract	An oral cephalosporin, or a quinolone	Extended-spectrum penicillin
Septicaemia	An aminoglycoside (intravenous) or cefuroxime	Imipenem or a quinolone
Shigella (dysentery)	A quinolone	Ampicillin or trimethoprim
Salmonella (typhoid, paratyphoid)	A quinolone or ceftriaxone	Amoxicillin or chloramphenicol or trimethoprim
Haemophilus influenzae (infections of the respiratory tract, ear, sinuses; meningitis)	Ampicillin or cefuroxime	Cefuroxime (not for meningitis) or chloramphenicol
Bordetella pertussis (whooping cough)	A macrolide	Ampicillin
Pasteurella multocida (wound infections, abscess)	Amoxicillin + clavulanic acid	Ampicillin
Vibrio cholerae (cholera)	A tetracycline	A quinolone
Legionella pneumophila (pneumonia, legionnaires disease)	A macrolide ± rifampicin	–
Helicobacter pylori (associated with peptic ulcer)	Metronidazole + amoxicillin + ranitidine[d] (2-week regimen)	Clarithromycin + metronidazole
Pseudomonas aeruginosa		
Urinary tract infection	A quinolone	Antipseudomonal penicillins
Other infections (of burns etc.)	Antipseudomonal penicillins + tobramycin[e]	Imipenem ± an aminoglycoside, or ceftazidime
Brucella (brucellosis)	Doxycycline + rifampicin	–
Bacteroides fragilis		
Oropharyngeal infection	Benzylpenicillin	Metronidazole or clindamycin
Gastrointestinal infection	Metronidazole, clindamycin	Imipenem
Gram-negative anaerobic rods (other than *B. fragilis*)	Benzylpenicillin or metronidazole	A cephalosporin or clindamycin
Campylobacter (diarrhoea)	A macrolide or a quinolone	A tetracycline or gentamicin
Spirochaetes		
Treponema (syphilis, yaws)	Benzylpenicillin	A macrolide or ceftriaxone

Table 46.1 (continued) General choice of antibiotics against common or important micro-organisms[a]

Micro-organism(s)[b]	First-choice antibiotic(s)[c]	Second-choice antibiotic(s)[c]
Borrelia recurrentis (relapsing fever)	A tetracycline	Benzylpenicillin
Borrelia burgdorferi (Lyme disease)	A tetracycline	–
Leptospira (Weil's disease)	Benzylpenicillin	A tetracycline
Rickettsiae (typhus, tick-bite fever, Q fever, etc.)	A tetracycline	A quinolone
Other organisms		
Mycoplasma pneumoniae	A tetracycline or a macrolide	Ciprofloxacin
Chlamydia (trachoma, psittacosis, urogenital infections)	A tetracycline	–
Actinomyces (abscesses)	Benzylpenicillin	A tetracycline
Pneumocystis (pneumonia, especially in AIDS patients)	Co-trimoxazole (high dose)	Pentamidine or atovaquone or trimetrexate
Nocardia (lung disease, brain abscess)	Co-trimoxazole	–

[a] This table is not meant to be a definitive guide for clinical treatment but a general indication of the main antimicrobial actions and thus of the overall usefulness of commonly used antibiotics. For a more comprehensive list, see Laurence et al. (1997).
[b] Only the main diseases caused by each organism are mentioned (in parentheses).
[c] ± signifies that an agent is to be used with or without another agent; if agents are to be used concomitantly, a plus sign only is used.
[d] An antiulcer drug, not an antibiotic (see Ch. 25).
[e] Not in the same syringe.

than Gram-positive bacteria. This is the basis of the extraordinary antibiotic resistance exhibited by *Pseudomonas aeruginosa*, a pathogen that can cause life-threatening infections in neutropenic patients and those with burns and wounds.

The cell wall lipopolysaccharide is also a major barrier to penetration. Antibiotics affected include **benzylpenicillin** (penicillin G), **methicillin**, the macrolides, **rifampicin** (**rifampin**), **fusidic acid**, **vancomycin**, **bacitracin** and **novobiocin**.

ANTIMICROBIAL AGENTS THAT INTERFERE WITH THE SYNTHESIS OR ACTION OF FOLATE

SULFONAMIDES

In a landmark discovery in the 1930s, Domagk demonstrated that it was possible for a drug to influence the course of a bacterial infection. The agent was **prontosil**, a dye that proved to be an inactive prodrug but which is metabolised in vivo to give the active product, **sulfanilamide** (Fig. 46.1). Many sulfonamides have been developed since, and some are still useful drugs although their importance has declined in the face of increasing resistance. Examples include **sulfadiazine** (Fig. 46.1), **sulfadimidine** (short acting), **sulfamethoxazole** (intermediate acting), **sulfametopyrazine** (long acting), **sulfasalazine** (poorly absorbed in the gastrointestinal tract; see also Chs 14 and 25) and sulfamethoxazole (in combination with **trimethoprim** as **co-trimoxazole**). In the UK, only sulfamethoxazole, sulfadiazine and trimethoprim are used clinically.

Mechanism of action

Sulfanilamide is a structural analogue of *p*-aminobenzoic acid (PABA; see Fig. 46.1), which is an essential precursor in the synthesis of folic acid in bacteria. As explained in Chapter 45, folate is required for the synthesis of the precursors of DNA and RNA both in bacteria and in mammals, but whereas bacteria need to synthesise folic acid, mammals can obtain it from dietary sources. Sulfonamides compete with PABA for the enzyme *dihydropteroate synthetase*, and the effect of the sulfonamide may be overcome by adding excess PABA. This is why some local anaesthetics, which are PABA esters (such as procaine; see Ch. 44), can antagonise the antibacterial effect of these agents.

The action of a sulfonamide is to inhibit *growth* of the bacteria, not to *kill* them; that is to say, it is *bacteriostatic* rather than *bactericidal*. The action is vitiated in the presence of pus or products of tissue breakdown, because these contain thymidine and purines, which bacteria utilise directly, bypassing the requirement for folic acid. Resistance to the drugs, which is common, is plasmid-mediated (see Ch. 45) and results from the synthesis of a bacterial enzyme insensitive to the drug.

Pharmacokinetic aspects

Most sulfonamides are readily absorbed in the gastrointestinal tract and reach maximum concentrations in the plasma in 4–6 hours. They are usually not given topically because of the risk of sensitisation or allergic reactions.

The drugs pass into inflammatory exudates and cross both placental and blood–brain barriers. They are metabolised mainly in the liver, the major product being an acetylated derivative that lacks antibacterial action.

Unwanted effects

Mild to moderate side effects include nausea and vomiting, headache and mental depression. Cyanosis caused by methaemoglobinaemia may occur but is a lot less alarming than it looks. Serious adverse effects necessitating cessation of therapy

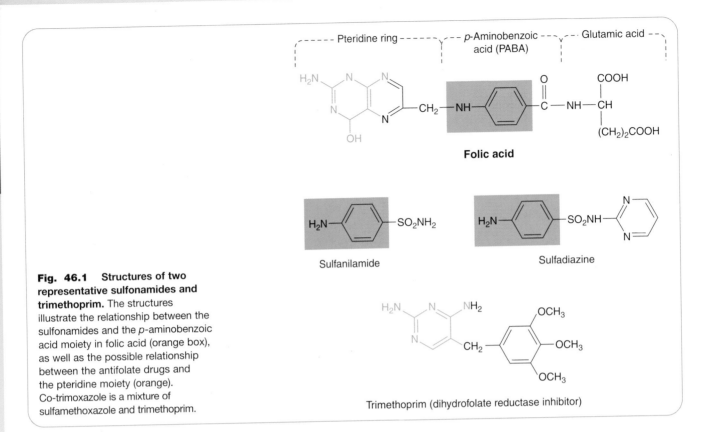

Fig. 46.1 Structures of two representative sulfonamides and trimethoprim. The structures illustrate the relationship between the sulfonamides and the *p*-aminobenzoic acid moiety in folic acid (orange box), as well as the possible relationship between the antifolate drugs and the pteridine moiety (orange). Co-trimoxazole is a mixture of sulfamethoxazole and trimethoprim.

include hepatitis, hypersensitivity reactions (rashes, fever, anaphylactoid reactions), bone marrow depression and crystalluria. This last effect results from the precipitation of acetylated metabolites in the urine.

TRIMETHOPRIM

Mechanism of action

Trimethoprim is chemically related to the antimalarial drug **pyrimethamine** (Fig. 49.3), both being folate antagonists. Struc-

turally (Fig. 46.1), it resembles the pteridine moiety of folate and the similarity is close enough to fool the bacterial *dihydrofolate reductase*, which is many times more sensitive to trimethoprim than the equivalent enzyme in humans (Table 45.1).

Trimethoprim is active against most common bacterial pathogens, and it too is bacteriostatic. It is sometimes given as a mixture with sulfamethoxazole in a combination called co-trimoxazole (Fig. 46.1). Because sulfonamides inhibit the same bacterial metabolic pathway, but upstream from dihydrofolate reductase, they can potentiate the action of trimethoprim (see Fig. 46.2). In the UK, its use is generally restricted to the treatment of *Pneumocystis carinii* pneumonia, toxoplasmosis and nocardiasis,

Pharmacokinetic aspects

Trimethoprim is given orally. It is fully absorbed from the gastrointestinal tract and widely distributed throughout the tissues and body fluids. It reaches high concentrations in the lungs and kidneys, and fairly high concentrations in the cerebrospinal fluid (CSF). When given with sulfamethoxazole, about half the dose of each is excreted within 24 hours. Because trimethoprim is a weak base, its elimination by the kidney increases with decreasing urinary pH.

Unwanted effects

Unwanted effects of trimethoprim include nausea, vomiting, blood disorders and skin rashes. Folate deficiency, with resultant *megaloblastic anaemia* (see Ch. 22)—a toxic effect related to the pharmacological action of trimethoprim—can be prevented by giving folinic acid.

Clinical uses of sulfonamides

- Combined with **trimethoprim (co-trimoxazole)** for *Pneumocystis carinii*.
- Combined with **pyrimethamine** for drug-resistant *malaria* (Table 49.1), and for toxoplasmosis.
- In *inflammatory bowel disease:* **sulfasalazine (sulfapyridine–aminosalicylate** combination) is used (see Ch. 14, clinical box on p. 242).
- For infected *burns* (silver *sulfadiazine* given topically).
- For some sexually transmitted infections (e.g. *trachoma, chlamydia, chancroid*).
- For respiratory infections: use now confined to a few special problems (e.g. infection with *Nocardia*).
- For acute urinary tract infection (now seldom used).

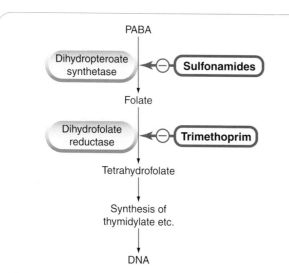

Fig. 46.2 **The action of sulfonamides and trimethoprim on bacterial folate synthesis.** See Figure 22.2 for more detail of tetrahydrofolate synthesis, and Table 45.1 for comparisons of antifolate drugs. PABA, *p*-aminobenzoic acid.

Clinical uses of trimethoprim/ co-trimoxazole

- For urinary tract and respiratory infections: **trimethoprim**, used on its own, is usually preferred.
- For infection with *Pneumocystis carinii*, which causes pneumonia in patients with AIDS: **co-trimoxazole** is used in high dose.

Antimicrobial agents that interfere with the synthesis or action of folate

- Sulfonamides are bacteriostatic; they act by interfering with folate synthesis and thus with nucleotide synthesis. Unwanted effects include crystalluria and hypersensitivities.
- Trimethoprim is bacteriostatic. It acts by antagonising folate.
- Co-trimoxazole is a mixture of trimethoprim with sulfamethoxazole, which affects bacterial nucleotide synthesis at two points in the pathway.

β-LACTAM ANTIBIOTICS

PENICILLIN

In 1928, Alexander Fleming, working at St Mary's Hospital in London, observed that a culture plate on which staphylococci were being grown had become contaminated with a mould of the genus *Penicillium*, and that bacterial growth in the vicinity of the mould had been inhibited. He isolated the mould in pure culture and demonstrated that it produced an antibacterial substance, which he called **penicillin**. This substance was subsequently extracted and its antibacterial effects analysed by Florey, Chain and their colleagues at Oxford in 1940. They showed that it had powerful chemotherapeutic properties in infected mice, and that it was non-toxic.

The remarkable antibacterial effects of penicillin in humans were clearly demonstrated in 1941. A small amount of penicillin, extracted laboriously from crude cultures in the laboratories of the Dunn School of Pathology in Oxford, was given to a policeman who had staphylococcal and streptococcal septicaemia with multiple abscesses, and osteomyelitis with discharging sinuses. He was in great pain and was desperately ill, and although sulfonamides were available, they would have had no effect in the presence of pus. Intravenous injections of penicillin were given to the policeman every 3 hours. All the patient's urine was collected, and each day the bulk of the excreted penicillin was extracted and reused. After 5 days, the patient's condition was vastly improved; his temperature was normal, he was eating well, and there was obvious resolution of the abscesses. Furthermore, there seemed to be no toxic effects of the drug. Unfortunately, when the supply of penicillin was finally exhausted his condition gradually deteriorated and he died a month later.

Although this was the first evidence of the dramatic antibacterial effect of penicillin when given systemically in humans, topical penicillin had actually been used with success in five patients with eye infections 10 years previously by Paine, a graduate of St Mary's who had obtained some penicillin mould from Fleming.

While the penicillins are extremely effective antibiotics and are very widely used, they may be destroyed by bacterial amidases and β-lactamases (penicillinases) (see Fig. 46.3).

Mechanisms of action

All β-lactam antibiotics interfere with the synthesis of the bacterial cell wall peptidoglycan (see Ch. 45, Fig. 45.3). After attachment to *penicillin-binding proteins* on bacteria (there may be seven or more types in different organisms), they inhibit the transpeptidation enzyme that cross-links the peptide chains attached to the backbone of the peptidoglycan.

The final bactericidal event is the inactivation of an inhibitor of autolytic enzymes in the cell wall, leading to lysis of the bacterium. Some organisms, referred to as 'tolerant', have defective autolytic enzymes and are inhibited but not lysed in the presence of the drug. Resistance to penicillin may result from a number of different causes and is discussed in detail in Chapter 45.

Types of penicillin and their antimicrobial activity

The first penicillins were the naturally occurring benzylpenicillin and its congeners, including **phenoxymethylpenicillin**. Benzylpenicillin is active against a wide range of organisms and is the drug of first choice for many infections (see Table 46.1 and the clinical box). Its main drawbacks are poor absorption in the gastrointestinal tract (which means it must be given by injection) and its susceptibility to bacterial β-lactamases.

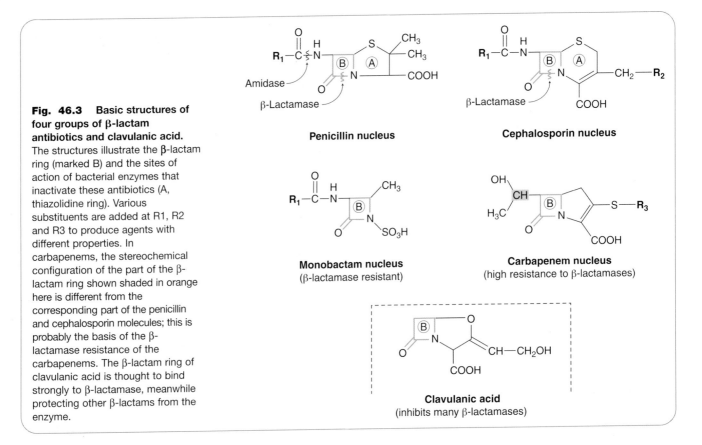

Fig. 46.3 Basic structures of four groups of β-lactam antibiotics and clavulanic acid. The structures illustrate the β-lactam ring (marked B) and the sites of action of bacterial enzymes that inactivate these antibiotics (A, thiazolidine ring). Various substituents are added at R1, R2 and R3 to produce agents with different properties. In carbapenems, the stereochemical configuration of the part of the β-lactam ring shown shaded in orange here is different from the corresponding part of the penicillin and cephalosporin molecules; this is probably the basis of the β-lactamase resistance of the carbapenems. The β-lactam ring of clavulanic acid is thought to bind strongly to β-lactamase, meanwhile protecting other β-lactams from the enzyme.

Various semisynthetic penicillins have been prepared by adding different side-chains to the penicillin nucleus (at R1 in Fig. 46.3). In this way, β-lactamase–resistant penicillins (e.g. **flucloxacillin**) and broad-spectrum penicillins (e.g. **ampicillin**, **pivampicillin** and **amoxicillin**) have been produced. Extended-spectrum penicillins (e.g. **ticarcilin**) with antipseudomonal activity have also been developed and have gone some way to overcoming the problem of serious infections caused by *P. aeruginosa*. Amoxicillin is sometimes combined with β-lactam inhibitor **clavulanic acid** as **co-amoxiclav**.

Pharmacokinetic aspects

When given orally, different penicillins are absorbed to differing degrees depending on their stability in acid and their adsorption to foodstuffs in the gut. Penicillins can be given by intramuscular or intravenous injection, but intrathecal administration is inadvisable, particularly in the case of benzylpenicillin, as it can cause convulsions.

The penicillins are widely distributed in body fluids, passing into joints; into pleural and pericardial cavities; into bile, saliva and milk; and across the placenta. Being lipid-insoluble, they do not enter mammalian cells and do not, therefore, cross the blood–brain barrier unless the meninges are inflamed, in which case they readily reach therapeutically effective concentrations in the CSF as well.

Elimination of most penicillins occurs rapidly and is mainly renal, 90% being through tubular secretion. The relatively short plasma half-life is a potential problem in the clinical use of benzylpenicillin, although because penicillin works by preventing cell wall synthesis

in dividing organisms, intermittent rather than continuous exposure to the drug can be an advantage.

Clinical use of the penicillins

Penicillins, often combined with other antibiotics, are crucially important in antibacterial chemotherapy. They are the drugs of choice for many infections. A list of clinical uses is given in the clinical box and also in Table 46.1.

Unwanted effects

Penicillins are relatively free from direct toxic effects (other than their proconvulsant effect when given intrathecally). The main unwanted effects are hypersensitivity reactions caused by the degradation products of penicillin, which combine with host protein and become antigenic. Skin rashes and fever are common; a delayed type of serum sickness occurs infrequently. Much more serious is acute anaphylactic shock, which although fortunately very rare, may in some cases be fatal. When given orally, penicillins, particularly the broad-spectrum type, alter the bacterial flora in the gut. This can be associated with gastrointestinal disturbances and in some cases with suprainfection by other, penicillin-insensitive, micro-organisms.

CEPHALOSPORINS AND CEPHAMYCINS

Cephalosporins N and C, which are chemically related to penicillin, and cephalosporin P, a steroidal antibiotic that resembles fusidic acid (see below), were first isolated from *Cephalosporium*

Clinical uses of the penicillins

- Penicillins are given by mouth or, in more severe infections, intravenously, and often in combination with other antibiotics.
- Uses are for sensitive organisms and may (but may not: individual sensitivity testing is often appropriate depending on local conditions—see below) include:
  - *bacterial meningitis* (e.g. caused by *Neisseria meningitidis, Streptococcus pneumoniae*): **benzylpenicillin**, high doses intravenously
  - *bone* and *joint* infections (e.g. with *Staphylococcus aureus*): **flucloxacillin**
  - *skin* and *soft tissue* infections (e.g. with *Strep. pyogenes* or *Staph. aureus*): **benzylpenicillin, flucloxacillin**; animal bites: **co-amoxiclav**
  - *pharyngitis* (from *Strep. pyogenes*): **phenoxymethylpenicillin**
  - *otitis media* (organisms commonly include *Strep. pyogenes, Haemophilus influenzae*): **amoxicillin**
  - *bronchitis* (mixed infections common): **amoxicillin**
  - *pneumonia*: **amoxicillin**
  - *urinary tract infections* (e.g. with *Escherichia coli*): **amoxicillin**
  - *gonorrhea*: **amoxicillin** (plus probenecid)
  - *syphilis*: **procaine benzylpenicillin**
  - *endocarditis* (e.g. with *Strep. viridans* or *Enterococcus faecalis*)
  - serious infections with *Pseudomonas aeruginosa*: **ticarcillin, piperacillin**.
- This list is not exhaustive. Treatment with penicillins is sometimes started empirically, if the likely causative organism is one thought to be susceptible to penicillin, while awaiting the results of laboratory tests to identify the organism and determine its antibiotic susceptibility.

Mechanism of action

The mechanism of action of these agents is similar to that of the penicillins: interference with bacterial peptidoglycan synthesis after binding to the β-lactam–binding proteins. This is described in detail in Chapter 45 and illustrated in Figure 45.3. Resistance to this group of drugs has increased because of plasmid-encoded or chromosomal β-lactamase. Nearly all Gram-negative bacteria have a chromosomal gene coding for a β-lactamase that is more active in hydrolysing cephalosporins than penicillins, and in several organisms a single mutation can result in high-level constitutive production of this enzyme. Resistance also occurs when there is decreased penetration of the drug as a result of alterations to outer membrane proteins, or mutations of the binding-site proteins.

Pharmacokinetic aspects

Some cephalosporins may be given orally (see Table 46.2), but most are given parenterally, intramuscularly (which may be painful) or intravenously. After absorption, they are widely distributed in the body and some, such as cefotaxime, cefuroxime and ceftriaxone, cross the blood–brain barrier. Excretion is mostly via the kidney, largely by tubular secretion, but 40% of ceftriaxone is eliminated in the bile.

Clinical use

Some clinical uses of the cephalosporins are given in Table 46.2 and in the clinical box.

Unwanted effects

Hypersensitivity reactions, very similar to those seen with penicillin, may occur, and there may be some cross-sensitivity; about 10% of penicillin-sensitive individuals will have allergic reactions to cephalosporins. Nephrotoxicity has been reported (especially with cefradine), as has drug-induced alcohol intolerance. Diarrhoea can occur with oral cephalosporins and **cefoperazone**.

---

fungus. The cephamycins are β-lactam antibiotics produced by *Streptomyces* organisms, and they are closely related to the cephalosporins.

Semisynthetic *broad-spectrum cephalosporins* have been produced by addition, to the cephalosporin C nucleus, of different side-chains at R1 and/or R2 (see Fig. 46.3). These agents are water-soluble and relatively acid-stable. They vary in susceptibility to β-lactamases. There are now a very large number of cephalosporins and cephamycins available for clinical use. Original members of the group such as cefradine, **cefalexin** and **cefradoxil** have largely been replaced with 'second-generation' drugs such as **cefuroxime**, **cefalcor** and **cefprozil**, or 'third-generation' drugs such as **cefotaxime**, **ceftazidime** and **ceftriaxone**. The actions and properties of some of these drugs are described in Table 46.2.

Clinical uses of the cephalosporins

- Cephalosporins are used to treat infections caused by sensitive organisms. As with other antibiotics, patterns of sensitivity vary geographically, and treatment is often started empirically. Many different kinds of infection may be treated, including:
  - *septicaemia* (e.g. **cefuroxime, cefotaxime**)
  - *pneumonia* caused by susceptible organisms
  - *meningitis* (e.g. **ceftriaxone, cefotaxime**)
  - *biliary tract infection*
  - *urinary tract infection* (especially in pregnancy or in patients unresponsive to other drugs)
  - *sinusitis* (e.g. **cefadroxil**).

Table 46.2 Cephalosporins and cephamycins

Categories, with example(s)	Important properties	Similar drug(s)
Oral drugs Cefalexin ($t_{1/2}$ 1 h)	An example of the first-generation compounds that have reasonable activity against Gram-positive organisms and modest activity against Gram-negative organisms	Cefachlor ($t_{1/2}$ 0.8 h) is a second-generation compound with greater potency against Gram-negative organisms, but it can cause unwanted cutaneous lesions
Parenteral drugs Cefuroxime ($t_{1/2}$ 1.5 h)	An example of the second-generation compounds that show only moderate activity against most Gram-positive organisms but reasonable potency against Gram-negative organisms	Cephamandole, cefoxitin ($t_{1/2}$ of both ~1 h), good activity against Gram-negative organisms, resistant to β-lactamase from Gram-negative rods, good potency against *Bacteroides fragilis,* bowel flora
Cefotaxime ($t_{1/2}$ 1 h)	An example of the third-generation compounds, which are less active against Gram-positive bacteria than those of the second generation but more active against Gram-negative bacteria. Has some activity against pseudomonads.	Ceftizoxime ($t_{1/2}$ 1.5 h); ceftriaxone ($t_{1/2}$ 8.5 h), excreted largely in the bile; cefperazone ($t_{1/2}$ 2 h), excreted mainly in the bile, can cause decrease of vitamin K–dependent clotting factors.

OTHER β-LACTAM ANTIBIOTICS

CARBAPENEMS AND MONOBACTAMS

Carbapenems and monobactams (see Fig. 46.3) were developed to deal with β-lactamase–producing Gram-negative organisms resistant to penicillins.

CARBAPENEMS

Imipenem, an example of a carbapenem, acts in the same way as the other β-lactams (see Fig. 46.3). It has a very broad spectrum of antimicrobial activity, being active against many aerobic and anaerobic Gram-positive and Gram-negative organisms. However, many of the 'methicillin-resistant' staphylococci (see p. 656) are less susceptible, and resistant strains of *P. aeruginosa* have emerged during therapy. Imipenem was originally resistant to all β-lactamases, but some organisms now have chromosomal genes that code for imipenem-hydrolysing β-lactamases. It is sometimes given together with **cilastatin**, which inhibits its inactivation by renal enzymes. **Meropenem** is similar but is not metabolised by the kidney. **Ertapenem** has a broad spectrum of antibacterial actions but is licensed only for a limited range of indications.

Unwanted effects are generally similar to those seen with other β-lactams, nausea and vomiting being the most frequently seen. Neurotoxicity can occur with high plasma concentrations.

MONOBACTAMS

The main monobactam is **aztreonam**, a simple monocyclic β-lactam with a complex substituent at R3 (see Fig. 46.3), which is resistant to most β-lactamases. It is given parenterally and has a plasma half-life of 2 hours. Aztreonam has an unusual spectrum of activity and is effective only against Gram-negative aerobic rods such as pseudomonads, *Neisseria meningitidis* and *Haemophilus influenzae*. It has no action against Gram-positive organisms or anaerobes.

Unwanted effects are, in general, similar to those of other β-lactam antibiotics, but this agent does not necessarily cross-react immunologically with penicillin and its products, and so does not usually cause allergic reactions in penicillin-sensitive individuals.

ANTIMICROBIAL AGENTS AFFECTING BACTERIAL PROTEIN SYNTHESIS

TETRACYCLINES

Tetracyclines are broad-spectrum antibiotics. The group includes **tetracycline, oxytetracycline, demeclocycline, lymecycline, doxycycline** and **minocycline**.

Mechanism of action

Following uptake into susceptible organisms by active transport, tetracyclines act by inhibiting protein synthesis. This action is described in detail in Chapter 45 (see Fig. 45.4). The tetracyclines are regarded as bacteriostatic, not bactericidal.

Antibacterial spectrum

The spectrum of antimicrobial activity of the tetracyclines is very wide and includes Gram-positive and Gram-negative bacteria, *Mycoplasma, Rickettsia, Chlamydia* spp., spirochaetes and some protozoa (e.g. amoebae). Minocycline is also effective against *N. eningitidis* and has been used to eradicate this organism from the nasopharynx of carriers. However, widespread resistance to these agents has decreased their usefulness (see p. 658). Resistance is transmitted mainly by plasmids and, because the genes controlling resistance to tetracyclines are closely associated with

β-Lactam antibiotics

- Bactericidal by interference with peptidoglycan synthesis.

Penicillins

- The first choice for many infections.
- Benzylpenicillin:
  - given by injection, short half-life and is destroyed by β-lactamases
  - spectrum: Gram-positive and Gram-negative cocci and some Gram-negative bacteria
  - many staphylococci are now resistant.
- β-Lactamase–resistant penicillins (e.g. flucloxacillin):
  - given orally
  - spectrum: as for benzylpenicillin
  - many staphylococci are now resistant.
- Broad-spectrum penicillins (e.g. amoxicillin):
  - given orally; they are destroyed by β-lactamases
  - spectrum: as for benzylpenicillin (although less potent); they are also active against Gram-negative bacteria.
- Extended-spectrum penicillins (e.g. ticarcillin):
  - given orally; they are susceptible to β-lactamases
  - spectrum: as for broad-spectrum penicillins; they are also active against pseudomonads.
- Unwanted effects of penicillins: mainly hypersensitivities.
- A combination of clavulanic acid plus amoxicillin or ticarcillin is effective against many β-lactamase–producing organisms.

Cephalosporins and cephamycins

- Second choice for many infections.
- Oral drugs (e.g. cefachlor) are used in urinary infections.
- Parenteral drugs (e.g. cefuroxime, which is active against *Staphylococcus aureus*, *Haemophilus influenzae*, Enterobacteriaceae).
- Unwanted effects: mainly hypersensitivities.

Carbapenems

- Imipenem is used with cilastin, which blocks its breakdown in the kidney.
- Imipenem is a broad-spectrum antibiotic.

Monobactams

- Aztreonam is active only against Gram-negative aerobic bacteria and is resistant to most β-lactamases.

Clinical uses of tetracyclines

- The usefulness of tetracyclines has declined because of widespread drug resistance. Most members of the group are microbiologically similar; **doxycycline** is given once daily and may be used in patients with renal impairment. Uses (sometimes in combination with other antibiotics) include:
  - *rickettsial* and *chlamydial* infections, *brucellosis*, *anthrax* and *Lyme disease*
  - as useful second choice, for example in patients with allergies, for several infections (see Table 46.1), including *mycoplasma* and *leptospira*
  - mixed *respiratory tract infections* (e.g. exacerbations of *chronic bronchitis*)
  - *acne*
  - *inappropriate secretion of antidiuretic hormone* (e.g. by some malignant lung tumours), causing hyponataemia: **demeclocycline** inhibits the action of this hormone (Ch. 28, p. 426).

magnesium, iron, aluminium), forming non-absorbable complexes, absorption is decreased in the presence of milk, certain antacids and iron preparations. Minocycline and doxycycline are virtually completely absorbed.

Unwanted effects

The commonest unwanted effects are gastrointestinal disturbances caused initially by direct irritation and later by modification of the gut flora. Vitamin B complex deficiency can occur, as can suprainfection. Because they chelate Ca^{2+}, tetracyclines are deposited in growing bones and teeth, causing staining and sometimes dental hypoplasia and bone deformities. They should therefore not be given to children, pregnant women or nursing mothers. Another hazard to pregnant women is hepatotoxicity. Phototoxicity (sensitisation to sunlight) has also been seen, particularly with demeclocycline. Minocycline can produce dose-related vestibular disturbances (dizziness and nausea). High doses of tetracyclines can decrease protein synthesis in host cells—an antianabolic effect that may result in renal damage. Long-term therapy can cause disturbances of the bone marrow.

CHLORAMPHENICOL

Chloramphenicol was originally isolated from cultures of *Streptomyces*. The drug binds to the same site of the 50S subunit of the bacterial ribosome as **erythromycin** and **clindamycin**, and acts to inhibit bacterial protein synthesis as described in Chapter 45 (see Fig. 45.4). The clinical use of chloramphenicol is given in the box.

Antibacterial spectrum

Chloramphenicol has a wide spectrum of antimicrobial activity, including Gram-negative and Gram-positive organisms and rickett-

genes for resistance to other antibiotics, organisms may develop resistance to many drugs simultaneously. The clinical use of the tetracyclines is given in the clinical box.

Pharmacokinetic aspects

The tetracyclines are generally given orally but can also be administered parenterally. The absorption of most preparations from the gut is irregular and incomplete but may be improved in the absence of food. Because tetracyclines chelate metal ions (calcium,

Clinical uses of chloramphenicol

- Chloramphenicol should be reserved for serious infections in which the benefit of the drug outweighs its uncommon but serious haematological toxicity. Such uses may include:
  — infections caused by *Haemophilus influenzae* resistant to other drugs
  — *meningitis* in patients in whom penicillin cannot be used.
- It is also safe and effective in *bacterial conjunctivitis* (given topically).
- It is effective in *typhoid fever*, but **ciprofloxacin** or **amoxicillin** and **co-trimoxazole** are similarly effective and less toxic.
- Other possible uses are given in Table 46.1.

siae. It is bacteriostatic for most organisms but kills *H. influenzae*. Resistance, caused by the production of *chloramphenicol acetyltransferase* (see p. 658), is plasmid-mediated.

Pharmacokinetic aspects

Given orally, chloramphenicol is rapidly and completely absorbed and reaches its maximum concentration in the plasma within 2 hours; it can also be given parenterally. The drug is widely distributed throughout the tissues and body fluids including the CSF, where its concentration may reach 60% of that in the blood. In the plasma, it is 30–50% protein-bound, and its half-life is approximately 2 hours. About 10% is excreted unchanged in the urine, and the remainder is inactivated in the liver.

Unwanted effects

The most important unwanted effect of chloramphenicol is severe, idiosyncratic depression of the bone marrow, resulting in *pancytopenia* (a decrease in all blood cell elements)—an effect that, although rare, can occur even with very low doses in some individuals. Chloramphenicol should also be used with great care in newborns, because inadequate inactivation and excretion of the drug (see Ch. 52) can result in the 'grey baby syndrome'—vomiting, diarrhoea, flaccidity, low temperature and an ashen-grey colour—which carries 40% mortality. If its use is essential, plasma concentrations should be monitored and the dose adjusted accordingly. Hypersensitivity reactions can occur with the drug, as can gastrointestinal disturbances secondary to alteration of the intestinal microbial flora.

AMINOGLYCOSIDES

The aminoglycosides are a group of antibiotics of complex chemical structure, resembling each other in antimicrobial activity, pharmacokinetic characteristics and toxicity. The main agents are **gentamicin**, streptomycin, **amikacin, tobramycin, netilmicin** and **neomycin.**

Mechanism of action

Aminoglycosides inhibit bacterial protein synthesis (see Ch. 45). Their penetration through the cell membrane of the bacterium depends partly on oxygen-dependent active transport by a polyamine carrier system, and they have minimal action against anaerobic organisms. Chloramphenicol blocks this transport system. The effect of the aminoglycosides is bactericidal and is enhanced by agents that interfere with cell wall synthesis. Some clinical uses of the aminoglycosides are given in Table 46.1.

Resistance

Resistance to aminoglycosides is becoming a problem. It occurs through several different mechanisms, the most important being inactivation by microbial enzymes, of which nine or more are known. Amikacin was purposefully designed as a poor substrate for these enzymes, but some organisms have developed enzymes that inactivate this agent as well. Resistance as a result of failure of penetration can be largely overcome by the concomitant use of penicillin and/or vancomycin.

Antibacterial spectrum

The aminoglycosides are effective against many aerobic Gram-negative and some Gram-positive organisms (see Table 46.1). They are most widely used against Gram-negative enteric organisms and in sepsis. They may be given together with a penicillin in streptococcal infections caused by *Listeria* sp. and *P. aeruginosa* (see Table 46.1). Gentamicin is the aminoglycoside most commonly used, although tobramycin is the preferred member of this group for *P. aeruginosa* infections. Amikacin has the widest antimicrobial spectrum and, along with netilmicin, can be effective in infections with organisms resistant to gentamicin and tobramycin.

Pharmacokinetic aspects

The aminoglycosides are polycations and therefore highly polar. They are not absorbed from the gastrointestinal tract and are usually given intramuscularly or intravenously. They cross the placenta but do not cross the blood–brain barrier, penetrate into the vitreous humour of the eye or into most other secretions or body fluids, although high concentrations can be attained in joint and pleural fluids. The plasma half-life is 2–3 hours. Elimination is virtually entirely by glomerular filtration in the kidney, 50–60% of a dose being excreted unchanged within 24 hours. If renal function is impaired, accumulation occurs rapidly, with a resultant increase in those toxic effects (such as ototoxicity and nephrotoxicity; see below) that are dose-related.

Unwanted effects

Serious, dose-related toxic effects, which may increase as treatment proceeds, can occur with the aminoglycosides, the main hazards being ototoxicity and nephrotoxicity.

The ototoxicity involves progressive damage to, and eventually destruction of, the sensory cells in the cochlea and vestibular organ of the ear. The result, usually irreversible, may manifest as vertigo, ataxia and loss of balance in the case of vestibular damage, and auditory disturbances or deafness in the case of cochlear damage. Any aminoglycoside may produce both types of effect, but streptomycin and gentamicin are more likely to interfere with vestibular function, whereas neomycin and amikacin mostly affect hearing. Netilmicin is less ototoxic than other aminoglycosides and is preferred when prolonged use is necessary. Ototoxicity is potentiated by the concomitant use of other ototoxic drugs (e.g. loop diuretics; Ch. 24).

The nephrotoxicity consists of damage to the kidney tubules, and can be reversed if the use of the drugs is stopped. Nephrotoxicity is more likely to occur in patients with pre-existing renal disease or in conditions in which urine volume is reduced, and concomitant use of other nephrotoxic agents (e.g. cephalosporins) increases the risk. Note that as the elimination of these drugs is almost entirely renal, their nephrotoxic action can impair their own excretion, and a vicious cycle may develop. Plasma concentrations should be monitored regularly. **Spectinomycin** is related to the aminoglycosides in structure, but its use is confined to the treatment of gonorrhoea in patients allergic to penicillin, or in those whose infections are caused by penicillin-resistant gonococci.

A rare but serious toxic reaction is paralysis caused by neuromuscular blockade. This is usually seen only if the agents are given concurrently with neuromuscular-blocking agents. It results from inhibition of the Ca^{2+} uptake necessary for the exocytotic release of acetylcholine (see Ch. 10).

MACROLIDES

For 40 years, erythromycin was the only macrolide antibiotic in general clinical use. (The term *macrolide* relates to the structure—a many-membered lactone ring to which one or more deoxy sugars are attached.) Several additional macrolide and related antibiotics are now available, the two most important of which are **clarithromycin** and **azithromycin. Spiramycin** and **telithromycin** are also macrolides but are of minor utility.

Mechanism of action

The macrolides inhibit bacterial protein synthesis by an effect on translocation (Fig. 45.4). Their action may be bactericidal or bacteriostatic, the effect depending on the concentration and on the type of micro-organism. The drugs bind to the same 50S subunit of the bacterial ribosome as chloramphenicol and clindamycin, and the three drugs may compete if given concurrently. The clinical use of the macrolides is given in Table 46.1.

Antimicrobial spectrum

The antimicrobial spectrum of erythromycin is very similar to that of penicillin, and it has proved to be a safe and effective alternative for penicillin-sensitive patients. Erythromycin is effective against Gram-positive bacteria and spirochaetes but not against most Gram-negative organisms, exceptions being *N. gonorrhoeae* and, to a lesser extent, *H. influenzae. Mycoplasma pneumoniae, Legionella* sp. and some chlamydial organisms are also susceptible (see Table 46.1). Resistance can occur and results from a plasmid-controlled alteration of the binding site for erythromycin on the bacterial ribosome (Fig. 45.4).

Azithromycin is less active against Gram-positive bacteria than erythromycin but is considerably more effective against *H. influenzae* and may be more active against *Legionella*. It has excellent action against *Toxoplasma gondii*, killing the cysts. Clarithromycin is as active, and its metabolite is twice as active,

against *H. influenzae* as erythromycin. It is also effective against *Mycobacterium avium-intercellulare* (which can infect immunologically compromised individuals and elderly patients with chronic lung disease), and it may also be useful in leprosy and against *Helicobacter pylori* (see Ch. 25). Both these macrolides are also effective in Lyme disease.

Pharmacokinetic aspects

The macrolides are administered orally, azithromycin and clarithromycin being more acid-stable than erythromycin. Erythromycin can also be given parenterally, although intravenous injections can be followed by local thrombophlebitis. All three diffuse readily into most tissues but do not cross the blood–brain barrier, and there is poor penetration into synovial fluid. The plasma half-life of erythromycin is about 90 minutes; that of clarithromycin is three times longer, and that of azithromycin 8–16 times longer. Macrolides enter and indeed are concentrated within phagocytes—azithromycin concentrations in phagocyte lysosomes can be 40 times higher than in the blood—and they can enhance intracellular phagocyte killing of bacteria.

Erythromycin is partly inactivated in the liver; azithromycin is more resistant to inactivation, and clarithromycin is converted to an active metabolite. Their effects on the P450 cytochrome system can affect the bioavailability of other drugs (see Ch. 52). The major route of elimination is in the bile.

Unwanted effects

Gastrointestinal disturbances are common and unpleasant but not serious. With erythromycin, the following have also been reported: hypersensitivity reactions such as skin rashes and fever, transient hearing disturbances and, rarely, following treatment for longer than 2 weeks, cholestatic jaundice. Opportunistic infections of the gastrointestinal tract or vagina can occur.

STREPTOGRAMINS

Quinupristin and **dalfopristin** are members of the streptogramin family of compounds isolated from *Streptomyces pristinaespiralis*. These agents are characterised by a cyclic peptide structure. They act by inhibiting bacterial protein synthesis. Individually, quinupristin and dalfopristin exhibit only very modest bacteriostatic activity, but combined together as an intravenous injection they are active against many Gram-positive bacteria.

Mechanism of action

Coadministration of quinupristin–dalfopristin (3 parts to 7 parts, weight for weight) is an effective approach to the treatment of serious infections, usually where no other antibacterial is suitable. For example, the combination is effective against methicillin-sensitive *Staphylococcus aureus* and is also active against vancomycin-resistant *Enterococcus faecium*. The mechanism of action is to inhibit protein formation by binding to the 50S subunit of the bacterial ribosome. Dalfopristin changes the structure of the ribosome so as to promote the binding of quinupristin, which probably explains the improved effectiveness of the drugs when administered together.

Pharmacokinetic aspects

Both quinupristin and dalfopristin are broken down in the liver and must therefore be given as an intravenous infusion. The half-life of each compound is 1–2 hours.

Unwanted effects

Unwanted effects include inflammation and pain at the infusion site, arthralgia, myalgia and nausea, vomiting and diarrhoea. To date, resistance to quinupristin and dalfopristin**e** does not seem to be a major problem.

LINCOSAMIDES

Clindamycin is active against Gram-positive cocci, including many penicillin-resistant staphylococci and many anaerobic bacteria such as *Bacteroides* species. Its mechanism of action involves inhibition of protein synthesis through an action similar to that of the macrolides and chloramphenicol (Fig. 45.4). In addition to its use in infections caused by *Bacteroides* organisms, it is used to treat staphylococcal infections of bones and joints. It is also given topically, as eye drops, for staphylococcal conjunctivitis.

Pharmacokinetics

Clindamycin may be given orally or parenterally and is widely distributed in tissues (including bone) and body fluids, although it does not cross the blood–brain barrier. There is active uptake into leucocytes. The half-life is 21 hours; some of the drug is metabolised in the liver, and the metabolites, which are active, are excreted in the bile and the urine.

Unwanted effects

Unwanted effects consist mainly of gastrointestinal disturbances, and a potentially lethal condition, *pseudomembranous colitis*, may develop. This is an acute inflammation of the colon caused by a necrotising toxin produced by a clindamycin-resistant organism, *Clostridium difficile*, which may form part of the normal faecal flora.[2] Vancomycin, given orally, and **metronidazole** (see below) are effective in the treatment of this condition.

OXALAZIDONONES

Hailed as the 'first truly new class of antibacterial agents to reach the marketplace in several decades' (Zurenko et al., 2001), the oxalizidonones boast a novel mechanism of action on bacterial protein synthesis: inhibition of *N*-formylmethionyl-tRNA binding to the 70S ribosome. **Linezolid** is the first member of this new antibiotic family to be introduced. It is active against a wide variety of Gram-positive bacteria and is particularly useful for the treatment of drug-resistant bacteria such as methicillin-resistant *Staph. aureus*, penicillin-resistant *Streptococcus pneumoniae* and vancomycin-resistant enterococci. The drug is also effective against some anaerobes, such as *C. difficile*. Most common Gram-negative organisms are not susceptible to the drug. Linezolid can be used

to treat pneumonia, septicaemia, and skin and soft tissue infections. The drug is usually restricted to serious bacterial infections where other antibiotics have failed.

It is encouraging to report that, so far, there have been few reports of linezolid resistance, although there is a risk this may develop if patients receive inadequate doses for extended periods.

Pharmacokinetics

Linezolid can be given orally or by intravenous infusion in serious infections. After oral administration, peak plasma concentrations are achieved quickly, and the drug has a half-life of 5–7 hours. Metabolism is through oxidation of the morpholine ring structure.

Unwanted effects

Unwanted effects include thrombocytopenia, diarrhoea, nausea and, rarely, rash and dizziness. Linezolid is a non-selective inhibitor of monoamine oxidase, and appropriate precautions need to be observed (see Ch. 37).

FUSIDIC ACID

Fusidic acid is a narrow-spectrum steroid antibiotic active mainly against Gram-positive bacteria. It acts by inhibiting bacterial protein synthesis (Fig. 45.4). As the sodium salt, the drug is well absorbed from the gut and is distributed widely in the tissues. Some is excreted in the bile and some metabolised.

Unwanted effects such as gastrointestinal disturbances are fairly common. Skin eruptions and jaundice can occur. It is also used topically for staphylococcal conjunctivitis.

ANTIMICROBIAL AGENTS AFFECTING TOPOISOMERASE

FLUOROQUINOLONES

The **fluoroquinolones** include the broad-spectrum agents **ciprofloxacin, levofloxacin, ofloxacin, norfloxacin** and **moxifloxacin**, as well as a narrow-spectrum drug used in urinary tract infections—**nalidixic acid** (the first quinolone and not fluorinated). These agents inhibit topoisomerase II (a bacterial DNA gyrase), the enzyme that produces a negative supercoil in DNA and thus permits transcription or replication (see Fig. 46.4).

Antibacterial spectrum and clinical use

Ciprofloxacin is the most commonly used fluoroquinolone and will be described as the type agent. It is a broad-spectrum antibiotic effective against both Gram-positive and Gram-negative organisms. It has excellent activity against the Enterobacteriaceae (the enteric Gram-negative bacilli), including many organisms resistant to penicillins, cephalosporins and aminoglycosides, and it is also effective against *H. influenzae*, penicillinase-producing *N. gonorrhoeae*, *Campylobacter* sp. and pseudomonads. Of the Gram-positive organisms, streptococci and pneumococci are only weakly inhibited, and there is a high incidence of staphylococcal resistance. Ciprofloxacin should be

[2]This may also occur with some penicillins and cephalosporins.

- *Tetracyclines* (e.g. minocycline). These are orally active, bacteriostatic, broad-spectrum antibiotics. Resistance is increasing. Gastrointestinal disorders are common. They chelate calcium and are deposited in growing bone. They are contraindicated in children and pregnant women.
- *Chloramphenicol*. This is an orally active, bacteriostatic, broad-spectrum antibiotic. Serious toxic effects are possible, including bone marrow depression, 'grey baby syndrome'. It should be reserved for life-threatening infections.
- *Aminoglycosides* (e.g. gentamicin). These are given by injection. They are bactericidal, broad-spectrum antibiotics (but with low activity against anaerobes, streptococci and pneumococci). Resistance is increasing. The main unwanted effects are dose-related nephrotoxicity and ototoxicity. Serum levels should be monitored. (Streptomycin is an antituberculosis aminoglycoside.)
- *Macrolides* (e.g. erythromycin). Can be given orally and parenterally. They are bactericidal/bacteriostatic. The antibacterial spectrum is the same as for penicillin. Erythromycin can cause jaundice. Newer agents are clarithromycin and azithromycin.
- *Clindamycin*. Can be given orally and parenterally. It can cause pseudomembranous colitis.
- *Quinupristin/dalfopristin*. Given by intravenous infusion as a combination. Considerably less active when administered separately. Active against several strains of drug-resistant bacteria.
- *Fusidic acid*. This is a narrow-spectrum antibiotic that acts by inhibiting protein synthesis. It penetrates bone. Unwanted effects include gastrointestinal disorders.
- *Linezolid*. Given orally or by intravenous injection. Active against several strains of drug-resistant bacteria.

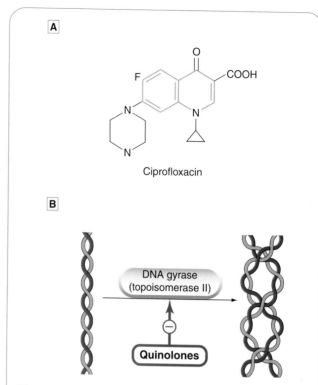

Fig. 46.4 **A simplified diagram of the mechanism of action of the fluoroquinolones.** **A** An example of a quinolone (the quinolone moiety is shown in orange). **B** Schematic diagram of (left) the double helix and (right) the double helix in supercoiled form (see also Fig. 45.6.). In essence, the DNA gyrase unwinds the RNA-induced positive supercoil (not shown) and introduces a negative supercoil.

Clinical uses of the fluoroquinolones

- Complicated *urinary tract infections* (**norfloxacin, ofloxacin**).
- *Pseudomonas aeruginosa* respiratory infections in patients with *cystic fibrosis*.
- *Invasive external otitis* ('malignant otitis') caused by *P. aeruginosa*.
- Chronic Gram-negative bacillary *osteomyelitis*.
- Eradication of *Salmonella typhi* in carriers.
- *Gonorrhoea* (**norfloxacin, ofloxacin**).
- *Bacterial prostatitis* (**norfloxacin**).
- *Cervicitis* (**ofloxacin**).
- *Anthrax*.

avoided in methicillin-resistant staphylococcal infections. Clinically, the fluoroquinolones are best used for infections with facultative and aerobic Gram-negative rods and cocci.[3] Resistant strains of *Staph. aureus* and *P. aeruginosa* have emerged. Further details of the clinical use of the fluoroquinolones are given in the box.

[3]When ciprofloxacin was introduced, clinical pharmacologists and microbiologists sensibly suggested that it should be reserved for organisms already resistant to other drugs so as to prevent emergence of resistance. However, by 1989 it was already estimated that it was prescribed for 1 in 44 of Americans, so it would seem that the horse had not only left the stable but had bolted off into the blue!

Pharmacokinetic aspects

Given orally, the fluoroquinolones are well absorbed. The half-life of ciprofloxacin and norfloxacin is 3 hours, and that of ofloxacin is 5 hours. The drugs accumulate in several tissues, particularly in the kidney, prostate and lung. All quinolones are concentrated in phagocytes. Most fail to cross the blood–brain barrier, but ofloxacin penetrates the CSF and attains 40% of its serum concentrations. Aluminium and magnesium antacids interfere with the absorption of the quinolones. Elimination of ciprofloxacin and norfloxacin is partly by hepatic metabolism by P450 enzymes (which they can inhibit, giving rise to interactions with other drugs; see below) and partly by renal excretion. Ofloxacin is excreted in the urine.

Unwanted effects

Unwanted effects are infrequent, usually mild, and disappear when the drugs are withdrawn. The most frequent manifestations are gastrointestinal disorders and skin rashes. Arthropathy has been reported in young individuals. Central nervous system symptoms—headache and dizziness—have occurred, as have, less frequently, convulsions associated with central nervous system pathology or concurrent use of **theophylline** or a non-steroidal anti-inflammatory drug.

There is a clinically important interaction between ciprofloxacin and this drug (through inhibition of P450 enzymes), which can lead to theophylline toxicity in asthmatics treated with the fluoroquinolones. The topic is discussed further in Chapter 23.

MISCELLANEOUS ANTIBACTERIAL AGENTS

Vancomycin is a glycopeptide antibiotic, and **teicoplanin** is similar but longer lasting. Vancomycin is bactericidal (except against streptococci) and acts by inhibiting cell wall synthesis (see Fig. 45.3). It is effective mainly against Gram-positive bacteria and has been used against methicillin-resistant staphylococci. Vancomycin is not absorbed from the gut and is only given by the oral route for treatment of gastrointestinal infection with *C. difficile*. For parenteral use, it is given intravenously and has a plasma half-life of about 8 hours.

The clinical use of vancomycin is limited mainly to pseudomembranous colitis (see clindamycin, p. 669) and the treatment of some multiresistant staphylococcal infections. It is also valuable in severe staphylococcal infections in patients allergic both to penicillins and cephalosporins, and in some forms of endocarditis.

Unwanted effects include fever, rashes and local phlebitis at the site of injection. Ototoxicity and nephrotoxicity can occur, and hypersensitivity reactions are occasionally seen.

Nitrofurantoin is a synthetic compound active against a range of Gram-positive and Gram-negative organisms. The development of resistance in susceptible organisms is rare, and there is no cross-resistance. Its mechanism of action is not known. It is given orally and is rapidly and totally absorbed from the gastrointestinal tract and just as rapidly excreted by the kidney. The clinical use of nitrofurantoin is confined to the treatment of urinary tract infections.

Unwanted effects such as gastrointestinal disturbances are relatively common, and hypersensitivity reactions involving the skin and the bone marrow (e.g. leucopenia) can occur. Hepatotoxicity and peripheral neuropathy have also been reported.

The *polymixin antibiotics* in use are **polymixin B** and **colistin** (polymixin E). They have cationic detergent properties and exert their antibacterial action by disrupting the cell membrane phospholipids (Ch. 45). They have a selective, rapidly bactericidal action on Gram-negative bacilli, especially pseudomonads and coliform organisms. They are not absorbed from the gastrointestinal tract. Clinical use of these drugs is limited by their toxicity (see below) and is confined largely to gut sterilisation and topical treatment of ear, eye or skin infections caused by susceptible organisms.

Unwanted effects may be serious and include neurotoxicity and nephrotoxicity.

Metronidazole was introduced as an antiprotozoal agent (see Ch. 49), but it is also active against anaerobic bacteria such as *Bacteroides*, *Clostridia* sp. and some streptococci. It is effective in the therapy of pseudomembranous colitis, a clostridial infection sometimes associated with antibiotic therapy (see above), and is important in the treatment of serious anaerobic infections (e.g. sepsis secondary to bowel disease).

Antimicrobial agents affecting DNA topoisomerase II

- The fluoroquinolones interfere with the supercoiling of DNA.
- Ciprofloxacin has a wide antibacterial spectrum, being especially active against Gram-negative enteric coliform organisms, including many organisms resistant to penicillins, cephalosporins and aminoglycosides; it is also effective against *Haemophilus influenzae*, penicillinase-producing *Neisseria gonorrhoeae*, *Campylobacter* sp. and pseudomonads. There is a high incidence of staphylococcal resistance. It is active orally, with a half life of 4.5 hours.
- Unwanted effects include gastrointestinal tract upsets, hypersensitivity reactions and, rarely, central nervous system disturbances.

Miscellaneous antibacterial agents

- *Glycopeptide antibiotics* (e.g. vancomycin). Vancomycin is bactericidal, acting by inhibiting cell wall synthesis. It is used intravenously for multiresistant staphylococcal infections and orally for pseudomembranous colitis. Unwanted effects include ototoxicity and nephrotoxicity.
- *Polymixins* (e.g. colistin). They are bactericidal, acting by disrupting bacterial cell membranes. They are highly neurotoxic and nephrotoxic, and are only used topically.

ANTIMYCOBACTERIAL AGENTS

The main mycobacterial infections in humans are *tuberculosis* and *leprosy*—typically chronic infections caused by *Mycobacterium tuberculosis* and *M. leprae*, respectively. A particular problem with both these organisms is that they can survive inside macrophages after phagocytosis, unless these cells are 'activated' by cytokines produced by T-helper 1 lymphocytes (see Ch. 13).

DRUGS USED TO TREAT TUBERCULOSIS

For centuries, tuberculosis was a major killer disease, but the introduction in the 1960s of **rifampicin** and **ethambutol** revolutionised therapy, and tuberculosis came to be regarded as an easily treatable condition. Regrettably, this is so no longer—the causative mycobacterium has returned to haunt us with a vengeance, and strains with increased virulence or exhibiting multidrug resistance strains are now common (Bloom & Small, 1998). Tuberculosis is again a major threat; the World Health Organization estimates that one-third of the world's population is currently infected with the bacillus and that 1 billion people will be newly infected in the period 2000–20, resulting in 35 million more deaths (1.75 million deaths in 2003). Africa bears the brunt of the disease, partly because of an ominous synergy between mycobacteria (e.g. *M. tuberculosis*, *M. avium-intercellulare*) and HIV. About 15% of HIV-associated deaths in the continent are caused by tuberculosis. The disease is out of control in many countries, and it is now the world's leading cause of death from a single agent.

Our counter-attack is led by the first-line drugs **isoniazid**, rifampicin, **rifabutin**, ethambutol and **pyrazinamide**. Some second-line drugs available are **capreomycin**, **cycloserine**, streptomycin (rarely used now in the UK), clarithromycin and ciprofloxacin. These are used to treat infections likely to be resistant to first-line drugs, or when the first-line agents have to be abandoned because of unwanted reactions.

To decrease the probability of the emergence of resistant organisms, compound drug therapy is a frequent strategy. This commonly involves:

- an initial phase of treatment (about 2 months) with a combination of isoniazid, rifampicin and pyrazinamide (plus ethambutol if the organism is suspected to be resistant)
- a second, continuation phase (about 4 months) of therapy with isoniazid and rifampicin; longer-term treatment is needed for patients with meningitis, bone/joint involvement or drug-resistant infection.

ISONIAZID

The antibacterial activity of isoniazid is limited to mycobacteria. It halts the growth of resting organisms (e.g. is bacteriostatic) but can kill dividing bacteria. It passes freely into mammalian cells and is thus effective against intracellular organisms. The mechanism of its action is not clear. There is evidence that it inhibits the synthesis of *mycolic acids*, important constituents of the cell wall peculiar to mycobacteria. It is also reported to combine with an enzyme that is uniquely found in isoniazid-sensitive strains of mycobacteria, disrupting cellular metabolism. Resistance to the drug, caused by reduced penetration into the bacterium, may be encountered, but cross-resistance with other tuberculostatic drugs does not occur.

Pharmacokinetic aspects

Isoniazid is readily absorbed from the gastrointestinal tract and is widely distributed throughout the tissues and body fluids, including the CSF. An important point is that it penetrates well into 'caseous' tuberculous lesions (i.e. necrotic lesions with a cheese-like consistency). Metabolism, which involves largely acetylation, depends on genetic factors that determine whether a person is a slow or rapid acetylator of the drug (see Chs 8 and 52), with slow inactivators enjoying a better therapeutic response. The half-life in slow inactivators is 3 hours and in rapid inactivators, 1 hour. Isoniazid is excreted in the urine partly as unchanged drug and partly in the acetylated or otherwise inactivated form.

Unwanted effects

Unwanted effects depend on the dosage and occur in about 5% of individuals, the commonest being allergic skin eruptions. A variety of other adverse reactions have been reported, including fever, hepatotoxicity, haematological changes, arthritic symptoms and vasculitis. Adverse effects involving the central or peripheral nervous systems are largely consequences of a deficiency of pyridoxine and are common in malnourished patients unless prevented by administration of this substance. Pyridoxal-hydrazone formation occurs mainly in slow acetylators. Isoniazid may cause haemolytic anaemia in individuals with glucose 6-phosphate dehydrogenase deficiency, and it decreases the metabolism of the antiepileptic agents **phenytoin**, **ethosuximide** and **carbamazepine**, resulting in an increase in the plasma concentration and toxicity of these drugs.

RIFAMPICIN

Rifampicin acts by binding to, and inhibiting, DNA-dependent RNA polymerase in prokaryotic but not in eukaryotic cells (Ch. 45). It is one of the most active antituberculosis agents known, and is also effective against most Gram-positive bacteria as well as many Gram-negative species. It enters phagocytic cells and can therefore kill intracellular micro-organisms including the tubercle bacillus. Resistance can develop rapidly in a one-step process and is thought to be caused by chemical modification of microbial DNA-dependent RNA polymerase, resulting from a chromosomal mutation (see Ch. 45).

Pharmacokinetic aspects

Rifampicin is given orally and is widely distributed in the tissues and body fluids, giving an orange tinge to saliva, sputum, tears and sweat. In the CSF, it reaches 10–40% of its serum concentration. It is excreted partly in the urine and partly in the bile, some of it undergoing enterohepatic cycling. The metabolite retains antibacterial activity but is less well absorbed from the gastrointestinal tract. The half-life is 1–5 hours, becoming shorter during treatment because of induction of hepatic microsomal enzymes.

Unwanted effects

Unwanted effects are relatively infrequent. The commonest are skin eruptions, fever and gastrointestinal disturbances. Liver damage with jaundice has been reported and has proved fatal in a very small proportion of patients, and liver function should be assessed before treatment is started. Rifampicin causes induction of hepatic metabolising enzymes, resulting in an increase in the degradation of **warfarin, glucocorticoids**, narcotic analgesics, oral antidiabetic drugs, **dapsone** and **oestrogens**, the last effect leading to failure of oral contraceptives.

ETHAMBUTOL

Ethambutol has no effect on organisms other than mycobacteria. It is taken up by the bacteria and exerts a bacteriostatic effect after a period of 24 hours, although the mechanism by which this occurs is unknown. Resistance emerges rapidly if the drug is used alone. Ethambutol is given orally and is well absorbed, reaching therapeutic concentrations in the plasma within 4 hours; it can also reach therapeutic concentrations in the CSF in tuberculous meningitis. In the blood, it is taken up by erythrocytes and slowly released. Ethambutol is partly metabolised and is excreted in the urine. The half-life is 3–4 hours.

Unwanted effects

Unwanted effects are uncommon, the most important being optic neuritis, which is dose-related and is more likely to occur if renal function is decreased. It results in visual disturbances manifesting initially as red–green colour blindness progressing to a decreased visual acuity. Colour vision should be monitored during prolonged treatment.

PYRAZINAMIDE

Pyrazinamide is inactive at neutral pH but tuberculostatic at acid pH. It is effective against the intracellular organisms in macrophages because, after phagocytosis, the organisms are contained in phagolysosomes where the pH is low. Resistance develops rather readily, but cross-resistance with isoniazid does not occur. The drug is well absorbed after oral administration and is widely distributed, penetrating well into the meninges. It is excreted through the kidney, mainly by glomerular filtration.

Unwanted effects

Unwanted effects include gout, which is associated with high concentrations of plasma urates. Gastrointestinal upsets, malaise and fever have also been reported. Historically high doses of this drug were used, and serious hepatic damage was a possibility; this is now less likely with lower dose/shorter course regimens but, nevertheless, liver function should be assessed before treatment.

CAPREOMYCIN

Capreomycin is a peptide antibiotic given by intramuscular injection. There is some cross-reaction with the aminoglycoside **kanamycin**.

Unwanted effects include kidney damage and injury to the eighth nerve, with consequent deafness and ataxia. The drug should not be given at the same time as streptomycin or other drugs that may damage the eighth nerve.

CYCLOSERINE

Cycloserine is a broad-spectrum antibiotic that inhibits the growth of many bacteria, including coliforms and mycobacteria. It is water-soluble and destroyed at acid pH. It acts by competitively inhibiting bacterial cell wall synthesis. It does this by preventing the formation of D-alanine and the D-Ala–D-Ala dipeptide that is added to the initial tripeptide side-chain on *N*-acetylmuramic acid, i.e. it prevents completion of the major building block of peptidoglycan (see Fig. 45.3). After oral administration, it is rapidly absorbed and reaches peak concentrations within 4 hours. It is distributed throughout the tissues and body fluids, and reaches concentrations in the CSF equivalent to those in the blood. Most of the drug is eliminated in active form in the urine, but approximately 35% is metabolised.

Cycloserine has *unwanted effects* mainly on the central nervous system. A wide variety of disturbances may occur, ranging from headache and irritability to depression, convulsions and psychotic states. Its use is limited to tuberculosis that is resistant to other drugs.

DRUGS USED TO TREAT LEPROSY

Leprosy is one of the most ancient diseases known to mankind and has been mentioned in texts dating back to 600 BC. It is a chronic disfiguring illness with a long latency, and historically sufferers have been ostracised and forced to live apart from their communities, although, in fact, the disease is not particularly contagious. Once viewed as incurable, the introduction in the 1940s of dapsone, and subsequently rifampicin and **clofazimine** in the 1960s, completely changed our perspective on leprosy. It is now considered relatively easy to diagnose and to cure, and the global figures show that the prevalence rates for the disease have dropped by 90% since 1985, and that the disease has been eliminated from 108 out of 122 countries where it was considered to be a major health problem. Today, some 650 000 new cases are reported each year (2002 figures). The bulk of these (70%) are in the Indian subcontinent.

Multidrug treatment regimens initiated by the World Health Organization in 1982 are now the mainstay of treatment. *Paucibacillary* leprosy, leprosy characterised by one to five numb patches, is mainly *tuberculoid*[4] in type and is treated for 6 months with dapsone and rifampicin. *Multibacillary* leprosy, characterised by more than five numb skin patches, is mainly *lepromatous* in type and is treated for at least 2 years with rifampicin, dapsone and clofazimine. The effect of therapy with minocycline or the fluoroquinolones is being investigated.

---

[4]The basis of the difference between tuberculoid and lepromatous disease appears to be that the T cells from patients with the former vigorously produce interferon-γ, which enables macrophages to kill intracellular microbes, whereas in the latter case the immune response is dominated by interleukin-4, which blocks the action of interferon-γ. See Chapter 13.

- To avoid the emergence of resistant organisms, *compound therapy* is used (e.g. three drugs initially, followed by a two-drug regimen later).

First-line drugs

- *Isoniazid* kills actively growing mycobacteria within host cells; mechanism of action unknown. Given orally, it penetrates necrotic lesions, also the cerebrospinal fluid (CSF). 'Slow acetylators' (genetically determined) respond well. It has low toxicity. Pyridoxine deficiency increases risk of neurotoxicity. No cross-resistance with other agents.
- *Rifampicin* (*rifampin*) is a potent, orally active drug that inhibits mycobacterial RNA polymerase. It penetrates CSF. Unwanted effects are infrequent (but serious liver damage has occurred). It induces hepatic drug-metabolising enzymes. Resistance can develop rapidly.
- *Ethambutol* inhibits growth of mycobacteria by an unknown mechanism. It is given orally and can penetrate CSF. Unwanted effects are uncommon, but optic neuritis can occur. Resistance can emerge rapidly.
- *Pyrazinamide* is tuberculostatic against intracellular mycobacteria by an unknown mechanism. Given orally, it penetrates CSF. Resistance can develop rapidly. Unwanted effects include increased plasma urate and liver toxicity with high doses.

Second-line drugs

- *Capreomycin* is given intramuscularly. Unwanted effects include damage to kidney and to eighth nerve.
- *Cycloserine* is a broad-spectrum agent. It inhibits an early stage of peptidoglycan synthesis. Given orally, it penetrates the CSF. Unwanted effects affect mostly central nervous system.
- *Streptomycin*, an aminoglycoside antibiotic, acts by inhibiting bacterial protein synthesis. It is given intramuscularly. Unwanted effects are ototoxicity (mainly vestibular) and nephrotoxicity.

DAPSONE

Dapsone is chemically related to the sulfonamides and, because its action is antagonised by PABA, probably acts through inhibition of bacterial folate synthesis. Resistance to the drug is increasing, and treatment with combinations of drugs is now recommended.

Dapsone is given orally; it is well absorbed and widely distributed through the body water and in all tissues. The plasma half-life is 24–48 hours, but some dapsone persists in certain tissues (liver, kidney, and to some extent skin and muscle) for much longer periods. There is enterohepatic recycling of the drug, but some is acetylated and excreted in the urine. Dapsone is also used to treat *dermatitis herpetiformis*, a chronic blistering skin condition associated with coeliac disease.

Unwanted effects

Unwanted effects occur fairly frequently and include haemolysis of red cells (usually not severe enough to lead to frank anaemia), methaemoglobinaemia, anorexia, nausea and vomiting, fever, allergic dermatitis and neuropathy. Lepra reactions (an exacerbation of lepromatous lesions) can occur, and a potentially fatal syndrome resembling infectious mononucleosis has occasionally been seen.

RIFAMPICIN

Rifampicin is discussed under *Drugs used to treat tuberculosis*.

CLOFAZIMINE

Clofazimine is a dye of complex structure. Its mechanism of action against leprosy bacilli may involve an action on DNA. It also has anti-inflammatory activity and is useful in patients in whom dapsone causes inflammatory side effects.

Clofazimine is given orally and accumulates in the body, being sequestered in the mononuclear phagocyte system. The plasma half-life may be as long as 8 weeks. The antileprotic effect is delayed and is usually not evident for 6–7 weeks.

Unwanted effects

Unwanted effects may be related to the fact that clofazimine is a dye. The skin and urine can develop a reddish colour and the lesions a blue-black discoloration. Dose-related nausea, giddiness, headache and gastrointestinal disturbances can also occur.

POSSIBLE NEW ANTIBACTERIAL DRUGS

The reader is referred to the notes at the conclusion of Chapter 45.

REFERENCES AND FURTHER READING

Antibacterial drugs

Allington D R, Rivey M P 2001 Quinupristine/dalfopristin: a therapeutic review. Clin Ther 23: 24–44

Ball P 2001 Future of the quinolones. Semin Resp Infect 16: 215–224 (*Good overview of this class of drugs*)

Blondeau J M 1999 Expanded activity and utility of the new fluoroquinolones: a review. Clin Ther 21: 3–15 (*Good overview*)

Blumer J L 1997 Meropenem: evaluation of a new generation carbapenem. Int J Antimicrob Agents 8: 73–92

Bryskier A 2000 Ketolides—telithromycin, an example of a new class of antibacterial agents. Clin Microbiol Infect 6: 661–669

Duran J M, Amsden G W 2000 Azithromycin: indications for the future? Expert Opin Pharmacother 1: 489–505

Finch R 1990 The penicillins today. Br Med J 300: 1289–1290

Fish D N, North D S 2001 Gatifloxacin, an advanced 8-methoxy fluoroquinolone. Pharmacotherapy 21: 35–59 (*Comprehensive evaluation of the effects of a novel fluoroquinolone*)

Greenwood D (ed) 1995 Antimicrobial chemotherapy, 3rd edn. Oxford University Press, Oxford

Jacoby G A, Medeiros A 1991b More extended-spectrum β-lactamases. Antimicrob Agents Chemother 35: 1697–1704

Laurence D R, Bennett P N, Brown M J 1997 Clinical pharmacology, 8th edn. Churchill Livingstone, Edinburgh

Lowy F D 1998 *Staphylococcus aureus* infections. N Engl J Med 339: 520–541 (*Basis of Staph. aureus pathogenesis of infection, resistance; extensive references; impressive diagrams*)

Moellering R C 1985 Principles of anti-infective therapy. In: Mandell G L, Douglas R G, Bennett J E (eds) Principles and practice of infectious disease. John Wiley, New York

Perry C M, Jarvis B 2001 Linezolid: a review of its use in the management of serious gram-positive infections. Drugs 61: 525–551

Quagliarello V J, Scheld W M 1997 Treatment of bacterial meningitis. N Engl J Med 336: 708–716

Raoult D, Drancourt M 1994 Antimicrobial therapy of rickettsial diseases. Antimicrob Agents Chemother 35: 2457–2462

Sato K, Hoshino K, Mitsuhashi S 1992 Mode of action of the new quinolones: the inhibitory action on DNA gyrase. Prog Drug Res 38: 121–132

Shimada J, Hori S 1992 Adverse effects of fluoroquinolones. Prog Drug Res 38: 133–143

Stojiljkovic I, Evavold B D, Kumar V 2001 Antimicrobial properties of porphyrins. Expert Opin Investig Drugs 10: 309–320

Tillotson G S 1996 Quinolones: structure activity relationships and future predictions. J Med Microbiol 44: 320–324

Zurenko G E, Gibson J K, Shinabarger D L et al. 2001. Oxazolidinones: a new class of antibacterials. Curr Opin Pharmacol 1: 470–476 (*Easy-to-assimilate review that discusses this relatively new group of antibacterials*)

Resistance

Bax R, Mullan N, Verhoef J 2000 The millennium bugs—the need for and development of new antibacterials. Int J Antimicrob Agents 16: 51–59 (*Good review that includes an account of the development of 'resistance' and a round-up of potential new drugs*)

Cohn D L, Bustreo F, Raviglioni M C 1997 Drug-resistant tuberculosis: review of the worldwide situation and the WHO/IUATLD global surveillance project. Clin Infect Dis 24: S121–S130

Courvalin P 1996 Evasion of antibiotic action by bacteria. J Antimicrob Chemother 37: 855–869 (*Covers recent developments in the understanding of the genetics and biochemical mechanisms of resistance*)

Gold H S, Moellering R C 1996 Antimicrobial drug resistance. N Engl J Med 335: 1445–1453 (*Excellent well-referenced review; covers mechanisms of resistance of important organisms to the main drugs; has useful table of therapeutic and preventive strategies, culled from the literature*)

Heym B, Honoré N et al. 1994 Implications of multidrug resistance for the future of short-course chemotherapy of tuberculosis: a molecular study. Lancet 344: 293–298

Iseman M D 1993 Treatment of multidrug-resistant tuberculosis. N Engl J Med 329: 784–791

Jacoby G A, Archer G L 1991a Mechanisms of disease: new mechanisms of bacterial resistance to antimicrobial agents. N Engl J Med 324: 601–612

Livermore D M 2000 Antibiotic resistance in staphylococci. J Antimicrob Agents 16: S3–S10 (*Overview of problems of bacterial resistance*)

Michel M, Gutman L 1997 Methicillin-resistant *Staphylococcus aureus* and vancomycin-resistant enterococci: therapeutic realities and possibilities. Lancet 349: 1901–1906 (*Excellent review article; good diagrams*)

Nicas T I, Zeckel M L, Braun D K 1997 Beyond vancomycin: new therapies to meet the challenge of glycopeptide resistance. Trends Microbiol 5: 240–249

Woodford N, Johnson A P et al. 1995 Current perspectives on glycopeptide resistance. Clin Microbiol Rev 8: 585–615 (*Comprehensive review*)

Bacterial evasion of host defences and miscellaneous

Bloom B R, Small P M 1998 The evolving relation between humans and *Mycobacterium* tuberculosis. Lancet 338: 677–678 (*Editorial comment*)

Loferer H 2000 Mining bacterial genomes for antimicrobial targets. Mol Med Today 6: 470–474 (*An interesting article focusing on the way in which a better understanding of the bacterial genome may lead to new drugs*)

Useful web sites

http://www.who.int (*Once again, the World Health Organization web site is a mine of information about the demographics and treatment of infectious diseases. The sections on leprosy and tuberculosis are especially worthwhile studying. The site includes photographs, maps and much statistical information, as well as information on drug resistance. Highly recommended.*)

Antiviral drugs 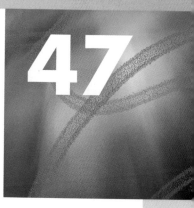 47

OVERVIEW

This chapter deals with drugs used to treat infections caused by viruses. We give first some necessary information about viruses: a simple outline of virus structure, a list of the main pathogenic viruses and a brief summary of the life history of an infectious virus. We then continue with a consideration of the host–virus interaction: the defences deployed by the human host against viruses and the strategies employed by viruses to evade these measures. We then describe the various types of antiviral drugs and their mechanisms of action, with particular reference to the treatment of AIDS, an infection caused by the human immunodeficiency virus (HIV).

BACKGROUND INFORMATION ABOUT VIRUSES

AN OUTLINE OF VIRUS STRUCTURE

Viruses are small (usually in the range 20–30 nm) infective agents that are incapable of reproduction outside their host cells. The free-living (e.g. outside its host) virus particle is termed a *virion*, and consists of segments of nucleic acid (either RNA or DNA) enclosed in a protein coat comprised of symmetrical repeating structural units and called a *capsid* (Fig. 47.1). The viral coat, together with the nucleic acid core, is termed the *nucleocapsid*. Some viruses have, in addition, a further external lipoprotein envelope, which may be decorated with antigenic viral glycoproteins or phospholipids acquired from its host when the nucleocapsid buds through the membranes of the infected cell. Certain viruses also contain enzymes that initiate their replication in the host cell.

Viruses are generally characterised either as *DNA* or *RNA viruses* depending on the nature of their nucleic acid content. These two broad categories are conventionally subdivided into some six subclasses, which classify viruses according to whether they contain single- or double-stranded nucleic acids and how this functions during replication.

EXAMPLES OF PATHOGENIC VIRUSES

Viruses can infect virtually all living organisms. Humans are no exception, and such infections are common.

▼ Some important examples of the diseases they cause are as follow.

- *DNA viruses*: poxviruses (smallpox), herpesviruses (chickenpox, shingles, cold sores, glandular fever), adenoviruses (sore throat, conjunctivitis) and papillomaviruses (warts).
- *RNA viruses*: orthomyxoviruses (influenza), paramyxoviruses (measles, mumps, respiratory tract infections), rubella virus (German measles), rhabdoviruses (rabies), picornaviruses (colds, meningitis, poliomyelitis), retroviruses (acquired immunodeficiency syndrome [AIDS], T-cell leukaemia), arenaviruses (meningitis, Lassa fever),

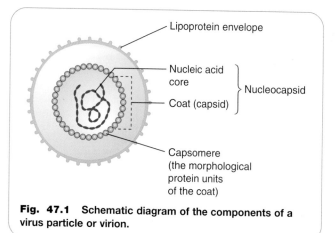

Fig. 47.1   Schematic diagram of the components of a virus particle or virion.

hepadnaviruses (serum hepatitis) and arboviruses (arthropod-borne encephalitis and various febrile illnesses, e.g. yellow fever).

VIRUS FUNCTION AND LIFE HISTORY

As viruses have no metabolic machinery of their own, they have to attach to and penetrate a living host cell—animal, plant or bacterial—and use the victim's own metabolic processes to replicate. The first step in this process is facilitated by polypeptide binding sites on the envelope or capsid, interacting with receptors on the host cell. These 'receptors' are normal membrane constituents—receptors for cytokines, neurotransmitters or hormones, ion channels, integral membrane glycoproteins, etc. Some examples of host cell receptors utilised by particular viruses are listed in Table 47.1.

Following attachment, the receptor–virus complex enters the cell (often by receptor-mediated endocytosis), during which time the virus coat may be removed by host cell enzymes (often lysosomal in nature). Some bypass this route. Once in the host cell, the nucleic acid of the virus then uses the host cell's machinery for synthesising nucleic acids and proteins that are assembled into new virus particles. The actual way in which this occurs varies between DNA and RNA viruses.

Table 47.1 Some host cell structures that can function as receptors for viruses

Host cell structure[a]	Virus(es)
Helper T-lymphocytes CD4 glycoprotein	HIV (causing AIDS)
CCR5 receptor for chemokines MCP-1 and RANTES	HIV (causing AIDS)
CXCR4 chemokine receptor for cytokine SDF-1	HIV (causing AIDS)
Acetylcholine receptor on skeletal muscle	Rabies virus
B-lymphocyte complement C3d receptor	Glandular fever virus
T-lymphocyte interleukin-2 receptor	T-cell leukaemia viruses
β-Adrenoceptors	Infantile diarrhoea virus
MHC molecules	Adenovirus (causing sore throat and conjunctivitis) T-cell leukaemia viruses

MCP-1, monocyte chemoattractant protein-1; MHC, major histocompatibility complex; RANTES, regulated on activation, normal T-cell–expressed and secreted; SDF-1, stromal cell–derived factor-1.
[a]For more detail on complement, interleukin-2, the CD4 glycoprotein on helper T lymphocytes, MHC molecules, etc., see Chapter 13. For SDF-1, see Chapter 22.

Replication in DNA viruses

Viral DNA enters the host cell nucleus, where transcription into mRNA occurs catalysed by the host cell RNA polymerase. Translation of the mRNA into virus-specific proteins then takes place. Some of these proteins are enzymes that then synthesise more viral DNA, as well as proteins comprising the viral coat and envelope. After assembly of coat proteins around the viral DNA, complete virions are released by budding or after host cell lysis.

Replication in RNA viruses

Enzymes within the virion synthesise its mRNA from the viral RNA template, or sometimes the viral RNA serves as its own mRNA. This is translated by the host cell into various enzymes, including RNA polymerase (which directs the synthesis of more viral RNA), and also into structural proteins of the virion. Assembly and release of virions occurs as explained above. With these viruses, the host cell nucleus is usually not involved in viral replication, although some RNA viruses (e.g. orthomyxoviruses) replicate exclusively within the host nuclear compartment.

Replication in retroviruses

The virion in retroviruses[1] contains a *reverse transcriptase* enzyme (virus RNA–dependent DNA polymerase), which makes a DNA copy of the viral RNA. This DNA copy is integrated into the genome of the host cell, and it is then termed a *provirus*. The provirus DNA is transcribed into both new viral genome RNA as well as mRNA for translation in the host into viral proteins, and the completed viruses are released by budding. Many retroviruses can replicate without killing the host cell.

The ability of several viruses to remain dormant within, and be replicated together with, the host genome is responsible for the periodic nature of some viral diseases, such as those caused by *herpes labialis* (cold sores) or the *varicella zoster* (chickenpox and shingles) virus, which recur when viral replication is reactivated by some factor (or when the immune system is compromised in some way). Some RNA retroviruses can transform normal cells into malignant cells.

THE HOST–VIRUS INTERACTION

HOST DEFENCES AGAINST VIRUSES

The first defence is the simple barrier function of intact skin, which most viruses are unable to penetrate. However, broken skin (e.g. at sites of wounds or insect bites) and mucous membranes are more vulnerable to viral attack. Should the virus gain entry to the body, then the host can deploy both the innate and subsequently the adaptive immune response (Ch. 13). The infected cell presents, on its surface, viral peptides complexed with major histocompatibility complex (MHC) class I molecules. This complex is recognised by T lymphocytes, which then kill the infected cell (Fig. 47.2). This may be accomplished by the release of lytic proteins (such as *perforins*, *granzymes*) or by

---

[1]A virus that can synthesise DNA from an RNA template—the reverse of the normal situation.

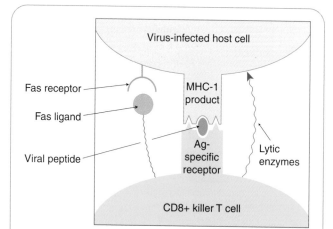

Fig. 47.2 **The mechanisms whereby a CD8⁺ T cell kills a virus-infected host cell.** The virus-infected host cell expresses a complex of virus peptides plus major histocompatibility complex class I product (MC H-I) on its surface. This is recognised by the CD8⁺ T cell, which then releases lytic enzymes into the virus-infected cell and also expresses a Fas ligand. This triggers apoptosis in the infected cell by stimulating its Fas 'death receptor'.

triggering the apoptotic pathway in the infected cell by activation of its Fas receptor ('death receptor'; see p. 79). The latter may also be triggered indirectly through the release of a cytokine such as tumour necrosis factor (TNF)-α. If the virus escapes immune detection by cytotoxic lymphocytes by modifying the expression of the peptide–MHC complex (see below), it may still fall victim to natural killer (NK) cells. This reaction to the absence of normal MHC molecules might be called the 'mother turkey' strategy (kill everything that does not sound exactly like a baby turkey; see footnote on p. 206). But some viruses also have a device for evading NK cells as well (see below).

Within the cell itself, a sophisticated mechanism known as *gene silencing* may also provide a further level of protection (see Schutze, 2004). Short double-stranded fragments of RNA, such as those that could arise as a result of the virus's attempts to recruit the host's transcription/translational machinery, actually cause the gene coding for the RNA to be 'silenced'—to be switched off, probably by DNA phosphorylation. This means that the gene is no longer able to direct further viral protein synthesis, thus interrupting the replication cycle. This mechanism can be exploited for experimental purposes in many areas of biology, and tailored siRNA (small—or short—interfering RNA) is a cheap and useful technique to suppress temporarily expression of a particular gene under investigation. Attempts to harness the technique for viricidal purposes have met with some success (see Barik, 2004).

VIRAL PLOYS TO CIRCUMVENT HOST DEFENCES

Viruses have evolved a variety of strategies to ensure successful infection, some entailing redirection of the host's response for the advantage of the virus (discussed by Tortorella et al., 2000).

Subversion of the immune response

Viruses can inhibit the action of the cytokines, such as interleukin-1, TNF-α and the antiviral interferons (IFNs; see p. 223), that normally coordinate the innate and adaptive immune responses. Following infection, for example, some poxviruses express proteins that mimic the extracellular ligand-binding domains of cytokine receptors. These *pseudoreceptors* bind cytokines, preventing them from reaching their natural receptors on cells of the immune system and thus moderating the normal immune response to virus-infected cells. Other viruses that can interfere with cytokine signalling include human cytomegalovirus, Epstein–Barr virus, herpesvirus and adenovirus.

Evasion of immune detection and attack by killer cells

Once within host cells, viruses may also escape immune detection and evade lethal attack by cytotoxic lymphocytes and NK cells in various ways, such as the following.

- *Interference with the surface protein markers on the infected cells essential for killer cell attack.* Some viruses inhibit generation of the antigenic peptide and/or the presentation of MHC–peptide molecules. This turns off the signal that the cells are infected, enabling the viruses to remain undetected. Examples of viruses that can do this are adenovirus, herpes simplex virus, human cytomegalovirus, Epstein–Barr virus and influenza virus.
- *Interference with the apoptotic pathway.* Some viruses (e.g. adenovirus, human cytomegalovirus, Epstein–Barr virus) can subvert this pathway for their own purposes.
- *Adopting the 'baby turkey' ploy.* Some viruses (e.g. cytomegalovirus) get round the mother turkey approach of NK cells by expressing a homologue of MHC class I (the equivalent of a turkey chick's chirping) that is close enough to the real thing to hoodwink NK cells.

It is evident that evolution has equipped pathogenic viruses with many efficacious tactics for circumventing host defences, and understanding these in more detail is likely to suggest new types of antiviral therapy. Fortunately, the biological arms race is not one-sided, and evolution has also equipped the host with sophisticated counter-measures. In most cases these prevail, with viral infections eventually generally resolving spontaneously, except in an immunocompromised host. The situation does not always end happily though; some viral infections, such as Lassa fever and Ebola virus infection, have a high mortality, and we now discuss a further, grave example of this group: the HIV virus. This is appropriate because HIV exhibits many of the features common to other viral infections, and the sheer scale of the global AIDS problem has pushed HIV to the top of the list of antiviral targets.

HIV AND AIDS

HIV is an RNA retrovirus. Two forms are known. *HIV-1* is the organism responsible for human AIDS. The *HIV-2* organism is

> **Viruses**
>
> - Viruses are small infective agents consisting of nucleic acid (RNA or DNA) enclosed in a protein coat.
> - They are not cells and, having no metabolic machinery of their own, are obligate intracellular parasites, utilising the metabolic processes of the host cell they infect to replicate.
> - *DNA viruses* usually enter the host cell nucleus and direct the generation of new viruses.
> - *RNA viruses* direct the generation of new viruses, usually without involving the host cell nucleus (the influenza virus is an exception in that it does involve the host cell nucleus).
> - *RNA retroviruses* (e.g. HIV, T-cell leukaemia virus) contain an enzyme, reverse transcriptase, which makes a DNA copy of the viral RNA. This DNA copy is integrated into the host cell genome and directs the generation of new virus particles.

similar to the HIV-1 virus in that it also causes immune suppression, but it is less virulent. HIV-1 is distributed around the world, whereas the HIV-2 virus is confined to parts of Africa. We will consider them together in this section.

▼ In 2004, the World Health Organization estimated that almost 40 million people were living with AIDS, and that women and children constituted approximately half that total number. During the same year, some 3 million people died of the disease (including 0.64 million children under 15 years), and there were a further 5 million new cases of AIDS infection reported. The epidemic is overwhelmingly centred on sub-Saharan Africa, which accounts for two-thirds of the total global number of infected persons, and where the adult prevalence is 7.4% (compared with 0.3% in Europe). For a review of the pathogenesis of AIDS, see Mindel & Tenant-Flowers (2001).

The interaction of HIV with the host's immune system is complex, and although it involves mainly cytotoxic T lymphocytes (CTLs, CD8⁺ T cells) and CD4⁺ helper T lymphocytes (CD4 cells), other immune cells, such as macrophages, dendritic cells and NK cells, also play a part. Antibodies are produced by the host to various HIV components, but it is the action of the CTLs and CD4 cells that initially prevents the spread of HIV.

Cytotoxic T lymphocytes directly kill virally infected cells and produce and release antiviral cytokines (Fig. 47.2). The lethal event is lysis of the target cell, but induction of apoptosis by interaction of Fas ligand ('death ligand'; see Fig. 5.5) on the CTL with Fas receptors on the virally infected cell can also play a part. **CD4⁺ cells** have an important role as helper cells, and it is the progressive loss of these cells that is the defining characteristic of HIV infection (Fig. 47.4). Recent work suggests that CD4 cells may themselves have a direct role (e.g. lysis of target cells) in the control of HIV replication (Norris et al., 2004).

Once within the cell, HIV is integrated with the host DNA (the provirus form), undergoing transcription and generating new virions when the cell is activated (Fig. 47.3). In an untreated subject, a

staggering 10^{10} new virus particles may be produced each day. Intracellular HIV can remain silent (latent) for a long time.

▼ The priming of naive T cells to become CTLs during the induction phase involves interaction of the T-cell receptor complex with antigenic HIV peptide in association with MHC class I molecules on the surface of antigen-presenting cells (APCs; see Figs 13.3 and 13.4). Priming also requires the presence and participation of CD4⁺ cells. It is thought that both types of cell need to recognise antigen on the surface of the same APC (Fig. 13.3).

The CTLs thus generated are effective during the initial stages of the infection but are not able to stop the progression of the disease. It is believed that this is because the CTLs have become 'exhausted' and dysfunctional. Two different mechanisms may be involved, and these are summarised in simple terms below.

- One possible mechanism has been suggested on the basis of recent research into a different viral infection. The study shows that the assistance of CD4⁺ cells *during the initial priming process* may be essential for the secondary expansion of CTLs on autonomous restimulation. The evidence is that, during priming, CD4⁺ cells help determine the development of the relevant CTL memory and the ability of CTLs to mount a secondary response. Without this, most CTL cells may, on interacting with antigen again, themselves become exhausted and enter apoptosis (Jansen et al., 2004). This throws new light on the role of CD4⁺ cells in the immune response to HIV.
- Another possible explanation for CD8⁺ T-cell exhaustion, also based on recent work with another viral infection, is that these cells over-express an apoptotic gene. Administration of an antibody that blocked the interaction between this factor and its receptor restored the ability of T cells to proliferate and kill infected cells, thus reducing the viral load. This notion also suggests a novel and potentially effective immunological strategy for treatment of chronic viral infections such as that caused by the HIV viruses (Barber et al., 2006).

The HIV virion cannily attaches to proteins on the host cell surface to gain entry to the cells. The main targets are CD4 (a glycoprotein marker of a particular group of helper T lymphocytes) and CCR5 (a coreceptor for certain chemokines, including monocyte chemoattractant protein-1 and RANTES [regulated on activation normal T-cell expressed and secreted]). CD4⁺ cells normally orchestrate the immune response to viruses, but by entering these cells and using them as virion factories, HIV virtually cripples this aspect of the immune response. Figure 47.3 shows an HIV virion infecting a CD4⁺ T cell. Infected activated CD4 T cells in lymphoid tissue form the major source of HIV production in HIV-infected individuals; infected macrophages are another source.

As for CCR5, evidence from exposed individuals who somehow evade infection indicates that this surface protein has a central role in HIV pathogenesis. Compounds that inhibit the entry of HIV into cells by blocking CCR5 are in phase III clinical trials and may soon be available commercially (Charo et al., 2006).

When immune surveillance breaks down, other strains of HIV arise that recognise other host cell surface molecules such as CD4 and CXCR4. A surface glycoprotein, gp120, on the HIV envelope binds to CD4 and also to the T-cell chemokine coreceptor CXCR4. Another viral glycoprotein, gp41, then causes fusion of the viral envelope with the plasma membrane of the cell (Fig. 47.3).

Viral replication is error-prone, and there are a large number of mutations daily at each site in the HIV genome, so HIV soon escapes recognition by the original cytotoxic lymphocytes. Although other cytotoxic lymphocytes arise that recognise the altered virus protein(s), further mutations, in turn, allow escape from surveillance by these cells too. It is suggested that wave after wave of cytotoxic lymphocytes act against new mutants as they arise, gradually depleting a T-cell repertoire already

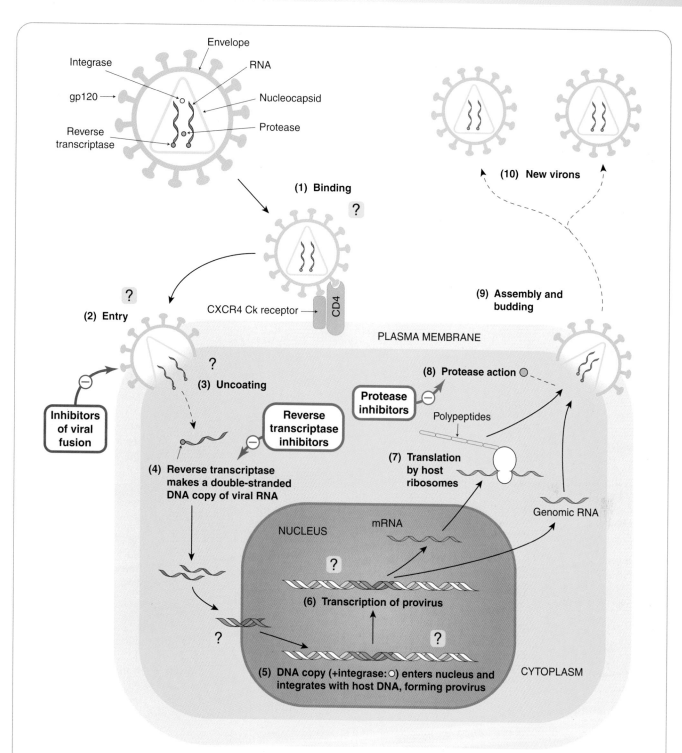

Fig. 47.3 **Schematic diagram of infection of a CD4+ T cell by an HIV virion, with the sites of action of the two main classes of anti-HIV drugs.** The 10 steps of HIV infection, from attachment to the cell to release of new virions, are shown. The virus uses the CD4 coreceptor and the chemokine (Ck) receptor CXCR4 as binding sites to facilitate entry into the cell, where it becomes incorporated into host DNA (steps 1–5). When transcription occurs (step 6), the T cell itself is activated and the transcription factor nuclear factor κB initiates transcription of both host cell and provirus DNA. A viral protease cleaves the nascent viral polypeptides (steps 7 and 8) into structural proteins and enzymes (integrase, reverse transcriptase, protease) for the new virion. The new virions are assembled and released from the cells, initiating a fresh round of infection (steps 9 and 10). The sites of action of the currently used anti-HIV drugs are shown.

seriously compromised by the loss of CD4⁺ helper T cells, until eventually the immune response fails.

There is considerable variability in the progress of the disease, but the usual clinical course of an untreated HIV infection is shown in Figure 47.4. An initial acute influenza-like illness is associated with an increase in the number of virus particles in the blood, their widespread dissemination through the tissues, and the seeding of lymphoid tissue with the virion particles. Within a few weeks, the *viraemia* is reduced by the action of cytotoxic lymphocytes as specified above.

The acute initial illness is followed by a symptom-free period during which there is reduction in the viraemia accompanied by silent virus replication in the lymph nodes, associated with damage to lymph node architecture and the loss of CD4⁺ lymphocytes and dendritic cells. Clinical latency (median, 10 years) comes to an end when the immune response finally fails and the signs and symptoms of AIDS appear—opportunistic infections (e.g. with *Pneumocystis carinii* or the tubercle bacillus), neurological disease (e.g. confusion, paralysis, dementia), bone marrow depression and cancers. Chronic gastrointestinal infections contribute to the severe weight loss. Cardiovascular damage and kidney damage can also occur. In an untreated patient, death usually follows within 2 years. The advent of complex combination drug regimens has changed the prognosis—at least in countries that are able to deploy them.

There is evidence that genetic factors play an important role in determining the susceptibility—or resistance—to HIV (see Flores-Villanueva et al., 2003).

ANTIVIRAL DRUGS

Because viruses hijack many of the metabolic processes of the host cell itself, it is difficult to find drugs that are selective for the pathogen. However, there are some enzymes that are virus-specific, and these have proved to be useful drug targets. Most currently available antiviral agents are effective only while the

virus is replicating. Because the initial phases of viral infection are often asymptomatic, treatment is often delayed until the infection is well established, and one therefore begins therapy at a tactical disadvantage. As is often the case with infectious diseases, an ounce of prevention is worth a pound of cure.

Many antiviral drugs are available, and we cannot discuss all these in detail for space reasons. However, most fall into only a few groups with similar mechanisms of action and often similar side effects too. Table 47.2 shows the commonest antiviral drugs, their mechanisms of action and some of the diseases they are used to treat. Some common side effects are shown in Table 47.3. We will discuss each group briefly.

NUCLEOSIDE REVERSE TRANSCRIPTASE INHIBITORS

This currently comprises a large group of nucleoside analogues all of which are phosphorylated by host cell enzymes to give the 5'-triphosphate derivative. This moiety competes with the equivalent host cellular triphosphate substrates for proviral DNA synthesis by viral reverse transcriptase (viral RNA–dependent DNA polymerase). Eventually, the incorporation of the 5'-triphosphate moiety into the growing viral DNA chain results in chain termination. Mammalian α-DNA polymerase is relatively resistant to the effect. However, γ-DNA polymerase in the host cell mitochondria is fairly sensitive to the compound, and this may be the basis of some unwanted effects. The main utility of these drugs is the treatment of HIV, but a number of them have useful activity against other viruses also. Some examples of nucleoside reverse transcriptase inhibitors are given below.

Zidovudine

Zidovudine is an analogue of thymidine. It can prolong life in HIV-infected individuals and diminish HIV-associated dementia. Given to the parturient mother and then to the newborn infant, it can reduce mother-to-baby transmission by more than 20%. It is

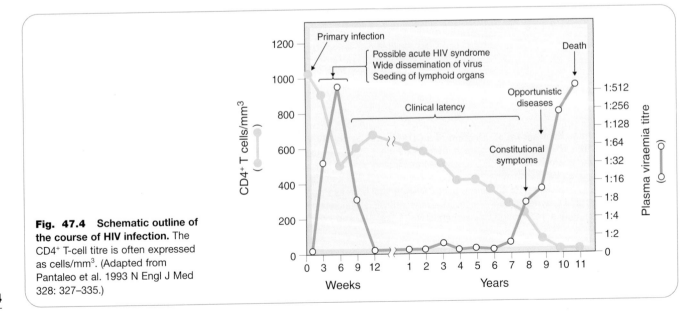

Fig. 47.4 Schematic outline of the course of HIV infection. The CD4⁺ T-cell titre is often expressed as cells/mm³. (Adapted from Pantaleo et al. 1993 N Engl J Med 328: 327–335.)

Table 47.2 Principal classes of antiviral drugs and some common therapeutic uses

Type	Common therapeutic indication(s)
Nucleoside reverse transcriptase inhibitors: *abacavir, adefovir dipivoxil, didanosine, emtricitabine, lamivudine, stavudine, tenofovir, zalcitabine, zidovudine*	Mainly HIV, generally in combination with other retrovirals Lamivudine and adefovir are also used in the treatment of hepatitis B
Non-nucleoside reverse transcriptase inhibitors: *efavirenz, nevirapine*	HIV, generally in combination with other retrovirals
Protease inhibitors: *amprenavir, atazanavir, indinavir, lopinavir, nelfinavir, ritonavir, saquinavir*	HIV, generally in combination with other retrovirals
Viral DNA polymerase inhibitors: *aciclovir[†], cidofovir*, famciclovir[†], foscarnet[†], ganciclovir*, idoxuridine[†], penciclovir[†], ribvarin[‡], valaciclovir*[†], valganciclovir**	Treatment of herpes[†], cytomegalovirus*, or hepatitis C and respiratory syncitial virus infections[‡]
Inhibitors of HIV fusion with host cells: *enfurvitide*	HIV, generally in combination with other retrovirals
Inhibitors of viral coat disassembly and neuraminidase inhibitors: *amantadine*, oseltamivir, zanamivir*	Influenza A* or A and B
Biologics and immunomodulators: *interferon-α, pegylated interferon-α, inosine pranobex*, palivizumab[†]*	Treatment of hepatitis B and C, herpes* and respiratory syncitial virus[†]

Table 47.3 Principal common unwanted effects of some antiviral drugs

Drug type	Principal common unwanted effects	Comments
Nucleoside reverse transcriptase inhibitors: *zidovudine, abacavir, didanosine, emtricitabine, lamivudine, stavudine, tenofovir, zalcatabine*	Gastrointestinal disturbances including nausea, vomiting, abdominal pain and diarrhoea Central nervous system and related effects including headache, insomnia and dizziness, and neuropathy Musculoskeletal and dermatological effects including fatigue, myalgia, arthralgia, rash, urticaria and fever Blood disorders including anaemia, neutropenia and thrombocytopenia Metabolic effects including pancreatitis, liver damage and lipodystrophy	–
Non-nucleoside reverse transcriptase inhibitors: *efavirenz, nevirapine*	Dermatological effects including rash and urticaria Central nervous system and related effects including fatigue, headache, sleep disturbances, depression and dizziness Gastrointestinal disturbances including nausea, vomiting, abdominal pain and diarrhoea Blood disorders including anaemia, neutropenia and thrombocytopenia[a] Metabolic effects including pancreatitis, raised cholesterol, liver dysfunction and lipodystrophy	High (15–25%) incidence of rash
Protease inhibitors: *amprenavir, atazanavir, indinavir, lopinavir, nelfinavir, ritonovir, saquinavir*	Gastrointestinal disturbances including nausea, vomiting, abdominal pain and diarrhoea Central nervous system and related effects including fatigue, headache, sleep disturbances and dizziness, taste disturbances and paraesthesia Musculoskeletal and dermatological effects including myalgia, arthralgia, rhabdomyolysis, rash, urticaria and fever Blood disorders including anaemia, neutropenia and thrombocytopenia Metabolic effects including pancreatitis, liver dysfunction and lipodystrophy	–

[a]Administration of epoietin (erythropoietin) and molgramostim (recombinant human granulocyte macrophage colony-stimulating factor; see Ch. 22, p. 354) may alleviate these problems.

generally administered orally twice daily but can also be given by intravenous infusion. The bioavailability is 60–80%, and the peak plasma concentration occurs at 30 minutes. Its half-life is 1 hour, and the intracellular half-life of the active trisphosphate is 3 hours. The concentration in cerebrospinal fluid (CSF) is 65% of the plasma level. Most of the drug is metabolised to the inactive glucuronide in the liver, only 20% of the active form being excreted in the urine.

Resistance to the antiviral action of zidovudine

Because of rapid mutation, the virus is a constantly moving target, thus the therapeutic response wanes with long-term use, particularly in late-stage disease. Furthermore, resistant strains can be transferred between individuals. Other factors that underlie the loss of efficacy of the drug are decreased activation of zidovudine to the trisphosphate and increased virus load owing to reduction in the host immune response.

Didanosine

Didanosine is an analogue of deoxyadenosine. It is given orally, is rapidly absorbed and is actively secreted by the kidney tubules. The level in the CSF reaches ~20% of the plasma concentration. The plasma half-life is 30 minutes, but the intracellular half-life is more than 12 hours.

Zalcitabine

Zalcitabine is a homologue of cytosine. It is activated in the T cell by a different phosphorylation pathway from zidovudine. It is given orally. Its plasma half-life is 20 minutes, and its intracellular half-life is nearly 3 hours; the CSF level is 20% of that in the plasma.

Lamivudine

Lamivudine is an analogue of cytosine. It is given orally, is well absorbed and most is excreted unchanged in the urine. The CSF level is 20% of the plasma concentration. Used alone, it could select for HIV mutants that are resistant to both the drug itself as well as other reverse transcriptase inhibitors. Lamivudine is also used in the therapy of hepatitis B infection.

Stavudine

Stavudine is a thymidine analogue. It is given orally, has a plasma half-life of 1 hour, and most is eliminated via the kidney by active tubular secretion. The CSF level is 55% of that in the plasma.

Abacavir

Abacavir is a guanosine analogue and has so far proved to be more effective than most other nucleoside reverse transcriptase inhibitors. It is well absorbed after oral administration and is metabolised in the liver to inactive compounds. The CSF level is 33% of that in the plasma.

NON-NUCLEOSIDE REVERSE TRANSCRIPTASE INHIBITORS

Non-nucleoside reverse transcriptase inhibitors are chemically diverse compounds that bind to the reverse transcriptase enzyme near the catalytic site and denature it. Most non-nucleoside reverse transcriptase inhibitors are inducers, substrates or inhibitors, to varying degrees, of the liver cytochrome P450 enzymes. Currently available drugs **nevirapine** are and **efavirenz**.

Nevirapine

Nevirapine is given orally, its bioavailability is >90%, and its CSF level is 45% of that in the plasma. It is metabolised in the liver, and the metabolite is excreted in the urine. Nevirapine can prevent mother-to-baby transmission of HIV if given to the parturient mother and the neonate.

Efavirenz

Efavirenz is given orally, once daily because of its plasma half-life (~50 hours). It is 99% bound to plasma albumin, and its CSF concentration is ~1% of that in the plasma. It is inactivated in the liver.

PROTEASE INHIBITORS

In HIV and many other viral infections, the mRNA transcribed from the provirus is translated into two biochemically inert *polyproteins*. A virus-specific protease then converts the polyproteins into various structural and functional proteins by cleavage at the appropriate positions (see Fig. 47.3). Because this protease does not occur in the host, it is a useful target for chemotherapeutic intervention. HIV-specific protease inhibitors bind to the site where cleavage occurs, and their use, in combination with reverse transcriptase inhibitors, has transformed the therapy of AIDS. Examples of current protease inhibitors are shown in Table 47.2 and are exemplified by drugs such as **saquinavir**, **nelfinavir**, **indinavir**, **ritonavir** and **amprenavir**.

Pharmacokinetic aspects

The drugs are generally given orally, saquinavir being subject to extensive first-pass metabolism. CSF levels are negligible with saquinavir and highest with indinavir (76% of the plasma concentration). Nelfinavir and ritonavir are best taken with food, and saquinavir within 2 hours of a meal.

Unwanted effects are also similar (see Table 47.3).

DNA POLYMERASE INHIBITORS

Aciclovir

The era of effective selective antiviral therapy began with **aciclovir**. This agent is a guanosine derivative with a high specificity for herpes simplex and varicella zoster viruses. Herpes simplex can cause cold sores, conjunctivitis, mouth ulcers, genital infections[2] and, rarely but very seriously, encephalitis; in immunocompromised patients, it is much more aggressive. Varicella zoster

---

[2]Venereologists (now called 'sexually transmitted disease physicians', references to Venus presumably being no longer acceptable) with a taste for cynical humour ask 'What is the difference between true love and genital herpes?', their answer being that genital herpes is for ever. It may not be.

viruses cause shingles and chickenpox. Herpes simplex is more susceptible to aciclovir than varicella zoster. Epstein–Barr virus (a herpesvirus that causes glandular fever) is also slightly sensitive. Aciclovir has a small but reproducible effect against cytomegalovirus—a herpesvirus that can affect the fetus with catastrophic consequences, can cause a glandular fever–like syndrome in adults and severe disease (e.g. retinitis, which can result in blindness) in immunocompromised individuals.

Mechanism of action

Aciclovir is converted to the monophosphate by thymidine kinase, and happily the virus-specific form of this enzyme is very much more effective in carrying out the phosphorylation than the enzyme of the host cell; it is therefore only activated adequately in infected cells. The host cell kinases then convert the monophosphate to the trisphosphate. It is the aciclovir trisphosphate that inhibits viral DNA polymerase, terminating the nucleotide chain. It is 30 times more potent against the herpesvirus enzyme than the host enzyme. Aciclovir trisphosphate is fairly rapidly broken down within the host cells, presumably by cellular phosphatases. Resistance caused by changes in the viral genes coding for thymidine kinase or DNA polymerase has been reported, and aciclovir-resistant herpes simplex virus has been the cause of pneumonia, encephalitis and mucocutaneous infections in immunocompromised patients.

Pharmacokinetic aspects

Aciclovir can be given orally, intravenously or topically. When it is given orally, only 20% of the dose is absorbed and peak plasma concentrations are reached in 1–2 hours. The drug is widely distributed, reaching concentrations in the CSF that are 50% of those in the plasma. It is excreted by the kidneys, partly by glomerular filtration and partly by tubular secretion.

Unwanted effects

These are minimal. Local inflammation can occur during intravenous injection if there is extravasation of the solution. Renal dysfunction has been reported when aciclovir is given intravenously; slow infusion reduces the risk. Nausea and headache can occur and, rarely, encephalopathy.

There are now many other drugs with a similar action to aciclovir (see Table 47.2). This group includes **valaciclovir**, a prodrug of aciclovir, and **famciclovir**, which is metabolised to the active compound **penciclovir** in vivo. Other viral DNA polymerase inhibitors include the following.

Ganciclovir

This acyclic analogue of guanosine is the drug of choice for *cytomegalovirus* infection. This is a frequent opportunistic infection in immunocompromised or AIDS patients and has been a formidable obstacle to successful transplantation of organs and bone marrow (which necessitates immunosuppressive therapy). Like aciclovir, **ganciclovir** has to be activated to the trisphosphate, and in this form it competes with guanosine trisphosphate for incorporation into viral DNA. It suppresses viral DNA replication, but unlike aciclovir it does not act as a chain terminator and has a longer duration of action, persisting in infected cells for 18–20 hours.

> **Clinical uses of drugs for herpes viruses (e.g. aciclovir, famciclovir, valaciclovir)**
>
> - *Varicella zoster* infections (chickenpox, shingles):
>   - orally in immunocompetent patients
>   - intravenously in immunocompromised patients.
> - *Herpes simplex* infections (*genital* herpes, *mucocutaneous* herpes and herpes *encephalitis*).
> - Prophylactically:
>   - patients who are to be treated with immunosuppressant drugs or radiotherapy and who are at risk of herpesvirus infection owing to reactivation of a latent virus
>   - in individuals who suffer from frequent recurrences of genital infection with herpes simplex virus.

Pharmacokinetic aspects

Ganciclovir is given intravenously. It is excreted in the urine and has a half-life of 4 hours.

Unwanted effects

Ganciclovir has serious unwanted actions, including bone marrow depression and potential carcinogenicity, and is consequently used only for life- or sight-threatening cytomegalovirus infections in patients who are immunocompromised. Oral administration can be used for maintenance therapy in AIDS patients.

Tribavirin (ribavirin)

Tribavirin is a synthetic nucleoside, similar in structure to guanosine. It is thought to act either by altering virus nucleotide pools or by interfering with the synthesis of viral mRNA. It inhibits a wide range of DNA and RNA viruses, including many that affect the lower airways. In aerosol form, it has been used to treat influenza and infections with *respiratory syncytial virus* (an RNA paramyxovirus). It has also been shown to be effective in hepatitis C as well as Lassa fever, an extremely serious *arenavirus* infection. When given promptly to victims of the latter disease, it has been shown to reduce to 9%, a case fatality rate previously 76%.

Foscarnet (phosphonoformate)

Foscarnet is a synthetic non-nucleoside analogue of pyrophosphate that inhibits viral DNA polymerase by binding directly to the pyrophosphate-binding site. It can cause serious nephrotoxicity. Given by intravenous infusion, it is a second-line drug in cytomegalovirus eye infection in immunocompromised patients.

INHIBITORS OF HIV FUSION WITH HOST CELLS

There is only one drug in this group: **enfurvirtide**. The drug is generally given by subcutaneous injection in combination with others to treat HIV when resistance becomes a problem or when the patient is intolerant of other antiretrovirals.

Unwanted effects

These include flu-like symptoms, central effects such as headache, dizziness, alterations in mood, gastrointestinal effects and sometimes hypersensitivity reactions.

NEURAMINIDASE INHIBITORS AND INHIBITORS OF VIRAL COAT DISASSEMBLY

Viral neuraminidase is one of three transmembrane proteins coded by the influenza genome. Infection with these RNA viruses begins with the attachment of the viral haemaglutinin to neuraminic (sialic) acid residues on host cells. The viral particle then enters the cell by an endocytic process. The endosome is acidified following influx of H⁺ through another viral protein, the *M2 ion channel*. This facilitates the disassembly of the viral structure, allowing the RNA to enter the host nucleus, thus initiating a round of viral replication. Newly replicated virions escape from the host cell by budding from the cell membrane. Viral neuraminidase promotes this by severing the bonds linking the particle coat and host sialic acid.

The neuraminidase inhibitors **zanamivir** and **oseltamivir** are active against both influenza A and B viruses, and are licensed for use at early stages in the infection or when use of the vaccine is impossible. Zanamivir is available as a powder for inhalation, and oseltamivir as an oral preparation. At the time of writing, governments around the world are stockpiling this latter drug in the expectation that it may offer some defence against 'bird flu', should this mutate into an organism capable of infecting humans.

Unwanted effects of both include gastrointestinal symptoms (nausea, vomiting, dyspepsia and diarrhoea), but these are less frequent and severe in the inhaled preparation.

Amantadine,[3] quite an old drug (1966) and seldom recommended today, effectively blocks the M2 ion channels, thus inhibiting viral disassembly. It is active against influenza A virus (an RNA virus) but has no action against influenza B virus. The closely related **rimantadine** is similar in its effects.

Pharmacokinetic aspects. Given orally, amantadine is well absorbed, reaches high levels in secretions (e.g. saliva) and most is excreted unchanged via the kidney. Aerosol administration is feasible.

Unwanted effects are relatively infrequent, occurring in 5–10% of patients, and are not serious. Dizziness, insomnia and slurred speech are the most common adverse effects.

BIOLOGICS AND IMMUNOMODULATORS

A number of other agents have been recruited in the fight against virus infections, including immunoglobulin preparations, IFNs, immunomodulators and monoclonal antibodies.

Immunoglobulin

Pooled immunoglobulin contains antibodies against various viruses present in the population. The antibodies are directed against the virus envelope and can 'neutralise' some viruses and prevent their attachment to host cells. If used before the onset of signs and symptoms, it may attenuate or prevent measles, infectious hepatitis, German measles, rabies or poliomyelitis. *Hyperimmune* globulin, specific against particular viruses, is used against hepatitis B, varicella zoster and rabies.

Palivisumab

Related in terms of its mechanism of action to immunoglobulins is **palivisumab**, a monoclonal antibody (see Chs 13 and 55) directed against a glycoprotein on the surface of respiratory syncytial virus. It is used (as an intramuscular injection) in infants to prevent infection by this organism.

Interferon

Interferons are a family of inducible proteins synthesised by mammalian cells and now generally produced commercially using recombinant DNA technology. There are at least three types, α, β, and γ, constituting a family of hormones involved in cell growth and regulation and the modulation of immune reactions. IFN-γ, termed *immune interferon* (see p. 223), is produced mainly by T lymphocytes as part of an immunological response to both viral and non-viral antigens, the latter including bacteria and their products, rickettsiae, protozoa, fungal polysaccharides and a range of polymeric chemicals and other cytokines. IFN-α and IFN-β are produced by B and T lymphocytes, macrophages and fibroblasts in response to the presence of viruses and cytokines. The general actions of the IFNs are described briefly in Chapter 13.

Mechanism of antiviral action

The IFNs bind to specific ganglioside receptors on host cell membranes. They induce, in host cell ribosomes, the production of enzymes that inhibit the translation of viral mRNA into viral proteins, thus halting viral replication. They have a broad spectrum of action and inhibit the replication of most viruses in vitro.

Pharmacokinetic aspects

Given intravenously, IFNs have a half-life of 2–4 hours. With intramuscular injections, peak blood concentrations are reached in 5–8 hours. They do not cross the blood–brain barrier.

Clinical use

Interferon-α-2a is used for treatment of hepatitis B infections and AIDS-related Kaposi sarcomas; **IFN-α-2b** is used for hepatitis C. There are reports that IFNs can prevent reactivation of herpes simplex after trigeminal root section and can prevent spread of herpes zoster in cancer patients. Preparations of IFNs conjugated with polyethylene glycol (**pegylated IFNs**) have a longer lifetime in the circulation.

Unwanted effects

Unwanted effects are common and include fever, lassitude, headache and myalgia. Repeated injections cause chronic malaise. Bone marrow depression, rashes, alopecia and disturbances in cardiovascular, thyroid and hepatic function can also occur.

Inosine pranobex

Immunomodulators are drugs that act by moderating the immune response to viruses or use an immune mechanism to target a virus

---

[3] Also used for its mildly beneficial effects in Parkinson's disease (see Ch. 35).

or other organism. **Inosine pranobex** may interfere with viral nucleic acid synthesis but also has immunopotentiating actions on the host. It is sometimes used to treat herpes infections in mucosal tissues or on the skin.

COMBINATION THERAPY FOR HIV

Two main classes of antivirals are used to treat HIV: reverse transcriptase inhibitors and protease inhibitors. As they have different mechanisms of action (Fig. 47.3), they can usefully be used in combinations and this technique has dramatically improved the prognosis of the disease. The combination treatment is known as <u>h</u>ighly <u>a</u>ctive <u>a</u>nti<u>r</u>etroviral <u>t</u>herapy (HAART). A typical HAART combination would involve two nucleoside reverse transcriptase inhibitors with either a non-nucleoside reverse transcriptase inhibitor or one or two protease inhibitors.

Using a HAART protocol, HIV replication is inhibited, the presence in the plasma of HIV RNA is reduced to undetectable levels, and patient survival is greatly prolonged. But the regimen is complex and has many unwanted effects. Compliance is difficult and treatment is lifelong. The virus is not eradicated but lies latent in the host genome of memory T cells, ready to reactivate if therapy is stopped.

Unwelcome interactions can occur between the three component drugs of HAART combinations, and there may be interindividual variations in absorption. Some drugs penetrate poorly into the brain, and this could lead to local proliferation of the virus. At present, there is no cross-resistance between the three groups of drugs, but it needs to be borne in mind that the virus has a high mutation rate—so resistance could be a problem in the future. The HIV virus has certainly not yet been outsmarted.

Antiviral drugs

- Most antiviral drugs generally fall into the following groups:
  - nucleoside analogues that inhibit the viral reverse transcriptase enzyme, preventing replication (e.g. lamivudine, zidovudine)
  - non-nucleoside analogues that have the same effect (e.g. efavirenz)
  - inhibitors of proteases that prevent viral protein processing (e.g. saquinavir, indinavir)
  - inhibitors of viral DNA polymerase that prevent replication (e.g. aciclovir, famciclovir)
  - inhibitors of viral capsule disassembly (e.g. amantidine)
  - inhibitors of neuraminidase that prevent viral escape from infected cells (e.g. oseltamivir)
  - immunomodulators that enhance host defences (e.g. interferons and inosine pranobex)
  - immunoglobulin and related preparations that contain neutralising antibodies to various viruses.

Drugs for HIV infections

- Reverse transcriptase inhibitors (RTIs):
  - *nucleoside RTIs* are phosphorylated by host cell enzymes to give the 5′-trisphosphate, which competes with the equivalent host cellular trisphosphates that are essential substrates for the formation of proviral DNA by viral reverse transcriptase (examples are zidovudine and abacavir); they are used in combination with protease inhibitors.
  - *non-nucleoside RTIs* are chemically diverse compounds that bind to the reverse transcriptase near the catalytic site and denature it; an example is nevirapine.
- Protease inhibitors inhibit cleavage of the nascent viral protein into functional and structural proteins. They are often used in combination with reverse transcriptase inhibitors. An example is saquinavir.
- Combination therapy is essential in treating HIV; this characteristically comprises two nucleoside RTIs with either a non-nucleoside RTI or one or two protease inhibitors.

Treatment of HIV/AIDS

- A consensus on the use of retroviral therapy in AIDS has emerged based on the following principles:
  - monitor plasma viral load and CD4$^+$ cell count
  - start treatment before immunodeficiency becomes evident
  - aim to reduce plasma viral concentration as much as possible for as long as possible
  - use combinations of at least three drugs (e.g. two reverse transcriptase inhibitors and one protease inhibitor)
  - change to a new regimen if plasma viral concentration increases.

The choice of drugs to treat pregnant or breast-feeding women is difficult. The main aims are to avoid damage to the fetus and to prevent transmission of the disease to the neonate. Therapy with zidovudine alone is often used in these cases. Another area that requires special consideration is prophylaxis for individuals who may have been exposed to the virus accidentally. Specific guidelines have been developed for such cases, but they are beyond the scope of this chapter.

PROSPECTS FOR NEW ANTIVIRAL DRUGS

At the beginning of the 1990s, there were only five drugs available to treat viral infections; 15 years later, this number has increased some sevenfold. New strategies—based on the growing understanding of the biology of pathogenic viruses and their action on and in host cells—could well, if vigorously implemented, have the potential to target the viruses causing most viral diseases (see de Clercq, 2002). However, the ultimate weapon in the fight against the virus is vaccination. This has proved to be stunningly effective in the past against diseases such as polio and smallpox, and more recently against influenza

(both types) and hepatitis B. However, while there have been many clinical trials, the prospect of a vaccine against HIV (or indeed many other viruses) still seems rather remote. Part of the problem is *antigenic drift*, a process whereby the virus mutates, thus presenting different antigenic structures and minimising the chance of an effective and long-lasting immune response or the production of a vaccine. The whole problem is the subject of numerous reviews (see Stratov et al., 2004; Tonini et al., 2005).

REFERENCES AND FURTHER READING

Viral infections in general

Hanazaki K 2004 Antiviral therapy for chronic hepatitis B: a review. Curr Drug Targets Inflamm Allergy 3: 63–70 (*Reviews the use of IFN and lamivudine, alone or in combination, in the treatment of this viral infection*)

Lauer G M, Walker B D 2001 Hepatitis C virus infection. N Engl J Med 345: 41–52 (*Comprehensive review of pathogenesis, clinical characteristics, natural history and treatment of hepatitis C infection*)

Lee W M 1997 Hepatitis B virus infection. N Engl J Med 337: 1733–1746 (*Detailed coverage of the epidemiology and pathogenesis of hepatitis B, the life cycle of the virus in the human host, and the treatment of the disease*)

Moomaw M D, Cornea P, Rathbun R C, Wendel K A 2003 Review of antiviral therapy for herpes labialis, genital herpes and herpes zoster. Expert Rev Antiinfect Ther 1: 283–295 (*Useful review focusing on the role of aciclovir, famcicolovir, penciclovir and valaciclovir in treating various manifestations of herpesvirus infections*)

Schmidt A C 2004 Antiviral therapy for influenza: a clinical and economic comparative review. Drugs 64: 2031–2046 (*A useful review of influenza biology, together with a comprehensive evaluation of drug treatments, their mechanisms of action and relative economic costs*)

Whitley R J, Roizman B 2001 Herpes simplex virus infections. Lancet 357: 1513–1518 (*A concise review of the viral replication cycle and the pathogenesis and treatment of herpes simplex virus infections*)

HIV infections

Barber D L, Wherry E J, Masopust D et al. 2006 Restoring function in exhausted CD8 T cells during chronic viral infection. Nature 439: 682–687 (*Deals with a potential mechanism whereby the exhaustion of T cells may be reversed*)

Cairns J S, D'Souza M P 1998 Chemokines and HIV-1 second receptors: the therapeutic connection. Nat Med 4: 563–568 (*Excellent review of therapeutic strategies that target the chemokine receptors used by HIV-1 to invade host cells*)

Charo I F, Ransohoff R M 2006 The many roles of chemokines and chemokine receptors in inflammation. N Engl J Med 354: 610–621 (*Useful review of the role of these receptors in facilitating HIV entry*)

Jansen C A, Piriou E, Bronke C et al 2004 Characterisation of virus-specific CD8(+) effector T cells in the course of HIV-1 infection: longitudinal analyses in slow and rapid progressors. Clin Immunol 11: 299–309.

Mindel A, Tenant-Flowers M 2001 Natural history and management of early HIV infection. Br Med J 322:

1290–1293 (*A clinical review covering the current classification of HIV disease, clinical manifestations of primary HIV infection and general treatment of HIV patients*)

Norris P J, Moffett H F, Brander C et al. 2004 Fine specificity and cross-clade reactivity of HIV type 1 Gag-specific CD4+ T cells. AIDS Res Hum Retroviruses 20: 315–325

Mechanisms of immune evasion by viruses and drug resistance

Hirsch M S 2002 HIV drug resistance: a chink in the armor. N Engl J Med 347: 438–439 (*Editorial on the challenge of drug-resistant HIV; see also Little S J et al. N Engl J Med 346: 385–394*)

Murphy P M 2001 Viral exploitation and subversion of the immune system through chemokine mimicry. Nat Immunol 2: 116–122 (*Excellent description of virus–immune system interaction*)

Tortorella D, Gewurz B E et al. 2000 Viral subversion of the immune system. Annu Rev Immunol 18: 861–926 (*A comprehensive and clearly written review of the various mechanisms by which viruses elude detection and destruction by the host immune system*)

Immune defences against viral attack

Guidotti L G, Chisari F V 2001 Noncytolytic control of viral infections by the innate and adaptive immune response. Annu Rev Immunol 19: 65–91 (*Detailed review emphasising the role of cytokines, for example IFN-α/β and TNF-α, in the endogenous control of viral infections*)

Levy J A 2001 The importance of the innate immune system in controlling HIV infection and disease. Trends Immunol 22: 312–316 (*Stresses the role of innate immunity in the response to HIV; clear exposition of the various components of the innate and adaptive immune systems, as well as the role of non-cytotoxic CD8+ cell response to HIV*)

Schutze N 2004 siRNA technology. Mol Cell Endocrinol 213: 115–119 (*An article explaining the siRNA concept*)

Mechanisms of antiviral drug action

Balfour H H 1999 Antiviral drugs. N Engl J Med 340: 1255–1268 (*An excellent and comprehensive review of antiviral agents other than those used for HIV therapy; describes their mechanisms of action, adverse effects and clinical use*)

de Clercq E 2002 Strategies in the design of antiviral drugs. Nat Rev Drug Discov 1: 13–24 (*Outstanding article describing the rationale behind current and future strategies for antiviral drug development*)

Flexner C 1998 HIV-protease inhibitors. N Engl J Med 338: 1281–1292 (*Excellent and comprehensive review

covering mechanisms of action, clinical and pharmacokinetic properties, potential drug resistance and possible treatment failure*)

Gubareva L, Kaiser L, Hayden F G 2000 Influenza virus neuraminidase inhibitors. Lancet 355: 827–835 (*Admirable coverage of this topic; lucid summary and clear diagrams of the influenza virus and its replication cycle; description of the structure and the action of, and resistance to, zanamivir and oseltamivir, and the relevant pharmacokinetic aspects and clinical efficacy*)

Patick A K, Potts K E 1998 Protease inhibitors as antiviral agents. Clin Microbiol Rev 11: 614–627 (*A useful review that summarises some of the general features of the viral proteases of the HIV virus, the human rhinovirus and the viruses causing herpes simplex and hepatitis C; the authors discuss the clinically useful inhibitors of HIV protease in some detail and outline the possible development of inhibitors of the proteases of the other viruses*)

Combination treatment for HIV

Carr A, Cooper D A 2000 Adverse effects of antiretroviral therapy. Lancet 356: 1423–1430 (*A review that focuses on the pathogenesis, clinical features and management of the main unwanted actions of current antiretroviral drugs*)

Flexner C 2000 Dual protease inhibitor therapy in HIV-infected patients: pharmacologic rationale and clinical benefits. Annu Rev Pharmacol Toxicol 40: 649–674 (*Review emphasising interactions between individual protease inhibitors and the potential benefits and disadvantages of dual therapy*)

Hammer S M 2002 Increasing choices for HIV therapy. N Engl J Med 346: 2022–2023 (*Succinct article; see also Walmsley et al. N Engl J Med 346: 2039–2046*)

Richman D D 2001 HIV chemotherapy. Nature 410: 995–1001 (*Outstanding article; covers pathogenesis and natural history of HIV infection and the impact on viral dynamics and immune function of antiretroviral therapy; discusses the main antiretroviral drugs, drug resistance of HIV and targets for new drugs; excellent figures and comprehensive references*)

Weller I V D, Williams I G 2001 Antiretroviral drugs. Br Med J 322: 1410–1412 (*Part of a British Medical Journal series on the ABC of AIDS; clear, succinct coverage of antiretroviral regimens, and a list of potential targets for new drug development*)

New leads in antiviral drug therapy

Barik S 2004 Control of nonsegmented negative-strand RNA virus replication by siRNA. Virus Res 102: 27–35 (*Interesting article explaining how siRNA technology might be used to inhibit viral replication*)

Flores-Villanueva P O, Hendel H, Caillat-Zucman S et al. 2003 Associations of MHC ancestral haplotypes with resistance/susceptibility to AIDS disease development. J Immunol 170: 1925–1929 (*A paper that deals with the hereditary component of HIV susceptibility/resistance; a bit complex for the non-geneticist but worth the effort*)

Kilby J M, Eron J J 2003 Novel therapies based on mechanisms of HIV-1 cell entry. N Engl J Med 348: 2228–2238 (*Excellent review on this innovative strategy*)

Kitabwalla M, Ruprecht R M 2002 RNA interference: a new weapon against HIV and beyond. N Engl J Med 347: 1364–1368 (*An article in the series* Clinical implications of basic research)

Moore J P, Stevenson M 2000 New targets for inhibitors of HIV-1 replication. Nat Rev Mol Cell Biol 1: 40–49 (*Excellent coverage of stages of the viral life cycle that might be susceptible to new drugs: attachment to host cell, membrane fusion, integration, accessory gene function, and assembly. Introduces various potentially promising chemical compounds.*)

Morgan R A 1999 Genetic strategies to inhibit HIV. Mol Med Today 5: 454–458 (*Discusses recent progress in gene therapy strategies; good diagram of potential targets for gene therapy*)

Stratov I, DeRose R, Purcell D F, Kent S J 2004 Vaccines and vaccine strategies against HIV. Curr Drug Targets 5: 71–88 (*Discusses the enormous challenges to the development of a successful vaccine against this disease*)

Tonini T, Barnett S, Donnelly J, Rappuoli R 2005 Current approaches to developing a preventative HIV vaccine. Curr Opin Investig Drugs 6: 155–162 (*An update on the issues surrounding the development of an effective HIV vaccine*)

Useful web resources

http://www.aidsinfo.nih.gov/ (*The official HIV/AIDS site of the US National Institutes of Health. This comprehensive web site carries authoritative and completely up-to-date information on every aspect of this disease and its treatment, including data on drugs and drug action as well as the results of recent clinical trials and the latest progress in developing a vaccine. Superb.*)

http://www.unaids.org/en/default.asp (*This is the official site of the United Nations Programme on HIV/AIDS. It deals with a wide range of issues but focuses on the demographics of the epidemic. It carries photographs, maps, slides and statistics, and other resources that bring home the enormous problems faced by the international community in dealing with this disease. Prepare to be appalled.*)

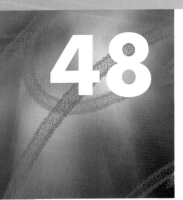

48

Antifungal drugs

OVERVIEW

Fungal infections (*mycoses*) are widespread in the population; they are generally associated with the skin (e.g. 'athlete's foot') or mucous membranes (e.g. 'thrush'). In temperate climates such as the UK, and in otherwise healthy people, they are mainly benign, being more of a nuisance than a threat. However, they become a more serious problem when the immune system is compromised or when they gain access to the systemic circulation. When this occurs, fungal infections can be fatal. In this chapter, we will briefly review the main types of fungal infections and discuss the drugs that can be used to treat them.

FUNGI AND FUNGI INFECTIONS

Fungi are eukaryotic cells and therefore represent a more complex and evolved organism than we have hitherto considered. Thousands of fungal species, predominantly parasitic in nature, have been characterised. Many are of economic importance, either because they are useful in manufacturing other products (e.g. yeast in brewing and the production of antibiotics) or because of the damage they cause to crops or to foodstuffs. Approximately 50 are pathogenic in humans. These organisms are present in the environment or may coexist with humans as *commensals* without causing any overt risks to health. However, since the 1970s, there has been a steady increase in the incidence of serious secondary systemic fungal infections. One of the contributory factors has been the widespread use of broad-spectrum antibiotics, which eliminate or decrease the non-pathogenic bacterial populations that normally compete with fungi. Other causes include the spread of AIDS and the use of immunosuppressant or cancer chemotherapy agents. The result has been an increased prevalence of *opportunistic infections*, i.e. infections that rarely cause disease in healthy individuals. Older people, diabetics, pregnant women and burn wound victims are particularly at risk of fungal infections such as *candidiasis*. Primary fungal infections, rare in many parts of the temperate world, are also now encountered more often because of the increase in international travel.

Clinically important fungi may be classified into four main types on the basis of their morphological and other characteristics. Of particular taxonomic significance is the presence of *hyphae*—filamentous projections that may knit together to form a complex *mycelium*, a mat-like structure giving the characteristic appearance of *moulds*. Drugs vary in their efficacy between the groups, and infective agents are remarkably specific for their preferred location. The main groups are:

- yeasts (e.g. *Cryptococcus neoformans*)
- yeast-like fungi that produce a structure resembling a mycelium (e.g. *Candida albicans*)
- filamentous fungi with a true mycelium (e.g. *Aspergillus fumigatus*)
- 'dimorphic' fungi that, depending on nutritional constraints, may grow as either yeasts or filamentous fungi (e.g. *Histoplasma capsulatum*).

Another organism, *Pneumocystis carinii*, shares characteristics of both protozoa (see Ch. 49) and fungi; however, it is not susceptible to antifungal drugs and will not be considered here even though it is an important opportunistic pathogen in patients with compromised immune systems (e.g. those suffering from AIDS).

Table 48.1 gives examples of each type of organism and lists some of the diseases caused by these agents and the most common choice of drug classes.

Superficial fungal infections can be classified into the *dermatomycoses* and *candidiasis*. Dermatomycoses include infections of the skin, hair and nails (onychomycosis). They are most commonly caused by *Trichophyton*, *Microsporum* or *Epidermophyton*, giving rise to various types of 'ringworm' (not to be confused with genuine helminth infections; see Ch. 50) or *tinea*. *Tinea capitis* affects the scalp; *Tinea cruris*, the groin ('Dhobie itch'); *Tinea pedis*, the feet (athlete's foot); and *Tinea*

Table 48.1 Some common fungal infections and their sensitivity to various classes of antifungals

Organism	Principal disease(s)	Most common treatment			
		Polyenes	Echinocandins	Azoles	Flucytosine[a]
Yeasts					
Cryptococcus neoformans	Meningitis	+++	−	+	+
Yeast-like fungus					
Candida albicans	Thrush, systemic candidiasis	++	Rarely	++	−
Filamentous fungi					
Trichophyton spp.	All these organisms cause skin and nail				
Microsporum spp.	infections and are referred to as tinea or	−	−	+++	−
Epidermophyton floccosum	'ringworm'				
Aspergillus fumigatus	Pulmonary aspergillosis	++	+	+	−
Dimorphic fungi					
Histoplasma capsulatum	Histoplasmosis	++	−	++	−
Coccidioides immitis	Coccidiomycosis	++	−	++	−
Blastomyces dermatides	Blastomycosis	++	−	+	−

[a]Generally used as an adjunct to amphotericin.

corporis, the body. In superficial candidiasis, the yeast-like organism may infect the mucous membranes of the mouth or vagina (thrush), or the skin. Secondary bacterial infections may complicate the course and treatment of these conditions.

In the UK, the commonest *systemic* (or 'disseminated') fungal disease is candidiasis. Other more serious conditions are cryptococcal meningitis, endocarditis, pulmonary aspergillosis, and rhinocerebral mucormycosis. Invasive pulmonary aspergillosis is now a leading cause of death in recipients of bone marrow transplants or those with neutropenia. Colonisation of the lungs of patients with asthma or cystic fibrosis by *Aspergillus* can lead to a similar condition termed *allergic bronchopulmonary aspergillosis*.

In other parts of the world, the commonest systemic fungal infections include blastomycosis, histoplasmosis, coccidiomycosis and paracoccidiomycosis; these are often primary infections, i.e. they are not secondary to reduced immunological function or altered commensal micro-organisms.

DRUGS USED TO TREAT FUNGAL INFECTIONS

The current therapeutic agents can be broadly classified into two groups: first, the naturally occurring antifungal antibiotics such as the *polyenes* and *echinocandins*, and second, synthetic drugs including *azoles* and *fluorinated pyrimidines*. Because many infections are superficial, there are many topical preparations. Many antifungal agents are quite toxic, and when systemic therapy is required these agents must often be used under strict medical supervision.

Figure 48.1 shows sites of action of common antifungal drugs.

ANTIFUNGAL ANTIBIOTICS
AMPHOTERICIN

Amphotericin (also called **amphotericin B**) is a mixture of antifungal substances derived from cultures of *Streptomyces*. Structurally, these are very large ('macrolide') molecules belonging to the polyene group of antifungal agents.

Mechanism of action
Like other polyene antibiotics (see Ch. 46), the site of amphotericin action is the fungal cell membranes, where it interferes with permeability and with transport functions. It probably has more than one mechanism of action, but its most important property is probably its ability to form large pores in the membrane. The hydrophilic core of the molecule creates a transmembrane ion channel, causing gross disturbances in ion balance including the loss of intracellular K^+. Amphotericin has a selective action, binding avidly to the membranes of fungi and some protozoa, less avidly to mammalian cells and not at all to bacteria. The basis of this relative specificity is the drug's greater avidity for *ergosterol*, a fungal membrane sterol that is not found in animal cells (where cholesterol is the principal sterol). Amphotericin is active against most fungi and yeasts, and is the gold standard for treating disseminated infections caused by several organisms including *Aspergillus* and *Candida*. Amphotericin also enhances the antifungal effect of **flucytosine** (see below), providing a useful synergistic combination.

Pharmacokinetic aspects
Amphotericin is very poorly absorbed when given orally, and this route is used only for treating fungal infections of the upper gastrointestinal tract. It can be used topically with success, but

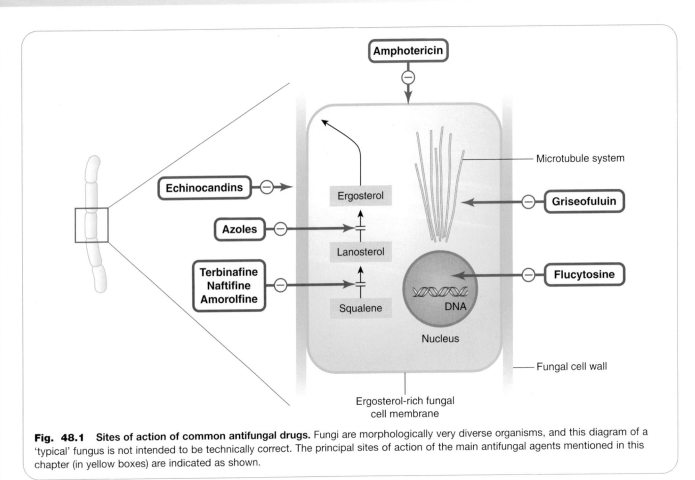

Fig. 48.1 **Sites of action of common antifungal drugs.** Fungi are morphologically very diverse organisms, and this diagram of a 'typical' fungus is not intended to be technically correct. The principal sites of action of the main antifungal agents mentioned in this chapter (in yellow boxes) are indicated as shown.

for systemic infections it is generally administered by slow intravenous injection complexed with liposomes or other lipid-containing preparations. This improves the pharmacokinetics and reduces the considerable burden of side effects. Long-circulating or so-called 'stealth' liposomes containing amphotericin have been used to good effect.

Amphotericin is very highly protein-bound. It penetrates tissues and membranes (such as the blood–brain barrier) poorly, although it is found in fairly high concentrations in inflammatory exudates and may cross the blood–brain barrier more readily when the meninges are inflamed, and intravenous amphotericin is used with flucytosine to treat *cryptococcal meningitis*. It is excreted very slowly via the kidney, traces being found in the urine for 2 months or more after administration has ceased.

Unwanted effects
The commonest and most serious unwanted effect of amphotericin is renal toxicity. Some degree of reduction of renal function occurs in more than 80% of patients receiving the drug; although this generally recovers after treatment is stopped, some impairment of glomerular filtration may remain. Hypokalaemia occurs in 25% of patients, requiring potassium chloride supplementation. Hypomagnesaemia also occurs, and anaemia can be a further problem. Other unwanted effects include impaired hepatic function, thrombocytopenia and anaphylactic reactions. Injection frequently results initially in chills, fever, tinnitus and

headache, and about one in five patients vomits. The drug is irritant to the endothelium of the veins, and local thrombophlebitis is sometimes seen after intravenous injection. Intrathecal injections can cause neurotoxicity, and topical applications cause a skin rash. The (considerably more expensive) liposome-encapsulated and lipid-complexed preparations have no greater efficacy than the native drug but cause fewer adverse reactions.

NYSTATIN

Nystatin (also called **fungicidin**) is a polyene macrolide antibiotic similar in structure to amphotericin and with the same mechanism of action. There is virtually no absorption from the mucous membranes of the body or from skin, and its use is mainly limited to *Candida* infections of the skin, mucous membranes and the gastrointestinal tract. *Unwanted effects* may include nausea, vomiting and diarrhoea.

GRISEOFULVIN

Griseofulvin is a narrow-spectrum antifungal agent isolated from cultures of *Penicillium griseofulvum*. It causes a fungistatic action by interacting with fungal microtubules and interfering with mitosis. It can be used to treat dermatophyte infections of skin or nails when local treatment is ineffective, but treatment needs to be very prolonged. It has largely been superseded by other drugs.

Pharmacokinetic aspects

Griseofulvin is given orally. It is poorly soluble in water, and absorption varies with the type of preparation, in particular with particle size. Peak plasma concentrations are reached in about 5 hours. It is taken up selectively by newly formed skin and concentrated in the keratin. The plasma half-life is 24 hours, but it is retained in the skin for much longer. It potently induces cytochrome P450 enzymes and causes several clinically important drug interactions.

Unwanted effects

Unwanted effects with griseofulvin use are infrequent, but the drug can cause gastrointestinal upsets, headache and photosensitivity. Allergic reactions (rashes, fever) may also occur. The drug should not be given to pregnant women.

ECHINOCANDINS

Echinocandins comprise a ring of six amino acids linked to a lipophilic side-chain. All drugs in this group are based on the structure of **echinocandin B**, which is found naturally in *A. nidulans*. The echinocandins inhibit the synthesis of 1,3-β-glucan, a glucose polymer that is necessary for maintaining the structure of fungal cell walls. In the absence of this polymer, fungal cells lose integrity and lysis quickly follows.

Caspofungin is active in vitro against a wide variety of fungi, and it has proved effective in the treatment of candidiasis and forms of invasive aspergillosis that are refractory to amphotericin. Oral absorption is poor, and caspofungin is extensively protein-bound in the bloodstream. It is given intravenously, once daily, and its plasma half-life in humans is 9–10 hours.

SYNTHETIC ANTIFUNGAL AGENTS

AZOLES

The azoles are a group of synthetic fungistatic agents with a broad spectrum of activity based on the *imidazole* (**clotrimazole, econazole, fenticonazole, ketoconazole, miconazole, tioconazole** and **sulconazole**) or *triazole* nucleus (**itraconazole, voriconazole** and **fluconazole**).

Mechanism of action of the azoles

The azoles inhibit the fungal cytochrome P450 3A enzyme, lanosine 14α-demethylase, which is responsible for converting lanosterol to ergosterol, the main sterol in the fungal cell membrane. The resulting depletion of ergosterol alters the fluidity of the membrane, and this interferes with the action of membrane-associated enzymes. The net effect is an inhibition of replication. Azoles also inhibit the transformation of candidal yeast cells into hyphae—the invasive and pathogenic form of the parasite. The depletion of membrane ergosterol reduces the binding sites for amphotericin.

Ketoconazole

Ketoconazole was the first azole that could be given orally to treat systemic fungal infections. It is effective against several different types of organism (see Table 48.1). It is, however, toxic (see below),

and relapse is common after apparently successful treatment. It is well absorbed from the gastrointestinal tract. It is distributed widely throughout the tissues and tissue fluids but does not reach therapeutic concentrations in the central nervous system unless high doses are given. It is inactivated in the liver and excreted in bile and in urine. Its half-life in the plasma is 8 hours.

Unwanted effects

The main hazard of ketoconazole is liver toxicity, which is rare but can prove fatal and must therefore be taken into account when deciding on a treatment regimen. Other side effects that occur are gastrointestinal disturbances and pruritus. Inhibition of adrenocortical steroid and testosterone synthesis has been recorded with high doses, the latter resulting in gynaecomastia in some male patients. There may be adverse interactions with other drugs. **Ciclosporin, terfenadine** and **astemizole** all interfere with drug-metabolising enzymes, causing increased plasma concentrations of ketoconazole or the interacting drug or both. **Rifampicin,** histamine H_2 receptor antagonists and antacids decrease the absorption of ketoconazole.

Fluconazole

Fluconazole is well absorbed and can be given orally or intravenously. It reaches high concentrations in the cerebrospinal fluid and ocular fluids, and may become the drug of first choice for most types of fungal meningitis. Fungicidal concentrations are also achieved in vaginal tissue, saliva, skin and nails. It has a half-life of ~25 hours; 90% is excreted unchanged in the urine and 10% in the faeces.

Unwanted effects

Unwanted effects, which are generally mild, include nausea, headache and abdominal pain. However, exfoliative skin lesions (including, on occasion, Stevens–Johnson syndrome[1]) have been seen in some individuals—primarily in AIDS patients who are being treated with multiple drugs. Hepatitis has been reported, although this is rare, and fluconazole, in the doses usually used, does not produce the inhibition of hepatic drug metabolism and of steroidogenesis that occurs with ketoconazole.

Itraconazole

Itraconazole is active against a range of dermatophytes. It may be given orally but, after absorption (which is variable), undergoes extensive hepatic metabolism. It is highly lipid-soluble (and water-insoluble), and a formulation in which the drug is retained within pockets of β-cyclodextrin is available. In this form, itraconazole can be administered intravenously, thereby overcoming the problem of variable absorption from the gastrointestinal tract. Administered orally, its half-life is about 36 hours, and it is excreted in the urine. It does not penetrate the cerebrospinal fluid.

---

[1]This is a severe and usually fatal condition involving blistering of the skin, mouth, eyes and genitalia, often accompanied by fever, polyarthritis and kidney failure.

Unwanted effects

Gastrointestinal disturbances, headache and dizziness can occur. Rare unwanted effects are hepatitis, hypokalaemia and impotence. Allergic skin reactions have been reported (including Stevens–Johnson syndrome; see above). Inhibition of steroidogenesis has not been reported. Drug interactions as a result of inhibition of cytochrome P450 enzymes occur (similar to those described above for ketoconazole). It has been associated with liver damage.

Miconazole

Miconazole is given orally for oral and other infections of the gastrointestinal tract. It has a short plasma half-life and needs to be given every 8 hours. It reaches therapeutic concentrations in bone, joints and lung tissue but not in the central nervous system, and it is inactivated in the liver.

Unwanted effects

Unwanted effects are relatively infrequent, those most commonly seen being gastrointestinal disturbances, but pruritus, blood dyscrasias and hyponatraemia are also reported. There are isolated reports of liver damage, and it should not be given to patients with impaired hepatic function.

Other azoles

Clotrimazole, econazole, tioconazole and sulconazole are used only for topical application. Clotrimazole interferes with amino acid transport into the fungus by an action on the cell membrane. It is active against a wide range of fungi, including candidal organisms.

FLUCYTOSINE

Flucytosine is a synthetic orally active antifungal agent that is effective against a limited range (mainly yeasts) of systemic fungal infections. If given alone, drug resistance commonly arises during treatment, so it is usually combined with amphotericin for severe systemic infections such as candidiasis and cryptococcal meningitis.

Mechanism of action

Flucytosine is converted to the antimetabolite 5-fluorouracil in fungal but not human cells. 5-Fluorouracil inhibits thymidylate synthetase and thus DNA synthesis (see Chs 5 and 51). Resistant mutants may emerge rapidly, so this drug should not be used alone.

Pharmacokinetic aspects

Flucytosine is usually given by intravenous infusion but can also be given orally. It is widely distributed throughout the body fluids, including the cerebrospinal fluid. About 90% is excreted unchanged via the kidneys, and the plasma half-life is 3–5 hours. The dosage should be reduced if renal function is impaired.

Unwanted effects

Unwanted effects are infrequent. Gastrointestinal disturbances, anaemia, neutropenia, thrombocytopenia and alopecia have occurred, but these are usually mild (but may be more significant in AIDS patients) and are easily reversed when therapy ceases.

Uracil is reported to decrease the toxic effects on the bone marrow without impairing the antimycotic action. Hepatitis has been reported but is rare.

TERBINAFINE

Terbinafine is a highly lipophilic, keratinophilic fungicidal compound active against a wide range of skin pathogens. It is particularly useful against nail infections. It acts by selectively inhibiting the enzyme *squalene epoxidase*, which is involved in the synthesis of ergosterol from squalene in the fungal cell wall. The accumulation of squalene within the cell is toxic to the organism.

When used to treat ringworm or fungal infections of the nails, it is given orally. The drug is rapidly absorbed and is taken up by skin, nails and adipose tissue. Given topically, it penetrates skin and mucous membranes. It is metabolised in the liver by the cytochrome P450 system, and the metabolites are excreted in the urine.

Unwanted effects

Unwanted effects occur in about 10% of individuals and are usually mild and self-limiting. They include gastrointestinal disturbances, rashes, pruritus, headache and dizziness. Joint and muscle pains have been reported and, more rarely, hepatitis.

Naftifine is similar in action to terbinafine. Among other developments, a morpholine derivative, **amorolfine**, which interferes with fungal sterol synthesis, is available as a nail lacquer, being effective against onchomycoses.

POTENTIAL NEW ANTIFUNGAL THERAPIES

Increasing numbers of fungal strains are becoming resistant to the current antifungal drugs (fortunately, drug resistance is not transferable in fungi), and toxicity and low efficacy also contribute to the need for better antifungal drugs. An additional problem is that new strains of commensal-turned-pathogenic fungi have emerged. Fungal infections are on the rise, partly because of the prevalence of cancer chemotherapy and transplant-associated immunosuppression. Encouragingly, new compounds are in development, some with novel mechanisms of action (for review, see Neely & Ghannoun, 2000), and the prospect of using combination therapies has been explored in more depth.

While not yet available in the UK, new echinocandins such as **micafungin** and **anidulafungin** have shown promise in treating infections caused by *Aspergillus* and *Candida* spp., even in patients who are immunocompromised with AIDS. Unwanted effects are mild, and their incidence less than that seen with amphotericin. Several 'new generation' triazoles are also in prospect. **Posaconazole** and **ravuconazole** both have good efficacy against a wide range of fungal pathogens. Other developments are beyond the scope of this chapter, and the interested reader is advised to consult the burgeoning literature on the subject (see, for example, Boucher et al., 2004).

Because fungal infections are often secondary to compromised host defence, attempts have been made to boost this by administration of the cytokine granulocyte macrophage colony stimulating factor (see Ch. 13) and other factors that increase host leucocyte numbers or function. The possibility of developing an antifungal vaccine, first mooted in the 1960s, has met with only very limited success in animals, and few fungal antigens have been characterised. It is hoped that advances in antibody technology will soon transform this dismal outlook.

REFERENCES AND FURTHER READING

Altamura M, Casale D, Pepe M, Tafaro A 2001 Immune responses to fungal infections and therapeutic implications. Curr Drug Targets Immune Endocr Metabol Disord 1: 189–197 (*This paper discusses the role of the host immune response in fungal infection and examines novel strategies for antifungal therapy drawing on these data*)

Blau I W, Fauser A A 2000 Review of comparative studies between conventional and liposomal amphotericin B (Ambisome) in neutropenic patients with fever of unknown origin and patients with systemic mycosis. Mycoses 43: 325–332 (*This review deals with a comparison between normal amphotericin and liposomal preparations*)

Boucher H W, Groll A H, Chiou C C, Walsh T J 2004 Newer systemic antifungal agents: pharmacokinetics, safety and efficacy. Drugs 64: 1997–2020 (*A useful review of the newer echinocandins and triazoles*)

Como J A, Dismukes W E 1994 Oral azole drugs as systemic antifungal therapy. N Engl J Med 330: 263–272 (*A bit dated now but still worth reading for the review of ketoconazole, fluconazole and itraconazole*)

Denning D W 2003 Echinocandin antifungal drugs. Lancet 362: 1142–1151 (*General review on the echinocandins, focusing on their clinical use*)

Dodds E S, Drew R H, Perfect J R 2000 Antifungal pharmacodynamics: review of the literature and clinical applications. Pharmacotherapy 20: 1335–1355 (*Good review of antifungals used to treat systemic infections; somewhat clinical in tone*)

Gruszecki W I, Gagos M, Herec M, Kernen P 2003 Organization of antibiotic amphotericin B in model lipid membranes. A mini review. Cell Mol Biol Lett 8: 161–170 (*If you are interested in understanding how amphotericin works, then this will be of interest*)

Gupta A K, Tomas E 2003 New antifungal agents. Dermatol Clin 21: 565–576 (*Quite a comprehensive review that deals mainly with the newer antifungals, their mechanisms of action and resistance*)

Hoeprich P D 1995 Antifungal chemotherapy. Prog Drug Res 44: 88–127 (*A bit dated now but contains very detailed coverage of the main classes of drug: chemical formulae, mode of action, pharmacokinetics, adverse effects*)

Kauffman C A 2001 Fungal infections in older adults. Clin Infect Dis 33: 550–555 (*Interesting account of fungal infections and their treatment*)

Neely M N, Ghannoun M A 2000 The exciting future of antifungal therapy. Eur J Clin Microbiol Infect Dis 19: 897–914

Van Spriel A B 2003 Novel immunotherapeutic strategies for invasive fungal disease. Curr Drug Targets Cardiovasc Haematol Disord 3: 209–217 (*Another paper that discusses the role of the host immune response in fungal infection and examines novel strategies for antifungal therapy drawing on these data*)

Vermes A, Guchelaar H J, Dankert J 2000 Flucytosine: a review of its pharmacology, clinical indications, pharmacokinetics, toxicity and drug interactions. J Antimicrob Chemother 46: 171–179 (*The title is self-explanatory!*)

Wiederhold N P, Lewis R E 2003 The echinocandin antifungals: an overview of the pharmacology, spectrum and clinical efficacy. Expert Opin Investig Drugs 12: 1313–1333 (*Another review of the echinocandins—very comprehensive*)

Useful web resources

http://www.doctorfungus.org (*This is an excellent site sponsored by a consortium of pharmaceutical companies. It covers all aspects of fungal infections and drug therapy, and has many compelling images and video clips. Highly recommended—and fun!*)

49

Antiprotozoal drugs

OVERVIEW

Protozoa (plural form of *protozoon*) are motile, unicellular eukaryotic organisms that have colonised virtually every habitat and ecological niche. They may be conveniently classified, on the basis of their method of locomotion, into four main groups: *amoebas, flagellates, sporozoa* and a further group comprising *ciliates* and other organisms of uncertain affiliation, such as the *Pneumocystis carinii* mentioned in the last chapter. The protozoa have diverse feeding behaviour, with some being parasitic. Many have extremely complex life cycles, sometimes involving several hosts, reminiscent of the helminths discussed in Chapter 50.

As a group, the protozoa are responsible for an enormous burden of disease among humans as well as domestic and wild animal populations. Table 49.1 lists some of these clinically important organisms, together with the diseases that they cause, as well an overview of the drugs used to combat infection. In this chapter, we will first

discuss some general features of protozoa–host interactions and then discuss the therapy of each group of diseases in turn. In view of its global importance, a discussion of malaria will occupy much of the chapter.

HOST–PARASITE INTERACTIONS

Mammals have developed very efficient mechanisms for dealing with invading parasites, and many of these parasites have, in turn, evolved clever tactics to evade the defensive responses of the host. Some of these gambits will be dealt with as we discuss each parasite in turn, but we also have some general comments.

One common parasite ploy is to take refuge within the cells of the host, where antibodies cannot reach them. Most protozoa do this, some (e.g. plasmodia species) taking up residence in red cells, some (*Leishmania* species) infecting macrophages exclusively, and some (various trypanosome species) invading many other cell types. The host has also evolved countermeasures to deal with these intracellular parasites, namely cell-mediated immune responses involving primarily the T-helper (Th) 1 pathway cytokines, such as interleukin (IL)-2, tumour necrosis factor-α and interferon-γ, that activate macrophages and cytotoxic CD8[+] T cells (Ch. 14). Activated macrophages kill intracellular parasites, and cytotoxic T cells collaborate with macrophages by producing macrophage-activating cytokines.

The Th1 pathway responses can be down-regulated by Th2 pathway cytokines such as transforming growth factor-β, IL-4 and IL-10. Some intracellular parasites have evolved mechanisms for manipulating the Th1–Th2 balance to their own advantage by stimulating production of the Th2 cytokines that down-regulate cell-mediated immune reactions. For example, the invasion of macrophages by *Leishmania* species is associated with induction of transforming growth factor-β, and the invasion of T cells, B cells and macrophages by trypanosomes is associated with induction of IL-10 (see Handman & Bullen, 2002, and Sacks & Toben-Trauth, 2002, for further details). Similar mechanisms occur during worm infestations (see Ch. 50).

Toxoplasma gondii has evolved a different ploy: up-regulation of some host responses. The definitive (i.e. where sexual recombination occurs) host of this protozoon is the cat, but humans can inadvertently become intermediate hosts, harbouring the asexual form of the parasite. In humans, *T. gondii* infects numerous cell types and has a highly virulent replicative stage;

Table 49.1 Principal protozoal infections and common drug treatments

Organism	Disease	Common drug treatment
Amoebas		
Entamoeba histolytica	Amoebic dysentery	Metronidazole, tinidazole, diloxanide
Flagellates		
Trypanosoma rhodesiense *Trypanosoma gambiense*	Sleeping sickness	Suramin, pentamidine, melarpasol, eflornithine, nifurtimox
Trypanosoma cruzi	Chagas' disease	Nifurtimox, benzindazole
Leishmania tropica *Leishmania donovani* *Leishmania braziliensis* *Leishmania mexicana*	Oriental sore Kala-azar Espundia Chiclero's ulcer	Sodium stibogluconate, amphotericin, pentamidine isethionate
Trichomonas vaginalis	Vaginitis	Metronidazole, tinidazole
Giardia lamblia	Diarrhoea, steatorrhoea	Metronidazole, tinidazole.
Sporozoa		
Plasmodium falciparum *Plasmodium vivax* *Plasmodium ovale* *Plasmodium malarariae*	Malignant tertian malaria Benign tertian malaria Benign tertian malaria Quartan malaria	Amodiaquine, artemisinin and derivatives, atovaquone, chloroquine, dapsone, doxycycline, halofantrine, lumefantrine, mefloquine, primaquine, proguanil, pyrimethamine, quinine, tafenoquine and tetracycline
Toxoplasma gondii	Encephalitis, congenital malformations, eye disease	Pyrimethamine, sulfadiazine pentamidine isethionate
Ciliates and others		
Pneumocystis carinii	Pneumonia	Co-trimoxazole, atovaquone, pentamidine isethionate

(After Greenwood, 1989.)

it is therefore important to the parasite that its host survives. To do this, it stimulates production of interferon-γ, thus modulating the host's cell-mediated responses, which then promote encystment of the parasite in the tissues.

Improved understanding of host–protozoon relationships has opened up new vistas for the development of antiprotozoal agents. The possibility of using cytokine analogues and/or antagonists to treat disease caused by protozoa is already being investigated (for review, see Odeh, 2001).

AMOEBIASIS AND AMOEBICIDAL DRUGS

The main organism in this group to concern us here is *Entamoeba histolytica*, the causative agent of *amoebiasis*, which may manifest as a severe colitis (*dysentery*) and sometimes liver abscesses.

▼ The infection is encountered around the world, although it is more often encountered in warmer climates. Approximately 500 million people are thought to harbour the disease, with 40 000–100 000 deaths occurring each year as a result (Stanley, 2003). It is considered to be the second leading cause of death from parasitic diseases worldwide.

The organism has a simple life cycle, and humans are the chief hosts. Infection, generally spread by poor hygiene, follows the ingestion of the mature cysts in water or food that is contaminated with human faeces.

The infectious cysts pass into the colon, where they develop into *trophozoites*. These motile organisms adhere to colonic epithelial cells, utilising a galactose-containing lectin on the host cell membrane, where the trophozoites feed, multiply, encyst and eventually pass out in the faeces, thus completing the life cycle. Some individuals are symptomless 'carriers'—they harbour the parasite without developing overt disease, but the cysts are present in their faeces and they can infect other individuals. The cysts can survive outside the body for at least a week in a moist and cool environment.

The trophozoite lyses the colonic mucosal cells (hence *histolytica*) using *amoebapores* (peptides that form pores in cell membranes) or by inducing host cell apoptosis. The organism then invades the submucosa, where it may secrete factors that modify the host response, which would otherwise prove lethal to the parasite. It is this process that produces the characteristic bloody diarrhoea and abdominal pain, although in many subjects a chronic intestinal infection may be present in the absence of dysentery. In some subjects, an amoebic granuloma (*amoeboma*) in the intestinal wall may be present. The trophozoites may also migrate through the damaged intestinal tissue into the portal blood and hence the liver, giving rise to the most common extraintestinal symptom of the disease—amoebic liver abscesses.

The use of drugs to treat this condition (see *Drugs used in amoebiasis box*) depends largely on the site and type of infection, as different drugs are differentially effective in acute amoebic dysentery, in chronic intestinal amoebiasis, in extraintestinal infection and in the carrier state. The main drugs currently used

---

Drugs used in amoebiasis

- Amoebiasis is caused by infection with *Entamoeba histolytica*, which causes dysentery and liver abcesses. The organism may be present in motile invasive form or as a cyst. The main drugs are as follow.
  — Metronidazole given orally (half-life 7 hours). Active against the invasive form in gut and liver but not the cysts. Unwanted effects (rare); gastrointestinal disturbances and central nervous system symptoms.
  — Diloxanide is given orally with no serious unwanted effects. It is active, while unabsorbed, against the non-invasive form in the gastrointestinal tract.

---

are **metronidazole**, **tinidazole** and **diloxanide**. These agents may be used in combination.

The drugs of choice for the various forms of amoebiasis are as follow:

- metronidazole (or tinidazole) followed by diloxanide for acute invasive intestinal amoebiasis resulting in acute severe amoebic dysentery
- diloxanide for chronic intestinal amoebiasis
- metronidazole followed by diloxanide for hepatic amoebiasis
- diloxanide for the carrier state.

Metronidazole

Metronidazole kills the trophozoites of *E. histolytica* but has no effect on the cysts. It is the drug of choice for invasive amoebiasis of the intestine or the liver, but it is less effective against organisms in the lumen of the gut. Metronidazole is activated by anaerobic organisms to a compound that damages parasite DNA, leading to parasite apoptosis.

Pharmacokinetic aspects

Metronidazole is usually given orally and is rapidly and completely absorbed, achieving peak plasma concentration in 1–3 hours, with a half-life of about 7 hours. Rectal and intravenous preparations are also available. It is distributed rapidly throughout the tissues, reaching high concentrations in the body fluids, including the cerebrospinal fluid. Some is metabolised, but most is excreted in urine.

Unwanted effects

The drug has a metallic, bitter taste in the mouth but causes few unwanted effects in therapeutic doses. Minor gastrointestinal disturbances have been reported, as have central nervous system (CNS) symptoms (dizziness, headache, sensory neuropathies). The drug interferes with alcohol metabolism, and concurrent use of the substance should be strictly avoided. Metronidazole should not be used in pregnancy.

Tinidazole is similar to metronidazole in its mechanism of action and unwanted effects, but is eliminated more slowly, having a half-life of 12–14 hours.

Diloxanide

Both diloxanide itself and, more particularly, an insoluble ester, **diloxanide furoate**, are the drugs of choice for the asymptomatic infected patient, and are often given as a follow-up after the disease has been reversed using metronidazole. Both drugs have a direct amoebicidal action, affecting the parasites before encystment. Diloxanide furoate is given orally, the unabsorbed moiety being the amoebicidal agent. It has an excellent safety profile.

Other drugs that are sometimes used outside the UK to treat this disease include **iodoquinol**, **dehydroemetine** and **paromomycin**.

FLAGELLATES

The principal disease-causing organisms in this group are species of *Trypanasoma*, *Leishmania*, *Trichomona* and *Giardia*. We will discuss each in turn.

TRYPANOSOMIASIS AND TRYPANICIDAL DRUGS

The three main species of trypanosome that cause disease in humans are *Trypanosoma gambiense* and *Trypanosoma rhodesiense*, which cause *sleeping sickness* in Africa, and *Trypanosoma cruzi*, which causes *Chagas' disease* in South America. About 100 000 new cases of sleeping sickness are reported each year, and 60 million people in 36 countries are classed as at risk of contracting the disease. *T. rhodesiense* causes the more aggressive form of sleeping sickness. All forms of the disease have shown signs of resurgence, because civil unrest, famine and AIDS have reduced the chances of receiving adequate medication or because patients are immunocompromised. Related trypanosome infections also pose a major risk to livestock and thus have a secondary impact on human health and well-being.

▼ The vector is the tsetse fly. In both types of disease, there is an initial local lesion at the site of entry, which may (in the case of *T. rhodesiense*) develop into a painful chancre. This is followed by bouts of parasitaemia and fever as the parasite enters the haemolymphatic system. Damage to organs is caused by the parasites and the toxins they release during the second phase of the disease. This manifests as somnolence and progressive neurological breakdown when the parasites reach the CNS (sleeping sickness), or damage to the heart, muscles and sometimes liver, spleen, bone and intestine (Chagas' disease). Left untreated, such infections are fatal.

The main drugs used for African sleeping sickness are **suramin**, with **pentamidine** as an alternative, in the haemolymphatic stage of the disease, and the arsenical **melarsoprol** for the late stage with CNS involvement (see Burchmore et al., 2002; Burri & Brun, 2003). Other agents include **nifurtimox** and **eflornithine**. Nifurtimox is also used in Chagas' disease as is **benznidazole** (but in the acute disease only and not in the UK); however, there is, in essence, no really effective treatment for this form of trypanosomiasis.

Suramin

Suramin was introduced into the therapy of trypanosomiasis in 1920. The drug binds firmly to host plasma proteins, and the complex enters the trypanosome by endocytosis from where it is liberated by lysosomal proteases. It does not kill the parasites immediately but inhibits parasite enzymes, inducing gradual destruction of organelles, such that the organisms are cleared from the circulation after a short interval.

The drug is given by slow intravenous injection. The blood concentration drops rapidly during the first few hours and then more slowly over the succeeding days. A residual concentration remains for 3–4 months. Suramin tends to accumulate in the mononuclear phagocyte system of the host and is also found in the cells of the proximal tubule in the kidney.

Unwanted effects

Suramin is relatively toxic, particularly in a malnourished patient, the main toxic effect being in the kidney. Other slowly developing adverse effects reported include optic atrophy, adrenal insufficiency, skin rashes, haemolytic anaemia and agranulocytosis. A small proportion of individuals have an immediate idiosyncratic reaction to suramin injection that may include nausea, vomiting, shock, seizures and loss of consciousness.

Pentamidine isethionate

Pentamidine has a direct trypanocidal action in vitro. It is rapidly taken up in the parasites by a high-affinity energy-dependent carrier and is thought to interact with the DNA. The drug is administered intravenously or by deep intramuscular injection, usually daily for 10–15 days. After absorption from the injection site, it binds strongly to tissues (especially the kidney) and is eliminated slowly, only 50% of a dose being excreted over 5 days. Fairly high concentrations of the drug persist in the kidney, the liver and the spleen for several months, but it does not penetrate the blood–brain barrier. Its usefulness is limited by its unwanted effects—an immediate decrease in blood pressure, with tachycardia, breathlessness and vomiting, and later serious toxicity, such as kidney damage, hepatic impairment, blood dyscrasias and hypoglycaemia.

A relatively new drug, eflornithine (the only new drug to be registered over the past 50 years) has shown good activity against *T. gambiense* and is used as a back-up for melarsoprol, although unfortunately it has limited activity against *T. rhodesiense*. The drug targets parasite ornithine metabolism. Side effects are common and may be severe, but are readily reversed when treatment is discontinued. A new drug candidate, **DB 289**, has shown promise (Legros et al., 2002), but **megazol**, another useful trypanocidal that was under development, has been dropped because of genotoxicity (Nesslany et al., 2004). Unfortunately, there are few (if any) other new drugs in the pipeline, and as resistance develops to the standard agents, the number of deaths from this condition is set to rise. Despite work into likely parasite antigens, the current prospects for a vaccine look bleak (Naula & Burchmore, 2003).

LEISHMANIASIS AND LEISHMANICIDAL DRUGS

There are a variety of *Leishmania* organisms that cause disease (sometimes fatal) afflicting about 12 million people in 90 countries; there are about 2 million new cases each year, mainly in tropical and subtropical regions. With increasing international travel, leishmaniasis is being imported into areas where it was not previously seen, and opportunistic infections are now being reported (particularly in AIDS patients).

▼ The insect vector in this case is the sandfly, and the parasite exists in two forms, a flagellated form (*promastigote*) found in the gut of the infected sandfly, and a non-flagellated intracellular form (*amastigote*) that occurs in the infected mammalian host, where it is harboured by mononuclear phagocytes. Within this cell, the parasites thrive in modified phagolysosomes and protect themselves from the usual intracellular killing mechanisms by modifying the macrophage's microbiocidal systems, apparently by deploying a lipophosphoglycan on their surface (Handman & Bullen, 2002). The amastigotes multiply, and eventually the infected cell releases a new crop of parasites into the haemolymphatic system, where they can infect further macrophages and possibly other cells.

The different species of *Leishmania* occur in different geographical zones and cause different clinical manifestations (see Table 49.1). Typical presentations include:

- a simple skin infection giving rise to an unpleasant chancre ('oriental sore', 'Chiclero's ulcer' and other names) that may heal spontaneously
- a mucocutaneous form ('espundia' and other names), in which there may be large ulcers of the mucous membranes
- a serious visceral form ('kala-azar' and other names), where the parasite spreads through the bloodstream and causes hepatomegaly, splenomegaly, anaemia and intermittent fever.

The main drugs used in visceral leishmaniasis are pentavalent antimony compounds such as **sodium stibogluconate** and **meglumine antimoniate** (not in the UK), but resistance to these agents is increasing and their toxicity is high. **Amphotericin** (see Ch. 48) is a useful back-up, and **pentamidine isethionate** (see above) is also used in antimony-resistant leishmaniasis. In some countries, **miltefosine**, originally developed as an antitumour drug, has been used with success to treat the disease.

Sodium stibogluconate

Sodium stibogluconate is given intramuscularly or by slow intravenous injection in a 10-day course. It is rapidly eliminated in the urine, 70% being excreted within 6 hours. More than one course of treatment may be required. Unwanted effects include anorexia, vomiting, bradycardia and hypotension. Treatment may also be associated with increased incidence of herpes zoster. Coughing and substernal pain may occur during intravenous infusion. The mechanism of action of sodium stibogluconate is not clear, but the drug may increase production of oxygen free radicals, which are toxic to the parasite.

Miltefosine (hexadecylphosphocholine) is also effective in the treatment of both cutaneous and visceral leishmaniasis. The drug may be given orally and is well tolerated. Side effects are mild and include nausea and vomiting. In vitro, the drug induces DNA fragmentation and apoptosis in the parasites (Verma & Dey, 2004).

Other drugs such as antibiotics and antifungals may be given concomitantly with the above agents. They may have some action on the parasite in their own right, but their main utility is to control the spread of secondary infections. Current drug usage and possible future approaches to the treatment of leishmaniasis are discussed by Murrey (2000). At present, there is no vaccine for leishmaniasis; an approach to this problem using recombinant *Leishmania* proteins is discussed by Kubar & Fragaki (2005).

TRICHOMONIASIS AND TRICHOMANICIDAL DRUGS

The principal *Trichomonas* organism that produces disease in humans is *Trichomonas vaginalis*. Virulent strains cause inflammation of the vagina in females and sometimes of the urethra in males. The main drug used in therapy is metronidazole (p. 699), although resistance to this drug is on the increase. High doses of tinidazole are also effective, with few side effects.

GIARDIASIS

The final flagellate we will discuss is *Giardia lamblia*. The trophozoite form of this parasite colonises the upper gastrointestinal tract, and the cysts pass out in the faeces. Infection is then spread by ingestion of food or water contaminated with faecal matter containing the cysts. It is encountered worldwide, and epidemics caused by bad sanitation are not uncommon. Metronidazole is the drug of choice, and treatment is usually very effective.

SPOROZOA

MALARIA

Malaria was once considered to arise from marshy land (hence the name 'mal aria'—bad or poisonous air), but we now recognise that the disease is caused by parasites belonging to the genus *Plasmodium*. Four species of plasmodia infect humans: *Plasmodium vivax*, *Plasmodium falciparum*, *Plasmodium ovale* and *Plasmodium malariae*. The insect vector is the female *Anopheles* mosquito, which breeds in stagnant water, and the disease it spreads is one of the major killers on our planet.

The statistics are staggering. According to the World Health Organization (WHO), malaria is a significant public health problem in more than 90 countries inhabited by some 2400 million people (about 40% of the world's population). The disease causes an estimated 300 million acute illnesses each year and at least 1 million deaths. More than 90% of these occur in sub-Saharan Africa, and it is estimated that the disease kills an African child every 30 seconds. Even those who survive may suffer from lasting mental impairment. Other high-risk groups include pregnant women, refugees and labourers entering endemic regions. Malaria also imposes a huge economic burden on countries where the disease is rife.[1]

The symptoms of malaria include fever, shivering, pain in the joints, headache, repeated vomiting, generalised convulsions and coma. Symptoms become apparent only 7–9 days after being bitten by an infected mosquito. By far the most dangerous parasite is *P. falciparum*.

Malaria was eradicated from most temperate countries in the 20th century, and the WHO attempted to eradicate malaria elsewhere using the powerful 'residual' insecticides and the highly effective antimalarial drugs that had become available. By the end of the 1950s, the incidence of malaria had dropped dramatically. However, during the 1970s it became clear that the attempt at eradication had failed—largely owing to the increasing resistance of the mosquito to the insecticides and of the parasite to the drugs. Sadly, it is now the case that malaria has re-emerged in several countries where it was previously under control or indeed eradicated. Sporadic cases—the result of air travel—are already quite common in Western Europe and the USA, where the actual risk of transmission is negligible.[2]

THE LIFE CYCLE OF THE MALARIA PARASITE

The mosquito, not the human, is the definitive host for plasmodia, and it has been said that the only function of humans is to enable the parasite to infect more mosquitoes so that further sexual recombination can occur. The life cycle of the parasites consists of a *sexual cycle*, which takes place in the female anopheline mosquito, and an *asexual cycle*, which occurs in humans (Fig. 49.1 and the *Malaria* box).

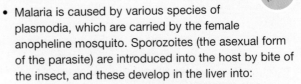

Malaria

- Malaria is caused by various species of plasmodia, which are carried by the female anopheline mosquito. Sporozoites (the asexual form of the parasite) are introduced into the host by bite of the insect, and these develop in the liver into:
  - schizonts (the pre-erythrocytic stage), which liberate merozoites—these infect red blood cells, forming motile trophozoites, which, after development, release another batch of erythrocyte-infecting merozoites, causing fever; this constitutes the erythrocytic cycle
  - dormant hypnozoites, which may liberate merozoites later (the exoerythrocytic stage).
- The main malarial parasites causing *tertian* ('every third day') malaria are:
  - *P. vivax*, which causes benign tertian malaria
  - *P. falciparum*, which causes malignant tertian malaria; unlike *P. vivax*, this plasmodium has no exoerythrocytic stage.
- Some merozoites develop into gametocytes, the sexual forms of the parasite. When ingested by the mosquito, these give rise to further stages of the parasite's life cycle within the insect.

---

[1]Taking into account factors such as initial poverty and economic policy, it has been calculated that countries with intensive malaria grow 1.3% less per person per year than malaria-free zones, and that a 1.1% reduction in malaria is associated with a 0.3% higher rate of economic growth.

[2]As an example of such 'airport malaria', the UK registered 2364 cases of malaria in 1997, all of them imported by travellers. 'Weekend malaria', which occurs when city dwellers in Africa spend weekends in the countryside, is also becoming more of a problem.

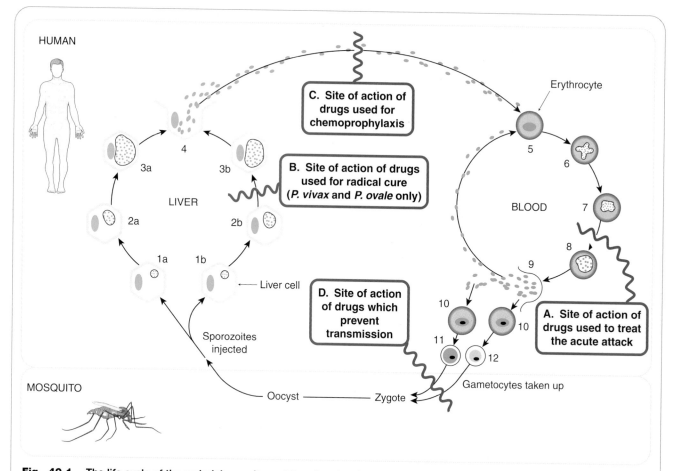

Fig. 49.1 **The life cycle of the malarial parasite and the site of action of antimalarial drugs.** The pre- or exoerythrocytic cycle in the liver and the erythrocytic cycle in the blood are shown: **1a** Entry of sporozoite into liver cell (the parasite is shown as a small circle containing dots, and the liver cell nucleus as a blue oval). **2a** and **3a** Development of the schizont in liver cell. **4** Rupture of liver cell with release of merozoites (some may enter liver cells to give resting forms of the parasite, hypnozoites). **5** Entry of merozoites into a red cell. **6** Trophozoite in red cell. **7** and **8** Development of schizont in red cell. **9** Rupture of red cell with release of merozoites, most of which parasitise other red cells. **10–12** Entry of merozoites into red cells and development of male and female gametocytes. **1b** Resting form of parasite in liver (hypnozoite). **2b** and **3b** Growth and multiplication of hypnozoites. Sites of drug action are as follow. **A** Drugs used to treat the acute attack (also called 'blood schizonticidal agents' or 'drugs for suppressive or clinical cure'). **B** Drugs that affect the exoerythrocytic hypnozoites and result in a 'radical' cure of *P. vivax* and *P. ovale*. **C** Drugs that block the link between the exoerythrocytic stage and the erythrocytic stage; they are used for chemoprophylaxis (also termed *causal prophylactics*) and prevent the development of malarial attacks. **D** Drugs that prevent transmission and thus prevent increase of the human reservoir of the disease.

▼ With the bite of an infected female mosquito, *sporozoites*—usually few in number—are inoculated into the bloodstream. Within 30 minutes, they disappear from the blood and enter the parenchymal cells of the liver, where, during the next 10–14 days, they undergo a *pre-erythrocytic stage* of development and multiplication. At the end of this stage, the parasitised liver cells rupture, and a host of fresh *merozoites* are released. These bind to and enter the red cells of the blood and form motile intracellular parasites termed *trophozoites*. The development and multiplication of the plasmodia within these cells constitutes the *erythrocytic stage*. During maturation within the red cell, the parasite remodels the host cell, inserting parasite proteins and phospholipids into the red cell membrane. The host's haemoglobin is digested and transported to the parasite's food vacuole, where it provides a source of amino acids. Free haem, which would be toxic to the plasmodium, is rendered harmless by polymerisation to *haemozoin*. Some antimalarial drugs act by inhibiting the haem polymerase enzyme responsible for this step (see below).

Following mitotic replication of its nucleus, the parasite in the red cell is termed a *schizont*, and its rapid growth and division, *schizogony*. Another phase of multiplication results in the production of further merozoites, which are released when the red cell ruptures. These merozoites then bind to and enter fresh red cells, and the erythrocytic cycle starts all over again. In certain forms of malaria, some sporozoites entering the liver cells form *hypnozoites*, or 'sleeping' forms of the parasite, which can be reactivated months or years later to continue an *exoerythrocytic cycle* of multiplication.

Malaria parasites can multiply in the body at a phenomenal rate—a single parasite of *P. vivax* can give rise to 250 million merozoites in 14 days. To appreciate the action required of an antimalarial drug, note that destruction of 94% of the parasites every 48 hours will serve only to maintain equilibrium and will not further reduce their number or their propensity for proliferation.

Some merozoites, on entering red cells, differentiate into male and female forms of the parasite, called *gametocytes*. These can complete their cycle only when taken up by the mosquito, when it sucks the blood of the infected host.

▼ The cycle in the mosquito involves fertilisation of the female gametocyte by the male gametocyte, with the formation of a *zygote*, which develops into an *oocyst* (*sporocyst*). A further stage of division and multiplication takes place, leading to rupture of the sporocyst with release of sporozoites, which then migrate to the mosquito's salivary glands and enter another human host with the mosquito's bite.

The periodic episodes of fever that characterise malaria result from the synchronised rupture of red cells with release of merozoites and cell debris. The rise in temperature is associated with a rise in the concentration of tumour necrosis factor-α in the plasma. Relapses of malaria are likely to occur with those forms of malaria that have an exoerythrocytic cycle, because the dormant hypnozoite form in the liver can emerge after an interval of weeks or months to start the infection again.

The characteristic presentations of the different forms of human malaria are as follow (see Fig. 49.1 for details).

• *P. falciparum*, which has an erythrocytic cycle of 48 hours in humans, produces *malignant tertian malaria*—'tertian' because the fever was believed to recur every third day (actually, it varies), 'malignant' because it is the most severe form of malaria and can be fatal. The plasmodium induces, on the infected red cell membrane, receptors for the adhesion molecules on vascular endothelial cells (see p. 000). These parasitised red cells then stick to uninfected red cells, forming clusters (rosettes), and also adhere to and pack the vessels of the microcirculation, interfering with tissue blood flow and causing organ dysfunction including renal failure and encephalopathy (cerebral malaria). *P. falciparum* does not have an exoerythrocytic stage, so if the erythrocytic stage is eradicated, relapses do not occur.

• *P. vivax* produces *benign tertian malaria*—'benign' because it is less severe than falciparum malaria and is rarely fatal. Exoerythrocytic forms may persist for years and cause relapses.

• *P. ovale*, which has a 48-hour cycle and an exoerythrocytic stage, is the cause of a rare form of malaria.

• *P. malariae* has a 72-hour cycle, causes *quartan malaria* and has no exoerythrocytic cycle.

Individuals living in areas where malaria is endemic may acquire a natural immunity, but this may be lost if the individual is absent from the area for more than 6 months.

ANTIMALARIAL DRUGS

The best way to deal with malaria is to avoid the disease in the first place by preventing mosquito bites.

▼ Travellers to infected areas should always take simple precautions such as wearing clothes that cover much of the skin and using insect repellents in living, and especially in sleeping, areas, because mosquitoes tend to bite between dusk and dawn. Bed nets sprayed with insecticides such as **permethrin** can be very effective.

Some drugs can be used prophylactically to prevent malaria, while others are directed towards treating acute attacks. In general,

---

> **Antimalarial therapy and the parasite life cycle** 🔑
>
> • Drugs used in the treatment of malaria may have several sites of action:
> — drugs used to treat the acute attack of malaria act on the parasites in the blood; they can cure infections with parasites (e.g. *Plasmodium falciparum*) that have no exoerythrocytic stage
> — drugs used for chemoprophylaxis (causal prophylactics) act on merozoites emerging from liver cells
> — drugs used for radical cure are active against parasites in the liver
> — some drugs act on gametocytes and prevent transmission by the mosquito.

---

antimalarial drugs are classified in terms of the action against the different stages of the life cycle of the parasite (Fig. 49.1).

Drugs used to treat the acute attack

Blood schizonticidal agents (Fig. 49.1, site A) are used to treat the acute attack—they are also known as drugs that produce a 'suppressive' or 'clinical' cure. They act on the erythrocytic forms of the plasmodium. In infections with *P. falciparum* or *P. malariae*, which have no exoerythrocytic stage, these drugs effect a cure; with *P. vivax* or *P. ovale*, the drugs suppress the actual attack, but exoerythrocytic forms can re-emerge later to cause relapses.

This group of drugs includes *quinoline–methanols* (e.g. **quinine** and **mefloquine**), various *4-aminoquinolines* (e.g. **chloroquine**), the phenanthrene **halofantrine**, and agents that interfere either with the synthesis of folate (e.g. **sulfones**) or with its action (e.g. **pyrimethamine** and **proguanil**), as well as the hydroxy-naphthoquinone compound **atovaquone**. Combinations of these agents are frequently used. Some antibiotics, such as **tetracycline** and **doxycycline** (see Ch. 46), have proved useful when combined with the above agents. Compounds derived from *qinghaosu*, for example **artemether**, **arteflene** and **artesunate**, have also proved effective.

For a brief summary of currently recommended treatment regimens, see the *Antimalarial drugs* box and Table 49.2. A more detailed coverage of the treatment of malaria is given by Newton & White (1999) and Baird (2005).

Drugs that effect a radical cure

Tissue schizonticidal agents effect a 'radical' (in the sense of striking at the root of the infection) cure by acting on the parasites in the liver (Fig. 49.1, site B). Only the 8-aminoquinolines (e.g. **primaquine** and **tafenoquine**) have this action. These drugs also destroy gametocytes and thus reduce the spread of infection.

Drugs used for chemoprophylaxis

Drugs used for chemoprophylaxis (also known as *causal prophylactic* drugs) block the link between the exoerythrocytic

Table 49.2 Summary of drugs used for treatment and chemoprophylaxis of malaria[a]

Infections	Typical drug choices for acute attacks	Typical drug choices for chemoprophylaxis
All plasmodial infections except chloroquine-resistant *Plasmodium falciparum*	Oral chloroquine or sulfadoxine–pyrimethamine	Oral chloroquine and/or proguanil
Infection with chloroquine-resistant *P. falciparum*	Oral quinine plus: (i) tetracycline or (ii) doxycycline, oral halofantrine or mefloquine	Oral chloroquine plus: (i) proguanil or (ii) doxycycline or (iii) pyrimethamine, Malarone[b] or oral mefloquine

(Source: British National Formulary.)

[a]It must be appreciated that this is only a summary, not a definitive guide to prescription, as the recommended drug combinations vary depending on the patient, the area visited, the overall risk of infection, the presence of resistant forms of the disease and so on.
[b]Malarone is a proprietary combination of atovaquine and proguanil hydrochloride.

stage and the erythrocytic stage, and thus prevent the development of malarial attacks. True causal prophylaxis—the prevention of infection by the killing of the sporozoites on entry into the host—is not feasible with the drugs at present in use, although it may be achieved in the future with vaccines. Prevention of the development of clinical attacks can, however, be effected by chemoprophylactic drugs that kill the parasites when they emerge from the liver after the pre-erythrocytic stage (Fig. 49.1, site C). The drugs used for this purpose are mainly those listed above: chloroquine, mefloquine, proguanil, pyrimethamine, **dapsone** and doxycycline. They are often used in combinations.

▼ Chemoprophylactic agents are given to individuals who intend travelling to an area where malaria is endemic. Administration should start 1 week before entering the area and should be continued throughout the stay and for at least a month afterwards. No chemoprophylactic regimen is 100% effective, and the choice of drug is difficult. In addition to the normal criteria used in selecting a drug, the unwanted effects of some antimalarial agents need to be borne in mind and weighed against the risk of a serious, possibly fatal, parasitaemia. A further problem is the complexity of the regimens, which require different drugs to be taken at different times, and the fact that different agents may be required for different travel destinations. For a brief summary of currently recommended regimens of chemoprophylaxis, see Table 49.2.

Drugs used to prevent transmission

Some drugs (e.g. primaquine, proguanil and pyrimethamine) have the additional action of destroying the gametocytes (Fig. 49.1, site D), preventing transmission by the mosquito and thus preventing the increase of the human reservoir of the disease— but they are rarely used for this action alone.

We will now look at some of these drugs in more detail.

4-AMINOQUINOLINES

The main 4-aminoquinoline used clinically is chloroquine (Fig. 49.2). **Amodiaquine** has very similar action to chloroquine. It was withdrawn several years ago because it caused agranulocytosis, but has now been reintroduced in several areas of the world where chloroquine resistance is endemic.

Chloroquine

Chloroquine is an old drug (1940s) but is still a very potent blood schizonticidal agent (Fig. 49.1, site A), effective against the erythrocytic forms of all four plasmodial species (if sensitive to the drug), but it does not have any effect on sporozoites, hypnozoites or gametocytes. It has a complex mechanism of action that is not fully understood. It is uncharged at neutral pH and can therefore diffuse freely into the parasite lysosome. At the acid pH of the lysosome, it is converted to a protonated, membrane-impermeable form and is 'trapped' inside the parasite. At high concentrations, chloroquine inhibits protein, RNA and DNA synthesis, but these effects are unlikely to be involved in its antimalarial activity. Probably, chloroquine acts mainly on haem disposal by preventing digestion of haemoglobin by the parasite and thus reducing the supply of amino acids necessary for parasite viability. It also inhibits haem polymerase—the enzyme that polymerises toxic free haem to haemozoin—rendering it harmless to the parasite. Chloroquine is also used as a disease-modifying antirheumatoid drug (Ch. 14) and also has some **quinidine**-like actions on the heart. The *clinical use* of chloroquine is summarised in Tables 49.1 and 49.2 and the *Antimalarial drugs* box.

Resistance

Plasmodium falciparum is now resistant to chloroquine in most parts of the world. Resistance appears to result from enhanced efflux of the drug from parasitic vesicles as a result of mutations in plasmodia transporter genes (Baird, 2005). Resistance of *P. vivax* to chloroquine is also a growing problem in many parts of the world.

Administration and pharmacokinetic aspects

Chloroquine is generally administered orally, but severe falciparum malaria may be treated by frequent intramuscular or subcutaneous injection of small doses, or by slow continuous intravenous infusion. Following oral dosing, it is completely absorbed, extensively distributed throughout the tissues and concentrated in parasitised red cells. Release from tissues and infected erythrocytes is slow. The drug is metabolised in the liver

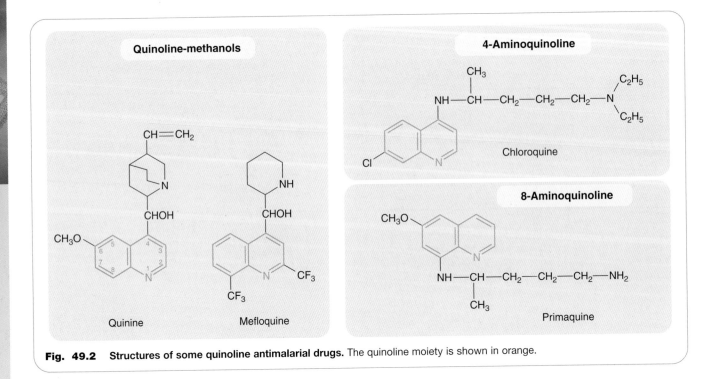

Fig. 49.2 **Structures of some quinoline antimalarial drugs.** The quinoline moiety is shown in orange.

and excreted in the urine, 70% as unchanged drug and 30% as metabolites. Elimination is slow, the major phase having a half-life of 50 hours, and a residue persists for weeks or months.

Unwanted effects

Chloroquine has few adverse effects when given for chemo-prophylaxis. However, unwanted effects, including nausea and vomiting, dizziness and blurring of vision, headache and urticarial symptoms, can occasionally occur when larger doses are administered to treat acute attacks of malaria. Large doses have also sometimes resulted in retinopathies. Bolus intravenous injections of chloroquine may cause hypotension and, if high doses are used, fatal dysrhythmias. Chloroquine is considered to be safe for use by pregnant women.

QUINOLINE–METHANOLS

The two most widely used quinoline–methanols are quinine and mefloquine (Fig. 49.2).

Quinine

Quinine is an alkaloid derived from cinchona bark. It has been used for the treatment of 'fevers' since the 16th century, when the bark was bought to Europe from Peru by Jesuit missionaries. It is a blood schizonticidal drug effective against the erythrocytic forms of all four species of plasmodium (Fig. 49.1, site A), but it has no effect on exoerythrocytic forms or on the gametocytes of *P. falciparum*. Its mechanism of action, like that of chloro-quine, is associated with inhibition of the parasite haem polymerase, but quinine is not so extensively concentrated in the plasmodium as chloroquine, so other mechanisms could also be involved. With the emergence and spread of chloroquine resistance, quinine is now the main chemotherapeutic agent for *P. falciparum*. Other

pharmacological actions on host tissue include a depressant action on the heart, a mild oxytocic effect on the uterus in pregnancy, a slight blocking action on the neuromuscular junction and a weak antipyretic effect. The *clinical use* of quinine is given in Tables 49.1 and 49.2 and in the box.

Pharmacokinetic aspects

Quinine is well absorbed and is usually administered orally as a 7-day course, but it can also be given by slow intravenous infusion for severe *P. falciparum* infections and in patients who are vomiting. A loading dose may be required, but bolus intravenous administration is contraindicated because of the risk of cardiac dysrhythmias. The half-life of the drug is 10 hours; it is metab-olised in the liver and the metabolites are excreted in the urine within about 24 hours.

Unwanted effects

Quinine has a bitter taste, and oral compliance is often poor.[3] It is irritant to the gastric mucosa and can cause nausea and vomiting. If the concentration in the plasma exceeds 30–60 μmol/l, 'cinchonism'—characterised by nausea, dizziness, tinnitus, head-ache and blurring of vision—is likely to occur. Excessive plasma levels of quinine can result in hypotension, cardiac dysrhythmias and severe CNS disturbances such as delirium and coma.

Other, infrequent, unwanted reactions that have been reported are blood dyscrasias (especially thrombocytopenia) and hyper-sensitivity reactions. Quinine can stimulate insulin release. Patients

---

[3]Hence the invention of palatable drinks containing the drug, including, of course, the 'tonic' drunk together with gin and other beverages.

with marked falciparum parasitaemia can have low blood sugar for this reason and also because of glucose consumption by the parasite. This makes a differential diagnosis—between a coma caused by cerebral malaria and hypoglycaemic coma—difficult. A rare result of treating malaria with quinine, or of erratic and inappropriate use of quinine, is *Blackwater fever*, a severe and often fatal condition in which acute haemolytic anaemia is associated with renal failure.

Resistance

Some degree of resistance is developing. Like chloroquine, resistance to quinine is conferred by increased expression of plasmodial drug efflux transporters.

Mefloquine

Mefloquine (Fig. 49.2) is a blood schizonticidal quinoline–methanol compound active against *P. falciparum* and *P. vivax* (Fig. 49.1, site A); however, it has no effect on hepatic forms of the parasites, so treatment of *P. vivax* infections should be followed by a course of primaquine (see below) to eradicate the hypnozoites. Mefloquine is frequently combined with pyrimethamine. The antiparasite action is associated with inhibition of the haem polymerase; however, because mefloquine, like quinine, is not as extensively concentrated in the parasite as chloroquine, other mechanisms might also be involved.

Resistance has occurred in *P. falciparum* in some areas—particularly in South-east Asia—and is thought to be caused, as with quinine, by increased expression in the parasite of drug efflux transporters. The *clinical use* of mefloquine is given in Tables 49.1 and 49.2 and the *Antimalarial drugs* box.

Pharmacokinetic aspects

Mefloquine is given orally and is rapidly absorbed. It has a slow onset of action and a very long plasma half-life (up to 30 days), which may be the result of enterohepatic cycling or tissue storage.

Unwanted effects

When mefloquine is used for treatment of the acute attack, about 50% of subjects complain of gastrointestinal disturbances. Transient CNS toxicity—giddiness, confusion, dysphoria and insomnia—can occur, and there have been a few reports of aberrant atrioventricular conduction and serious, but rare, skin diseases. Rarely, mefloquine may provoke severe neuropsychiatric reactions. Mefloquine is contraindicated in pregnant women or in those liable to become pregnant within 3 months of stopping the drug, because of its long half-life and uncertainty about its teratogenic potential. When used for chemoprophylaxis, the unwanted actions are usually milder, but the drug should not be used in this way unless there is a high risk of acquiring chloroquine-resistant malaria.

PHENANTHRENE–METHANOLS

Halofantrine

Halofantrine is a blood schizonticidal drug. It is one of a group of compounds that were studied during the Second World War and found to have antimalarial activity but were not developed further when chloroquine was brought out of retirement. However, as chloroquine resistance developed, halofantrine

came in from the cold. It is active against strains of *P. falciparum* that are resistant to chloroquine, pyrimethamine and quinine. It is effective against the erythrocytic form of *P. vivax* (Fig. 49.1, site A) but not the hypnozoites. However, it is not usually used for *P. vivax* malaria because this is generally susceptible to chloroquine. Cross-resistance between halofantrine and mefloquine in falciparum infections has been reported. Its mechanism of action is not known. The *clinical use* of halofantrine is given in Tables 49.1 and 49.2 and the box.

Pharmacokinetic aspects

Halofantrine is given orally. It is slowly and rather irregularly absorbed, with a peak plasma concentration achieved approximately 4–6 hours after ingestion. The half-life is 1–2 days, although its main metabolite, which has equal potency, has a half-life of 3–5 days. Absorption is substantially increased by a fatty meal, and elimination is in the faeces.

Unwanted effects

Abdominal pain, gastrointestinal disturbances, headache, a transient rise in hepatic enzymes and cough occur. Pruritus is reported but is less marked than with chloroquine. Halofantrine can produce changes in cardiac rhythm (most notably a lengthening of the QT interval), particularly if given with other similar drugs, and it should be used with caution in patients with a history of dysrhythmia. It has caused sudden cardiac death. Rarer reactions include haemolytic anaemia and convulsions. Because of such unwanted actions, halofantrine is no longer used for 'standby' treatment of malaria, and it is now reserved for infections caused by resistant organisms. However, even in this case, decreasing sensitivity and resistance of *P. falciparum* have been reported.

DRUGS AFFECTING THE SYNTHESIS OR UTILISATION OF FOLATE

Antifolate drugs are classified into type 1 and type 2 compounds. The type 1 antifolates are the sulfonamides and the sulfones, which inhibit the synthesis of folate by competing with *p*-aminobenzoic acid (see Chs 45 and 46). The type 2 antifolates include drugs such as pyrimethamine and proguanil, which prevent the utilisation of folate in the conversion of dihydrofolate to tetrahydrofolate by inhibiting *dihydrofolate reductase*. Combinations of folate antagonists (type 2) with drugs inhibiting folate synthesis (type 1) cause sequential blockade, affecting the same pathway at different points; these combinations thus have synergistic action.

Pyrimethamine is a 2,4-diaminopyrimidine (see Fig. 49.3) and is similar in structure to **trimethoprim** (see Ch. 46). The structure of proguanil is different, but it can assume a configuration similar to that of pyrimethamine (see Fig. 49.3). These compounds inhibit the formation of tetrahydrofolate and hence DNA synthesis as outlined in Chapter 51, but both drugs have a greater affinity for the plasmodial enzyme than for the human enzyme. They have a slow action against the erythrocytic forms of the parasite (Fig. 49.1, site A), and proguanil is believed to have an additional effect on the initial hepatic stage (1a to 3a in Fig. 49.1) but not on the hypnozoites of *P. vivax* (Fig. 49.1, site B). Pyrimethamine is used only in combination with either dapsone or a sulfonamide.

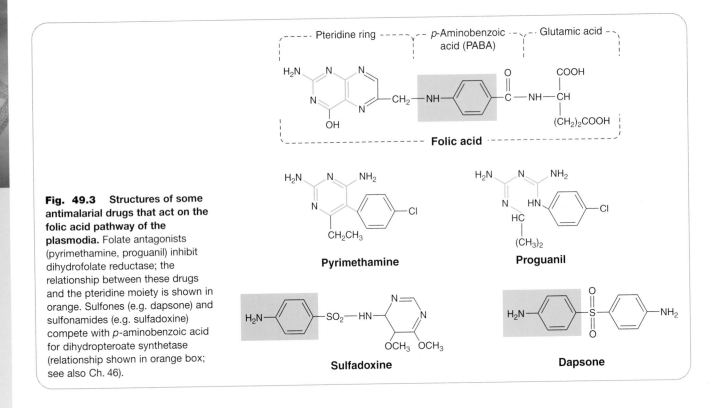

Fig. 49.3 **Structures of some antimalarial drugs that act on the folic acid pathway of the plasmodia.** Folate antagonists (pyrimethamine, proguanil) inhibit dihydrofolate reductase; the relationship between these drugs and the pteridine moiety is shown in orange. Sulfones (e.g. dapsone) and sulfonamides (e.g. sulfadoxine) compete with *p*-aminobenzoic acid for dihydropteroate synthetase (relationship shown in orange box; see also Ch. 46).

The main sulfonamide used in malaria treatment is **sulfadoxine**, and the only sulfone used is dapsone (see Fig. 49.3). Details of these drugs are given in Chapter 46. The sulfonamides and sulfones are active against the erythrocytic forms of *P. falciparum* but are less active against those of *P. vivax*; they have no activity against the sporozoite or hypnozoite forms of the plasmodia. Pyrimethamine–sulfadoxine has been extensively used for chloroquine-resistant malaria, but resistance to this combination has developed in many areas.

Pharmacokinetic aspects

Both pyrimethamine and proguanil are given orally and are well, although slowly, absorbed. Pyrimethamine has a plasma half-life of 4 days, and effective 'suppressive' plasma concentrations may last for 14 days; it is taken once a week. The half-life of proguanil is 16 hours. It is a prodrug and is metabolised in the liver to its active form, cycloguanil, which is excreted mainly in the urine. It must be taken daily. Details of the pharmacokinetics of dapsone are given in Chapter 46.

Unwanted effects

These drugs have few untoward effects if used carefully in therapeutic doses. Larger doses of the pyrimethamine–dapsone combination can cause serious reactions such as haemolytic anaemia, agranulocytosis and eosinophilic alveolitis. The pyrimethamine–sulfadoxine combination can cause serious skin reactions, blood dyscrasias and allergic alveolitis; it is no longer recommended for chemoprophylaxis. In high doses, pyrimethamine may inhibit mammalian dihydrofolate reductase and cause a megaloblastic anaemia (see Ch. 22); folic acid supplements should be given if this drug is used during pregnancy. Resistance to antifolate drugs arises from single-point mutations in the genes encoding parasite dihydrofolate reductase.

8-AMINOQUINOLINES

The only 8-aminoquinoline licensed for current use is primaquine (see Fig. 49.2). **Etaquine** and tafenoquine are more active and slowly metabolised analogues of primaquine. The mechanism of action of these comparatively new compounds is not known.

The antimalarial action of this class of drugs is exerted against the liver hypnozoites, and they can effect a radical cure of those forms of malaria in which the parasites have a dormant stage in the liver—*P. vivax* and *P. ovale*. Primaquine does not affect sporozoites and has little if any action against the erythrocytic stage of the parasite. However, it has a gametocidal action and is the most effective antimalarial drug for *preventing transmission* of the disease in all four species of plasmodia. It is almost invariably used in combination with another drug, usually chloroquine. Resistance to primaquine is rare, although evidence of a decreased sensitivity of some *P. vivax* strains has been reported. The pharmacology of primaquine and like drugs has been reviewed by Shanks et al. (2001).

Pharmacokinetic aspects

Primaquine is given orally and is well absorbed. Its metabolism is rapid, and very little drug is present in the body after 10–12 hours. The half-life is 3–6 hours. Tafenoquine is broken down much more slowly and therefore has the advantage that it can be given on a weekly basis.

Unwanted effects

Primaquine has few unwanted effects in most patients when used in normal therapeutic dosage. Dose-related gastrointestinal symptoms can occur, and large doses may cause methaemoglobinaemia with cyanosis. This antimalarial drug can, however, cause haemolysis in individuals with an X chromosome–linked genetic metabolic condition—*glucose 6-phosphate dehydrogenase deficiency*—in red cells. When this deficiency is present, the red cells are not able to regenerate NADPH, its concentration being reduced by the oxidant metabolic derivatives of primaquine. As a consequence, the metabolic functions of the red cells are impaired and haemolysis occurs. Primaquine metabolites have greater haemolytic activity than the parent compound. The deficiency of the enzyme occurs in up to 15% of black males and is also fairly common in some other ethnic groups. Glucose 6-phosphate dehydrogenase activity should be estimated before giving primaquine.

ANTIBIOTICS USED IN MALARIA

Some antibiotics, for example doxycycline and tetracycline, have a place in the treatment of the acute attack of malaria and in chemoprophylaxis; see Table 49.2. Details of these antibiotics are given in Chapter 46.

QINGHAOSU (ARTEMISININ) AND RELATED COMPOUNDS

The qinghaosu-based compounds are derived from the herb *qing hao*, a traditional Chinese remedy for malaria. The scientific name, conferred on the herb by Linnaeus, is *Artemisia*.[4] **Artemisinin**, a poorly soluble chemical extract from *Artemisia*, is a fast-acting blood schizonticide effective in treating the acute attack of malaria (including chloroquine-resistant and cerebral malaria). Artesunate, a water-soluble derivative, and the synthetic analogues artemether and **artether** have higher activity and are better absorbed. The compounds are concentrated in parasitised red cells. The mechanism of action is not known; it may involve damage to the parasite membrane by carbon-centred free radicals (generated by the breakdown of ferrous protoporphyrin IX) or covalent alkylation of proteins. These drugs are without effect on liver hypnozoites and are not useful for chemoprophylaxis. **Artemisinin** can be given orally, intramuscularly or by suppository, artemether orally or intramuscularly, and artesunate intramuscularly or intravenously. They are rapidly absorbed and widely distributed, and are converted in the liver to the active metabolite dihydroartemisinin. The half-life of **artemisinin** is about 4 hours, of artesunate 45 minutes and of artemether 4–11 hours.

Unwanted effects

There have been few unwanted effects reported to date. Transient heart block, decrease in blood neutrophil count, and brief episodes of fever have been reported. In animal studies, **artemisinin** causes an unusual injury to some brain stem nuclei, particularly those involved in auditory function; however, there have been no reported incidences of neurotoxicity in humans. So far, there have also been no reported cases of resistance.

---

[4]The herbs are noted for their extreme bitterness, and their name derives from *Artemisia*, wife and sister of the fourth century king of Halicarnassus; her sorrow on his death led her to mix his ashes with whatever she drank to make it bitter.

In rodent studies, **artemisinin** potentiated the effects of mefloquine, primaquine and tetracycline; was additive with chloroquine; and antagonised the sulfonamides and the folate antagonists. For this reason, **artemisinin** derivatives are frequently used in combination with other antimalarial drugs; for example, artemether is often given in combination with the aminoalcohol **lumefantrine**.

In randomised trials, the qinghaosu compounds have cured attacks of malaria, including cerebral malaria, more rapidly and with fewer unwanted effects than other antimalarial agents. **Artemisinin** and derivatives are effective against multidrug-resistant *P. falciparum* in sub-Saharan Africa and, combined with mefloquine, against multidrug-resistant *P. falciparum* in Southeast Asia. However, the preclinical and clinical data are at present insufficient to satisfy the drug regulatory requirements in many countries. For a review of this topic, see Olliaro et al. (2001).

HYDROXYNAPHTHOQUINONE DRUGS

Atavaquone is used for the treatment of malaria and can prevent its development. It acts primarily to inhibit the parasite's mitochondrial electron transport chain, possibly by mimicking the natural substrate *ubiquinone*. Atavaquone is usually used in combination with the antifolate drug proguanil, because they act together to cause a synergistic antimalarial effect. The mechanism underlying this effect is not known, but synergy is specific for this particular pair of drugs, because other antifolate drugs or electron transport inhibitors have no such effect. When combined with proguanil, atavaquone is highly effective and well tolerated. Few side effects of such combination treatment have been reported, but abdominal pain, nausea and vomiting can occur. Pregnant or breast-feeding women should not take atavaquone. Resistance to atavaquone is rapid and results from a single point mutation in the gene for cytochrome *b*. Resistance to combined treatment with **atavaquone** and proguanil is less common.

POTENTIAL NEW ANTIMALARIAL DRUGS

Several new drugs are currently under test for antimalarial activity, with positive results in animals and in preliminary trials in humans. One of these, **pyronaridine**, has been used in China for almost 10 years. It is active against *P. falciparum* and *P. vivax*, and is also active in chloroquine-resistant *P. falciparum*. It is effective orally and has low toxicity. The mechanism of action is unknown. Lumefantrine is structurally related to quinine and is effective against *P. falciparum*, particularly when combined with either mefloquine or artemisinin derivatives.

TOXOPLASMOSIS AND TOXOPLASMOCIDAL DRUGS

The cat is the definitive host of *Toxoplasma gondii* (i.e. it is the only host in which the sexual cycle can occur), and it expels the infectious cysts in its faeces; humans can inadvertently become intermediate hosts, harbouring the asexual form of the parasite. Ingested oocysts develop into sporozoites, then to

Antimalarial drugs

- Chloroquine is a blood schizonticide that is concentrated in the parasite and inhibits the haem polymerase. Orally active; half-life 50 hours. Unwanted effects: gastrointestinal disturbances, dizziness and urticaria. Bolus intravenous injections can cause dysrhythmias.
- Quinine is a blood schizonticide. It may be given orally or intravenously; half-life 10 hours. Unwanted effects: gastrointestinal tract disturbances, tinnitus, blurred vision and, in large doses, dysrhythmias and central nervous system disturbances. It is usually given in combination therapy with:
  — pyrimethamine, a folate antagonist that acts as a slow blood schizonticide (orally active; half-life 4 days) and either
  — dapsone, a sulfone (orally active; half-life 24–48 hours), or
  — sulfadoxine, a long-acting sulfonamide (orally active; half-life 7–9 days).
- Proguanil, a folate antagonist, is a slow blood schizonticide with some action on the primary liver forms of *P. vivax*. Orally active; half-life 16 hours.
- Mefloquine is a blood schizonticidal agent active against *P. falciparum* and *P. vivax*, and acts by inhibiting the parasite haem polymerase. Orally active; half-life 30 days. The onset of action is slow. Unwanted effects: gastrointestinal disturbances, neurotoxicity and psychiatric problems.

- Halofantrine is a blood schizonticidal agent active against all species of malarial parasite, including multiresistant *P. falciparum*. Orally active; half-life 1–2 days (active metabolite half-life 3–5 days). Unwanted effects: abdominal pain, gastrointestinal disturbances, headache. Serious cardiac problems sometimes occur.
- Primaquine is effective against the liver hypnozoites and is also active against gametocytes. Orally active; half-life 36 hours. Unwanted effects: gastrointestinal tract disturbances and, with large doses, methaemoglobinaemia. Erythrocyte haemolysis in individuals with genetic deficiency of glucose 6-phosphate dehydrogenase.
- Artemisinin derivatives are widely used in Asia and Africa but are not licensed in some other countries. They are fast-acting blood schizonticidal agents that are effective against both *P. falciparum* and *P. vivax*. Artesunate is water-soluble and can be given orally or by intravenous, intramuscular or rectal administration. Side effects are rare.
- Atavaquone (in combination with proguanil) is used for the treatment of acute, uncomplicated *P. falciparum* malaria. The drug combination is effective orally. It is given at regular intervals over 3–4 days. Unwanted effects: diarrhoea, nausea and vomiting. Resistance to atavaquone develops rapidly if it is given alone.

trophozoites, and finally encyst in the tissues. In most individuals, the disease is asymptomatic or self-limiting, although intrauterine infections can severely damage the developing fetus and it may cause fatal generalised infection in immuno-suppressed patients or those with AIDS, in whom toxoplasmic encephalitis may occur. In humans, *T. gondii* infects numerous cell types and has a highly virulent replicative stage.

The treatment of choice is pyrimethamine–**sulfadiazine** (to be avoided in pregnant patients); trimethoprim–**sulfamethoxazole** or parenteral pentamidine is also used and, more recently, **azithromycin** has shown promise.

CILIATES AND OTHERS

First recognised in 1909, *Pneumocystis carinii* was presumed to belong to the protozoa, but recent studies have shown that it shares structural features with both protozoa and fungi, leaving its precise classification uncertain. Previously considered to be a widely distributed but largely innocuous micro-organism, it now causes opportunistic infections in immunocompromised patients. It is common in AIDS, where *P. carinii* pneumonia is often the presenting symptom as well as a leading cause of death.

High-dose **co-trimoxazole** (Ch. 46) is the drug of choice, with parenteral pentamidine (see above) as an alternative. Other treatment regimens include trimethoprim–dapsone, or atavaquone or **clindamycin**–primaquine.

NEW APPROACHES TO ANTIPROTOZOAL THERAPY

This field is a huge challenge, with each protozoa species posing its own distinct problems to the would-be designer of new anti-protozoal drugs. Where appropriate in this chapter, we have indicated possible future avenues for research and development, but the interested reader is referred to the reading list and web sites listed below for further information. While there are undoubtedly many technical issues to be surmounted, ironically these do not represent the major challenge to the eradication of protozoal diseases. There are a host of socioeconomic problems that also need to be addressed first.

It is abundantly clear that the diseases caused by the protozoa constitute a major global challenge, but the problems of provision and distribution of new drugs are daunting. Managing the costs of research and development in this area is complex. Transnational initiatives (e.g. *Drugs for Neglected Diseases Initiative*) and philanthropic foundations (e.g. *Institute for OneWorld Health*) are proving helpful, but it is not simply a lack of new drugs that is the problem. For economic reasons, the very countries and populations one would most like to target often lack an efficient infrastructure for the distribution and safe administration of the drugs that we already possess. Cultural attitudes, civil wars, famine, the circulation of counterfeit or defective drugs, drought and natural disasters also exacerbate this problem. At the moment, there seems no easy way out of this dilemma.

REFERENCES AND FURTHER READING

Host–parasite interactions

Brenier-Pinchart M-P, Pelloux H, Derouich-Guergour D et al. 2001 Chemokines in host–parasite interactions. Trends Parasitol 17: 292–296 (*Good review of role of immune system*)

Amoebiasis

Haque R, Huston C D, Hughes M et al. 2003 Amebiasis. N Engl J Med 348: 1565–1573 (*Good review; concentrates on the pathogenesis of the disease but has a useful table of drugs and their side effects*)

Martinez-Palomo A, Espinosa-Cantellano M 1998 Amoebiasis: new understandings and new goals. Parasitol Today 14: 1–3

Stanley S L 2001 Pathophysiology of amoebiasis. Trends Parasitol 17: 280–285 (*A good account of the human disease that incorporates some results from animal models also*)

Stanley S L 2003 Amoebiasis. Lancet 361: 1025–1034 (*Comprehensive and easy-to-read account of this disease, covering all aspects from diagnosis to treatment—excellent*)

Trypanosomiasis

Aksoy S, Gibson W C, Lehane M J 2003 Interactions between tsetse and trypanosomes with implications for the control of trypanosomiasis. Adv Parasitol 53: 1–83 (*A very substantial and comprehensive article covering the biology of the tsetse fly, which also discusses alternative methods from controlling the insect population. Less good on drug therapy, but if you are interested in the biology of the insect vector of trypanosomiasis then this is for you.*)

Burchmore R J, Ogbunude P O, Enanga B, Barrett M P 2002 Chemotherapy of human African trypanosomiasis. Curr Pharm Des 8: 256–267 (*Very good concise article; nice discussion of future therapeutic possibilities*)

Burri C, Brun R 2003 Eflornithine for the treatment of human African trypanosomiasis. Parasitol Res 90(suppl 1): S49–S52

Denise H, Barrett M P 2001 Uptake and mode of action of drugs used against sleeping sickness. Biochem Pharmacol 61: 1–5 (*Good coverage of drug therapy*)

Keiser J, Stich A, Burri C 2001 New drugs for the treatment of human African trypanosomiasis: research and development. Trends Parasitol 17: 42–49 (*Excellent review on an increasingly threatening disease*)

Legros D, Ollivier G, Gastellu-Etchegorry M et al. 2002 Treatment of human African trypanosomiasis—present situation and needs for research and development. Lancet Infect Dis 2: 437–440

Naula C, Burchmore R 2003 A plethora of targets, a paucity of drugs: progress towards the development of novel chemotherapies for human African trypanosomiasis. Expert Rev Antiinfect Ther 1: 157–165

Nesslany F, Brugier S, Mouries M A et al. 2004 In vitro and in vivo chromosomal aberrations induced by megazol. Mutat Res 560: 147–158

Leishmaniasis

Berman J 2003 Current treatment approaches to leishmaniasis. Curr Opin Infect Dis 16: 397–401 (*Good general review that includes some data on new clinical trials*)

Handman E, Bullen D V R 2002 Interaction of *Leishmania* with the host macrophage. Trends Parasitol 18: 332–334 (*Very good article describing how this parasite colonises macrophages and evades intracellular killing; easy to read*)

Jayanarayan K G, Dey C S 2002. Microtubules: dynamics, drug interaction and drug resistance in *Leishmania*. J Clin Pharm Ther 27: 313–320 (*Deals with the action on parasite microtubules of antileishmanial drugs—very specialised*)

Kubar J, Fragaki K 2005 Recombinant DNA derived *Leishmania* proteins: from the laboratory to the field. Lancet Infect Dis 5: 107–114 (*Some interesting discussion and observations on possible drug targets but a bit specialised*)

Murrey H W 2000 Treatment of visceral leishmaniasis (kala-azar): a decade of progress and future approaches. Int J Infect Dis 4: 158–177 (*Clear account of present clinical therapy and potential new drugs*)

Sacks D, Toben-Trauth N 2002 The immunology of susceptibility and resistance to *Leishmania major* in mice. Nat Rev Immunol 2: 845–858 (*A lengthy article that explores the host response to* Leishmania *parasite infection using mouse models of the disease; fascinating and authoritative—but only attempt it if your immunology is up to scratch!*)

Verma N K, Dey C S 2004 Possible mechanism of miltefosine-mediated death of *Leishmania donovani*. Antimicrob Agents Chemother 48: 3010–3015

Malaria

Ashley E A, White N J 2005 Artemisinin based combinations. Curr Opin Infect Dis 18: 531–536 (*This review details the results of successful clinical trials of artemisinin combinations in South-east Asia*)

Baird J K 2005 Effectiveness of antimalarial drugs. N Engl J Med 352: 1565–1577 (*An excellent overview covering many aspects of drug therapy, drug resistance and the socioeconomic factors affecting the treatment of this disease—thoroughly recommended*)

Berent A R, Craig A G 1997 *Plasmodium falciparum*— sticky jams and PECAM pie. Nat Med 3: 1315–1316 (*Deals with malaria parasites and host adhesion molecules*)

Foley M, Tilley L 1997 Quinoline antimalarials: mechanisms of action and resistance. Int J Parasitol 27: 231–240 (*Good, short review; useful diagrams*)

Holt R A, Subramanian G M et al. 2002 The genome sequence of the malaria mosquito *Anopheles gambiae*. Science 298: 129–149 (*For those who want to explore the genomic aspects more thoroughly*)

Krishna S 1997 Malaria. Br Med J 315: 730–732 (*Good, short review in the series* Science, medicine and the future; *useful diagram*)

Lell B, Luckner D et al. 1998 Randomised placebo-controlled study of atovaquone plus proguanil for malaria prophylaxis in children. Lancet 351: 709–713 (*States that this combination is highly effective and well tolerated*)

Newton P, White N 1999 Malaria: new developments in treatment and prevention. Annu Rev Med 50: 179–192 (*Excellent review of drug treatment and management of malaria*)

O'Brien C 1997 Beating the malaria parasite at its own game. Lancet 350: 192 (*Clear, succinct coverage of mechanisms of action and resistance of current antimalarials and potential new drugs; useful diagram*)

Odeh M 2001 The role of tumour necrosis factor-alpha in the pathogenesis of complicated falciparum malaria. Cytokine 14: 11–18

Olliaro P L, Haynes R K, Meunier B et al. 2001 Possible modes of action of artemisin-type compounds. Trends Parasitol 17: 266–268

Shanks G D, Kain K C, Keystone J S 2001 Malaria chemoprophylaxis in the age of drug resistance. II Drugs that may be available in the future. Clin Infect Dis 33: 381–385 (*A useful look ahead to new drugs*)

Targett G A 1998 Malaria—variety is the price of life. Nat Med 4: 267–268 (*The biological roles of the surface proteins of malaria-infected red cells*)

Pneumocystis pneumonia

Warren E, George S et al. 1997 Advances in the treatment and prophylaxis of *Pneumocystis carinii* pneumonia. Pharmacotherapy 17: 900–916

Future drugs for protozoal infections and general

Croft S L 1997 The current status of antiparasite chemotherapy. Parasitology 114: S3–S15 (*Comprehensive coverage of current drugs and outline of approaches to possible future agents*)

Rosenblatt J E 1999 Antiparasitic agents. Mayo Clin Proc 74: 1161–1175 (*Broad review article, wide coverage*)

Useful web resources

http://archive.bmn.com/supp/part/swf012.html (*An interactive animation showing the infection of a human host with* Leishmania *by a tsetse fly vector— fun*)

http://mosquito.who.int/cmc_upload/0/000/015/372/RB MInfosheet_1.htm (*2001–10 is the decade of the United Nations Roll Back Malaria programme, and this site contains a wealth of statistics, photographs, maps and explanatory text covering every aspect of this depressing disease. Together with the other web sites shown below, it forms the nucleus of a comprehensive resource for exploring the implications of the global malaria problem more closely.*)

http://www.oneworldhealth.org (*The web page of the visionary 'non profit pharmaceutical company', with details of their current programmes dealing with global health issues*)

http://www.who.int/en/ (*The WHO home page, with links to all other sites relevant to this chapter*)

http://www.who.int/mediacentre/factsheets/fs094/en/ (*This web site is a subsite of the WHO home page and contains links to all the major information on the site dealing with malaria, including the sites above—a terrific starting point for further investigation*)

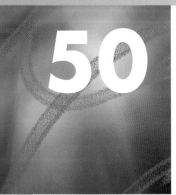

50 Antihelminthic drugs

OVERVIEW

Among the most widespread of all chronic infections
are those caused by various species of parasitic
helminths (worms). For example, it is estimated
that over half the world's population may be
infected with gastrointestinal helminths. Inhabitants
of tropical or subtropical low-income countries are
most at risk; children often become infected with
one or more species almost as soon as they are
born and may remain infected throughout their
lives. In some cases (e.g. *threadworms*), these
infections result mainly in discomfort and do not
cause substantial ill health, but others, such as
schistosomiasis (*bilharzia*) and *hookworm* disease,
can produce very serious morbidity. Because of its
prevalence, the problem of the treatment of
helminthiasis is therefore one of very great
practical therapeutic importance. Worm infections
are also a major cause for concern in veterinary
medicine, affecting both domestic pets and farm
animals. In some parts of the world, *fascioliasis* is
associated with significant loss of livestock.

HELMINTH INFECTIONS

The helminths comprise two major groups of multicellular worms
that evolved from a common ancestor some 600 million years
ago and diverged into two rather different groups: the
nemathelminths (nematodes, roundworms) and the *platyhelminths*
(flatworms). The latter group is subdivided into the *trematodes*
(flukes) and the *cestodes* (tapeworms). Almost 350 species of

helminths have been found in humans, and most colonise the
gastrointestinal tract.

Helminths have a complex life cycle, often involving several
species. Infection by helminths may occur in many ways, and
poor hygiene is a major contributory factor. Many enter by mouth
in unpurified drinking water or in badly cooked meat from infected
animals or fish. However, other types can enter through the skin
following a cut, an insect bite or even after swimming or walking
on infected soil. Humans are generally the *primary* (or definitive)
host for helminth infections, in the sense that they harbour the
sexually mature form that reproduces. Eggs or larvae then pass
out of the body and infect the secondary (intermediate) host. In
some cases, the eggs or larvae may persist in the human host and
become *encysted*, covered with granulation tissue, giving rise to
cysticercosis. This is characterised by encysted larvae in the
muscles and the viscera or, more seriously, in the eye or the brain.
Approximately 20 helminth species are considered to be clinically significant, and these fall into two main categories—those
in which the worm lives in the host's alimentary canal, and those
in which the worm lives in other tissues of the host's body.

The main examples of worms that live in the host's alimentary
canal are as follow.

- *Tapeworms: Taenia saginata, Taenia solium, Hymenolepis
  nana and Diphyllobothrium latum.* Some 85 million people
  in Asia, Africa and parts of America harbour one or other of
  these tapeworm species. Only the first two are likely to be
  seen in the UK. The usual intermediate hosts of the two most
  common tapeworms (*Taenia saginata and Taenia solium*) are
  cattle and pigs, respectively. Humans become infected by
  eating raw or undercooked meat containing the larvae, which
  have encysted in the animals' muscle tissue. *H. nana* may
  exist as both the adult (the intestinal worm) and the larval
  stage in the same host, which may be human or rodent,
  although some insects (fleas, grain beetles) can also serve as
  intermediate hosts. The infection is usually asymptomatic.
  Diphyllobothrium latum has two sequential intermediate
  hosts: a freshwater crustacean and a freshwater fish. Humans
  become infected by eating raw or incompletely cooked fish
  containing the larvae, and vitamin B_{12} deficiency sometimes
  occurs (see Ch. 22).
- *Intestinal roundworms: Ascaris lumbricoides* (common
  roundworm), *Enterobius vermicularis* (threadworm, called
  pinworm in the USA), *Trichuris trichiura* (whipworm),
  Strongyloides stercoralis (threadworm in the USA), *Necator*

americanus and *Ankylostoma duodenale* (hookworms). Again, undercooked meat or contaminated food is an important cause of infection by roundworm, threadworm and whipworm, whereas hookworm is generally acquired when their larvae penetrate the skin.

The main examples of worms that live in the tissues of the host are as follow.

- *Flukes: Schistosoma haematobium, Schistosoma mansoni,* and *Schistosoma japonicum.* These cause *schistosomiasis* (bilharzia). The adult worms of both sexes live and mate in the veins or venules of the gut wall or the bladder. The female lays eggs that pass into the bladder or gut and produce inflammation of these organs, resulting in haematuria in the former case and, occasionally, loss of blood in the faeces in the latter. The eggs hatch in water after discharge from the body and thus enter the secondary host— a particular species of snail. After a period of development in this host, free-swimming *cercariae* emerge. These are capable of infecting humans by penetration of the skin. About 200 million people are infected with one or other of the schistosomes.
- *Tissue roundworms: Trichinella spiralis, Dracunculus medinensis* (guinea worm) and the *filariae,* which include *Wuchereria bancrofti, Loa loa, Onchocerca volvulus* and *Brugia malayi.* The adult filariae live in the lymphatics, connective tissues or mesentery of the host and produce live embryos or *microfilariae,* which find their way into the bloodstream. They may be ingested by mosquitoes or similar biting insects when they feed. After a period of development within this secondary host, the larvae pass to the mouthparts of the insect and are reinjected into humans. Major filarial diseases are caused by *Wuchereria* or *Brugia,* which cause obstruction of lymphatic vessels, producing *elephantiasis.* Other related diseases are *onchocerciasis* (in which the presence of microfilariae in the eye causes 'river blindness') and *loiasis* (in which the microfilariae cause inflammation in the skin and other tissues). *Trichinella spiralis* causes trichinosis; the larvae from the viviparous female worms in the intestine migrate to skeletal muscle, where they become encysted. In guinea worm infection, larvae released from crustaceans in wells and waterholes are ingested and migrate from the intestinal tract to mature and mate in the tissues; the gravid female then migrates to the subcutaneous tissues of the leg or the foot, where she may protrude through an ulcer in the skin. The worm may be up to a metre in length and has to be removed surgically or by slow mechanical winding of the worm on to a stick over a period of days.
- *Hydatid tapeworm.* These are cestodes of the *Echinococcus* species for which canines are the primary hosts, and sheep the intermediate hosts. The primary, intestinal stage does not occur in humans, but under certain circumstances humans can function as the intermediate host, in which case the larvae develop into hydatid cysts within the tissues.

Some nematodes that usually live in the gastrointestinal tract of animals may infect humans and penetrate tissues. A skin infes-

tation, termed *creeping eruption* or *cutaneous larva migrans,* is caused by the larvae of dog and cat hookworms. *Toxocariasis* or visceral larva migrans is caused by larvae of cat and dog roundworms of the *Toxocara* genus.

ANTIHELMINTHIC DRUGS

Mankind has attempted to treat helminth infections since antiquity. Extracts of herbs or plants such as extracts of male fern formed the basis of many early 'cures', but the 20th century saw the advent of a new group of drugs based on heavy metals such as arsenic (atoxyl) or antimony (tartar emetic), which were effective in trypanosome and schistosome infestations.

Generally speaking, the current antihelminthic therapies act by incapacitating the parasite by paralysis (e.g. by preventing muscular contraction), damaging the worm such that the immune system can eliminate it, or by altering its metabolic processes (e.g. by affecting microtubule function). Because the metabolic requirements of these parasites vary greatly from one species to another, drugs that are highly effective against one type of worm may be ineffective against others. Clearly, to be an effective antihelminthic, a drug must be able to penetrate the tough exterior *cuticle* of the worm or gain access to its alimentary tract in sufficient concentrations to be effective. This in itself may present difficulties, because some worms are exclusively *haemophagous* (blood eating), while others are best described as 'tissue grazers'. A further complication is that many helminths contain active drug efflux pumps that reduce the concentration of the drug in the parasite. The route and dose of antihelminthic are therefore important and must be chosen carefully, because parasitic worms cannot be relied on to consume sufficient amounts of the drug to be effective.

Some individual antihelminthic drugs are described briefly below, and indications for their use are given in Table 50.1. For a more comprehensive coverage of antiparasitic drugs and their use in humans and animals, you are directed to the literature cited in the bibliography. Several of these drugs (i.e. **niclosamide**, **albendazole**, **tiabendazole**, **levamisole** and **praziquantel**) are available in the UK only on a 'named patient' basis.[1]

BENZIMIDAZOLES

One of the principal groups of antihelminthics used clinically are the substituted benzimidazoles. This group of broad-spectrum agents includes **mebendazole**, tiabendazole and albendazole. They are thought to act by inhibiting the polymerisation of helminth β-tubulin, thus interfering with microtubule-dependent functions such as glucose uptake. They have a selective inhibitory action,

---

[1] A relatively rare situation in which the physician seeks approval from a pharmaceutical company to use one of their drugs in a named individual. The drug is either a 'newcomer' that has shown particular promise in clinical trials but has not yet been licensed or, as in these instances, an established drug that has not been licensed because the company has not applied for a product licence (possibly for commercial reasons).

Table 50.1   Principal drugs used in helminth infections

Helminth(s)	Drug(s) used
Threadworm (pinworm)	
Enterobius vermicularis	Mebendazole, albendazole, piperazine
Strongyloides stercoralis (threadworm in the USA)	Albendazole, tiabendazole, ivermectin
Common roundworm	
Ascaris lumbricoides	Levamisole, mebendazole, piperazine
Other roundworm (filariae)	
Wuchereria bancrofti, Loa loa	Diethylcarbamazine, ivermectin
Onchocerca volvulus	Ivermectin
Guinea worm (*Dracunculus medinensis*)	Praziquantel, mebendazole
Trichiniasis (*Trichinella spiralis*)	Tiabendazole, mebendazole
Cysticercosis (infection with larval *Taenia solium*)	Praziquantel, albendazole
Tapeworm (*Taenia saginata, Taenia solium*)	Praziquantel, niclosamide
Hydatid disease (*Echinococcus granulosus*)	Albendazole, praziquantel
Hookworm (*Ankylostoma duodenale, Necator americanus*)	Mebendazole, albendazole
Whipworm (*Trichuris trichiura*)	Mebendazole, albendazole, diethylcarbamazine
Blood flukes (*Schistosoma* spp.)	
S. haematobium	Praziquantel
S. mansoni	Praziquantel
S. japonicum	Praziquantel
Cutaneous larva migrans	
Ankylostoma caninum	Albendazole, ivermectin, tiabendazole
Visceral larva migrans	
Toxacara canis	Albendazole, tiabendazole, diethylcarbamazine

(Sourced mainly from the *British National Formulary 2004*.)

being 250–400 times more effective in producing this effect in helminth than in mammalian tissue. However, the effect takes time to develop and the worms may not be expelled for several days. Cure rates are generally between 60 and 100% with most parasites.

Only 10% of mebendazole is absorbed after oral administration, but a fatty meal increases absorption. It is rapidly metabolised, the products being excreted in the urine and the bile within 24–48 hours. It is generally given as a single dose for threadworm, and twice daily for 3 days for hookworm and roundworm infestations. Tiabendazole is rapidly absorbed from the gastrointestinal tract, very rapidly metabolised and excreted in the urine in conjugated form. It is given twice daily for 3 days for guinea worm and *Strongyloides* infestations, and for up to 5 days for hookworm and roundworm infestations. Albendazole is also poorly absorbed but, like mebendazole, this may be increased by food, especially fats. It is metabolised extensively by first-pass metabolism to the sulfoxide and sulfone metabolites. The former is likely to be the pharmacologically active species.

Unwanted effects are few with albendazole or mebendazole, although gastrointestinal disturbances can occasionally occur. Unwanted effects with tiabendazole are more frequent but usually transient, the commonest being gastrointestinal disturbances, although headache, dizziness and drowsiness have been reported and allergic reactions (fever, rashes) can occur. Mebendazole should not be given to pregnant women or children less than 2 years old.

PRAZIQUANTEL

Praziquantel is a highly effective broad-spectrum antihelminthic drug that was introduced over 20 years ago. It is the drug of choice for all forms of schistosomiasis and is the agent generally used in large-scale schistosome eradication programmes. It is also effective in cysticercosis, for which there was previously no effective therapy. The drug affects not only the adult schistosomes but also the immature forms and the cercariae—the form of the parasite that infects humans by penetrating the skin.

The drug apparently disrupts Ca^{2+} homeostasis in the parasite by binding to consensus protein kinase C–binding sites in a β subunit of schistosome voltage-gated calcium channels (Greenberg, 2005). This induces an influx of the ion, a rapid and prolonged contraction of the musculature, and eventual paralysis and death of the worm. Praziquantel also disrupts the tegument of the parasite, unmasking novel antigens, and as a result it may become more susceptible to the host's normal immune responses.

Given orally, praziquantel is well absorbed; much of the drug is rapidly metabolised to inactive metabolites on first passage through the liver, and the metabolites are excreted in the urine. The plasma half-life of the parent compound is 60–90 minutes.

Praziquantel is considered to be a very safe drug with minimal side effects in therapeutic dosage. Such effects as do occur are usually transitory and rarely of clinical importance. They include gastrointestinal disturbance, dizziness, aching in muscles and joints, skin eruptions and low-grade fever. Some effects are more marked in patients with a heavy worm load and may be caused by products released from the dead worms. Praziquantel is considered safe for pregnant and lactating women, an important property for a drug that is commonly used in national disease control programmes. Some resistance has developed to the drug.

PIPERAZINE

Piperazine can be used to treat infections with the common roundworm (*Ascaris lumbricoides*) and the threadworm (*Enterobius vermicularis*). It reversibly inhibits neuromuscular transmission in the worm, probably by acting like GABA, the inhibitory neurotransmitter, or GABA-gated chloride channels in nematode muscle. The paralysed worms are expelled alive by normal intestinal peristaltic movements.

Piperazine is given orally and some, but not all, is absorbed. It is partly metabolised, and the remainder is eliminated, unchanged, via the kidney. The drug has little pharmacological action in the host. When used to treat roundworm, piperazine is effective in a single dose. For threadworm, a longer course (7 days) at lower dosage is necessary.

Unwanted effects are uncommon, but gastrointestinal disturbances, urticaria and bronchospasm occur occasionally, and some patients experience dizziness, paraesthesias, vertigo and incoordination. The drug should not be given to pregnant patients or to those with compromised renal or hepatic function.

NICLOSAMIDE

Niclosamide is widely used for the treatment of tapeworm infections together with praziquantel. The *scolex* (the head of the worm with the parts that attach to the host intestinal cells) and a proximal segment are irreversibly damaged by the drug; the worm separates from the intestinal wall and is expelled. For *Taenia solium*, the drug is given in a single dose after a light meal, followed by a purgative 2 hours later; this is necessary because the damaged tapeworm segments may release ova, which are not affected by the drug, so there is a theoretical possibility that cysticercosis may develop. For other tapeworm infections, it is not necessary to give a purgative after administration of niclosamide. There is negligible absorption of the drug from the gastrointestinal tract.

Unwanted effects are few, infrequent and transient. Nausea and vomiting can occur.

DIETHYLCARBAMAZINE

Diethylcarbamazine is a piperazine derivative that is active in filarial infections caused by *W. bancrofti* and *L. loa*. Diethylcarbamazine rapidly removes the microfilariae from the blood circulation and has a limited effect on the adult worms in the lymphatics, but it has little action on microfilariae in vitro. It has been suggested that it modifies the parasite so that it becomes susceptible to the host's normal immune responses. It may also interfere with helminth arachidonate metabolism.

The drug is absorbed following oral administration and is distributed throughout the cells and tissues of the body, excepting adipose tissue. It is partly metabolised, and both the parent drug and its metabolites are excreted in the urine, being cleared from the body within about 48 hours.

Unwanted effects are common but transient, subsiding within a day or so even if the drug is continued. Side effects from the drug itself include gastrointestinal disturbances, arthralgias, headache and a general feeling of weakness. Allergic side effects referable to the products of the dying filariae are common and vary with the species of worm. In general, these start during the first day's treatment and last 3–7 days; they include skin reactions, enlargement of lymph glands, dizziness, tachycardia, and gastrointestinal and respiratory disturbances. When these symptoms disappear, larger doses of the drug can be given without further problem. The drug is not used in patients with onchocerciasis, in whom it can have serious unwanted effects.

LEVAMISOLE

Levamisole is effective in infections with the common roundworm (*Ascaris lumbricoides*). It has a nicotine-like action, stimulating and subsequently blocking the neuromuscular junctions. The paralysed worms are then expelled in the faeces. Ova are not killed. The drug is given orally, is rapidly absorbed and is widely distributed. It crosses the blood–brain barrier. It is metabolised in the liver to inactive metabolites, which are excreted via the kidney. Its plasma half-life is 4 hours.

When single-dose therapy is used, *unwanted effects* are generally few and soon subside. They include gastrointestinal disturbances, dizziness and skin eruptions. High concentrations can have nicotinic actions on autonomic ganglia in the mammalian host. There are some reports of encephalopathy associated with levamisole usage, but this seems to be a rare side effect.

IVERMECTIN

First introduced in 1981 as a veterinary drug, **ivermectin** has been used with enormous success in humans as a safe and highly effective broad-spectrum antiparasitic. It is the first choice of drug for the treatment of filarial infections and is very effective in onchocerciasis. Over 250 million doses of the drug have been administered around the world since 1990, and it is frequently used in global public health campaigns. Chemically, ivermectin is a semisynthetic agent derived from a group of natural substances, the avermectins, obtained from an actinomycete organism. It has potent antihelminthic activity against filaria in humans, being the drug of choice for onchocerciasis, which causes river blindness; it has also given good results against *W. bancrofti*, which causes elephantiasis. A single dose kills the immature microfilariae of *O. volvulus* but not the adult worms. Ivermectin reduces the incidence of onchocercal blindness by up to 80%. The drug also has activity against infections with some roundworms: common roundworms, whipworms, and threadworms of both the UK (*Enterobius vermicularis*) and the US variety (*Strongyloides stercoralis*), but not hookworms. It is given orally and has a half-life of 11 hours.

Ivermectin is thought to kill the worm by opening glutamate-gated chloride channels (found only in invertebrates) and increasing Cl⁻ conductance; by binding to a novel allosteric site on the acetylcholine nicotinic receptor to cause an increase in transmission, leading to motor paralysis; or by binding to aminobutyric acid receptors.

Unwanted effects include skin rashes, fever, giddiness, headaches and pains in muscles, joints and lymph glands. In general, the drug is very well tolerated.

RESISTANCE TO ANTIHELMINTHIC DRUGS

Resistance to antihelminthic drugs is a widespread and growing problem affecting not only humans but also the animal health market. During the 1990s, helminth infections in sheep (and to a lesser extent cattle) developed varying degrees of resistance to a number of different antihelminthic drugs. Parasites that develop such resistance pass this ability on to their offspring, leading in quick succession to treatment failure and the persistence of the worm infection. The widespread use of antihelminthic agents in farming has been blamed for the spread of resistant species.

There are probably several factors that contribute to the molecular mechanisms involved in drug resistance. The presence of the P-glycoprotein transporter in some species of nematode has already been mentioned, and it has been demonstrated that the use of agents such as **verapamil** that block the transporter can partially reverse **benzimidazole** resistance in trypanosomes. However, some aspects of benzimidazole resistance may be attributed to an impairment of high-affinity binding to parasite β-tubulin. Likewise, resistance to levamisole is associated with changes in the structure of the target acetylcholine nicotinic receptor. Whether such changes are the result of random genetic polymorphisms or some other facet of parasite biology is not clear.

Of great significance is the way in which helminths evade the host's immune system. Even though they may thrive in immunologically exposed sites such as the lymphatics or the bloodstream, many are long-lived and may coexist with their hosts for many years without seriously affecting their health, or in some cases without even being noticed. It is striking that the two major families of helminths, while evolving separately, deploy similar strategies to evade destruction by the immune system. Clearly, this must be of major survival value for the species.

In Chapter 14, we discussed the two main types of inflammatory/immune strategies, termed the *Th1* and the *Th2* responses, the latter being characterised by the development of an antibody-mediated response rather than the development of a cell-mediated immune response. It appears that many helminths can actually exploit this mechanism by steering the immune system away from a local Th1 response, which would be potentially more damaging to the parasite, and promoting instead a modified systemic Th2 type of response. This is associated with the production of 'anti-inflammatory' cytokines such as interleukin-10, and is therefore favourable to, or at least better tolerated by, the parasites. The mechanism by which this is achieved is complex and is only marginally relevant to the present discussion, so the interested reader is encouraged to pursue the subject separately if wished (Pearce & MacDonald, 2002; Maizels et al., 2004).

Ironically, the ability of helminths to modify the host immune response in this way may confer some survival value on the hosts themselves. For example, in addition to the local anti-inflammatory effect exerted by helminth infections, rapid wound healing is also seen. Clearly, this is of advantage to parasites that must penetrate tissues without killing the host but may also be beneficial to the host as well. It has been proposed that the presence of helminth infections may mitigate some forms of malaria and other diseases, possibly conferring survival advantages in populations where these diseases are endemic. The deliberate infestation of Crohn's disease patients with nematodes has even been suggested as a strategy to induce remission of the disease, presumably because the Th2 pathways that are activated during parasite infection down-regulate the Th1 responses that drive this type of intestinal inflammation (see Hunter & McKay, 2004). Certainly, this can be demonstrated experimentally in mice, and there is some evidence arising from human studies using the whipworm *Trichuris suis* that this may indeed be a viable therapeutic option. On the basis that Th2 responses can reciprocally inhibit the development of Th1 diseases, it has also been hypothesised that the comparative absence of Crohn's, as well as some other autoimmune diseases, in the developing world may be associated with the high incidence of parasite infection, and that the rise of these disorders in the west is associated with the high level of sanitation and reduced helminth infection! This type of argument is generally known as the 'hygiene hypothesis'.

VACCINES AND OTHER NOVEL APPROACHES TO ANTIHELMINTHIC THERAPY

Despite the enormity of the clinical problem, there have been few recent small-molecule additions to the antihelminthic arsenal. On a more positive note, the sequencing of the genome of the free-living nematode *Caenorhabditis elegans* is now complete, and the genomes of several other helminths have been partially sequenced. This exciting new resource may make it possible in the future to create a transgenic species that expresses mutations found in resistant parasitic worms, thus providing a better understanding of the mechanisms underlying resistance. In addition, genome databases can be searched for likely opportunities for therapeutic intervention. The availability of such information also opens the way for other types of antihelmithic agent, such as those based on antisense DNA or small interfering RNA (see Boyle & Yoshino, 2003).

But it is in the field of antihelminthic vaccines that the most exciting progress has been made (see Dalton et al., 2003). The key here has been the development of recombinant DNA technology. Antigens such as the proteins present on the surface of the (highly infectious) larval stage have been identified, the genes cloned, and the transcripts expressed in high abundance in *Escherichia coli* and used as an immunogen. Using this approach, considerable success has been achieved in the veterinary field with vaccines to organisms such as *Taenia ovis* and *Enterobius granulosus* (in sheep) as well as *Taenia saginata* (in cattle) and *Taenia solium* (in pigs), with cure rates of 90–100% often reported (see Dalton & Mulcahy, 2001; Lightowlers et al., 2003). Qualified success has also been obtained with vaccines to other helminth species. Other potential targets for this type of strategy might include secreted proteins crucial to parasite survival (e.g. the cathepsin protease of *Fasciola hepatica* and the aspartate peptidase of schistosomes and hookworms).

While it is true that helminth infections caused by *Taenia ovis* and *Taenia saginata* lie at the margins of economic or medical importance, this progress is encouraging because, if it can be replicated in the case of the more serious helminth diseases such as schistosomiasis, it would revolutionise the treatment of these widespread infections, as well as minimising the problem of developing drug resistance and reducing the environmental burden of residual pesticide residues, which sometimes occurs as a consequence of overenthusiastic antihelminth control campaigns. Looking further into the future, it may be possible to develop DNA vaccines against these organisms without having to produce any protein-based immunogen at all.

REFERENCES AND FURTHER READING

General papers on helminths and their diseases
Drake L J, Bundy D A 2001 Multiple helminth infections in children: impact and control. Parasitology 122 (suppl):S73–S81 (*The title is self-explanantory*)
Horton J 2003 Human gastrointestinal helminth infections: are they now neglected diseases? Trends Parasitol 19: 527–531 (*Accessible review on helminth infections and their treatments*)

Antihelminthic drugs
Boyle J P, Yoshino T P 2003 Gene manipulation in parasitic helminths. Int J Parasitol 33: 1259–1268 (*Deals with approaches such as antisense therapy; for the interested reader only*)
Burkhart C N 2000 Ivermectin: an assessment of its pharmacology, microbiology and safety. Vet Hum Toxicol 42: 30–35 (*Useful paper that focuses on ivermectin pharmacology*)
Croft S L 1997 The current status of antiparasite chemotherapy. Parasitology 114: S3–S15 (*Comprehensive coverage of current drugs and outline of approaches to possible future agents*)
Dayan A D 2003 Albendazole, mebendazole and praziquantel. Review of non-clinical toxicity and pharmacokinetics. Acta Trop 86: 141–159 (*Comprehensive review of the pharmacokinetics and toxicity of these important drugs*)
Fisher M H, Mrozik H 1992 The chemistry and pharmacology of the avermectins. Annu Rev Pharmacol Toxicol 32: 537–553

Geary T G, Sangster N C, Thompson D P 1999 Frontiers in anthelmintic pharmacology. Vet Parasitol 84: 275–295 (*Thoughtful account of the difficulties associated with drug treatment*)
Greenberg R M 2005 Are Ca²⁺ channels targets of praziquantel action? Int J Parasitol 35: 1–9 (*Interesting review on praziquantal action for those who wish to go into it in depth*)
Liu L X, Weller P F 1996 Antiparasitic drugs. N Engl J Med 334: 1178–1184 (*Excellent coverage of antiparasitic drugs and their clinical use*)
Prichard R, Tait A 2001 The role of molecular biology in veterinary parasitology. Vet Parasitol 98: 169–194 (*Excellent review of the application of molecular biology to understanding the problem of drug resistance and to the development of new anthelminthic agents*)
Robertson A P, Bjorn H E, Martin R J 2000 Pyrantel resistance alters nematode nicotinic acetylcholine receptor single channel properties. Eur J Pharmacol 394: 1–8
World Health Organization 1995 WHO model prescribing information: drugs used in parasitic diseases, 2nd edn. WHO, Geneva

Antihelminth vaccines
Dalton J P, Brindley P J, Knox D P et al. 2003 Helminth vaccines: from mining genomic information for vaccine targets to systems used for protein expression. Int J Parasitol 33: 621–640 (*Very comprehensive but may be overcomplicated in parts for the non-specialist*)
Dalton J P, Mulcahy G 2001 Parasite vaccines—a reality? Vet Parasit 98: 149–167 (*Interesting discussion of the promise and pitfalls of vaccines*)
Lightowlers M W, Colebrook A L, Gauci C G et al. 2003 Vaccination against cestode parasites: anti-helminth vaccines that work and why. Vet Parasitol 115: 83–123 (*Very comprehensive review for the dedicated reader!*)

Immune evasion by helminths and its potential therapeutic uses
Hunter M M, McKay D M 2004 Review article: helminths as therapeutic agents for inflammatory bowel disease. Aliment Pharmacol Ther 19:167–177 (*Fascinating review on potential therapeutic uses of helminths and why they work*)
Maizels R M, Balic A, Gomez-Escobar N et al. 2004 Helminth parasites—masters of regulation. Immunol Rev 201: 89–116 (*Excellent and very comprehensive review dealing with mechanisms of immune evasion; complicated in parts for the non-specialist*)
Pearce E J, MacDonald A S 2002 The immunobiology of schistosomiasis. Nat Rev Immunol 2: 499–512 (*Deals mainly with the immunology of schistosome infections in mice*)

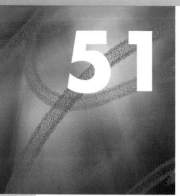

51 Cancer chemotherapy

OVERVIEW

In this chapter, we deal with cancer and anticancer therapy, emphasising first the pathogenesis of cancer before proceeding to describe the drugs that can be used therapeutically. Finally, we consider the extent to which our new knowledge of cancer biology is leading to new treatments.

BACKGROUND

Cancer is a disease characterised by uncontrolled multiplication and spread of abnormal forms of the body's own cells. It is one of the major causes of death in the developed nations: one in three people will be diagnosed with cancer during their lifetime, and in 2001 (for example) 270 000 new cases were reported in the UK. Cancer is also responsible for approximately one-quarter of all deaths in the UK, with lung and bowel cancer comprising the largest category, closely followed by breast and prostate cancer. At first sight, incidence figures for the past 100 years or so give the impression that the disease is increasing in developed countries, but cancer is largely a disease of later life, and with advances in public health and medical science many more people now live to an age where they are more liable to contract cancer.

The terms *cancer*, *malignant neoplasm* (neoplasm simply means 'new growth') and *malignant tumour* are synonymous. Both *benign* and *malignant* tumours manifest uncontrolled proliferation, but the latter are distinguished by their capacity for *dedifferentiation*, their *invasiveness* and their ability to *metastasise* (spread to other parts of the body). In this chapter, we shall be concerned only with the therapy of malignant neoplasia or cancer. The appearance of these abnormal characteristics reflects altered patterns of gene expression in the cancer cells, resulting from genetic mutations.

There are three main approaches to treating established cancer—*surgical excision*, *irradiation* and *chemotherapy*—and the relative value of each of these approaches depends on the type of tumour and the stage of its development. Chemotherapy may be used on its own or as an adjunct to other forms of therapy. Other approaches to cancer treatment, based, for example, on our increasing knowledge of the pathobiology of cancer, are being pursued (see below) and are beginning to produce results of real value.

Chemotherapy of cancer, as compared with that of bacterial disease, presents a difficult problem. In biochemical terms, micro-organisms are both quantitatively and qualitatively different from human cells (see Ch. 45), but cancer cells and normal cells are so similar in most respects that it is more difficult to find general, exploitable, biochemical differences between them.

THE PATHOGENESIS OF CANCER

To understand the action and drawbacks of current anticancer agents and to appreciate the therapeutic hurdles that must be surmounted by putative new drugs, it is important to consider in more detail the pathobiology of this disease.

Cancer cells manifest, to varying degrees, four characteristics that distinguish them from normal cells. These are:

- uncontrolled *proliferation*
- *dedifferentiation* and loss of function

- *invasiveness*
- *metastasis*.

THE GENESIS OF A CANCER CELL

A normal cell turns into a cancer cell because of one or more mutations in its DNA, which can be acquired or inherited. A good example is breast cancer; women who inherit a single defective copy of either of the tumour suppressor genes *BRCA1* and *BRCA2* (see below) have a significantly increased risk of developing breast cancer. However, carcinogenesis is a complex multistage process, usually involving more than one genetic change as well as other, *epigenetic* factors (hormonal, cocarcinogen and tumour promoter effects, etc.) that do not themselves produce cancer but which increase the likelihood that the genetic mutation(s) will result eventually result in cancer.

There are two main categories of genetic change that are important.

- The activation of *proto-oncogenes* to *oncogenes*. Proto-oncogenes are genes that normally control cell division, apoptosis and differentiation, but which can be converted to oncogenes that induce malignant change by viral or carcinogen action.
- The inactivation of *tumour suppressor genes*. Normal cells contain genes that have the ability to suppress malignant change—termed *tumour suppressor genes* (antioncogenes)—and there is now good evidence that mutations of these genes are involved in many different cancers. The loss of function of tumour suppressor genes can be the critical event in carcinogenesis.

About 30 tumour suppressor genes and 100 dominant oncogenes have been identified. The changes that lead to malignancy are a result of point mutations, gene amplification or chromosomal translocation, often caused by viruses or chemical carcinogens.

THE SPECIAL CHARACTERISTICS OF CANCER CELLS

UNCONTROLLED PROLIFERATION

Some healthy cells (such as neurons) have little or no capacity to divide and proliferate, whereas others, in the bone marrow and the epithelium of the gastrointestinal tract for example, have the property of continuous rapid division. Some cancer cells multiply slowly (e.g. those in plasma cell tumours) and some much more rapidly (e.g. the cells of Burkitt's lymphoma). It is therefore not generally true that cancer cells proliferate faster than normal cells. The significant issue is that cancer cells have *escaped from the mechanisms that normally regulate cell division and tissue growth*. It is this, rather than their *rate* of proliferation, that distinguishes them from normal cells.

What are the changes that lead to the uncontrolled proliferation of tumour cells? Inactivation of tumour suppressor genes or transformation of proto-oncogenes into oncogenes can confer autonomy of growth on a cell and thus result in uncontrolled proliferation by producing changes in several cellular systems (see Fig. 51.1), including:

- *growth factors*, their receptors and signalling pathways
- the *cell cycle transducers*, for example cyclins, cyclin-dependent kinases (*cdks*) or the *cdk* inhibitors
- the *apoptotic machinery* that normally disposes of abnormal cells
- *telomerase expression*
- *local blood vessels*, resulting from tumour-directed angiogenesis.

Potentially all the genes coding for the above components could be regarded as oncogenes or tumour suppressor genes (see Fig. 51.2), although not all are equally prone to malignant transformation. It should be understood that malignant transformation of several components is needed for the development of cancer.

Apoptosis and the genesis of a cancer cell

Apoptosis is programmed cell death (Ch. 5), and genetic mutations in the antiapoptotic genes are usually a prerequisite for cancer; indeed, resistance to apoptosis is a hallmark of the disease. It can be brought about by inactivation of proapoptotic factors or by activation of antiapoptotic factors.

Telomerase expression

Telomeres are specialised structures that cap the ends of chromosomes—like the small metal tubes on the end of shoelaces—protecting them from degradation, rearrangement and fusion with other chromosomes. Put simply, DNA polymerase cannot easily duplicate the last few nucleotides at the ends of DNA, and telomeres prevent loss of the 'end' genes. With each round of cell division, a portion of the telomere is eroded, so that eventually it becomes non-functional. At this point, DNA replication ceases and the cell becomes senescent.

Rapidly dividing cells, such as stem cells and those of the bone marrow, the germline, and the epithelium of the gastrointestinal tract, express *telomerase*, an enzyme that maintains and stabilises telomeres. While it is absent from most fully differentiated somatic cells, about 95% of late-stage malignant tumours do express the enzyme, and it is this that may confer 'immortality' on cancer cells.

The control of tumour-related blood vessels

The factors described above lead to the uncontrolled proliferation of individual cancer cells, but we also need to consider factors that influence the total tumour mass. The actual growth of a solid tumour depends absolutely on the development of its own blood supply. Tumours 1–2 mm in diameter can obtain nutrients by diffusion, but any further expansion requires *angiogenesis*, the development of new blood vessels (see p. 77). Angiogenesis occurs in response to growth factors produced by the growing tumour (see Carmeliet & Jain, 2000; Griffioen & Molema, 2000).

DEDIFFERENTIATION AND LOSS OF FUNCTION

The multiplication of normal cells in a tissue begins with division of the undifferentiated stem cells giving rise to *daughter* cells. These daughter cells eventually differentiate to become the mature cells of the relevant tissue, ready to perform their programmed functions. For example, when fibroblasts mature, they secrete

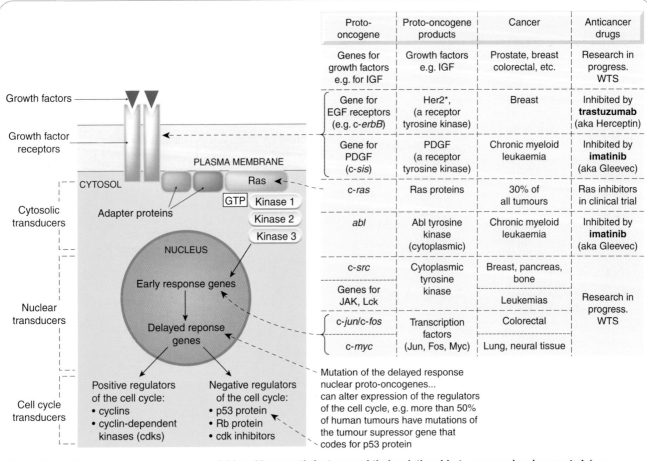

Fig. 51.1 **Signal transduction pathways initiated by growth factors and their relationship to cancer development.** A few examples of proto-oncogenes and the products they code for are given in the table, with examples of the cancers that are associated with their conversion to oncogenes. Drugs (some available, others in the pipeline) are also shown. Many growth factor receptors are receptor tyrosine kinases, the cytosolic transducers including adapter proteins that bind to phosphorylated tyrosine residues in the receptors. Ras proteins are guanine nucleotide–binding proteins and have GTPase action; decreased GTPase action means that Ras remains activated. EGF, epidermal growth factor; IGF, insulin-like growth factor; PDGF, platelet-derived growth factor; WTS, watch this space. *Her2 is also termed *her2/neu*.

and organise extracellular matrix; mature muscle cells are capable of contraction. One of the main characteristics of cancer cells is that they dedifferentiate to varying degrees. In general, poorly differentiated cancers multiply faster and carry a worse prognosis than well-differentiated cancers.

INVASIVENESS

Normal cells are not found outside their 'designated' tissue of origin; for example, liver cells are not found in the bladder and pancreatic cells are not found in the testis. This is because, during differentiation and tissue or organ growth, normal cells develop certain spatial relationships with respect to each other. These relationships are maintained by various tissue-specific survival factors that prevent apoptosis (see Ch. 5). In this way, any cells that escape accidentally lose these survival signals and die.

Consequently, although the cells of the normal mucosal epithelium of the rectum proliferate continuously as the lining is shed, they remain as a lining epithelium. A cancer of the rectal

mucosa, by comparison, invades other tissues forming the rectum and may even invade the tissues of other pelvic organs. Cancer cells have not only lost, through mutation, the restraints that act on normal cells, but they also secrete enzymes (e.g. metalloproteinases; see Ch. 5) that break down the extracellular matrix, enabling them to move around.

METASTASES

Metastases are secondary tumours formed by cells that have been released from the initial or *primary tumour* and have reached other sites through blood vessels or lymphatics, or as a result of being shed into body cavities. Metastases are the principal cause of mortality and morbidity in most cancers and constitute a major problem for cancer therapy.

As discussed above, dislodgment or aberrant migration of normal cells would lead to programmed cell death as a result of withdrawal of the necessary antiapoptotic factors. Cancer cells that metastasise have undergone a series of genetic changes that alter their responses

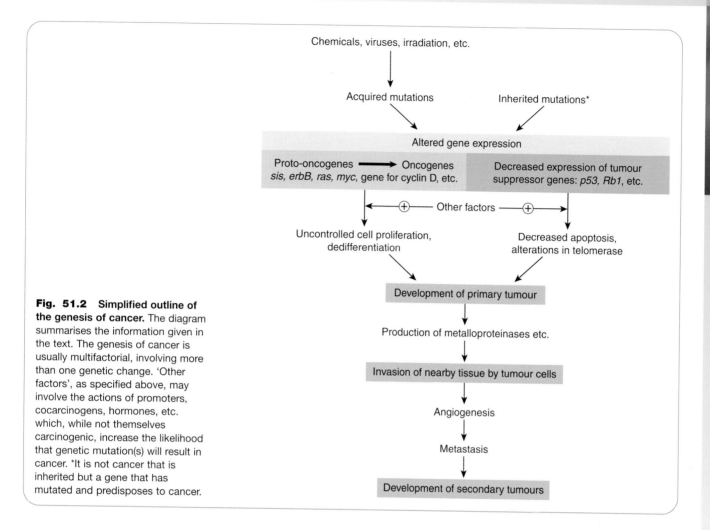

Fig. 51.2 Simplified outline of the genesis of cancer. The diagram summarises the information given in the text. The genesis of cancer is usually multifactorial, involving more than one genetic change. 'Other factors', as specified above, may involve the actions of promoters, cocarcinogens, hormones, etc. which, while not themselves carcinogenic, increase the likelihood that genetic mutation(s) will result in cancer. *It is not cancer that is inherited but a gene that has mutated and predisposes to cancer.

to the regulatory factors that control the cellular architecture of normal tissues, enabling them to establish themselves 'extra-territorially'. Tumour-induced growth of new blood vessels locally (see above) makes metastasis easier and more likely.

Secondary tumours occur more frequently in some tissues than in others. For example, metastases of mammary cancers are often found in lung, bone and brain. The reason for this is that breast cancer cells express chemokine receptors such as CXR4 on their surfaces, and chemokines that recognise these receptors are expressed at high level in these tissues but not in others (e.g. kidney), facilitating the selective accumulation of cells at these sites.

GENERAL PRINCIPLES OF ACTION OF CYTOTOXIC ANTICANCER DRUGS

In experiments with rapidly growing transplantable leukaemias in mice, it has been found that a given therapeutic dose of a cytotoxic drug[1] destroys a constant fraction of the malignant

cells. Thus a dose that kills 99.99% of cells, if used to treat a tumour with 10^{11} cells, will still leave 10 million (10^7) viable malignant cells. As the same principle holds for fast-growing tumours in humans, schedules for chemotherapy are aimed at producing as near a total cell kill as possible because, in contrast to the situation that occurs in micro-organisms, little reliance can be placed on the host's immunological defence mechanisms against the remaining cancer cells.

One of the major difficulties in treating cancer is that tumour growth is usually far advanced before cancer is diagnosed. Let us suppose that a tumour arises from a single cell and that the growth is exponential, as it may well be during the initial stages. 'Doubling' times vary, being, for example, approximately 24 hours with Burkitt's lymphoma, 2 weeks in the case of some leukaemias, and 3 months with mammary cancers. Approximately 30 doublings would be required to produce a cell mass with a diameter of 2 cm, containing 10^9 cells. Such a tumour is within the limits of diagnostic procedures, although it might go unnoticed if it arose in a tissue such as the liver. A further 10 doublings would produce 10^{12} cells, a tumour mass that is likely to be lethal, and which would measure about 20 cm in diameter if it were one solid mass.

However, continuous exponential growth of this sort does not usually occur. In the case of most solid tumours (for example of

---

[1]The term *cytotoxic drug* applies to any drug that can damage or kill cells. In practice, it is used more restrictively to refer to drugs that inhibit cell division and are therefore potentially useful in cancer chemotherapy.

Cancer pathogenesis and cancer chemotherapy: general principles

- The term *cancer* refers to a malignant neoplasm (new growth).
- Cancer arises as a result of a series of genetic and epigenetic changes, the main genetic lesions being:
  — inactivation of tumour suppressor genes (e.g. p53)
  — the activation of oncogenes (mutation of the normal genes controlling cell division and other processes).
- Cancer cells have four characteristics that distinguish them from normal cells:
  — uncontrolled proliferation
  — loss of function because of lack of capacity to differentiate
  — invasiveness
  — the ability to metastasise.
- Cancer cells have uncontrolled proliferation because of changes in:
  — growth factors and/or their receptors
  — intracellular signalling pathways, particularly those controlling the cell cycle and apoptosis
  — telomerase expression
  — tumour-related angiogenesis.
- Most anticancer drugs are antiproliferative—most damage DNA and thereby initiate apoptosis. They also affect rapidly dividing normal cells and are thus likely to depress bone marrow, impair healing and depress growth. Most cause nausea, vomiting, sterility, hair loss and teratogenicity.

biology—cell division—but have no specific inhibitory effect on invasiveness, the loss of differentiation, or the tendency to metastasise. In many cases, the antiproliferative action results from an action during S phase of the cell cycle, and the resultant damage to DNA initiates apoptosis (see above and p. 77). Furthermore, because their main target is cell division, they will affect all rapidly dividing normal tissues, and thus they are likely to produce, to a greater or lesser extent, the following general toxic effects:

- *bone marrow toxicity* (myelosuppression) with decreased leucocyte production and thus decreased resistance to infection
- *impaired wound healing*
- *loss of hair* (alopecia)
- damage to *gastrointestinal epithelium*
- *depression of growth* in children
- *sterility*
- *teratogenicity.*

They can also, in certain circumstances, be themselves carcinogenic. Rapid cell destruction also entails extensive purine catabolism, and urates may precipitate in the renal tubules and cause kidney damage. Finally, virtually all cytotoxic drugs produce severe nausea and vomiting, which has been called the 'inbuilt deterrent' to patient compliance in completing a course of treatment with these agents (see p. 732). Some compounds have particular toxic effects that are specific for them. These will be dealt with when we come to discuss individual drugs.

DRUGS USED IN CANCER CHEMOTHERAPY

The main anticancer drugs can be divided into the following general categories.

- *Cytotoxic drugs.* The mechanism of action of these drugs is discussed more fully below and summarised in Figure 51.3; they include:
  —*alkylating agents* and related compounds, which act by forming covalent bonds with DNA and thus impeding replication
  —*antimetabolites,* which block or subvert one or more of the metabolic pathways involved in DNA synthesis
  —*cytotoxic antibiotics,* i.e. substances of microbial origin that prevent mammalian cell division
  —*plant derivatives* (vinca alkaloids, taxanes, campothecins) —most of these specifically affect microtubule function and hence the formation of the mitotic spindle.
- *Hormones,* of which the most important are steroids, namely glucocorticoids, oestrogens and androgens, as well as drugs that suppress hormone secretion or antagonise hormone action.
- *Miscellaneous agents* that do not fit into the above categories. This group includes a number of recently developed drugs designed to affect specific tumour-related targets.

The clinical use of anticancer drugs is the province of the specialist oncologist, who selects treatment regimens appropriate to the patient with the objective of curing, prolonging life or

lung, stomach, uterus and so on), as opposed to *leukaemias* (tumours of white blood cells), the growth rate falls as the neoplasm grows. This is partly because the tumour partially necroses as it outgrows its ability to maintain its blood supply, and partly because not all the cells proliferate continuously. The cells of a solid tumour can be considered as belonging to three compartments:

- *compartment A* consists of dividing cells, possibly being continuously in cell cycle (p. 72)
- *compartment B* consists of resting cells (G_0 phase) which, although not dividing, are potentially able to do so
- *compartment C* consists of cells that are no longer able to divide but which contribute to the tumour volume.

Essentially, only cells in compartment A, which may form as little as 5% of some solid tumours, are susceptible to the main current cytotoxic drugs, as is explained below. The cells in compartment C do not constitute a problem, but it is the existence of compartment B that makes cancer chemotherapy difficult, because these cells are not very sensitive to cytotoxic drugs and are liable to re-enter compartment A following chemotherapy.

Most current anticancer drugs, particularly those that are 'cytotoxic', affect only one characteristic aspect of cancer cell

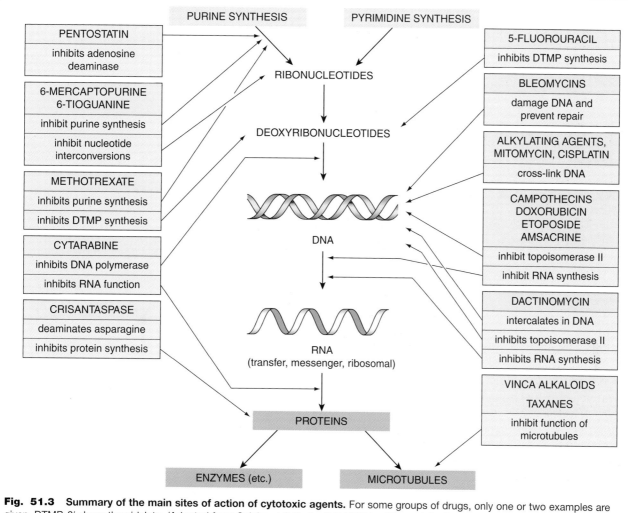

Fig. 51.3 **Summary of the main sites of action of cytotoxic agents.** For some groups of drugs, only one or two examples are given. DTMP, 2'-deoxythymidylate. (Adapted from Calabresi P, Parks R E 1980 In: Gilman A G, Goodman L S, Gilman A (eds) The pharmacological basis of therapeutics, 6th edn. Macmillan, New York.)

providing palliative therapy. Such matters are not addressed here; instead, we concentrate on more pharmacological matters such as mechanisms of action and the main unwanted effects of commonly used anticancer agents.

ALKYLATING AGENTS AND RELATED COMPOUNDS

Alkylating agents and related compounds contain chemical groups that can form covalent bonds with particular nucleophilic substances in the cell. With alkylating agents themselves, the main step is the formation of a *carbonium ion*—a carbon atom with only six electrons in its outer shell. Such ions are highly reactive and react instantaneously with an electron donor such as an amine, hydroxyl or sulfhydryl group. Most of the cytotoxic anticancer alkylating agents are *bifunctional*, i.e. they have two alkylating groups (Fig. 51.4).

The nitrogen at position 7 (N7) of guanine, being strongly nucleophilic, is probably the main molecular target for alkylation in DNA (Fig. 51.5), although N1 and N3 of adenine and N3 of

cytosine may also be affected. A bifunctional agent, being able to react with two groups, can cause intra- or interchain cross-linking (Fig. 51.4). This interferes not only with transcription but also with replication, which is probably the critical effect of anticancer alkylating agents. Other effects of alkylation at guanine N7 are excision of the guanine base with main chain scission, or pairing of the alkylated guanine with thymine instead of cytosine, and eventual substitution of the GC pair by an AT pair. Their main impact is seen during replication (S phase), when some zones of the DNA are unpaired and more susceptible to alkylation. This results in a block at G_2 (see Fig. 5.3) and subsequent apoptotic cell death.

All alkylating agents depress bone marrow function and cause gastrointestinal disturbances. With prolonged use, two further unwanted effects occur: depression of gametogenesis (particularly in men), leading to sterility, and an increased risk of acute non-lymphocytic leukaemia and other malignancies.

Alkylating agents are among the most commonly employed of all anticancer drugs. A large number are available for use in cancer chemotherapy (some dozen are approved in the UK at

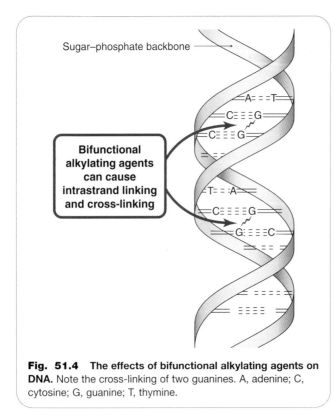

Fig. 51.4   The effects of bifunctional alkylating agents on DNA. Note the cross-linking of two guanines. A, adenine; C, cytosine; G, guanine; T, thymine.

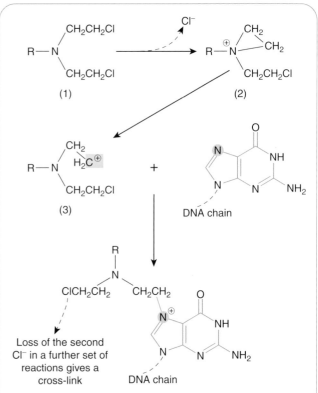

Fig. 51.5   An example of alkylation and cross-linking of DNA by a nitrogen mustard. A bis(chloroethyl)amine (1) undergoes intramolecular cyclisation, forming an unstable ethylene immonium cation (2) and releasing Cl⁻, the tertiary amine being transformed to a quaternary ammonium compound. The strained ring of the ethylene immonium intermediate opens to form a reactive carbonium ion (in yellow box) (3), which reacts immediately with N7 of guanine (in green circle) to give 7-alkylguanine (bond shown in blue), the N7 being converted to a quaternary ammonium nitrogen. These reactions can then be repeated with the other –CH₂CH₂Cl to give a cross-link.

the time of writing). Only a few commonly used ones will be dealt with here.

Nitrogen mustards

Nitrogen mustards are related to the 'mustard gas' used during the First World War; their basic formula (R-*N*-*bis*-(2-chloroethyl)) is shown in Figure 51.5. In the body, each 2-chloroethyl side-chain undergoes an intramolecular cyclisation with the release of a Cl⁻. The highly reactive *ethylene immonium* derivative so formed can interact with DNA (see Figs 51.4 and 51.5) and other molecules.

Cyclophosphamide is probably the most commonly used alkylating agent. It is inactive until metabolised in the liver by the P450 mixed function oxidases (see Fig. 51.6 and Ch. 8). It has a pronounced effect on lymphocytes and can also be used as an immunosuppressant (see Ch. 14). It is usually given orally or by intravenous injection but may also be given intramuscularly. Important toxic effects are nausea and vomiting, bone marrow depression and haemorrhagic cystitis. This last effect (which also occurs with the related drug **ifosfamide**) is caused by the metabolite *acrolein* and can be ameliorated by increasing fluid intake and administering compounds that are sulfhydryl donors, such as ***N*-acetylcysteine** or **mesna** (sodium-2-mercaptoethane sulfonate). These agents interact specifically with acrolein, forming a non-toxic compound. See also Chapters 8 and 53.

Estramustine is a combination of chlormethine (mustine) with an oestrogen. It has both cytotoxic and hormonal action, and is generally used for the treatment of prostate cancer. Other nitrogen mustards used are **melphalan** and **chlorambucil**.

Nitrosoureas

Examples of the nitrosoureas are the chloroethylnitrosoureas **lomustine** and **carmustine**. As they are lipid-soluble and cross the blood–brain barrier, they may be used against tumours of the brain and meninges. However, most nitrosoureas have a severe cumulative depressive effect on the bone marrow that starts 3–6 weeks after initiation of treatment.

Busulfan

Busulfan has a selective effect on the bone marrow, depressing the formation of granulocytes and platelets in low dosage and of red cells in higher dosage. It has little or no effect on lymphoid tissue or the gastrointestinal tract. It is used in chronic granulocytic leukaemia.

Other alkylating agents

Other alkylating agents in clinical use include **thiotepa** and **treosulfan**.

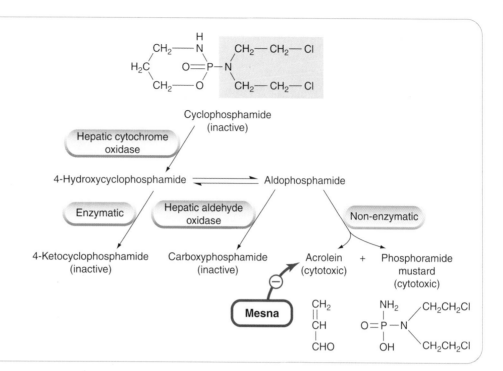

Fig. 51.6 The metabolism of cyclophosphamide.
Cyclophosphamide is inactive until metabolised in the liver by P450 mixed function oxidases to 4-hydroxycyclophosphamide, which (reversibly) forms aldophosphamide. Aldophosphamide is conveyed to other tissues, where it is converted to phosphoramide mustard, the actual cytotoxic molecule, and acrolein, which is responsible for unwanted effects. The part of the cyclophosphamide molecule that gives rise to the active metabolites is shown in the blue box. Mesna (sodium 2-mercaptoethane sulfonate) interacts with acrolein, forming a non-toxic compound.

Anticancer drugs: alkylating agents and related compounds

- Alkylating agents have groups that form covalent bonds with cell substituents; a carbonium ion is the reactive intermediate. Most have two alkylating groups and can cross-link two nucleophilic sites such as the N7 of guanine in DNA. Cross-linking can cause defective replication through pairing of alkylguanine and thymine, leading to substitution of AT for GC, or it can cause excision of guanine and chain breakage.
- Their principal effect occurs during DNA synthesis and the resulting damage triggers apoptosis.
- Unwanted effects include myelosuppression, sterility and risk of non-lymphocytic leukaemia.
- The main alkylating agents are:
  - *nitrogen mustards*, for example cyclophosphamide, which is activated to give aldophosphamide, then converted to phosphoramide mustard (the cytotoxic molecule) and acrolein (which causes bladder damage that can be ameliorated by mesna). Cyclophosphamide myelosuppression affects particularly the lymphocytes.
  - *nitrosoureas*, for example lomustine, may act on non-dividing cells, can cross the blood–brain barrier, and cause delayed, cumulative myelotoxicity.
- Cisplatin causes intrastrand linking in DNA. It has low myelotoxicity but causes severe nausea and vomiting, and can be nephrotoxic. It has revolutionised the treatment of germ cell tumours.

Platinum compounds

Cisplatin is a water-soluble planar coordination complex containing a central platinum atom surrounded by two chlorine atoms and two ammonia groups. Its action is analogous to that of the alkylating agents. When it enters the cell, Cl^- dissociates, leaving a reactive complex that reacts with water and then interacts with DNA. It causes intrastrand cross-linking, probably between N7 and O6 of adjacent guanine molecules, which results in local denaturation of DNA.

Cisplatin has revolutionised the treatment of solid tumours of the testes and ovary. Therapeutically, it is given by slow intravenous injection or infusion. It is seriously nephrotoxic, and strict regimens of hydration and diuresis must be instituted. It has low myelotoxicity but causes very severe nausea and vomiting. The 5-HT$_3$ receptor antagonists (e.g. **ondansetron**; see Chs 12 and 25) are very effective in preventing this and have transformed cisplatin-based chemotherapy. Tinnitus and hearing loss in the high-frequency range may occur, as may peripheral neuropathies, hyperuricaemia and anaphylactic reactions.

Carboplatin is a derivative of cisplatin. Because it causes less nephrotoxicity, neurotoxicity, ototoxicity, nausea and vomiting than cisplatin (although it is more myelotoxic), it is sometimes given on an outpatient basis. **Oxaliplatin** is another platinum-containing compound with a restricted application.

Dacarbazine

Dacarbazine, a prodrug, is activated in the liver, and the resulting compound is subsequently cleaved in the target cell to release an alkylating derivative. Unwanted effects include myelotoxicity and severe nausea and vomiting. **Temozolimide** is a related compound with a restricted usage (malignant glioma).

ANTIMETABOLITES

Folate antagonists

The main folate antagonist is **methotrexate**, one of the most widely used antimetabolites in cancer chemotherapy. Folates are essential for the synthesis of purine nucleotides and thymidylate, which in turn are essential for DNA synthesis and cell division. (This topic is also dealt with in Chs 22, 45 and 49.) The main action of the folate antagonists is to interfere with thymidylate synthesis.

In structure, folates consist of three elements: a *pteridine ring*, p-*aminobenzoic acid* and *glutamic acid* (Fig. 51.7). Folates are actively taken up into cells, where they are converted to polyglutamates. In order to act as coenzymes, folates must be reduced to tetrahydrofolate (FH_4). This two-step reaction is catalysed by *dihydrofolate reductase*, which converts the substrate first to dihydrofolate (FH_2), then to FH_4 (Fig. 51.8). FH_4 functions as an essential cofactor carrying the methyl groups necessary for the transformation of 2′-deoxyuridylate (DUMP) to the 2′-deoxythymidylate (DTMP) required for the synthesis of DNA and purines. During the formation of DTMP from DUMP, FH_4 is converted back to FH_2, enabling the cycle to repeat. Methotrexate has a higher affinity than FH_2 for dihydrofolate reductase and thus inhibits the enzyme (Fig. 51.8), depleting intracellular FH_4. The binding of methotrexate to dihydrofolate reductase involves an additional bond not present when FH_2 binds. The reaction most sensitive to FH_4 depletion is DTMP formation.

Methotrexate is usually given orally but can also be given intramuscularly, intravenously or intrathecally. The drug has low lipid solubility and thus does not readily cross the blood–brain barrier. It is, however, actively taken up into cells by the folate transport system and is metabolised to polyglutamate derivatives, which are retained in the cell for weeks (or even months in some cases) in the absence of extracellular drug. Resistance to methotrexate may develop in tumour cells by a variety of mechanisms (see below, p. 731).

Unwanted effects include depression of the bone marrow and damage to the epithelium of the gastrointestinal tract.

Pneumonitis can occur. In addition, when high-dose regimens are used, there may be nephrotoxicity caused by precipitation of the drug or a metabolite in the renal tubules. High-dose regimens (doses 10 times greater than the standard doses), sometimes used in patients with methotrexate resistance, must be followed by 'rescue' with *folinic acid* (a form of FH_4).

Pyrimidine analogues

Fluorouracil, an analogue of uracil, also interferes with DTMP synthesis (Fig. 51.8). It is converted into a 'fraudulent' nucleotide, *fluorodeoxyuridine monophosphate* (FDUMP). This interacts with thymidylate synthetase but cannot be converted into DTMP. The result is inhibition of DNA but not RNA or protein synthesis. **Raltitrexed** also inhibits thymidylate synthetase and **pemetrexed**, thymidylate transferase.

Fluorouracil is usually given parenterally. The main *unwanted effects* are gastrointestinal epithelial damage and myelotoxicity. Cerebellar disturbances can also occur. Another drug, **capecitabine**, is metabolised to fluorouracil.

Cytarabine (cytosine arabinoside) is an analogue of the naturally occurring nucleoside 2′-deoxycytidine. The drug enters the target cell and undergoes the same phosphorylation reactions as the endogenous nucleoside to give *cytosine arabinoside trisphosphate*, which inhibits DNA polymerase (see Fig. 51.9). The main unwanted effects are on the bone marrow and the gastrointestinal tract. It also causes nausea and vomiting.

Gemcitabine, a relatively new analogue of cytarabine, has fewer unwanted actions, mainly an influenza-like syndrome and mild myelotoxicity. It is often given in combination with other drugs such as cisplatin.

Purine analogues

The main anticancer purine analogues include **fludarabine**, **pentostatin**, **cladribine**, **mercaptopurine** and **tioguanine**.

Fludarabine is metabolised to the trisphosphate and inhibits DNA synthesis by actions similar to those of cytarabine. It is myelosuppressive. Pentostatin has a different mechanism of action. It inhibits *adenosine deaminase*, the enzyme that transforms adenosine to inosine. This action interferes with

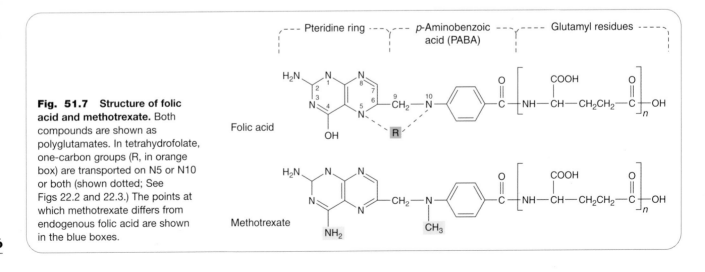

Fig. 51.7 Structure of folic acid and methotrexate. Both compounds are shown as polyglutamates. In tetrahydrofolate, one-carbon groups (R, in orange box) are transported on N5 or N10 or both (shown dotted; See Figs 22.2 and 22.3.) The points at which methotrexate differs from endogenous folic acid are shown in the blue boxes.

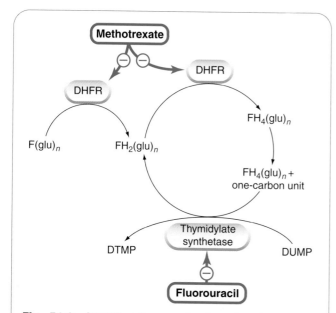

Fig. 51.8 Simplified diagram of action of methotrexate and fluorouracil on thymidylate synthesis. Tetrahydrofolate polyglutamate FH_4 (glu)$_n$ functions as a carrier of a one-carbon unit, providing the methyl group necessary for the conversion of 2′-deoxyuridylate (DUMP) to 2′-deoxythymidylate (DTMP) by thymidylate synthetase. This one-carbon transfer results in the oxidation of FH_4 (glu)$_n$ to FH_2 (glu)$_n$. Fluorouracil is converted to FDUMP, which inhibits thymidylate synthetase. DHFR, dihydrofolate reductase.

critical pathways in purine metabolism and can have significant effects on cell proliferation. Cladribine, mercaptopurine and tioguanine are used mainly in the treatment of leukaemia.

CYTOTOXIC ANTIBIOTICS

This is a widely used group of drugs that mainly produce their effects through direct action on DNA. As a rule, they should not be given together with radiotherapy, as the cumulative burden of toxicity is very high.

The anthracyclines

The main anticancer anthracycline antibiotic is **doxorubicin**. Other related compounds include **idarubicin**, **daunorubicin**, **epirubicin**, **aclarubicin**, and **mitoxantrone** (mitozantrone).

Doxorubicin has several cytotoxic actions. It binds to DNA and inhibits both DNA and RNA synthesis, but its main cytotoxic action appears to be mediated through an effect on topoisomerase II (a DNA gyrase; see Ch. 45), the activity of which is markedly increased in proliferating cells. The significance of the enzyme lies in the fact that, during replication of the DNA helix, reversible swivelling needs to take place around the replication fork in order to prevent the daughter DNA molecule becoming inextricably entangled during mitotic segregation. The 'swivel' is produced by topoisomerase II, which nicks both DNA strands and subsequently reseals the breaks. Doxorubicin intercalates in the DNA, and its effect is, in essence, to stabilise the DNA–topoisomerase II complex after the strands have been nicked, thus halting the process at this point.

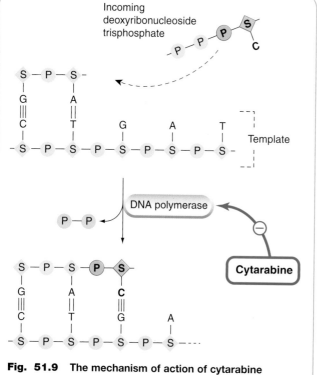

Fig. 51.9 The mechanism of action of cytarabine (cytosine arabinoside). For details of DNA polymerase action, see Figure 45.8. Cytarabine is an analogue of cytosine.

> **Anticancer drugs: antimetabolites**
>
> - Antimetabolites block or subvert pathways of DNA synthesis.
> - *Folate antagonists*. Methotrexate inhibits dihydrofolate reductase, preventing generation of tetrahydrofolate interfering with thymidylate synthesis. Methotrexate is taken up into cells by the folate carrier and, like folate, is converted to the polyglutamate form. Normal cells affected by high doses can be 'rescued' by folinic acid. Unwanted effects are myelosuppression and possible nephrotoxicity.
> - *Pyrimidine analogues*. Fluorouracil is converted to a 'fraudulent' nucleotide and inhibits thymidylate synthesis. Cytarabine in its trisphosphate form inhibits DNA polymerase. They are potent myelosuppressives.
> - *Purine analogues*. Mercaptopurine is converted into fraudulent nucleotide. Fludarabine in its trisphosphate form inhibits DNA polymerase and is myelosuppressive. Pentostatin inhibits adenosine deaminase—a critical pathway in purine metabolism.

Doxorubicin is given by intravenous infusion. Extravasation at the injection site can cause local necrosis. In addition to the general unwanted effects (p. 722), the drug can cause cumulative, dose-related cardiac damage, leading to dysrhythmias and heart failure. This action may be the result of generation of free radicals. Marked hair loss frequently occurs.

Dactinomycin

Dactinomycin intercalates in the minor groove of DNA between adjacent guanosine–cytosine pairs, interfering with the movement of RNA polymerase along the gene and thus preventing transcription. There is also evidence that it has a similar action to that of the anthracyclines on topoisomerase II. It produces most of the toxic effects outlined above, except cardiotoxicity. It is mainly used for treating paediatric cancers.

Bleomycins

The bleomycins are a group of metal-chelating glycopeptide antibiotics that degrade preformed DNA, causing chain fragmentation and release of free bases. This action is thought to involve chelation of ferrous iron and interaction with oxygen, resulting in the oxidation of the iron and generation of superoxide and/or hydroxyl radicals. **Bleomycin** is most effective in the G_2 phase of the cell cycle and mitosis, but it is also active against non-dividing cells (i.e. cells in the G_0 phase; Fig. 5.4). It is often used to treat germline cancer. In contrast to most anticancer drugs, bleomycin causes little myelosuppression: its most serious toxic effect is pulmonary fibrosis, which occurs in 10% of patients treated and is reported to be fatal in 1%. Allergic reactions can also occur. About half the patients manifest mucocutaneous reactions (the palms are frequently affected), and many develop hyperpyrexia.

Mitomycin

Following enzymic activation, **mitomycin** functions as a bifunctional alkylating agent, binding preferentially at O6 of the guanine nucleus. It cross-links DNA and may also degrade DNA through the generation of free radicals. It causes marked delayed myelosuppression and can also cause kidney damage and fibrosis of lung tissue.

Procarbazine

Procarbazine inhibits DNA and RNA synthesis and interferes with mitosis at interphase. Its effects may be mediated by the production of active metabolites. It is given orally, and its main use is in Hodgkin's disease. It causes disulfiram-like actions with alcohol (see Ch. 52), exacerbates the effects of central nervous system depressants and, because it is a weak monoamine oxidase inhibitor, can produce hypertension if given with certain sympathomimetic agents (see Ch. 39). It causes the usual unwanted effects (p. 722), thus it can be leukaemogenic, carcinogenic and teratogenic. Allergic skin reactions may necessitate cessation of treatment.

Hydroxycarbamide

Hydroxycarbamide (hydroxyurea) is a urea analogue that inhibits ribonucleotide reductase, thus interfering with the conversion of ribonucleotides to deoxyribonucleotides. It is mainly used to treat leukaemia but has the familiar spectrum of unwanted effects (p. 722), bone marrow depression being significant.

PLANT DERIVATIVES

Several naturally occurring substances exert potent cytotoxic effects and have earned a place in the arsenal of anticancer drugs on that basis.

VINCA ALKALOIDS

The vinca alkaloids are derived from the *Madagascar periwinkle*. The principal members of the group are **vincristine**, **vinblastine** and **vindesine**. **Vinorelbine** is a semisynthetic vinca alkaloid with similar properties that is mainly used in breast cancer. The drugs bind to tubulin and inhibit its polymerisation into microtubules, preventing spindle formation in dividing cells and causing arrest at metaphase. Their effects become manifest only during mitosis. They also inhibit other cellular activities that involve the microtubules, such as leucocyte phagocytosis and chemotaxis, as well as axonal transport in neurons.

The vinca alkaloids are relatively non-toxic. Vincristine has very mild myelosuppressive activity but causes paraesthesias (sensory changes), abdominal pain and muscle weakness fairly frequently. Vinblastine is less neurotoxic but causes leucopenia, while vindesine has both moderate myelotoxicity and neurotoxicity. All members of the group can cause reversible alopecia.

Taxanes

Paclitaxel and **docetaxel** are derived from a naturally occurring compound found in the bark of the yew tree. They act on microtubules, stabilising them (in effect 'freezing' them) in the

---

Anticancer drugs: cytotoxic antibiotics

- *Doxorubicin* inhibits DNA and RNA synthesis; the DNA effect is mainly through interference with topoisomerase II action. Unwanted effects include nausea, vomiting, myelosuppression and hair loss. It is cardiotoxic in high doses.
- *Bleomycin* causes fragmentation of DNA chains. It acts on non-dividing cells. Unwanted effects include fever, allergies, mucocutaneous reactions and pulmonary fibrosis. There is virtually no myelosuppression.
- *Dactinomycin* intercalates in DNA, interfering with RNA polymerase and inhibiting transcription. It also interferes with the action of topoisomerase II. Unwanted effects include nausea, vomiting and myelosuppression.
- *Mitomycin* is activated to give an alkylating metabolite.

polymerised state, achieving a similar effect to that of the vinca alkaloids. Paclitaxel is given by intravenous infusion and docetaxel by mouth. Both have a place in the treatment of breast cancer, and paclitaxel, given with carboplatin, is the treatment of choice for ovarian cancer.

Unwanted effects, which can be serious, include bone marrow suppression and cumulative neurotoxicity. Resistant fluid retention (particularly oedema of the legs) can occur with docetaxel. Hypersensitivity to both compounds is liable to occur and requires pretreatment with corticosteroids and antihistamines.

Etoposide

Etoposide is derived from mandrake root. Its mode of action is not clearly known, but it may act by inhibiting mitochondrial function and nucleoside transport, as well as having an effect on topoisomerase II similar to that seen with doxorubicin (see above). *Unwanted effects* include nausea and vomiting, myelosuppression and hair loss.

Campothecins

The campothecins **irinotecan** and **topotecan**, isolated from the stem of the tree *Camptotheca acuminata*, bind to and inhibit topoisomerase I, high levels of which occur throughout the cell cycle. Diarrhoea and reversible bone marrow depression occur but, in general, these alkaloids have fewer unwanted effects than most other anticancer agents.

HORMONES

Tumours derived from hormone-sensitive tissues may be *hormone-dependent*, an effect related to the presence of steroid receptors in the malignant cells. Their growth can be inhibited by hormones with opposing actions, by hormone antagonists or by agents that inhibit the endogenous hormone synthesis. Hormones or their analogues that have inhibitory actions on target tissues can be used in treatment of tumours of those tissues. Such procedures alone rarely effect a cure but do mitigate the symptoms of the cancer and thus play an important part in the clinical management of sex hormone–dependent tumours.

Glucocorticoids

Glucocorticoids such as **prednisolone** and **dexamethasone** have marked inhibitory effects on lymphocyte proliferation (see Chs 14 and 28) and are used in the treatment of leukaemias and lymphomas. Their ability to lower raised intracranial pressure, and to mitigate some of the side effects of anticancer drugs, makes them useful as supportive therapy when treating other cancers, as well as in palliative care.

Oestrogens

Diethylstilbestrol and **ethinyloestradiol** are two oestrogens used clinically in the palliative treatment of androgen-dependent prostatic tumours. The latter compound has fewer side effects. These tumours are also treated with gonadotrophin-releasing hormone analogues (see below).

Oestrogens can be used to recruit resting mammary cancer cells (i.e. cells in compartment B; see above) into the proliferating pool of cells (i.e. into compartment A), thus facilitating killing by other, cytotoxic drugs.

Progestogens

Progestogens such as **megestrol**, **norehisterone** and **medroxy-progesterone** have been useful in endometrial neoplasms and in renal tumours.

Gonadotrophin-releasing hormone analogues

As explained in Chapter 30, analogues of the gonadotrophin-releasing hormones, such as **goserelin**, **buserelin**, **leuprorelin** and **triptorelin**, can, under certain circumstances, inhibit gonadotrophin release. These agents are therefore used to treat advanced breast cancer in premenopausal women and prostate cancer. The transient surge of testosterone secretion that can occur in patients treated in this way for prostate cancer can be prevented by an antiandrogen such as **cyproterone**.

Analogues of somatostatin such as **octreotide** and **lanreotide** (see p. 422) are used to relieve the symptoms of neuroendocrine tumours, including hormone-secreting tumours of the gastrointestinal tract such as VIPomas, glucagonomas, carcinoid syndrome and gastrinomas. These tumours express somatostatin receptors, activation of which inhibits cell proliferation as well as hormone secretion.

HORMONE ANTAGONISTS

In addition to the hormones themselves, hormone antagonists can also be effective in the treatment of several types of hormone-sensitive tumours.

Antioestrogens

An antioestrogen, **tamoxifen**, is remarkably effective in some cases of hormone-dependent breast cancer and may have a role in preventing these cancers. In breast tissue, tamoxifen competes with endogenous oestrogens for the oestrogen receptors and therefore inhibits the transcription of oestrogen-responsive genes. Tamoxifen is also reported to have cardioprotective effects, partly by virtue of its ability to protect low-density lipoproteins against oxidative damage.

Anticancer drugs: plant derivatives

- *Vincristine* inhibits mitosis at metaphase by binding to tubulin. It is relatively non-toxic but can cause unwanted neuromuscular effects.
- *Etoposide* inhibits DNA synthesis by an action on topoisomerase II and also inhibits mitochondrial function. Common unwanted effects include vomiting, myelosuppression and alopecia.
- *Paclitaxel* stabilises microtubules, inhibiting mitosis; it is relatively toxic, and hypersensitivity reactions occur.
- *Irinotecan* inhibits topoisomerase I; it has relatively few toxic effects.

Unwanted effects are similar to those experienced by women following the menopause. Potentially more serious are hyperplastic events in the endometrium, which may progress to malignant changes, and the risk of thromboembolism.

Other oestrogen receptor antagonists include **toremifene** and **fulvestrant**. Aromatase inhibitors such as **anastrozole**, **letrozole** and **exemestane**, which suppress the synthesis of oestrogen from androgens, are also effective in the treatment of breast cancer. **Aminoglutethimide**, which blocks the generation of all steroids, has been largely replaced by the aromatase inhibitors.

Antiandrogens

The androgen antagonists, **flutamide**, cyproterone and **bicalutamide**, may be used either alone or in combination with other agents to treat tumours of the prostate. They are also used to control the 'flare' that is seen when treating patients with gonadorelin analogues (see above).

Adrenal hormone synthesis inhibitors

Several agents that inhibit synthesis of adrenal hormones have effects in postmenopausal breast cancer. The drugs used are **trilostane** and (rarely today) aminoglutethimide (see Fig. 28.5), which inhibit the early stages of sex hormone synthesis. Replacement of corticosteroids is necessary with these latter two agents.

RADIOACTIVE ISOTOPES

Radioactive isotopes have an important place in the therapy of certain tumours; for example, **radioactive iodine** (^{131}I) is used in treating thyroid tumours (discussed in Ch. 29).

MISCELLANEOUS AGENTS

Crisantaspase

Crisantaspase is a preparation of the enzyme *asparaginase*, given intramuscularly or intravenously. It breaks down asparagine to aspartic acid and ammonia, and is active against tumour cells, such as those of acute lymphoblastic leukaemia, that have lost the capacity to synthesise asparagine and therefore require an exogenous source. As most normal body cells are able to synthesise asparagine, the drug has a fairly selective action and has very little suppressive effect on the bone marrow, the mucosa of the gastrointestinal tract or hair follicles. It may cause nausea and vomiting, central nervous system depression, anaphylactic reactions and liver damage.

Amsacrine

Amsacrine has a mechanism of action similar to that of doxorubicin (p. 727). Bone marrow depression and cardiac toxicity have been reported.

Monoclonal antibodies

Monoclonal antibodies are immunoglobulins, of one molecular type,[2] produced by hybridoma cells in culture, that react with defined target proteins expressed on cancer cells. Some are *humanised*, meaning that they are hybrids or *chimerae* of human antibodies with a murine or primate backbone (and hence are less likely to be immunogenic in their own right; see Ch. 55 for more details). In some cases, binding of the antibody to its target activates the host's immune mechanisms and the cancer cell is killed by complement-mediated lysis (see p. 204) or by killer cells (see p. 210). Other monoclonal antibodies attach to and inactivate growth factor receptors on cancer cells, thus inhibiting the survival pathway and promoting apoptosis (Fig. 5.5).

Two monoclonal antibodies are currently in clinical use: **rituximab** and **trastuzumab**.

Rituximab

Rituximab is a monoclonal antibody that is licensed (in combination with other chemotherapeutic agents) for treatment of certain types of *lymphoma*. It lyses B lymphocytes by binding to the calcium channel–forming CD20 protein and activating complement. It also sensitises resistant cells (see below) to other chemotherapeutic drugs. It is effective in 40–50% of cases when combined with standard chemotherapy.

The drug is given by infusion, and its plasma half-life is approximately 3 days when first given, increasing with each administration to about 8 days by the fourth administration.

Unwanted effects include hypotension, chills and fever during the initial infusions and subsequent hypersensitivity reactions. A *cytokine release* reaction can occur and has been fatal. The drug may exacerbate cardiovascular disorders.

Alemtuzumab is another monoclonal antibody that lyses B lymphocytes, and is used in the treatment of resistant chronic lymphocytic leukaemia. It may also cause a similar cytokine release reaction to that with rituximab.

Trastuzumab

Trastuzumab (Herceptin) is a humanised murine monoclonal antibody that binds to a protein termed *HER2* (the human epidermal growth factor receptor 2), a member of the wider family of receptors with integral tyrosine kinase activity (Fig. 51.1). There is some evidence that, in addition to inducing host immune

---

> **Anticancer agents: hormones and radioactive isotopes**
>
> • Hormones or their antagonists are used in hormone-sensitive tumours:
> - *glucocorticoids* for leukaemias and lymphomas
> - *tamoxifen* for breast tumours
> - *gonadotrophin-releasing* hormone analogues for prostate and breast tumours
> - *antiandrogens* for prostate cancer
> - *inhibitors of sex hormone synthesis* for postmenopausal breast cancer.
> • Radioactive iostopes can be targeted at specific tissues, for example ^{131}I for thyroid tumours.

---

[2]As opposed to the 'polyclonal' antibodies generally produced by the body in response to a foreign antigen, which comprise a complex (and variable) mixture of molecular species.

responses, trastuzumab induces cell cycle inhibitors p21 and p27 (Fig. 5.2). Tumour cells, in about 25% of breast cancer patients, overexpress this receptor and the cancer proliferates rapidly. Early results show that trastuzumab given with standard chemotherapy has resulted in a 79% 1-year survival rate in treatment-naive patients with this aggressive form of breast cancer. The drug is often given with a taxane such as docetaxel.

Unwanted effects are similar to those with rituximab.

Imatinib mesylate

Hailed as a conceptual breakthrough in targeted chemotherapy, **imatinib mesylate** is a small-molecule inhibitor of signalling pathway kinases. It not only inhibits platelet-derived growth factor (a receptor tyrosine kinase; Fig. 51.1), but also a cytoplasmic kinase (Bcr/Abl kinase, see Fig. 51.1) considered to be a unique factor in the pathogenesis of chronic myeloid leukaemia. It is licensed for the treatment of this tumour when this has proved to be resistant to other therapeutic strategies, as well as for the treatment of some gastrointestinal tumours not susceptible to surgery.

The drug is given orally. Absorption is almost complete, but plasma protein binding is high (95%). The half-life is long, about 18 hours, and the main site of metabolism is in the liver, where approximately 75% of the drug is converted to a metabolite that is also biologically active. The bulk (81%) of the metabolised drug is excreted is the faeces.

Unwanted effects include gastrointestinal symptoms (pain, diarrhoea, nausea), fatigue, headaches and sometimes rashes.

Biological response modifiers

Agents that enhance the host's response are referred to as *biological response modifiers*. Some, for example **interferon-α** (and its pegylated derivative), are used in treating some solid tumours and lymphomas, and **aldesleukin** (recombinant interleukin-2) is used in some cases of renal tumours. **Tretinoin** (a form of vitamin A) is a powerful inducer of differentiation in leukaemic cells and is used as an adjunct to chemotherapy to induce remission.

RESISTANCE TO ANTICANCER DRUGS

The resistance that neoplastic cells manifest to cytotoxic drugs is said to be *primary* (present when the drug is first given) or *acquired* (developing during treatment with the drug). Acquired resistance may result from either adaptation of the tumour cells or mutation, with the emergence of cells that are less susceptible or resistant to the drug and consequently have a selective advantage over the sensitive cells. The following are examples of various mechanisms of resistance.

- *Decreased accumulation of cytotoxic drugs* in cells as a result of the increased expression of cell surface, energy-dependent drug transport proteins. These are responsible for multidrug resistance to many structurally dissimilar anticancer drugs (e.g. doxorubicin, vinblastine and dactinomycin; see Gottesman et al., 2002). An important member of this group is *P-glycoprotein* (PGP/MDR1). The

---

Anticancer drugs: miscellaneous agents

- *Procarbazine* inhibits DNA and RNA synthesis and interferes with mitosis.
- *Crisantaspase* is active against acute lymphoblastic leukaemia cells, which cannot synthesise asparagine.
- *Hydroxycarbamide* (hydroxyurea) inhibits ribonucleotide reductase.
- *Amsacrine* acts on topoisomerase II.
- *Mitoxantrone* (mitozantrone) causes DNA chain breakage.
- *Trilostane* inhibits adrenocortical steroid synthesis.
- *Monoclonal antibodies*: rituximab and alemtuzumab lyse B lymphocytes and are used for B-cell lymphomas. Trastuzumab targets epidermal growth factor receptor and is used for breast cancer.
- *Imatinib* inhibits tyrosine kinase signalling pathways and is used for chronic myeloid leukaemia.

---

physiological role of P-glycoprotein is thought to be the protection of cells against environmental toxins. It functions as a hydrophobic 'vacuum cleaner', picking up foreign chemicals, such as drugs, as they enter the cell membrane and expelling them. Non-cytotoxic agents that reverse multidrug resistance are being investigated as potential adjuvants to treatment.

- *A decrease in the amount of drug taken up by the cell* (e.g. in the case of methotrexate).
- *Insufficient activation of the drug* (e.g. mercaptopurine, fluorouracil and cytarabine). Some drugs require metabolic activation to manifest their antitumour activity. If this fails, they may be unable to block the metabolic pathways required to exert their effects. For example, fluorouracil may not be converted to FDUMP, cytarabine may not undergo phosphorylation, and mercaptopurine may not be converted into a fraudulent nucleotide.
- *Increase in inactivation* (e.g. cytarabine and mercaptopurine).
- *Increased concentration of target enzyme* (methotrexate).
- *Decreased requirement for substrate* (crisantaspase).
- *Increased utilisation of alternative metabolic pathways* (antimetabolites).
- *Rapid repair of drug-induced lesions* (alkylating agents).
- *Altered activity of target*, for example modified topoisomerase II (doxorubicin).
- *Mutations* in various genes, giving rise to resistant target molecules. For example, the p53 gene and overexpression of the *Bcl-2* gene family (several cytotoxic drugs).

TREATMENT SCHEDULES

Treatment with combinations of several anticancer agents increases the cytotoxicity against cancer cells without necessarily increasing the general toxicity. For example, methotrexate, with mainly myelosuppressive toxicity, may be used in a regimen with vincristine, which has mainly neurotoxicity. The few drugs we possess with low myelotoxicity, such as cisplatin and bleomycin, are good candidates for combination regimens. Treatment with combinations of drugs also decreases the possibility of the development of resistance to individual agents. Drugs are often given in large doses intermittently in several courses, with intervals of 2–3 weeks between courses, rather than in small doses continuously, because this permits the bone marrow to regenerate during the intervals. Furthermore, it has been shown that the same total dose of an agent is more effective when given in one or two large doses than in multiple small doses.

The possible clinical applications of drug action during the cell cycle

Cells that are constantly replicating constitute the 'growth fraction' of the tumour. Anticancer drugs may be classified in terms of their actions at particular phases on the cell cycle, as shown below, and it has been proposed that this information could be of value in selecting individual agents or combinations for clinical use. However, not all authorities agree that treatment schedules based on these principles are better than purely empirical schedules.

- *Phase-specific agents.* Many cytotoxic drugs act at different points in the cycle. For example, the vinca alkaloids act in mitosis, whereas cytarabine, hydroxycarbamide, fluorouracil, methotrexate and mercaptopurine act in S phase. Some of these compounds also have some action during G_1 phase and thus may slow the entry of a cell into S phase, where it would be more susceptible to the drug.
- *Cycle-specific agents.* These act at all stages of the cell cycle but do not have much effect on cells out of cycle (e.g. alkylating agents, dactinomycin, doxorubicin and cisplatin).
- *Cycle non-specific agents.* These act on cells whether in cycle or not (e.g. bleomycin and nitrosoureas).

TECHNIQUES FOR DEALING WITH EMESIS AND MYELOSUPPRESSION

EMESIS

The nausea and vomiting induced by many cancer chemotherapy agents constitute an inbuilt deterrent to patient compliance (see also Ch. 25, p. 391). It is a particular problem with cisplatin but also complicates therapy with many other compounds, such as the alkylating agents. 5-HT$_3$ receptor antagonists such as ondansetron or **granisetron** (see Chs 12 and 25) are effective against cytotoxic drug–induced vomiting and have revolutionised cisplatin chemotherapy. Of the other antiemetic agents available (see p. 391), **metoclopramide**, given intravenously in high dose, has proved useful and is often combined with dexamethasone (Ch. 28) or **lorazepam** (Ch. 37), both of which further mitigate the unwanted effects of chemotherapy. As metoclopramide commonly causes extrapyramidal side effects in children and young adults, **diphenhydramine** (Ch. 14) can be used instead.

MYELOSUPPRESSION

Myelosuppression limits the use of many anticancer agents. Regimens contrived to surmount the problem have included removal of some of the patient's own bone marrow prior to treatment, purging it of cancer cells (using specific monoclonal antibodies; see below) and replacing it after cytotoxic therapy is finished. A protocol in which aliquots of stem cells, harvested from the blood following administration of the growth factor **molgramostim**, are expanded in vitro using further haemopoietic growth factors (Ch. 22) is now frequently used. The use of such growth factors after replacement of the marrow has been successful in some cases. A further possibility is the introduction, into the extracted bone marrow, of the mutated gene that confers multidrug resistance, so that when replaced, the marrow cells (but not the cancer cells) will be resistant to the cytotoxic action of the anticancer drugs.

POSSIBLE FUTURE STRATEGIES FOR CANCER CHEMOTHERAPY

As the reader will have judged by now, our current approach to cancer chemotherapy embraces an eclectic mixture of drugs and techniques, all designed to target selectively cancer cells. Real therapeutic progress has been achieved, although 'cancer' as a disease (actually many different diseases with a similar outcome) has not been defeated and remains a massive challenge for future generations of researchers. In this therapeutic area, probably more than in any other, the debate about the risk–benefit of treatment and the patient quality of life issues has taken centre stage and remains a major area of concern. Many advanced cancers (such as metastasised lung cancer) remain essentially incurable, and there is a common perception that chemotherapy, with its distressing unwanted effects and minor increases in longevity, is largely superfluous in such cases. This is not necessarily the case: chemotherapy, although often unpleasant for the patient, may be a superior alternative to conventional palliative care. In the case of breast cancer, even extremely modest increases in life expectancy are sufficient to persuade women to a course of chemotherapy (in addition to surgical resection), although this is also influenced by other domestic factors, such as dependents. These difficult issues have been explored in several recent publications, including Duric & Stockler (2001) and Klastersky & Paesmans (2001).

The quest for less toxic forms of therapy is, of course, central to anticancer initiatives, and there is a bewildering array of new (or usually modified) drugs or novel combination regimens in clinical trial or at earlier stages of development (see for example Kurtz et al., 2003, and Socinski, 2004). What follows is a selection of new and different approaches to the treatment of cancer that may bear fruit over the next decade.

Tyrosine kinase inhibitors

The conceptual—and clinical—success of imatinib has prompted many to develop further useful compounds of this type (see Krause & Van Etten, 2005). So far, success has been thin on the ground, but there is no doubt that this is an important area of pharmaceutical endeavour that may well impact on future therapies.

Angiogenesis and metalloproteinase inhibitors

Tumour cells produce metalloproteinases and angiogenic factors that facilitate tumour growth, invasion of normal tissue and metastases (see p. 77). Targeting the mechanisms involved could provide us with drugs that block metastases. Several inhibitors of angiogenesis or metalloproteinases are in clinical trial (see Griffioen & Molema, 2000; Rosen, 2000).

Cyclo-oxygenase inhibitors

There is strong epidemiological evidence that chronic use of cyclo-oxygenase (COX) inhibitors (see Ch. 14) protects against cancer of the gastrointestinal tract and possibly other sites as well. The COX-2 isoform is overexpressed in about 85% of cancers, and prostanoids originating from this source may activate signalling pathways that enable cells to escape from apoptotic death. The COX-2 inhibitor **celecoxib** reduces mammary and gastrointestinal cancer incidence in animal models and causes regression of existing tumours, and it is in trial in humans as an inhibitor of a familial type of colon tumour. Overall, COX-2 is now considered to be a potentially important target for anticancer drug development. The recent literature is daunting and includes some debate about their precise mechanism of action; see Marnett & DuBois (2002), Karamouzis & Papavassiliou (2004) and Amir & Agarwal (2004) for recent comment.

p53 as anticancer target

More than 50% of human tumours carry a mutation of the p53 tumour suppressor gene (see p. 719 and Fig. 51.1), and there have been many attempts to capitalise on this. Virally mediated introduction of the wild-type (normal) *p53* gene (see below) has not been very successful, but therapy with oncolytic virus ONYX-015, given into the tumour in conjunction with standard chemotherapy, has given good preliminary results. ONYX-015 replicates in and lyses tumour cells but not cells expressing normal p53 protein.

Antisense oligonucleotides

Antisense oligonucleotides are synthetic sequences of single-stranded DNA complementary to specific coding regions of mRNA, which can inhibit gene expression. An antisense drug, *augmerosen*, down-regulates the antiapoptotic factor Bcl-2. In an early clinical trial, it sensitised malignant melanoma to standard anticancer drugs. These 'drugs' have to be delivered by viruses or other 'vectors' (see below).

Gene therapy

This approach to therapy in general is dealt with in Chapter 55. Conceptually, it offers enormous advantages to conventional approaches in terms of selective toxicity to cancer cells. There are a number of technical problems yet to be solved with the delivery of the gene or antisense construct (e.g. p53 or growth factor antisense DNA) into the target tissue, but there have

already been clinical trials, some of which showed modest success (see for example Wolf & Jenkins, 2002, on ovarian cancer trials).

Reversal of multidrug resistance

Several non-cytotoxic drugs (e.g. **verapamil**) that inhibit P-glycoprotein can reverse multidrug resistance. Development of related compounds could overcome this type of resistance. In addition, the use of antibodies, immunotoxins, antisense oligonucleotides (see above) or liposome-encapsulated agents may be useful in the elimination of cells with multidrug resistance (reviewed by Gottesman & Pastan, 1993).

> ### General approaches to cancer therapy
>
> - Kill or remove malignant cells:
>   — cytotoxic drugs[a]
>   — surgery[a]
>   — irradiation[a]
>   — targeted cytotoxic agents (e.g. antibody-linked toxins or radioactive agents).[b]
> - Inactivate components of oncogene signalling pathway:
>   — inhibitors of growth factor receptors (e.g. receptor tyrosine kinases)[a]
>   — inhibitors of adapter proteins (e.g. Ras), cytoplasmic kinases, cyclins, cyclin-dependent kinases, etc.[c]
>   — antisense oligonucleotides[b]
>   — inhibitors of antiapoptotic factors or stimulators of proapoptotic factors[c]
> - Restore function of tumour suppressor genes:
>   — gene therapy.[b]
> - Employ tissue-specific proliferation inhibitors:
>   — oestrogens, antioestrogens, androgens, antiandrogens, glucocorticoids, gonadotrophin-releasing hormone analogues.
> - Inhibit tumour growth, invasion, metastasis:
>   — inhibitors of angiogenesis[b]
>   — matrix metalloproteinase inhibitors.[b]
> - Enhance host immune response:
>   — cytokine-based therapies[b]
>   — gene therapy-based approaches[b]
>   — cell-based approaches (e.g. antitumour T cells).[c]
> - Reverse drug resistance:
>   — inhibitors of multidrug resistance transport.[b]
>
> [a]Therapies in general use.
> [b]Therapies in development.
> [c]Potential approaches.

REFERENCES AND FURTHER READING

Mechanisms of carcinogenesis

Blume-Jensen P, Hunter T 2001 Oncogenic kinase signalling. Nature 411: 355–365 (*Excellent article. Emphasises oncogenic receptor tyrosine kinases and cytoplasmic tyrosine kinases. Useful figures and tables. Note that there are eight other relevant articles in the same issue of* Nature)

Buys C H C M 2000 Telomeres, telomerase and cancer. N Engl J Med 342: 1282–1283 (*Clear, concise coverage*)

Carmeliet P, Jain R K 2000 Angiogenesis in cancer and other diseases. Nature 407: 249–257 (*Gives details of mechanisms involved in angiogenesis; lists biological activators and inhibitors, and agents in clinical trials; excellent figures*)

Chambers A F, Groom A C, MacDonald I C 2002 Dissemination and growth of cancer cells in metastatic sites. Nat Rev Cancer 2: 557–563 (*Review; stresses the importance of metastases in most cancer deaths, discusses the mechanisms involved in metastasis and raises the possibility of targeting these in anticancer drug development*)

Greider C W, Blackburn E H 1996 Telomeres, telomerase and cancer. Sci Am Feb: 80–85 (*Simple, clear overview with high-quality figures*)

Griffioen A, Molema G 2000 Angiogenesis: potentials for pharmacologic intervention in the treatment of cancer, cardiovascular diseases and chronic inflammation. Pharmacol Rev 52: 237–268 (*Comprehensive review covering virtually all aspects of angiogenesis and the potential methods of modifying it to produce an antineoplastic effect*)

Haber D A, Fearon E R 1998 The promise of cancer genetics. Lancet 351: 1–8 (*Excellent coverage; detailed tables of mutations in proto-oncogenes and tumour suppressor genes in human cancers*)

Streiter R M 2001 Chemokines: not just leukocyte attractants in the promotion of cancer. Nat Immunol 2: 285–286 (*Elegant, crisp article on the role of chemokines in tumour growth, invasion and metastasis; good diagram*)

Talapatra S, Thompson C B 2001 Growth factor signalling in cell survival: implications for cancer treatment. J Pharmacol Exp Ther 298: 873–878 (*Succinct overview of death receptor-induced apoptosis, the role of growth factors in preventing it and potential drugs that could be used to promote cell death*)

Weinberg R A 1996 How cancer arises. Sci Am Sept: 42–48 (*Simple, clear overview, listing main oncogenes, tumour suppressor genes and the cell cycle; excellent diagrams*)

Yarden Y, Sliwkowski M X 2001 Untangling the ErbB signalling network. Nat Mol Cell Biol 2: 127–137 (*Describes ErbBs epidermal growth factor receptors, their ligands and their signalling pathways, their involvement in cancer and their potential as targets for anticancer drugs*)

Zörnig M, Hueber A-O et al. 2001 Apoptosis regulators and their role in tumorigenesis. Biochim Biophys Acta 1551: F1–F37 (*Extensive review describing the genes and mechanisms involved in apoptosis, and summarising the evidence that impaired apoptosis is a prerequisite for cancer development*)

Anticancer therapy

Gottesman M M, Fojo T, Bates S E 2002 Multidrug resistance in cancer: role of ATP-dependent transporters. Nat Rev Cancer 2: 48–56 (*Outlines cellular mechanisms of resistance; describes ATP-dependent transporters, emphasising those in human cancer; considers resistance reversal strategies*)

Houghton A N, Scheinberg D 2000 Monoclonal antibody therapies—a 'constant' threat to cancer. Nat Med 6: 373–374 (*Lucid article; very useful diagram*)

Hurwitz H, Fehrenbacher L, Novotny W et al. 2004 Bevacizumab plus irinotecan, fluorouracil, and leucovorin for metastatic colorectal cancer. N Engl J Med 350: 2335–2342 (*Reports the results of an encouraging clinical trial using combination therapy*)

Krause D S, Van Etten R 2005 Tyrosine kinases as targets for cancer therapy. N Engl J Med 353: 172–187 (*Excellent review on tyrosine kinases as targets; good diagrams and tables as well as a highly readable style*)

Kurtz J-E, Emmanuel A, Natarajan-Ame S et al. 2003 Oral chemotherapy in colorectal cancer treatment: review of the literature. Eur J Int Med 14: 18–25 (*Discusses potential new leads in colorectal cancer; good tables summarising recent advances and clinical trials*)

Norman K L, Farassati F, Lee P W K 2001 Oncolytic viruses and cancer therapy. Cytokine Growth Factor Rev 12: 271–282 (*Describes mechanisms of action and efficacy of three oncolytic viruses in clinical trial*)

Overall C M, López-Otin C 2002 Strategies for MMO inhibition in cancer: innovations for the post-trial era. Nat Rev Cancer 2: 6577–7672 (*Review of matrix metalloproteinases and their role in tumour metastasis; also discusses various approaches that could be used to target metalloproteinases, thus producing new anticancer drugs*)

Reed J C 2002 Apoptosis-based therapies. Nat Rev Drug Discov 1: 111–121 (*Excellent coverage, useful tables, good diagrams*)

Rosenberg S A 2001 Progress in human tumour immunology and immunotherapy. Nature 411: 380–384 (*Commendable coverage of current status*)

Savage D G, Antman K H 2002 Imatinib mesylate—a new oral targeted therapy. N Engl J Med 346: 683–693 (*Review with detailed coverage of this relatively new drug for chronic myelogenous leukaemia; very good diagrams*)

Senderowicz A M, Sausville E A 2000 Preclinical and clinical development of cyclin-dependent kinase modulators. J Natl Cancer Inst 92: 376–387 (*Outlines cell cycle control and targets for intervention, and discusses preclinical pharmacology of several agents in clinical trial*)

Socinski M A 2004 Cytotoxic chemotherapy in advanced non-small cell lung cancer: a review of standard treatment paradigms. Clin Cancer Res 10: 4210s–4214s (*A discussion of the role of combination regimens in treating this form of cancer*)

White C A, Weaver R L, Grillo-López 2001 Antibody-targeted immunotherapy for treatment of malignancy. Annu Rev Med 52: 125–145 (*Clear, comprehensive review; includes tables of monoclonals and radiolabelled monoclonals in clinical trial*)

Workman P, Kaye S B (eds) 2002 Cancer therapeutics. A *Trends Guide* with eleven reviews on various new potential approaches to the development of anticancer drugs. Trends Mol Med Suppl 8: S1–S73 (*A series of short reviews covering the main approaches to developing novel anticancer drugs*)

New directions and miscellaneous

Adjei A A 2001 Blocking oncogenic Ras signaling for cancer therapy. J Natl Cancer Inst 93: 1062–1074 (*Gives details of Ras processing, activation, mutations, cytoplamsic targets and physiological role, and outlines therapeutic implications*)

Amir M, Agarwal H K 2004 Role of COX-2 selective inhibitors for prevention and treatment of cancer.

Pharmazie 60: 563–570 (*Review of the role of COX inhibitors in cancer therapy; discusses various mechanisms by which they might act*)

Anderson W F 2000 Gene therapy scores against cancer. Nat Med 6: 862–863 (*Short crisp article*)

Armstrong A C, Eaton D, Ewing J C 2001 Cellular immunotherapy for cancer. Br Med J 323: 1289–1293 (*Brief discussion of rationale and possible future exploitation of tumour cell and dendritic cell vaccines and T cell therapy*)

Carter P 2001 Improving the efficacy of antibody-based cancer therapies. Nat Rev Cancer 1: 118–128 (*Review considering the possible future use of monoclonal antibodies to treat cancer; lists antibodies in advanced clinical trials*)

Dempke W, Rie C et al. 2001 Cyclooxygenase-2: a novel target for cancer chemotherapy. J Cancer Res Clin Oncol 127: 411–417 (*Discusses role of COX-2 in apoptosis, angiogenesis and invasiveness*)

Duric V, Stockler M 2001 Patients' preferences for adjuvant chemotherapy in early breast cancer. Lancet Oncol 2: 691–697 (*The title is self-explanatory; deals with patients' assessment of quality of life issues*)

English J M, Cobb M H 2002 Pharmacological inhibitors of MAPK pathways. Trends Pharmacol Sci 23: 40–45 (*Lists mitogen-activated protein kinases and discusses small-molecule inhibitors under investigation*)

Favoni R E, de Cupis A 2000 The role of polypeptide growth factors in human carcinomas: new targets for a novel pharmacological approach. Pharmacol Rev 52: 179–206 (*Thorough review that describes 14 growth factor families, their signalling pathways and their possible role in cancer; it also deals with drug action on signalling pathways*)

Gottesman M M, Pastan I 1993 Biochemistry of multidrug resistance mediated by the multidrug transporter. Annu Rev Biochem 62: 385–427

Gupta R A, Dubois R N 2001 Colorectal cancer prevention and treatment by inhibition of cyclooxygenase-2. Nat Rev Cancer 1: 11–21 (*Reviews evidence from human, animal and cell culture studies that COX-2 may be implicated in the development of colorectal cancer, and discusses inhibition of COX-2 as a viable strategy for cancer prevention and/or therapy*)

Karamouzis M V, Papavassiliou A G 2004 COX-2 inhibition in cancer therapeutics: a field of controversy or a magic bullet? Expert Opin Investig Drugs 13: 359–372 (*Good review of the field of COX inhibitors in cancer therapy*)

Klastersky J, Paesmans M 2001 Response to chemotherapy, quality of life benefits and survival in advanced non-small lung cancer: review of literature results. Lung Cancer 34: S95–S101 (*Another paper that addresses quality of life issues surrounding chemotherapy*)

Marnett L J, DuBois R N 2002 COX-2: a target for colon cancer prevention. Annu Rev Pharmacol Toxicol 42: 55–80 (*Colon cancer was one of the first tumours to be investigated in the context of anti-COX therapy; the field is reviewed here by two of the researchers who were responsible for much of the original work*)

Rosen L 2000 Antiangiogenic strategies and agents in clinical trial. Oncologist 5: 20–27 (*Succinct coverage; useful summary tables*)

Sikic B I 1999 New approaches in cancer treatment. Ann Oncol 10: S149–S153 (*Pithy coverage of monoclonal antibodies, angiogenic inhibitors, agents for supportive care; very useful tables*)

Smith I E 2002 New drugs for breast cancer. Lancet 360: 790–792 (*Succinct coverage*)

Various authors. (*Nature Insight 2006 441, is a compendium volume devoted to* Signalling in Cancer, *and contains many useful and interesting papers relevant to future directions in anti-cancer therapy. Strongly recommended if you are interested in the latest ideas on the subject*).

Wolf J K, Dwayne Jenkins A 2002 Gene therapy for ovarian cancer (review). Int J Oncol 21: 461–468 (*Very readable review of ovarian cancer and basic concepts in gene therapy, coupled with a round-up of data on compounds in clinical trial*)

Zwick E, Baaange J, Ullrich A 2002 Receptor tyrosine kinases as targets for anticancer drugs. Trends Mol Med 8: 17–23 (*Review of receptor tyrosine kinases, RTKs, highlighting their crucial role as main mediators of extracellular signals for cell proliferation. It also discusses strategies for targeting RTKs in anticancer therapy. Lists RTK-based anticancer drugs in clinical trial.*)

Useful web sites

http://www.cancer.org/ (*The US equivalent of the UK site below. The best sections for you are those marked* Health Information Seekers *and* Professionals)

http://www.cancerresearchuk.org (*The web site of Cancer Research UK, the largest cancer charity in the UK. Contains valuable data on the epidemiology and treatment of cancer, including links to clinical trials. An excellent resource.*)

SPECIAL TOPICS

Individual variation and drug interaction

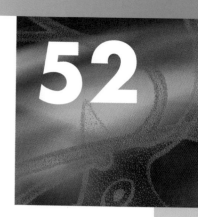

52

- ethnicity
- age
- pregnancy
- genetic factors
- idiosyncratic reactions
- disease
- drug interactions.

EFFECTS OF ETHNICITY

Ethnic means 'pertaining to race' (*Oxford English Dictionary*), and many anthropologists are sceptical as to the value of this concept (see for example Cooper et al., 2003). Citizens of several modern societies are asked to define their race or ethnicity from a list of options (e.g. 'white', 'black', 'mixed', 'Chinese', 'Asian' or 'other' were the options provided by the UK Office of National Statistics for the 2001 National Census). Members of self-defined groups arrived at in such ways share some characteristics on the basis of shared genetic and cultural heritage, but there is obviously also enormous diversity within each group.

Despite the crudeness of such categorisation, it can give some pointers to drug responsiveness. A topical example is the evidence discussed in Chapter 19 (p. 314) that African-Americans with

OVERVIEW

Therapeutics would be a great deal easier if responses to the same dose of drug were always the same. In reality, inter- and even intraindividual variation is often substantial. Physicians need to be aware of the sources of such variation to prescribe drugs safely and effectively. Variation can be caused by different concentrations at sites of drug action or by different responses to the same drug concentration. The first kind is called pharmacokinetic variation and can occur because of differences in absorption, distribution, metabolism or excretion (Chs 7 and 8). The second kind is called pharmacodynamic variation.

Variation is usually quantitative in the sense that the drug produces a larger or smaller effect, or acts for a longer or shorter time, while still exerting qualitatively the same effect. In other cases, the action is qualitatively different. These are known as idiosyncratic reactions (the *Oxford English Dictionary* defines an idiosyncrasy as 'the physical constitution peculiar to an individual or class') and are often caused by genetic or immunological differences between individuals.

Effects on drug absorption and elimination of bioavailability, food intake, and gastric and urinary pH were discussed in Chapters 7 and 8. In this chapter, we describe other important factors responsible for variation in drug response, namely:

> **Individual variation**
>
> - Variability is a serious problem; if not taken into account, it can result in:
>   - lack of efficacy
>   - unexpected side effects.
> - Types of variability may be classified as:
>   - pharmacokinetic
>   - pharmacodynamic
>   - idiosyncratic.
> - The main causes of variability are:
>   - age
>   - genetic factors
>   - immunological factors (Ch. 53)
>   - pathological states (e.g. kidney or liver disease)
>   - drug interactions.

heart failure gain a mortality benefit from treatment with a combination of **hydralazine** plus a nitrate, whereas white Americans do not.

Some adverse effects may also be predicted on the basis of race; for example, many Chinese subjects differ from white people in the way that they metabolise ethanol, producing a higher plasma concentration of acetaldehyde, which can cause flushing and palpitations (Ch. 53). Chinese subjects are considerably more sensitive to the cardiovascular effects of **propranolol** (Ch. 11) than white people, whereas Afro-Caribbean individuals are less sensitive. Despite their increased sensitivity to β-adrenoceptor antagonists, Chinese subjects metabolise propranolol faster than white people, implying that the difference relates to pharmacodynamic differences in sensitivity at or beyond the β adrenoceptors.

Overall effectiveness of **gefitinib** in treating patients with advanced lung tumours has been disappointing, but in about 10% of patients lung tumours shrink rapidly. Japanese patients are three times as likely as whites to fall into this group. The underlying difference is that patients who respond well have specific mutations in the receptor for epidermal growth factor (see Wadman, 2005, for comment). It is probable that many such ethnic differences are genetic in origin, but environmental factors, for example relating to diet, may also contribute. It is important not to abandon the much more sophisticated search for ways to individualise medicine on the basis of pharmacogenomics (see below, p. 742) just because the much simpler and cheaper process of asking patients to define their ethnic group has had some success: this should rather act as a spur. If such a crude and imperfect approach has had some success, think how much better we ought to be able to do with genomic testing!

EFFECTS OF AGE

The main reason that age affects drug action is that drug elimination is less efficient in newborn babies and in old people,

so that drugs commonly produce greater and more prolonged effects at the extremes of life. Other age-related factors, such as variations in pharmacodynamic sensitivity, are also important with some drugs. Physiological factors (e.g. altered cardiovascular reflexes) and pathological factors (e.g. hypothermia), which are common in elderly people, also influence drug effects. Body composition changes with age, fat contributing a greater proportion to body mass in the elderly, with consequent changes in distribution volume of drugs. Elderly people consume more drugs than do younger adults, so the potential for drug interactions (see below) is also increased.

EFFECT OF AGE ON RENAL EXCRETION OF DRUGS

Glomerular filtration rate (GFR) in the newborn, normalised to body surface area, is only about 20% of the adult value, and tubular function is also reduced. Accordingly, plasma elimination half-lives of renally eliminated drugs are longer in neonates than in adults (Table 52.1). In babies born at term, renal function increases to values similar to those in young adults in less than a week, and indeed continues to increase to a maximum of approximately twice the adult value at 6 months of age. The improvement in renal function occurs more slowly in premature infants. Renal immaturity in premature infants can have a substantial effect on drug elimination. For example, in premature newborn babies the antibiotic **gentamicin** has a plasma half-life of 18 hours or greater, compared with 1–4 hours for adults and approximately 10 hours for babies born at term. It is therefore necessary to reduce and/or space out doses to avoid toxicity in premature babies.

Glomerular filtration rate declines slowly from about 20 years of age, falling by about 25% at 50 years and by 50% at 75 years. Figure 52.1 shows that the renal clearance of **digoxin** in young and old subjects is closely correlated with creatinine clearance, a measure of GFR. Consequently, chronic administration over the years of the same daily dose of digoxin to an individual as he or

---

Table 52.1   **Effect of age on plasma elimination half-lives of various drugs**

Drug	Mean or range of half-life (h)		
	Term neonate[a]	Adult	Elderly person
Drugs that are mainly excreted unchanged in the urine			
Gentamicin	10	2	4
Lithium	120	24	48
Digoxin	200	40	80
Drugs that are mainly metabolised			
Diazepam	25–100	15–25	50–150
Phenytoin	10–30	10–30	10–30
Sulfamethoxypyridazine	140	60	100

[a]Even greater differences from mean adult values occur in premature babies.
(Data from Reidenberg 1971 Renal function and drug action. Saunders, Philadelphia; and Dollery 1991 Therapeutic drugs. Churchill Livingstone, Edinburgh.)

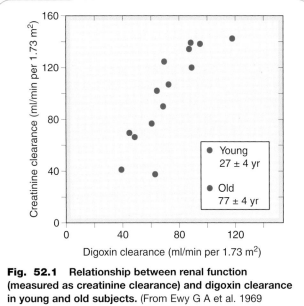

Fig. 52.1   Relationship between renal function (measured as creatinine clearance) and digoxin clearance in young and old subjects. (From Ewy G A et al. 1969 Circulation 34: 452.)

The activity of hepatic microsomal enzymes declines slowly (and very variably) with age, and the distribution volume of lipid-soluble drugs increases, because the proportion of the body that is fat increases with advancing age. The increasing half-life of the anxiolytic drug **diazepam** with advancing age (Fig. 52.2) is one consequence of this. Some other benzodiazepines and their active metabolites show even greater age-related increases in half-life. Because half-life determines the time course of drug accumulation during repeated dosing (Ch. 8), insidious effects, developing over days or weeks, can occur in elderly people and may be misattributed to age-related memory impairment rather than to drug accumulation. The effect of age is less marked for many other drugs, but even though the mean half-life may not change much, there is often a striking increase in the *variability* of half-life between individuals with increasing age. This is important, because a population of old people will contain some individuals with grossly reduced rates of drug metabolism, whereas such extremes do not occur so commonly in young adult populations. Drug regulatory authorities therefore usually require studies in elderly patients as part of drug evaluation.

AGE-RELATED VARIATION IN SENSITIVITY TO DRUGS

The same plasma concentration of a drug can cause different effects in young and old subjects. Benzodiazepines (Ch. 37) exemplify this, producing more confusion and less sedation in elderly than in young subjects; similarly, hypotensive drugs (Ch. 19) cause postural hypotension more commonly in elderly than in younger adult patients.

EFFECTS OF PREGNANCY

Pregnancy causes physiological changes that can influence drug disposition in mother and fetus. Maternal plasma albumin concentration is reduced, influencing drug protein binding

she ages leads to a progressive increase in plasma concentration, and this is a common cause of glycoside toxicity in elderly people (see Ch. 18).

▼ The age-related decline in GFR is not reflected by an increase in plasma creatinine concentration, as distinct from creatinine clearance. Plasma creatinine typically remains within the normal adult range in elderly persons despite substantially diminished GFR. This is because creatinine *synthesis* is reduced in elderly persons because of their reduced muscle mass. Consequently, a 'normal' plasma creatinine in an elderly person does not indicate that they have a normal GFR. Failure to recognise this and reduce the dose of drugs that are eliminated by renal excretion can lead to drug toxicity.

EFFECT OF AGE ON DRUG METABOLISM

Several important enzymes, including hepatic microsomal oxidase, glucuronyltransferase, acetyltransferase and plasma esterases, have low activity in neonates, especially if premature. These enzymes take 8 weeks or longer to reach the adult level of activity. The relative lack of conjugating activity in the newborn can have serious consequences, as in kernicterus caused by drug displacement of bilirubin from its binding sites on albumin (see below) and in the 'grey baby' syndrome caused by the antibiotic **chloramphenicol** (see Ch. 46). This sometimes fatal condition, at first thought to be a specific biochemical sensitivity to the drug in young babies, actually results simply from accumulation of very high tissue concentrations of chloramphenicol because of slow hepatic conjugation. Chloramphenicol is no more toxic to babies than to adults provided the dose is reduced to make allowance for this. Slow conjugation is also one reason why **morphine** (which is excreted mainly as the glucuronide) is not used as an analgesic in labour, because drug transferred via the placenta has a long half-life in the newborn baby and can cause prolonged respiratory depression.

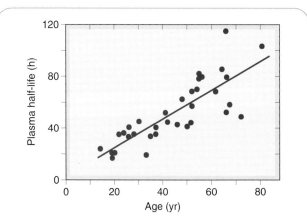

Fig. 52.2   Increasing plasma half-life for diazepam with age in 33 normal subjects. Note the increased variability as well as increased half-life with ageing. (From Klotz U et al. 1975 J Clin Invest 55: 347.)

(Ch. 7). Cardiac output is increased, leading to increased renal blood flow and GFR, and increased renal elimination of drugs (Ch. 8). Lipophilic molecules rapidly traverse the placental barrier, whereas transfer of hypdrophilic drugs is slow, limiting fetal drug exposure following a single maternal dose. The placental barrier excludes some drugs (e.g. *low-molecular-weight heparins*; Ch. 21) so effectively that they can be administered chronically to the mother without causing effects in the fetus. However, drugs that *are* transferred to the fetus are *slowly* eliminated. The activity of most drug-metabolising enzymes in fetal liver is much less than in the adult. Furthermore, the fetal kidney is not an efficient route of elimination because excreted drug enters the amniotic fluid, which is swallowed by the fetus.

GENETIC FACTORS

Studies on identical and non-identical twins have shown that much individual variability is genetically determined. Thus half-life values for **antipyrene**, a probe of hepatic drug oxidation (Ch. 8), and for **warfarin**, an oral anticoagulant (Ch. 21), are 6–22 times less variable in identical than in fraternal twins. Genes influence pharmacokinetics, pharmacodynamics and the susceptibility to idiosyncratic reactions. To understand this better, it is necessary to recall some elementary genetics.

Mutations change the base sequence of DNA. This may, or may not,[1] result in a change in the amino acid sequence of the protein for which the gene codes. Most changes in protein structure are deleterious, and so the altered gene dies out in future generations as a result of natural selection. Some changes may confer advantages, however, at least under some environmental circumstances. An example is the X-linked gene for *glucose 6-phosphate dehydrogenase* (*G6PD*); deficiency of this enzyme may confer partial resistance to malaria (a considerable selective advantage in parts of the world where this disease is common) at the expense of susceptibility to haemolysis in response to oxidative stress in the form of exposure to various dietary constituents, including drugs (see below and Ch. 53, also Ch. 49, p. 709). This ambiguity gives rise to the abnormal gene being preserved in future generations, at a frequency that depends on the balance of selective pressures in the environment. Therefore the frequency of G6PD deficiency is similar to the geographical distribution of malaria.

The situation where several functionally distinct genes are common in a population is called a 'balanced polymorphism'. Now that genes can be sequenced readily, it has become apparent that such balanced polymorphisms are very common, although it is seldom known what is the selective advantage conferred by the mutant gene.

---

[1]The genetic code is 'redundant', i.e. more than one set of nucleotide base triplets code for each amino acid. If a mutation results in a base change that leads to a triplet that codes for the same amino acid as the original, there is no change in the protein and consequently no change in function. Such mutations are neither advantageous nor disadvantageous, so they will neither be eliminated by natural selection nor accumulate in the population at the expense of the wild-type gene.

PERSONALISED MEDICINE: GENETIC INFLUENCES

Polymorphisms can affect individual susceptibility to both dose-dependent and dose-independent adverse drug reactions. Determinants of susceptibility include pharmacokinetic factors (e.g. polymorphisms in the genes encoding cytochrome P450 enzymes) and pharmacodynamic factors (e.g. polymorphisms in drug targets such as receptors and enzymes). More than one gene may be involved. There is therefore great excitement over the potential of the approach of profiling the whole genome for *single nucleotide polymorphisms* as a means of predicting individual susceptibility to adverse effects. It is probable that genes for, for example, carrier mechanisms will need to be considered in combination with ones for, say, the receptor on which the drug acts, so to be useful *haplotypes* (groups of closely linked alleles that tend to be inherited together) will probably need to be defined. The only way to prove the usefulness of such an approach will be via appropriately powered (and necessarily large) clinical studies. If successful, this could ultimately replace the current empirical approach to drug selection in diseases such as hypertension: instead of using one of a range of antihypertensive drugs on a trial-and-error basis, and changing if there is lack of efficacy or poor tolerability, one would profile DNA from the individual and select a drug accordingly—an aspiration known as 'personalised medicine'.

During drug development, blood samples are now often stored in the hope of testing this approach retrospectively, but it has yet to prove its value. Meanwhile, there are several clear-cut examples of single gene variations that do cause variations in drug responsiveness, and these are considered below.

Figure 52.3 contrasts the approximately Gaussian distribution of plasma concentrations achieved 3 hours after administration of a dose of **salicylate** with the bimodal distribution of plasma concentrations after a dose of **isoniazid**. The isoniazid concentration was < 20 μmol/l in about half the population, and in this group the mode was approximately 9 μmol/l. In the other half of the population (plasma concentration > 20 μmol/l), the mode was approximately 30 μmol/l. Elimination of isoniazid depends mainly on acetylation, involving acetyl-CoA and an acetyltransferase enzyme (Ch. 46). White populations contain roughly equal numbers of 'fast acetylators' and 'slow acetylators' (i.e. a 'balanced polymorphism', as described above). The characteristic of fast or slow acetylation is controlled by a single recessive gene associated with low hepatic acetyltransferase activity. Other ethnic groups have different proportions of fast and slow acetylators. Isoniazid causes two distinct forms of toxicity. One is peripheral neuropathy, which is produced by isoniazid itself and is commoner in slow acetylators. The other is hepatotoxicity, which has been related to conversion of the acetylated metabolite to acetylhydrazine and is commoner in fast acetylators, at least in some populations. This type of genetic variation thus produces a qualitative change in the pattern of toxicity caused by the drug in different populations. Acetyltransferase is also important in the metabolism of other drugs, including **hydralazine** (Ch. 19), procainamide (Ch. 18) and various sulfonamides (Ch. 46).

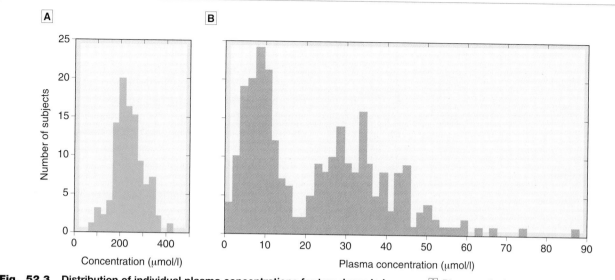

Fig. 52.3 Distribution of individual plasma concentrations for two drugs in humans. [A] Plasma salicylate concentration 3 hours after oral dosage with sodium salicylate at 0.19 mmol/kg. [B] Plasma isoniazid concentration 6 hours after oral dosage. Note the normally distributed values for salicylate, compared with the bimodal distribution of isoniazid. (From: (A) Evans & Clarke 1961 Br Med Bull 17: 234–280; (B) Price-Evans D A 1963 Am J Med 3: 639.)

Ten isoforms of cytochrome P450 (Ch. 8) account for the oxidative metabolism of most therapeutic drugs. The effect of polymorphic variation on catalytic activity is greatest for three isoforms (CYP2C9, CYP2C19 and CYP2D6), which together account for approximately 40% of cytochrome P450–mediated drug oxidation (Caraco, 2004). CYP2D6 has been studied intensively and is involved in the metabolism of many important drugs, including many β-adrenoceptor antagonists (Ch. 11), antidysrhythmic drugs (Ch. 18), opioids (Ch. 41) and other central nervous system drugs. It has more than 80 allelic variants (http://www.imm.ki.se/CYPalleles/cyp2d6.htm), some of which code for proteins with reduced or absent activity and which are found in very different frequencies in different geographical regions. Conversely, some individuals express additional copies of the *CYP2D6* gene, resulting in ultrarapid metabolism (see for example Gasche et al., 2004). The situation is further complicated because, whereas most cytochrome P450–mediated metabolism results in inactivation, some *prodrugs* (e.g. **codeine**; Ch. 7, p. 111) are activated by CYP2D6, and because of interactions between different genes (e.g. polymorphism of the gene encoding codeine glucuronidation influences the amount of codeine available as substrate for CYP2D6 for conversion to morphine, and there is also functional polymorphism in the gene coding the μ receptor on which morphine acts; Ch. 41). At present, it is still not possible to predict the phenotype (in terms of drug response) precisely from the genotype, and we are still some way from getting clinically useful information on safety and efficacy from such genetic tests.

Suxamethonium provides a well-studied example of genetic variation in the rate of drug metabolism as a result of a Mendelian autosomal recessive trait. This short-acting neuromuscular-blocking drug is widely used in anaesthesia and is normally rapidly hydrolysed by plasma cholinesterase (Ch. 10). About 1 in 3000 individuals fail to inactivate suxamethonium rapidly and experience prolonged neuromuscular block if treated with it; this is because a recessive gene gives rise to an abnormal type of plasma cholinesterase. The abnormal enzyme has a modified pattern of substrate and inhibitor specificity. It is detected by measuring the effect of the inhibitor **dibucaine**, which inhibits the abnormal enzyme less than the normal enzyme. Heterozygotes hydrolyse suxamethonium at a more or less normal rate, but their plasma cholinesterase has reduced sensitivity to dibucaine, intermediate between normal subjects and homozygotes (Fig. 52.4). There are other, non-genetic, reasons why suxamethonium hydrolysis may be impaired in an individual patient (see p. 161), so it is important to discover whether this genetic abnormality is present in patients who experience prolonged paralysis following treatment with this drug, and to test family members who may be affected.

Genetic factors

- Genetic variation is an important source of pharmacokinetic variability.
- There are several clear examples where genetic variation influences drug response, including:
  - fast/slow acetylators (hydralazine, procainamide, isoniazid)
  - plasma cholinesterase variants (suxamethonium)
  - hydroxylase polymorphism (debrisoquine).
- In future, profiling an individual's DNA (e.g. for combinations of single nucleotide polymorphisms) could provide a way to anticipate drug responsiveness.

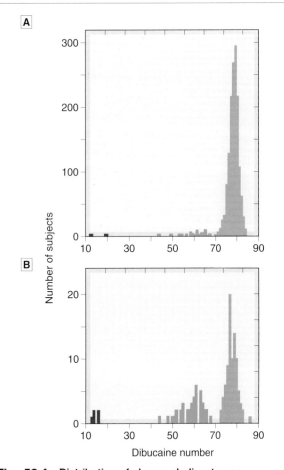

Fig. 52.4 Distribution of plasma cholinesterase phenotypes in humans. Dibucaine number is a measure of the percentage inhibition of plasma cholinesterase by 10^{-5} mol/l dibucaine. The abnormal enzyme has, in addition to low enzymic activity, a low dibucaine number. **A** Normal population. **B** Families of subjects with low or intermediate dibucaine numbers. (From Kalow 1962 Pharmacogenetics. Saunders, Philadelphia.)

This was described in antiquity in Mediterranean countries and in China. G6PD is needed to maintain the content of reduced glutathione (GSH) in red cells, GSH being necessary to prevent haemolysis. Primaquine and related substances reduce red cell GSH harmlessly in normal cells but enough to cause haemolysis in G6PD-deficient cells. As explained above, heterozygote females, who show no tendency to haemolysis, have an increased resistance to malaria, providing a selective advantage that accounts for the persistence of the gene in regions where malaria is endemic.

The hepatic *porphyrias* are prototypic pharmacogenetic disorders. Although individually rare, they are clinically important. The well-intentioned use of sedative, antipsychotic or analgesic drugs in patients with undiagnosed hepatic porphyria can be lethal, whereas with appropriate supportive management most patients recover completely.[2] These disorders are characterised by absence of one of the enzymes required for haem synthesis, with the result that various porphyrin-containing haem precursors accumulate, giving rise to acute attacks of gastrointestinal, neurological and behavioural disturbances. Many drugs, especially but not exclusively those that induce hepatic mixed function P450 oxidase enzymes (e.g. barbiturates, **griseofulvin**, **carbamazepine**, oestrogens), can precipitate acute attacks in susceptible individuals. Porphyrins are synthesised from δ-amino laevulinic acid (ALA), formed by ALA synthase in the liver. This enzyme is induced, like various other hepatic enzymes, by drugs such as barbiturates, resulting in increased ALA production and hence increased porphyrin accumulation.

Various other diseases cause genetically determined idiosyncratic reactions. These include *malignant hyperthermia*, a metabolic reaction to drugs including **suxamethonium** and various inhalational anaesthetic and antipsychotic drugs. It is caused by an inherited abnormality in the Ca^{2+} release channel of the sarcoplasmic reticulum in striated muscle, which is known as the ryanodine receptor (Ch. 4).

Immunological mechanisms underlie many idiosyncratic reactions. They are considered further in Chapter 53.

IDIOSYNCRATIC REACTIONS

An idiosyncratic reaction is a qualitatively abnormal, and usually harmful, drug effect that occurs in a small proportion of individuals. For example, **chloramphenicol** causes aplastic anaemia in approximately 1 in 50 000 patients (p. 670). In many cases, genetic anomalies are responsible, although the mechanisms are often poorly understood. G6PD deficiency (see above) is the basis for the most common known form of genetically determined adverse reaction to drugs, a discovery that stemmed from investigation of the antimalarial drug **primaquine** (Ch. 49), which, while well tolerated in most individuals, causes haemolysis leading to severe anaemia in 5–10% of Afro-Caribbean men. This reaction, in sensitive individuals, also occurs with other drugs, including **dapsone**, **doxorubicin** and some sulfonamide drugs, and after eating the bean *Vicia fava* or inhaling its pollen. This underlies the condition known as favism.

> **Idiosyncratic reactions**
>
> - Harmful, sometimes fatal, reactions that occur in a small minority of individuals.
> - Reactions may occur with low doses.
> - Genetic factors may be responsible (e.g. **primaquine** sensitivity, malignant hyperthermia), although often the cause is poorly understood (e.g. bone marrow depression with **chloramphenicol**).
> - Immunological factors are also important (see Ch. 53).

[2]Life expectancy, obtained from parish records, of patients with porphyria diagnosed retrospectively within large kindreds in Scandinavia was normal until the advent and widespread use of barbiturates and opioids in the 19th century, when it plummeted.

EFFECTS OF DISEASE

Detailed consideration of the many diseases that are important as a cause of individual variation is beyond the scope of this book. Disease can cause pharmacokinetic or pharmacodynamic variation. Common disorders such as impaired renal or hepatic function predispose to toxicity by causing unexpectedly intense or prolonged drug effects as a result of increased drug concentration following a standard dose. Drug absorption is slowed in conditions causing gastric stasis (e.g. *migraine, diabetic neuropathy*) and may be incomplete in patients with malabsorption owing to ileal or pancreatic disease or to oedema of the ileal mucosa caused by heart failure or nephrotic syndrome. *Nephrotic syndrome* (characterised by heavy proteinuria, oedema and a reduced concentration of albumin in plasma) alters drug absorption because of oedema of intestinal mucosa; alters drug disposition through changes in binding to plasma albumin; and causes insensitivity to diuretics such as **furosemide** (frusemide) that act on ion transport mechanisms on the lumenal surface of tubular epithelium (Ch. 24), through binding to albumin in tubular fluid. *Hypothyroidism* is associated with increased sensitivity to several widely used drugs (e.g. **pethidine**), for reasons that are poorly understood. *Hypothermia* (to which elderly persons, in particular, are predisposed) markedly reduces the clearance of many drugs.

Other disorders, although unusual, are important because they illustrate mechanisms that may prove to be of more general applicability. Examples include:

- diseases that influence receptors:
  —*myasthenia gravis,* an autoallergic disease characterised by antibodies to nicotinic acetylcholine receptors (Ch.10)
  —*X-linked nephrogenic diabetes insipidus,* characterised by abnormal antidiuretic hormone (vasopressin) receptors (Ch.24)
  —*familial hypercholesterolaemia,* an inherited disease of low-density lipoprotein receptors (Ch.20).

- diseases that influence signal transduction mechanisms:
  —*pseudohypoparathyroidism,* which stems from impaired coupling of receptors with adenylate cyclase
  —*familial precocious puberty* and *hyperthyroidism caused by functioning thyroid adenomas,* which are each caused by mutations in G-protein–coupled receptors that result in the receptors remaining 'turned on' even in the absence of the hormones that are their natural agonists.

DRUG INTERACTIONS

Many patients, especially the elderly, are treated continuously with one or more drugs for chronic diseases such as hypertension, heart failure, osteoarthritis and so on. Acute events (e.g. infections, myocardial infarction) are treated with additional drugs. The potential for drug interactions is therefore substantial. Drugs can also interact with other dietary constituents (e.g. grapefruit juice, which down-regulates expression of CYP3A4 in the gut) and herbal remedies (such as St John's wort). The

---

Variation due to disease

Pharmacokinetic alterations in:
- Absorption:
  - gastric stasis (e.g. migraine)
  - malabsorption (e.g. steatorrhoea from pancreatic insufficiency)
  - oedema of ileal mucosa (e.g. heart failure, nephrotic syndrome).
- Distribution:
  - altered plasma protein binding (e.g. of phenytoin in chronic renal failure)
  - impaired blood–brain barrier (e.g. to penicillin in meningitis).
- Metabolism:
  - chronic liver disease
  - hypothermia.
- Excretion:
  - acute and/or chronic renal failure.

Pharmacodynamic alterations in:
- Receptors (e.g. myasthenia gravis, familial hypercholesterolaemia).
- Signal transduction (e.g. pseudohypoparathyroidism, familial precocious puberty).
- Unknown mechanisms (e.g. increased sensitivity to pethidine in hypothyroidism).

---

administration of one drug (A) can alter the action of another (B) by one of two general mechanisms:[3]

- modification of the pharmacological effect of B without altering its concentration in the tissue fluid (pharmacodynamic interaction)
- alteration of the concentration of B that reaches its site of action (pharmacokinetic interaction).

For such interactions to be important clinically, it is necessary that the therapeutic range of drug B is narrow (i.e. that a small reduction in effect will lead to loss of efficacy and/or a small increase in effect will lead to toxicity). For pharmacokinetic interactions to be clinically important, it is also necessary that the concentration–response curve of drug B is steep (so that a small change in plasma concentration leads to a substantial

---

[3]A third category of pharmaceutical interactions should be mentioned, in which drugs interact in vitro so that one or both are inactivated. No pharmacological principles are involved, just chemistry. An example is the formation of a complex between **thiopental** and **suxamethonium**, which must not be mixed in the same syringe. Heparin is highly charged and interacts in this way with many basic drugs; it is sometimes used to keep intravenous lines or cannulae open and can inactivate basic drugs if they are injected without first clearing the line with saline.

change in effect). For many drugs, these conditions are not met: even quite large changes in plasma concentrations of relatively non-toxic drugs such as **penicillin** are unlikely to give rise to clinical problems, because there is usually a comfortable safety margin between plasma concentrations produced by usual doses and those resulting in either loss of efficacy or toxicity. Several drugs do have steep concentration–response relationships and a narrow therapeutic margin and, for these, drug interactions can cause major problems, for example with *antithrombotic*, *antidysrhythmic* and *antiepileptic* drugs; *lithium*; and several *antineoplastic* and *immunosuppressant* drugs.

PHARMACODYNAMIC INTERACTION

Pharmacodynamic interaction can occur in many different ways (including those discussed under *Drug antagonism* in Ch. 2). There are many mechanisms, and some examples of practical importance are probably more useful than attempts at classification.

- β-Adrenoceptor antagonists diminish the effectiveness of β-adrenoceptor agonists such as **salbutamol** (Ch. 11).
- Many diuretics lower plasma K^+ concentration (see Ch. 24), and thereby predispose to **digoxin** toxicity and to toxicity with *type III antidysrhythmic drugs* (Ch. 18).
- **Sildenafil** inhibits the isoform of phosphodiesterase (type V) that inactivates cGMP (Chs 17 and 30); consequently, it potentiates organic nitrates, which activate guanylate cyclase, and can cause severe hypotension in patients taking these drugs.
- *Monoamine oxidase inhibitors* increase the amount of noradrenaline (norepinephrine) stored in noradrenergic nerve terminals and interact dangerously with drugs, such as **ephedrine** or **tyramine**, that release stored noradrenaline. This can also occur with tyramine-rich foods—particularly fermented cheeses such as Camembert (see Ch. 39).
- **Warfarin** competes with vitamin K, preventing hepatic synthesis of various coagulation factors (see Ch. 21). If vitamin K production in the intestine is inhibited (e.g. by antibiotics), the anticoagulant action of warfarin is increased.
- The risk of bleeding, especially from the stomach, caused by warfarin is increased by drugs that cause bleeding by different mechanisms (e.g. **aspirin**, which inhibits platelet thromboxane A_2 biosynthesis and which can damage the stomach; Ch. 14).
- Sulfonamides prevent the synthesis of folic acid by bacteria and other micro-organisms; **trimethoprim** inhibits its reduction to tetrahydrofolate. Given together, the drugs have a synergistic action of value in treating *Pneumocystis carinii* (Ch. 49).
- Non-steroidal anti-inflammatory drugs (NSAIDs; Ch. 14), such as **ibuprofen** or **indometacin**, inhibit biosynthesis of prostaglandins, including renal vasodilator/natriuretic prostaglandins (prostaglandin E_2, prostaglandin I_2). If administered to patients receiving treatment for hypertension, they cause a variable but sometimes marked increase in blood pressure. If given to patients being treated with diuretics for chronic heart failure, they can cause salt and water retention and hence cardiac decompensation.[4]

- Histamine H_1 receptor antagonists, such as **promethazine**, commonly cause drowsiness as an unwanted effect. This is more troublesome if such drugs are taken with alcohol, and it may lead to accidents at work or on the road.

PHARMACOKINETIC INTERACTION

All the four major processes that determine pharmacokinetics—absorption, distribution, metabolism and excretion—can be affected by drugs. Pharmacokinetic interactions have received a great deal of attention, and examples have sprouted in the literature like mushrooms. Some of the more important mechanisms are given here, with examples.

Absorption

Gastrointestinal absorption is slowed by drugs that inhibit gastric emptying, such as **atropine** or opiates, or accelerated by drugs that hasten gastric emptying (e.g. **metoclopramide**; see Ch. 25). Alternatively, drug A may interact with drug B in the gut in such a way as to inhibit absorption of B (cf. pharmaceutical interactions; see footnote 3, p. 745). For example, Ca^{2+} (and also iron) forms an insoluble complex with **tetracycline** and retards its absorption; **colestyramine**, a bile acid–binding resin, binds several drugs (e.g. **warfarin**, **digoxin**), preventing their absorption if administered simultaneously. Another example is the addition of **adrenaline** (epinephrine) to local anaesthetic injections; the resulting vasoconstriction slows the absorption of the anaesthetic, thus prolonging its local effect (Ch. 44).

Drug distribution

One drug may alter the distribution of another, but such interactions are seldom clinically important. Displacement of a drug from binding sites in plasma or tissues transiently increases the concentration of free (unbound) drug, but this is followed by increased elimination, so a new steady state results in which total drug concentration in plasma is reduced but the free drug concentration is similar to that before introduction of the second 'displacing' drug. There are several consequences of potential clinical importance:

- toxicity from the transient increase in concentration of free drug before the new steady state is reached
- if dose is being adjusted according to measurements of total plasma concentration, it must be appreciated that the target therapeutic concentration range will be altered by coadministration of a displacing drug

---

[4]The interaction with diuretics may involve a pharmacokinetic interaction in addition to the pharmacodynamic effect described here, because NSAIDs can compete with weak acids, including diuretics, for renal tubular secretion; see below.

- when the displacing drug additionally reduces elimination of the first, so that the free concentration is increased not only acutely but also chronically at the new steady state, severe toxicity may ensue.

Although many drugs have appreciable affinity for plasma albumin and therefore might potentially be expected to interact in these ways, there are rather few instances of clinically important interactions of this type. Protein-bound drugs that are given in large enough dosage to act as displacing agents include various **sulfonamides** and **chloral hydrate**; trichloracetic acid, a metabolite of chloral hydrate, binds very strongly to plasma albumin. Displacement of *bilirubin* from albumin by such drugs in jaundiced premature neonates could have clinically disastrous consequences: bilirubin metabolism is undeveloped in the premature liver, and unbound bilirubin can cross the immature blood–brain barrier and cause *kernicterus* (staining of the basal ganglia by bilirubin). This causes a distressing and permanent disturbance of movement known as choreoathetosis, characterised by involuntary writhing and twisting movements in the child.

Phenytoin dose is adjusted according to measurement of its concentration in plasma, and such measurements do not routinely distinguish bound from free phenytoin (that is, they reflect the total concentration of drug). Introduction of a displacing drug in an epileptic patient whose condition is stabilised on phenytoin (Ch. 40) reduces the total plasma phenytoin concentration owing to increased elimination of free drug, but there is no loss of efficacy because the concentration of unbound (active) phenytoin at the new steady state is unaltered. If it is not appreciated that the therapeutic range of plasma concentrations has been reduced in this way, an increased dose may be prescribed, resulting in toxicity.

There are several instances where drugs that alter protein binding additionally reduce elimination of the displaced drug, causing clinically important interactions. **Phenylbutazone** displaces **warfarin** from binding sites on albumin, and more importantly selectively inhibits metabolism of the pharmacologically active (*S*) isomer (see below), prolonging prothrombin time and resulting in increased bleeding (Ch. 21). **Salicylates** displace **methotrexate** from binding sites on albumin and reduce its secretion into the nephron by competition with the anion secretory carrier (Ch. 8). **Quinidine** and several other antidysrhythmic drugs including **verapamil** and **amiodarone** (Ch. 18) displace **digoxin** from tissue-binding sites while simultaneously reducing its renal excretion; they consequently can cause severe dysrhythmias through digoxin toxicity.

Drug metabolism

Drugs can either inhibit (Table 52.2) or induce (Table 52.3) drug-metabolising enzymes.

Enzyme induction

Enzyme induction (e.g. by barbiturates, ethanol or **rifampicin**; see Ch. 8, p. 116) is an important cause of drug interaction. Over 200 drugs cause enzyme induction and thereby decrease the pharmacological activity of a range of other drugs. Some examples are given in Table 52.3. Because the inducing agent is normally itself a substrate for the induced enzymes, the process

Table 52.2 Examples of drugs that inhibit drug-metabolising enzymes

Drugs inhibiting enzyme action	Drugs with metabolism affected
Allopurinol	Mercaptopurine, azathioprine
Chloramphenicol	Phenytoin
Cimetidine	Amiodarone, phenytoin, pethidine
Ciprofloxacin	Theophylline
Corticosteroids	Tricyclic antidepressants, cyclophosphamide
Ciprofloxacin	Theophylline
Disulfiram	Warfarin
Erythromycin	Ciclosporin, theophylline
Monoamine oxidase inhibitors	Pethidine
Ritonavir	Saquinavir

Table 52.3 Examples of drugs that induce drug-metabolising enzymes

Drugs inducing enzyme action	Drugs with metabolism affected
Phenobarbital	Warfarin
Rifampicin	Oral contraceptives
Griseofulvin	Corticosteroids
Phenytoin	Ciclosporin
Ethanol Carbamazepine	Drugs listed in left-hand column will also be affected

can result in slowly developing tolerance. This pharmacokinetic kind of tolerance is generally less marked than pharmacodynamic tolerance, for example to opioids (Ch. 41), but it is clinically important in starting treatment with **carbamazepine** (Ch. 40, p. 583). This is initiated at a low dose to avoid toxicity (because liver enzymes are not induced initially) and gradually increased over a period of a few weeks, during which it induces its own metabolism.

Figure 52.5 shows how the antibiotic **rifampicin**, given for 3 days, reduces the effectiveness of **warfarin** as an anticoagulant. Conversely, enzyme induction can increase toxicity

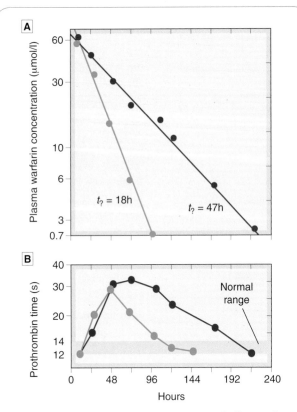

Fig. 52.5 **Effect of rifampicin on the metabolism and anticoagulant action of warfarin.** **A** Plasma concentration of warfarin (log scale) as a function of time following a single oral dose of 5 μmol/kg body weight. After the subject was given rifampicin (600 mg daily for a few days), the plasma half-life of warfarin decreased from 47 hours (red curve) to 18 hours (green curve). **B** The effect of a single dose of warfarin on prothrombin time under normal conditions (red curve) and after rifampicin administration (green curve). (Redrawn from O'Reilly 1974 Ann Intern Med 81: 337.)

patients with HIV infection with triple and quadruple therapy, because some protease inhibitors are potent inhibitors of P450 enzymes (Ch. 47). Another example is the interaction between the non-sedating antihistamine **terfenadine** and imidazole antifungal drugs such as **ketoconazole** and other drugs that inhibit the CYP3A subfamily of P450 enzymes (Ch. 8). This can result in prolongation of the *QT interval*[5] on the electro-cardiogram and a form of ventricular tachycardia in susceptible individuals. *Grapefruit juice* reduces the metabolism of terfenadine and other drugs, including **ciclosporin** and several calcium channel antagonists. To make life even more difficult, several inhibitors of drug metabolism influence the metabolism of different stereoisomers selectively. Examples of drugs that inhibit the metabolism of the active (*S*) and less active (*R*) isomers of warfarin in this way are shown in Table 52.4.

The therapeutic effects of some drugs are a direct consequence of enzyme inhibition (e.g. the xanthine oxidase inhibitor **allopurinol**, used to prevent gout; Ch. 14, pp. 238–239). Xanthine oxidase metabolises several cytotoxic and immunosuppressant drugs, including **mercaptopurine** (the active metabolite of azathioprine), the action of which is thus potentiated and prolonged by allopurinol. **Disulfiram**, an inhibitor of aldehyde dehydrogenase used to produce an aversive reaction to ethanol (see Ch. 43), also inhibits metabolism of other drugs, including **warfarin**, which it potentiates. **Metronidazole**, an antimicrobial used to treat anaerobic bacterial infections and several protozoal diseases (Chs 46 and 49), also inhibits this enzyme, and patients prescribed it are advised to avoid alcohol for this reason.

In other instances, inhibition of drug metabolism is less expected because enzyme inhibition is not the main mechanism of action of the offending agents. Thus **steroids** and **cimetidine**

of a second drug if the toxic effects are mediated via an active metabolite. **Paracetamol** toxicity is a case in point (see Fig. 53.1): it is caused by *N*-acetyl-*p*-benzoquinone imine, which is formed by cytochrome P450. Consequently, the risk of serious hepatic injury following paracetamol overdose is increased in patients whose cytochrome P450 system has been induced, for example by chronic use of alcohol. It is likely that part of the variability in rates of drug metabolism between individuals results from varying exposure to environmental contaminants, some of which are strong enzyme inducers.

Enzyme induction is exploited therapeutically by administering **phenobarbital** to premature babies to induce glucuronyltransferase, thereby increasing bilirubin conjugation and reducing the risk of kernicterus (see above).

Enzyme inhibition

Enzyme inhibition, particularly of the P450 system, slows the metabolism and hence increases the action of other drugs metabolised by the enzyme. Such effects can be clinically important and are major considerations in the treatment of

Table 52.4 **Stereoselective and non-stereoselective inhibition of warfarin metabolism**

Inhibition of metabolism	Drug(s)
Stereoselective for (*S*) isomer	Phenylbutazone Metronidazole Sulfinpyrazone Trimethoprim–sulfamethoxazole Disulfiram
Stereoselective for (*R*) isomer	Cimetidine[a] Omeprazole[a]
Non-stereoselective effect on both isomers	Amiodarone

[a]Minor effect only on prothrombin time.
(From Hirsh 1991 N Engl J Med 324: 1865–1875.)

[5]The QT interval (see Fig. 18.1) normally varies physiologically with the heart rate; this is corrected for by calculating a corrected QT interval (QTc) by dividing by the square root of the RR interval.

enhance the actions of a range of drugs including some antidepressant and cytotoxic drugs. The only rule for prescribers is this: if in doubt about the existence of a possible interaction, look it up (e.g. in the *British National Formulary*, which has an invaluable appendix on drug interactions indicating which are of known clinical importance).

Haemodynamic effects

Variations in hepatic blood flow influence the rate of inactivation of drugs that are subject to extensive presystemic hepatic metabolism (e.g. **lidocaine**, **propranolol**). A reduced cardiac output reduces hepatic blood flow, so negative inotropes (e.g. propranolol) reduce the rate of metabolism of lidocaine by this mechanism.

Drug excretion

The main mechanisms by which one drug can affect the rate of renal excretion of another are by:

- altering protein binding, and hence filtration
- inhibiting tubular secretion
- altering urine flow and/or urine pH.

Inhibition of tubular secretion

Probenecid (Ch. 24) was developed to inhibit **penicillin** secretion and thus prolong its action. It also inhibits the excretion of other drugs, including **zidovudine** (see Ch. 47). Other drugs have an incidental probenecid-like effect and can enhance the actions of substances that rely on tubular secretion for their elimination. Table 52.5 gives some examples. Because diuretics act from within the tubular lumen, drugs that inhibit their secretion into the tubular fluid, such as NSAIDs, reduce their effect.

Alteration of urine flow and pH

Diuretics tend to increase the urinary excretion of other drugs, but this is seldom clinically important. Conversely, loop and thiazide diuretics indirectly increase the proximal tubular reabsorption of **lithium** (which is handled in a similar way as Na^+), and this can cause lithium toxicity in patients treated with lithium carbonate for mood disorders (Ch. 39). The effect of urinary pH on the excretion of weak acids and bases is put to use in the treatment of poisoning with **salicylate** (see Ch. 7, p. 100 and p. 119), but is not a cause of accidental interactions.

Table 52.5 Examples of drugs that inhibit renal tubular secretion

Drug(s) causing inhibition	Drug(s) affected
Probenecid	
Sulfinpyrazone	
Phenylbutazone	Penicillin
Sulfonamides	Azidothymidine
Aspirin	Indometacin
Thiazide diuretics	
Indometacin	
Verapamil	
Amiodarone	Digoxin
Quinidine	
Indometacin	Furosemide (frusemide)
Aspirin	
Non-steroidal anti-inflammatory drugs	Methotrexate

Drug interactions

- These are many and varied: if in doubt, look it up.
- Interactions may be pharmacodynamic or pharmacokinetic.
- Pharmacodynamic interactions are often predictable from the actions of the interacting drugs.
- Pharmacokinetic interactions can involve effects on:
  - absorption
  - distribution (e.g. competition for protein binding)
  - hepatic metabolism (induction or inhibition)
  - renal excretion.

REFERENCES AND FURTHER READING

Further reading

Bailey D G, Malcolm J, Arnold O, Spence J D 1998 Grapefruit juice–drug interactions. Br J Clin Pharmacol 46: 101–110 (*Review*)

Barry M, Mulcahy F, Merry C et al. 1999 Pharmacokinetics and potential interactions amongst antiretroviral agents used to treat patients with HIV infection. Clin Pharmacokinet 36: 289–304 (*Multidrug combinations have transformed the outlook for patients with HIV infection; drug interactions are one of the main problems associated with these*)

Carmichael D J S 2005 Handling of drugs in kidney disease. In: Davison A M et al. (eds) Oxford textbook of clinical nephrology, 3rd edn. Oxford University Press, Oxford, pp. 2599–2618 (*Principles and practice of dose adjustment in patients with renal failure*)

Cooper R S, Kaufman J S, Ward R 2003 Race and genomics. N Engl J Med 348: 1166–1170 (*Scholarly and appropriately sceptical analysis*)

Fugh-Berman A, Ernst E 2001 Herb–drug interactions: review and assessment of report reliability. Br J Clin Pharmacol 52: 587–595 (*Warfarin the most common drug, St John's wort the most common herb; more data needed! See also Fugh-Berman A 2000 Lancet 355: 134–138*)

Hanratty C G, McGlinchey P, Johnston G D, Passmore A P 2000 Differential pharmacokinetics of digoxin in elderly patients. Drugs Aging 17: 353–362 (*Reviews pharmacokinetics of digoxin in relation to age, concomitant disease and interacting drugs*)

Ito K, Iwatsubo T, Kanamitsu S et al. 1998 Prediction of pharmacokinetic alterations caused by drug–drug interactions: metabolic interactions in the liver. Pharmacol Rev 50: 387–411 (*Can one predict pharmacokinetic changes from findings in isolated human hepatocytes? Reviews influences of plasma protein binding, hepatic uptake, transport systems, etc.*)

Lin J H, Liu A Y H 2001 Interindividual variability in inhibition and induction of cytochrome P450 enzymes. Annu Rev Pharmacol Toxicol 41: 535–567 (*Examines sources of interindividual variability in inhibition and induction of P450 enzymes*)

Morgan D J 1997 Drug disposition in mother and fetus. Clin Exp Pharmacol Physiol 24: 869–873 (*Review*)

Pirmohamed M, Park B K 2001 Genetic susceptibility to adverse drug reactions. Trends Pharmacol Sci 22: 298–304 (*Review, with sensibly sceptical approach to the possibility that genotyping will prove useful in preventing adverse drug reactions, which 'needs to be proven by use of prospective controlled clinical trials'*)

Price-Evans D A 1993 Genetic factors in drug therapy, clinical and molecular pharmacogenetics. Cambridge University Press, Cambridge (*A classic*)

Ritter J M, Lewis L D, Mant T G K 1999 A textbook of clinical pharmacology, 4th edn. Edward Arnold, London (*Chapters on drugs at extremes of age, pregnancy and drug interactions provide an introduction*)

Roden D M, George A L 2002 The genetic basis of variability in drug responses. Nat Rev Drug Discov 1: 37–44 (*Discusses the concept that genetic variants determine much of the variability in response to drugs*)

Rowland M, Tozer T N 1995 Clinical pharmacokinetics, concepts and applications. Williams & Wilkins, Baltimore, pp. 203–312 (*See section IV: Individualisation*)

Sproule B A, Hardy B G, Shulman K I 2000 Differential pharmacokinetics in elderly patients. Drugs Aging 16: 165–177 (*Reviews age-related changes in pharmacodynamics as well as pharmacokinetics and drug interactions, all of which are clinically important*)

Weinshilboum R, Liewei Wang 2004 Pharmacogenomics: bench to bedside. Nat Rev Drug Discov 3: 739–748 (*Reviews convergence of pharmacogenetics with human genomics, and influences on translation to the clinical arena*)

Westphal J F 2000 Macrolide-induced clinically relevant drug interactions with cytochrome P450A (CYP) 3A4: an update focused on clarithromycin, azithromycin and dirithromycin. Br J Clin Pharmacol 50: 285–295 (*Review: theophylline, ciclosporine, warfarin, involvement of P-glycoprotein as well as metabolism*)

Wood A J J 2001 Racial differences in response to drugs—pointers to genetic differences. N Engl J Med 344: 1393–1396

Xie H-G, Kim R B, Wood A J J, Stein C M 2001 Molecular basis of ethnic differences in drug disposition and response. Annu Rev Pharmacol Toxicol 41: 815–850 (*Recent developments in understanding genetic variations that may underlie ethnic differences in drug-metabolising enzymes, transporters, receptors and second messenger systems*)

Zevin S, Benowitz N L 1999 Drug interactions with tobacco smoking—an update. Clin Pharmacokinet 36: 425–438 (*Polycyclic aromatic hydrocarbons in tobacco smoke induce various P450 enzymes. 'Cigarette smoking should be specifically studied in clinical trials of new drugs'*)

References

Caraco Y 2004 Genes and the response to drugs. N Engl J Med 351: 2867–2869 (*Beautifully clear succinct account, especially focused on CYP2D6*)

Gasche Y et al. 2004 Codeine intoxication associated with ultrarapid CYP2D6 metabolism. N Engl J Med 351: 2827–2831 (*Multiple functional alleles of CYP2D6 associated with ultrarapid metabolism of codeine and consequent morphine intoxication*)

Wadman M 2005 Drug targeting: is race enough? Nature 435: 1008–1009 (*No*)

Harmful effects of drugs

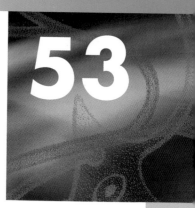

53

- teratogenesis
- allergic reactions to drugs.

OVERVIEW

Clinically important adverse drug reactions are common, costly and avoidable (see Pirmohamed et al., 2004). Any organ can be the principal target, and several systems can be involved simultaneously. The time course of an adverse drug effect sometimes closely shadows drug administration and discontinuation, but in other cases adverse effects are delayed, first appearing months or years after treatment is started. Delayed adverse events represent a huge challenge in terms of their initial recognition, especially if they are an increased frequency of a common problem such as malignancy or myocardial infarction. Even when such an adverse event has been convincingly demonstrated epidemiologically, causality can be impossible to establish in individual patients. Some adverse effects occur typically at the end of treatment, when drug administration is stopped. Consequently, anticipating, avoiding, recognising and responding to adverse drug reactions are among the most challenging and important parts of clinical practice. In this chapter we discuss:

- **types of adverse drug reaction**
- **toxicity testing in animals**
- **general mechanisms of toxin-induced cell damage and cell death**
- **mutagenesis and carcinogenesis**

TYPES OF ADVERSE DRUG REACTION

All drugs can produce harmful as well as beneficial effects. These are either related or unrelated to the principal pharmacological action of the drug. Adverse effects are of great concern to drug regulatory authorities, which are charged with establishing the safety as well as the efficacy of drugs before these are licensed for marketing. Unpredictable events are of particular concern, as are events that are masked by a high background incidence unrelated to drug exposure.

Adverse effects related to the main pharmacological action of the drug

Many adverse effects related to the main pharmacological action of the drug are predictable, at least if this action is well understood. They are sometimes referred to as type A ('augmented') adverse reactions (Rawlins & Thomson, 1985). Many such reactions have been described in previous chapters. For example, postural hypotension occurs with α_1-adrenoceptor antagonists, bleeding with anticoagulants, sedation with anxiolytics and so on. In many instances, this type of unwanted effect is reversible, and the problem can often be dealt with by reducing the dose. Such effects are sometimes serious (e.g. intracerebral bleeding caused by anticoagulants, hypoglycaemic coma from insulin), and occasionally they are not easily reversible, for example drug dependence produced by opiate analgesics (see Ch. 43).

Drugs that block cyclo-oxygenase-2 ('coxibs', for example **rofecoxib, celecoxib, valdecoxib**) predictably increase the risk of thrombotic events such as myocardial infarction (Ch. 14, p. 236). This potential was apparent from the pharmacology of these drugs, in particular their ability to inhibit prostacyclin biosynthesis, and early studies gave a hint of such problems. The effect was difficult to prove because of the high background incidence of coronary thrombosis, and it was only when placebo-controlled trials were performed for another indication (it is hoped that these drugs may prevent bowel cancer) that a prothrombotic action was confirmed unequivocally. The absolute level of thrombotic risk is quite low unless coxibs are taken by individuals at high risk of such events. Such risks need to be quantified, and drug regulators will need to take a more proactive stance in this regard if they are to protect the public.

Adverse effects unrelated to the main pharmacological action of the drug

Adverse effects unrelated to the main pharmacological effect may be predictable when a drug is taken in *excessive dose* (e.g. **paracetamol** hepatotoxicity, **aspirin**-induced tinnitus, aminoglycoside ototoxicity), during *pregnancy* (e.g. **thalidomide** teratogenicity) or by patients with a *predisposing disorder* (e.g. **primaquine**-induced haemolysis in patients with glucose 6-phosphate dehydrogenase deficiency, as described in Ch. 52, p. 742).

Sometimes a predictable subsidiary pharmacological effect can have serious implications for rare susceptible individuals; there is concern over effects of drugs on the electrocardiographic QT interval for this reason (e.g. the antihistamine **terfenadine**, see p. 748, and for the predictable interaction of such drugs with drugs that lower plasma K^+ concentration).

Rare but severe unpredictable adverse effects have been mentioned in earlier chapters, including aplastic anaemia from **chloramphenicol**, anaphylaxis in response to **penicillin**, and oculomucocutaneous syndrome with **practolol**, a β_1-selective antagonist that had to be withdrawn because of this problem. These idiosyncratic reactions are termed type B ('bizarre') in the Rawlins & Thomson (1985) classification. They are usually severe—otherwise they would go unrecognised—and their existence is important in establishing the safety of medicines.

▼ If the incidence of an adverse reaction is 1 in 6000 patients exposed, approximately 18 000 patients would have to be exposed to the drug for three events to occur, and approximately double that number for three events to be detected and their possible relationship to the drug recognised and reported, even if there were no background incidence of the event in question. Consequently, such reactions cannot be excluded by early-phase clinical trials (which might typically expose only a few thousand individuals to the drug), and the association may come to light only after years of use, so there is a need for continued monitoring by regulatory authorities after drugs have been licensed and marketed. An example is the association between pulmonary hypertension and valvular heart disease with **fenfluramine**, an appetite suppressant that had been used for several years, and with **dexfenfluramine**, its pharmacologically active isomer. Such experiences call for a conservative approach to prescribing new drugs if there are adequate existing alternatives. This conflicts with the culture of drug marketing, especially when this involves advertising the product direct to the consumer.

Idiosyncratic reactions are often initiated by a chemically reactive metabolite rather than the parent drug. Such indirect toxicity may be direct or immunological in nature. Examples include liver or kidney damage, bone marrow suppression, carcinogenesis and disordered fetal development. Such effects (which are by no means confined to drugs, being liable to occur with any kind of chemical) fall conventionally into the area of toxicology rather than pharmacology.

DRUG TOXICITY

TOXICITY TESTING

Toxicity testing in animals is carried out on new drugs to identify potential hazards before administering them to humans. It involves the use of a wide range of tests in different species, with long-term administration of the drug, regular monitoring for physiological or biochemical abnormalities, and a detailed postmortem examination at the end of the trial to detect any gross or histological abnormalities. Recently, use of non-mammalian species, notably the transparent zebra fish, has shown promise as an intermediate stage between toxicity studies on cells and tissues in vitro and mammalian toxicity testing (see Parng, 2005, for a review). Toxicity testing is performed with doses well above the expected therapeutic range, and establishes which tissues or organs are likely 'targets' of toxic effects of the drug. Recovery studies are performed to assess whether toxic effects are reversible, and particular attention is paid to irreversible changes such as carcinogenesis or neurodegeneration. The basic premise is that toxic effects caused by a drug are similar in humans and other animals. This is inherently reasonable in view of the similarities between higher organisms at the cellular and molecular levels. There are, nevertheless, wide interspecies variations, especially in metabolising enzymes; consequently, a toxic metabolite formed in one species may not be formed in another, and so toxicity testing in animals is not always a reliable guide. **Pronethalol**, the first β-adrenoceptor antagonist synthesised (by James Black) at ICI, was not developed because it caused carcinogenicity in mice; it subsequently emerged that carcinogenicity occurred *only* in the ICI strain—but by then other β-blockers were already in development.

Toxic effects can range from negligible to so severe as to preclude further development of the compound. Intermediate levels of toxicity are more acceptable in drugs intended for severe illnesses (e.g. AIDS or cancers), and decisions on whether or not to continue development are often difficult. If development does proceed, safety monitoring can be concentrated on the system 'flagged' as a poten-

---

Types of drug toxicity

- Toxic effects of drugs can be:
  - related to the principal pharmacological action (e.g. bleeding with anticoagulants)
  - unrelated to the principal pharmacological action (e.g. liver damage with **paracetamol**).
- Some adverse reactions that occur with ordinary therapeutic dosage are unpredictable, serious and uncommon (e.g. agranulocytosis with **carbimazole**). Such *idiosyncratic* reactions are almost inevitably detected only after widespread use of a new drug.
- Adverse effects unrelated to the main action of a drug are often caused by reactive metabolites and/or immunological reactions.

tial target of toxicity by the animal studies.[1] *Safety* of a drug (as opposed to toxicity) can be established only during use in humans.

GENERAL MECHANISMS OF TOXIN-INDUCED CELL DAMAGE AND CELL DEATH

Toxic concentrations of drugs or drug metabolites can cause *necrosis*; however, programmed cell death (*apoptosis*; see Ch. 5) is increasingly recognised to be of paramount importance, especially in chronic toxicity (see for example Pirmohamed, 2003).

Chemically reactive drug metabolites can form covalent bonds with target molecules or alter the target molecule by non-covalent interactions. Some metabolites do both. The liver is of great importance in drug metabolism (Ch. 8), and hepatocytes are exposed to high concentrations of nascent metabolites as these are formed by cytochrome P450–dependent drug oxidation. Drugs and their polar metabolites are concentrated in renal tubular fluid as water is reabsorbed, so renal tubules are exposed to higher concentrations than are other tissues. Furthermore, renal vascular mechanisms are critical to the maintenance of glomerular filtration, and are vulnerable to drugs that interfere with the control of afferent and efferent arteriolar contractility. It is therefore not surprising that hepatic or renal damage are common reasons for abandoning development of drugs during toxicity testing.

NON-COVALENT INTERACTIONS

Reactive metabolites of drugs can be involved in several related, potentially cytotoxic, non-covalent interactions, including:

- lipid peroxidation
- generation of toxic reactive oxygen species
- reactions causing depletion of glutathione (GSH)
- modification of sulfhydryl groups.

Some of these effects are also produced by covalent reactions.

Lipid peroxidation

Peroxidation of unsaturated lipids can be initiated either by reactive metabolites or by reactive oxygen species (see below). Lipid peroxyradicals (ROO•) can produce lipid hydroperoxides (ROOH), which produce further lipid peroxyradicals. This chain reaction—a peroxidative cascade—may eventually affect much of the membrane lipid. Defence mechanisms, for example GSH peroxidase and vitamin E, protect against this. Cell damage results from alteration of membrane permeability or from reactions of the products of lipid peroxidation with proteins.

Reactive oxygen species

Reduction of molecular oxygen to superoxide anion ($O_2^{-•}$) may be followed by enzymic conversion to hydrogen peroxide (H_2O_2), hydroperoxy (HOO•) and hydroxyl (OH•) radicals or singlet oxygen. These reactive oxygen species are cytotoxic, both directly and through lipid peroxidation (see above), and are important in excitotoxicity and neurodegeneration (Ch. 35, Fig. 35.1 and p. 512).

Depletion of glutathione

The GSH redox cycle protects cells from oxidative stress. GSH can be depleted by accumulation of normal oxidative products of cell metabolism, or by the action of toxic chemicals. GSH is normally maintained in a redox couple with its disulfide, GSSG. Oxidising species convert GSH to GSSG, GSH being regenerated by NADPH-dependent GSSG reductase. When cellular GSH falls to about 20–30% of normal, cellular defence against toxic compounds is impaired and cell death can result.

Modification of sulfhydryl groups

Modification of sulfhydryl groups can be produced either by oxidising species that alter sulfhydryl groups reversibly or by covalent interaction. Free sulfhydryl groups have a critical role in the catalytic activity of many enzymes. Important targets for sulfhydryl modification by reactive metabolites include the cytoskeletal protein actin, GSH reductase (see above) and Ca^{2+}-transporting ATPases in the plasma membrane and endoplasmic reticulum. These maintain cytoplasmic Ca^{2+} concentration at approximately 0.1 μmol/l in the face of an extracellular Ca^{2+} concentration of more than 1 mmol/l. A sustained rise in cell Ca^{2+} occurs with inactivation of these enzymes (or with increased membrane permeability; see above), and this compromises cell viability. Lethal processes leading to cell death after acute Ca^{2+} overload include activation of degradative enzymes (neutral proteases, phospholipases, endonucleases) and protein kinases, mitochondrial damage and cytoskeletal alterations (e.g. modification of association between actin and actin-binding proteins).

COVALENT INTERACTIONS

Targets for covalent interactions include DNA, proteins/peptides, lipids and carbohydrates. Covalent bonding to DNA is a basic mechanism of mutagenic chemicals; this is dealt with below. Several non-mutagenic chemicals also form covalent bonds with macromolecules, but the relationship between this and cell damage is incompletely understood. For example, the cholinesterase inhibitor **paraoxon** binds acetylcholinesterase at the neuromuscular junction and causes necrosis of skeletal muscle. One toxin from an exceptionally poisonous toadstool, *Amanita phalloides*, binds actin, and another binds RNA polymerase, interfering with actin depolymerisation and protein synthesis, respectively.

HEPATOTOXICITY

Many therapeutic drugs cause liver damage, manifested clinically as hepatitis or (in less severe cases) only as laboratory abnormalities (e.g. increased activity of plasma aspartate transaminase, an enzyme released from damaged liver cells). **Paracetamol, isoniazid,**

---

[1] The value of toxicity testing is illustrated by experience with **triparanol**, a cholesterol-lowering drug marketed in the USA in 1959. Three years later, a team from the Food and Drug Administration, acting on a tip-off, paid the manufacturer a surprise visit that revealed falsification of toxicology data demonstrating cataracts in rats and dogs. The drug was withdrawn, but some patients who had been taking it for a year or more also developed cataracts. Regulatory authorities now require that toxicity testing is performed under a tightly defined code of practice (*Good Laboratory Practice*), which incorporates many safeguards to minimise the risk of error or fraud.

> **General mechanisms of cell damage and cell death** 🔑
>
> - Drug-induced cell damage/death is usually caused by reactive metabolites of the drug, involving non-covalent and/or covalent interactions with target molecules. Cell death is often 'self-inflicted', via triggering apoptosis.
> - Non-covalent interactions include:
>   — lipid peroxidation via a chain reaction
>   — generation of cytotoxic reactive oxygen species
>   — depletion of reduced glutathione
>   — modification of sulfhydryl groups on key enzymes (e.g. Ca^{2+}-ATPase) and structural proteins.
> - Covalent interactions, for example adduct formation between a metabolite of **paracetamol** (NAPBQI: *N*-acetyl-*p*-benzoquinone imine) and cellular macromolecules (Fig. 53.1). Covalent binding to protein can produce an immunogen; binding to DNA can cause carcinogenesis and teratogenesis.

iproniazid and **halothane** cause hepatotoxicity by the mechanisms of cell damage outlined above. Genetic differences in drug metabolism (see Ch. 52) have been implicated in some instances (e.g. **isoniazid, phenytoin**). Mild drug-induced abnormalities of liver function are not uncommon, but the mechanism of liver injury is often uncertain (e.g. statins; Ch. 20). It is not always necessary to discontinue a drug when such mild laboratory abnormalities occur, but the occurrence of irreversible liver disease (cirrhosis) as a result of long-term low-dose **methotrexate** treatment (Ch. 14, p. 241) for arthritis or psoriasis (a chronic scaling skin disease of unknown cause that is usually mild, if tiresome, but can rarely be very severe[2]) argues for caution. Hepatotoxicity of a different kind, namely reversible obstructive jaundice, occurs with **chlorpromazine** (Ch. 38) and **androgens** (Ch. 30).

Hepatotoxicity caused by **paracetamol** overdose remains a common cause of death following self-poisoning. An outline is given in Chapter 14 (pp. 235–236). Because the body's handling of this drug exemplifies many of the general mechanisms of cell damage outlined above, the story is taken up again here. With toxic doses of paracetamol, the enzymes catalysing the normal conjugation reactions are saturated, and mixed-function oxidases convert the drug to the reactive metabolite *N*-acetyl-*p*-benzoquinone imine (NAPBQI). As explained in Chapters 8 (p. 117) and 52 (p. 748), paracetamol toxicity is increased in patients in whom P450 enzymes have been induced, for instance by chronic excessive consumption of alcohol. NAPBQI initiates several of the covalent and non-covalent interactions described above and illustrated in Figure 53.1. Oxidative stress from GSH

depletion is important in leading to cell death. Regeneration of GSH from GSSG depends on the availability of cysteine, the intracellular availability of which can be limiting. *Acetylcysteine* or *methionine* can substitute for cysteine, increasing GSH availability and reducing mortality in patients with paracetamol poisoning.

Liver damage can also be produced by immunological mechanisms (see below), which have been particularly implicated in **halothane** hepatitis (see Ch. 36).

NEPHROTOXICITY

Drug-induced nephrotoxicity is a common clinical problem: non-steroidal anti-inflammatory drugs (NSAIDs; Table 53.1) and angiotensin-converting enzyme (ACE) inhibitors are among the commonest causes of acute renal failure. This is usually caused by the principal pharmacological actions of these drugs, which, although well tolerated in healthy people, cause renal failure in patients with diseases that jeopardise glomerular filtration. In patients with heart or liver disease, glomerular filtration rate (GFR) depends critically on vasodilator prostaglandin biosynthesis. This is inhibited by NSAIDs (Ch. 14), and hence these drugs reduce renal perfusion in such patients. Similarly, in patients with bilateral renal artery stenosis (i.e. narrowings of the renal arteries, most often caused by fibromuscular tissue in young women or by atheromatous disease in older people), GFR depends on angiotensin II–mediated efferent arteriolar vasoconstriction (which is inhibited by ACE inhibitors; Ch. 19); acute renal impairment occurs on starting an ACE inhibitor drug and is reversible if the drug is discontinued promptly. Additionally, NSAIDs indirectly depress renin and aldosterone secretion by inhibiting renal prostaglandin I_2 biosynthesis, and ACE inhibitors depress angiotensin II–stimulated aldosterone secretion, leading to low renin/low aldosterone states ('hyporeninaemic hypoaldosteronism') that are particularly notable in diabetic patients. Reduced aldosterone can cause hyperkalaemia, especially if GFR is also reduced.

In addition to these effects related to their main pharmacological action, NSAIDs can also cause an allergic interstitial nephritis. This rare problem usually occurs several months to 1 year after starting treatment. It manifests clinically as acute renal failure, often accompanied by eosinophil leucocytes in the urine and proteinuria, or as nephrotic syndrome (heavy proteinuria, hypoalbuminuria and oedema). **Fenoprofen** is particularly liable to cause this type

> **Hepatotoxicity** 🔑
>
> - Hepatocytes are exposed to reactive metabolites of drugs as these are formed by P450 enzymes.
> - Liver damage is produced by several mechanisms of cell injury; **paracetamol** exemplifies many of these (see Fig. 53.1).
> - Some drugs (e.g. **chlorpromazine**) can cause reversible cholestatic jaundice.
> - Immunological mechanisms are sometimes implicated (e.g. **halothane**).

---

[2]Aficionados of Dennis Potter will recall the protagonist in the television drama *The Singing Detective*; Potter was himself afflicted by the most severe form of the disease.

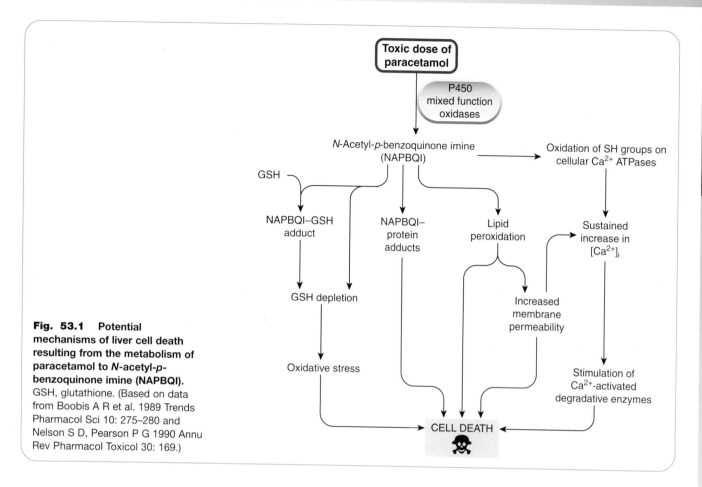

Fig. 53.1 Potential mechanisms of liver cell death resulting from the metabolism of paracetamol to *N*-acetyl-*p*-benzoquinone imine (NAPBQI). GSH, glutathione. (Based on data from Boobis A R et al. 1989 Trends Pharmacol Sci 10: 275–280 and Nelson S D, Pearson P G 1990 Annu Rev Pharmacol Toxicol 30: 169.)

Table 53.1 Adverse effects of non-steroidal anti-inflammatory drugs on the kidney

Cause	Adverse effects
Principal pharmacological action (i.e. inhibition of prostaglandin biosynthesis)	Acute ischaemic renal failure. Sodium retention (leading to or exacerbating hypertension and/or heart failure) Water retention Hyporeninaemic hypoaldosteronism (leading to hyperkalaemia)
Unrelated to principal pharmacological action (allergic-type interstitial nephritis) Unknown whether or not related to principal pharmacological action (analgesic nephropathy)	Renal failure Proteinuria Papillary necrosis Chronic renal failure

(Adapted from Murray & Brater 1993.)

of renal damage, possibly because its metabolites bind irreversibly to albumin. Penicillins (Ch. 46), especially **meticillin**, also cause interstitial nephritis.

Analgesic nephropathy is a third kind of renal damage in which NSAIDs are implicated. This consists of renal papillary necrosis[3]

and chronic *interstitial nephritis*. The clinical course is typically insidious but leads ultimately to end-stage chronic renal failure. It is associated with prolonged and massive overuse of analgesics. **Phenacetin** has particularly been incriminated, but **paracetamol** and NSAIDs have not been exonerated. The role of **caffeine** (often included with analgesics and NSAIDs in combined preparations for migraine) is uncertain but could be important. It is possible that such analgesic-associated nephropathy is causally related to inhibition of renal prostaglandin synthesis, but its pathogenesis is not understood.

---

[3]It is worth re-emphasising that the renal papilla is the part of the kidney exposed to the highest concentration of solutes, including drug metabolites; it also has a lower blood flow than other parts as a result of counter-current exchange in the vasa recta.

Captopril, in higher doses than are currently recommended, can cause heavy proteinuria (Ch. 19). This is the result of glomerular injury, which is also caused by some other drugs that, like captopril, contain a sulfhydryl group (e.g. **penicillamine**, a copper-chelating agent introduced originally to treat Wilson's disease but more widely used because of its disease-modifying effect in rheumatoid arthritis; Ch. 14, p. 241). It is therefore believed that it is this chemical feature rather than ACE inhibition per se that is responsible for this adverse effect.

Ciclosporin, used to prevent transplant rejection (Ch. 14), causes renal damage via renal vasoconstriction, which reduces GFR and causes hypertension. It alters renal prostaglandin biosynthesis.

Many hepatotoxic drugs (e.g. **paracetamol**) also damage the kidney, producing necrosis of renal tubular cells. Mechanisms are described above (pp. 754–755).

MUTAGENESIS AND CARCINOGENICITY

Mutation changes the genotype of a cell, and the change is passed on when the cell divides. Chemical agents cause mutation by covalent modification of DNA. Certain kinds of mutation result in carcinogenesis, because the affected DNA sequence codes for a protein that is involved in growth regulation. It usually requires more than one mutation in a cell to initiate the changes that result in malignancy, mutations in proto-oncogenes (which regulate cell growth) and tumour suppressor genes (which code for products that inhibit the transcription of oncogenes) being particularly implicated (see Ch. 5). Some oncogenes code for modified growth factors or growth factor receptors, or for elements of the intracellular transduction mechanism by which growth factors regulate cell proliferation (see p. 719). Growth factors are polypeptide mediators that stimulate cell division; examples are *epidermal growth factor* and *platelet-derived growth factor*. The receptors for these growth factors regulate a number of cellular processes through tyrosine phosphorylation (see Fig. 3.15). Although there are many details to be filled in, the complex connection between exposure to a mutagenic chemical and the development of a cancer is beginning to be understood.

BIOCHEMICAL MECHANISMS OF MUTAGENESIS

▼ Most chemical carcinogens act by modifying bases in DNA, particularly guanine, the O6 and N7 positions of which readily combine covalently with reactive metabolites of chemical carcinogens. Substitution at the O6 position is the more likely to produce a permanent mutagenic effect, because N7 substitutions are usually quickly repaired.

The accessibility of bases in DNA to chemical attack is greatest when DNA is in the process of replication (i.e. during cell division). The likelihood of genetic damage by many mutagens is therefore related to the frequency of cell division. The developing fetus is particularly susceptible, and mutagens are also potentially teratogenic (see below). This is also important in relation to mutagenesis of germ cells, particularly in girls, because in humans the production of primary oocytes occurs by a rapid succession of mitotic divisions very early in embryogenesis. Each primary oocyte then undergoes only two further divisions much later in life, at the time of ovulation. It is consequently during early pregnancy that germ cells of the developing female embryo are most likely to undergo mutagenesis, the mutations being transmitted to progeny conceived many years after exposure to the mutagen. In the male, germ cell divisions occur throughout life, and sensitivity to mutagens is continuously present.

Nephrotoxicity 🔑

- Renal tubular cells are exposed to high concentrations of drugs and metabolites as urine is concentrated.
- Renal damage can cause papillary and/or tubular necrosis.
- Inhibition of prostaglandin synthesis by non-steroidal anti-inflammatory drugs causes vasoconstriction and lowers glomerular filtration rate.

Mutagenesis and carcinogenicity 🔑

- Mutagenesis involves modification of DNA.
- Mutation of proto-oncogenes or tumour suppressor genes leads to carcinogenesis
  — More than one mutation is usually required.
- Drugs are relatively uncommon (but not unimportant) causes of birth defects and cancers.

The importance of drugs, in comparison with other chemicals such as pollutants and food additives, as a causative factor in mutagenesis has not been established, and such epidemiological evidence as exists suggests that they are uncommon (but not unimportant) causes of fetal malformations and cancers.

CARCINOGENESIS

Alteration of DNA is the first step in the complex, multistage process of carcinogenesis (see Ch. 5). Carcinogens are chemical substances that cause cancer, and can interact directly with DNA or act at a later stage to increase the likelihood that mutation will result in a tumour (Fig. 53.2). Carcinogens are divided into two groups.

- *Genotoxic carcinogens* (i.e. mutagens, see above) or 'initiators', further divided into:
  —primary carcinogens that act directly on DNA
  —secondary carcinogens, which must be converted to a reactive metabolite before they affect DNA; most clinically important carcinogens are secondary.
- *Epigenetic carcinogens* (i.e. agents that do not themselves cause genetic damage but increase the likelihood that such damage will cause cancer). The most important types are as follow.
  —Promoters: these produce cancers when given *after* a genotoxic agent; examples include *phorbol esters* and *cigarette smoke* (in addition to carcinogenic aromatic hydrocarbons).
  —Cocarcinogens: these enhance the effect of genotoxic agents when given simultaneously; examples include *phorbol esters* (again) and various aromatic and aliphatic hydrocarbons. It will be appreciated that some chemicals have genotoxic, promoter and cocarcinogenic activity.

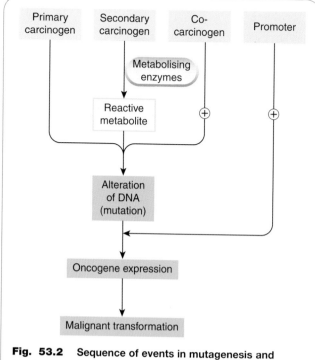

Fig. 53.2 Sequence of events in mutagenesis and carcinogenesis.

—Hormones: some tumours are hormone-dependent (see Ch. 51), for example oestrogen-dependent breast and uterine cancers and androgen-dependent prostatic cancers.

MEASUREMENT OF MUTAGENICITY AND CARCINOGENICITY

Much effort has gone into developing assays to detect mutagenicity and carcinogenicity. These can be broadly divided into:

- *In vitro tests for mutagenicity.* These are suitable for screening large numbers of compounds but can give false positive or false negative results in terms of carcinogenicity.
- *Whole-animal tests for carcinogenicity.* Such tests are expensive and time-consuming but are usually required by regulatory authorities before a new drug is licensed for use in humans. The main limitation of this kind of study is that there are important species differences, mainly to do with the metabolism of the foreign compound and the formation of reactive products.
- *Whole-animal tests for teratogenesis (reproductive toxicity testing).* Tests on pregnant animals are required for drugs that are to be used by women of reproductive potential, especially (obviously) if they are to be used during pregnancy. Similar limitations of such tests apply as with carcinogenicity testing.

In vitro tests for genotoxic carcinogens

Bacteria have great advantages as a test system for measuring mutagenicity because of their high replication rate. The most widely used assays are variations on the *Ames* test, which measures the rate of back-mutation (i.e. reversion from mutant to wild-type form) in *Salmonella typhimurium*.

▼ The wild-type strain can grow in a medium containing no added amino acids, because it can synthesise all the amino acids it needs from simple carbon and nitrogen sources. The test makes use of the fact that a mutant form of the organism cannot make histidine in this way and therefore grows only on a medium containing this amino acid. The test involves growing the mutant form on a medium containing a small amount of histidine, the drug to be tested being added to the culture. After several divisions, the histidine becomes depleted, and the only cells that continue dividing are those that have back-mutated to the wild type. A count of colonies following subculture on plates deficient in histidine gives a measure of the mutation rate.

Primary carcinogens cause mutation by a direct action on bacterial DNA, but most carcinogens have to be converted to an active metabolite (see above). Therefore it is necessary to include, in the culture, enzymes that catalyse the necessary conversion. An extract of liver from a rat treated with **phenobarbital** to induce liver enzymes is usually employed. There are many variations based on the same principle.

Other short-term in vitro tests for genotoxic chemicals include measurements of mutagenesis in mouse lymphoma cells, and assays for chromosome aberrations and sister chromatid exchanges in Chinese hamster ovary cells. However, all the in vitro tests give some false positives and some false negatives.

In vivo tests for carcinogenicity

In vivo tests for carcinogenicity entail detection of tumours in groups of test animals. Carcinogenicity tests are inevitably slow, because there is usually a latency of months or years before tumours develop. Furthermore, tumours can develop spontaneously in control animals, and the results often provide only equivocal evidence of carcinogenicity of the test drug, making it difficult for industry and regulatory authorities to decide on further development and possible licensing of a product. None of the tests so far described can reliably detect epigenetic carcinogens. To do this, it is necessary to measure the effect of the test substance on tumour production with a threshold dose of a genotoxic agent. Such tests are being evaluated.

Few therapeutic drugs are known to increase the risk of cancer, the most important groups being drugs that act on DNA, i.e. *cytotoxic* and *immunosuppressant* drugs (Chs 51 and 14, respectively), and sex hormones (e.g. **oestrogens**, Ch. 30). **Pyrimethamine** (Ch. 49) is mutagenic in high concentrations, and carcinogenicity testing in strain A mice (but not other strains or species) was positive for a threefold increase in lung tumours. **Methoxsalen** (a psoralen used together with ultraviolet light, PUVA, in specialist skin disease centres for treatment of psoriasis) is both mutagenic and carcinogenic in animal models and may increase the incidence of skin cancer in humans.

TERATOGENESIS AND DRUG-INDUCED FETAL DAMAGE

Teratogenesis signifies the production of gross structural malformations during fetal development, in distinction from other kinds of drug-induced fetal damage such as growth retardation, dysplasia (e.g. iodide-associated goitre), or the asymmetrical limb reduction resulting from vasoconstriction caused by **cocaine** (see Ch. 43) in

Carcinogens

- Carcinogens can be:
  - *genotoxic,* i.e. causing mutations directly (primary carcinogens) or after conversion to reactive metabolites (secondary carcinogens)
  - *epigenetic,* i.e. increasing the possibility that a mutagen will cause cancer, although not themselves mutagenic.
- Epigenetic carcinogens include 'promoters', which increase cancer rate if given after the mutagen, and 'cocarcinogens', which increase the rate if given with it. Phorbol esters have both actions.
- New drugs are tested for mutagenicity and carcinogenicity.
- The main test for mutagenicity measures back-mutation, in histidine-free medium, of a mutant *Salmonella typhimurium* (which, unlike the wild type, cannot grow without histidine) in the presence of:
  - the chemical to be tested
  - a liver microsomal enzyme preparation for generating reactive metabolites.
- Colony growth indicates that mutagenesis has occurred. The test is rapid and inexpensive, but some false positives and false negatives occur.
- Carcinogenicity testing:
  - involves chronic dosing of groups of animals
  - is expensive and time-consuming
  - there is no really suitable test for epigenetic carcinogens.

an otherwise normally developing limb. Examples of drugs that affect fetal development adversely are given in Table 53.2.

It has been known that external agents can affect fetal development since the 1920s, when it was discovered that X irradiation during pregnancy causes fetal malformation. The importance of rubella infection was recognised two decades later, but it was not until 1960 that drugs were implicated as causative agents in teratogenesis: the shocking experience with **thalidomide** led to a widespread reappraisal of many other drugs in clinical use, and to the setting up of drug regulatory bodies in many countries. Most birth defects (about 70%) occur with no recognisable causative factor. Drug or chemical exposure during pregnancy is believed to account for only about 1% of all fetal malformations. While this percentage is *relatively* small (fetal malformations such as cleft lip are extremely common), the *absolute* numbers of children affected are substantial.

MECHANISM OF TERATOGENESIS

The timing of the teratogenic insult in relation to fetal development is critical in determining the type and extent of damage. Mammalian fetal development passes through three phases (Table 53.3):

- blastocyst formation
- organogenesis
- histogenesis and maturation of function.

Cell division is the main process occurring during blastocyst formation. During this phase, drugs can kill the embryo by inhibiting cell division, but provided the embryo survives, its subsequent development does not generally seem to be compromised. Ethanol is an exception, affecting development at this very early stage (Ch. 43).

Drugs can cause gross malformations if administered during organogenesis (days 17–60). The structural organisation of the embryo occurs in a well-defined sequence: eye and brain, skeleton and limbs, heart and major vessels, palate, genitourinary system. The type of malformation produced thus depends on the time of exposure to the teratogen.

The cellular mechanisms by which teratogenic substances produce their effects are not at all well understood. There is a considerable overlap between mutagenicity and teratogenicity. In one large survey, among 78 compounds, 34 were both teratogenic and mutagenic, 19 were negative in both tests, and 25 (among them thalidomide) were positive in one but not the other. Damage to DNA is important but, as with carcinogenesis, is not the only factor. The control of morphogenesis is poorly understood; *vitamin A derivatives* (retinoids) are involved and are potent teratogens (see below). Known teratogens also include several drugs (e.g. **methotrexate** and **phenytoin**) that do not react directly with DNA but which inhibit its synthesis by their effects on *folate metabolism* (see Ch. 22, p. 350). Administration of **folate** during pregnancy reduces the frequency of both spontaneous and drug-induced malformations, especially *neural tube defects*.

The fetus depends on an adequate supply of nutrients during the final stage of histogenesis and functional maturation, and development is regulated by a variety of hormones. Gross structural malformations do not arise from exposure to mutagens at this stage, but drugs that interfere with the supply of nutrients or with the hormonal milieu may have deleterious effects on growth and development. Exposure of a female fetus to androgens at this stage can cause masculinisation. **Stilbestrol** was commonly given to pregnant women with a history of recurrent miscarriage during the 1950s (for unsound reasons) and causes dysplasia of the vagina of the infant and an increased incidence of carcinoma of the vagina in the teens and twenties. Angiotensin II plays an important part in the later stages of fetal development and in renal function in the fetus, and ACE inhibitors and angiotensin receptor antagonists ('sartans') cause oligohydramnios and renal failure if administered during later stages of pregnancy. They have been associated with skull defects in experimental animals.

TESTING FOR TERATOGENICITY

The **thalidomide** disaster dramatically brought home the need for routine teratogenicity studies on new therapeutic drugs. Assessment of teratogenicity in humans is a particularly difficult problem for various reasons. One is that the 'spontaneous' malformation rate is high (3–10% depending on the definition of a significant malformation) and highly variable between different regions, age groups and social classes. Large-scale studies are required, which take

Table 53.2 Some drugs reported to have adverse effects on human fetal development

Agent	Effect(s)	Teratogenicity[a]	See Chapter
Thalidomide	Phocomelia, heart defects, gut atresia, etc.	K	53
Penicillamine	Loose skin etc.	K	14
Warfarin	Saddle nose; retarded growth; defects of limbs, eyes, central nervous system	K	21
Corticosteroids	Cleft palate and congenital cataract—rare	–	28
Androgens	Masculinisation in female	–	30
Oestrogens	Testicular atrophy in male	–	30
Stilbestrol	Vaginal adenosis in female fetus, also vaginal or cervical cancer	20+ years later	30
Phenytoin	Cleft lip/palate, microcephaly, mental retardation	K	40
Valproate	Neural tube defects (e.g. spina bifida)	K	40
Carbamazepine	Retardation of fetal head growth	S	40
Cytotoxic drugs (especially folate antagonists)	Hydrocephalus, cleft palate, neural tube defects, etc.	K	51
Aminoglycosides	Deafness	–	46
Tetracycline	Staining of bones and teeth, thin tooth enamel, impaired bone growth	S	46
Ethanol	Fetal alcohol syndrome	K	43
Retinoids	Hydrocephalus etc.	K	52
Angiotensin-converting enzyme inhibitors	Oligohydramnios, renal failure	K	19

[a]K, known teratogen (in experimental animals and/or humans); S, suspected teratogen (in experimental animals and/or humans). (Adapted from Juchau 1989 Annu Rev Pharmacol Toxicol 29: 165.)

Table 53.3 The nature of drug effects on fetal development

Stage	Gestation period in humans	Main cellular process(es)	Affected by
Blastocyst formation	0–16 days	Cell division	Cytotoxic drugs, ?alcohol
Organogenesis	17–60 days approximately	Division	Teratogens
		Migration	Teratogens
		Differentiation	Teratogens
		Death	Teratogens
Histogenesis and functional maturation	60 days to term	As above	Miscellaneous drugs (e.g. alcohol, nicotine, antithyroid drugs, steroids)

many years and much money to perform, and they usually give suggestive, rather than conclusive, results.

Studies using embryonic stem cells in assessing developmental toxicity are showing some promise (see Bremer & Hartung, 2004, for a review from a regulatory perspective). In vitro methods, based on the culture of cells, organs or whole embryos, have, however, not so far been developed to a level where they satisfactorily predict teratogenesis in vivo, and most regulatory authorities require teratogenicity testing in a rodent plus in one non-rodent species

(e.g. rabbit). The visceral yolk sac and development of the chorioallantoic placenta of the rabbit resemble those of humans more so than do rodents', in some respects (Foote & Carney, 2000). Pregnant females are dosed at various levels during the critical period of organogenesis, and the fetuses are examined for structural abnormalities. However, poor cross-species correlation means that tests of this kind are not reliably predictive in humans, and it is usually recommended that new drugs are not used in pregnancy unless it is essential.

SOME DEFINITE AND PROBABLE HUMAN TERATOGENS

Although many drugs have been found to be teratogenic in varying degrees in experimental animals, relatively few are known to be teratogenic in humans (see Table 53.2). Some of the more important are discussed below.

Thalidomide

Thalidomide is virtually unique in producing, at therapeutic dosage, virtually 100% malformed infants when taken in the first 3–6 weeks of gestation. It was introduced in 1957 as a hypnotic and sedative with the special feature that it was much less hazardous in overdosage than barbiturates, and it was even recommended specifically for use in pregnancy (with the advertising slogan 'the safe hypnotic'). As was then normal, it had been subjected only to acute toxicity testing, and not to chronic toxicity[4] or teratogenicity testing. Thalidomide was marketed energetically and successfully, and the first suspicion of its teratogenicity arose early in 1961 with reports of a sudden increase in the incidence of phocomelia. This abnormality ('seal limbs') consists of an absence of development of the long bones of the arms and legs, and had hitherto been virtually unknown. At this time, approximately 1 000 000 tablets were being sold daily in West Germany. Reports of phocomelia came simultaneously from Hamburg and Sydney, and the connection with thalidomide was made. The drug was withdrawn late in 1961, by which time an estimated 10 000 malformed babies had been born (Fig. 53.3). Despite intensive study, its mechanism remains poorly understood, although epidemiological investigation showed very clearly the correlation between the time of exposure and the type of malfunction produced (Table 53.4).

Cytotoxic drugs

Many alkylating agents (e.g. **chlorambucil** and **cyclophosphamide**) and antimetabolites (e.g. **azathioprine** and **mercaptopurine**) cause malformations when used in early pregnancy but more often lead to abortion (see Ch. 51). Folate antagonists (e.g. **methotrexate**) produce a much higher incidence of major malformations, evident in both live-born and stillborn fetuses. (Conversely, folic acid taken before conception and for the first 12 weeks of a pregnancy reduces the risk of 'spontaneous' neural tube defects; see Ch. 22, clinical box p. 351.)

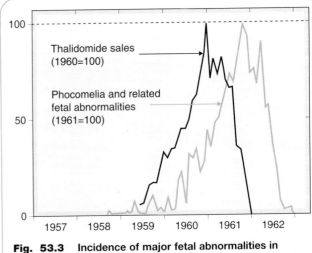

Fig. 53.3 Incidence of major fetal abnormalities in Western Europe following the introduction and withdrawal of thalidomide.

Table 53.4 Thalidomide teratogenesis

Day of gestation	Type of deformity
21–22	Malformation of ears Cranial nerve defects
24–27	Phocomelia of arms
28–29	Phocomelia of arms and legs
30–36	Malformation of hands Anorectal stenosis

Retinoids

Etretinate, a retinoid (i.e. vitamin A derivative) with marked effects on epidermal differentiation, is a known teratogen and causes a high proportion of serious abnormalities (notably skeletal deformities) in exposed fetuses. Dermatologists use retinoids to treat skin diseases including several, such as acne and psoriasis, that are common in young women. Etretinate accumulates in subcutaneous fat and is eliminated extremely slowly, detectable amounts persisting for many months after chronic dosing is discontinued. Because of this, women should avoid pregnancy for at least 2 years after treatment. **Acitretin** is an active metabolite of etretinate. It is equally teratogenic, but tissue accumulation is less pronounced and elimination may therefore be more rapid.

Heavy metals

Lead, cadmium and *mercury* all cause fetal malformations in humans. The main evidence comes from *Minamata disease*, named after the locality in Japan where an epidemic occurred when the local population ate fish contaminated with methylmercury that had been used as an agricultural fungicide. This impaired brain development in exposed fetuses, resulting in cerebral palsy and mental retardation, often with microcephaly.

---

[4]A severe peripheral neuropathy, leading to irreversible paralysis and sensory loss, was reported within a year of the drug's introduction and subsequently confirmed in many reports. The drug company responsible was less than punctilious in acting on these reports (see Sjostrom & Nilsson, 1972), which were soon eclipsed by the discovery of teratogenic effects, but the neurotoxic effect was severe enough in its own right to have necessitated withdrawal of the drug from general use. Today, use of thalidomide has had a small resurgence related to several highly specialised applications. It is prescribed by specialists (in dermatology and in HIV infection, among others) under tightly controlled and restricted conditions.

Mercury, like other heavy metals, inactivates many enzymes by forming covalent bonds with sulfhydryl and other groups, and this is believed to be responsible for these developmental abnormalities.

Antiepileptic drugs

Congenital malformations are increased two- to threefold in babies of epileptic mothers. Interestingly, all existing antiepileptic drugs have been implicated, including **phenytoin** (particularly cleft lip/palate), **valproate** (neural tube defects) and **carbamazepine** (spina bifida and hypospadias, a malformation of the male urethra), as well as newer agents (Ch. 40).

Warfarin

Administration of **warfarin** (Ch. 21) in the first trimester is associated with nasal hypoplasia and various central nervous system abnormalities, affecting roughly 25% of exposed babies. In the last trimester, it must not be used because of the risk of intracranial haemorrhage in the baby during delivery.

Antiemetics

Antiemetics have been widely used to treat morning sickness in early pregnancy, and some are teratogenic in animals. Results of surveys in humans are inconclusive, providing no clear evidence of teratogenicity. Nevertheless, it is prudent to avoid the use of these drugs in pregnant patients if possible.

ASSESSMENT OF GENOTOXIC POTENTIAL

Registration of pharmaceuticals requires a comprehensive assessment of their genotoxic potential. Because no single test is adequate, the usual approach recommended by the International Conference

> ### Teratogenesis and drug-induced fetal damage
>
> - Teratogenesis means production of gross structural malformations of the fetus (e.g. the absence of limbs after thalidomide). Less comprehensive damage can be produced by several drugs (see Table 53.2). Less than 1% of congenital fetal defects are attributed to drugs given to the mother.
> - Gross malformations are produced only if teratogens act during organogenesis. This occurs during the first 3 months of pregnancy but after blastocyst formation. Drug-induced fetal damage is rare during blastocyst formation (exception: fetal alcohol syndrome) and after the first 3 months (exception: angiotensin-converting enzyme inhibitors and sartans).
> - The mechanisms of action of teratogens are not clearly understood, although DNA damage is a factor.
> - New drugs are usually tested in pregnant females of at least one rodent and one non-rodent (e.g. rabbit) species.

on Harmonisation (ESRA Rapporteur 1997 4: 5–7) is to carry out a battery of in vitro and in vivo tests for genotoxicity. The following battery is often used:

- a test for gene mutation in bacteria
- an in vitro test with cytogenetic evaluation of chromosomal damage
- an in vivo test for chromosomal damage using rodent haemopoietic cells
- reproductive toxicity testing
- carcinogenicity testing.

ALLERGIC REACTIONS TO DRUGS

Allergic reactions of various kinds are a common form of adverse response to drugs. Most drugs, being low-molecular-weight substances, are not immunogenic in themselves. A drug or its metabolites can, however, act as a *hapten* by interacting with protein to form a stable conjugate that is immunogenic (Ch. 13). The immunological basis of some allergic drug reactions has been well worked out, but often it is inferred from the clinical characteristics of the reaction, and direct evidence of an immunological mechanism is lacking. The main criteria that are suggestive of an immune response are as follow.

- The time course differs from the main action of the drug; it is either delayed in onset or occurs only with repeated exposure to the drug
- Allergy may result from doses that are too small to elicit pharmacodynamic effects.
- The reaction conforms to one of the clinical syndromes associated with allergy—types I, II, III and IV of the Gell and Coombs classification (below and Ch. 13)—and is unrelated to the pharmacodynamic effect of the drug.

The overall incidence of allergic drug reactions is variously reported as being between 2 and 25%. Most are minor skin eruptions. Serious reactions (e.g. anaphylaxis, haemolysis and bone marrow depression), which can be fatal, are rare. **Penicillins**, which are the commonest cause of drug-induced anaphylaxis, produce this response in an estimated 1 in 50 000 patients exposed. Skin eruptions can be severe, and fatalities occur with Stevens–Johnson syndrome (provoked, for example, by sulfonamides) and with toxic epidermal necrolysis (which can be caused by **allopurinol**).

Immunological mechanisms

The formation of an immunogenic conjugate between a small molecule and an endogenous protein requires covalent bonding. In most cases, reactive metabolites, rather than the drug itself, are responsible. Such reactive metabolites can be produced during drug oxidation or by photoactivation in the skin. They may also be produced by the action of toxic oxygen metabolites generated by activated leucocytes. Rarely (e.g. in drug-induced lupus erythematosus), the reactive moiety interacts to form an immunogen with nuclear components (DNA, histone) rather than proteins (see below). Conjugation with a macromolecule is usually essential, although penicillin is an exception because it can form sufficiently large polymers in solution to elicit an anaphylactic reaction in a sensitised individual even without conjugation to protein. Conjugates of penicillin and its metabolites with protein are also formed and can also act as immunogens.

Clinical types of allergic response to drugs

In the Gell and Coombs classification of hypersensitivity reactions (Ch. 13), types I, II and III are antibody-mediated reactions and type IV is cell-mediated. Unwanted reactions to drugs involve both antibody- and cell-mediated reactions. The more important clinical manifestations of hypersensitivity include anaphylactic shock, haematological reactions, allergic liver damage and other hypersensitivity reactions.

Anaphylactic shock

Anaphylactic shock—see also Chapter 23—is a type I hypersensitivity response. It is a sudden and life-threatening reaction that results from the release of *histamine, leukotrienes* and other mediators (Ch. 13). The main features include urticarial rash, swelling of soft tissues, bronchoconstriction and hypotension.

Penicillins are the drugs most likely to cause anaphylactic reactions and account for about 75% of anaphylactic deaths, reflecting the frequency with which they are used in clinical practice. Other drugs that can cause anaphylaxis include various enzymes, for example **streptokinase** (Ch. 21), **asparaginase** (Ch. 51); hormones, for example **corticotropin** (adrenocorticotrophic hormone; Ch. 28); **heparin** (Ch. 21); *dextrans; radiological contrast agents; vaccines;* and other *serological products.* Anaphylaxis with local anaesthetics (Ch. 44), the antiseptic chlorhexidine and with many other drugs has been reported but is uncommon. Treatment of anaphylaxis is given in Chapter 23.

It is sometimes feasible to carry out a skin test for the presence of anaphylactic hypersensitivity, which involves injecting a minute dose intradermally. This is sometimes done if a patient reports that she or he is allergic to a particular drug. However, the test is not completely reliable and may itself may elicit a severe reaction. The use of penicilloylpolylysine as a skin test reagent for penicillin allergy is an improvement over the use of penicillin itself, because it bypasses the need for conjugation of the test substance, thereby reducing the likelihood of a false negative. Other specialised tests are available to detect the presence of specific immunoglobulin E in the plasma, or to measure histamine release from the patient's basophils, but these are not used routinely.

Other drug-induced type I hypersensitivity reactions include bronchospasm (Ch. 23) and urticaria.

Haematological reactions

Drug-induced haematological reactions can be produced by type II, III or IV hypersensitivity. Type II reactions can affect any or all of the formed elements of the blood, which may be destroyed by effects either on the circulating blood cells themselves or on their progenitors in the bone marrow. They involve antibody binding to a drug–macromolecule complex on the cell surface membrane. The antigen–antibody reaction activates complement, leading to lysis (Fig. 13.1) or provokes attack by killer lymphocytes or phagocytic leucocytes. *Haemolytic anaemia* has

been most commonly reported with sulfonamides and related drugs (Ch. 46) and with an antihypertensive drug, **methyldopa** (Ch. 11), which is still widely used to treat hypertension during pregnancy. With methyldopa, significant haemolysis occurs in less than 1% of patients, but the appearance of antibodies directed against the surface of red cells is detectable in 15% by the Coombs test. The antibodies are directed against Rh antigens, but it is not known how methyldopa produces this effect.

Drug-induced agranulocytosis (complete absence of circulating neutrophils) is usually delayed 2–12 weeks after beginning drug treatment but may then be sudden in onset. It often presents with mouth ulcers, a severe sore throat or other infection. Serum from the patient lyses leucocytes from other individuals, and circulating antileucocyte antibodies can usually be detected immunologically. Drugs associated with agranulocytosis include NSAIDs, especially **phenylbutazone** (Ch. 14); **carbimazole** (Ch. 29); **clozapine** (Ch. 38); and **sulfonamides** and related drugs (e.g. thiazides and sulfonylureas). Agranulocytosis is rare but life-threatening. Recovery when the offending drug is stopped is often slow or absent. Antibody-mediated leucocyte destruction must be distinguished from the direct effect of cytotoxic drugs (see Ch. 51), which cause granulocytopenia that is rapid in onset, predictably related to dose and reversible.

Thrombocytopenia (reduction in platelet numbers) can be caused by type II reactions to **quinine** (Ch. 49), **heparin** (Ch. 21) and thiazide diuretics (Ch. 24).

Some drugs (notably **chloramphenicol**) can suppress all three haemopoietic cell lineages, giving rise to *aplastic anaemia* (anaemia with associated agranulocytosis and thrombocytopenia).

The distinction between type III and type IV hypersensitivity reactions in the causation of haematological reactions is not clear-cut, and either or both mechanisms can be involved.

Allergic liver damage

Most drug-induced liver damage results from the direct toxic effects of drugs or their metabolites, as described above. However, hypersensitivity reactions are sometimes involved, a particular example being **halothane**-induced hepatic necrosis (see Ch. 36). *Trifluoracetylchloride*, a reactive metabolite of halothane, couples to a macromolecule to form an immunogen. Most patients with halothane-induced liver damage have antibodies that react with halothane–carrier conjugates. Halothane–protein antigens can be expressed on the surface of hepatocytes. Destruction of the cells occurs by type II hypersensitivity reactions involving killer T cells, and type III reactions can also contribute.

Other hypersensitivity reactions

The clinical manifestations of type IV hypersensitivity reactions are diverse, ranging from minor skin rashes to generalised autoimmune disease. Fever may accompany these reactions. Skin rashes can be antibody-mediated but are usually cell-mediated. They range from mild eruptions to fatal exfoliation. *Stevens–Johnson syndrome* is a very severe generalised rash that extends into the alimentary tract and carries an appreciable mortality. In some cases, the lesions are photosensitive, probably because ultraviolet light converts the drug to reactive products.

Some drugs (notably **hydralazine** and **procainamide**) can produce an autoimmune syndrome resembling *systemic lupus erythematosus*. This is a multisystem disorder in which there is immunological damage to many organs and tissues (including joints, skin, lung, central nervous system and kidney) caused particularly, but not exclusively, by type III hypersensitivity reactions. The prodigious array of antibodies directed against 'self' components has been termed 'an autoimmune thunderstorm'. The antibodies react with determinants shared by many molecules, for example the phosphodiester backbone of DNA, RNA and phospholipids. In drug-induced systemic lupus erythematosus, the immunogen may result from the reactive drug moiety interacting with nuclear material, and joint and pulmonary damage is common. The condition usually resolves when treatment with the offending drug is stopped.

Allergic reactions to drugs

- Drugs or their reactive metabolites can bind covalently to proteins to form immunogens. **Penicillin** (which can also form immunogenic polymers) is an important example.
- Drug-induced allergic (hypersensitivity) reactions may be antibody-mediated (types I, II, III) or cell-mediated (type IV). Important clinical manifestations include the following.
  - anaphylactic shock (type I): many drugs can cause this, and most deaths are caused by penicillin
  - haematological reactions (type II, III or IV): including haemolytic anaemia (e.g. **methyldopa**), agranulocytosis (e.g. **carbimazole**), thrombocytopenia (e.g. **quinine**) and aplastic anemia (e.g. **chloramphenicol**)
  - hepatitis (types II, III): for example **halothane, phenytoin**
  - rashes (type I, IV): are usually mild but can be life-threatening (e.g. Stevens–Johnson syndrome)
  - drug-induced systemic lupus erythematosus (mainly type II): antibodies to nuclear material are formed (e.g. **hydralazine**).

REFERENCES AND FURTHER READING

Bhogal N, Grindon C, Combes R, Balls M 2005 Toxicity testing: creating a revolution based on new technologies. Trends Biotechnol 23: 299–307 (*Reviews current and likely future value of new technologies in relation to toxicological evaluation*)

Bremer S, Hartung T 2004 The use of embryonic stem cells for regulatory developmental toxicity testing in vitro—the current status of test development. Curr Pharm Des 10: 2733–2747 (*Summarises requirements for an in vitro embryotoxicity test needed for regulatory toxicity testing*)

Briggs G G, Freeman R K, Sumner J Y 2001 Drugs in pregnancy and lactation, 6th edn. Williams & Wilkins, Baltimore (*Invaluable reference guide to fetal and neonatal risk for clinicians caring for pregnant women*)

Brimblecombe R W, Dayan A D 1993 Preclinical toxicity testing. In: Burley D M, Clarke J M, Lasagna L (eds) Pharmaceutical medicine, 2nd edn. Edward Arnold, London, pp. 12–32 (*Scholarly review*)

Collins M D, Mayo G E 1999 Teratology of retinoids. Annu Rev Pharmacol Toxicol 39: 399–430 (*Overviews principles of teratology as they apply to the retinoids, describes signal transduction of retinoids and toxikinetics*)

Davila J C, Rodriguez R J, Melchert R B, Acosta D 1998 Predictive value of in vitro model systems in toxicology. Annu Rev Pharmacol Toxicol 38: 63–96 (*Overviews in vitro model systems to investigate target organ toxicity, with examples of cutaneous and ocular toxicity and the role of drug metabolism in hepatotoxicity, plus use of in vitro model systems in drug development*)

Farrar H C, Blumer J L 1991 Fetal effects of maternal drug exposure. Annu Rev Pharmacol 31: 525–547 (*Reviews teratology, fetal drug effects, teratogenesis and fetal pharmacology*)

Foote R H, Carney E W 2000 The rabbit as a model for reproductive and developmental toxicity studies. Reprod Toxicol 14: 477–493 (*Discusses the use of the rabbit in developmental toxicity and teratology studies*)

Glassman A H, Bigger J T 2001 Antipsychotic drugs: prolonged QTc interval, torsade de pointes, and sudden death. Am J Psychiat 158: 1774–1782 (*Reviews mechanisms and risks of torsade and sudden death with antipsychotic drugs; the greatest risk is with thioridazine*)

Hanson J W, Streissguth A P, Smith D W 1978 The effects of moderate alcohol consumption during pregnancy on fetal growth and morphogenesis. J Paediatr 92: 457–460

Hay A 1988 How to identify a carcinogen. Nature 332: 782–783

Hinson J A, Roberts D W 1992 Role of covalent and noncovalent interactions in cell toxicity: effects on proteins. Annu Rev Pharmacol Toxicol 32: 471–510

Huff J, Haseman J, Rall D 1991 Scientific concepts, value, and significance of chemical carcinogenesis studies. Annu Rev Pharmacol Toxicol 31: 621–652

Kenna J G, Knight T L, van Pelt F N A M 1993 Immunity of halothane metabolite–modified proteins in halothane hepatitis. Ann NY Acad Sci 685: 646–661

Lutz W K, Maier P 1988 Genotoxic and epigenetic chemical carcinogens: one process, different mechanisms. Trends Pharmacol Sci 9: 322–326

Moss A J 1993 Measurement of the QT interval and the risk of QTc prolongation: a review. Am J Cardiol 72: 23B–25B

Murray M D, Brater D C 1993 Renal toxicity of the nonsteroidal anti-inflammatory drugs. Annu Rev Pharmacol Toxicol 33: 435–465

Nicotera P, Bellomo G, Orrenius S 1992 Calcium-mediated mechanisms in chemically-induced cell death. Annu Rev Pharmacol Toxicol 32: 449–470 (*Discusses the role of Ca²⁺ in the early development of cell damage*)

Park B K, Kitteringham N R, Maggs J L et al. 2005 The role of metabolic activation in drug-induced hepatotoxicity. Annu Rev Pharmacol Toxicol 45: 177–202 (*Reviews evidence for reactive metabolite formation from hepatotoxic drugs such as paracetamol, tamoxifen, diclofenac and troglitazone, and the current hypotheses of how this leads to liver injury*)

Parng C 2005 In vivo zebrafish assays for toxicity testing. Curr Opin Drug Discov Devel 8: 100–106 (*Effective in vivo toxicity screening early in development can reduce the number of compounds that progress to laborious and costly late-stage animal testing. The transparent zebra fish provides accessibility to internal organs, tissues and even cells, and has emerged as a model organism for toxicity testing. Straightforward in vivo zebra fish assays can serve as an intermediate step between cell-based and mammalian testing, thus streamlining the drug development timeline*)

Pirmohamed M 2003 Drug-induced apoptosis: clinical significance. Drug Metab Rev 35: 24–24 48(suppl 1)

Pirmohamed M 2004 Role of the immune system in idiosyncratic drug reactions. Drug Metab Rev 36: 29–29; 58(suppl 1)

Pirmohamed M, James S, Meakin S et al. 2004 Adverse drug reactions as cause of admission to hospital: prospective analysis of 18,820 patients. Br Med J 329: 15–19 (*There were 1225 admissions related to an adverse drug reaction. The median bed stay was 8 days, accounting for 4% of the hospital bed capacity. The projected annual cost is £466 million. Most reactions were avoidable. Drugs most commonly implicated were aspirin and other NSAIDs, diuretics, warfarin; the most common reaction was gastrointestinal bleeding.)*

Plante I, Charbonneau M, Cyr D G 2002 Decreased gap junctional intercellular communication in hexachlorobenzene-induced gender-specific hepatic tumor formation in the rat. Carcinogenesis 23: 1243–1249 (*Hexachlorobenzene, an epigenetic carcinogen, induces gender-specific long-term alterations in intercellular gap junctional communication in female rat liver; this effect appears to be a critical mechanism in liver carcinogenesis and tumor promotion)*

Pohl L R, Satoh H, Christ D D, Kenna J G 1988 The immunologic and metabolic basis of drug hypersensitivities. Annu Rev Pharmacol 28: 367–387

Pumford N R, Halmes N C 1997 Protein targets of xenobiotic reactive intermediates. Annu Rev Pharmacol Toxicol 37: 91–117 (*Intrinsic versus idiosyncratic toxicity*)

Raffray M, Cohen G M 1997 Apoptosis and necrosis in toxicology: a continuum or distinct modes of cell death? Pharmacol Ther 75: 153–177 (*Essentially distinct processes with only limited molecular overlap*)

Rawlins M D, Thomson J W 1985 Mechanisms of adverse drug reactions. In: Davies D M (ed) Textbook of adverse drug reactions, 3rd edn. Oxford University Press, Oxford, pp. 12–38 (*Type A/type B classification*)

Scales M D C 1993 Toxicity testing. In: Griffin J P, O'Grady J, Wells F O (eds) The textbook of pharmaceutical medicine. Queen's University Press, Belfast, pp. 53–79 (*Thoughtful review*)

Sjostrom H, Nilsson R 1972 Thalidomide and the power of the drug companies. Penguin Books, London

Svensson C K, Cowen E W, Gaspari A A 2001 Cutaneous drug reactions. Pharmacol Rev 53: 357–380 (*Covers epidemiology, clinical morphology and mechanisms. Assesses current knowledge of four types of cutaneous drug reaction: immediate-type immune-mediated, delayed-type immune-mediated, photosensitivity and autoimmune. Also reviews the role of viral infection as predisposing factor.*)

Uetrecht J 2003 Screening for the potential of a drug candidate to cause idiosyncratic drug reactions. Drug Discov Today 8: 832–837 (*Highlights current mechanistic hypotheses of idiosyncratic drug reactions and discusses future directions in the development of better predictive tests*)

Walker D K 2004 The use of pharmacokinetic and pharmacodynamic data in the assessment of drug safety in early drug development. Br J Clin Pharm 58: 601–608 (*Pharmacokinetic profile is a factor in assessing safety during early drug development, especially in relation to safety parameters such as QT interval prolongation, where free plasma concentrations are predictive; procedures are available that allow this on the microdose scale— potential limitations are discussed*)

Weisburge J H, Williams G M 1984 New, efficient approaches to test for carcinogenicity of chemicals based on their mechanisms of action. In: Zbinden G et al. (eds) Current problems in drug toxicology. Libbey, Paris (*Scheme of classification of carcinogens*)

Lifestyle drugs and drugs in sport

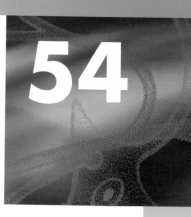

54

OVERVIEW

The term *lifestyle drugs* refers to an eclectic group of drugs that are used for non-medical purposes. It includes drugs of abuse, drugs used to enhance athletic performance, and those taken for cosmetic purposes or for purely social reasons. The pharmacology of these agents, many of which are also used as conventional therapeutic agents, is dealt with elsewhere in this book. In this chapter, we present an overall summary of the classes of drugs that are used for non-medical purposes, and discuss some of the social and medico-legal problems associated with their growing use. Drugs, officially prohibited, that are used to enhance sporting performance represent a special category of lifestyle drugs. A wide range of drugs are used for this purpose, and their pharmacological properties are described in other chapters. Here we discuss specific issues relating to their use in competitive sports.

WHAT IS A LIFESTYLE DRUG?

The term *lifestyle drugs* is of fairly recent origin and not precisely defined. The most commonly accepted definition refers to a drug or medicine that is used to satisfy an aspiration or a non-health related goal, or alternatively a drug or medicine used for treating problems that lie at the margins of health and well-being. Examples include the use of the antihypertensive **minoxidil** for treating baldness and

sildenafil for erectile difficulties in the absence of underlying disease. Oral contraceptives, which clearly lie in the domain of mainstream medicine, could be considered lifestyle drugs. The term is also used to describe medicines that are used to treat 'lifestyle illnesses', that is to say diseases that arise through 'lifestyle choices' such as smoking, alcoholism or overeating, and there are many other shades of meaning as well. Some also include in this category food supplements and other related preparations that are taken by the general public from choice, even when there is no good evidence that they are effective.

CLASSIFICATION OF LIFESTYLE DRUGS

To classify all the different drugs or medicines that might fall into the lifestyle category, and provide a standard universally acceptable definition, is therefore difficult, and cuts across the pharmacological classification used throughout this book. The classification scheme summarised in Table 54.1 is based on the work of Gilbert et al. (2000) and Young (2003). This scheme embraces drugs that have been used for lifestyle choices based on historical precedent, such as oral contraceptives, as well as agents used to manage potentially debilitating lifestyle illnesses such as addiction to smoking (e.g. **bupropion**). It also includes drugs such as **caffeine** and **alcohol** that are consumed on a mass scale around the world, and drugs of abuse such as **cocaine** as well as nutritional supplements.

Drugs can, over time, switch from 'lifestyle' to 'mainstream' use. For example, atropine (Ch. 10) was first used as a beauty aid based on its ability to dilate the pupil. Cocaine (see Fig. 54.1) was first described as a lifestyle drug in use by the Indians in South America. Early explorers commented that it 'satisfies the hungry, gives new strength to the weary and exhausted and makes the unhappy forget their sorrows'. Subsequently assimilated into European medicine as a local anaesthetic (Ch. 44), it is now largely returned to lifestyle drug status and, regrettably, is the basis of an illegal multimillion dollar international drugs industry. **Cannabis** is another good example of a drug that has been considered (in the west at least) as a purely recreational drug but which is now (as **tetrahydrocannabinol**) in clinical trial for the relief of chronic pain and nausea (see Chs 15 and 43).

Many widely used lifestyle drugs consist of natural products (e.g. ginkgo extracts, melatonin, St John's wort, cinchona extracts), whose manufacture and sale is not generally controlled by regulatory bodies. Their composition is therefore highly variable, and their efficacy and safety are often not adequately tested. Many

Table 54.1 Lifestyle drugs and medicines, excluding drugs in sport

Category	Example(s)	Chapter	Primary clinical use	'Lifestyle' use
Medicines approved for specific indications that can also be used to satisfy 'lifestyle choices' or to treat 'lifestyle diseases'	Sildenafil	30	Erectile dysfunction	Erectile dysfunction
	Oral contraceptives	30	Preventing conception	Preventing conception
	Orlistat	27	Obesity	Weight loss
	Sibutramine	27	Anorectic agent	Weight loss
	Bupropion	37	Managing nicotine addiction	Managing nicotine addiction
	Methadone	41	Managing opiate addiction	Managing opiate addiction
Medicines approved for specific indications but that can also be used for for other 'lifestyle' purposes	Minoxidil	19	Hypertension	Regrowth of hair
	Finasteride	24	Prostatic hypertrophy	Regrowth of hair
	Opiates	41	Analgesia	Recreational
Drugs that have slight or no current clinical use but which fall into the lifestyle category	Alcohol	43	None as such	Widespread as a component of drinks
	Botulinum toxin	10	Relief of muscle spasm	Cosmetic alteration
	Caffeine	42	Migraine treatment	Widespread as a component of drinks
	Cannabis	15, 43	Managing chronic pain and muscle spasm (under investigation)	'Recreational' usage
Drugs (generally illegal) that have no clinical utility but which are used to satisfy lifestyle requirements	Methylenedioxymethamphetamine (MDMA, 'ecstasy')	42	None as such	Recreational usage
	Tobacco (nicotine)	43	Patches for tobacco addiction only	Recreational use
	Cocaine (some formulations)	44	Local anaesthesia (largely obsolete)	Recreational use
Natural products, largely unregulated but with many (often anecdotal and unsubstantiated) claims about their action or safety but which often cater to lifestyle needs or desires	Fish oils	–	Slight—perhaps as nutritional supplements	Widespread, for many conditions
	Ascorbic acid	–	Slight—perhaps as nutritional supplements	Widespread, for many conditions
	Melatonin	–	None	Widespread, for many conditions
	Numerous herbal and other preparations	–	None	Widespread, for many conditions

(After Gilbert et al. 2000 and Young 2003.)

contain active substances that, like synthetic drugs, can produce adverse as well as beneficial effects.

DRUGS IN SPORT

The use of drugs to enhance sporting performance is evidently widespread although officially prohibited. The World Anti-Doping Agency (http://www.wada-ama.org) publishes an annually updated list of prohibited substances that may not be used by sportsmen or sportswomen either in or out of competition. Drug testing is based mainly on analysis of blood or urine samples according to strictly defined protocols. The chemical analyses, which rely mainly on gas chromatography/mass spectrometry or immunoassay techniques, must be carried out by approved laboratories.

Table 54.2 summarises the main classes of drugs that are prohibited for use in sports. Athletes are easily persuaded of the potential of a wide variety of drugs to increase their chances of winning, but it should be emphasised that in very few cases have controlled trials shown that the drugs actually improve sporting performance, and indeed many such trials have proved negative. However, marginal improvements in performance (often 1% or less), which are difficult to measure experimentally, make the difference between

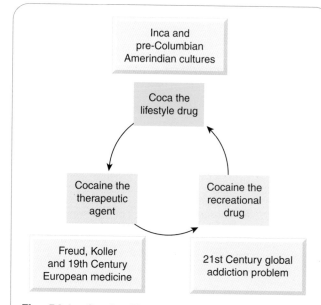

Fig. 54.1 Cocaine: lifestyle drug, therapeutic drug and now recreational drug.

winning and losing, and the competitive instincts of athletes and their trainers generally carry more weight than scientific evidence.

A brief account of some of the more important drugs in common use follows. For a broader and more complete coverage, see British Medical Association (2002) and Mottram (2005).

ANABOLIC STEROIDS

Anabolic steroids (Ch. 30) include a large group of compounds with testosterone-like effects, including about 50 named compounds on the prohibited list. New chemical derivatives ('designer steroids') are regularly developed and offered illicitly to athletes, which represents a continuing problem to the authorities charged with detecting and identifying them. A further problem is that some drugs in use are endogenous compounds or their metabolites, making it difficult to prove that the substance had been administered illegally. Isotope ratio techniques, based on the fact that endogenous and

exogenous steroids have slightly different $^{12}C:^{13}C$ ratios, may enable the two to be distinguished analytically.

Anabolic steroids produce long-term effects and are normally used throughout training, rather than during competition, so out-of-competition testing is necessary.

Although anabolic steroids, when given in combination with training and high protein intake, undoubtedly increase muscle mass and body weight, there is little evidence that they increase muscle strength over and above the effect of training, or that they improve sporting performance. On the other hand, have serious long-term effects, including male infertility, female masculinisation, liver and kidney tumours, hypertension and increased cardiovascular risk, and in adolescents premature skeletal maturation causing irreversible cessation of growth. Anabolic steroids produce a feeling of physical well-being and increased aggressiveness, sometimes progressing to actual psychosis. Depression is common when the drugs are stopped, sometimes leading to long-term psychiatric problems.

Clenbuterol, a β-adrenoceptor antagonist (see Ch. 11), has recently come into use by athletes. Through an unknown mechanism of action, it produces anabolic effects similar to those of androgenic steroids, with apparently fewer adverse effects. It can be detected in urine and is banned for use in sport.

There is little evidence that anabolic drugs, despite their clear-cut physical effects, enhance sporting performance.

HUMAN GROWTH HORMONE

The use of human growth hormone (hGH; see Ch. 28) by athletes followed the availability of the recombinant form of hGH, used to treat endocrine disorders. It must be given by injection, carrying a risk of transmission of infections such as HIV and hepatitis. Its effects appear to be similar to those of anabolic steroids, and hGH is reported to produce a similar feeling of well-being, although without the accompanying aggression and changes in sexual development and behaviour. It increases lean body mass and reduces body fat, but its effects on muscle strength and athletic performance are unclear. It is claimed to increase the rate of recovery from tissue injury, allowing more intensive training routines to be followed.

The main adverse effect of hGH is the development of acromegaly, causing overgrowth of the jaw and thickening of the fingers (Ch. 28), but it may also lead to cardiac hypertrophy and cardiomyopathy, and possibly also an increased cancer risk.

Detection of hGH administration is difficult because physiological secretion is pulsatile, so normal plasma concentrations vary widely. The plasma half-life is short (20–30 min), and only trace amounts are excreted in urine. However, secreted hGH consists of three isoforms varying in molecular weight, whereas recombinant hGH contains only one, so measuring the relative amounts of the isoforms can be used to detect the exogenous material.

Growth hormone acts partly by releasing insulin-like growth factor from the liver, and insulin-like growth factor itself is coming into use by athletes.

Another hormone, **erythropoietin,** which increases erythrocyte production (see Ch. 22) is given by injection for days or weeks to increase the erythrocyte count and hence the O_2-carrying

Table 54.2 Drugs used in sport

Drug class	Example(s)	Effects	Detection	Notes
Anabolic agents	Androgenic steroids (testosterone, nandrolone and many others; Ch. 30)	Mainly increased muscle development. Increases aggression. Serious long-term side effects (see text).	Urine or blood samples	Many are endogenous compounds, so results significantly outside the physiological range are required.
	Clenbuterol (Ch. 11)	Combined anabolic and agonist action on β_2 adrenoceptors, which may increase muscle strength.		Human chorionic gonadotrophin sometimes used by athletes to increase androgen secretion.
Hormones and related substances	Erythropoietin (Ch. 22)	Increased erythrocyte formation, leading to increased oxygen transport. Increased blood viscosity, causing hypertension and risk of strokes and coronary attacks. Used mainly for endurance sports.	Plasma half-life is short, so detection is difficult	Use of other plasma markers indicating erythropoietin administration may be possible. 'Blood doping' (removal of 1–2 l of blood in advance, followed by retransfusion before competition) has similar effect, even more difficult to detect.
	Human growth hormone (Ch. 28)	Increases lean body mass and reduces body fat. May accelerate recovery from tissue injury. Adverse effects include cardiac hypertrophy, acromegaly, liver damage, increased cancer risk.	Blood testing. Distinguishing endogenous (highly variable) from exogenous human growth factor is difficult	–
	Insulin (Ch. 26)	Sometimes used (with glucose so as to avoid hypoglycaemia) to promote glucose uptake and energy production in muscle. Probably ineffective in improving performance.	Plasma samples	–
β_2-adrenoceptor agonists (Ch. 11)	Salbutamol and others	Used by runners, cyclists, swimmers, etc. with the aim of increasing oxygen uptake (by bronchodilatation) and cardiac function. Controlled studies show no improvement in performance.	Urine samples	–
β-adrenoceptor antagonists (Ch. 11)	Propranolol etc.	Used to reduce tremor and anxiety in certain 'precision' sports (shooting, gymnastics, diving, etc.)	Urine samples	Not banned in most sports where they impair, rather than improve performance.
'Stimulants' (Ch. 42)	Ephedrine and derivatives Amphetamines Cocaine Caffeine	Many trials show slight increase in muscle strength and performance in non-endurance events (sprint, swimming, field events, etc.)	Urine samples	The most widely used group, along with anabolic steroids.
Diuretics (Ch. 24)	Thiazides, furosemide	Used mainly to achieve rapid weight loss before weighing in. Also to mask presence of other agents in urine by dilution.	Urine samples	–
Narcotic analgesics (Ch. 41)	Codeine, morphine, etc.	Used to mask injury-associated pain.	Urine samples	–

capacity of blood. The development of recombinant erythropoietin has made it widely available, and detection of its use is difficult. It carries a risk of neurologic disease and thrombosis.

STIMULANT DRUGS

The main drugs of this type used by athletes and officially prohibited are ephedrine and methylephedrine; various amphetamines and similar drugs, such as fenfluramine and methylphenidate; cocaine; and a variety of other CNS stimulants such as nikethamide, amiphenazole and strychnine (see Ch. 42). Caffeine is also used.

In contrast to steroids, some trials have shown these drugs to improve performance in events such as sprinting and weightlifting, and under experimental conditions they increase muscle strength and reduce muscle fatigue significantly. The psychological effect of stimulants is probably more relevant than their physiological effects. Surprisingly, caffeine appears to be more consistently effective in improving muscle performance than other more powerful stimulants.

Several deaths have occurred among athletes taking amphetamines and ephedrine-like drugs in endurance events. The main causes are coronary insufficiency, associated with hypertension; hyperthermia, associated with cutaneous vasoconstriction; and dehydration.

CONCLUSION

The recent lifestyle drugs debate is one aspect of the broader long-standing question of what constitutes 'disease' and how far medical science should go in attempting to alleviate human distress and dysfunction in the absence of pathological disease, or to enhance the perceived well-being of healthy individuals. Discussion of these issues is beyond the scope of this book but can be found in articles cited at the end of this chapter.

There are several reasons why the lifestyle drug phenomenon—no matter how we choose to define it—is of increasing concern. The increasing availability of information about illness through the Internet, as well as the direct advertising by the pharmaceutical industry to the public that occurs in some countries, will ensure that demand is kept buoyant, and the pharmaceutical sector will undoubtedly develop more lifestyle agents. The lobbying power of patients for particular drugs regardless of the potential costs or proven utility is causing major problems for drug regulators and those who set healthcare priorities for state-funded systems of social medicine.

From a pharmacological perspective, it is fair to say that the use of drugs to enhance sporting performance carries many risks and is of very doubtful efficacy. Its growing prevalence reflects many of the same pressures as those driving the introduction of lifestyle drugs, namely the desire to improve on human attributes that are not impaired by disease, coupled with disregard for scientific evidence relating to efficacy and risk.

> **Drugs in sport**
>
> - Many drugs of different types are commonly used by sportsmen and sportswomen with the aim of improving performance in competition.
> - The main types used are:
>   - anabolic agents, mainly androgenic steroids and clenbuterol
>   - hormones, particularly erythropoietin and human growth hormone
>   - stimulants, mainly amphetamine and ephedrine derivatives and caffeine
>   - β-adrenoceptor antagonists, to reduce anxiety and tremor in 'accuracy' sports.
> - The use of drugs in sport is officially prohibited—in most cases, in or out of competition.
> - Detection depends mainly on analysis of the drug or its metabolites in urine or blood samples. Detection of abuse is difficult for endogenous hormones such as erythropoietin, growth hormone and testosterone.
> - Controlled trials have mostly shown that drugs produce no improvement in sporting performance. Anabolic agents increase body weight and muscle volume without clearly increasing strength. The effect of stimulants is psychological rather than physiological.

REFERENCES AND FURTHER READING

Lifestyle drugs and medicines, and general reading

Atkinson T 2002 Lifestyle drug market booming. Nat Med 8: 909 (*Interesting comments on the financial value of this sector*)

Flower R J 2004 Lifestyle drugs: pharmacology and the social agenda. Trends Pharmacol Sci 25: 182–185 (*Accessible review that enlarges on some of the issues raised in this chapter*)

Gilbert D, Walley T, New B 2000 Lifestyle medicines. Br Med J 321: 1341–1344. (*Short but focused review dealing mainly with the clinical implications of the 'lifestyle medicine' phenomenon*)

Lexchin J 2001 Lifestyle drugs: issues for debate. CMAJ 164: 1449–1451 (*Excellent review highlighting many important issues*)

Walley T 2002 Lifestyle medicines and the elderly. Drugs Aging 19: 163–168 (*Excellent review of the whole area and its relevance to the treatment of the elderly*)

Young S N 2003 Lifestyle drugs, mood, behaviour and cognition. J Psychiatry Neurosci 28: 87–89

Drugs in sport

British Medical Association 2002 Drugs in sport: the pressure to perform. BMJ Publications, London (*Useful coverage of the whole topic*)

Mottram D R (ed) 2005 Drugs in sport, 4th edn. Routledge, London (*Comprehensive description of pharmacological and regulatory aspects of drugs in sport, with balanced discussion of evidence relating to efficacy and risk*)

55

Biopharmaceuticals and gene therapy

OVERVIEW

In this chapter, we review the impact of two therapeutic concepts based on our growing understanding and skill in manipulating genes. *Biopharmaceuticals* is an umbrella term applied to the use of nucleic acids or 'engineered' proteins and antibodies in medicine, while *gene therapy* refers specifically to attempts to use those nucleic acids to reprogram cells to prevent, alleviate or cure disease. Of the two, the former has already proved itself in the clinic, whereas the latter has not yet led to licensed products, although there are many ongoing trials, and it is clear that once the last remaining technical hurdles have been surmounted, it will hold great promise. In addition to introducing the central concepts in this chapter, we consider the considerable technical problems associated with these therapies, discuss safety issues, and review the progress made to date.

INTRODUCTION

The 'molecular biology revolution', which had its roots in the discovery of the structure of DNA in the 1950s, and the advances in cell biology that followed in its train, has provided us with the knowledge and ability to manipulate the genetic material from cells in ways that are useful in practical therapeutics. The seductive notion that a gene of interest can be isolated and prepared in such a way that it can be expressed in vitro to generate useful proteins that could not be prepared synthetically or, more daringly, that a gene could be directly introduced in vivo and persuaded to synthesise some crucial cellular component, has driven this field at breakneck speed.

Biopharmaceuticals (considered for the purposes of this chapter to comprise genetically engineered proteins) are already a well-recognised part of therapy, and we have already encountered some of them elsewhere in this book (see for example the 'humanised monoclonal' anti–tumour necrosis factor antibodies in Ch. 14). There are still many problems that have to be surmounted in this area, not the least of which is the cost of manufacture, but the technology is established and maturing fast. Reviewing the area in 2004, Walsh noted that some 140 biopharmaceuticals had been licensed around the world by the previous year, and that 250 million patients were receiving these products at a cost of some US $30 billion.

While the same basic concepts and technologies underpin both these approaches, gene therapy is the more considerable challenge. However, the idea commands such appeal that vast resources (both public and private) have been committed to its development. There are several reasons for this appeal. First, the approach offers the potential for radical cure of single-gene diseases such as *cystic fibrosis* and the *haemoglobinopathies*, which are collectively responsible for much misery throughout the world. Second, many other more common conditions, including malignant, neurodegenerative and infectious diseases, have a large genetic component. Conventional treatment of such disorders is, as readers of this book will appreciate, woefully inadequate, so the promise of a completely new approach has enormous attraction. Finally, an ability to control gene expression could revolutionise the management of diseases in which there is no genetic component at all.

The gurus are emphatic that 'the conceptual part of the gene therapy revolution has indeed occurred...'—so where are the therapies? The devil, of course, is in the detail: in this case, the details of:

- pharmacokinetics, delivery of the gene to appropriate target cells
- pharmacodynamics, the controlled expression of the gene in question
- safety
- clinical efficacy and long-term practicability.

But perhaps the most fundamental hurdle is the delivery problem; here, modern virology has helped with techniques borrowed from viruses that can be used to introduce functional nucleic acids into mammalian cells. The principle is so simple that any broadsheet reader can apprehend it, and the potential rewards (humanitarian, scientific and commercial) so great, that it has led inevitably to great expectations and, perhaps equally inevitably, to frustration at the lack of practical progress.

There is a broad consensus that attempts at gene therapy should focus on somatic cells, and a moratorium has been agreed on therapies intended to alter the DNA of germ cells and hence influence future generations.

BIOPHARMACEUTICALS

We consider first the use of proteins as therapeutic agents. Of course, this in itself is not a novel idea; insulin, extracted from animal pancreas tissue (Ch. 26), and human growth hormone, extracted from human cadaver pituitary glands (Ch. 28), were among the first therapeutic proteins to be used, and for many years provided the only option for treating hormone deficiency disorders. However, there were problems. First, there were difficulties in extraction and the problem of low yields. Second, in the case of the insulin, administration of animal hormones to humans could evoke an

---

Biopharmaceuticals and gene therapy: definition and potential uses 🔑

- *Biopharmaceuticals* include proteins, antibodies (and oligonucleotides) used as drugs.
  - *First-generation* biopharmaceuticals are mainly copies of endogenous proteins or antibodies, produced by recombinant DNA technology.
  - *Second-generation* biopharmaceuticals have been 'engineered' to improve the performance of the protein or antibody.
- Applications:
  - therapeutic monoclonal antibodies
  - recombinant hormones.
- *Gene therapy* is the genetic modification of cells to prevent, alleviate or cure disease.
- Potential applications:
  - radical cure of monogenic diseases (e.g. cystic fibrosis, haemoglobinopathies)
  - amelioration of diseases with or without a genetic component, including many malignant, neurodegenerative and infectious diseases.

---

immune response. Third, there was always a danger of the transmission of infectious agents across species, or between people. This was highlighted in the 1970s, when cases of Creutzfeldt–Jakob disease (see Ch. 35) occurred in patients treated with human growth hormone obtained from cadavers. This serious problem was later traced to contamination of the donor pituitary glands with infectious prions (Ch. 35). The advent of 'genetic engineering' techniques offered a new way to deal with these perennial problems.

PROTEINS AND POLYPEPTIDES

The biopharmaceuticals in use today are generally classified as 'first-' or 'second-' generation agents. *First-generation* biopharmaceuticals are usually simply straightforward copies of human hormones or other proteins prepared by *transfecting* the human gene into a suitable *expression system* (a cell line that produces the protein in good yield), harvesting and purifying the *recombinant* protein produced and using this as the drug. The first agent to be produced in this way was human recombinant insulin in 1982; some others are given in Table 55.1.

Second-generation biopharmaceuticals are those that have been *engineered;* either the gene has been deliberately altered prior to transfection such that the structure of the expressed protein is changed, or some alteration is made to the purified end product. The reasons for making these changes are generally to improve some aspect of the protein's activity profile. Human insulins designed to act faster or last longer (p. 404) were among the first in this class to be marketed; Table 55.1 contains other examples. *Third-generation* agents would be those in which proteins are designed from scratch to do a particular biological function. This technology is still some way off.

PROBLEMS IN MANUFACTURE

There are several problems associated with the manufacture of any type of recombinant protein, and one of the most pressing is the choice of expression system. Many recombinant proteins are expressed in bacterial systems (*Escherichia coli* for example), which are useful because cultures grow quickly and they are generally easy to manipulate. Disadvantages include the fact that they may contain bacterial endotoxins, which must be scrupulously removed before administration to patients, and that bacterial cells do not accomplish the same type of *post-translational processing* (e.g. glycosylation) as mammalian cells. This could pose problems if the protein's action is crucially dependent on this modification. To circumvent these problems, mammalian (e.g. Chinese hamster ovary, CHO) cells are also used as expression systems, although here the problem is often one of yield. Such cells require more careful culture, grow more slowly and produce less product, all of which contribute to the expense of the final medicine.

There are, however, a number of emergent technologies that could revolutionise the production process. The use of plants to produce recombinant proteins has attracted considerable interest (see Daniell et al., 2001, and Fischer et al., 2004). Several species have shown promise, including the tobacco plant. Human genes of interest can readily be transfected into the plant using tobacco mosaic virus as a vector; the crop grows rapidly (yields a high biomass) and

Table 55.1   Some examples of 'second-generation' biopharmaceuticals

Type of change	Protein	Indication	Reason for change
Altered amino acid sequence	Insulin	Diabetes	Faster-acting hormone
	Tissue plasminogen activator analogues	Thrombolysis	Longer circulating half-life
	Interferon analogue	Antiviral	Superior antiviral action
	Factor VIII analogue	Haemophilia	Smaller molecule with good activity
	Diphtheria toxin–interleukin-2 fusion protein	T-cell lymphoma	Targets toxin to appropriate cells
	Tumour necrosis factor receptor–human immunoglobulin G F_c fusion protein	Rheumatoid disease	Inhibits tumour necrosis factor, long half-life
Altered carbohydrate residues	Glucocerebrosidase enzyme	Gaucher's disease	Promotes phagocyte uptake of enzyme
	Erythropoietin analogue	Anaemia	Prolongs half-life
Covalent attachment to polyethylene glycol	Interferon	Hepatitis C	Prolongs half-life
	Human growth hormone	Acromegaly	Prolongs half-life

(Modified from Walsh, 2004.)

offers a number of other advantages. But attention has also focused on edible plants such as lettuce and bananas. The advantage here is that some orally active proteins, such as vaccines, expressed in the plant could be consumed directly without the need for prior purification. Several proteins have already been produced in plants, and some are in an advanced stage of clinical trial.

Another technology that could dramatically increase the yield of human recombinant proteins is the use of transgenic cattle. A dairy cow can produce some 10 000 litres of milk per year, and recombinant proteins introduced into the genome, and under the control of promoters that regulate production of other milk proteins, can generate yields as high as 1 g/l (see Brink et al., 2000).

'ENGINEERED' PROTEINS

There are several ways in which proteins can be altered prior to expression. Alteration of the nucleotide sequence of the gene coding for the protein in question can be used to change single amino acids or, indeed, whole regions of the polypeptide chain. Alternatively, the protein could be altered after expression by the addition of other chemical groups, such as polyethylene glycol (PEG), that alter its behaviour in vivo. There are good reasons why it is an advantage to 'engineer' proteins prior to expression:

- modification of pharmacokinetic properties
- generation of novel *fusion* or other proteins
- reducing immunogenicity.

It is frequently advantageous to modify the pharmacokinetic properties of recombinant proteins. Changes in the structure of human insulin, for example, provided diabetics with a form of the hormone that did not self-associate during storage and was thus faster acting and easier to manage. The half-life of proteins in the blood can often be extended by *PEGylation*, the addition of PEG

to the molecule. This *post-translational engineering* approach has been applied to some human hormones, such as recombinant growth hormone, interferons and others. Prolonging half-life is not merely a convenience to patients; it also reduces the overall cost of the treatment, and economic factors are important in the adoption of this type of therapy.

Fusion proteins comprise two or more proteins engineered to be expressed as one single polypeptide chain, sometimes joined by a short linker. An example is **etanercept**, an anti-inflammatory used in the treatment of rheumatoid arthritis and other conditions (see Ch. 14). This consists of the ligand-binding domain taken from the tumour necrosis factor receptor, joined to the F_c domain of a human immunoglobulin G antibody. The latter moiety increases its persistence in the blood. The question of reducing immunogenicity through bioengineering will be dealt with below.

MONOCLONAL ANTIBODIES

Although antibodies have always been used clinically (and still are) to confer *passive immunity*, there are a number of disadvantages inherent in their production and use that limit their utility. Conventionally, antisera are produced from the blood of immunised humans (e.g. to collect antitetanus serum) or from animals immunised with the antigen in question (e.g. with inactivated snake toxins). These are converted into serum containing high levels of specific antibodies, which can then be used clinically to neutralise pathogens or other dangerous substances in the blood of the patient.

Such preparations contain *polyclonal antibodies*—that is, a mixture of antibodies from all the plasma cell clones that reacted to that particular antigen. The actual composition and efficacy of these varies over time, and obviously there is a limit to how much plasma one can collect on any one occasion. The development in 1975 of a method of producing from immunised mice an immortalised *hybridoma*, a fusion of one particular lymphocytic clone with an immortalised tumour cell, provided us for the first time with a method of producing *monoclonal antibodies*, comprising a single species of defined antibody at high abundance in vitro. Because these hybridomas were immortal, the cell line could be retained indefinitely and expanded to any density while preserving the integrity of its product.

FIRST-GENERATION MONOCLONAL ANTIBODIES

The monoclonals can also be classified into first- or second-generation reagents along similar lines to other proteins discussed above. First-generation monoclonals were essentially murine monoclonals (or fragments thereof), but these suffered from several drawbacks. As mouse-based proteins, they provoked an immune response in between half and three-quarters of all recipients. Other limiting factors were the short half-life in the circulation and the inability of the mouse antibodies to activate human complement.

Most of these problems have been surmounted by using either *chimeric* or *humanised* monoclonals. The two terms refer to the degree to which the monoclonals have been engineered. Figure 55.1 shows how this is done; the antibody molecule consists of a *constant* domain (F_c) and the *antibody-binding* domain (F_{ab}), with *hypervariable regions* that recognise and bind to the antigen in question. The genes for chimeric monoclonals are engineered to contain the cDNA of the murine F_{ab} domain coupled with the human F_c domain sequences. This greatly (around fivefold) extends the plasma half-life and improves the ability of the antibody to activate human defence mechanisms. A further development (and now the preferred approach) is to replace the entire F_c and F_{ab} region with the human equivalent with the exception of the hypervariable regions, giving a molecule that, while essentially human in nature, contains the murine antibody-binding sites. The anticancer monoclonal **herceptin** (trastuzumab; see Ch. 51) is an example of such a therapeutically useful antibody, and some others are given in Table 55.2.

GENE THERAPY
GENE DELIVERY

The transfer of recombinant nucleic acid into target cells—a special instance of the 'drug distribution' problem—is critical to the success of gene therapy. Nucleic acid must pass from the extracellular

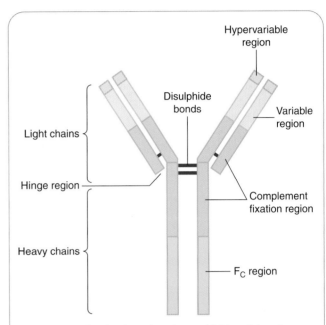

Fig. 55.1   Production of engineered 'chimeric' and 'humanised' monoclonal antibodies. The Y-shaped antibody molecule consists of two main domains: the F_c (constant) domain and the F_{ab} (antibody-binding) domain. At the tip of the F_{ab} regions (on the arms of the 'Y') are the *hypervariable regions* that actually bind the antigen. Chimeric antibodies are produced by replacing the murine F_c region with its human equivalent by altering and splicing the gene. For humanised antibodies, only the murine hypervariable regions are retained, the remainder of the molecule being human in origin. (After Walsh, 2004.)

Table 55.2   Some 'second-generation' therapeutic monoclonal antibodies

Antibody	Type	Target	Use
Infliximab	Chimeric monoclonal	Tumour necrosis factor	Crohn's disease, rheumatoid disease
Adalimumab	Human recombinant monoclonal	Tumour necrosis factor	Rheumatoid disease
Trastuzumab	Humanised monoclonal	Epidermal growth factor receptor	Breast cancer
Palivizumab	Humanised monoclonal	Respiratory syncitial virus	Respiratory infections in young children
Omalizumab	Humanised monoclonal	Immunoglobulin E	Immunoglobulin E–mediated asthma
Basiliximab	Chimeric monoclonal	Interleukin 2 (α chain)	Kidney transplant rejection

(Source: Walsh 2004 and British National Formulary.)

space across the plasma and nuclear membranes, and it must then be incorporated into the chromosomes. Because DNA is highly negatively charged and single genes have molecular weights around 10^4 times greater than conventional drugs, the problem is of a different order from the equivalent stage of routine drug development.

There are several important considerations in choosing a delivery system; these include:

- the *capacity* of the system (e.g. how much DNA it can carry)
- the *transfection efficiency* (how many cells it can infect)
- the *lifetime* of the transfected material (depends on the cell type)
- the *safety issue*, especially important in the case of viral systems.

Various approaches have been developed (see Table 55.3) in an attempt to produce the optimal system.

There are two main strategies for delivering genes into patients: the in vivo and ex vivo approach. Using the former strategy, the *vector* containing the therapeutic gene is injected into the patient, either intravenously (in which case some form of organ or tissue targeting is required) or directly into the target tissue (e.g. a malignant tumour). The ex vivo strategy is to remove cells from the patient (e.g. stem cells from marrow or circulating blood, or myoblasts from a biopsy of striated muscle), treat them with the vector and inject the genetically altered cells back into the patient.

An ideal vector should be *safe*, highly *efficient* (i.e. insert the therapeutic gene into a high proportion of target cells) and *selective* in that it would lead to expression of the therapeutic protein in the target cells but not to the expression of viral proteins. Provided that the cell into which it is inserted is itself long-lived, the vector should ideally cause persistent expression, avoiding the need for repeated treatment. The latter consideration can be a problem in some tissues. In the autosomal recessive disorder *cystic fibrosis*, for example, the airway epithelium malfunctions because it lacks a membrane Cl^- transporter known as the *cystic fibrosis transport regulator* (CFTR). Epithelial cells in the airways are continuously dying off and being replaced, so even if the *CFTR* gene were stably transfected into the epithelium, there would still be a periodic need for further treatment unless the gene could be inserted into the progenitor (stem) cells. Similar problems are anticipated in other cells that turn over continuously, such as gastrointestinal epithelium and skin.

VIRAL VECTORS

Many contemporary gene delivery strategies aim to capitalise on the capacity of viruses to subvert the transcriptional machinery of the cells they invade and their ability (in some cases) to fuse with the host genome. While producing a tantalising glimpse of the possible, there remain substantial practical problems with this approach, partly because as viruses have evolved the means to invade human cells, so humans have evolved immune responses and other protective mechanisms to thwart them. Although irritating in some respects, this is not all bad news from the point of view of safety.

Retroviruses

If introduced into stem cells, retroviral vectors have the attraction that their effects are persistent because they are incorporated into, and replicate with, host DNA, and so the 'therapeutic' gene is passed down to each daughter cell during division. Against this, retroviruses randomly insert into chromosomes, so they may cause damage (see below), and because they show little specificity they could infect germ or non-target cells and produce undesired effects if administered in vivo. For this reason, retroviruses are mainly used for ex vivo gene therapy.

The life cycle of naturally occurring retroviruses may be exploited to create useful vectors for gene therapy (see Fig. 55.2). In the future, it is hoped to alter the retroviral envelope to increase specificity, so that the vector could be administered systemically but would target only the desired cell population. An example of this approach is the substitution of the envelope protein of a non-pathogenic vector (e.g. mouse leukaemia virus) with the envelope protein of human vesicular stomatitis virus, in order specifically to target human epithelial cells. Most retrovirus vectors are unable

Table 55.3 Delivery systems for gene therapy

Vector	Advantages	Disadvantages
Liposomes	Virus-free	Low efficiency, sometimes cytotoxic
DNA cassettes	Virus-free	Low efficiency, expression temporary
Herpes simplex virus type I	Highly infective, persistent expression	No integration with host DNA, cytotoxic, difficult to handle
Adenovirus	Highly infective in epithelia	Immunogenic and temporary
Adeno-associated virus	Stable	Low capacity, requires a helper virus
Retrovirus	Efficient, permanent	Low capacity, unstable, must integrate into host DNA

(After Wolf & Jenkins, 2002.)

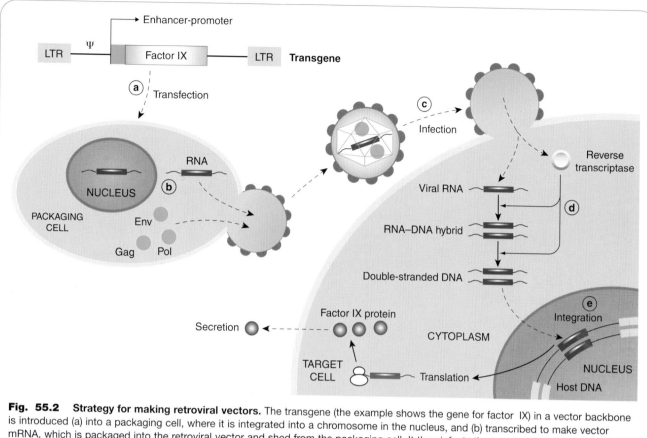

Fig. 55.2 Strategy for making retroviral vectors. The transgene (the example shows the gene for factor IX) in a vector backbone is introduced (a) into a packaging cell, where it is integrated into a chromosome in the nucleus, and (b) transcribed to make vector mRNA, which is packaged into the retroviral vector and shed from the packaging cell. It then infects the target cell (c). Virally encoded reverse transcriptase (d) converts vector RNA into an RNA–DNA hybrid, and then into double-stranded DNA, which is integrated (e) into the genome of the target cell. It can then be transcribed and translated to make factor IX protein. (Redrawn from Verma I M, Somia N 1997 Nature 389: 239–242.)

to penetrate the nuclear envelope, and because the nuclear membrane dissolves during cell division, only infect dividing cells and not non-dividing cells such as adult neurons.

Adenovirus

Adenovirus vectors are popular because of the high transgene expression that can be achieved. They transfer genes to the nucleus of the host cell, but (unlike retroviruses) these are not inserted into the host genome and so do not produce effects that outlast the lifetime of the transfected cell. This property also obviates the risk of disturbing the function of other cellular genes and the theoretical risk of carcinogenicity, although at the cost of producing only a temporary effect. Because of these favourable properties, adenovirus vectors have been used for in vivo gene therapy. The vectors are genetically modified by making deletions in the viral genome, rendering it unable to replicate or cause widespread infection in the host while at the same time creating space in the viral genome for the therapeutic transgene to be inserted.

One of the first adenoviral vectors to be used lacked part of a growth-controlling region called E_1. This defective virus was grown in a cell line that substitutes for the missing E_1 function. Recombinant virus was produced by infecting target cells with a plasmid containing the cloned DNA of therapeutic interest plus an expression cassette and portions of adenoviral DNA.

Recombination between this and the 'backbone' of the E_1-deficient adenoviral genome resulted in a virus encoding the desired transgene. This approach led to seemingly spectacular results, demonstrating gene transfer to cell lines and animal models of disease, but it has been disappointing (e.g. in cystic fibrosis) in humans. The main problem is that low doses (administered by aerosol to patients with this disease) produce only a very low-efficiency transfer, whereas higher doses cause inflammation, a host immune response and short-lived gene expression. Furthermore, treatment cannot be repeated because of neutralising antibodies. This has led to recent attempts to manipulate adenoviral vectors to mutate or remove the genes that are most strongly immunogenic.

Other viral vectors

Other potential viral vectors under investigation include *adeno-associated virus*, *herpes virus* and disabled versions of *human immunodeficiency virus* (*HIV*). Adeno-associated virus associates with host DNA but is not activated unless the cell is infected with an adenovirus. It is less immunogenic than other vectors but is hard to mass produce and cannot be used to carry large transgenes. Herpes virus does not associate with host DNA but is very long-lived in nervous tissue and could have a specific application in treating neurological disease. HIV, unlike most other retroviruses (see above), can infect non-dividing cells such as neurons. It is possible to remove the genes from HIV that control replication and substitute other genes. Alternatively, it may prove possible to transfer to other non-pathogenic retroviruses those genes that permit HIV to penetrate the nuclear envelope.

NON-VIRAL VECTORS

Liposomes

Non-viral vectors include a variant of liposomes (Ch. 7). Plasmids (diameter up to approximately 2 μm) are too big to package in regular liposomes (diameter 0.025–0.1 μm), but larger particles can be made from positively charged lipids ('lipoplexes'), which interact with both negatively charged cell membranes and DNA, improving delivery into the cell nucleus and incorporation into the host chromosome. Such particles have been used to deliver the genes for HLA-B7, interleukin-2 and CFTR. They are much less efficient than viruses, and attempts are currently under way to improve this by incorporating various viral signal proteins (membrane fusion proteins, for example) in their outer coat. Direct injection of these complexes into solid tumours (e.g. melanoma, breast, kidney and colon cancers) can, however, achieve high local concentrations within the tumour.

Microspheres

Biodegradable microspheres made from polyanhydride copolymers of fumaric and sebacic acids (see Ch. 7) can be loaded with plasmid DNA. A plasmid with bacterial β-galactosidase activity formulated in this way and given by mouth to rats has resulted in systemic absorption and expression of the bacterial enzyme in the rat liver, raising the possibility of oral gene therapy!

Plasmid DNA

Surprisingly, it has emerged that plasmid DNA itself ('naked DNA') enters the nucleus of some cells and is expressed, albeit much less efficiently than when it is packaged in a vector. Such DNA carries no risk of viral replication and is not usually immunogenic (although autoantibodies to DNA do occur in systemic lupus erythematosus), but it cannot be targeted to a cell of interest. There is considerable interest in the possibility of using naked DNA for vaccines, because even very small amounts of foreign protein can stimulate an immune response. Such a vaccine for influenza is in clinical development, and more ambitious long-term targets include malaria, tuberculosis, *Chlamydia*, *Helicobacter* and hepatitis.

CONTROLLING GENE EXPRESSION

To realise the full potential of gene therapy, it is not enough to transfer the gene selectively to the desired target cells and maintain acceptable expression of its product—difficult though these goals are—it is also essential that the activity of the gene is controlled. Historically, it was the realisation of the magnitude of this task that diverted attention from the haemoglobinopathies (which were the first projected targets of gene therapy). Correction of these disorders demands an appropriate balance of normal α- and β-globin chain synthesis to be effective and for this, and many other potential applications, precisely controlled gene expression will be essential.

It has not yet proved possible to control transgenes in human recipients, but there are techniques that may enable us to achieve this goal. One hinges on the use of a *tetracycline-inducible expression system*. This was first applied in cultured cells and subsequently in vivo in the mouse. Myoblasts were engineered for doxycycline-inducible and skeletal muscle–specific expression of erythropoietin by the use of two retroviral vectors. After intramuscular injection of these cells, transgene expression was detectable in skeletal muscle of the recipient, and it was possible to 'switch' erythropoietin production 'on' or 'off' by treatment with, or withdrawal of, doxycycline (Fig. 55.3). To pursue this strategy further, it will be necessary to discover how physiological stimuli might control expression of the therapeutic gene. This will clearly be a great deal more difficult for situations where very rapid responses (e.g. to changing blood glucose in a diabetic) are required.

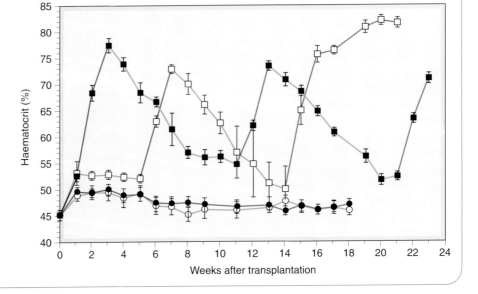

Fig. 55.3 Control of erythropoietin secretion by doxycycline in mice. The mice were transplanted with myoblasts containing an erythropoietin transgene with (squares) or without (circles) a second transgene that confers doxycycline inducibility. Intermittent administration of doxycycline in the drinking water (indicated in red) 'turned on' the secretion of erythropoietin (and hence increased haematocrit) over a 5-month period in the animals that had received the doxycycline inducibility gene. (From Bohl D, Naffakh N, Heard J M 1997 Nat Med 3: 299–305.)

The control of transfected genes is important in gene targeting as well. If it were possible to splice the gene of interest with a tissue-specific promoter, then it would be possible, in theory at least, to inject the vector systemically in the knowledge that the gene would be expressed only in the target tissue. Such an approach has been used in the design of gene therapy constructs for use in ovarian cancer that express several proteins at high abundance, including the proteinase inhibitor SLP1. By using the SLP1 promoter, plasmids carrying various genes were successfully and selectively expressed in ovarian cancer cell lines (Wolf & Jenkins, 2002).

SAFETY

In addition to safety concerns specific to any particular therapy (e.g. polycythaemia, thrombosis and hypertension from overexpression of erythropoietin; see above and Fig. 55.3), a number of concerns relate generally to the use of viral vectors. These are usually selected because they are non-pathogenic, or modified to render them innocuous, but there is a concern that such agents might still acquire virulence during use. Retroviruses, which insert randomly into host DNA, could damage the genome and interfere with the protective mechanisms that normally regulate the cell cycle (see Ch. 5), and if they happen to disrupt essential cellular functions this could increase the risk of malignancy. This risk is more than a theoretical possibility; a child treated for severe combined immunodeficiency (SCID; see below) developed a leukaemia-like illness. The retroviral vector was shown to have inserted itself into a gene called *LMO-2*. Mutations of *LMO-2* are associated with childhood cancers.

Another problem is that immunogenic viral proteins may be expressed that elicit an inflammatory response, and this could be harmful in some situations (e.g. in the airways of patients with cystic fibrosis). Initial clinical experience was reassuring, but the tragic death of Jesse Gelsinger, an 18-year-old volunteer in a gene therapy trial for the non-fatal disease *ornithine transcarbamylase deficiency* (which can be controlled by diet and drugs) led to the appreciation that safety concerns related to immune-mediated responses to vectors are very real. Protocol violations were exposed, and subsequently six further linked, but previously unreported, deaths were discovered in two other gene therapy programmes. The possible influence of commercial interests on reporting of such events was much discussed at the time (see *References and further reading*), and the issue of the appropriate level of public scrutiny of such studies is still under debate.

SOME THERAPEUTIC ASPECTS

SINGLE-GENE DEFECTS

Single-gene (*monogenic*) disorders are individually relatively uncommon, but because of their nature seemed to be the obvious starting point for gene therapy trials. The haemoglobinopathies were the first projected targets, but early attempts (in the 1980s) were put 'on hold' because of the problem, mentioned above, posed by the need to control precisely the expression of the genes encoding

---

Gene delivery and expression

- Gene delivery is one of the main hurdles to practical gene therapy.
- Recombinant genes are transferred using a *vector*, often a suitably modified virus.
- There are two main strategies for delivering genes into patients:
  - *in vivo* injection of the vector directly into the patient (e.g. into a malignant tumour)
  - *ex vivo* treatment of cells from the patient (e.g. stem cells from marrow or circulating blood), which are then returned to the patient.
- An *ideal vector* would be safe, efficient, selective and produce long-lasting expression of the therapeutic gene.
- *Viral vectors* include retroviruses, adenoviruses, adeno-associated virus, herpesvirus and disabled human immunodeficiency virus (HIV).
  - *Retroviruses* infect many different types of dividing cells and become incorporated randomly into host DNA.
  - *Adenoviruses* are genetically modified to prevent replication and accommodate the therapeutic transgene. They transfer genes to the nucleus but not to the genome of the host cell. Problems include a strong host immune response, inflammation and short-lived expression. Treatment cannot be repeated because of neutralising antibodies.
  - *Adeno-associated* virus associates with host DNA and is non-immunogenic but is hard to mass produce and has a small capacity.
- Herpesvirus does not associate with host DNA but persists in nervous tissue and may be useful in treating neurological disease.
- Disabled versions of HIV differ from most other retroviruses in that they infect non-dividing cells, including neurons.
- Non-viral vectors include:
  - a variant of liposomes, made using positively charged lipids and called 'lipoplexes'
  - biodegradable microspheres, which may offer orally active gene therapy
  - plasmid DNA ('naked DNA'), which can be used as a vaccine.
- A *tetracycline-inducible expression system* or similar technique can control the activity of the therapeutic gene.

---

the different polypeptide chains of the haemoglobin molecule. Patients with thalassaemia (the commonest monogenic disease) exhibit enormous phenotypic diversity and hence variable clinical symptoms, because even in monogenic disorders other genes as well as environmental factors are also important. The focus

Safety

- There are those safety concerns that are *specific* to any particular therapy (e.g. polycythaemia from overexpression of erythropoietin) and additional general concerns relating, for example, to the nature of vectors.
- Viral vectors:
  — might acquire virulence during use
  — contain viral proteins, which may be immunogenic
  — can elicit an inflammatory response
  — could damage the host genome and interfere with the cell cycle, provoking malignancy.
- The limited clinical experience to date has not so far provided evidence of insurmountable problems.

then shifted to a rare genetic disorder called *adenine deaminase deficiency*, which results in SCID. This led to the first therapeutic gene transfer protocol to be approved by the US National Institutes of Health, and subsequently a French team has treated 11 children with another form of SCID. The results provided the first proof that gene therapy can cure a life-threatening disease but also, less happily, evidence that retroviral vectors can cause malignancy.

Precise regulation of therapeutic protein expression may not be essential in the management of some other disorders (e.g. cystic fibrosis and the haemophilias). Attempts to utilise gene therapy for these and for other single-gene disorders continue; protocols that have been approved by the recombinant DNA advisory committee include clinical trials for *α1-antitrypsin deficiency* (which causes chronic lung disease), *chronic granulomatous disease* (an X-linked disease in which neutrophils malfunction), *familial hypercholesterolaemia* (see Ch. 20), *Duchenne muscular dystrophy* (another X-linked disease, in which affected boys become progressively disabled), and various lysosomal storage disorders including *Gaucher's disease* and *Hunter's syndrome* (in which abnormal lipids or mucopolysaccharides accumulate in various organs).

GENE THERAPY FOR CANCER

Approximately half of all current clinical gene therapy research relates to its use in cancer. The first gene transfer experiment to be approved by the National Institutes of Health was a non-therapeutic protocol in the late 1980s designed to introduce a marker gene (conferring resistance to an analogue of neomycin) into a class of lymphocytes that infiltrate various tumours. Gene transfer was performed ex vivo and the cells reinjected into the patient in order to track their subsequent redistribution. This strategy was useful in tracking other cells and hence identifying the cause of relapse following bone marrow transplantation for various leukaemias. Several therapeutic approaches are under investigation, and there is excellent evidence from animal models of their potential utility, although experience with conventional antineoplastic drugs

(Ch. 51) cautions against extrapolation to the clinical situation. Promising approaches include:

- restoring 'protective' proteins such as the tumour suppressor gene p53 (see Ch. 5)
- inactivating oncogene expression (e.g. by using a retroviral vector bearing an antisense transcript RNA to the *k-ras* oncogene; see below)
- delivering a gene to malignant cells that renders them sensitive to drugs (e.g. thymidylate kinase, which activates **ganciclovir**)
- delivery of proteins to healthy host cells in order to protect them (e.g. addition of the multidrug resistance channel to bone marrow cells ex vivo, thereby rendering them resistant to drugs used in chemotherapy)
- tagging cancer cells with genes expressing proteins that render malignant cells more visible to the immune system (e.g. for antigens such as HLA-B7 or cytokines such as granulocyte macrophage colony-stimulating factor and interleukin-2).

Gap junctions between malignant cells may propagate the desired effect, enabling vectors to pass between neighbouring cells. Trials based on these approaches are in progress for head and neck cancer, involving injection into the tumour of recombinant adenoviral vectors containing the human p53 gene, and trials in *glioblastoma* (a brain tumour that affects 4000–5000 people in the UK each year) involving herpesvirus vectors bearing a gene to activate a prodrug. The most clinically advanced programme for glioblastoma currently is a phase III trial using a retroviral vector encoding the herpes simplex virus gene for *thymidylate kinase*, which is administered into the tumour at the time of surgery and may render the tumour susceptible to drugs such as ganciclovir.

Ovarian cancer is considered to be a good target for gene therapy because the vector can be directly introduced into the peritoneal cavity, where it is retained in a 'closed' environment. Several clinical trials are in progress or have been completed (see Wolf & Jenkins, 2002) with a variety of genes including p53 and the multidrug resistance gene, and utilising retroviral, adenoviral and liposome vectors.

Gene therapy for cancer

- Promising approaches include:
  — restoring protective proteins such as p53
  — inactivating oncogenes
  — delivering a gene to malignant cells that renders them sensitive to drugs
  — delivering a gene to healthy host cells to protect them from chemotherapy
  — tagging cancer cells with genes that make them immunogenic.

GENE THERAPY AND INFECTIOUS DISEASE

In addition to DNA vaccines mentioned above, there is considerable interest in the potential of gene therapy for HIV infection. Some 10% of all clinical gene therapy research is focused on this area and, by rendering stem cells (which differentiate into immune cells) resistant to HIV before they mature, aims to prevent HIV replication as well as its spread to uninfected cells. Various strategies are under investigation, including the use of genes that code for variants of HIV-directed proteins that serve as blocking agents (so-called 'dominant-negative' mutations, e.g. *rev*, which began clinical testing in 1995), RNA decoys and soluble forms of CD4 (the cellular receptor used by HIV to enter lymphocytes; Ch. 47) that will bind, and it is hoped inactivate, HIV extracellularly.

GENE THERAPY AND CARDIOVASCULAR DISEASE

Vascular gene transfer is attractive not least because cardiologists and vascular surgeons routinely perform invasive studies that offer the opportunity to administer gene therapy vectors ex vivo (e.g. to a blood vessel that has been removed to use as an autograft) or locally in vivo (e.g. by injection through a catheter directly into a diseased coronary or femoral artery). Vascular gene transfer offers potential new treatments for several cardiovascular diseases (see Ylä-Herttuala & Martin, 2000). The nature of many vascular disorders, such as restenosis following angioplasty (stretching up a narrowed artery using a balloon that can be inflated via a catheter), is such that transient gene expression might be all that is needed therapeutically. There is no shortage of attractive candidates for therapeutic overexpression in blood vessels, including nitric oxide synthase, prostacyclin synthase, thymidylate kinase, cyclin, growth arrest homeobox and many others. Some of these have been studied in animal models of restenosis, finding that overexpression of vascular endothelial growth factor and fibroblast growth factor increases blood flow and collateral vessel growth in ischaemic leg muscle and myocardium. This is a promising area; for a review on angiogenic gene therapy, see Hammond & McKirnan (2001).

OTHER GENE-BASED APPROACHES

So far, we have largely been considering the addition of entire genes, but there are other, related nucleic acid–based therapeutic strategies. One such attempt is to correct a gene that has been adversely altered by mutation. This has the enormous theoretical advantage that the corrected gene would remain under physiological control, avoiding many of the problems discussed above. This approach is in its infancy and is beyond the scope of this book.

Other therapeutic approaches that are, in effect, gene therapies are conventionally excluded from this category. These include organ transplantation to correct a gene deficiency (e.g. liver transplantation to correct low-density lipoprotein receptor deficiency in homozygous familial hypercholesterolaemia; Ch. 20) or the use of conventional drugs to alter gene expression, for example the use of steroids (which can regulate the expression of many genes) or

of **hydroxycarbamide (hydroxyurea)** to increase the expression of γ-chain globin, and hence fetal haemoglobin, thus ameliorating sickle cell anaemia.

Another technique, known as the *antisense oligonucleotide* approach alluded to above, also has enormous theoretical appeal. This uses short (15–25mer) oligonucleotides that are complementary to part of a gene or gene product that it is desired to inhibit. These snippets of genetic material can be designed to influence the expression of a gene either by forming a triplex (three-stranded helix) with a regulatory component of chromosomal DNA, or by complexing a region of mRNA. Oligonucleotides can cross plasma and nuclear membranes by endocytosis as well as by direct diffusion, despite their molecular size and charge. However, there are abundant enzymes that cleave foreign DNA in plasma and in cell cytoplasm, so *methylphosphorate* analogues have been synthesised in which a methyl group substitutes for an oxygen atom in the nucleotide backbone. Another approach is the use of *phosphothiorate* analogues in which a negatively charged sulfur atom substitutes for oxygen (so-called 'S oligomers'). This increases water solubility as well as conferring resistance to enzymic degradation. The oligomer needs to be at least 15 bases long to confer specificity and tight binding.

Following parenteral administration, such oligomers distribute widely (although not to the central nervous system) and work in part by interfering with the transcription of mRNA and in part by stimulating its breakdown by ribonuclease H, which cleaves the bound mRNA. This approach is being used in clinical studies in patients with viral disease (including HIV infection) and malignancy (including the use of *Bcl-2* antisense therapy administered subcutaneously in patients with non-Hodgkin's lymphoma). The use of 'gene silencing' sRNAi constructs also lends itself to this type of approach.

Other gene-based approaches

- Correction of a mutated gene. This is in its infancy.
- *Antisense oligonucleotides* are short (15–25) oligonucleotides that are complementary to part of the target gene and influence expression by forming a triplex (three-stranded helix) with a regulatory component of chromosomal DNA or by complexing a region of mRNA. sRNAi can be used in the same way.
- Oligonucleotides can cross plasma and nuclear membranes but there are abundant enzymes that cleave foreign DNA, so water-soluble methylphosphorate or phosphothiorate analogues, which are resistant to enzymic degradation, are used. This approach is being used in clinical trials in HIV infection and malignancy.

REFERENCES AND FURTHER READING

General reviews on biopharmaceuticals, gene therapy and utilities

Scientific American published an issue devoted to gene therapy in June 1997, which is an excellent introduction, including articles by T Friedmann (on 'overcoming the obstacles to gene therapy'), P L Felgner (on non-viral strategies for gene therapy), R M Blaese (on gene therapy for cancer) and D Y Ho and R M Sapolsky (on gene therapy for the nervous system).

Brink M F, Bishop M D, Pieper F R 2000 Developing efficient strategies for the generation of transgenic cattle which produce biopharmaceuticals in milk. Theriogenology 53: 139–148 (*A bit specialised, as it focuses mainly on the husbandry of transgenic cattle, but interesting nonetheless*)

Daniell H, Streatfield S J, Wycoff K 2001 Medical molecular farming: production of antibodies, biopharmaceuticals and edible vaccines in plants. Trends Plant Sci 6: 219–226 (*Interesting paper with some good examples*)

Fischer R, Stoger E, Schillberg S et al. 2004 Plant-based production of biopharmaceuticals, Curr Opin Plant Biol 7: 152–158. (*Interesting general review on the use of plants for the production of biopharmaceuticals*).

Guttmacher A E, Collins F S 2002 Genomic medicine: a primer. N Engl J Med 347: 1512–1520 (*First in a series on genomic medicine*)

Reichert J M, Healy E M 2001 Biopharmaceuticals approved in the EU 1995–1999: a European Union–United States comparison. Eur J Pharm Biopharm 51: 1–7 (*Lists recently approved biopharmaceuticals*)

Verma I M, Somia N 1997 Gene therapy—promises, problems and prospects. Nature 389: 239–242 (*The authors, from the Salk Institute, describe the principle of getting corrective genetic material into cells to alleviate disease, the practical obstacles to this, and the hopes that better delivery systems will overcome them*)

Walsh G 2004 Second-generation biopharmaceuticals. Eur J Pharm Biopharm 58: 185–196 (*Excellent overview of therapeutic proteins and antibodies; some good tables and figures*)

Weatherall D J 2000 Single gene disorders or complex traits: lessons from the thalassaemias and other monogenic diseases. Br Med J 321: 1117–1120 (*Argues that relating genotype to phenotype is the challenge for genetic medicine over the next century*)

Problems

Anson D S 2004 The use of retroviral vectors for gene therapy—what are the risks? A review of retroviral pathogenesis and its relevance to retroviral vector–mediated gene delivery. Genet Vaccines Ther 2: 9 (*Comprehensive review*)

Check E 2002 A tragic setback. Nature 420: 116–118 (*News feature describing efforts to explain the mechanism underlying a leukaemia-like illness in a child previously cured of SCID by gene therapy*)

Marshall E 1999 Gene therapy death prompts review of adenovirus vector. Science 286: 2244–2245 (*Deals with the tragic 'Gelsinger affair'*)

Patten P A, Schellekens H 2003 The immunogenicity of biopharmaceuticals. Lessons learned and consequences for protein drug development. Dev Biol (Basel) 112: 81–97 (*Deals with several aspects relating to the immunogenicity question; good tables*)

Therapeutic uses

Athanasopoulos T, Fabb S, Dickson G 2000 Gene therapy vectors based on adeno-associated virus: characteristics and applications to acquired and inherited diseases (review). Int J Mol Med 6: 363–375 (*Good review*)

Bauerschmitz G J, Barker S D, Hemminki A 2002 Adenoviral gene therapy for cancer: from vectors to targeted and replication competent agents (review).

Int J Oncol 21: 1161–1174 (*Superb review: very comprehensive*)

Coutelle C, Themis M, Waddington S et al. 2003 The hopes and fears of in utero gene therapy for genetic disease—a review. Placenta 24(suppl B): S114–S121 (*Review of rather a specialised form of gene therapy; for aficionados only*)

Hammond H K, McKirnan M D 2001 Angiogenic gene therapy for heart disease: a review of animal studies and clinical trials. Cardiovasc Res 49: 561–567 (*Comprehensive review spanning animal and human trials of gene therapy for myocardial ischaemia*)

Klink D T, Glick M C, Scanlin T F 2001 Gene therapy of cystic fibrosis (CF) airways: a review emphasizing targeting with lactose. Glycoconj J 18: 731–740 (*A bit specialist but contains some interesting material relative to cystic fibrosis*)

Li F, Hayes J K, Wong K C 2000 Gene therapy: a novel method for the treatment of myocardial ischemia and reperfusion injury—mini-review. Acta Anaesthesiol Sin 38: 207–215 (*The title is self-explanatory*)

Nathwani A C, Davidoff A M, Linch D C 2005 A review of gene therapy for haematological disorders. Br J Haematol 128: 3–17 (*The title is self-explanatory; easy to read and comprehensive in scope*)

Roth J A, Grammer S F 2004 Gene replacement therapy for non-small cell lung cancer: a review. Hematol Oncol Clin North Am 18: 215–229 (*Useful and readable paper on 'replacement therapy' in cancer therapy*)

Wolf J K, Jenkins A D 2002 Gene therapy for ovarian cancer (review). Int J Oncol 21: 461–468 (*Excellent review and general introduction to gene therapy*)

Ylä-Herttuala S, Martin J F 2000 Cardiovascular gene therapy. Lancet 355: 213–222 (*Reviews rationale, vectors, delivery, therapeutic targets, human trials, ethics and future directions*)

Drug discovery and development

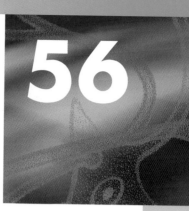

56

OVERVIEW

With the development of the pharmaceutical industry towards the end of the 19th century, drug discovery became a highly focused and managed process. Discovering new drugs moved from the domain of inventive doctors to that of scientists hired for the purpose. Today, the bulk of modern therapeutics, and of modern pharmacology, is based on drugs that came from the laboratories of pharmaceutical companies, without which neither the practice of therapeutics nor the science of pharmacology would be more than a pale fragment of what they have become.

In this chapter, we describe in outline the main stages of the process, namely (i) the discovery phase, i.e. the identification of a *new chemical entity* as a potential therapeutic agent; and (ii) the development phase, during which the compound is tested for safety and efficacy in one or more clinical indications, and suitable formulations and dosage forms devised. The aim is to achieve registration by one or more regulatory authorities, to allow the drug to be marketed legally as a medicine for human use.

Our account is necessarily brief and superficial, and more detail can be found elsewhere (Drews, 1998; Rang 2006).

THE STAGES OF A PROJECT

Figure 56.1 shows in an idealised way the stages of a 'typical' project, aimed at producing a marketable drug that meets a particular medical need (e.g. to retard the progression of Parkinson's disease or cardiac failure, or to prevent migraine attacks).

Broadly, the process can be divided into three main components, namely:

- *drug discovery*, during which candidate molecules are chosen on the basis of their pharmacological properties
- *preclinical development*, during which a wide range of non-human studies (e.g. toxicity testing, pharmacokinetic analysis and formulation) are performed
- *clinical development*, during which the selected compound is tested for efficacy, side effects and potential dangers in volunteers and patients.

These phases do not necessarily follow in strict succession as indicated in Figure 56.1, but generally overlap.

THE DRUG DISCOVERY PHASE

Given the task of planning a project to discover a new drug to treat, say, Parkinson's disease, where does one start? Assuming that we are looking for a novel drug rather than developing a slightly improved 'me too' version of a drug already in use,[1] we first need to choose a new molecular target.

TARGET SELECTION

As discussed in Chapter 2, drug targets are, with few exceptions, functional proteins (e.g. receptors, enzymes, transport proteins). Although, in the past, drug discovery programmes were often based—successfully—on measuring a complex response in vivo, such as prevention of experimentally induced seizures, lowering

---

[1]Many commercially successful drugs have in the past emerged from exactly such 'me too' projects, examples being the dozen or so β-adrenoceptor–blocking drugs developed in the wake of propranolol, or the plethora of 'triptans' that followed the introduction of sumatriptan to treat migraine. Quite small improvements (e.g. in pharmacokinetics or side effects), coupled with aggressive marketing, have often proved enough, but the barriers to registration are getting higher, so the emphasis has shifted towards developing innovative (first in class) drugs aimed at novel molecular targets.

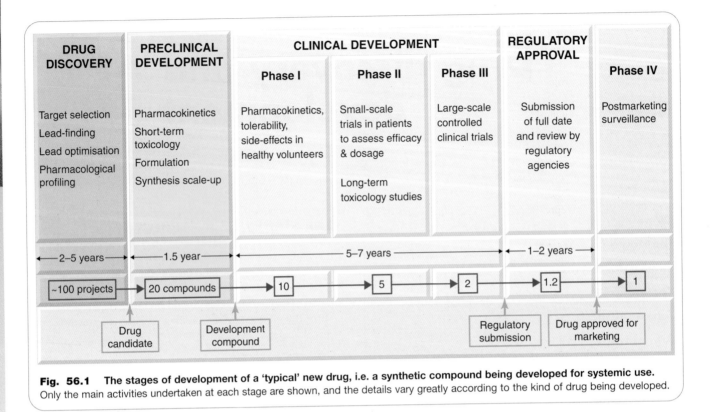

Fig. 56.1 **The stages of development of a 'typical' new drug, i.e. a synthetic compound being developed for systemic use.** Only the main activities undertaken at each stage are shown, and the details vary greatly according to the kind of drug being developed.

of blood sugar, or suppression of an inflammatory response, without the need for prior identification of a drug target, nowadays it is rare to start without a defined protein target, so the first step is *target identification*. This most often comes from biological intelligence. It was known, for example, that inhibiting angiotensin-converting enzyme lowers blood pressure by suppressing angiotensin formation, so it made sense to look for antagonists of the vascular angiotensin II receptor—hence the successful 'sartan' series of antihypertensive drugs (Ch. 19). Similarly, the knowledge that breast cancer is often oestrogen-sensitive led to the development of aromatase inhibitors such as **anastrazole**, which prevents oestrogen synthesis. Current therapeutic drugs address about 120 distinct targets (see Hopkins & Groom, 2002; Rang, 2006), but there are still many proteins that are thought to play a role in disease for which we still have no cognate drug, and many of these represent potential starting points for drug discovery. Estimates range from a few hundred to several thousand potential drug targets that remain to be exploited therapeutically (see Betz, 2005).

Conventional biological wisdom, drawing on a rich fund of knowledge of disease mechanisms and chemical signalling pathways, remains the basis on which novel targets are most often chosen. However, looking ahead, there is no doubt that genomics will play an increasing role by revealing new proteins involved in chemical signalling and new genes involved in disease. Space precludes discussion here of this burgeoning area; interested readers are referred to more detailed accounts (Lindsay, 2003; Kramer & Cohen, 2004; Betz, 2005; Rang, 2006).

Overall, it is evident that in the foreseeable future there is ample biological scope in terms of novel drug targets for

therapeutic innovation. The limiting factor is not the biology and pharmacology, but rather the cost and complexity of drug discovery and development in relation to healthcare economics.

LEAD FINDING

When the biochemical target has been decided and the feasibility of the project has been assessed, the next step is to find *lead compounds*. The usual approach involves cloning of the target protein—normally the human form, because the sequence variation among species is often associated with pharmacological differences, and it is essential to optimise for activity in humans. An assay system must then be developed, allowing the functional activity of the target protein to be measured. This could be a cell-free enzyme assay, a membrane-based binding assay or a cellular response assay. It must be engineered to run automatically, if possible with an optical read-out (e.g. fluorescence or optical absorbance), and in a miniaturised multiwell plate format for reasons of speed and economy. Robotically controlled assay facilities capable of testing tens of thousands of compounds per day in several parallel assays are now commonplace in the pharmaceutical industry, and have become the standard starting point for most drug discovery projects. For an update on how the technology is developing, see Sundberg (2000).

To keep such hungry monsters running requires very large compound libraries. Large companies will typically maintain a growing collection of a million or more synthetic compounds, which will be routinely screened whenever a new assay is set up. Whereas, in the past, compounds were generally synthesised and purified one by one, often taking a week or more for each, the present tendency is to use *combinatorial chemistry*, which allows families of several hundreds or thousands of related compounds to be made simultaneously. By coupling such high-speed chemistry to high-throughput assay systems, the time taken over the initial lead-finding stage of projects has been reduced to a few months in most cases, having previously often taken several years. Despite the apparent mindlessness of the high-throughput random screening approach, it is often successful in identifying lead compounds that have the appropriate pharmacological activity and are amenable to further chemical modification. Building and maintaining huge compound libraries is, however, a costly business, and it has to be realised that even the largest practicable compound collection represents only a minute fraction of the number of 'drug-like' molecules that exists in theory—estimated at about 10^{60}.

One problem with random screening is that many of the 'hits' detected in the initial screen turn out to be molecules that have features undesirable in a drug, such as too high a molecular weight, excessive polarity, and possession of groups known to be associated with toxicity. Computational 'prescreening' of compound libraries is often used to eliminate such compounds.

The hits identified from the primary screen are used as the basis for preparing sets of homologues by combinatorial chemistry so as to establish the critical structural features necessary for binding selectively to the target. Several such iterative cycles of synthesis and screening are usually needed to identify one or more lead compounds for the next stage.

Natural products as lead compounds

Historically, natural products, derived mainly from fungal and plant sources, have proved to be a fruitful source of new therapeutic agents, particularly in the field of anti-infective, anticancer and immunosuppressant drugs. Familiar examples include **penicillin**, **streptomycin** and many other antibiotics; vinca alkaloids; **taxol**; **ciclosporin**; and **sirolimus** (rapamycin). These substances presumably serve a specific protective function, having evolved so as to recognise with great precision vulnerable target molecules in their enemies or competitors. The surface of this resource has barely been scratched, and many companies are actively engaged in generating and testing natural product libraries for lead-finding purposes. Fungi and other microorganisms are particularly suitable for this, because they are ubiquitous, highly diverse, and easy to collect and grow in the laboratory. Compounds obtained from plants, animals or marine organisms are much more troublesome to produce commercially. The main disadvantage of natural products as lead compounds is that they are often complex molecules that are difficult to synthesise or modify by conventional synthetic chemistry, so that lead optimisation may be difficult and commercial production very expensive.

LEAD OPTIMISATION

Lead compounds found by random screening are the basis for the next stage, *lead optimisation*, where the aim (usually) is to increase the potency of the compound on its target and to optimise it with respect to other properties, such as selectivity and metabolic stability. In this phase, the tests applied include a broader range of assays on different test systems, including studies to measure the activity and time course of the compounds in vivo (where possible in animal models mimicking aspects of the clinical condition), and checking for unwanted effects in animals, evidence of genotoxicity, and usually for oral absorption. The objective of the lead optimisation phase is to identify one or more *drug candidates* suitable for further development.

As shown in figure 56.1, only about one project in four succeeds in generating a drug candidate, and it can take up to 5 years. The most common problem is that lead optimisation proves to be impossible; despite much ingenious and back-breaking chemistry, the lead compounds, like antisocial teenagers, refuse to give up their bad habits. In other cases, the compounds, although they produce the desired effects on the target molecule, and have no other obvious defects, fail to produce the expected effects in animal models of the disease, implying that the target is probably not a good one. The virtuous minority proceed to the next phase, *preclinical development*.

PRECLINICAL DEVELOPMENT

The aim of preclinical development is to satisfy all the requirements that have to be met before a new compound is deemed ready to be tested for the first time in humans. The work falls into four main categories.

- Pharmacological testing to check that the drug does not produce any obviously hazardous acute effects, such as bronchoconstriction, cardiac dysrhythmias, blood pressure changes and ataxia. This is termed Safety Pharmacology.
- Preliminary toxicological testing to eliminate genotoxicity and to determine the maximum non-toxic dose of the drug (usually when given daily for 28 days, and tested in two species). As well as being checked regularly for weight loss and other gross changes, the animals so treated are examined minutely post mortem at the end of the experiment to look for histological and biochemical evidence of tissue damage.
- Pharmacokinetic testing, including studies on the absorption, metabolism, distribution and elimination (ADME studies) in laboratory animals.
- Chemical and pharmaceutical development to assess the feasibility of large-scale synthesis and purification, to assess the stability of the compound under various conditions, and to develop a formulation suitable for clinical studies.

Much of the work of preclinical development, especially that relating to safety issues, is done under a formal operating code, known as *Good Laboratory Practice* (GLP), which covers such aspects as record-keeping procedures, data analysis, instrument calibration and staff training. The aim of GLP is to eliminate human error as far as possible, and to ensure the reliability of the data submitted to the regulatory authority, and laboratories are regularly monitored for compliance to GLP standards. The strict discipline involved in working to this code is generally ill-suited to the creative research needed in the earlier stages of drug discovery, so GLP standards are not usually adopted until projects get beyond the discovery phase.

Roughly half the compounds identified as drug candidates fail during the preclinical development phase; for the rest, a detailed dossier is prepared for submission to the regulatory authority such as the European Medicines Evaluation Agency or the US Food and Drugs Administration, whose permission is required to proceed with studies in humans. This is not lightly given, and the regulatory authority may refuse permission or require further work to be done before giving approval.

Non-clinical development work continues throughout the clinical trials period, when much more data, particularly in relation to long-term toxicity in animals, has to be generated. If a drug is intended for long-term use in the clinic, the toxicology studies may have to be extended for up to 2 years, and may include time-consuming studies for possible effects on fertility and fetal development. Failure of a compound at this stage is very costly, and considerable efforts are made to eliminate potentially toxic compounds much earlier in the drug discovery process by the use of in vitro, or even in silico, methods.

CLINICAL DEVELOPMENT

Clinical development proceeds through four distinct phases (see Friedman et al., 1996, for details).

- Phase I trials are performed on a small group (normally 20–80) of normal healthy volunteers, and their aim is to check for *safety* (does the drug produce any potentially dangerous effects, for example on cardiovascular, respiratory, hepatic or renal function?), *tolerability* (does the drug produce any unpleasant symptoms, for example headache, nausea, drowsiness?) and *pharmacokinetic properties* (is the drug well absorbed? What is the time course of the plasma concentration? Is there evidence of cumulation or non-linear kinetics?). Phase I studies may also test for pharmacodynamic effects in volunteers (e.g. does a novel analgesic compound block experimentally induced pain in humans? How does the effect vary with dose?).
- Phase II studies are performed on groups of patients (normally 100–300) and are designed to test for efficacy in the clinical situation, and if this is confirmed, to establish the dose to be used in the definitive phase III study. Often, such studies will cover several distinct clinical disorders (e.g. depression, anxiety states and phobias) to identify the possible therapeutic indications for the new compound and the dose required. When new drug targets are being studied, it is not until these phase II trials are completed that the team finds out whether or not its initial hypothesis was correct, and lack of the expected efficacy is a common reason for failure.
- Phase III studies are the definitive double-blind randomised trials, commonly performed as multicentre trials on 1000–3000 patients, aimed at comparing the new drug with commonly used alternatives. These are extremely costly, difficult to organise, and often take years to complete, particularly if the treatment is designed to retard the progression of a chronic disease. It is not uncommon for a drug that seemed highly effective in the limited patient groups tested in phase II to look much less impressive under the more rigorous conditions of phase III trials.

Increasingly, phase III trials are being required to include a pharmacoeconomic analysis (see Ch. 1), such that not only clinical but also economic benefits of the new treatment are assessed. The whole process has to comply with an elaborate code known as *Good Clinical Practice*, covering every detail of the patient group, data collection methods, recording of information, statistical analysis and documentation.[2]

At the end of phase III, the drug will be submitted to the relevant regulatory authority for licensing. The dossier required for this is a massive and detailed compilation of preclinical and clinical data. Evaluation by the regulatory authority normally takes a year or more, and further delays often arise when aspects of the submission have to be clarified or more data are required. Eventually, about two-thirds of submissions gain marketing approval.

- Phase IV studies comprise the obligatory *postmarketing surveillance* designed to detect any rare or long-term adverse effects resulting from the use of the drug in a clinical setting in many thousands of patients. Such events may necessitate limiting the use of the drug to particular patient groups, or even withdrawal of the drug.[3]

BIOPHARMACEUTICALS

'Biopharmaceuticals', i.e. therapeutic agents produced by biotechnology rather than conventional synthetic chemistry, are discussed in Chapter 55. Such therapeutic agents comprise an increasing proportion—currently about 30%—of new products registered each year. The principles underlying the development and testing of biopharmaceuticals are basically the same as for synthetic drugs. In practice, biopharmaceuticals generally run into fewer toxicological problems than synthetic drugs but more problems relating to production, quality control and drug delivery. Walsh (2003) covers this specialised field in more detail.

COMMERCIAL ASPECTS

Figure 56.1 shows the approximate time taken for such a project and the attrition rate (at each stage and overall) based on recent data from several large pharmaceutical companies. The key messages are (i) that it is a high-risk business, with only about one drug discovery project in 50 reaching its goal of putting a new drug on the market, (ii) that it takes a long time—about 12 years on average, and (iii) that it costs a lot of money to develop one

---

[2]Similar highly detailed codes must be followed in laboratory tests to determine safety (*Good Laboratory Practice*; see text) and drug manufacture (*Good Manufacturing Practice*).

[3]Recent high-profile cases include the withdrawal of rofecoxib (a cyclo-oxygenase-2 inhibitor; see Ch. 14) when it was found to increase the frequency of heart attacks, and of cerivastatin (Ch. 20), a cholesterol-lowering drug found to cause severe muscle damage in a few patients.

drug (about £500 million to £1 billion and increasing, according to recent estimates; see Betz, 2005).[4] For any one project, the costs escalate rapidly as development proceeds, phase III trials and long-term toxicology studies being particularly expensive. The time factor is crucial, because the new drug has to be patented, usually at the end of the discovery phase, and the period of exclusivity (20 years in most countries) during which the company is free from competition in the market starts on that date. After 20 years, the patent expires, and other companies, which have not supported the development costs, are free to make and sell the drug much more cheaply, so the revenues for the original company decrease rapidly thereafter. Reducing the development time after patenting is a major concern for all companies, but so far it has remained stubbornly fixed at around 10 years, partly because the regulatory authorities are demanding more clinical data before they will grant a license. In practice, only about one drug in three that goes on the market brings in enough revenue to cover its development costs. Success for the company relies on this one drug generating enough profit to pay for the rest.[5]

Figure 56.2 illustrates the steady decline in the number of new drugs launched in the major markets worldwide, despite escalating costs and improved technology. There has been much speculation as to the causes, the optimistic view (see below) being that fewer but better drugs are being introduced, and that the recent technological jump has yet to make its impact.

---

[4]These cost estimates have been strongly challenged by commentators (see Angell, 2004) who argue that the pharmaceutical companies overestimate their costs several-fold in order to justify high drug prices.

[5]Actually, companies spend about twice as much on marketing and administration as on research and development.

FUTURE PROSPECTS

Since about 1990, the drug discovery process has been in the throes of a substantial methodological revolution, following the rapid ascendancy of molecular biology, genomics and informatics, amid high expectations that this would bring remarkable dividends in terms of speed, cost and success rate. High-throughput screening has undoubtedly emerged as a powerful lead-finding technology, but overall, the benefits are not yet clear: costs have risen steadily, the success rate has drifted downwards (fig. 56.2) and development times have not decreased. None of this matters, of course, if the new drugs that are being developed improve the quality of medical care, and here there is room for optimism. In recent years, synthetic drugs aimed at new targets (e.g. selective serotonin reuptake inhibitors, statins and the kinase inhibitor imatinib) have made major contributions to patient care. These are 'prerevolutionary' drugs. It may be too soon for the new technologies to have made an impact on new drug registrations, but we can reasonably expect that their ability to make new targets available to the drug discovery machine will have a real effect on patient care.

Trends to watch include the growing armoury of biopharmaceuticals, particularly monoclonal antibodies such as trastuzumab (an oestrogen receptor antibody used to treat breast cancer) and infliximab (a tumour necrosis factor antibody used to treat inflammatory disorders; see Ch. 14); these are successful recent examples, and more are in the pipeline. Another likely change will be the use of genotyping to 'individualise' drug treatments, so as to reduce the likelihood of administering drugs to 'non-responders' (see Ch. 52). There are already well-documented examples of genetic polymorphism affecting the characteristics of drug-metabolising enzymes, receptors and protein kinases, which mean that drugs may be selected for particular

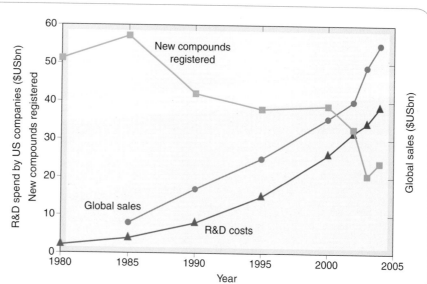

Fig. 56.2 **Research and development (R & D) spend, sales and new drug registrations, 1980–2004.** Registrations refer to new chemical entities (including biopharmaceuticals, excluding new formulations and combinations of existing registered compounds). (Data from various sources, including the Centre for Medicines Research, Pharmaceutical Research and Manufacturers Association of America.)

individuals on the basis of genotyping, and some predict that this approach to individualising therapy will quickly gain ground, heralding a 'pharmacogenomics revolution'. For a balanced view, see Evans & Relling (2004). The implications for drug discovery will be profound, for the resulting therapeutic compartmentation of the patient population will mean that markets will decrease, bringing to an end the reliance on the 'blockbusters' referred to earlier. At the same time, clinical trials will become more complex (and expensive), as different genotypic groups will have to be included in the trial design. The hope is that therapeutic efficacy will be improved, not that it will be a route to developing drugs more cheaply and quickly.

A FINAL WORD

The pharmaceutical industry in recent years has attracted much adverse publicity, some of it well deserved, concerning drug pricing and profits, non-disclosure of adverse clinical trials data, reluctance to address major global heath problems such as tuberculosis and malaria, aggressive marketing practices, and much else (see Angell, 2004). It needs to be remembered though that, despite its faults, the industry has been responsible for most of the therapeutic advances of the past half-century, without which medical care would effectively have stood still.

REFERENCES AND FURTHER READING

Angell M 2004 The truth about the drug companies. Random House, New York (*A powerful broadside directed against the commercial practices of pharmaceutical companies*)

Betz U A K 2005 How many genomics targets can a portfolio afford? Drug Discov Today 10: 1057–1063 (*Interesting analysis—despite its odd title—of approaches to target identification in drug discovery programmes*)

Drews J 1998 In quest of tomorrow's medicines. Springer, New York (*Thoughtful and non-technical account of the history, principles and future directions of drug discovery*)

Evans W E, Relling M V 2004 Moving towards individualised medicine with pharmacogenomics.

Nature 429: 464–468 (*Good review article discussing the likely influence of pharmacogenomics on therapeutics*)

Friedman L M, Furberg C D, DeMets D L 1996 Fundamentals of clinical trials, 3rd edn. Mosby, St Louis (*Standard textbook*)

Hopkins A L, Groom C R 2002 The druggable genome. Nat Rev Drug Discov 1: 727–730 (*Interesting analysis of the potential number of drug targets represented in the human genome*)

Kramer R, Cohen D 2004 Functional genomics to new drug targets. Nat Rev Drug Discov 3: 965–972 (*Describes the various approaches for finding new drug targets, starting from genomic data*)

Lindsay M A 2003 Target discovery. Nat Rev Drug

Discov 2: 831–836 (*Well-balanced discussion of the application of genomics approaches to discovering new drug targets; more realistic in its stance than many*)

Rang H P (ed) 2006 Drug discovery and development. Elsevier, Amsterdam (*Short textbook describing the principles and practice of drug discovery and development at the beginning of the 21st century*)

Sundberg S A 2000 High-throughput and ultra-high-throughput screening: solution and cell-based approaches. Curr Opin Biotechnol 11: 47–53

Walsh G 2003 Biopharmaceuticals, 2nd edn. Wiley, Chichester (*Comprehensive textbook covering all aspects of discovery, development and applications of biopharmaceuticals*)

Appendix
Some important pharmacological agents

Students may feel overwhelmed by the number of drugs described in pharmacology textbooks. We would emphasise that it is more important to understand general pharmacological principles, and to appreciate the pharmacology of the main classes of drug, than to attempt to memorise details of individual agents. Specific drugs are best learned about when they are encountered in the setting of particular topics (e.g. noradrenergic transmission), during practical classes or (for therapeutic drugs) near a patient's bedside. The following list gives examples of some of the more important pharmacological agents. It is not intended as a starting point to learning pharmacology, and we would caution against attempting to memorise lists of names and properties. The examples we provide here are divided into agents of primary and secondary importance. For students of some subjects, and in different geographical areas, one or another class of drug will have more or less importance (e.g. antihelminthics are very important for veterinarians and for all clinicians in regions where helminthiasis is common), so these categories are meant only as a broad guide. The list includes not only drugs used therapeutically, but also endogenous mediators/transmitters (med/trnsm) and certain important drugs used mainly as experimental tools (exp.tool)—especially important for students studying basic or applied pharmacology as a science subject—and drugs used for recreational (recreat) rather than therapeutic purposes. Some endogenous mediators (e.g. adrenaline [epinephrine]) are also important therapeutic drugs. A working knowledge of drugs in the 'primary importance' category, including effects and mode of action, and (for those used therapeutically) pharmacokinetic properties, side effects, toxicity and main uses, should be built up gradually as they are encountered during training. For drugs in the second category, it is usually sufficient to be aware of the mechanism of action, supplemented by understanding how they differ from those in the primary category when relevant.

The choice of drugs in clinical use is somewhat arbitrary. Hospital formulary committees (on which pharmacists play a crucial role) grapple with choosing which individual drugs to stock in the pharmacy. There is a play-off between stocking several individual drugs of one category, for each of which there is good evidence of efficacy for distinct indications, and stocking a more restricted choice based on indirect evidence that efficacy is likely to be a common feature of different members of a class of drugs. Local variations will be encountered (e.g. as to which angiotensin-converting enzyme inhibitor or non-steroidal anti-inflammatory drugs are stocked in the hospital pharmacy). If the

student or clinician (e.g. doctor, dentist, veterinarian or nurse) comes to these (e.g. when changing to a job in a new hospital) with a sound appreciation of the general principles of pharmacology and of the specifics of the various classes of agent involved, he or she will be able to look up and understand the details of agents favoured locally and use them sensibly. (Learning how to cope with change is one of the main educational objectives defined in the General Medical Council's recommendations on undergraduate medical training in *Tomorrow's Doctors*, and this is one example of its importance.)

Drugs are grouped broadly as in the chapters of the text, and some appear more than once in the lists.

KEY

med/trnsm = mediators/transmitter
exp.tool = experimental tool
recreat = drug used for recreational purposes
antag = antagonist

Primary	Secondary
1. Cholinergic transmission (see Ch. 10)	
Agonists	
acetylcholine (med/trnsm)	carbachol
suxamethonium	pilocarpine
nicotine (recreat)	
Antagonists	
atropine	tropicamide
tubocurarine (exp.tool)	pirenzepine
hexamethonium (exp.tool)	atracurium
vecuronium (see Ch. 36)	α-bungarotoxin (exp.tool)
oxybutinin (see Ch. 24)	
Anticholinesterases and related drugs	
neostigmine	pyridostigmine
edrophonium	pralidoxime:
	cholinesterase
	reactivator

Primary   Secondary   Primary   Secondary

2. Noradrenergic transmission (Ch. 11)

Agonists

adrenaline (epinephrine) (med/trnsm) — clonidine

noradrenaline (norepinephrine) (med/trnsm) — phenylephrine

isoprenaline (isoproterenol)

salbutamol

Antagonists

propranolol — prazosin

atenolol — doxazosin

metoprolol

bisoprolol

Drugs affecting noradrenergic neurons

cocaine (and see Ch. 43) — guanethidine (exp.tool)

tyramine (exp.tool) — reserpine (exp.tool)

methyldopa (Ch. 19) — imipramine (Ch. 39)

amphetamine (recreat) (Ch. 43) — α-methyltyrosine (exp.tool) phenelzine (Ch. 39)

3. 5-Hydroxytryptamine (serotonin) and purines (Ch. 12)

Drugs acting on 5-HT receptors (see Ch.39 for 5-HT reuptake inhibitors)

5-HT (serotonin) (med/trnsm) — ergotamine/ dihydroergotamine

LSD (recreat) — metoclopramide (high dose; see also Ch. 25)

ondansetron (Ch. 25) — granisetron

methysergide — pizotifen

triptans (e.g. sumatriptan) — ketotifen

Drugs/mediators acting on purinoceptors or purine uptake

adenosine (med/trnsm) (and Ch. 18)

theophylline (and Ch. 23) — dipyridamole

caffeine (recreat)

ATP (med/trnsm)

ADP (med/trnsm) (Ch. 21)

clopidogrel (Ch. 21)

5-HT, 5-hydroxytryptamine; LSD, lysergic acid diethylamide.

4. Local hormones (Ch. 13; see also Tables 7 and 8 for peptides and nitric oxide)

Eicosanoids and related substances (all med/trnsm)

prostaglandins E and F — platelet activating factor

prostaglandin I_2 (prostacyclin, epoprostenol)

thromboxane A_2

leukotrienes

Leukotriene antagonists (e.g. montelukast; Ch. 23)

histamine (med/trnsm)

Histamine antagonists (see Table 5 below)

kinins (bradykinin, tachykinins; see Table 7 below) (med/trnsm) — icatibant (bradykinin antagonist) (exp. tool)

Cytokines (all: med/trnsm)

interleukins

chemokines

tumour necrosis factor

Tumour necrosis factor antagonists: etanercept, infliximab

interferons (med/trnsm)

colony-stimulating factors (Ch. 22) (med/trnsm)

Primary　　　　　　　　Secondary　　　　　　　Primary　　　　　　　　Secondary

5. Anti-inflammatory and immunosuppressant drugs (Ch. 14)

Cyclo-oxygenase inhibitors (NSAIDs)

Primary	Secondary
aspirin (see also Ch. 21)	naproxen
paracetamol (acetaminophen)	
ibuprofen	coxibs (e.g. celecoxib)
indometacin	

Histamine antagonists

Primary	Secondary
mepyramine	terfenadine
promethazine	fexofenadine
ranitidine	cimetidine

Drugs used in gout

Primary	Secondary
NSAIDs (see above)	colchicine
allopurinol (prophylaxis)	probenecid (prophylaxis)
	sulfinpyrazone

Immunosuppressant drugs

Primary	Secondary
azathioprine	anakinra (interleukin-1 antagonist)
ciclosporin	
tacrolimus	
methotrexate	
prednisolone	

Tumor necrosis factor antagonists

infliximab
etanercept

Other disease-modifying antirheumatic drugs

Primary	Secondary
	auranofin
	hydroxychloroquine
	penicillamine
	sulfasalazine

NSAID, non-steroidal anti-inflammatory drug.

6. Cannabinoids and related drugs (Ch. 15)

Primary	Secondary
Δ^9-tetrahydrocannabinol (recreat)	nabilone
anandamide (med/trnsm)	

Antagonist/inverse agonist

rimonabant

7. Peptides and proteins (Ch. 16, and see Table 10 below)

Renin–angiotensin system

angiotensin II (med/trnsm)
angiotensin-converting enzyme inhibitors (e.g. captopril)
AT_1 antagonists ('sartans', e.g. losartan)

Various peptides

Primary	Secondary
bradykinin (med/trnsm)	icatibant (exp.tool)
natriuretic peptides (atrial natriuretic peptide, B-type natriuretic hormone, C-type natriuretic hormone) (med/trnsm)	
endothelin (med/trnsm)	bosentan (see also Ch. 19)
calcitonin (med/trnsm)	calcitonin gene–related peptide (med/trnsm)
oxytocin (med/trnsm)	atosiban (see also Ch. 30)
substance P (med/trnsm)	aprepitant (see also Ch. 25)
vasopressin (med/trnsm)	tolvaptan (see also Ch. 19)
	cholecystokinin (med/trnsm)
	octreotide (see also Ch. 25)

8. Nitric oxide (Ch. 17)

nitric oxide (med/trnsm)
L-N^G-monomethyl arginine (L-NMMA) (exp.tool)
glyceryl trinitrate (see also Chs 18 and 19)
nitroprusside (see also Ch. 19)

9. The heart (Ch. 18)

Antidysrhythmic drugs (Vaughan–Williams classification)

	Primary	Secondary
Class I	lidocaine	flecainide
Class II	metoprolol	
Class III	amiodarone	sotalol
Class IV	verapamil	
Unclassified	adenosine	
	digoxin	

Antianginal drugs
Nitrates
glyceryl trinitrate
isosorbide mononitrate
β-Blockers
metoprolol
Calcium antagonists
diltiazem

Primary   Secondary

10. The vascular system (Ch. 19)

Antihypertensive drugs (A, B, C and D)
A: angiotensin-converting enzyme inhibitors and angiotensin II (AT$_1$ receptor) antagonists

Primary	Secondary
captopril	lisinopril
enalapril	trandolapril
losartan	irbesartan
candesartan	

B: β-adrenoceptor antagonists
metoprolol

C: calcium antagonists
amlodipine
nifedipine

D: thiazides and related diuretics
bendroflumethiazide
hydrochlorothiazide
indapamide
chlortalidone

α$_1$-Adrenoceptor antagonists
doxazosin

Other vasodilators

Primary	Secondary
hydralazine	minoxidil
	nitroprusside (see also Ch. 17)

Centrally acting drugs

Primary	Secondary
	methyldopa
	moxonidine

Drugs used in heart failure and shock
Diuretics (see also Ch. 24)
furosemide
amiloride
spironolactone
eplerenone

Angiotensin-converting enzyme inhibitors and AT$_1$ antagonists: see antihypertensives table above for important drugs

Cardiac glycoside
digoxin

Drugs acting on adrenoceptors

Primary	Secondary
carvedilol	dobutamine
bisoprolol	dopamine
metoprolol	

Vasodilators
hydralazine
isosorbide mononitrate

Pulmonary hypertension
epoprostenol
iloprost
sildenafil
bosentan

11. Atherosclerosis and dyslipidaemia (Ch. 20)

Primary	Secondary
simvastatin	
atorvastatin	pravastatin
ezetimibe	
	gemfibrozil
	fenofibrate
	nicotinic acid
	colestyramine
	fish oil

12. Haemostasis and thrombosis (Ch. 21)

Oral anticoagulants and related drugs

Primary	Secondary
warfarin	ximelagatran
vitamin K (antag)	

Heparin-related drugs and related drugs

Primary	Secondary
heparin	protamine (antag)
enoxaparin	fondaparinux

Antiplatelet drugs

Primary	Secondary
aspirin	dipyridamole
clopidogrel	epoprostenol
abciximab	

Fibrinolytic drugs and inhibitors of fibrinolysis
streptokinase
tissue plasminogen activator
tranexamic acid (inhibitor)

13. Haematinics and related drugs (Ch. 22)

Primary	Secondary
ferrous sulfate	filgrastim
desferrioxamine (iron chelator)	
folic acid	
hydroxocobalamin	
epoietin	

Primary	Secondary

14. Respiratory system (Ch. 23)

β_2-adrenoceptor agonists

Primary	Secondary
salbuterol	terbutaline
salmeterol	formeterol

Inhaled glucocorticoids

beclometasone
mometasone

Inhaled muscarinic antagonists

Primary	Secondary
ipratropium	tiotropium

Xanthine alkaloids

theophylline

Leukotriene antagonists and 5-lipoxygenase inhibitors

Primary	Secondary
	montelukast
	zileutin

Anti-immunoglobulin E

Primary	Secondary
	omalizumab

Antitussive drug

codeine

15. The kidney (Ch. 24)

Thiazides and related diuretics
See Table 10 above on the vascular system

Loop diuretics

Primary	Secondary
furosemide	bumetanide

K^+-sparing diuretics

Primary	Secondary
spironolactone	triamterene
amiloride	eplerenone

Osmotic diuretics

mannitol

Carbonic anhydrase inhibitors

acetazolamide

Antidiuretic hormone (vasopressin) V_2 agonists and antagonists

Primary	Secondary
desmopressin	demeclocycline (antag)

Anion exchange resin

Primary	Secondary
	sevelamer

16. Gastrointestinal system (Ch. 25)

Ulcer-healing drugs
H_2 receptor antagonists

Primary	Secondary
ranitidine	cimetidine

Proton pump inhibitors

omeprazole
lansoprazole

Antibiotics for *Helicobacter pylori*

amoxicillin
clarithromycin
metronidazole

Prostaglandin analogues

Primary	Secondary
	misoprostol

Aluminium complexes

Primary	Secondary
	sucralfate

Laxatives

Primary	Secondary
lactulose	sodium picosulfate
senna	

Antiemetics

Primary	Secondary
phenothiazines (see also Ch. 38)	
antihistamines (see also Ch. 14)	
domperidone	granisetron
metoclopramide	nabilone
ondansetron	aprepitant

Antidiarrhoeal drugs

codeine
loperamide

Drugs for inflammatory bowel disease

Primary	Secondary
prednisolone (also Ch. 28)	
sulfasalazine	mesalazine

Antispasmodics

hyoscine
cyclizine

Gastric Secretagogues

Primary	Secondary
gastrin (med/trnsm)	pentagastrin

Primary   Secondary

Primary   Secondary

17. Endocrine pancreas and related drugs (Ch. 26)

Hormones
insulin
insulin glargine   amylin (med/trnsm)
insulin lispro   somatostatin (med/trnsm)
glucagon

Drugs that act on the sulfonylurea receptor
tolbutamide   nateglinide
glibenclamide   gliburide

Biguanides
metformin

α-Glucosidase inhibitor
acarbose

Thiazolidinediones
rosiglitazone
pioglitazone

18. Obesity (Ch. 27)

leptin (med/trnsm)   neuropeptide Y
                          (med/trnsm)
                          orlistat
                          sibutramine
                          fenfluramine
                          rimonabant (see also
                          Ch. 15)

19. Adrenal cortex and pituitary (Ch. 28)

Glucocorticoids and related drugs (see also Ch. 23 for inhaled preparations)
hydrocortisone   metyrapone
                         (blocks synthesis)

prednisolone (med/trnsm)
dexamethasone

Mineralocorticoids (and their antagonists)
fludrocortisone
spironolactone (antag)   eplerenone (antag)

Pituitary hormones and related drugs
corticotropin
(adrenocorticotrophic
hormone) (med/trnsm)
growth hormone (med/trnsm)   sermorelin (growth
                             hormone– releasing
                             hormone analogue)

somatostatin (med/trnsm)
octreotide   lanreotide
vasopressin (med/trnsm)   desmopressin
oxytocin (med/trnsm)
prolactin (med/trnsm)
gonadorelin
bromocriptine (Ch. 35)

20. Thyroid (Ch. 29)

Hormones and precursors
thyroxine (med/trnsm)
liothyronine (med/trnsm)
calcitonin (med/trnsm) (see also Ch. 31)
iodine/iodide

Antithyroid drugs
carbimazole
propylthiouracil
radioiodine (^{131}I)

21. Reproductive system (Ch. 30)

Oestrogens
oestradiol (med/trnsm)

Antioestrogens
tamoxifen   clomiphene

Progestins
progesterone (med/trnsm)   norethisterone

Antiprogestogens
mifepristone

Androgens
testosterone (med/trnsm)

Antiandrogens and related drugs
cyproterone   bicalutamide
flutamide   finasteride (5-α
                         reductase inhibitor)

Gonadotrophin-releasing hormone analogues
buserelin
goserelin

Drugs acting on the uterus
ergometrine
oxytocin   atosiban
dinoprostone (prostaglandin E$_2$)

Erectile dysfunction
sildenafil
tadalafil

22. Drugs and bone (Ch. 31)

parathyroid hormone (med/trnsm)   calcitonin
vitamin D   teriparatide
calcium salts
oestrogen (med/trnsm)
raloxifene
alendronate   etidronate
risedronate   strontium ranelate

Primary | Secondary | Primary | Secondary

23. Chemical mediators in the central nervous system (Ch. 32)

Neurotransmitters and related drugs

Primary	Secondary
glutamate	
NMDA (exp.tool)	ketamine (NMDA channel blocker) (recreat)
glycine (med/trnsm)	strychnine (exp.tool) (glycine antag)
GABA (med/trnsm)	baclofen
	bicuculline (GABA$_A$ antag)

Amines

Primary	Secondary
noradrenaline (norepinephrine) (med/trnsm)	melatonin (med/trnsm)
dopamine (med/trnsm)	
5-hydroxytryptamine (med/trnsm)	
acetylcholine (med/trnsm)	
histamine (med/trnsm)	

24. Neurodegenerative diseases (Ch. 35)

Parkinson's disease

Primary	Secondary
levodopa	selegiline
carbidopa	benzatropine (benztropine)
bromocriptine	amantadine
	apomorphine
	MPTP (exp.tool)

Amyotrophic lateral sclerosis

Primary	Secondary
	riluzole

Alzheimer's disease

Primary	Secondary
donepezil	rivastigmine
memantine	galantamine

25. General anesthetics (Ch. 36)

Inhalational

Primary	Secondary
halothane	ether
fluranes (enflurane, isoflurane, desflurane, sevoflurane)	chloroform
nitrous oxide	

Intravenous

Primary	Secondary
propofol	
etomidate	
thiopental	ketamine

26. Anxiolytic, hypnotic and related drugs (Ch. 37)

Benzodiazepines and related drugs

Primary	Secondary
temazepam	nitrazepam
diazepam	lorazepam
midazolam	flumazenil (antag)

Barbiturates

Primary	Secondary
	phenobarbital

Other

buspirone (5-HT$_{1A}$ receptor agonist)

27. Antipsychotic drugs (Ch. 38)

Classic

Primary	Secondary
chlorpromazine	fluphenazine
haloperidol	thioridazine

Atypical

Primary	Secondary
clozapine	risperidone
olanzapine	sulpiride

28. Drugs used in affective disorders (Ch. 39)

Tricyclic antidepressants

Primary	Secondary
amitriptyline	imipramine

Selective serotonin (5-HT) reuptake inhibitors

Primary	Secondary
fluoxetine	fluvoxamine
sertraline	

Monoamine oxidase inhibitors

Primary	Secondary
moclobemide ('RIMA')	phenelzine
	tranylcypromine

Miscellaneous antidepressants

Primary	Secondary
venlafaxine	trazodone
	bupropion

Mood stabilisers

Primary	Secondary
lithium	
carbamazepine	

Primary   Secondary

29. Antiepileptic drugs and centrally acting muscle relaxants (Ch. 40)

phenytoin   phenobarbital
carbamazepine   diazepam
valproate   clonazepam
vigabatrin   ethosuximide
gabapentin
lamotrigine
baclofen

30. Analgesics and related substances (Ch. 41)

Opioids and related drugs
morphine
codeine
fentanyl   methadone
pethidine   diamorphine
naloxone (antag)   naltrexone (antag)

Mild analgesics (see also Ch. 14)
aspirin
paracetamol

Other analgesic drugs
tramadol
carbamazepine
gabapentin
amitriptyline

Other compounds involved in nociception
enkephalins and endorphins: dynorphin (med/trnsm)
substance P (med/trnsm)
capsaicin (exp.tool)

31. Central nervous system stimulants and psychotomimetics (Ch. 42)

amphetamine (recreat)   methylphenidate
cocaine (recreat)   *MDMA* ('ecstasy')
caffeine (recreat)   *LSD* (recreat)
                           phencyclidine (recreat)
                           strychnine (exp.tool)
                           bicuculline (exp.tool)
                           pentylenetetrazol
(exp.tool)

LSD, lysergic acid diethylamide; MDMA,
methylenedioxymethamphetamine.

32. Drug dependence and drug abuse (Ch. 43)

opiates (morphine, heroin) Δ^9-tetrahydrocannabinol
                             (recreat)
nicotine (recreat)   amphetamine (recreat)
ethanol (recreat)   solvents (recreat)
cocaine (recreat)   benzodiazepines

33. Local anaesthetics and other drugs that affect sodium or potassium channels (Ch. 44)

Local anaesthetics
lidocaine   tetracaine (amethocaine)
bupivacaine (and levobupivacaine) ropivacaine

Selective sodium channel blocker
tetrodotoxin (exp.tool)

Potassium channel antagonists
tetraethylammonium (exp.tool)
sulfonylureas (see Ch. 26)

Potassium channel activators
nicorandil (see Ch. 19)   minoxidil
                                   cromakalim

34. Antibacterial agents (Ch. 46)

Bacterial cell wall inhibitors
benzylpenicillin   piperacillin
amoxicillin
flucloxacillin
cephalosporins (cefadroxil, cefotaxime,
ceftriaxone)
vancomycin

Topoisomerase inhibitor
ciprofloxacin

Folate inhibitors
trimethoprim   sulfonamides

Bacterial protein synthesis inhibitors
gentamicin
amikacin
tetracycline
chloramphenicol
erythromycin
clarithromycin

Antianaerobe drug
metronidazole

Antimycobacterial agents
isoniazid   ethambutol
rifampicin   streptomycin
pyrazinamide   dapsone

Primary Secondary   Primary Secondary

35. Antiviral agents (Ch. 47)

DNA polymerase inhibitors
aciclovir   foscarnet
                             ganciclovir
                             tribavirin (ribavirin)

Reverse transcriptase inhibitors
zidovudine (AZT)   didanosine
efavirenz (non-nucleoside inhibitor)   zalcitabine

Protease inhibitor
saquinavir

Immunomodulators
interferons (med/trnsm) (see Ch. 13)

Neuraminidase inhibitors
zanamavir

Inhibitor of HIV fusion with host cells
enfurvitide

36. Antifungal drugs (Ch. 48)

Polyene antibiotics
amphotericin B   nystatin

Azoles
fluconazole   miconazole

Antimetabolites
                             flucytosine

Others
                             terbinafine
                             echinocandin B

37. Antiprotozoal drugs (Ch. 49)

Antimalarials
chloroquine   pyrimethamine plus
                             sulfadoxine
quinine
artemesenin
primaquine

For *Pneumocystis pneumoniae*
co-trimoxazole (high dose)   pentamidine

Amoebicidal drugs
metronidazole

Leishmanicidal drugs
antimonials (e.g. stibogluconate)
pentamidine

Trypanosomicidal drugs
suramin   pentamidine

Toxoplasmicidal drugs
pyrimethamine–sulfadiazine

38. Anthelminthic drugs (Ch. 50)

Broad spectrum
mebendazole

Roundworm, threadworm
piperazine
levamisole (roundworm)

Schistosomes
praziquantel

River blindness
ivermectin

Primary   Secondary

39. Cancer chemotherapy (Ch. 51)

Alkylating agents and related compounds
cyclophosphamide	lomustine
melphalan	busulfan
cisplatin	chlorambucil

Antimetabolites
cytarabine	fluorouracil
methotrexate	mercaptopurine
thioguanine	
pentostatin	gemcitabine

Cytotoxic antibiotics
doxorubicin	
bleomycin	dactinomycin

Plant derivatives
vinca alkaloids (vincristine, vinblastine)	etoposide
taxanes (paclitaxel, docetaxel)	

Hormones and related drugs
prednisolone	
dexamethasone	
flutamide	
buserelin	anastrazole
tamoxifen	

Monoclonal antibodies
rituximab
trastuzumab

(This appendix was originally adapted from that in Dale M M, Dickenson A H, Haylett D G 1996 Companion to pharmacology, 2nd edn. Churchill Livingstone, Edinburgh, with permission.)

Index

P

827